Essentials of Interventional Cancer Pain Management

Amitabh Gulati • Vinay Puttanniah
Brian M. Bruel • William S. Rosenberg
Joseph C. Hung
Editors

Essentials of Interventional Cancer Pain Management

Springer

Editors
Amitabh Gulati
Department of Anesthesiology and Critical Care
Memorial Sloan Kettering Cancer Center
New York, NY
USA

Vinay Puttanniah
Anesthesiology and Critical Care Medicine
Memorial Sloan Kettering Cancer Center
New York, NY
USA

Brian M. Bruel
Physical Medicine and Rehabilitation
Baylor College of Medicine
Houston, TX
USA

William S. Rosenberg
Midwest Neuroscience Institute
Center for the Relief of Pain
Kansas City, MO
USA

Joseph C. Hung
Anesthesiology and Critical Care Medicine
Memorial Sloan Kettering Cancer Center
New York, NY
USA

ISBN 978-3-319-99682-0 ISBN 978-3-319-99684-4 (eBook)
https://doi.org/10.1007/978-3-319-99684-4

Library of Congress Control Number: 2018964427

This Springer imprint is published by the registered company Springer Nature Switzerland AG
The registered company address is: Gewerbestrasse 11, 6330 Cham, Switzerland

Preface

The writing of this manuscript has been a remarkable experience that started 4 years ago and has now finally reached its completion phase. My decision to pursue this project was not only to share my thoughts in the field of interventional cancer pain medicine but also to educate myself on how various disciplines both encounter and treat their cancer pain patients. The manuscript is not meant to diminish the incredible work, education, and research that have improved pharmacotherapeutic options for our patients, but rather serve as a supplement to these therapies.

All too often, it is easy to assess one problem and quickly "Google" it for a searchable solution. We find ourselves piecing together answers from a handful of incomplete resources. These fragmented answers don't tell the complete story. Thus, I do believe that a larger compendium, a "textbook," can be quite helpful. Our many specialties – radiation oncology, neurosurgery, rehabilitation, supportive care, oncologists, radiologists, psychiatrists, integrative medicine, and anesthesiologists, among others – address only a part of the cancer pain story. But as far as I have seen, we have been missing one collective resource that surveys the broad knowledge of these fields. I pursued this project specifically because I wanted to help create something meaningful for all of us struggling to successfully treat cancer pain.

The first part of the book addresses the lack of consistency seen in the literature regarding interventional treatment options for specific cancer pain syndromes. Initially, we discuss both primary cancer and treatment-related cancer pain syndromes that we may encounter as physicians managing cancer patients. What follows is our initial attempt to implement paradigms we can use in treating specific groups of cancer, such as breast cancer. This is a daunting task made even more difficult as new treatment options emerged during the writing of the textbook. I hope this will be a starting point for future paradigms to develop for our patients.

The remainder of the text divides into a more common approach to addressing interventional cancer pain medicine. After discussing interventional options that are commonly employed by physicians, we begin to investigate how our surgical colleagues may address some of our more severe pain syndromes. We continue with an extended section on perhaps the most important interventional available for our patients, intrathecal drug delivery.

Next, an emerging field of interventional oncology has led to many therapeutic advances in treating focal cancer lesions. We highlight radiologic options in targeted neurolysis and ablative techniques, specifically for bone metastasis. Furthermore, with newer modalities in radiation delivery, I feel that it is important to develop collaboration with our radiation oncology colleagues to develop paradigms involving radiation therapies.

As we begin to see how cancer pain affects our patient's quality of life and function, we introduce our rehabilitation section to address these concerns. The effects of exercise and physical therapy should not be underappreciated especially when addressing fatigue and oncologic outcomes. I have personally seen the improvements of our bracing and manipulation techniques in improving our patient's mobility and pain. I think this section's significance is highlighted in the care the subject is given in our text. The final section echoes this sentiment as we introduce our integrative and psychological therapies. Taken together, we can globally assess and address our patient's needs throughout the cancer journey.

I hope this reference will serve as a special guide for our readers. The large breadth and scope of this project exemplifies our need to coalesce knowledge to truly deliver a multispecialty approach for managing our cancer pain patients. This is our first step in this field and hopefully will expand ideas for our patients on this foundation we present to you.

In the end, I hope this manuscript serves to help and guide many future physicians, as it has helped me, establish a better framework to manage our complex patients.

New York, NY, USA Amitabh Gulati

Acknowledgments

From Amitabh Gulati:

Throughout this journey, I have been fortunate to have the support of many people but none more important than my wife, Rati, and my two young children, Ariya and Taran (both of whom were born during this project).

Furthermore, I would like to take a moment to commend my mentors during my journey as a cancer pain physician. As a resident, I was exposed to the caring and compassion required to support our cancer patient's journey. Under Dr. Michael Byas-Smith's tutelage, I came to realize that for patients suffering from cancer-related pain, their fight is surviving and beating cancer, but this pain is a constant reminder of their struggle. While "treating the cancer will treat the pain" works, lessening suffering during the process should be both an admirable goal and a necessity. While I was a fellow, Dr. Kenneth Cubert exemplified this as a mentor and friend. We play a small, yet vital role to help our fellow patients overcome their disease. I want to personally thank both and many of my other esteemed colleagues for their inspiration and everlasting knowledge.

Furthermore, in the last few years, I have cherished the exchange of ideas with the Cancer Pain Resource Consortium. This may very well be the first group of people with the diversity of experiences allowing all of us to collaborate and treat our patients with a new sense of completeness. Many of the authors are eager members who share the same passion as I do. I hope that this project is a testament to the group's ideals in pursuing the best care for all of our patients.

While I hope we have contributed to this field, I feel that this project is just the beginning of our goal to improve our patient's care. Our patient's lives are changing because of newer oncologic treatments and promise. Maybe we will be lucky one day, and cancer will be treated quickly and without suffering. Until then, I hope all of us in this field adapt and treat our patients with the best of our abilities, using the growing collaboration among us.

From Vinay Puttanniah:

To my mentors and teachers in science and medicine who encouraged me to ask the difficult questions and pursue profound answers.

To my father who instilled in me the value of hard work and dedication entirely through his actions.

To my mother who showed me what it meant to practice compassionate medicine.

To my children, Arun, Devan, and Vera, whose curiosity and persistence inspire me daily to be the best father and teacher I can be.

And most of all, to my wife, Lukshmi, for believing in me. Your relentless encouragement, guidance, and unconditional love have allowed, inspired, and motivated all of my actions.

Contents

Part I Perspectives on Cancer Pain Medicine

1 **Perspectives on Interventional Cancer Pain Management** 3
Arvider Gill and Oscar A. de Leon-Casasola

2 **The Practice of Cancer Pain: A Case Series** 5
Sana Shaikh

Part II Cancer Pain Syndromes

3 **Pathophysiology of Cancer Pain** 13
Stephen Lawrence Thorp

4 **Chemotherapy** 19
Karina Gritsenko and Michael Lubrano

5 **Postsurgical Pain Syndromes** 29
Thomas J. Van de Ven and Amitabh Gulati

6 **Radiation-Induced Pain Syndromes** 39
Jasmit Brar, Grant H. Chen, and Amitabh Gulati

Part III Paradigms in Cancer Pain Syndromes

7 **General Pain Management Concepts** 47
Dhanalakshmi Koyyalagunta, Maureen J. Simmonds, and Diane M. Novy

8 **Head and Neck Cancer Pain** 55
Vinay Puttanniah and Elena V. Zininberg

9 **Breast Cancer Pain: A Review of Pathology and Interventional Techniques** 63
Ali Valimahomed, Jennifer Zocca, and Amitabh Gulati

10 **Thoracic Cancer Pain** 85
Joseph C. Hung, Rajiv Shah, and Amitabh Gulati

11 **Gastrointestinal Cancer Pain** 97
Daniel Pak and Joseph C. Hung

12 **Genitourinary Cancer Pain Syndromes** 107
Ilan Margulis and Amitabh Gulati

13 **Pediatric Cancer Pain Management** 113
Stephen L. Long and Anurag K. Agrawal

14 **Pain in Hematologic Malignancies** 123
Kanu Sharan

15 **Dermatologic Cancer Pain Syndromes** 133
Katerina Svigos, Viswanath Reddy Belum, and Mario E. Lacouture

Part IV Percutaneous Pain Techniques and Anatomy

16 **Ablative Techniques** 141
Simon Guo and Jack W. Lam

17 **Sympathetic Nervous System Blocks for the Treatment of Cancer Pain** 145
Nadya M. Dhanani, Wilson A. Almonte, and Mitchell P. Engle

18 **Peripheral Nerve Blocks** 167
Nantthasorn Zinboonyahgoon, Christopher R. Abrecht, and Sanjeet Narang

19 **Cranial Nerve Targets** 183
Jill E. Sindt

20 **Vertebroplasty, Kyphoplasty, and Sacroplasty** 201
Dawood Sayed and Shervin Razavian

21 **Treatment Considerations for Cancer Pain Syndromes** 213
Devin Peck and Gendai J. Echezona

Part V Surgical Techniques and Neuromodulation

22 **Intracranial Neuroablation** 225
Roy Hwang, Ashwin Viswanathan, Ahmed M. Raslan, and Erich Richter

23 **Spinal Neuroablation for Cancer Pain** 231
William S. Rosenberg, Parag G. Patil, and Ahmed M. Raslan

24 **Radiosurgery** 235
Simon S. Lo, Tithi Biswas, Rodney J. Ellis, and Peter C. Gerszten

25 **Deep Brain Stimulation and Motor Cortical Stimulation for Malignant Pain** . . . 241
Joshua M. Rosenow and Jonathan Miller

26 **Spinal Cord Stimulation and Oncologic Pain Management** 247
Neel D. Mehta and Mohammad M. Piracha

27 **Peripheral Nerve Stimulation for the Treatment of Cancer Pain** 255
Jennifer A. Sweet and Nicholas M. Boulis

28 **Transcutaneous Electrical Nerve Stimulation for Cancer Pain** 261
Jeffrey Loh

Part VI Intrathecal Drug Delivery

29 **Indications for Intrathecal Pump Therapy** 269
Mercy A. Udoji and Helen M. Blake

30 **Intrathecal Drug Delivery System Trialing for Cancer Pain Management** 273
Namrata Khimani and Sanjeet Narang

31 **Intrathecal Pump Implantation Technique** 277
Shane E. Brogan and Christina Bokat

32 **Medications in Intrathecal Pumps** 287
Grant H. Chen

33 **Compounding Drugs for Intrathecal Use** 293
Shalini Shah

Part VII Interventional Oncology

34 **Image Guidance and Planning** 301
Ramon Go and Jeffrey Prinsell Jr.

35 **Ablative Techniques for Painful Metastasis (Radiofrequency ablation, Microwave ablation, Cryoablation, Chemical ablation, and HIFU)** 307
Hooman Yarmohammadi

36 **Introduction to Radiation Therapy** 319
Shayna E. Rich and Kavita V. Dharmarajan

37 **Palliative Radiation Therapy** 329
Shayna E. Rich and Kavita V. Dharmarajan

38 **External Beam Radiotherapy in the Treatment of Painful Bone Metastases** 339
Candice Johnstone, Amol J. Ghia, and Anussara Prayongrat

39 **Non-opioid Intravenous Infusions for Management of Cancer-Associated Pain** 353
Yury Khelemsky and Mourad M. Shehabar

Part VIII Interventional Physiatry

40 **Cancer Rehabilitation** 363
Ameet Nagpal, Jacob Fehl, Brittany Bickelhaupt, Maxim S. Eckmann, Brian Boies, and Jon Benfield

41 **Neuromuscular Medicine: Cancer Pain** 375
Eric Leung

42 **Cancer-Related Pelvic Pain** 385
Sarah Hwang and Megan Clark

43 **Exercise Therapy and Fatigue Management** 395
Jack B. Fu and Arash Asher

44 **Physical Therapy** 403
Monica Verduzco-Gutierrez, Roy Rivera Jr., and Prathap Jayaram

45 **Occupational Therapy** 417
Meilani Mapa and Jason Chen

46 **Cancer Pain and Physical Modalities** 427
Joel Frontera and Amy Cao

47 **Osteopathic Treatment for Cancer-Related Pain** 433
Ryan K. Murphy and Jonas M. Sokolof

48 **Rehabilitation-Bracing as a Conservative Treatment Option** 443
Lisa Marie Ruppert and Michelle Yakaboski

Part IX Complementary and Psycho-Behavioral Therapies

49 Psychosocial Assessment and Treatment for Patients with Cancer Pain 451
Laura M. van Veldhoven and Diane M. Novy

50 Relaxation Techniques and Biofeedback for Cancer Pain Management 463
Asimina Lazaridou and Robert R. Edwards

51 Mood and Anxiety in Cancer Pain 473
R. Garrett Key and William S. Breitbart

52 Acupuncture and Cancer Pain 485
Yan Cui Magram and Gary E. Deng

53 Creative Therapies and Mind-Body Health Systems 489
Veena Sankar

54 Botanical Treatments in Cancer Pain Management 503
Helen M. Blake

55 Integrative Therapies for Pain Modulation 507
Joan Pope and Aron Legler

Index 513

Contributors

Christopher R. Abrecht, MD Department of Anesthesiology, Perioperative and Pain Medicine, Brigham and Women's Hospital, Harvard Medical School, Boston, MA, USA

Anurag K. Agrawal, MD Department of Hematology/Oncology, UCSF Benioff Children's Hospital Oakland, Oakland, CA, USA

Wilson A. Almonte, MD Victoria Pain and Rehabilitation Center, Victoria, TX, USA

Arash Asher, MD Samuel Oschin Comprehensive Cancer Institute at Cedars-Sinai Medical Center, Los Angeles, CA, USA

Viswanath Reddy Belum, MD Department of Medicine, Memorial Sloan Kettering Cancer Center, New York, NY, USA

Jon Benfield, DO South Texas Spinal Clinic, San Antonio, TX, USA

Brittany Bickelhaupt, MD University of Texas Health Science Center at San Antonio (UTHSCSA), Department of Physical Medicine and Rehabilitation, San Antonio, TX, USA

Tithi Biswas, MD University Hospitals Seidman Cancer Center, Case Comprehensive Cancer Center, Department of Radiation Oncology, Cleveland, OH, USA

Helen M. Blake, MD Pain and Rehabilitation Specialists of Saint Louis, LLC, St. Louis, MO, USA

Brian Boies, MD University of Texas Health Science Center at San Antonio (UTHSCSA), UT Medicine Pain Consultants, Department of Anesthesiology, San Antonio, TX, USA

University of Texas Health Science Center at San Antonio (UTHSCSA), Department of Anesthesiology, San Antonio, TX, USA

Christina Bokat, MD, MPhil University of Utah, Department of Anesthesiology, Salt Lake City, UT, USA

Nicholas M. Boulis, MD Neurosurgery, Emory University Hospital, Atlanta, GA, USA

Jasmit Brar, MD New York Presbyterian-Weill Cornell Medicine, Department of Anesthesiology, New York, NY, USA

William S. Breitbart, MD Department of Psychiatry and Behavioral Sciences, Memorial Sloan Kettering Cancer Center, New York, NY, USA

Shane E. Brogan, MD, MPhil University of Utah, Department of Anesthesiology, Salt Lake City, UT, USA

Amy Cao Baylor St. Luke's Medical Center, Physical medicine and rehabilitation, Houston, TX, USA

Grant H. Chen, MD Memorial Sloan Kettering Cancer Center, Department of Anesthesiology and Critical Care Medicine, New York, NY, USA

Jason Chen, DO McGovern Medical School at UT Health, Department of Physical Medicine and Rehabilitation, The University of Texas Health Science Center at Houston, Houston, TX, USA

Megan Clark, MD University of Kansas, Department of Physical Medicine and Rehabilitation, Kansas City, KS, USA

Yan Cui Magram, MD New York Presbyterian Hospital-Weill Cornell Medicine, Department of Anesthesiology, New York, NY, USA

Oscar A. de Leon-Casasola, MD The Jacobs School of Medicine and Biomedical Sciences, Department of Anesthesiology, Buffalo, NY, USA

Division of Pain Medicine, Roswell Park Cancer Institute, Buffalo, NY, USA

Gary E. Deng, MD, PhD Memorial Sloan Kettering Cancer Center, Department of Integrative Medicine Service, New York, NY, USA

Nadya M. Dhanani, MD Memorial Hermann Hospital/Mischer Neuroscience Institute, Department of Pain Management/Neurosurgery, Houston, TX, USA

Kavita V. Dharmarajan, MD, MSc Icahn School of Medicine at Mount Sinai, New York, NY, USA

Gendai J. Echezona, MD Eagle Consulting Services,White Plains, NY, USA

Maxim S. Eckmann, MD University of Texas Health Science Center at San Antonio (UTHSCSA), UT Medicine Pain Consultants, Department of Anesthesiology, San Antonio, TX, USA

University of Texas Health Science Center at San Antonio (UTHSCSA), Department of Anesthesiology, San Antonio, TX, USA

Robert R. Edwards, PhD Department of Anesthesiology, Perioperative, and Pain Medicine, Brigham & Women's Hospital and Harvard Medical School, BWH Pain Management Center, Chestnut Hill, MA, USA

Rodney J. Ellis, MD University Hospitals Seidman Cancer Center, Case Comprehensive Cancer Center, Department of Radiation Oncology, Cleveland, OH, USA

Mitchell P. Engle, MD, PhD Institute of Precision Pain Medicine, Corpus Christi, TX, USA

Jacob Fehl, MD Kansas City VA Medical Center, Kansas City, MO, USA

Joel Frontera, MD McGovern Medical School at The University of Texas Health Science Center at Houston (UTHealth), Houston, TX, USA

Jack B. Fu, MD Department of Palliative Care & Rehabilitation Medicine, University of Texas MD Anderson Cancer Center, Houston, TX, USA

R. Garrett Key, MD University of Texas at Austin Dell Medical School, Austin, TX, USA

Peter C. Gerszten, MD, MPH, FACS University Hospitals Seidman Cancer Center, Case Comprehensive Cancer Center, Department of Radiation Oncology, Cleveland, OH, USA

Amol J. Ghia, MD University of Texas MD Anderson Cancer Center, Department of Radiation Oncology, Houston, TX, USA

Arvider Gill, DO The Jacobs School of Medicine and Biomedical Sciences, Department of Anesthesiology, Buffalo, NY, USA

Ramon Go, MD Pain Management, Memorial Sloan Kettering Cancer Center, New York, NY, USA

Karina Gritsenko, MD Montefiore Medical Center – Albert Einstein College of Medicine, Bronx, NY, USA

Amitabh Gulati, MD, FIPP Department of Anesthesiology and Critical Care, Memorial Sloan Kettering Cancer Center, New York, NY, USA

Simon Guo, MD Northport Veterans Affairs Medical Center, Department of Anesthesia, Northport, NY, USA

Joseph C. Hung, MD Memorial Sloan Kettering Cancer Center, Anesthesiology and Critical Care Medicine, New York, NY, USA

Roy Hwang West Virginia University, Department of Neurosurgery, Morgantown, WV, USA

Sarah Hwang, MD Shirley Ryan AbilityLab, Chicago, IL, USA

Prathap Jayaram, MD Baylor College of Medicine, Department of Physical Medicine and Rehabilitation, Houston, TX, USA

Candice Johnstone, MD, MPH Department of Radiation Oncology, Medical College of Wisconsin, Milwaukee, WI, USA

Yury Khelemsky, MD Icahn School of Medicine at Mount Sinai, Department of Anesthesiology, New York, NY, USA

Namrata Khimani, MD Department of Anesthesiology, Perioperative and Pain Medicine, The Pain Management Center at Brigham and Women's Hospital, Chestnut Hill, MA, USA

Dhanalakshmi Koyyalagunta, MD Department of Pain Medicine, UTMD Anderson Cancer Center, Houston, TX, USA

Mario E. Lacouture, MD Department of Medicine, Memorial Sloan Kettering Cancer Center, New York, NY, USA

Jack W. Lam, MD Rex Hospital, Wake Med Cary Hospital, Duke Raleigh Hospital, Department of Anesthesia, Raleigh, NC, USA

Asimina Lazaridou, PhD Department of Anesthesiology, Brigham & Women's Hospital and Harvard Medical School, BWH Pain Management Center, Chestnut Hill, MA, USA

Aron Legler, MD Memorial Sloan Kettering, Department of Anesthesiology, New York, NY, USA

Eric Leung, MD Department of Physical Medicine and Rehabilitation, Northwell Health, Manhasset, NY, USA

Jeffrey Loh, MD, MS Queen's Medical Center, Department of Anesthesiology & Pain Management, Honolulu, HI, USA

Stephen L. Long, MD Department of Anesthesiology, UCSF Benioff Children's Hospital Oakland, Oakland, CA, USA

Simon S. Lo, MD, FACR University of Washington School of Medicine, Department of Radiation Oncology, Seattle, WA, USA

Michael Lubrano, MD, MPH Department of Anesthesia & Perioperative Care, University of California San Francisco (UCSF) Medical Center, San Francisco, CA, USA

Meilani Mapa, MD Memorial Rehabilitation Institute, Memorial Healthcare Systems, Division of Physical Medicine and Rehabilitation, Hollywood, FL, USA

Ilan Margulis Department of Anesthesiology, New York-Presbyterian Hospital/Weill Cornell Medicine, New York, NY, USA

Neel D. Mehta, MD Joan and Sanford I. Weill Cornell Medical College of Cornell University, New York Presbyterian Hospital, Division of Pain Management, Department of Anesthesiology, New York, NY, USA

Jonathan Miller, MD, FAANS, FACS University Hospitals Case Medical Center, Case Western Reserve University, Cleveland, OH, USA

Ryan K. Murphy, DO Valley Medical Group, Waldwick, NJ, USA

Ameet Nagpal, MD, MS, MEd University of Texas Health Science Center at San Antonio (UTHSCSA), UT Medicine Pain Consultants, Department of Anesthesiology, San Antonio, TX, USA

University of Texas Health Science Center at San Antonio (UTHSCSA), Department of Anesthesiology, San Antonio, TX, USA

Sanjeet Narang, MD Department of Anesthesiology, Perioperative and Pain Medicine, The Pain Management Center at Brigham and Women's Hospital, Harvard Medical School, Chestnut Hill, MA, USA

Diane M. Novy, PhD Department of Pain Medicine, The University of Texas MD Anderson Cancer Center, Houston, TX, USA

Daniel Pak, MD Massachusetts General Hospital, Boston, MA, USA

Parag G. Patil, MD, PhD University of Michigan Medical Center, Ann Arbor, MI, USA

Devin Peck, MD Physician, Austin Interventional Pain, Austin, TX, USA

Mohammad M. Piracha, MD Joan and Sanford I. Weill Cornell Medical College of Cornell University, New York Presbyterian Hospital, Division of Pain Management, Department of Anesthesiology, New York, NY, USA

Joan Pope, MSN Memorial Sloan Kettering, New York, NY, USA

Anussara Prayongrat, MD King Chulalongkorn Memorial Hospital and Chulalongkorn University, Department of Radiation Oncology, Bangkok, Thailand

Jeffrey Prinsell Jr., MD Pain Management, Memorial Sloan Kettering Cancer Center, New York, NY, USA

Vinay Puttanniah, MD Memorial Sloan Kettering Cancer Center, Anesthesiology and Critical Care Medicine, New York, NY, USA

Ahmed M. Raslan, MD Oregon Health & Science University, Department of Neurosurgery, Portland, OR, USA

Portland VA Medical Center, Neurological Surgery, Portland, OR, USA

Shervin Razavian, MD Anesthesia Associates of Kansas City, Overland Park, KS, USA

Shayna E. Rich, MD, PhD, MA Haven Hospice, Gainesville, FL, USA

Erich Richter, MD, FAANS New Orleans Neurosurgical Associates, Marrero, LA, USA

Roy Rivera Jr., PT, PhD, DPT, CHES Crom Rehabilitation, LLC, Department of Outpatient Sports Medicine, Houston, TX, USA

William S. Rosenberg, MD, FAANS Center for the Relief of Pain, Kansas City, MO, USA

Joshua M. Rosenow, MD Northwestern Memorial Hospital, Department of Neurosurgery, Neurology and Physical Medicine and Rehabilitation, Chicago, IL, USA

Lisa Marie Ruppert, MD Memorial Sloan Kettering Cancer Center, New York, NY, USA

Veena Sankar, MD Austin Anesthesiology Group, Austin, TX, USA

Dawood Sayed, MD University of Kansas Medical Center, Department of Anesthesiology and Pain Medicine, Kansas City, KS, USA

Rajiv Shah, MD Washington University School of Medicine, Saint Louis, MO, USA

Shalini Shah, MD University of California, Irvine, Department of Anesthesiology and Perioperative Care, Irvine, CA, USA

Sana Shaikh, MD Memorial Sloan Kettering Cancer Center, New York, NY, USA

Kanu Sharan, MD MD Anderson Cancer Center at Cooper, Department of Hematology/Oncology, Camden, NJ, USA

Mourad M. Shehabar, MD Icahn School of Medicine at Mount Sinai, Department of Anesthesiology, New York, NY, USA

Maureen J. Simmonds, PhD, PT University of Texas, Physical Therapy Department, San Antonio, TX, USA

Jill E. Sindt, MD University of Utah, Department of Anesthesiology, Salt Lake City, UT, USA

Jonas M. Sokolof, DO Department of Rehabilitative Medicine, Weill College of Medicine Cornell University, New York, NY, USA

Department of Neurology – Rehabilitation Services, Memorial Sloan-Kettering Cancer Center, New York, NY, USA

Katerina Svigos, BA New York University School of Medicine, New York, NY, USA

Jennifer A. Sweet, MD University Hospitals Case Medical Center, Cleveland, OH, USA

Stephen Lawrence Thorp, MD Pain Medicine, Northwell Health Phelps Hospital, Sleepy Hollow, NY, USA

Mercy A. Udoji, MD Emory University/Atlanta Veterans' Administration, Department of Anesthesiology, Decatur, GA, USA

Ali Valimahomed, MD Department of Physical Medicine and Rehabilitation, New York-Presbyterian Hospital, Weill Cornell Medical College/Columbia University Vagelos College of Physicians and Surgeons, New York, NY, USA

Laura M. van Veldhoven, PhD, MPH Department of Physical Medicine and Rehabilitation, Baylor College of Medicine, Houston, TX, USA

Thomas J. Van de Ven, MD, PhD Duke University Medical Center and Durham VAMC, Department of Anesthesiology, Durham, NC, USA

Monica Verduzco-Gutierrez, MD Department of Physical Medicine and Rehabilitation, University of Texas Health Science Center, Houston, TX, USA

Ashwin Viswanathan Baylor College of Medicine, Department of Neurosurgery, Houston, TX, USA

Michelle Yakaboski, CPO Certified Prosthetist Orthotist at Boston Orthotics and Prosthetics, Stony Brook, NY, USA

Hooman Yarmohammadi, MD Certified Prosthetist Orthotist at Boston Orthotics and Prosthetics, Stony Brook, NY, USA

Nantthasorn Zinboonyahgoon, MD Department of Anesthesiology, Faculty of Medicine Siriraj Hospital, Mahidol University, Bangkok, Thailand

Department of Anesthesiology, Perioperative and Pain Medicine, Brigham and Women's Hospital, Harvard Medical School, Boston, MA, USA

Elena V. Zininberg, MD Weill Cornell School of Medicine, Department of Anesthesiology, New York, NY, USA

Department of Anesthesiology/Pain Management, Memorial Sloan Kettering, New York, NY, USA

Jennifer Zocca, MD Department of Anesthesiology, New York-Presbyterian Hospital, Weill Cornell Medical College, New York, NY, USA

Part I

Perspectives on Cancer Pain Medicine

1 Perspectives on Interventional Cancer Pain Management

Arvider Gill and Oscar A. de Leon-Casasola

As of January 2012, approximately 13.7 million Americans with a history of cancer were alive [1]. It is unclear how many of these individuals were cancer-free and how many had evidence of cancer and may have been undergoing treatment. Regardless, the burden of disease is significant; about 1,665,540 new cancer cases, not including cancer in situ, are expected to be diagnosed in 2014 [1]. If 30–50% of individuals with advanced cancer experience significant pain, then one can understand the high prevalence of pain affecting this population. Moreover, the 5-year relative survival rate for all cancers diagnosed between 2003 and 2009 is 68%, up from 49% in 1975–1977 [1]. These numbers explain the high number of patients experiencing pain due to their cancer treatments, including chemotherapy-induced peripheral neuropathy, postradiation visceral and neuropathic pain, and postsurgical pain syndromes. These survivors have increased the need for resources to treat these patients at cancer centers, as they have complex pain syndromes that are not managed by community physicians.

Despite advances in the understanding of the neurobiology of pain in cancer, the translation of this information to multimodal pharmacologic analgesic therapy and the advent of new interventional techniques for the management of cancer pain have not shown a dramatic reduction in the prevalence of patients experiencing cancer pain. Recently, a group in the Netherlands reported that 55% of the 1429 respondents with a diagnosis of cancer had experienced moderate to severe pain in the week prior to the survey and that 42% of patients were experiencing pain despite receiving pharmacological treatment for it [2]. In the United States, 3,123 ambulatory patients with breast, prostate, colorectal, or lung cancer were evaluated for pain at their first visit and then 4–5 weeks later. Of those patients, 67% had pain and ongoing pharmacological treatment with opioids at the first visit. However, 33% did not have adequate pain control at that time despite their treatment with opioids [3]. At the follow-up visit, though they continued treatment with opioids, there was no reduction in the number of patients experiencing inadequate pain control [3]. This study also showed that the prevalence of pain due to solid tumors has not changed in the United States in more than 20 years, despite the wide availability and increased consumption of opioids [3]. In contrast, a randomized clinical trial comparing intrathecal therapy (IT) to comprehensive medical management (CMM) in the treatment of refractory cancer pain showed that once the patients were enrolled into the study, and then treated by a pain specialist, there was a further 39% pain reduction in patients allocated to the CMM group versus a 51% in those receiving IT therapy [4]. The difference was not statistically significant illustrating the power of pharmacological therapy in the hands of pain specialists.

These findings suggest that the involvement of a pain specialist may have a significant impact in the quality of pain control experienced by cancer patients. This difference may be the result of the implementation of multimodal therapy with topical analgesics [5], judicious opioid use [6], anticonvulsants with modulating capabilities of the voltage-gated calcium channel [7], tricyclic antidepressants [7], and titration to doses associated with therapeutic effects [8]. The importance of adequate pain management in cancer patients needs to be underscored because there is evidence in the oncology literature that survival rates are proportionally related to symptom control and that pain management contributes to better psychosocial functioning and quality of life [9]. Because of the interactions of psychosocial issues and

A. Gill
The Jacobs School of Medicine and Biomedical Sciences, Department of Anesthesiology, Buffalo, NY, USA

O. A. de Leon-Casasola (✉)
The Jacobs School of Medicine and Biomedical Sciences, Department of Anesthesiology, Buffalo, NY, USA

Division of Pain Medicine, Roswell Park Cancer Institute, Buffalo, NY, USA
e-mail: Oscar.deleon@roswellpark.org

A. Gulati et al. (eds.), *Essentials of Interventional Cancer Pain Management*, https://doi.org/10.1007/978-3-319-99684-4_1

pain, care for these patients is best provided in a multidisciplinary environment where psychological support includes emotional support, coping skills training, and cognitive behavioral therapy [10].

As noted, evaluation of pain is critically important in the oncology patient. Pain intensity must be quantified, and quality must be characterized by the patient (whenever possible based on patient communication capacity). The brief pain inventory is an appropriate tool for this purpose [11], while the short form McGill Pain Questionnaire may be used in cancer patient to evaluate the multidimensionality of pain [12]. A comprehensive pain assessment should be performed if new pain is present and regularly performed for persisting pain. Moreover, the quality of pain must be evaluated to determine if there is a neuropathic pain component. There are several neuropathic pain scales that may be implemented for this purpose, including the Douleur Neuropathique (DN4) [13] and the Leeds assessment of neuropathic symptoms and signs (LANSS) [14], which are easy to use, and may be applied in a short period of time. The patient impression of adequate pain relief and the healthcare provider assessment of adequacy of function, and any special issues for the patient relevant to pain treatment, is also necessary to have a complete evaluation of the success of therapy. Because patients with cancer pain will likely need opioid therapy, it is also important to evaluate the patient for the risk of abuse and diversion. Several tools have been created for this purpose and can be easily implemented [15, 16].

Pharmacological pain therapy is very successful in cancer pain [6, 17]. However, invasive techniques are sometimes needed because patients cannot tolerate pharmacologic titration to therapeutic levels or because inadequate analgesia is achieved despite maximum doses of these agents. In these individuals, there are several options. These include neurolytic blocks of the sympathetic axis for those patients with a visceral pain component [18, 19], intrathecal therapy for both somatic and neuropathic pain components [20–22], peripheral and spinal cord stimulation [23], and other interventional procedures performed in the non-cancer population, as non-cancer-related pain may also occur in this population.

In summary, the use of pharmacological multimodal therapy and interventional procedures may result in successful pain control in the great majority of patients afflicted by cancer-related pain when implemented by practitioners well versed in the use of these alternative therapies.

References

1. American Cancer Society. Cancer facts & figures 2014. Atlanta: American Cancer Society; 2014.
2. van den Beuken-van Everdingen MHJ, de Rijke JM, Kessels AG, Schouten HC, van Kleef M, Parjin J. High prevalence of pain in patients with cancer in a large population-based study in the The Netherlands. Pain. 2007;132:312–20.
3. Fisch MJ, Lee J-W, Weiss M, Wagner LI, Chang VT, Cella V, Manola JB, Minasian LM, McCaskill-Stevens W, Mendoza TR, Cleeland CS. Prospective, observational study of pain and analgesic prescribing in medical oncology outpatient with breast, colorectal, lung, or prostate cancer. J Clin Oncol. 2012;30:1980–91.
4. Smith TJ, Staats PS, Deer T, Stearns LJ, Rauck RL, Boortz-Marx RL, Buchser E, Catala E, Bryce DA, Coyne PJ, Pool GE. Randomized clinical trial of an implantable drug delivery sytem compared with comprehensive medical management for refractory cancer pain: impact on pain, drug-related toxicity, and survival. J Clin Oncol. 2002;20:4040–9.
5. de Leon-Casasola OA. Multimodal approaches to the management of neuropathic pain: the role of topical analgesia. J Pain and Symp Manag. 2007;33:356–64.
6. de Leon-Casasola OA. Current developments in opioid therapy for the management of cancer pain. Clin J Pain. 2008;24(Suppl 10):S3–7.
7. O'Connor AB, Dworkin RH. Treatment of neuropathic pain: an overview of recent guidelines. Am J Med. 2009;122:S22–32.
8. de Leon-Casasola OA. Multimodal, multiclass, multidisciplinary therapy: the key to better analgesia in the 21st century? Clin J Pain. 2010;26(Suppl 10):S1–2.
9. Temel JS, Greer JA, Muzikansky A. Early palliative care for patients with metastatic non-small-cell lung cancer. N Engl J Med. 2010;363:733–42.
10. Morley S, Eccleston C, Williams A. Systematic review and meta-analysis of randomized controlled trials of cognitive behavior therapy and behavior therapy for chronic pain in adults, excluding headache. Pain. 1999;80:1–13.
11. Cleeland CS, Ryan KM. Pain assessment: global use of the brief pain inventory. Ann Acad Med Singapore. 1994;23:129–38.
12. Gauthier LR, Young A, Dworkin RH, Rodin G, Zimmermann C, Warr D, Librach SL, Moore M, Sheperd FA, Riddell RP, Macpherson A, Melzack R, Gagliese L. Validation of the short-form Mc Gill pain questionnaire-1 in younger and older people with cancer pain. J Pain. 2014;15:756–70.
13. Bouhassira D, Attal N, Alchaar H, Boureau F, Brochet B, Bruxelle J, Cunin G, Fermanian J, Ginies P, Grun-Overdyking A, Jafari-Schluep H, Lanteri-Minet M, Laurent B, Mick G, Serrie A, Valade D, Vicaut E. Comparison of pain syndromes associated with nervous or somatic lesions and development of a new neuropathic pain diagnostic questionnaire (DN4). Pain. 2005;114:29–36.
14. Bennett M. The LANSS pain scale: the Leeds assessment of neuropathic symptoms and signs. Pain. 2001;92:147–57.
15. Moore TM, Jones T, Browder JH, Daffron S, Passik SD. A comparison of common screening methods for predicting aberrant drug-related behavior among patients receiving opioids for chronic pain management. Pain Med. 2009;10:1426–33.
16. Webster LR, Webster RM. Predicting aberrant behaviors in opioid-treated patients: preliminary validation of the opioid risk tool. Pain Med. 2005;6:432–42.
17. de Leon-Casasola OA. Implementing therapy with opioids in cancer pain. Oncol Nurs Forum. 2008;35(6):S1–6.
18. Wong GY, Schroeder DR, Carns PE, Wilson JI, Martin DP, Kinney MO, Mantilla CB, Warner DO. Effect of neurolytic celiac plexus block on pain relief, quality of life, and survival in patients with unresectable pancreatic cancer. A randomized controlled trial. JAMA. 2004;291:1092–9.
19. de Leon-Casasola OA, Kent E, Lema MJ. Neurolytic superior hypogastric plexus block for chronic pelvic pain associated with cancer. Pain. 1993;54:145–51.
20. Lozano J, de Leon-Casasola OA. Indications for intrathecal therapy in cancer patients. Tech Reg Anesth Pain Manag. 2011;15:147–9.
21. de Leon-Casasola OA. Implementing and managing intrathecal pumps. Tech Reg Anesth Pain Manag. 2011;15:155–7.
22. Sparlin J, de Leon-Casasola OA. Intrathecal pump implantation techniques. Tech Reg Anesth Pain Manag. 2011;15:158–61.
23. de Leon-Casasola OA. Spinal cord and peripheral nerve stimulation techniques for neuropathic pain. J Pain Symp Manag. 2009;38:S28–38.

The Practice of Cancer Pain: A Case Series

2

Sana Shaikh

Introduction

Surviving cancer is just the beginning. Often the struggle for many patients is thriving after treatment which may be limited by pain. While strategies to treat pain in the chronic pain population exist, implementing pharmacologic and interventional therapies for the cancer pain patient may be challenging. The following case series illustrate a framework that chronic pain physicians may use to treat cancer pain syndromes.

The clinical practice of pain management can vary from one practice to another based on patient population and referrals. In community-based practices, practitioners may have a consistent population base with similar anatomy and pathophysiology. A distinct challenge to the practice of cancer pain medicine is that each patient's tumor pathology and metastatic disease leads to evolving sources of pain. It is important to consistently reevaluate imaging as the primary and secondary diseases result in changing pain syndromes. Choosing interventions is often balanced with oncologic treatment protocols and life expectancy.

Case 1: Oncologic Diagnosis in the Community Setting The incidence of cancer is 454.8 cases per 100,000 men and women per year (based on 2008–2012 cases) [1]. The epidemiology of cancer pain among diagnosed cases of cancer is variable depending on the source. A systematic review of 52 articles showed that pain was prevalent in 64% of patients with metastatic or advanced-stage disease, 59% in patients on anticancer treatment, and 33% in patients after curative treatment [2]. Another study estimated the prevalence of pain in cancer at 25% for those newly diagnosed, 33% for those undergoing active treatment, and greater than 75% for those with advanced-stage disease[3, 4]. Due to the high prevalence of pain as a symptom in cancer patients, it is important to consider an underlying oncologic process in the differential diagnosis when evaluating the initial presentation of pain.

Case 1: A 75-year-old female with a distant history of non-small cell lung cancer presents with right shoulder pain. The pain in the right-sided shoulder is a constant, sharp pain with radiation to the lateral aspect of the deltoid, elbow, and anterior chest wall over the right pectoralis muscle. She denies any numbness or tingling in the arm. Upon initial presentation of pain, the patient was evaluated at a community-based pain practice where she was given a prescription for physical therapy for the right shoulder and an intraarticular steroid injection.

The patient noted that physical therapy exacerbated her shoulder pain and that the injection resulted in minimal improvement of her symptoms. Multiple opioid regimens were tried with dose-limiting nausea noted and a lack of adequate pain relief achieved. Despite the addition of steroids, nerve pain-modulating medications, and muscle relaxants, the pain progressively worsened at which time she presented to the hospital with severe pain and limited ability to move the right shoulder.

CT examination of the right shoulder revealed a lytic lesion in the glenoid process of the right scapula along with a complete supraspinatus tear (Fig. 2.1). A PET scan showed a large lytic lesion within the right coracoid process extending into the glenoid process. She was started on a regimen of steroids and radiation therapy to the right glenoid process. After 2 weeks of radiation with minimal improvement in symptoms, both the interventional pain service and orthopedic surgery were consulted for possible interventions to improve patient's shoulder pain.

Given her the anatomy and location of her pathology, the patient would unlikely benefit from an additional intraarticular shoulder joint injection. A consultation and discussion with orthopedic surgery led to a recommendation of

S. Shaikh (✉)
Memorial Sloan Kettering Cancer Center, New York, NY, USA
e-mail: shaikhs@mskcc.org

A. Gulati et al. (eds.), *Essentials of Interventional Cancer Pain Management*, https://doi.org/10.1007/978-3-319-99684-4_2

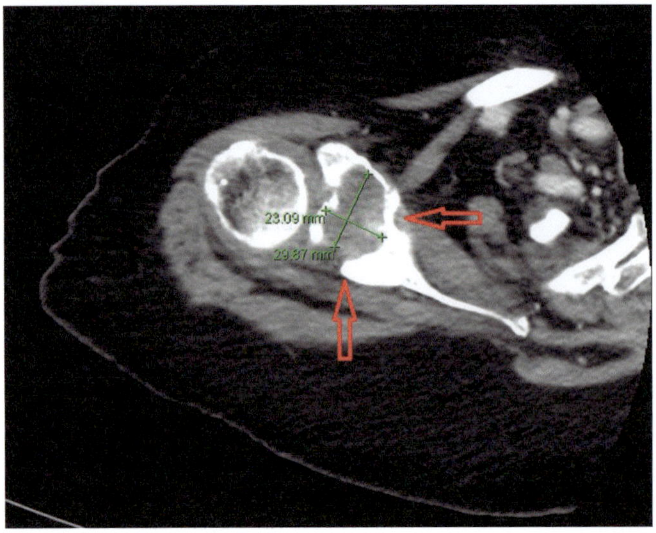

Fig. 2.1 CT scan of the right upper extremity is demonstrating a lytic metastasis in the superior glenoid (arrows) with new cortical breakthrough and an extraosseous soft tissue component and new probable nondisplaced, pathologic fracture

surgical resection of the coracoid and scapula fracture along with rotator cuff tendon repairs. After pain management, anesthesia, and surgical discussion, it was decided to proceed with the surgery with preoperative nerve blocks to help with postoperative pain control and rehabilitation. Ultrasound guidance was used to target right cervical C5 and C6 for neural blockade in combination with the PECSII nerve block. Perioperatively, the patient was noted to have excellent pain relief with regional analgesia lending to an overall perceived decrease in oral opioid regimen requirements.

Patients undergoing orthopedic surgery for tumor resection often have anatomical considerations unique to their tumor location. Surgical incisions and planning can often be unpredictable and cross multiple dermatomes in comparison with orthopedic surgery for nonmalignant pain. Careful planning between the acute pain specialist, anesthesiologist, and surgical teams is important to ensure adequate perioperative pain relief.

Case 2: Symptom Management in Oncologic Pain Treatment A systematic review of palliative symptoms in cancer patients showed that their most prevalent symptoms were fatigue, excretory symptoms, urinary incontinence, asthenia, pain, constipation, and anxiety which occurred in at least 50% of patients [5]. In a comparison between palliative care in cancer and non-cancer geriatric patients, cancer patients were found to have more pain, digestive symptoms, psychological symptoms, and fatigue than non-cancer patients. The study also found that the prevalence of digestive symptoms, pain, and psychological symptoms was higher in younger and in cancer patients than in the elderly and the non-cancer patients [6]. A systematic review demonstrated that home, hospital, and inpatient specialist palliative care significantly improved patient outcomes in the domains of pain and symptom control, anxiety, and reduced hospital admissions [7]. Overall the treatment of palliative and pain symptoms is crucial to the quality of life patients experience as part of their cancer treatment.

Case 2: A 57-year-old male with metastatic colon cancer involving the liver and lungs presents with intractable hiccups. His hiccups started after a CT scan and have occurred every few minutes consistently with some periods of pause not lasting longer than 20 min. As an outpatient, his oncologist tried a regimen of baclofen twice a day dosing with no change in symptoms. He was also given a single dose of fluconazole to empirically treat esophageal candidiasis. As part of the workup for this patient's new onset of hiccups, the patient had reimaging of the body including CT of the chest, abdomen, and pelvis (Fig. 2.2). This imaging showed an increase in size and number of multiple bilateral pulmonary metastases and persistent splenomegaly, with portal venous hypertension. It was suspected that diaphragmatic irritation secondary to pulmonary metastatic disease was the likely etiology of the patient's persistent hiccups.

A trial of bilateral sphenopalatine ganglion blocks was performed which resulted in only a 20 min resolution of the hiccups. A trial of gabapentin 300 milligrams daily was initiated and titrated to three times a day dosing along with a regimen of oral viscous lidocaine to be swallowed instead of rinsed three times a day. The patient had complete resolution of hiccups after therapeutic titration of oral viscous lidocaine and Neurontin at three times a day. The patient was discharged on maintenance gabapentin therapy and oral viscous lidocaine on an as-needed basis.

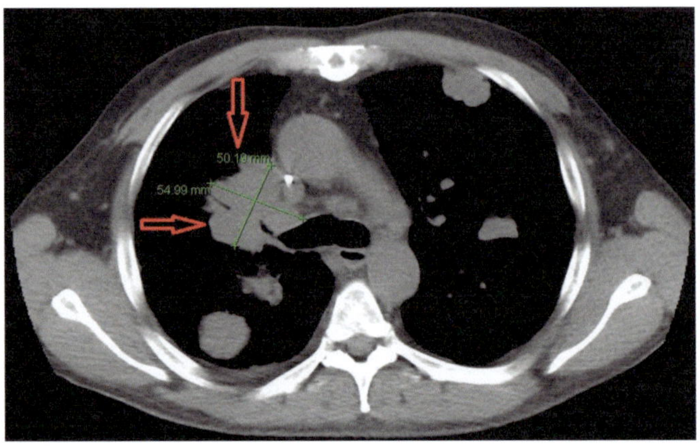

Fig. 2.2 CT of the chest, abdomen, and pelvis with contrast showed slightly increased size of bilateral pulmonary metastases in the right upper and lower lobes. The picture above showed the right peri-hilar mass increased marked narrowing of the right upper lobe bronchus (arrows)

Localized treatments for pain including directed topical treatments can often be helpful to treat novel causes of pain.

Case 3: Changing Pain States in Oncologic Patients The symptoms of cancer often change over time, and there is a need for practitioners to have a low threshold for reevaluation of the underlying disease process. New symptoms can manifest from treatment or from progression of cancer, either locally or to distant sites. Diagnostic workup of these possibilities is important in determining the treatment plan. Collaboration between interventional pain and other service may offer patients a wide variety of options to treat different pain and non-pain symptoms during cancer treatment. Ultimately, it is most important to consider a wide array of therapies to optimize symptom manage and quality of life.

Case 3: A 41-year-old male with multifocal peripheral schwannoma involving the pleura and liver presents with right-sided chest wall pain. Interventional radiology recommended cryoablation of this lesion on the anterior aspect of the seventh rib. The patient was also referred for consultation with the pain service for possible interventional options for pain relief.

On initial assessment, patient noted pain as a sharp, tingling, and burning in the right upper quadrant of the abdomen. Despite the use of opioids, the patient found the pain to cause significant daily disability. Upon physical exam, there was tenderness to palpation across the right seventh and eighth rib in an anterolateral location This correlated with a seventh rib schwannoma (Fig. 2.3). A right-sided intercostal nerve block of the seventh and eighth ribs under ultrasound guidance was performed.

The patient's noted significant improvement from baseline and that relief lasted for 11 weeks. At that time, pain returned with the same presentation and severity. Given the positive response from first procedure, the intercostal nerve blocks were repeated; however the patient had minimal relief from this procedure. Given this response, imaging with an MRI of the thoracolumbar spine was repeated to evaluate for extension of disease into the spinal cord. MRI of the spine revealed paraspinal masses abutting exiting nerve roots at the right T7–T8 level. A thoracic epidural was performed with significant relief of the patient's pain. Patient's pain relief lasted for 6 weeks with significant progression of the original disease. Due to the rate of disease growth, we planned for intrathecal pump placement to treat the neuraxial source of the pain.

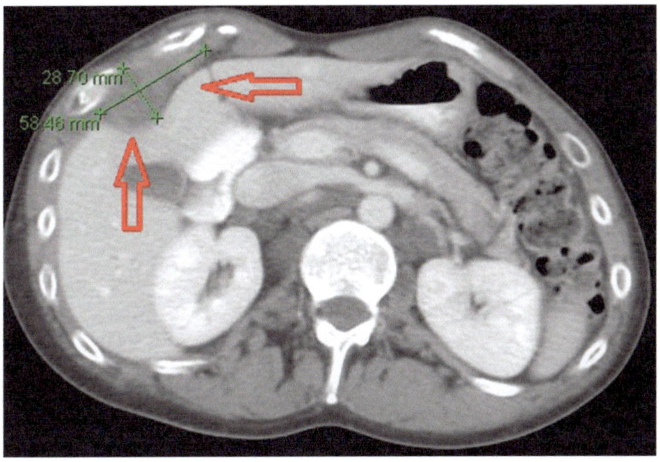

Fig. 2.3 CT of the chest and abdomen with contrast showing right-sided chest wall mass responsible for patient's first onset of chest wall pain (arrows)

Though various nerve blocks can make sense clinically based on the history and physical exam, it is often necessary to correlate these findings with relevant and up-to-date imaging in order to optimize efficacy and safety of a planned intervention. It's important to consider the possibility that an initial intervention that was helpful may not be possible given changes in anatomy related to progression of disease. It is crucial to always reassess patients given the aggressive nature of some of the baseline etiologies.

Case 4 and 5: Considerations for Intrathecal Drug Delivery in the Oncologic Population The goal of interventional pain physician is to consider intervening in someone's pain outcome as early as possible to treat a patient's pain and improve their quality of life and function. The intrathecal delivery of opioids and other adjuvant medications is an effective way to treat refractory cancer pain while minimizing systemic side effects and allowing for a greater ability to address increased pain medication requirements. A randomized clinical trial of implantable drug systems showed better clinical pain relief, less systemic side effects, and a tendency toward increased survival in the treatment of cancer pain [8].

The following two cases describe clinical scenarios where directed drug delivery via an intrathecal pump would be indicated and how the progression of disease ultimately was the reason to proceed or the reason to not proceed with an intrathecal pump placement. Intrathecal drug delivery is an especially useful method to very quickly adjust and meet increasing opioid requirements while minimizing side effects.

Case 4: A 35-year-old woman who was recently diagnosed with adenocarcinoma of the rectum in the setting of Crohn's disease presents for consultation with the interventional pain team 6 months after being diagnosed. The patient's pain first started with increasing perineal discomfort and pain. She underwent imaging studies with MRI of the abdomen and pelvis which showed enlarged perirectal lymph nodes and three irregular hypodense masses in the liver which were suspicious for metastatic disease. Liver biopsy would confirm metastatic disease and rectal cancer. Further imaging showed perirectal nodal disease and distant mets to the liver, pleura, left adrenal, and bone.

The patient's perirectal pain progressed to include saddle anesthesia, with pain in the right buttock radiating around laterally into the right groin and intermittent right first toe paresthesia. Additional workup was consistent with extensive disease from T12 through the sacrum, an L5 fracture, left foraminal narrowing due to metastasis at L4–L5 and L5–S1, and presacral extraosseous disease with right S2–S3 sacral nerve root impingement (Fig. 2.4a and b). She denies bowel or bladder incontinence and noted no weakness in the lower extremities. Interventional radiology and the pain service were consulted for on input on symptomatic treatment of the pain in conjunction with ongoing chemotherapy. Radiation therapy to the sacral spine was started along with an oral steroid regimen.

The patient and pain practitioner's initial goal was to alleviate as much of the patient's perineal paresthesias and radicular pain as possible. Review of the MRI showed no disease at the sacral hiatus, and a caudal epidural steroid injection was planned. The patient's INR was elevated likely due to hepatic involvement and was treated with vitamin K. Once the coagulopathy improved, a caudal epidural steroid injection was performed with moderate relief of radicular pain. She continued to have midline sacral pain. Directed drug delivery via an intrathecal pump was discussed given the fast progression of the disease after completion of radiation therapy. Unfortunately, the patient's disease would continue to progress aggressively and left her with a limited prognosis affecting her risk and benefit profile for intrathecal pump placement. The benefits of the procedure did not outweigh the risks and costs for placement of an intrathecal pump. Further goals of care were discussed with the patient, and a plan for hospice initiation was determined. The patient's pain was managed with hydromorphone PCA.

Patient's may often have pain that is amenable to directed drug delivery via intrathecal pump; however it is important to reconcile the patient's wishes and beliefs regarding palliation with the risks and benefits of the procedure. An intrathecal pump placement can improve patient's ability to be functional, and often pain is a short-term setback before the benefits are achieved.

Case 5: A 36-year-old male with a history of sacral spindle cell sarcoma metastatic to the pelvis presented to the inpatient pain service after having had a left-sided hind-quarter amputation (Fig. 2.5). The consultation is called for acutely worsened pain in the left groin and pelvis on an inpatient basis. An epidural catheter had been placed perioperatively for acute pain control, but a plan for intrathecal drug delivery had simultaneously been discussed with the patient. The epidural was dosed with a combination of hydromorphone and bupivacaine solution. An epidural trial of medica-

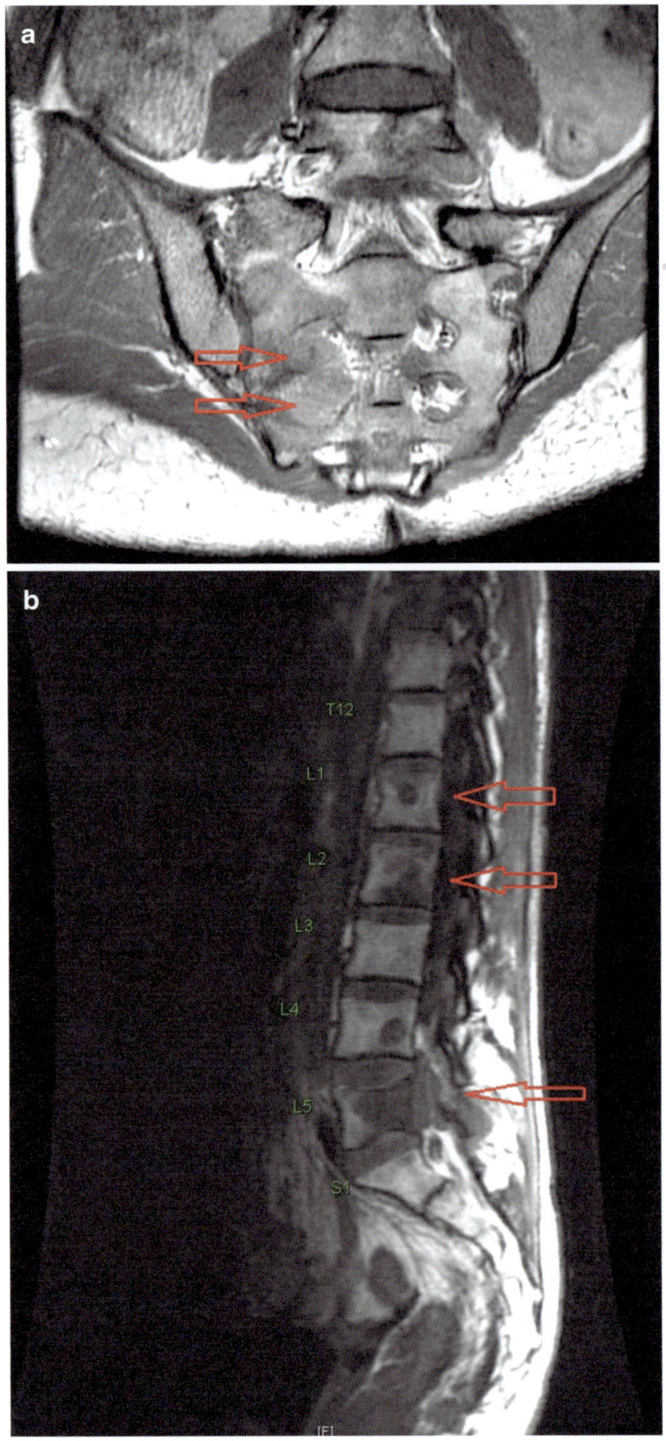

Fig. 2.4 (**a**) *Left* MRI sacrum showing bilateral sacral metastases have increased with bilateral presacral extraosseous disease. The right sacral ala with metastasis infiltrates into the S2 and to a greater extent the S3 neural foramina (arrows). (**b**) *Right* MRI lumbar spine consistent with osseous metastases involving almost every level throughout the cervical, thoracic, and lumbar spine (arrows at L1, L2, and L5 vertebral disease with epidural extension at L5)

tion can often be considered when considering the efficacy of neuraxial medicine prior to intrathecal pump placement. The patient noted improved pain control and side effect pro-

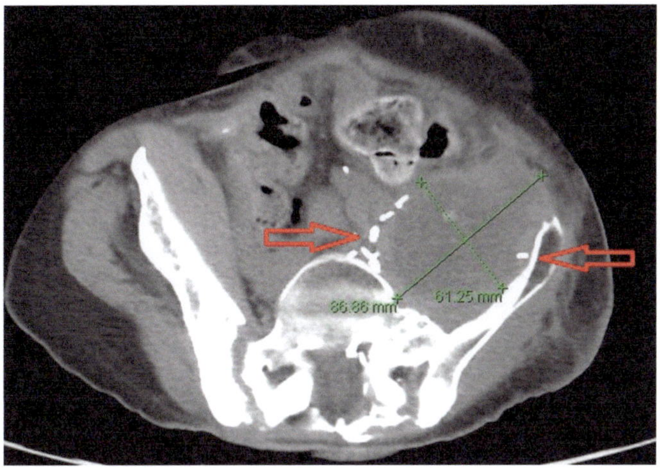

Fig. 2.5 CT of the chest, abdomen, and pelvis shows necrotic left pelvic mass centered at the left iliopsoas muscle and extending into the peritoneum (arrows)

file from decrease in systemic opioid treatment. An intrathecal pump was placed without any side effects or complications, and the patient returned for subsequent outpatient visits and for adjustment of dose over the next few months. Ultimately the cancer progressed, and various combinations and doses of intrathecal medications were titrated to alleviate the pain.

A retrospective case study of 46 cancer patients who had an epidural trial discussed how to use a patient's pre-pump systemic opioid requirements to calculate an appropriate intrathecal dose without having to do an epidural trial [8]. There are several ways to trial a patient for neuraxial directed drug delivery, but epidural trial can be a reasonable option for patients who are in the hospital.

Conclusion

This chapter highlights several different cases that can represent challenges to interventional pain physicians when treating cancer patients. It is crucial to continuously challenge and adjust the therapeutic plan as patients' underlying pathology, treatments, and goals of care change. Most important is having a low threshold to consider that an initial underlying pathology has changed and may require new diagnostics or a change in management. Ultimately the goal is optimal pain relief and to give patients a chance to enhance their quality of life and functionality. Each patient has personal goals, and it is these benchmarks that should guide therapy. Each patient's case provides an opportunity for reflection and reminds pain practitioners to learn, advance, and develop algorithms to best treat each patient.

References

1. NIH: National Cancer Institute. Cancer statistics. https://www.cancer.gov/about-cancer/understanding/statistics
2. Van den Beuken-van Everdingen MH, de Rijke JM, Kessels AG, et al. Prevalence of pain in patients with cancer: a systematic review of the past 40 years. Ann Oncol. 2007;18(9):1437–49.
3. American Pain Society (APS). Principles of analgesic use in the treatment of acute pain and cancer pain. 6th ed. Glenview: American Pain Society; 2008.
4. National Comprehensive Cancer Network. Clinical practice guidelines in oncology for adult cancer pain. V. 1.2010. Fort Washington: National Comprehensive Cancer Network. 2010. Available at: www.nccn.org. Accessed 1 Nov 2010.
5. Van Lancker A, Velghe A, Van Hecke A, Verbrugghe M, Van Den Noortgate N, Grypdonck M, Verhaeghe S, Bekkering G, Beeckman D. Prevalence of symptoms in older cancer patients receiving palliative care: a systematic review and meta-analysis. J Pain Symptom Manag. 2014;47(1):90–104. https://doi.org/10.1016/j.jpainsymman.2013.02.016.
6. Borgsteede SD, et al. Symptoms in patients receiving palliative care: a study on patient-physician encounters in general practice. Palliat Med. 2007;21:417–23.
7. Higginson IJ, Evans CJ. What is the evidence that palliative care teams improve outcomes for cancer patients and their families? Cancer J. 2010;16(5):423–35. https://doi.org/10.1097/PPO.0b013e3181f684e5.
8. Malhotra VT, Root J, Kesselbrenner J, Njoku I, Cubert K, Gulati A, Puttanniah V, Bilsky M, Kaplitt M. Intrathecal pain pump infusions for intractable cancer pain: an algorithm for dosing without a neuraxial trial. Anesth Analg. 2013;116(6):1364–70.

Part II

Cancer Pain Syndromes

Pathophysiology of Cancer Pain

3

Stephen Lawrence Thorp

Introduction

The International Association for the Study of Pain defines pain as "an unpleasant sensory and emotional experience associated with actual or potential tissue damage, or described in terms of such damage" [1]. Pain is prevalent among patients with cancer, with a systematic review finding pain prevalence to be 66.4% in advanced metastatic or terminal disease, 55% during anticancer treatment, 39.3% after curative treatment, and moderate to severe pain being reported in 38.0% of all patients [2]. Adequate control of pain can improve patient's quality of life through improved mood, functional status, and rest, among other things. Pain may even be related to survival [3]. Cancer-related pain is unique and may be related to the anatomic location of the tumor, pathophysiology of the tumor, or treatment of the tumor. Similarly, the origin of the pain itself can be somatic, visceral, neuropathic, or mixed in nature. Given the complexity of cancer pain and its multiple etiologies, it is critical to assess the pathophysiology of the cancer and its role in creating a pain syndrome.

Anatomic Location of Tumors

Pathophysiology of Bone Tumor Pain

The location of a tumor is often the direct cause of significant pain for patients. As an example, tumors in the bone are one of the most common sources of pain in patients with cancer. There are multiple types of primary benign and malignant bone tumors, and metastasis to bone is common [4]. When tumors metastasize to the bone, the route is most commonly hematogenous but can also be due to contiguous spread or via lymphatics. The vertebrate is the most common site of metastasis; however the pelvis, ribs, femur, and skull are also common sites. Patients typically present with well-localized pain that worsens with weight bearing and activity and is tender to palpation on physical examination.

The etiology of bone pain is complex and not fully understood [5]. The periosteum and marrow cavity are both innervated by peripheral nociceptors capable of causing pain. In animal studies, it has been shown that sensory and sympathetic neurons innervate the bone, with the periosteum having the densest innervation followed by the bone marrow [6]. The sensory fibers that innervate the bone differ from more well-characterized afferents that innervate the skin. Bone is innervated primarily by A-delta fibers, and there is very little innervation by either C-fibers or A-β fibers [7]. Sharp nociceptive bone pain is likely transmitted by the A-δ fibers, and the dull ache is transmitted from the C-fibers that become sensitized. Bone pain likely has a neuropathic component as well, as invading tumor cells injure sensory fibers [8].

When bone is invaded by cancer cells, a release of inflammatory mediators such as prostaglandin E_2 (PGE2) sensitizes the peripheral nociceptors. This mechanism underlies the role for nonsteroidal anti-inflammatory (NSAIDS) agents in treating bone pain. Metastasis and primary tumors can be lytic, due to increased osteoclastic activity, or sclerotic, due to increased osteoblastic activity, both of which induce mechanical instability in the bone [9]. The instability in the bone may eventually manifest as a vertebral compression fractures (VCF) if the tumor is located in the vertebral body. Fractures localized within the vertebral body may be treated with vertebral augmentation techniques such as kyphoplasty; however, more severe fractures resulting in neurological dysfunction and severe pain may require surgical stabilization.

S. L. Thorp (✉)
Pain Medicine, Northwell Health Phelps Hospital,
Sleepy Hollow, NY, USA
e-mail: sthorp@northwell.edu

A. Gulati et al. (eds.), *Essentials of Interventional Cancer Pain Management*, https://doi.org/10.1007/978-3-319-99684-4_3

Etiologies of Neuropathic Pain

Accordingly, tumor location in close proximity to neural structures can lead to neurological impairment and neuropathic pain. Neoplastic plexopathy represents a severe and difficult to treat form of cancer pain. Neoplastic plexopathy arises when a tumor progresses to involve one of the main plexuses; the cervical, brachial, or lumbosacral plexus. Treatment for tumor-induced plexopathies may involve surgical or radiation therapy, in addition to neuropathic pain medications.

The cervical plexus contains contributions from the C1, C2, C3, and C4 spinal nerves and provides innervation for the muscles of the neck as well as the prevertebral muscles. Impingement upon this plexus by tumor can result in cervical plexopathy, which typically presents with pain in the neck, shoulder, or throat. Weakness in the shoulder is related to weakness in the trapezius and sternocleidomastoid muscles, which are innervated by the spinal accessory nerve. The patient may also have shortness of breath, particularly if there is underlying pulmonary pathology, due to involvement of the phrenic nerve and hemidiaphragmatic paralysis. Cervical plexopathy is most commonly associated with head and neck tumors and lymphomas but may also be due to lung and breast cancers [10]. The cervical plexus can be blocked superficially resulting in cutaneous analgesia, or by anesthetizing the C2, C3, and C4 spinal nerves as they exit their respective cervical foramina, or the deep cervical plexus.

Far more common than tumors impacting the cervical plexus are tumors compressing the brachial plexus. The brachial plexus is composed of the ventral rami of C5–T1 in most individuals, with occasional contributions from C4 and T2 spinal nerves. The nerve roots exit the foramina and travel anterolateral between the anterior and middle scalene muscles, where they combine to form superior, middle, and interior trunks. At approximately the level of the first rib, these trunks again divide into an anterior and posterior division, which then form the lateral, medial, and posterior cords, so-named for their relation to the axillary artery. The three cords then divide into the peripheral nerves which supply innervation to the upper extremities.

Brachial plexopathy is most commonly associated with lung and breast cancer. Superior sulcus, or Pancoast, tumors are located at the apex of the lung and may impinge upon the brachial plexus. The clinical presentation of the plexopathy is related to where the plexus is impacted. The most commonly affected portion of the brachial plexus is the lower roots, and patients often present with radicular pain and radiculopathies in an ulnar nerve distribution. When head and neck neoplasms impact the brachial plexus, they typically affect the upper cervical roots and superior trunk, causing pain more commonly in a median or radial nerve distribution.

The lumbar and sacral plexus provide innervation to the lower extremity. The lumbar plexus is comprised of the ventral rami of the L1–L4 spinal nerves, with variable contributions from the T12 and L5 spinal nerves. The plexus lies in the psoas compartment located between the quadratus lumborum and psoas muscles and is composed of dorsal and ventral divisions. The main branches of the lumbar plexus include the femoral, obturator, and lateral femoral cutaneous nerves as well as the iliohypogastric, ilioinguinal, and genitofemoral nerves. The sacral plexus arises from S1–S3 giving rise to the sciatic nerve posteriorly, which then forms the common peroneal and tibial nerves, as well as the pudendal nerve which provides sensation to the perineal area.

The most common tumors invading this plexus are colorectal, sarcomas, and genito-ureteral tumors, with the sacral plexus being involved more commonly than the lumbar plexus. When the lumbar plexus is involved, the most common presenting symptom is leg pain, followed by numbness and weakness [11]. As the plexus lies in the psoas compartment, tumors affecting the psoas muscle can cause significant pain, termed malignant psoas syndrome [12]. When the sacral plexus is involved, the clinical picture can present with pain down the posterior aspect of the leg and weakness in the foot, similar to an S1 radiculopathy. The patient may also present with perineal pain and incontinence in later stages. Diagnosis of neoplastic plexopathy is confirmed with magnetic resonance imaging (MRI) and positron emission tomography (PET) to identify areas of active neoplasm in or abutting the plexus. Electromyography (EMG) can be used to further elucidate which nerves are most affected and guide treatment.

Other Associated Pathophysiology for Anatomic Cancer-Related Pain

While pain related to tumor in the bone and nervous system structures is the most common cause of anatomical pain, other anatomical locations may generate pain as well. Tumors in the brain are well known to cause headaches, as are metastasis to the spinal meninges [13]. Distension of capsular organs is another well-known cause of tumor-related pain as occurs when liver tumors distend Glisson's capsule causing abdominal pain [14]. In all of these examples, the primary treatment of cancer pain is treatment of the cancer and any therapies that remove or reduce the size of the tumor.

Chemical Mediators of Pain

The tumor microenvironment (TME) is composed of tumor cells and stromal cells and has a substantial role in tumor progression and cancer-mediated pain [15]. Tumor and stromal cells communicate with each other, their microenvironment, as well as the tissue they are invading by secreting multiple noxious chemical factors, inflammatory mediators, and immunomodulators. These stimuli are transduced at peripheral nociceptors and transmitted via an action potential to the spinal cord and travel via ascending tracts to the supraspinal processing centers. While this likely plays a role in all cancers, the details of a few specific examples have been elucidated.

Pathophysiology of Pain in Patients with Multiple Myeloma

Multiple myeloma is a malignant cancer of plasma cells that results in a unique pain syndrome referred to as myeloma bone disease. Bone pain is the most common symptom reported at presentation, in more than two-thirds of patients, and 80–90% of patients with multiple myeloma will develop bone lesions during their disease [16]. The etiology of this bone pain is likely dysregulation in bone remodeling. Normal bone remodeling is a continuous process of old bone resorption stimulated by osteoclasts and new bone formation through collagen synthesis and mineralization by osteoblasts. When multiple myeloma metastasizes to the bone, it induces bone resorption by activating osteoclasts. The myeloma cells release and stimulate cells in the bone marrow microenvironment to release osteoclastogenic activating factors such as RANKL, MIP-1α, TNF-α, interleukin 3 (IL-3), and IL-6 [17]. In addition to the stimulation of osteoclast formation and activity, many of these factors are also involved in the inhibition of osteoblastic activity as well as a supportive role for myeloma cells themselves.

Pathophysiology of Cancer Pain in Patients with Breast Cancer

Breast cancer, in addition to causing pain with metastasis to sites such as the bone and compressing neural structures as discussed previously, causes pain through the release of chemical mediators as well. The tumor and stromal cells release and induce host release of numerous mediators of pain. The amount and content of circulating cytokines have been shown to be not only distinct to subtype of breast cancer but potentially to the amount of pain suffered by patients as well. Luminal type A and B breast cancers exhibit higher levels of TGF-β1 and TNF-α than healthy controls, and TGF-β1 levels are higher in HER2-amplified tumors than luminal types [18]. In contradistinction, triple-negative tumors have lower circulating levels of TGF-β1 when compared with other subtypes and healthy volunteers. While the different cytokine profiles of tumors are currently under investigation, the direct relationship with pain is still being elucidated.

In addition to inflammatory cytokines inducing inflammation and sensitization of peripheral nociceptors, cytokines may also be involved in noninflammatory pain. TGF-β is a cytokine that has been implicated in regulating osteoclasts and mediating bone resorption, as occurs with metastasis to bone. TGF-β is released by chondrocytes during bone injury and may mediate the production of nerve growth factor (NGF) in chondrocytes as well [19]. Further, TGF-β has been shown to be inhibited by proinflammatory cytokines and, as such, may be a noninflammatory mediator of pain in metastatic bone pain. The stimulation of osteoclastogenesis may also lead to the release of growth factors and other mediators that may cause the growth of the invading tumor cells.

Novel Therapies for Cancer-Related Pain

The treatment of cancer pain is multifaceted and discussed throughout this text. The most important treatment of cancer pain is treatment of the cancer itself. Treatments in the form of surgery, radiation therapy, chemotherapy, interventional treatments, and medication management are at the forefront of treatment. These treatments may be the cause of, or contribute to, the patient's pain as well, as with chronic postsurgical pain, radiation-induced neuritis, or chemotherapy-induced peripheral neuropathy, to name a few examples. In recent years there has been increased interest in treatments that target the pathophysiology of the cancer. These same molecular targets are also potential targets for the treatment of pain, as these therapies that target the cytokine and inflammatory mediators released by tumors and inhibit tumor growth also decrease tumor-related pain.

Bone-related pain and the molecular causes of the pain are now being targeted as pain therapies. One such molecule is Src, a protein tyrosine kinase non-receptor that is associated with the N-methyl-D-aspartate (NMDA) receptor complex. Found in neurons, Src has been shown to be associated with pain and maintaining inflammatory hyperalgesia [20]. Further, Src has a vital role in osteoclast activity. By targeting this molecule involved in bone resorption, there is potential to decrease the breakdown of bone and thus one aspect of the bone pain itself. Bisphosphates are another well-known treatment that inhibits osteoclast-mediated bone resorption by reducing osteoclast activity [21]. While effective in reducing osteoclastic activity, bisphosphonates do not impact osteoblastic activity and have numerous potential side effects including renal impairment and osteonecrosis of the jaw. Further, bisphosphonates have been shown to inhibit the ability of the metastasis to interact with the osteoblasts and inhibit their secretion of chemokine CCL2 [22].

The treatment of myeloma bone disease is multifaceted and involves mediation management, radiation therapy, chemotherapy, vertebral augmentation, and surgery. The under-

Table 3.1 Potential targets for the treatment of myeloma bone disease

Osteoclast mediators	Osteoblast mediators
OPG	WIF-1
RANK	SFRPs
MIP-1 alpha	Dkk
VEGF	Runx2
SDF-1 alpha	TGF-beta

OPG osteoprotegerin, *RANK* receptor activator of nuclear factor kappa-B, *MIP-1 alpha* macrophage inflammatory protein-1 alpha, *VEGF* vascular endothelial growth factor, *SDF-1 alpha* stromal-derived factor-1 alpha, *WIF-1* wnt inhibitory factor-1, *SFRPs* secreted frizzled-related proteins, *Dkk* Dickkorf family of secreted proteins, *Runx2* runt-related transcription factor 2, *TGF-beta* transforming growth factor-beta

lying pathophysiology discussed previously has also become a target for therapy. Bisphosphonates, discussed previously, are a mainstay of therapy for multiple myeloma. In addition to bisphosphonates, a number of mediators known to be involved in the pathogenesis of myeloma bone pain are currently being investigated as potential therapeutic targets, and there is tremendous potential for such agents (Table 3.1). One such agent, bortezomib, is a proteasome inhibitor that has been found to improve the survival of patients with multiple myeloma [23].

Pain related to breast cancer may be related to many of the topics discussed previously, including compression of neural structures and metastasis to bone. As in the treatment of myeloma bone pain, there are many potential novel therapies being investigated that may be used to not only treat the cancer but the pain it causes as well. It has been shown that altered glutamatergic signaling can disrupt the normal cycle of bone remodeling and cause significant pain [24]. Utilizing inhibitors of glutamate release from the cancer cells is one such novel therapeutic approach. Sulfasalazine is an inhibitor of glutamate release that has been shown to reduce nociceptive behavior in a mouse model of breast cancer bone pain [25]. The continued investigation of further treatments related to the pathophysiology of breast cancer pain will continue to change the management of the cancer itself and the pain it causes.

Conclusion

Cancer pain is difficult to treat and a terrible malady for those suffering from cancer. Traditional therapies continue to be the standard of care and involve medication management, radiation therapy, chemotherapy, vertebral augmentation, and surgery, among other therapies. New studies that elucidate the pathophysiology of individual cancers open the door for novel therapies that may target the cancers as never done before. As new therapies evolve, the treatment of cancer-related pain will evolve as well, ushering in a new paradigm of treatment for our patients.

References

1. Merskey H, Bogduk N. Classification of chronic pain: descriptions of chronic pain syndromes and definitions of pain terms. Seattle: IASP; 1994. Print.
2. Van Den Beuken-Van Everdingen MHJ, Hochstenbach LMJ, Joosten BEAJ, Tjan-Heijnen VCG, Janssen DJA. Update on prevalence of pain in patients with Cancer: systematic review and meta-analysis. J Pain Symptom Manag. 2016;51(6):1070–90. n. pag. Web.
3. Koizumi M, Yoshimoto M, Kasumi F, Iwase T, Ogata E. Post-operative breast Cancer patients diagnosed with skeletal metastasis without bone pain had fewer skeletal-related events and deaths than those with bone pain. BMC Cancer. 2010;10(1):423. Web.
4. Fletcher CDM. WHO classification of tumours of soft tissue and bone. Lyon: IARC; 2013. Print.
5. Nencini S, Ivanusic JJ. The physiology of bone pain. How much do we really know? Front Physiol Front Physiol. 2016;7:157. n. pag. Web.
6. Mach DB, Rogers SD, Sabino MC, Luger NM, Schwei MJ, Pomonis JD, Keyser CP, Clohisy DR, Adams DJ, O'Leary P, Mantyh PW. Origins of skeletal pain: sensory and sympathetic innervation of the mouse femur. Neuroscience. 2002;113(1):155–66. Web.
7. Jimenez-Andrade JM, Mantyh WG, Bloom AP, Haili X, Ferng AS, Dussor G, Vanderah TW, Mantyh PW. A phenotypically restricted set of primary afferent nerve fibers innervate the bone versus skin: therapeutic opportunity for treating skeletal pain. Bone. 2010;46(2):306–13. Web.
8. Ohtori S, Orita S, Yamashita M, Ishikawa T, Ito T, Shigemura T, Nishiyama H, Konno S, Ohta H, Takaso M, Inoue G, Eguchi Y, Ochiai N, Kishida S, Kuniyoshi K, Aoki Y, Arai G, Miyagi M, Kamoda H, Suzkuki M, Nakamura J, Furuya T, Kubota G, Sakuma Y, Oikawa Y, Suzuki M, Sasho T, Nakagawa K, Toyone T, Takahashi K. Existence of a neuropathic pain component in patients with osteoarthritis of the knee. Yonsei Med J Yonsei Med J. 2012;53(4):801. Web.
9. Arrington SA, Schoonmaker JE, Damron TA, Mann KA, Allen MJ. Temporal changes in bone mass and mechanical properties in a murine model of tumor osteolysis. Bone. 2006;38(3):359–67. Web.
10. Jaeckle K. Neurologic manifestations of neoplastic and radiation-induced Plexopathies. Semin Neurol. 2010;30(03):254–62. Web.
11. Jaeckle KA, Young DF, Foley KM. The natural history of lumbosacral plexopathy in cancer. Neurology. 1985;35(1):8. Web.
12. Stevens MJ, Atkinson C, Broadbent AM. The malignant psoas syndrome revisited: case report, mechanisms, and current therapeutic options. J Palliat Med. 2010;13(2):211–6. Web.
13. Fizazi K, Asselain B, Vincent-Salomon A, Jouve M, Dieras V, Palangie T, Beuzeboc P, Dorval T, Pouillart P. Meningeal Carcinomatosis in patients with breast carcinoma: clinical features, prognostic factors, and results of a high-dose intrathecal methotrexate regimen. Cancer. 1996;77(7):1315–23. Web.
14. Mehrabi A, Kashfi A, Fonouni H, Schemmer P, Schmied BM, Hallscheidt P, Schirmacher P, Weitz J, Friess H, Buchler MW, Schmidt J. Primary malignant hepatic epithelioid Hemangioendothelioma. Cancer. 2006;107(9):2108–21. Web.
15. Quail DF, Joyce JA. Microenvironmental regulation of tumor progression and metastasis. Nat Med. 2013;19(11):1423–37. Web.
16. Hameed JB, Dowling P, Clynes M, O'Gorman P. Bone disease in multiple myeloma: pathophysiology and management. CGM Cancer Growth Metastasis. 2014;7:33. Web.
17. Edwards CM, Zhuang J, Mundy GR. The pathogenesis of the bone disease of multiple myeloma. Bone. 2008;42(6):1007–13. Web.
18. Panis C, Pavanelli WR. Cytokines as mediators of pain-related process in breast cancer. Mediat Inflamm. 2015;2015:1–6. Web.

19. Davidson ENB, Van Caam APM, Vitters EL, Bennink MB, Thijssen E, Van Den Berg WB, Koenders MI, Van Lent PLEM, Van De Loo FAJ, Van Der Kraan PM. TGF-β is a potent inducer of nerve growth factor in articular cartilage via the ALK5-Smad2/3 pathway. Potential role in OA related pain? Osteoarthr Cartil. 2015;23(3):478–86. Web.
20. De Felice M, Lambert D, Holen I, Escott KJ, Andrew D. Effects of Src-kinase inhibition in cancer-induced bone pain. Mol Pain. 2016;12(0): n. pag. Web.
21. Rodan GA, Fleisch HA. Bisphosphonates: mechanisms of action. J Clin Invest. 1996;97(12):2692–6. Web.
22. Kaiser T, Teufel I, Geiger K, Vater Y, Aicher WK, Klein G, Fehm T. Bisphosphonates modulate vital functions of human osteoblasts and affect their interactions with breast Cancer cells. Breast Cancer Res Treat. 2013;140(1):35–48. Web.
23. Kumar SK, Rajkumar SV, Dispenzieri A, Lacy MQ, Hayman SR, Buadi FK, Zeldenrust SR, Dingli D, Russell SJ, Lust JA, Greipp PR, Kyle RA, Gertz MA. Improved survival in multiple myeloma and the impact of novel therapies. Blood. 2007;111(5):2516–20. Web.
24. Fazzari J, Lin H, Murphy C, Ungard R, Singh G. Inhibitors of glutamate release from breast Cancer cells; new targets for Cancer-induced bone-pain. Sci Rep Sci Rep. 2015;5:8380. Web.
25. Ungard RG, Seidlitz EP, Singh G. Inhibition of breast Cancer-cell glutamate release with sulfasalazine limits Cancer-induced bone pain. Pain. 2014;155(1):28–36. Web.

Chemotherapy

4

Karina Gritsenko and Michael Lubrano

Introduction

In this chapter, the most common chemotherapeutic agents, a number of their uses, and most of their relevant side effects are addressed. For some compounds, their uses may extend further than just neoplastic therapies as a number of inflammatory diseases benefit from immune modulation. For the purposes of our review, only antineoplastic uses and their adverse effects will be mentioned.

Chemotherapeutic Classes

Chemotherapeutic agents are subdivided into major classes and then subcategories. Therapies are grouped according to which component of the cell cycle they impair and the mechanism by which this occurs. Tumor cells are rapidly growing, and dividing entities thus are more susceptible to interventions that impair cellular division, triggering a cascade toward cell destruction. The cycle for somatoform non-gamete developing cells begins with G1 phase. The cell prepares for division by expressing RNA and proteins which allow the cell to grow in anticipation of future cell division. The next phase, S, allows for DNA replication. G2 phase subsequently occurs with a number of checkpoints to assure the cell is ready to appropriately divide. The final phase is M phase, which occurs directly before cell division, with its hallmark mitotic spindle that develops down the center of a cell prior to division, aligning and separating chromosomes to opposite, cellular poles [1]. Chemotherapeutic agents may affect all phases of the cell cycle, with the majority focusing on S phase (antimetabolites) or M phase (taxanes and vinca alkaloids) [2–5]. A summary of antineoplastic agents, by class, is included in Table 4.1.

K. Gritsenko (✉)
Montefiore Medical Center – Albert Einstein College of Medicine, Bronx, NY, USA

M. Lubrano
Department of Anesthesia & Perioperative Care, University of California San Francisco (UCSF) Medical Center, San Francisco, CA, USA
e-mail: Michael.Lubrano@ucsf.edu

Alkylating Agents

Alkylating agents are a large and diverse class of agents that actively cross-link DNA strands in order to reduce the synthesis of DNA during all steps of the cell cycle. Subcategories include alkyl sulfonates, bioreductives, nitrogen mustards, nitrosoureas, and triazenes. *Alkyl sulfonate* (*busulfan*) primarily interacts with guanosine at the N-7 position in order to disrupt RNA transcription and the replication of DNA. It is especially effective in hematologic cells with considerable efficacy on myeloid cells compared to lymphoid cells. *Alkyl bioreductives* (*mitomycin C*) are most active during late-G1 and early-S phases of the cell cycle. It is converted to an alkylating metabolite and functions as such by cross-linking nucleotides, primarily guanine and cytosine, thus disrupting cell activity. DNA and RNA syntheses are also impaired. Reduced environments, such as hypoxic tumor cells, increase the effectiveness of this agent. *Nitrogen mustards* (*cyclophosphamide*, *mechlorethamine*, *melphalan*, *chlorambucil*) include a myriad of agents that are effective in cross-linking DNA strands to impair DNA synthesis. As such, they are active during all phases of the cell cycle. *Nitrosoureas* (*carmustine*, *lomustine*, *semustine*, *streptozocin*) also cross-link DNA and RNA strands but may have a secondary function of modifying and disrupting proteins as well. Given their lipid-soluble nature, nitrosoureas are able to cross the blood-brain barrier in order to treat tumors of the central nervous system.

Busulfan is an *alkylating agent* used in chronic myelogenous leukemia with up to 90% remission. Seizures have been reported in patients who are predisposed to them, and prophylactic anticonvulsants may be administered prior to

A. Gulati et al. (eds.), *Essentials of Interventional Cancer Pain Management*, https://doi.org/10.1007/978-3-319-99684-4_4

Table 4.1 Summary of agents

Class	Agent	Uses	Adverse effects
Alkyl sulfonate	Busulfan	CML	Adrenal insufficiency, bone marrow suppression, seizures, pulmonary fibrosis, hepatic sinusoidal obstruction syndrome, cardiac tamponade
Bioreductive	Mitomycin C	Adenocarcinomas of the stomach/pancreas, anal carcinoma, bladder cancer, cervical cancer, esophageal cancer, non-small cell lung cancer	Bladder fibrosis, hemolytic uremic syndrome, pulmonary toxicity
Nitrogen mustard	Cyclophosphamide	Breast cancer, ALL/AML/CLL/CML, Ewing's sarcoma, Hodgkin's/non-Hodgkin's lymphoma, multiple myeloma, mycosis fungoides, pheochromocytoma, small-cell lung cancer, Wilm's tumor	Acute respiratory distress syndrome, bladder cancer, cardiotoxicity, hemorrhagic cystitis, infertility, pneumonitis
Nitrosourea	Carmustine	Astrocytomas, ependymomas, glioblastomas, medulloblastomas, multiple myeloma, Hodgkin's/non-Hodgkin's lymphoma, mycosis	Bone marrow suppression, ocular toxicity, pulmonary toxicity, renal impairment
Nitrosourea	Streptozocin	Adrenal carcinoma, pancreatic islet cell carcinoma	Bone marrow suppression, glucose intolerance, confusion/lethargy, depression
Triazene	Dacarbazine	Melanoma, Hodgkin's lymphoma, medullary carcinoma pheochromocytoma, medullary carcinoma	Anaphylaxis, extravasation
Triazene	Temozolomide	Gliomas, refractory astrocytoma	*Pneumocystis jirovecii* pneumonia
Folate	Methotrexate	Acute lymphoblastic leukemia, breast cancer, central nervous system tumors, head and neck cancer, lung cancers, meningeal leukemia, trophoblastic neoplasms	Acute kidney injury, bone marrow suppression, dermatologic reactions, diarrhea/stomatitis, infertility, hepatotoxicity, neurotoxicity, pneumonitis, tumor lysis syndrome
Folate	Pemetrexed	Bladder cancer, cervical cancer, ovarian cancer, pleural mesothelioma, non-squamous non-small cell lung cancer, thymus cancer	Bone marrow suppression, dermal reactions, GI toxicity, hepatotoxicity, interstitial pneumonitis
Platinum analog	Cisplatin	Bladder cancer, breast cancer, cervical cancer, endometrial cancer, esophageal and gastric cancer, hepatobiliary cancer, Hodgkin's lymphoma, testicular cancer, ovarian cancer, neuroblastoma, neuroendocrine tumors	Anaphylaxis, extravasation, hyperuricemia, gastroenteric toxicity, neurotoxicity, ototoxicity, renal toxicity, posterior reversible leukoencephalopathy syndrome (PRES)
Platinum analog	Carboplatin	Advanced ovarian cancer, Merkel cell carcinoma, small-cell lung cancer, thymic malignancies, others similar to cisplatin	Similar to cisplatin with less gastrointestinal and renal toxicity
Platinum analog	Oxaliplatin	Colorectal cancer, esophageal cancer, gastric cancer, pancreatic cancer, hepatobiliary cancer, ovarian/testicular cancer	Anaphylaxis, GI toxicity, neuropathy, hepatic toxicity, pulmonary fibrosis, posterior reversible leukoencephalopathy syndrome (PRES)
Purine analog	Mercaptopurine	Acute lymphoblastic leukemia, acute promyelocytic leukemia, non-Hodgkin's lymphoma	Bone marrow suppression, hepatotoxicity, immunosuppression, secondary malignancies
Purine analog	Thioguanine	Adult acute myelogenous leukemia	Bone marrow suppression, hepatotoxicity, malignancies, tumor lysis syndrome
Purine analog	Hydroxyurea	Chronic myelocytic leukemia, ovarian cancer, melanoma, meningiomas, squamous head and neck cancer	Bone marrow suppression, megaloblastic erythropoiesis, vascular ulceration, gangrene, secondary malignancy, tumor lysis syndrome
Pyrimidine analog	5-Fluorouracil (5-FU)	Breast cancer, bladder cancer, colon cancer, gastric cancer, head and neck cancers, hepatobiliary cancers, neuroendocrine cancers, pancreatic cancer	Palmar-plantar erythrodysesthesia (hand-foot) syndrome, diarrhea, neurotoxicity, neutropenia
Pyrimidine analog	Capecitabine	Metastatic colon cancer, similar tumor profile as 5-FU	Bone marrow suppression, cardiotoxicity, gastrointestinal toxicity, hand-foot syndrome, hepatotoxicity
Pyrimidine analog	Cytarabine	Acute lymphocytic leukemia, acute myelocytic leukemia, chronic myelocytic leukemia in blast phase, chronic lymphocytic leukemia, meningeal leukemia, refractory Hodgkin's lymphoma	Acute pancreatitis, bone marrow suppression, hypersensitivity, respiratory arrest, tumor lysis syndrome

Table 4.1 (continued)

Class	Agent	Uses	Adverse effects
Pyrimidine analog	Gemcitabine	Bladder cancer, cervical cancer, Hodgkin's/non-Hodgkin's lymphoma, metastatic breast cancer, non-small cell lung cancer, ovarian cancer, pancreatic adenocarcinoma, renal cell cancer, small-cell lung cancer, sarcomas, testicular cancer, thymic malignancies	Bone marrow suppression, capillary leak syndrome (CLS), hemolytic uremic syndrome (HUS), pulmonary toxicity
Anthracycline	Doxorubicin	Acute lymphocytic leukemia, acute myeloid leukemia, breast cancer, sarcomas of the soft tissues and bone, thyroid cancer, small-cell lung cancer, gastric cancer, neuroblastoma, Wilm's tumor	Bone marrow suppression, cardiac toxicity, secondary malignancy, skin extravasation, tumor lysis syndrome
Antibiotic	Bleomycin	Cervical cancer, penis carcinoma, head and neck squamous cell carcinoma, Hodgkin's/non-Hodgkin's lymphoma, ovarian germ cell tumors, testicular carcinoma	Hepatotoxicity, renal toxicity, pulmonary toxicity, idiosyncratic reaction
Vinca alkaloid	Vincristine	Acute lymphocytic leukemia, chronic lymphocytic leukemia, Ewing's sarcoma, gestational trophoblastic tumors, Hodgkin's/non-Hodgkin's lymphoma, multiple myeloma, small-cell lung cancer, Wilm's tumor, neuroblastoma, retinoblastoma, rhabdomyosarcoma	Gastrointestinal toxicity, neurotoxicity, respiratory complications, uric acid nephropathy
Vinca alkaloid	Vinblastine	Bladder cancer, breast cancer, choriocarcinoma desmoid tumors, Hodgkin's/non-Hodgkin's lymphoma, Kaposi's sarcoma, melanoma, ovarian cancer, testicular cancer	Disabling neurotoxicity, peripheral sensory neuropathy
Taxane	Paclitaxel	Adenocarcinoma, bladder cancer, breast cancer, head and neck cancers, Kaposi's sarcoma, non-small cell lung cancer, ovarian cancer, small-cell lung cancer	Bone marrow suppression, cardiovascular toxicity, hypersensitivity reactions, peripheral neuropathy

therapy initiation in cases where high doses may be anticipated. Pulmonary fibrosis and bronchopulmonary dysplasia can occur with an average of 4 years after treatment in up to 4% of patients. Hepatic sinusoidal obstruction syndrome may occur and is associated with high concentrations as a result of rapid infusion. This risk is increased with doses over 16 mg/kg based on ideal body weight. With pulmonary symptoms, it is important to rule out opportunistic infections as well as leukemic infiltrates before diagnosing busulfan toxicity. This may require biopsy of the lung. If toxicity is diagnosed, busulfan should be discontinued immediately.

Mitomycin C is an *alkylating agent* effective against a number of GI adenocarcinomas. It can be used alongside 5-fluorouracil for squamous cell cancer of the anus. As a vesicular infusion, it may also be used to topically treat bladder cancer. Bladder fibrosis is a common side effect. Patient may also experience pulmonary toxicity and hemolytic uremic syndrome.

Cyclophosphamide is a *nitrogen mustard* most frequently utilized clinically in a large number of oncologic and inflammatory settings, including hematologic, adrenal, and lung cancers. Hepatocytes metabolize cyclophosphamide to aldophosphamide, which is further converted into toxic compounds by cells throughout the body, including target tumor cells. These toxic compounds thus function as alkylating agents. High doses of cyclophosphamide may cause cardiotoxicity by damaging endothelial capillaries. This can lead to pericarditis or pericardial effusions and may eventually develop into a cardiac tamponade [6]. ACE inhibitors, inotropes, beta-blockers, and diuretics can help to manage cardiotoxicity. Pneumonitis is rare and can be reversed with early discontinuation within the first several months of use. Pleural thickening is associated with late-onset pneumonitis which may become a chronic, progressive condition [7]. Interstitial cystitis and bladder cancer are additional concerns, as acrolein (a toxic metabolite of cyclophosphamide) may accumulate in the bladder, thus predisposing transitional bladder cells to oncogenicity. In order to avoid these toxic side effects, clinicians should consider pulse doses as well as giving 2-mercaptoethanesulfonate, a compound that conjugates acrolein in the urine. Patients should also be advised to drink fluids to maintain adequate hydration. Of note, some individuals with a G516 T variant of CYP2B6 metabolize cyclophosphamide much more rapidly and therefore may require lower doses in order to avoid the toxic effects of this agent.

Carmustine is similar to other *nitrosoureas* as it cross-links DNA and RNA strands. It may also carbamylate amino acids which modify proteins. This agent is lipid soluble, thus allowing it to cross the blood-brain barrier in order to combat malignancies in the central nervous system (including astrocytomas, ependymomas, glioblastomas, and medulloblastomas). Cumulative doses greater than 1400 mg/m^2 place patient at risk for delayed-onset pulmonary fibrosis typically in those who have had prolonged treatment.

Streptozocin is a *nitrosourea* that functions similarly to carmustine by cross-linking DNA, modifying proteins, and crossing the blood-brain barrier. It is typically used to treat metastatic islet cell carcinoma of the pancreas and metastatic adrenal carcinomas. Patients experience less bone marrow suppression for this agent than for carmustine, although it has been associated with psychiatric side effects such as depression and confusion.

Dacarbazine is a *triazene* that is activated by the cytochrome P450 system by conversion to methyl-triazene-1-l-imidazole-4-carboxamide (MTIC). As MTIC, it functions by methylating the O6 and N6 positions of guanine in DNA. This subsequently causes breaks in the DNA double strand and eventual triggers apoptosis. It may be used for treating melanoma and adrenal malignancies. Extravasation is a serious consequence that results in extreme pain and tissue damage.

Temozolomide: This prodrug is converted to MTIC nonenzymatically through a spontaneous and rapid process in bodily tissues after redistributing. It functions similar to dacarbazine as a *triazene*. Typically, this agent is reserved for refractory astrocytoma and a number of additional, off-label uses in the central nervous system tumors. Radiotherapy in conjunction with this agent increases risk for *Pneumocystis jirovecii* pneumonia, thus warranting prophylactic antibiotics in select patient populations.

Folates

Folates participate in a disruption of the folate cycle (*methotrexate, pemetrexed)*. These agents irreversibly inhibit dihydrofolate reductase (DHFR), an enzyme that donates methyl groups to folate, thus impairing an essential step for intracellular production of purines and thymidylic acid. DNA, RNA, and various proteins require this in order to function. While folates may also be used in inflammatory diseases, the mechanism of action is unknown.

Methotrexate is a *folate* that is especially useful in treating solid tumors found in a myriad of organ systems. It is often the agent of choice for trophoblastic neoplasms and may be given as a sole agent for hydatidiform moles or ectopic pregnancies of small enough sizes. The hepatotoxic side effects of methotrexate are related to a cumulative dose of greater than 1.5 grams. Hepatic biopsies are recommended in patients with prolonged exposure. Other hepatotoxic risk factors include ethanol consumption, diabetes, hyperlipidemia, family history of liver disease, and obesity. Methotrexate elimination is renal based, with greater than 50% not metabolized. Neurotoxicity includes seizures that occur predominantly in children who are being treated for ALL, as well as encephalopathy from high doses or concurrent radiation. Intrathecal administration raises concerns for arachnoiditis, chronic leukoencephalopathy, and myelopathy. Administering leucovorin (5-formyltetrahydrofolate) may reduce the toxicity of methotrexate and spares nontumor cells. Another treatment modality for overexposure includes glucarpidase, an enzyme that rapidly hydrolyzes methotrexate in the extracellular space into an inactive metabolite that allows for its elimination. Tumor lysis syndrome is another severe side effect that may lead to acute kidney injury and/or failure, especially when tumor burden is high.

Pemetrexed functions similarly to methotrexate but also inhibits thymidylate synthase and two other enzymes that play roles in the reduction of folate. Its uses include treating pleural mesothelioma and thymus cancer. Bone marrow suppression and interstitial pneumonitis are concerning adverse effects; however, hepatic toxicity is especially concerning with pemetrexed with several case reports identifying this as a cause of mortality. Folate and vitamin B12 are essential for reducing bone marrow and gastrointestinal toxicity.

Nucleotide and Platinum Analogs

Nucleotide analogs are broken down into two subgroups. *Purine analogs* (*mercaptopurine*, *thioguanine*, *hydroxyurea*) **mimic** adenosine and guanine. They typically deceive intracellular machinery in order to be inappropriately placed into DNA. Once present, DNA replication is impaired, and tumor cells are unable to undergo S phase and replicate. This triggers a number of mechanisms that lead to apoptosis. *Pyrimidine analogs* (*fluorouracil*, *capecitabine*, *cytaragine*, *gemcitabine*) either mimic cytosine, thymine, and uracil or entirely block pyrimidine synthesis within cells. These agents commonly are administered as prodrugs that require activation by either hepatic cells or cellular machinery within the tumor of interest.

Platinum analogs (*carboplatin*, *cisplatin*, and *oxaliplatin*) effectively treat malignancies by interacting with tumors in a number of ways. They actively bind the DNA of target cells and form intra-strand and inter-strand DNA covalent cross-links. These cross-links inhibit DNA synthesis and denature the double helix.

Mercaptopurine is a *purine analog* converted by hypoxanthine-guanine phosphoribosyl transferase (HGPRT) into monophosphate and triphosphate forms. The monophosphate form inhibits purine synthesis. The triphosphate form is falsely incorporated into DNA and RNA by cellular machinery to inhibit replication. Xanthine oxidase (XO) is the enzyme that metabolizes its active forms, as well as purines themselves. By co-administering allopurinol, a XO inhibitor, the dose of mercaptopurine can be reduced by 50–70%. Mercaptopurine is mainly used for hematologic cancers and thus has a number of side effects involving the manipulation of hematologic cell lines. This includes bone marrow suppression, immunosuppression, and subsequent secondary malignancies. Hepatotoxicity occurs at any dose, but increased risk occurs above 2.5 mg/kg/day. Discontinuation may resolve hepatic symptoms after about 1–2 months. Secondary malignancies are a major concern, especially hepatosplenic T-cell lymphomas (HSTCL) which are a rare and frequently fatal cancer.

Thioguanine is a *purine analog* closely related to mercaptopurine and has a similar function and metabolism. Its primary use is for adult acute myelogenous leukemia. Side effects parallel those of mercaptopurine with concern for tumor lysis syndrome. Some patients have genetic polymorphism that results in a deficiency of thiopurine methyltransferase (TPMT). Medications that are salicylic acid derivatives are able to inhibit TPMT and may lead to significant myelosuppression while taking this agent for some patients. This would require considerable dose reduction to avoid serious toxicity.

Hydroxyurea is another *purine* analog that disrupts DNA synthesis by inhibiting ribonucleoside-diphosphate reductase. This blocks the development of deoxyribonucleotides from ribonucleotides, thus freezing target cells in the G1 phase. It is effective in leukemias, melanoma, and squamous cancers. In addition to tumor lysis syndrome, concerning adverse effects include bone marrow suppression, megaloblastic erythropoiesis, vascular ulceration, and gangrene. Erythrocyte abnormalities may erupt displaying megaloblastic erythropoiesis that is typically self-limiting. Hydroxyurea has also been associated with the development of skin cancer with long-term use.

5-Fluorouracil (5-FU) is a *pyrimidine analog* requiring activation in order to inhibit thymidylate synthase. This enzyme is necessary for generating thymidine triphosphate, an essential factor for synthesizing DNA. A second metabolite of 5-FU is generated that may be inappropriately incorporated in RNA and effectively disrupt translation. This is a very useful agent to treat solid tumors found throughout multiple organ systems. Palmar-plantar erythrodysesthesia (hand-foot) syndrome is a side effect that 5-FU may precipitate that involves tingling in the hands and feet. It has the potential for developing into pain associated with erythema. The resolution typically occurs within a week of discontinuing 5-FU. Toxicity can also occur in the 5% of patients who are deficient in dihydropyrimidine dehydrogenase (DPD), the enzyme responsible for metabolizing 5-FU. Without DPD, 5-FU toxicity can cause neutropenia, diarrhea, and neurotoxicity. Overdose of 5-FU may be treated with uridine triacetate if administered within 4 days, with multiple, small cohort studies showing full recovery in all patients who received this rescue agent [8, 9].

Capecitabine is another *pyrimidine analog* (prodrug) that must be hydrolyzed by the liver as well as other bodily tissues to become 5-FU. Its uses are therefore similar to 5-FU, but it is capable of oral administration. Its side effect profile is similar; although bone marrow suppression is significant, patients with platelets less than 100,000 or neutrophils less than 1500 are not candidates for this medication. Dysrhythmia, angina, myocardial infarction, cardiac arrest, cardiac myopathy, and sudden death have all occurred in patients receiving capecitabine.

Cytarabine, a *pyrimidine analog*, utilizes cellular transporters to enter tumors prior to being converted to aracytidine triphosphate. In this phosphorylated form, it may be placed into DNA. Unlike other analogs, cytarabine functions by directly inhibiting DNA polymerase, both alpha and beta, thus impairing DNA replication and repair, primarily useful to treat hematologic malignancies. In addition to acute pancreatitis and tumor lysis syndrome, a hypersensitivity reaction with acute cardiopulmonary arrest is a rare side effect. Sudden respiratory arrest syndrome is also a subsequent concern that may take up to 12 h to precipitate following treatment. This involves malaise, maculopapular rash, fever, myalgia, bone pain, and chest pain and requires immediate administration of corticosteroids to manage. Patients receiving doses that exceed 1.5 g/m^2 may experience conjunctivitis.

Gemcitabine is also a *pyrimidine analog* that functions similarly to cytarabine. It is metabolized to gemcitabine diphosphate and works to inhibit ribonucleotide reductase and DNA synthesis. Its triphosphate form is effective in incorporating itself into DNA directly to inhibit DNA polymerase. This agent is used to treat metastatic breast cancer and solid and hematopoietic tumors from a number of organ systems. Capillary leak syndrome (CLS) and hemolytic uremic syndrome (HUS) are serious, adverse events. Gemcitabine should be discontinued if CLS precipitates. HUS may result in considerable morbidity and mortality. Any patient on this agent must therefore have an established renal baseline that is continuously monitored. Adult respiratory distress syndrome and pneumonitis and fibrosis are other observed effects although symptoms may not precipitate for 2 weeks after a patient's gemcitabine dose.

Cisplatin is a *platinum analog* that exists in two isomer forms, with the cis form actively functioning at 14 times the cytotoxic level as its trans-isomer counterpart. Both isomers function similarly, but cellular mechanisms are less capable of recognizing and repairing the cis-isomer form. It is effective in eradicating a number of tumor cells, most notably solid tumors. Adverse effects are also numerous and considerable – perhaps the most notable including ototoxicity and renal toxicity. Neurotoxicity is an additional concern for all platinum agents. Hyperuricemia may also occur with cisplatin due to tumor lysis. Neuropathies that are severe and potentially irreversible can occur when administration is too frequent or recommended doses are exceeded. A number of neurologic sequelae have been described, including posterior reversible leukoencephalopathy syndrome (PRES), seizures, and loss of taste or motor function. Children with thiopurine S-methyltransferase (TPMT) polymorphisms are more susceptible to ototoxicity, which is also dose dependent and perpetuated by aminoglycoside use.

Carboplatin is another *platinum analog*, with a similar mechanism of action to cisplatin. In addition to tumors treated by cisplatin, carboplatin also treats Merkel cell carcinoma and thymic malignancies. It has a similar side effect profile but with less renal and gastrointestinal toxicity.

Oxaliplatin is an additional *platinum analog* that functions synonymously to other agents in its class. Oxaliplatin is a staple medication for use in colorectal cancer as well as a number of other gastrointestinal cancers. Like cisplatin, patients receiving oxaliplatin treatments also are subject to PRES and gastrointestinal toxicity, although anaphylaxis is an especially significant side effect. Anaphylactic hypersensitivity is very dangerous and may precipitate anywhere from 5 to 70 min after the initiation of a treatment. Patients experience symptoms distinctive of hypersensitivity, urticaria, erythema, flushing, hypotension, bronchospasm, and syncope.

Typically, these reactions occur after a patient has received several cycles with a median of seven to nine cycles. Premedication with antihistamines may allow for an additional two to four cycles without serious complications [10]. Oxaliplatin has a major side effect of neuropathy that may be categorized as either acute or persistent. The acute phenomenon begins within hours of treatment and typically resolves within 2 weeks. Symptoms are frequently peripheral and reoccur with additional doses. The persistent form of platinum neuropathy continued for more than 2 weeks and can inhibit activities like writing and swallowing. Discontinuing treatment may ameliorate symptoms. Calcium infusion (pre-/post-infusion) was initially thought to reduce the rate of these neuropathic symptoms; however, a recent randomized, double-blinded, and placebo-controlled trial indicated that there is no benefit to using these molecules as prevention [11].

Anthracyclines

Anthracyclines have numerous methods of action within tumor cells to inhibit proliferation and promote cellular death. They are capable of intercalating into DNA and RNA, thus halting their production in addition to obstructing topoisomerase II. They also chelate iron prior to binding DNA and cell membranes, subsequently releasing free radicals that destroy both of these structures (*dactinomycin*, *doxorubicin (Adriamycin)*, *daunorubicin (idarubicin)*).

Doxorubicin (Adriamycin) is an *anthracycline* with a myriad of uses, mainly for cancers found in the blood, bone, and endocrine tissue. Cardiotoxicity is a major concern for this agent due to damage from free radical formation and is directly correlated with dosing. A cumulative dose beyond 450–500 mg/m2 increases the risk for irreversible myocardial toxicity. Acute cardiotoxicity may happen in 10% of cases and may resolve by 2 months after discontinuing the agent. About 2% of patients will get a more severe cardiotoxicity with a prognosis of 60% mortality within 3 weeks of the onset of symptoms. Acute myelogenous leukemia has been a reported adverse outcome. Extravasation is also a concern as this can damage local tissue causing pain and necrosis.

Bleomycin is an *antibiotic* with antineoplastic properties that bind to DNA and causes both single- and double-strand breaks. RNA and protein syntheses are also inhibited. Patients may experience what is referred to as an "idiosyncratic reaction" that is similar to anaphylaxis and takes place after the first or second doses. It may precipitate with fever, chills, hypotension, wheezing, and confusion in about 1% of lymphoma patients receiving bleomycin. More than 400 cumulative units increase the risk for pneumonitis and progression to pulmonary fibrosis. Smoking, age greater than 40, and renal impairment with a glomerular filtration rate below 80 ml/min all increase risk for bleomycin toxicity [12]. Lung pathology can range from eosinophilic hypersensitivity to interstitial pneumonitis that may progress to pulmonary fibrosis. Pulmonary capillary endothelial damage may subsequently take place with necrosis of type I alveolar cells. Management of this complication includes excessive crystalloid infusion, and high FiO2 may actually contribute to pulmonary damage, which has been replicated in animal models [13]. Given the data in the literature, it is therefore recommended that inspired oxygen be maintained below 30%.

Antimitotic Drugs

Antimitotic drugs primarily function during the M phase of the cell cycle and disrupt the formation of the mitotic spindle necessary for aligning and separating chromosomes prior to cellular division. Two major subgroups exist in this class. The *vinca alkaloids* (*vinblastine*, *vincristine*) occur naturally and are effective in stopping the formation of microtubule formation by binding tubulin directly, thus freezing cell cycles in metaphase. *Taxanes* (*paclitaxel*, *docetaxel*) actively encourage microtubule elongation by further activating tubulin dimers and stabilizing the already existing microtubules. This enhancement does not incorporate guanosine triphosphate; thus, division is not possible. Chromosomes are subject to breakage during the inappropriate elongation of the mitotic spindle.

Vincristine is a *vinca alkaloid* that may be used to treat a number of solid and hematopoietic tumors including Ewing's sarcoma, gestational trophoblastic tumors, and retinoblastoma. Gastrointestinal effects include paralytic ileus and constipation that may result in necrosis and perforation. Given the potential for gastric catastrophe, a prophylactic plan for gastric motility and laxatives to manage the bowel should always be considered. Neurotoxicity occurs with a variety of symptoms that include depression, insomnia, or general mental confusion. Peripheral sensory neuropathy also occurs. These effects are typically dose limiting, and some may be reversible. *Vinblastine has* a similar mechanism of action and may also functionally treat Kaposi's sarcoma, melanoma, and desmoid tumors. Patients may experience disabling neurotoxicity, similar to vincristine, but this is typically reversible.

Paclitaxel is a *taxane* that is effective in treating a number of squamous cell, lung, and hormonal cancers. Due to bone marrow toxicity, it is not advised that this agent be used if absolute neutrophil counts are <1500 cells/mm^3. Cardiovascular effects are typically related to the infusion of the treatment. Hypotension/hypertension and bradycardia have been documented during infusion. Premedication with immune modulators is sometimes advisable in order to prevent hypersensitivity reactions. Hypertension, dyspnea, and angioedema are considered reactions that warrant immediate cessation of treatment without consideration for future challenge with the agent. Peripheral neuropathy in a glove and stocking distribution occurs in patients with diabetes or preexisting neuropathies. If severe neuropathy is experienced, reducing doses by 20% is recommended. Myopathic side effects typically precipitate 2–3 days after treatment and may resolve by day 6 posttreatment.

Monoclonal Antibodies

Monoclonal antibodies take advantage of host immune systems, by binding antibodies to a slew of oncogenic factors on cell surfaces in order to trigger immune responses. *Cetuximab*, for example, targets epidermal growth factor receptors (EGFR), which are overexpressed in a number of solid tumor cells. Some of the more frequently used monoclonal antibodies include *bevacizumab* (binds VEGF), *trastuzumab* (binds HER-2), *rituximab* (binds CD20 antigen), and tyrosine kinase inhibitors such as *imatinib* (binds Bcr-Abl tyrosine kinase) and its newer version *gefitinib*. These factors are all essential for treating cancers that range from breast to blood cell and have side effects that include hypomagnesemia and hypersensitivity infusion reactions.

Chemotherapeutic Pain

As reviewed in this chapter, chemotherapeutic agents have a variety of adverse side effects that patients may endure including pain. These drugs are especially toxic to the areas of the body with a high mitotic index, such as the bone marrow and gastrointestinal tract. For example, one of the most common and painful gastrointestinal adverse effects is oral mucositis, which occurs in as many as 40% of patients receiving cytotoxic agents causing discomfort, mucosal irritation, and ulceration. Nearly 3/4 of patients receiving chemotherapeutic doses considered "high" experience extreme pain from oral mucositis that may interfere with their ability to talk or swallow [14]. A number of chemotherapy associated with pain symptoms are classified as infusion or toxicity related and are listed in Table 4.2.

Many chemotherapeutic agents are neurotoxic and may precipitate mono- or polyneuropathies commonly from the *taxanes*, *vinca alkaloids*, and *platinum analogs*. Usually, neuropathic symptoms from chemotherapeutic agents will resolve several weeks after conclusion of therapy, but chronic neuropathies may develop. Drug-induced neurologic pain is associated with nerve disruption or direct damage. Some platinum agents, like oxaliplatin, create nerve disruption by chelating calcium, resulting in hyperexcitation [15]. All of these effects tend to be dose dependent. Preexisting neuropathy is a risk factor for chemotherapeutic-induced neuropathy even doses that are not considered "high" for any given agents. Diabetes as a predisposing factor for neuropathy remains a controversy in the literature [16].

Neuropathies can occur in any segment of the nervous system, although sensory neuropathy is the most common. Sensory neuropathic symptoms with taxanes present as burning paresthesias along the longest sensory nerves, predominantly hands and feet [17]. An acute pain syndrome is associated with paclitaxel occurring a few days after therapy. Symptoms include myalgias, arthralgias, numbness, and tingling [18].

Platinum agents may generate numbness, paresthesias, and pain in a similar stocking-glove pattern, affecting large myelinated sensory fibers by damaging the dorsal root ganglion. Temperature sensation and motor strength are usually spared, while proprioception and reflexes are usually damaged [19, 20]. Oxaliplatin may precipitate two different neurologic syndromes. One is an acute neurotoxicity characterized by distinct dysesthesias in over 80% of

Table 4.2 Chemotherapeutic pain

Infusion related	Venous spasm Extravasation Phlebitis IV infusion pain Perineal burning from IV steroid administration Intravesicular or intraperitoneal pain from direct instillation
Toxicity related	Oral mucositis Arthralgia/myalgia Hand-foot syndrome 5-FU-induced angina Intrathecal administration (headache) Peripheral neuropathy Acute limb ischemia (Raynaud's) Diffuse bone pain from retinoic acid or hematopoietic stimulators

patients with potential neuropathy in their hands, feet, and perioral region. A cold-induced pharyngolaryngeal dysesthesia is also present [21]. A second syndrome includes a late-onset axonal neuropathy that is symmetric but without motor neuropathy.

Vinca alkaloids generate a distal sensory loss of the lower extremities usually sparing the upper extremities. Neurologic symptoms are similar to taxanes and platinum agents, primarily paresthesias with muscle cramps. Unlike the taxanes with which symptoms develop within days, neuropathy from vinca alkaloids may take several months, and patients may no longer be receiving therapy at the time [22].

Motor neuropathies are less common for all of the chemotherapeutic agents but are of significant concern. The taxanes are responsible for motor neuropathies in 10–20% of patients receiving them, usually presenting as a proximal weakness. The symptoms may occur at any time, regardless of treatment stage, with a highly variable course. Taxanes are associated with either distal axonopathy or proximal denervation at the nerve root/anterior horn cell on nerve conduction analysis [17]. Less commonly, vinca alkaloids may cause distal, symmetric weakness that may progress to foot and wrist drop. These patients are subsequently found to have neurophysiologic studies indicating a primarily axonal neuropathy [23].

Autonomic neuropathy is rare. If it occurs, it typically presents as constipation in patients being treated with vinca alkaloids. Approximately half of patients receiving vincristine may experience colicky abdominal pain in addition to constipation. Orthostatic hypotension and other autonomic symptoms may occur [24].

Treating chemotherapeutic pain from neuropathy is difficult and primarily involves risk reduction and symptomatic management. This involves dose limitation as well as eventual agent cessation in the presence of severe symptoms. Analgesics, anticonvulsants, and antidepressants have become the mainstays of symptom management. Agents for prophylactic treatment of neurotoxicity have been studied, and none are shown to be efficacious thus far in the literature. To this extent, L-carnitine is an oral supplement that has shown to increase neurotoxicity; therefore, its avoidance is highly recommended [25].

Of Special Note

As treatment options change in the field of oncology, newer therapies emerge and have their own host of side effects. Immunotherapy, or specifically checkpoint inhibitors, has an effect of increasing an immune response [26]. Research in this field has revolutionized treatment options for various oncologic diseases, and now newer targets and combinational therapy may be a therapeutic option in the future [27]. The pain syndromes are varied and may be related to the increased immune response, similar to rheumatologic disease [28]. An increased emphasis on the side effects from immunotherapy and other novel modalities will be a focus in the future of cancer pain medicine.

Summary

Modern medicine has a docket of potent antineoplastic agents at its fingertips, yet utilization of these by physicians comes at a price. Each medication has side effect profiles that are less than ideal. Mechanisms for generating chemotherapeutic agent-induced pain include a disruption of cells with a high mitotic index with subsequent, local irritation and electrolyte disruption or by damaging neurons directly. The taxanes, vinca alkaloids, and platinum agents are more likely to cause neuropathies in patients, especially at higher doses. Appropriate clinical care includes adequate preparation for managing any significant side effect, especially when severe pain may occur.

References

1. Cooper G. The cell: a molecular approach. 2nd ed. Washington, DC: ASM Press; 2000.
2. Brunton LL, et al. Goodman & Gilman's pharmacologic basis of therapeutics. 12th ed. New York: McGraw Hill Companies; 2011.
3. Katsung BG, Masters SB, Trevor AJ. Basic and clinical pharmacology. 11th ed. New York: McGraw Hill Medical; 2009.
4. NCCN Clinical Practice Guidelines in Oncology. NCCN.org
5. Stoelting RK, Hillier SC. Pharmacology and physiology in anesthetic practice. 4th ed. Philadelphia: Lippincott Williams & Wilkins; 2006. p. 551–68.
6. Floyd J, Mirza I, Sachs B, Perry MC. Hepatotoxicity of chemotherapy. Semin Oncol. 2006;33(1):50–67. https://doi.org/10.1053/j.seminoncol.2005.11.002.
7. Malik SW, Myers JL, DeRemee RA, Specks U. Lung toxicity associated with cyclophosphamide use. Two distinct patterns. Am J Respir Crit Care Med. 1996;154(6 Pt 1):1851–6. https://doi.org/10.1164/ajrccm.154.6.8970380.
8. Bamat M, Tremmel R, O'Neil J. Uridine triacetate: an investigational orally administered, life-saving antidote for 5FU oversode. Annual Meeting of the American Society of Clinical Oncologists, Chicago. 2010.
9. McEvilly M, Popelas C, Tremmel B. Use of uridine triacetate for the management of fluorouracil overdose. Am J Health Syst Pharm. 2011;68(19):1806–9. https://doi.org/10.2146/ajhp100434.
10. Polyzos A, Tsavaris N, Gogas H, Souglakos J, Vambakas L, Vardakas N, et al. Clinical features of hypersensitivity reactions to oxaliplatin: a 10-year experience. Oncology. 2009;76(1):36–41. https://doi.org/10.1159/000178163.
11. Loprinzi CL, Qin R, Dakhil SR, et al. Phase III randomized, placebo (PL)-controlled, double-blind study of intravenous calcium/magnesium (CaMg) to prevent Oxaliplatin-induced sensory neurotoxicity (sNT), N08CB: an alliance for clinical trials in oncology study. J Clin Oncol. 2013;31:3501.
12. Sleijfer S. Bleomycin-induced pneumonitis. Chest. 2001;120(2):617–24.
13. Hay JG, Haslam PL, Dewar A, et al. Development of acute lung injury after the combination of intravenous bleomycin and exposure to hyperoxia in rats. Thorax. 1987;42:374–82.

14. Sonis ST, Elting LS, Keefe D, Peterson DE, Schubert M, Hauer-Jensen M, Bekele BN, Raber-Durlacher J, Donnelly JP. Rubenstein EB; mucositis study section of the multinational Association for Supportive Care in Cancer; International Society for Oral Oncology. Perspectives on cancer therapy-induced mucosal injury: pathogenesis, measurement, epidemiology, and consequences for patients. Cancer. 2004;100(9 Suppl):1995–2025.
15. Park SB, Lin CS, Krishnan AV, Goldstein D, Friedlander ML, Kiernan MC. Oxaliplatin-induced neurotoxicity: changes in axonal excitability precede development of neuropathy. Brain. 2009;132(Pt 10):2712–23. https://doi.org/10.1093/brain/awp219. Epub 2009 Sep 10
16. Windebank AJ, Grisold W. Chemotherapy-induced neuropathy. J Peripher Nerv Syst. 2008;13(1):27–46. https://doi.org/10.1111/j.1529-8027.2008.00156.x. Review
17. Freilich RJ, Balmaceda C, Seidman AD, Rubin M, DeAngelis LM. Motor neuropathy due to docetaxel and paclitaxel. Neurology. 1996;47(1):115–8.
18. Reeves BN, Dakhil SR, Sloan JA, Wolf SL, Burger KN, Kamal A, Le-Lindqwister NA, Soori GS, Jaslowski AJ, Kelaghan J, Novotny PJ, Lachance DH, Loprinzi CL. Further data supporting that paclitaxel-associated acute pain syndrome is associated with development of peripheral neuropathy: north central Cancer treatment group trial N08C1. Cancer. 2012;118(20):5171–8. https://doi.org/10.1002/cncr.27489. Epub 2012 Mar 13. PubMed PMID: 22415454; PubMed Central PMCID: PMC3376686
19. Krarup-Hansen A, Helweg-Larsen S, Schmalbruch H, Rørth M, Krarup C. Neuronal involvement in cisplatin neuropathy: prospective clinical and neurophysiological studies. Brain. 2007;130(Pt 4):1076–88. Epub 2007 Feb 14
20. von Schlippe M, Fowler CJ, Harland SJ. Cisplatin neurotoxicity in the treatment of metastatic germ cell tumour: time course and prognosis. Br J Cancer. 2001;85(6):823–6. PubMed PMID: 11556831; PubMed Central PMCID: PMC2375074
21. Argyriou AA, Cavaletti G, Briani C, Velasco R, Bruna J, Campagnolo M, Alberti P, Bergamo F, Cortinovis D, Cazzaniga M, Santos C, Papadimitriou K, Kalofonos HP. Clinical pattern and associations of oxaliplatin acute neurotoxicity: a prospective study in 170 patients with colorectal cancer. Cancer. 2013;119(2):438–44. https://doi.org/10.1002/cncr.27732. Epub 2012 Jul 11
22. Verstappen CC, Koeppen S, Heimans JJ, Huijgens PC, Scheulen ME, Strumberg D, Kiburg B, Postma TJ. Dose-related vincristine-induced peripheral neuropathy with unexpected off-therapy worsening. Neurology. 2005;64(6):1076–7. PubMed PMID: 15781834
23. McLeod JG, Penny R. Vincristine neuropathy: an electrophysiological and histological study. J Neurol Neurosurg Psychiatry. 1969;32(4):297–304. PubMed PMID: 4309019; PubMed Central PMCID: PMC496516
24. Legha SS. Vincristine neurotoxicity. Pathophysiology and management. Med Toxicol. 1986;1(6):421–7.
25. Hershman DL, Unger JM, Crew KD, Minasian LM, Awad D, Moinpour CM, Hansen L, Lew DL, Greenlee H, Fehrenbacher L, Wade JL 3rd, Wong SF, Hortobagyi GN, Meyskens FL, Albain KS. Randomized double-blind placebo-controlled trial of acetyl-L-carnitine for the prevention of taxane-induced neuropathy in women undergoing adjuvant breast cancer therapy. J Clin Oncol. 2013;31(20):2627–33. https://doi.org/10.1200/JCO.2012.44.8738. Epub 2013 Jun 3. PubMed PMID: 23733756; PubMed Central PMCID: PMC3699727
26. Alsaab HO, Sau S, Alzhrani R, Tatiparti K, Bhise K, Kashaw SK, Iyer AK. PD-1 and PD-L1 checkpoint signaling inhibition for cancer immunotherapy: mechanism, combinations, and clinical outcome. Front Pharmacol. 2017;8:561.
27. Fang F, Xiao W, Tian Z. NK cell-based immunotherapy for cancer. Semin Immunol. 2017;31:37–54.
28. De Velasco G, Je Y, Bossé D, Awad MM, Ott PA, Moreira RB, Schutz F, Bellmunt J, Sonpavde GP, Hodi FS, Choueiri TK. Comprehensive meta-analysis of key immune-related adverse events from CTLA-4 and PD-1/PD-L1 inhibitors in cancer patients. Cancer Immunol Res. 2017;5(4):312–8.

5 Postsurgical Pain Syndromes

Thomas J. Van de Ven and Amitabh Gulati

Introduction

Currently, 12 million people in the United States are living with a previous diagnosis of cancer, and two out of three newly diagnosed cancer patients will survive for at least 5 years (http://www.cdc.gov/cancer/survivorship/basic_info/). As more efficacious primary cancer therapy is developed, these numbers should only improve over time. Many of these cancer survivors have undergone major surgical resection. A large database analysis of cancer patients from the UK National Health Service (NHS) revealed almost 10% of patients with prostate, bladder, lung, and pancreas cancers underwent major surgical resection, while more than 50% of patients with uterine, breast, kidney, and ovarian cancers had major surgical resection. With the growing realization that many surgical procedures are associated with a significant incidence of chronic, sometimes disabling, neuropathic pain, it follows that chronic postsurgical pain is becoming an important survivorship issue (http://www.ncin.org.uk/publications/data_briefings/major_resection).

The past two decades have seen increased interest in understanding the burden of chronic postsurgical pain (CPSP), while prevention of this growing problem has been named the "holy grail" of anesthesiology [1–4]. Many of the main cancer-related surgical procedures, including mastectomy, amputation, and thoracotomy, necessarily involve damage to the major peripheral nerves. In the case of thoracotomy, even with thoracoscopic techniques, intercostal nerve injury is almost assured. Each of these surgical procedures has been associated with a very high rate of chronic pain incidence at 3–6 months after surgery (Table 5.1). Severe chronic pain occurs in 5–10% of patients, but with the large and increasing numbers of these procedures performed annually, tens of thousands of severe chronic pain suffering cancer survivors are likely being created every year.

T. J. Van de Ven
Duke University Medical Center and Durham VAMC, Department of Anesthesiology, Durham, NC, USA
e-mail: Thomas.vandeven@duke.edu

A. Gulati (✉)
Department of Anesthesiology and Critical Care, Memorial Sloan Kettering Cancer Center, New York, NY, USA

Chronic Postmastectomy Pain

Breast cancer accounts for 14.1% of new cancer diagnoses in the United States, and 41% of those diagnosed with breast cancer will undergo either partial or total mastectomy. The incidence of chronic pain following mastectomy, as for most other surgical procedures, has proven to be highly variable in the literature which is not surprising since the outcome measures used in these studies are also highly variable. Chronic postmastectomy pain incidence is often reported as somewhere in the range of 15–58% [5]. However, if only trials that consider pain scores of greater than 3 or 4 in the area of mastectomy incision persisting at least 2 months after surgery are considered as significant, this range decreases to 30–40%. It is estimated that there are currently 2.5 million breast cancer survivors, which means that likely hundreds of thousands of these survivors have significant chronic pain after mastectomy.

Table 5.1 Estimated incidence of chronic postsurgical pain and estimated annual surgical volume in the United States of selected procedures

Type of operation	Incidence of chronic pain (severe, >5/10 pain)	Number of procedures in the United States[a]
Mastectomy [7]	20–30% (5–10%)	87,000
Amputation [99, 100]	50–80% (5–10%)	138,000
Thoracotomy [101]	30–40% (10%)	~ 30,000–65,000[b]

[a]CDC Health Data Interactive 2009
[b]Agency for Healthcare Research and Quality

A. Gulati et al. (eds.), *Essentials of Interventional Cancer Pain Management*, https://doi.org/10.1007/978-3-319-99684-4_5

A recent questionnaire-based study by Gartner et al. evaluating prevalence of and risk factors for chronic post-mastectomy pain in a cohort of Danish women found 47% of more than 3200 respondents had pain in the area of surgery at 2–3 years after surgery, with 13% of those reporting severe pain (pain scores of 8–10) [6]. This agrees well with previously reported incidence from multiple sources [7–9] including an incidence of 52% in a prospective cohort study published by Alves Nogueira Fabro et al. in 2012 [10]. This questionnaire-based study also identified multiple predisposing risk factors. Axillary node dissection was associated with increased risk of chronic post-mastectomy pain. This agrees with recent evidence from a study by de Menezes Couceiro et al. that found an increased risk of chronic pain in women with quadrantectomy, a procedure almost always accompanied by lymph node dissection at their institution [11].

Chronic Post-thoracotomy Pain

Post-thoracotomy pain syndrome (PTPS) may have an incidence even higher than chronic pain after mastectomy with most studies reporting pain 3 months after surgery in 30–80% of patients [12–16]. A recent prospective cross-sectional study of patients who had previously undergone thoracotomy for lung cancer between 2 and 12 months prior to enrollment revealed that 40% of patients had significant pain (pain score greater than 3) and 17% of patients had severe pain (pain score greater than 7) at the surgical site. In these patients, significant pain was also associated with decreased quality of life and increased anxiety and depression.

Chronic Postamputation Pain

Limb amputation, though less prevalent than thoracotomy or mastectomy, is still carried out in 4–5000 patients each year often for soft tissue and osseous sarcomas. The incidence of chronic pain after amputation is the highest of all types of cancer-related surgery – a fact that is not especially surprising as this surgery involves actual transection of large peripheral nerves. Also, while phantom pain is occasionally seen after mastectomy, a very large proportion of amputees (up to 80%) suffer phantom limb pain at some point during surgical recovery. Also, while chronic post-thoracotomy pain and postmastectomy pain are often mostly neuropathic in nature (with accompanying allodynia and burning paresthesias), postamputation pain is often more complex and includes neuroma formation, stump irritation from prostheses, poor wound healing, heterotopic ossification, and complex regional pain syndrome.

Risk Factors for CPSP

One of the enigmas of CPSP is that patients who appear very similar, undergoing almost identical surgical procedures, often develop widely divergent pain phenotypes months after surgery. In the case of patients undergoing thoracotomy, for example, half will have almost no pain near the incision in the year following surgery, and 20% will have severe, life-altering pain. Because of this variability in pain outcomes, there has been increasing efforts to understand what clinical and genetic factors alter a patient's risk for developing CPSP. There is a large amount of evidence that comorbid psychosocial factors are strongly associated with CPSP [17, 18]. The presence of catastrophizing, especially, is highly prevalent in patients with CPSP [19, 20]. Perhaps the most useful, sensitive, and strong predictor of CPSP is the presence of severe pain perioperatively [21–23]. The risk of chronic pain in patients with severe perioperative pain is the main reason, so many early attempts at prevention involved short-term perioperative regional anesthesia techniques.

Attempts at Prevention in Clinical Studies

Already established chronic neuropathic pain following surgical nerve injury is difficult to treat and/or reverse with current therapies, so prevention has been the major goal of a variety of small studies since the early 1990s. These initial efforts at prevention were designed around the hypothesis that abnormal nociceptor signaling at the time of surgical nerve injury led to chronic sensitization through a process similar to NMDA receptor-dependent long-term potentiation. Three main approaches were used: (1) blockade of nociceptor signaling through regional anesthesia techniques or lidocaine infusions, (2) NMDA receptor antagonism to help prevent synaptic strengthening and central sensitization, and (3) gabapentinoid treatments to reduce synaptic neurotransmitter release (Table 5.2).

Nerve Blockade with Regional and Neuraxial Anesthetic Techniques

Because chronic neuropathic pain becomes more difficult to treat as duration of pain increases, there have been a number of attempts to prevent this type of postsurgical pain before it becomes entrenched. Most of these studies have targeted either nociceptor signaling or inflammation during the immediate perioperative period. Regional or neuraxial techniques preventing neuronal signaling from the surgical site with local anesthetics provided an obvious initial strategy for

Table 5.2 Selected clinical studies attempting preventive analgesia for chronic postamputation and post-thoracotomy pain

Study	Number of patients	Single-blinded RCT	Intervention tested for significance	Significant reduction in chronic pain (per study authors)	Ref.
Amputation					
Fisher et al.	11	No	Continuous sciatic nerve sheath block	Yes	26
Bach et al.	25	No	Perioperative epidural vs. multimodal analgesia	Yes	25
Borghi et al.	71	No	Prolonged continuous regional analgesia	Yes	32
Nikolajsen et al.	60	Yes	Preemptive vs. postoperative epidural analgesia	No	27
Karanikolas et al.	65 (randomized to 5 groups)	Yes	Perioperative epidural analgesia vs. perioperative IV PCA	No	28
Pinzur et al.	21	Yes	Continuous perineural bupivacaine infusion	No	29
Hayes et al.	45	Yes	72 h ketamine infusion	No	34
Nikolajsen et al.	46	Yes	30 days gabapentin	No	35
Schley et al.	19	Yes	4 weeks memantine	Yes at 6 months No at 12 months	36
Thoracotomy					
Tiippana et al.	114	No	Thoracic epidural	Yes	12
Ju et al.	107	Yes	Thoracic epidural vs. intercostal cryoanalgesia	No	30
Lu et al.	105 (divided into 3 groups)	Yes	Thoracic epidural	Yes	24
Suzuki et al.	50	Yes	Ketamine infusion	No at 6 months	38
Kinney et al.	120	Yes	Gabapentin	No	16

pain prevention. If chronic pain occurs simply because of abnormal nociceptor signaling, blocking that signaling could prevent the development of chronic pain by blocking the initiation of the peripheral and central sensitization. Initial small studies, in thoracotomy and amputation patients, for example, were encouraging [12, 14, 24–26]. For example, Bach et al. in a small prospective but unblinded trial showed that 72 h of preoperative epidural analgesia before amputation continued through the end of surgery prevented postoperative phantom limb for every patient in the treatment group [25]. Also, a small prospective observational study by Fisher et al. in 1991 showed that perioperative bupivacaine through a regional anesthesia catheter placed intraoperatively and continued for 72 h completely prevented postoperative phantom limb pain [26]. These initial positive results, however, were followed by a number of somewhat larger randomized prospective trials of either epidural analgesia or regional analgesia that were less encouraging [27–31]. Nikolajsen et al. randomized patients before amputation to either epidural analgesia throughout the perioperative period or epidural analgesia postoperatively only and found no significant improvement in phantom limb pain or residual limb pain [27]. More recently, Karanikolas et al. showed that epidural analgesia was no more efficacious than intravenous patient-controlled opioid administration for prevention of chronic phantom limb pain [28]. Interestingly, Borghi et al. reported reduced phantom limb pain when regional analgesia was continued for up to 80 days after amputation [32]. This study, however, was observational only. More promisingly, a recent Cochrane systematic review of regional anesthesia for the prevention of chronic pain after mastectomy and thoracotomy showed a significant improvement in chronic post-thoracotomy pain with perioperative epidural analgesia and a significant improvement in chronic postmastectomy pain with perioperative paravertebral blockade [14, 33]. Unfortunately, only three studies fit inclusion criteria for thoracotomy and two studies for mastectomy, so limited patient number reduced the impact of the analysis.

Pharmacological Modulation of Neurotransmission

Multiple attempts have also been made to use existing pharmacotherapy perioperatively to block the transition from acute to chronic postsurgical pain [16, 34–38]. A recent Cochrane review examined all trials attempting to use pharmacotherapy for prevention of chronic postsurgical pain [39]. The inclusion criteria accepted all trials using double blinding and randomization to administer systemic pharmacologic therapy perioperatively with pain scores measured 3 months or more after surgery. The review included 40 trials, but only ketamine and gabapentinoids had been studied sufficiently to attempt a conclusion about efficacy as preventive therapy. Ketamine, studied in 14 randomized controlled trials, was found by the authors to have "modest" but significant efficacy as a preventive analgesic. Gabapentinoids (including ten RCTs of gabapentin and five RCTs of pregabalin) were found to have no significant preventive analgesic efficacy. Studies evaluating the preventive potential of corticosteroids, nonsteroidal anti-inflammatory drugs, NMDA receptor antagonists, local anesthetics, opioids, and venlafaxine were included, but no other class of therapeutic had been studied sufficiently for a meta-analysis to be completed. Another systematic review evaluating the preventive analgesic efficacy of gabapentinoids [40] was published concurrently, concluding gabapentinoids were effective at preventing CPSP though the exclusion of one negative trial [35], and a number of large pharmaceutical company-funded trials have been cited as significant weaknesses [41].

Limitations of Current Preventive Strategies

It is not surprising that researchers addressing the problem of chronic postsurgical pain turned first to existing analgesics and anesthetic techniques for the initial attempts at prevention. Practical considerations and the short time many patients remain in the hospital where investigators and study coordinators have easy access to them limited the therapeutic complexity and duration of treatment. Mechanistic understanding of the factors causing transition from acute pain to chronic pain was also limited at the time. Central sensitization due to abnormal nociceptor activity was thought to be the most likely candidate for causing chronic neuropathic pain [42], and it seemed rational that reducing nociceptor signaling intensity at the time of the nerve injury and during the most acute phase of postsurgical pain would be sufficient for prevention [43, 44]. It is clear, however, that single-agent treatment with drugs designed to reduce action potential frequency applied either systemically or regionally has not provided the dramatic preventive option hoped for 20 years ago. Recent evidence suggests inflammatory response to nerve injury (i.e., neuroinflammation) remains active both peripherally and centrally for months and even years after injury [45]. The intrinsic function of nociceptors and CNS neurons is significantly altered after injury (neural plasticity in the PNS and CNS) [46, 47], contributing to failure of single-agent, short-term, preventive therapies.

Mechanisms Underlying CPSP

Neuroinflammation, including inflammation of both peripheral and central neural tissue, has been increasingly recognized as an important driver of the abnormal neuronal signaling leading to neuropathic pain after surgical nerve injury [48, 49]. Prolonged neuroinflammation and neuronal plasticity are so intimately intertwined during the time following peripheral nerve injury that it is difficult to describe them as separate processes. The next section will attempt to do this, but the reader is encouraged to keep in mind that both processes are happening simultaneously.

CPSP and Neuronal Plasticity

Peripheral Sensitization

Surgical trauma always involves nerve damage – whether large named nerves like intercostal nerve damage in thoracotomy or small unnamed sensory nerves in an abdominal incision. When damaged, all peripheral nerves begin to spontaneously fire even without distal activation [46] due to hyperactivity of sodium channels present in the axon. After injury, sodium channels are rapidly distributed to a midaxonal location at high density, allowing this spontaneous firing [47]. This intrinsic pacemaker activity occurs in both A and C fibers, but large Aβ fibers develop this ability within a day of injury [50], and, though they likely don't carry nociceptive signals themselves, they can depolarize and sensitize postsynaptic neurons [46] (Fig. 5.1).

Central Sensitization

Peripheral sensitization inevitably leads to increased activity at central terminals through release of neurotransmitters and growth factors. This central sensitization is responsible for the hyperalgesia and allodynia that develop months after nerve injury. This central sensitization is largely NMDA receptor dependent [51]. NMDA receptor subunit expression and phosphorylation change quickly with increased peripheral input [52, 53]. In addition to NMDA receptor changes, altered AMPA receptor expression and the loss of GABA and glycine inhibitory control all drive the development of central sensitization and lasting neuropathic pain [54–56].

CPSP and Neuroinflammation

Postsurgical tissue damage leads to local release of multiple inflammatory mediators including prostaglandins, bradykinins, cytokines, hydrogen ions, bacterial peptides, and miRNAs [49]. Peripheral nociceptors contain receptors for these compounds on each distal terminal, and binding of these receptors causes depolarization and increased action potential generation. In a positive feedback loop, the increased nociceptor activity itself causes the release of mediators that attract immune cells (neutrophils, macrophages, and T cells) to the injured nerve which in turn release inflammatory mediators and cause more nociceptor firing [48, 57, 58] (Fig. 5.2).

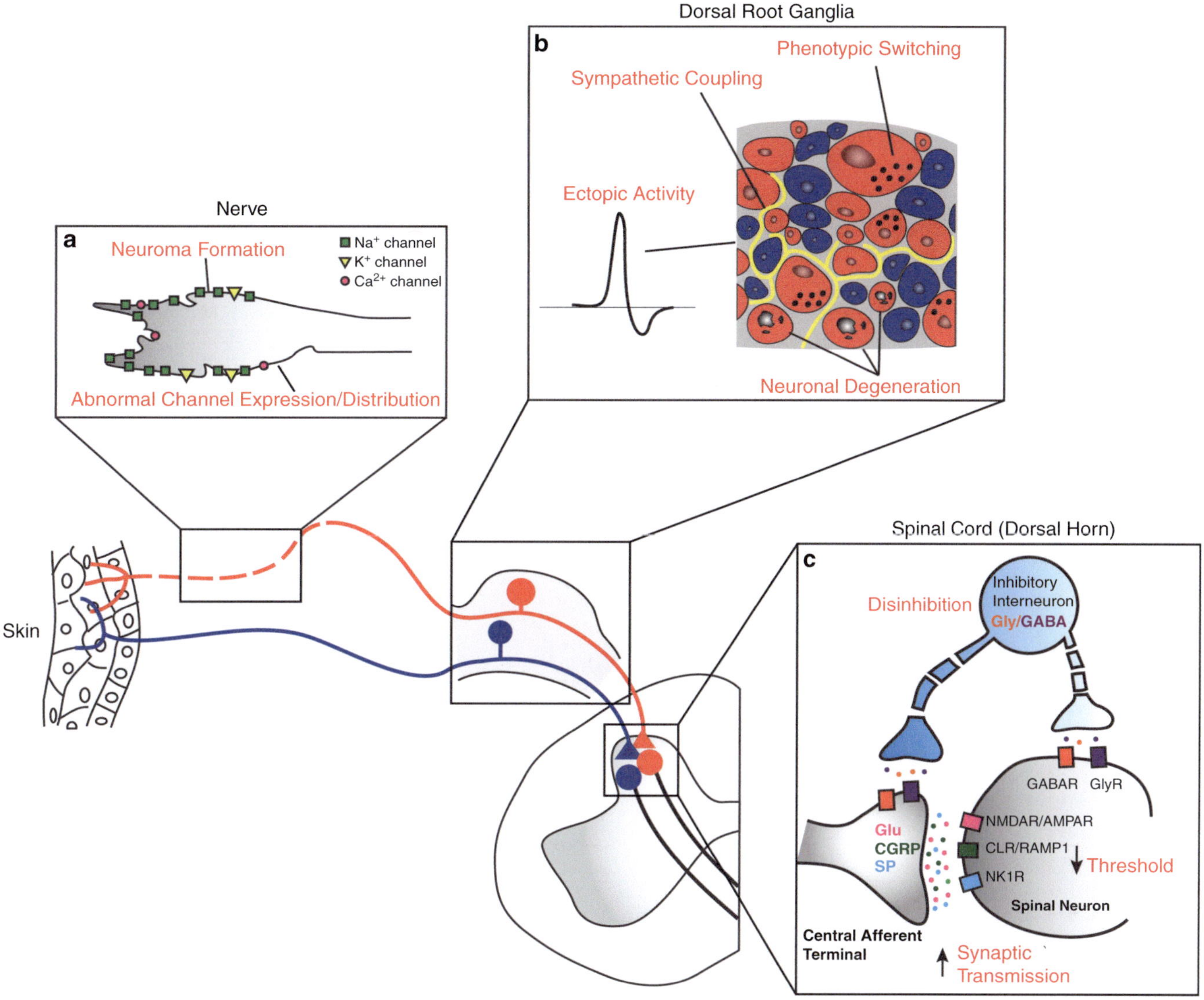

Fig. 5.1 (**a**) At the site of nerve injury, disorganized attempts at regrowth result in the formation of a neuroma. A principal feature of the neuroma is the abnormal expression and distribution of electrogenic ion channels at the neuroma end bulb. In particular, there is an abnormal accumulation of sodium channels and also calcium and potassium channels (downregulation), which enable both spontaneous and evoked *ectopic activity*. (**b**) At the level of the dorsal root ganglia (DRGs), several key changes occur after injury that contribute to neuropathic pain. Like the distal neuroma, the somata of injured sensory neurons take on the ability to generate ectopic activity, even in the absence of a stimulus. Another prominent change is *phenotypic switching*, wherein a portion of the large-sized A fibers, which normally transmit low-threshold, non-noxious stimuli, begin to express nociceptive neuropeptides such as calcitonin gene-related peptide (CGRP) and substance P (SP), which are only produced by nociceptors under normal conditions. This alteration in neurotransmitter content of low-threshold "touch fibers" may be partly responsible for the perception of the pain evoked by light touch – mechanical allodynia – that is characteristic after nerve injury. Under normal conditions, sympathetic fibers are not associated with the somata of the DRG, but after nerve injury, particularly transection, sympathetic fibers invade the DRG and enmesh the somata in process called *sympathetic coupling*. The clinical efficacy of sympathetic blockade is likely due to interference with this coupling process. Finally, as a result of distal injury and reduced access to trophic factors such as nerve growth factor (NGF), some neuronal cell bodies undergo *degeneration*, which itself can lead to pain by causing neuronal hyperexcitability or producing oxidants and pro-inflammatory mediators. (**c**) In the dorsal horn of the spinal cord, two major consequences of nerve injury are increased *excitatory synaptic transmission* and *disinhibition*, both of which lead to enhanced transmission of pain signals through the CNS. The central terminals of nociceptors demonstrate an increase in the release of neurotransmitters such as glutamate, SP, and CGRP onto postsynaptic spinal neurons. In concert with increased neurotransmitter release, the dorsal horn spinal neurons also upregulate neurotransmitter receptors, notably AMPA and NMDA receptors, which results in hyperactivity and hyperexcitability of nociceptive neurons. Further enhancement of pain signal transmission occurs due to a reduction in tonic inhibitory activity – disinhibition – from GABAergic and glycinergic interneurons, which are key modulators of synaptic transmission and neuronal activity in the spinal cord. Collectively, these changes lead to central amplification of pain signals arriving from the periphery (Figure prepared by Alexander Chamessian)

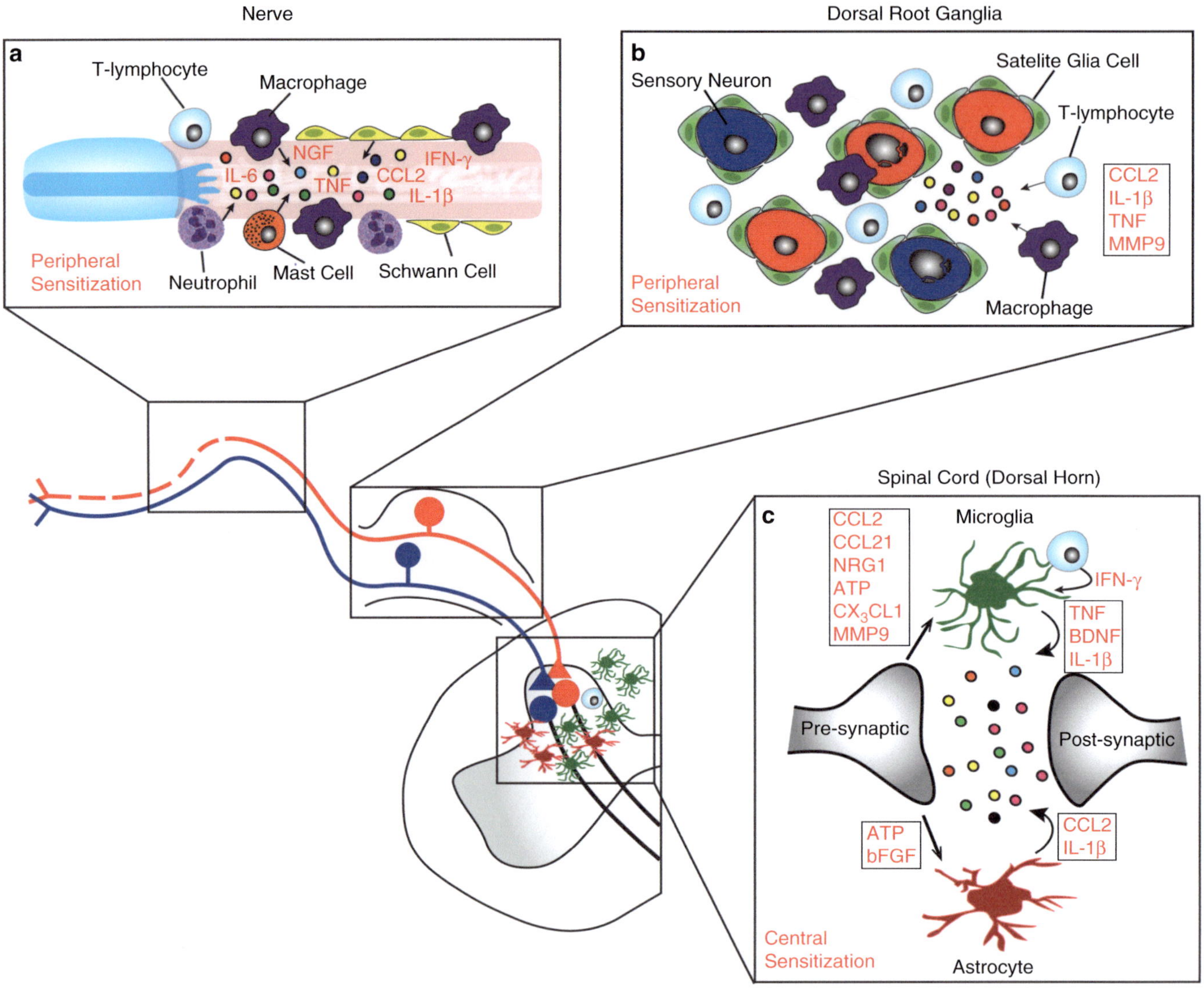

Fig. 5.2 After nerve trauma, a robust inflammatory response occurs at the site of injury. Immediately after injury, resident macrophages, mast cells, and Schwann cells release inflammatory mediators such as TNF, IL-1β, and CCL2, leading to the recruitment of neutrophils within the first 24 h. As Wallerian degeneration progresses over subsequent days, macrophages infiltrate the nerve to remove debris, further contributing to the release of chemokines and cytokines. Later in the course of injury, T lymphocytes also invade the injured nerve and release pro-inflammatory mediators such as IFN-γ. Collectively, the production and release of pro-inflammatory mediators by resident and infiltrating immune cells result in *peripheral sensitization* through direct and indirect interactions with injured (red) and intact (blue) neurons. (**b**) In the dorsal root ganglia (DRG), an inflammatory response also occurs. Macrophages and T lymphocytes infiltrate the DRG and release pro-inflammatory mediators around the somata of sensory neurons. Satellite glial cells also release mediators such as TNF and IL-1β that also interact with DRG somata and immune cells. As in the injured nerve, the inflammatory response in the DRG results in sensitization of injured and intact neurons, which contributes to pain hypersensitivity. (**c**) Peripheral nerve injury produces a dramatic inflammatory response in the spinal cord that is mediated principally by microglia and astrocytes (but we should not exclude oligodendrocytes[134]). Microglia respond to nerve injury with characteristic changes in morphology, gene expression, and proliferation and assume a pro-inflammatory or "reactive" state. Mediators released by injured and intact afferents such as ATP, CCL2, CX_3CL1, and MMP-9 contribute to this characteristic microglial change. The reactive microglia in turn release inflammatory mediators, namely, TNF, IL-1β, and growth factor BDNF which then act on central afferent terminals (presynaptic) and second-order spinal neurons (postsynaptic) to enhance and amplify afferent signals, or *central sensitization*. In addition, mediators released by microglia can also recruit T lymphocytes to the spinal cord, where they interact with the microglia and release mediators such as IFN-γ, helping to maintain the microglial reactive state and neuropathic pain. Astrocytes, while not immune cells themselves, are immunocompetent and assume a reactive state after nerve injury, undergoing morphological and transcriptional changes, as well as proliferation. Like microglia, they release pro-inflammatory chemokines, namely, CXCL1 and CCL2, which directly interact with spinal neurons and primary afferent terminals as neuromodulators. Collectively, microglia, astrocytes, and T lymphocytes work in concert to amplify the afferent signals arriving from the periphery, driving neuropathic pain (Figures prepared by Alexander Chamessian)

Dorsal Root Ganglion

A similar but longer-lasting immune response occurs in ipsilateral dorsal root ganglion (DRG) after peripheral nerve injury. Three days after nerve injury, circulating monocytes infiltrate the DRG and become macrophages. These macrophages phagocytose the dying DRG neurons and remain active in the DRG for months [45, 59–61]. T lymphocytes and neutrophils also invade the DRG beginning at about 7 days after injury likely in response to chemokine signaling events (CCL2) triggered by injury [62]. This long-lasting neuroinflammatory response, and corresponding increase in neuronal signaling, likely allows the creation and maintenance of the central signaling and inflammatory events that lead to chronic CPSP.

Central Inflammatory Responses in the Spinal Cord

Activation of microglia and astrocytes in the spinal cord is crucial to the creation and maintenance of chronic pain after nerve injury [49, 63]. Three days after peripheral nerve injury, microglia undergo dramatic changes in the genes they express and in their morphology [64].These activated microglia wrap themselves around the synapse between primary and secondary nociceptors, producing multiple inflammatory mediators and growth factors that lead to both sensitization and disinhibition [65–67].

Astrocyte activation occurs following the peak of microglial activation and lasts much longer (up to 150 days post-injury) [63, 68]. It is likely that signaling molecules released at primary afferent central terminals cause microglial activation since long-lasting blockade of peripheral input was able to prevent microglial activation [69]. In addition, neuronal signaling alone appears to be able to activate the spinal cord microglia [70].

Emerging Preventive Therapeutics

The recent realization that the events leading to peripheral and central sensitization after nerve injury last a very long time and involve a complex inflammatory reaction likely explains why the success of current attempts at prevention of CPSP has largely failed. It is likely that effective prevention will have to address both the neuroplastic and inflammatory events that occur with nerve injury in addition to the temporal nature of those events.

Neurotransmission Modulation

Modulation of neurotransmission will continue to be an important goal of preventive therapies though the risks and difficulties of long-term peripheral and neuraxial catheter placement make this method less useful than hoped. There are, however, a number of neurotransmission modulators with strong preclinical evidence that may provide a way to reduce nociceptor activity for the entire multiple month-long inflammatory process that occurs after surgical nerve injury. Possible pharmacologic modulators include the potent capsaicin analogue resiniferatoxin (RTX) [71], novel TRPV1 antagonists [72], and monoclonal antibodies specific to the sodium channel subtype Na_V 1.7 [73].

Neuroinflammatory Modulation

As the importance of neuroinflammation in the initiation and maintenance of neuropathic pain after nerve injury becomes more clear, modulators of inflammation at all levels have been studied more and more intensely and for longer periods of time as potential preventive therapeutics [48, 49, 74–79]. Pharmacologic modifiers of glia (minocycline and propentofylline) [80–84], cytokine and chemokine inhibitors [85–88], treatment with anti-inflammatory cytokines (IL-10, TGF-b) [89], and protease inhibitors (MMP-9, cathepsin S, and caspase 6) [49, 63, 90–92] have all shown effectiveness at reducing neuropathic pain at least in preclinical models of peripheral nerve injury.

Pro-resolution Lipid Mediators

Perhaps most intriguing are a class of small lipids derived from the fish-oil constituents DHA and EPA called pro-resolution lipid mediators. This class includes the resolvins, neuroprotectins, and maresins. There is more and more evidence that inflammation does not just passively end. It is an active process requiring mediators that promote resolution of inflammation [93–95]. The PRLMs appear to be central to this process and in multiple studies have also been shown to be powerful analgesics. Resolvins, maresins, and neuroprotectins at very low doses (nanogram range) have been shown to reduce inflammatory pain. In addition, resolvins and neuroprotectin have been shown to block spinal cord synaptic plasticity such as long-term potentiation following intense sciatic nerve stimulation [96, 97]. The resolvins and protectins represent a group termed the pro-resolution lipid mediators (PRLMs) and are derived from the omega-3 fatty acids docosahexaenoic acid (DHA) and eicosapentaenoic acid (EPA) enriched in fish oil.

Protectin D1 or neuroprotectin D1 (PD1/NPD1) is one of the few new compounds that have shown potential for not only treatment but prevention of chronic neuropathic pain after surgery. Perioperative and perineural application of NPD1 at one time point has been shown to prevent mechanical allodynia in a mouse chronic constriction injury model of neuropathic pain. In addition, NPD1 given 2 weeks after nerve injury was able to transiently reverse mechanical allodynia in a similar manner to gabapentin but at a much lower dose [98]. NPD1 also inhibits the formation of neuroma after amputation (transection of the sciatic nerve) and protects axonal injury and spinal cord neuroinflammation (glial activation and cytokine/chemokine expression) after nerve injury [98]. Therefore, NPD1 and other pro-resolution lipid mediators (PRLMs) may possess the rare ability to prevent CPSP following nerve trauma because of a unique combination of attributes including promotion of inflammation resolution (unlike corticosteroids that block both inflammatory and anti-inflammatory processes) and the ability to normalize neuronal potentiation and sensitization (unlike local anesthetics that completely block signaling).

Conclusion

Awareness of the toll that chronic neuropathic pain after cancer surgery takes on the quality of life of cancer survivors has increased significantly over the past 20 years. Initial efforts at preventing the transition to chronic pain after surgical nerve injury were disappointing. Recent rapid advances in our understanding of the complex neuronal signaling and neuroinflammatory events that occur after nerve injury have created new hope that multimodal-targeted therapies of adequate duration may help to prevent the transition from acute to chronic pain in the near future.

References

1. Sommer C, Kress M. Recent findings on how proinflammatory cytokines cause pain: peripheral mechanisms in inflammatory and neuropathic hyperalgesia. Neurosci Lett. 2004;361:184–7.
2. Cohen SP, Raja SN. Prevention of chronic postsurgical pain: the ongoing search for the holy grail of anesthesiology. Anesthesiology. 2013;118:241–3.
3. Calvo M, Dawes JM, Bennett DL. The role of the immune system in the generation of neuropathic pain. Lancet Neurol. 2012;11:629–42.
4. Gold MS, Gebhart GF. Nociceptor sensitization in pain pathogenesis. Nat Med. 2010;16:1248–57.
5. Schreiber KL, Kehlet H, Belfer I, Edwards RR. Predicting, preventing and managing persistent pain after breast cancer surgery: the importance of psychosocial factors. Pain Manag. 2014;4:445–59.
6. Gärtner R, Jensen MB, Nielsen J, Ewertz M. JAMA network | JAMA | prevalence of and factors associated with persistent pain following breast cancer surgery. JAMA. 2009;302(18):1985–92.
7. Jung BF, Ahrendt GM, Oaklander AL, Dworkin RH. Neuropathic pain following breast cancer surgery: proposed classification and research update. Pain. 2003;104:1–13.
8. Wallace MS, Wallace AM, Lee J, Dobke MK. Pain after breast surgery: a survey of 282 women. Pain. 1996;66:195–205.
9. Smith W, Bourne D, Squair J, Phillips DO, Chambers WA. A retrospective cohort study of post mastectomy pain syndrome. Pain. 1999;83:91–5.
10. Fabro EAN, Bergmann A, do Amaral E, Silva B, Ribeiro ACP, de Souza Abrahão K, da Costa Leite Ferreira MG, de Almeida Dias R, Thuler LCS. Post-mastectomy pain syndrome: incidence and risks. Breast. 2012;21:321–5.
11. de Menezes Couceiro TC, Valença MM, Raposo MCF, de Orange FA, Amorim MMR. Prevalence of post-mastectomy pain syndrome and associated risk factors: a cross-sectional cohort study. Pain Manag Nurs. 2013; https://doi.org/10.1016/j.pmn.2013.07.011.
12. Tiippana E, Nilsson E, Kalso E. Post-thoracotomy pain after thoracic epidural analgesia: a prospective follow-up study. Acta Anaesthesiol Scand. 2003;47:433–8.
13. Song JG, Shin JW, Lee EH, Choi DK, Bang JY, Chin JH, Choi IC. Incidence of post-thoracotomy pain: a comparison between total intravenous anaesthesia and inhalation anaesthesia. Eur J Cardiothorac Surg. 2012;41:1078–82.
14. Sentürk M, Ozcan PE, Talu GK, Kiyan E, Camci E, Ozyalçin S, Dilege S, Pembeci K. The effects of three different analgesia techniques on long-term postthoracotomy pain. Anesth Analg. 2002;94:11–5. –tableofcontents.
15. Yarnitsky D, Crispel Y, Eisenberg E, Granovsky Y, Ben-Nun A, Sprecher E, Best L-A, Granot M. Prediction of chronic post-operative pain: pre-operative DNIC testing identifies patients at risk. Pain. 2008;138:22–8.
16. Kinney MAO, Mantilla CB, Carns PE, Passe MA, Brown MJ, Hooten WM, Curry TB, Long TR, Wass CT, Wilson PR, Weingarten TN, Huntoon MA, Rho RH, Mauck WD, Pulido JN, Allen MS, Cassivi SD, Deschamps C, Nichols FC, Shen KR, Wigle DA, Hoehn SL, Alexander SL, Hanson AC, Schroeder DR. Preoperative gabapentin for acute post-thoracotomy analgesia: a randomized, double-blinded, active placebo-controlled study. Pain Pract. 2012;12:175–83.
17. Hanley MA, Jensen MP, Ehde DM, Hoffman AJ, Patterson DR, Robinson LR. Psychosocial predictors of long-term adjustment to lower-limb amputation and phantom limb pain. Disabil Rehabil. 2004;26:882–93.
18. Hinrichs-Rocker A, Schulz K, Järvinen I, Lefering R, Simanski C, Neugebauer EAM. Psychosocial predictors and correlates for chronic post-surgical pain (CPSP) – a systematic review. Eur J Pain. 2009;13:719–30.
19. Belfer I, Schreiber KL, Shaffer JR, Shnol H, Blaney K, Morando A, Englert D, Greco C, Brufsky A, Ahrendt G, Kehlet H, Edwards RR, Bovbjerg DH. Persistent postmastectomy pain in breast cancer survivors: analysis of clinical, demographic, and psychosocial factors. J Pain. 2013;14:1185–95.
20. Jensen MP, Ehde DM, Hoffman AJ, Patterson DR, Czerniecki JM, Robinson LR. Cognitions, coping and social environment predict adjustment to phantom limb pain. Pain. 2002;95:133–42.
21. Katz J, Jackson M, Kavanagh BP, Sandler AN. Acute pain after thoracic surgery predicts long-term post-thoracotomy pain. Clin J Pain. 1996;12:50–5.
22. Nikolajsen L, Ilkjær S, Krøner K, Christensen JH, Jensen TS. The influence of preamputation pain on postamputation stump and phantom pain. Pain. 1997;72:393–405.
23. Van de Ven TJ, John Hsia H-L. Causes and prevention of chronic postsurgical pain. Curr Opin Crit Care. 2012;18:366–71.
24. Lu Y-L, Wang X-D, Lai R-C. Correlation of acute pain treatment to occurrence of chronic pain in tumor patients after thoracotomy. Ai Zheng. 2008;27:206–9.
25. Bach S, Noreng MF, Tjéllden NU. Phantom limb pain in amputees during the first 12 months following limb amputation, after preoperative lumbar epidural blockade. Pain. 1988;33:297–301.
26. Fisher A, Meller Y. Continuous postoperative regional analgesia by nerve sheath block for amputation surgery – a pilot study. Anesth Analg. 1991;72:300–3.
27. Nikolajsen L, Ilkjær S, Christensen JH, Krøner K, Jensen TS. Randomised trial of epidural bupivacaine and morphine in prevention of stump and phantom pain in lower-limb amputation. Lancet. 1997;350:1353–7.
28. Karanikolas M, Aretha D, Tsolakis I, Monantera G, Kiekkas P, Papadoulas S, Swarm RA, Filos KS. Optimized perioperative analgesia reduces chronic phantom limb pain intensity, prevalence, and frequency: a prospective, randomized, clinical trial. Anesthesiology. 2011;114:1144–54.

29. Pinzur MS, Garla PG, Pluth T, Vrbos L. Continuous postoperative infusion of a regional anesthetic after an amputation of the lower extremity. A randomized clinical trial. J Bone Joint Surg Am. 1996;78:1501–5.
30. Ju H, Feng Y, Yang B-X, Wang J. Comparison of epidural analgesia and intercostal nerve cryoanalgesia for post-thoracotomy pain control. Eur J Pain. 2008;12:378–84.
31. Kavanagh BP, Katz J, Sandler AN, Nierenberg H, Roger S, Boylan JF, Laws AK. Multimodal analgesia before thoracic surgery does not reduce postoperative pain. Br J Anaesth. 1994;73(2):184–9.
32. Borghi B, D'Addabbo M, White PF, Gallerani P, Toccaceli L, Raffaeli W, Tognù A, Fabbri N, Mercuri M. The use of prolonged peripheral neural blockade after lower extremity amputation: the effect on symptoms associated with phantom limb syndrome. Anesth Analg. 2010;111:1308–15.
33. Andreae MH, Andreae DA. Regional anaesthesia to prevent chronic pain after surgery: a Cochrane systematic review and meta-analysis. Br J Anaesth. 2013;111:711–20.
34. Hayes C, Armstrong-Brown A, Burstal R. Perioperative intravenous ketamine infusion for the prevention of persistent post-amputation pain: a randomized, controlled trial. Anaesth Intensive Care. 2004;32:330–8.
35. Nikolajsen L, Finnerup NB, Kramp S, Vimtrup A-S, Keller J, Jensen TS. A randomized study of the effects of gabapentin on postamputation pain. Anesthesiology. 2006;105:1008–15.
36. Schley M, Topfner S, Wiech K, Schaller HE, Konrad CJ, Schmelz M, Birbaumer N. Continuous brachial plexus blockade in combination with the NMDA receptor antagonist memantine prevents phantom pain in acute traumatic upper limb amputees. Eur J Pain. 2007;11:299–308.
37. Dualé C, Sibaud F, Guastella V, Vallet L, Gimbert Y-A, Taheri H, Filaire M, Schoeffler P, Dubray C. Perioperative ketamine does not prevent chronic pain after thoracotomy. Eur J Pain. 2009;13:497–505.
38. Suzuki M, Haraguti S, Sugimoto K, Kikutani T, Shimada Y, Sakamoto A. Low-dose intravenous ketamine potentiates epidural analgesia after thoracotomy. Anesthesiology. 2006;105:111–9.
39. Chaparro LE, Smith SA, Moore RA, Wiffen PJ, Gilron I. Pharmacotherapy for the prevention of chronic pain after surgery in adults. Cochrane Database Syst Rev. 2013;7:CD008307.
40. Clarke H, Wijeysundera DN, Bonin RP, Orser B, Englesakis M, Katz J. Pregabalin effective for the prevention of chronic postsurgical pain: really? Reply. Anesth Analg. 2013;116:508–9.
41. Chelly JE. Pregabalin effective for the prevention of chronic postsurgical pain: really? Anesth Analg. 2013;116:507–8.
42. Woolf CJ. Central sensitization: implications for the diagnosis and treatment of pain. Pain. 2011;152:S2–S15.
43. Wall PD. The prevention of postoperative pain. Pain. 1988;33:289–90.
44. Woolf CJ. Evidence for a central component of post-injury pain hypersensitivity. Nature. 1983;306:686–8.
45. Scholz J, Woolf CJ. The neuropathic pain triad: neurons, immune cells and glia. Nat Neurosci. 2007;10:1361–8.
46. Devor M. Ectopic discharge in Abeta afferents as a source of neuropathic pain. Exp Brain Res. 2009;196:115–28.
47. Devor M. Sodium channels and mechanisms of neuropathic pain. J Pain. 2006;7:S3–S12.
48. Ji RR, Xu ZZ, Gao YJ. Emerging targets in neuroinflammation-driven chronic pain. Nat Rev Drug Discov. 2014;13(7):533.
49. Ellis A, Bennett DLH. Neuroinflammation and the generation of neuropathic pain. Br J Anaesth. 2013;111:26–37.
50. Sun Q, Tu H, Xing G-G, Han J-S, Wan Y. Ectopic discharges from injured nerve fibers are highly correlated with tactile allodynia only in early, but not late, stage in rats with spinal nerve ligation. Exp Neurol. 2005;191:128–36.
51. Liu XJ, Gingrich JR, Vargas-Caballero M, Dong YN, Sengar A, Beggs S, Wang S-H, Ding HK, Frankland PW, Salter MW. Treatment of inflammatory and neuropathic pain by uncoupling Src from the NMDA receptor complex. Nat Med. 2008;14:1325–32.
52. Wilson JA, Garry EM, Anderson HA, Rosie R, Colvin LA, Mitchell R, Fleetwood-Walker SM. NMDA receptor antagonist treatment at the time of nerve injury prevents injury-induced changes in spinal NR1 and NR2B subunit expression and increases the sensitivity of residual pain behaviours to subsequently administered NMDA receptor antagonists. Pain. 2005;117:421–32.
53. Ultenius C, Linderoth B, Meyerson BA, Wallin J. Spinal NMDA receptor phosphorylation correlates with the presence of neuropathic signs following peripheral nerve injury in the rat. Neurosci Lett. 2006;399:85–90.
54. Kuner R. Central mechanisms of pathological pain. Nat Med. 2010;16:1258–66.
55. Lu Y, Dong H, Gao Y, Gong Y, Ren Y, Gu N, Zhou S, Xia N, Sun Y-Y, Ji R-R, Xiong L. A feed-forward spinal cord glycinergic neural circuit gates mechanical allodynia. J Clin Invest. 2013;123:4050–62.
56. Coull JAM, Boudreau D, Bachand K, Prescott SA, Nault F, Sík A, De Koninck P, De Koninck Y. Trans-synaptic shift in anion gradient in spinal lamina I neurons as a mechanism of neuropathic pain. Nature. 2003;424:938–42.
57. Gold MS, Gebhart GF. Nociceptor sensitization in pain pathogenesis. Nat Med. 2010;16:1248–57.
58. Hucho T, Levine JD. Signaling pathways in sensitization: toward a nociceptor cell biology. Neuron. 2007;55:365–76.
59. Hu P, McLachlan EM. Macrophage and lymphocyte invasion of dorsal root ganglia after peripheral nerve lesions in the rat. Neuroscience. 2002;112:23–38.
60. Kim CF, Moalem-Taylor G. Detailed characterization of neuro-immune responses following neuropathic injury in mice. Brain Res. 2011;1405:95–108.
61. Hu P, McLachlan EM. Distinct functional types of macrophage in dorsal root ganglia and spinal nerves proximal to sciatic and spinal nerve transections in the rat. Exp Neurol. 2003;184:590–605.
62. Zhuang Z-Y, Kawasaki Y, Tan P-H, Wen Y-R, Huang J, Ji R-R. Role of the CX3CR1/p38 MAPK pathway in spinal microglia for the development of neuropathic pain following nerve injury-induced cleavage of fractalkine. Brain Behav Immun. 2007;21:642–51.
63. Ji R-R, Berta T, Nedergaard M. Glia and pain: is chronic pain a gliopathy? Pain. 2013:1–19. https://doi.org/10.1016/j.pain.2013.06.022.
64. Calvo M, Bennett DLH. The mechanisms of microgliosis and pain following peripheral nerve injury. Exp Neurol. 2012;234:271–82.
65. Grace PM, Hutchinson MR, Maier SF, Watkins LR. Pathological pain and the neuroimmune interface. Nat Rev Immunol. 2014;14:217–31.
66. Kawasaki Y, Zhang L, Cheng J-K, Ji R-R. Cytokine mechanisms of central sensitization: distinct and overlapping role of interleukin-1beta, interleukin-6, and tumor necrosis factor-alpha in regulating synaptic and neuronal activity in the superficial spinal cord. J Neurosci. 2008;28:5189–94.
67. Coull JAM, Beggs S, Boudreau D, Boivin D, Tsuda M, Inoue K, Gravel C, Salter MW, De Koninck Y. BDNF from microglia causes the shift in neuronal anion gradient underlying neuropathic pain. Nature. 2005;438:1017–21.
68. Gwak YS, Kang J, Unabia GC, Hulsebosch CE. Spatial and temporal activation of spinal glial cells: role of gliopathy in central neuropathic pain following spinal cord injury in rats. Exp Neurol. 2012;234:362–72.
69. Wen Y-R, Suter MR, Kawasaki Y, Huang J, Pertin M, Kohno T, Berde CB, Decosterd I, Ji R-R. Nerve conduction blockade in

the sciatic nerve prevents but does not reverse the activation of p38 mitogen-activated protein kinase in spinal microglia in the rat spared nerve injury model. Anesthesiology. 2007;107:312–21.
70. Hathway GJ, Vega-Avelaira D, Moss A, Ingram R, Fitzgerald M. Brief, low frequency stimulation of rat peripheral C-fibres evokes prolonged microglial-induced central sensitization in adults but not in neonates. Pain. 2009;144:110–8.
71. Karai L, Brown DC, Mannes AJ, Connelly ST, Brown J, Gandal M, Wellisch OM, Neubert JK, Olah Z, Iadarola MJ. Deletion of vanilloid receptor 1-expressing primary afferent neurons for pain control. J Clin Invest. 2004;113:1344–52.
72. Peters CM, Ririe D, Houle TT, Aschenbrenner CA, Eisenach JC. Nociceptor-selective peripheral nerve block induces delayed mechanical hypersensitivity and neurotoxicity in rats. Anesthesiology. 2014;120:976–86.
73. Lee J-H, Park C-K, Chen G, Han Q, Xie R-G, Liu T, Ji R-R, Lee S-Y. A monoclonal antibody that targets a NaV1.7 channel voltage sensor for pain and itch relief. Cell. 2014;157:1393–404.
74. Obata K. Role of mitogen-activated protein kinase activation in injured and intact primary afferent neurons for mechanical and heat hypersensitivity after spinal nerve ligation. J Neurosci. 2004;24:10211–22.
75. Matsuoka Y, Yang J. Selective inhibition of extracellular signal-regulated kinases 1/2 blocks nerve growth factor to brain-derived neurotrophic factor signaling and suppresses the development of and reverses already established pain behavior in rats. Neuroscience. 2012;206:224–36.
76. Jin SX, Zhuang ZY, Woolf CJ, Ji RR. p38 mitogen-activated protein kinase is activated after a spinal nerve ligation in spinal cord microglia and dorsal root ganglion neurons and contributes to the generation of neuropathic pain. J Neurosci. 2003;23(10):4017–22.
77. Schäfers M, Brinkhoff J, Neukirchen S, Marziniak M, Sommer C. Combined epineurial therapy with neutralizing antibodies to tumor necrosis factor-alpha and interleukin-1 receptor has an additive effect in reducing neuropathic pain in mice. Neurosci Lett. 2001;310:113–6.
78. Sommer C, Petrausch S, Lindenlaub T, Toyka KV. Neutralizing antibodies to interleukin 1-receptor reduce pain associated behavior in mice with experimental neuropathy. Neurosci Lett. 1999;270:25–8.
79. Kiguchi N, Maeda T, Kobayashi Y, Fukazawa Y, Kishioka S. Macrophage inflammatory protein-1 alpha mediates the development of neuropathic pain following peripheral nerve injury through interleukin-1 beta up-regulation. Pain. 2010;149:305–15.
80. Padi SSV, Kulkarni SK. Minocycline prevents the development of neuropathic pain, but not acute pain: possible anti-inflammatory and antioxidant mechanisms. Eur J Pharmacol. 2008;601:79–87.
81. Lin C, Tsaur M, Chen C, Wang T, Lin C, Lai Y, Hsu T, Pan Y, Yang C, Cheng J. Chronic intrathecal infusion of minocycline prevents the development of spinal-nerve ligation–induced pain in rats. Reg Anesth Pain Med. 2007;32:209–16.
82. Raghavendra V. Inhibition of microglial activation attenuates the development but not existing hypersensitivity in a rat model of neuropathy. J Pharmacol Exp Ther. 2003;306:624–30.
83. Zhang J, Wu D, Xie C, Wang H, Wang W, Zhang H, Liu R, Xu L-X, Mei X-P. Tramadol and propentofylline coadministration exerted synergistic effects on rat spinal nerve ligation-induced neuropathic pain. Edited by Siegel A. PloS One. 2013;8:e72943.
84. Raghavendra V, Tanga F, Rutkowski MD, DeLeo JA. Anti-hyperalgesic and morphine-sparing actions of propentofylline following peripheral nerve injury in rats: mechanistic implications of spinal glia and proinflammatory cytokines. Pain. 2003;104:655–64.
85. Lu C-H, Chao P-C, Borel CO, Yang C-P, Yeh C-C, Wong C-S, Wu C-T. Preincisional intravenous pentoxifylline attenuating perioperative cytokine response, reducing morphine consumption, and improving recovery of bowel function in patients undergoing colorectal cancer surgery. Anesth Analg. 2004;99:1465–71. tableofcontents.
86. Wordliczek J, Szczepanik AM, Banach M, Turchan J, Zembala M, Siedlar M, Przewlocki R, Serednicki W, Przewlocka B. The effect of pentoxifylline on post-injury hyperalgesia in rats and postoperative pain in patients. Life Sci. 2000;66:1155–64.
87. Genevay S, Finckh A, Zufferey P, Viatte S, Balagué F, Gabay C. Adalimumab in acute sciatica reduces the long-term need for surgery: a 3-year follow-up of a randomised double-blind placebo-controlled trial. Ann Rheum Dis. 2012;71:560–2.
88. Thacker MA, Clark AK, Bishop T, Grist J, Yip PK, Moon LDF, Thompson SWN, Marchand F, McMahon SB. CCL2 is a key mediator of microglia activation in neuropathic pain states. Eur J Pain. 2009;13:263–72.
89. Wagner R, Janjigian M, Myers RR. Anti-inflammatory interleukin-10 therapy in CCI neuropathy decreases thermal hyperalgesia, macrophage recruitment, and endoneurial TNF-a expression. Pain. 1998;74:35–42.
90. Kawasaki Y, Xu Z-Z, Wang X, Park JY, Zhuang Z-Y, Tan P-H, Gao Y-J, Roy K, Corfas G, Lo EH, Ji R-R. Distinct roles of matrix metalloproteases in the early- and late-phase development of neuropathic pain. Nat Med. 2008;14:331–6.
91. Clark AK, Yip PK, Grist J, Gentry C, Staniland AA, Marchand F, Dehvari M, Wotherspoon G, Winter J, Ullah J, Bevan S, Malcangio M. Inhibition of spinal microglial cathepsin S for the reversal of neuropathic pain. Proc Natl Acad Sci U S A. 2007;104:10655–60.
92. Berta T, Park C-K, Xu Z-Z, Xie R-G, Liu T, Lü N, Liu Y-C, Ji R-R. Extracellular caspase-6 drives murine inflammatory pain via microglial TNF-α secretion. J Clin Invest. 2014;124:1173–86.
93. Ortega-Gómez A, Perretti M, Soehnlein O. Resolution of inflammation: an integrated view. EMBO Mol Med. 2013;5:661–74.
94. Serhan CN, Brain SD, Buckley CD, Gilroy DW, Haslett C, O'Neill LAJ, Perretti M, Rossi AG, Wallace JL. Resolution of inflammation: state of the art, definitions and terms. FASEB J. 2007;21:325–32.
95. Serhan CN, Chiang N, Van Dyke TE. Resolving inflammation: dual anti-inflammatory and pro-resolution lipid mediators. Nat Rev Immunol. 2008;8:349–61.
96. Park C-K, Lü N, Xu Z-Z, Liu T, Serhan CN, Ji R-R. Resolving TRPV1- and TNF-α-mediated spinal cord synaptic plasticity and inflammatory pain with neuroprotectin D1. J Neurosci. 2011;31:15072–85.
97. Park C-K, Xu Z-Z, Liu T, Lü N, Serhan CN, Ji R-R. Resolvin D2 is a potent endogenous inhibitor for transient receptor potential subtype V1/A1, inflammatory pain, and spinal cord synaptic plasticity in mice: distinct roles of resolvin D1, D2, and E1. J Neurosci. 2011;31:18433–8.
98. Xu Z-Z, Liu X-J, Berta T, Park C-K, Lü N, Serhan CN, Ji R-R. Neuroprotectin/protectin D1 protects against neuropathic pain in mice after nerve trauma. Ann Neurol. 2013;74:490–5.
99. Kooijman CM, Dijkstra PU, Geertzen JH, Elzinga A, van der Schans CP. Phantom pain and phantom sensations in upper limb amputees: an epidemiological study. Pain. 2000;87:33–41.
100. Kern U, Busch V, Rockland M, Kohl M, Birklein F. Prevalence and risk factors of phantom limb pain and phantom limb sensations in Germany. A nationwide field survey. Schmerz. 2009;23:479–88.
101. Steegers MAH, Snik DM, Verhagen AF, van der Drift MA, Wilder-Smith OHG. Only half of the chronic pain after thoracic surgery shows a neuropathic component. J Pain. 2008;9:955–61.

Radiation-Induced Pain Syndromes

6

Jasmit Brar, Grant H. Chen, and Amitabh Gulati

Introduction

As cancer therapies improve and survival rates increase, treatment-related pain syndromes are becoming more prevalent. Surgery, chemotherapy, and radiation therapy (RT) can all contribute to chronic pain years after treatment. Approximately one-third of patients with cancer experience chronic pain after curative therapy [1]. In particular, radiation therapy can produce a wide array of pain syndromes including chronic abdominal pain, neuropathies, osteoradionecrosis, chest pain, and myofascial pain (Table 6.1). This chapter will provide an overview of radiation-induced pain syndromes.

Principles of Radiotherapy

Ionizing radiation is a critical component of cancer treatment, with an estimated 50–75% of cancer patients exposed to a form of radiation during their therapy [2, 3]. Radiation is classified based on the rate of energy deposition into cells and can be divided into low-energy-transfer radiation (X-rays or gamma rays) or high-energy-transfer radiation (neutrons and heavy ions) [4]. The dose of radiation is measured based on the amount of energy in joules absorbed per unit of mass in kilograms, known as gray (Gy). RT utilized in cancer therapy is primarily in the form of low-energy-transfer radiation provided by linear accelerators. The therapeutic principle of radiotherapy relies on the ability to damage DNA in rapidly dividing cancer cells. Normal healthy cells withstand exposure to sublethal radiation via preserved DNA repair mechanisms. However, cancer cells have impaired DNA repair capabilities, and thus radiation results in the activation of apoptotic pathways or cell senescence.

The direct effect of ionizing radiation on DNA results in the splitting of chemical bonds of the DNA helix, creating both single-strand and double-strand breaks. Ionizing radiation also indirectly promotes the generation of reactive oxygen species (ROS) compounding the level of cellular stress [5]. Current evidence suggests the accumulation of ROS within the cell further compromises DNA integrity and serves as an important source of radiation-induced cell injury [4]. Local cellular signaling from irradiated cells may also produce increased cellular stress on non-irradiated adjacent cells. This phenomenon is known as radiation-induced bystander effects [6]. Given the risk of undesired injury to healthy neighboring tissue, radiation therapy is administered in divided doses known as fractions, with the intention of optimizing the ability of normal tissue to recover from radiation exposure while limiting the side effects of radiation therapy [7]. Figure 6.1 demonstrates approximate radiation doses for various radiation-induced pain syndromes.

Table 6.1 Radiation-induced pain syndromes

Plexopathies
Peripheral nerve entrapment
Myelopathy
Enteritis
Proctitis
Cystitis
Osteoradionecrosis
Pelvic fractures
Chest pain

J. Brar (✉)
New York Presbyterian-Weill Cornell Medicine, Department of Anesthesiology, New York, NY, USA
e-mail: jsb9014@nyp.org

G. H. Chen
Memorial Sloan Kettering Cancer Center, Department of Anesthesiology and Critical Care Medicine, New York, NY, USA
e-mail: cheng@mskcc.org

A. Gulati
Department of Anesthesiology and Critical Care, Memorial Sloan Kettering Cancer Center, New York, NY, USA

A. Gulati et al. (eds.), *Essentials of Interventional Cancer Pain Management*, https://doi.org/10.1007/978-3-319-99684-4_6

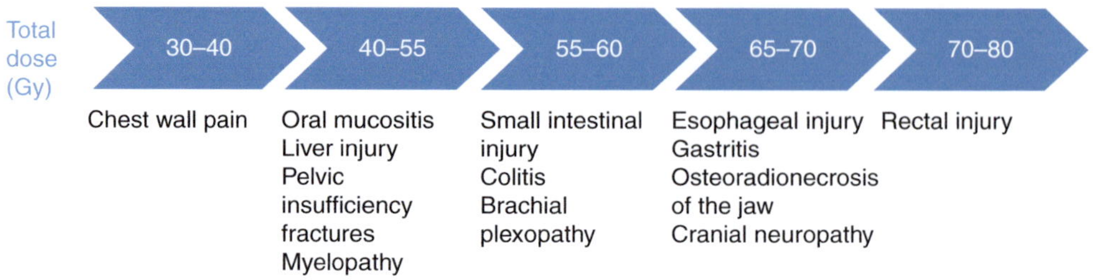

Fig. 6.1 Radiation doses for various radiation-induced pain syndromes

Radiation-Induced Head and Neck Pain

The treatment of head and neck malignancies commonly utilizes radiotherapy in conjunction with surgery and chemotherapy. Approximately 60% of patients with head and neck cancer are treated with standard radiation therapy, and 50% of patients may additionally receive chemotherapy [8]. Conventional radiation therapy involves daily fractions of 1.8–2 Gy administered over 6–7 weeks, with a total dose of 66–70 Gy [9]. Radiation exposure to the head and neck region produces both acute and late adverse effects that can result in significant pain and morbidity for patients. Acute effects commonly include mucositis, xerostomia, and dermatitis. Mucositis in head and neck cancer population is reported to affect 30–60% of patients [10]. The pathophysiology of radiation-induced injury occurs from the mitotic death of basal cells of the oral mucosa, which typically presents clinically 2 weeks posttreatment [11]. Following exposure to 20–30 Gy, with a fraction dose of 1.8–2 Gy, mucosal erythema develops, followed by signs of patchy pseudomembrane formation with an additional radiation dose of 10–20 Gy [11]. Cutaneous erythema and desquamation lag behind mucosal injury by 1–2 weeks, as cellular turnover is generally greater within the mucosa than the dermis. The development of oral ulcerations in nonkeratinized tissue of the soft palate, pharynx, and floor of the mouth can contribute significantly to mucositis pain. Symptoms tend to improve 2–4 weeks after the completion of radiation therapy [12]. The severity of mucositis depends on the radiation dose, field size, fractionation schedule, and combination of chemotherapy.

Head and Neck Osteoradionecrosis

Osteoradionecrosis as a consequence of head and neck radiation is a serious and painful condition. It predominately affects the mandible and presents with erythematous and ulcerative changes in the mucosa revealing necrotic bone underneath [11, 13]. Symptoms include severe continuous pain and drainage in the area of injury, which persists without evidence of healing for at least 3 months postradiation. Lytic lesions and periosteal thickening may be seen on radiographic imaging. Major risk factors include radiation doses greater than 60 Gy, use of brachytherapy, and dental extraction [13]. Generally, incidence can vary widely from 2% to 22% based on radiation techniques and fractionation schemes.

Radiation-Induced Abdominopelvic Pain

While radiation therapy is effective in targeting rapidly proliferating cancer cells, other tissues with high cellular turnover are particularly vulnerable. Intestinal epithelial cells are among the most prone to cellular damage from radiation, often demonstrating apoptotic or intermitotic cell death soon after exposure [14]. The acute effects of radiation-induced damage to gastrointestinal mucosa can lead to profound nausea, vomiting, and diarrhea. The development of radiation-induced gastrointestinal mucositis can often be the major dose-limiting factor for patients undergoing radiation therapy [15].

While acute radiation-induced gastrointestinal pain is generally reversible and resolves within 3 weeks of completion of radiation therapy, symptoms that persist for greater than 90 days are considered to be "chronic." Chronic abdominal pain often involves tissue changes resulting in transmural fibrosis and vascular sclerosis [16]. Chronic structural changes in the gastrointestinal mucosa contribute to dysmotility, stricture formation, obstruction, and abdominal pain. Factors influencing the radiation-induced side effects include the total radiation dose, dose per fraction, fractionation schedules, and the volume of tissue irradiated [17, 18].

Radiation treatment for prostate, uterine, cervical, and rectal malignancies can expose multiple tissues and organs to radiation toxicity. Radiation cystitis, enteritis, proctitis, and pelvic insufficiency fractures can all contribute to post-radiation pelvic pain [19]. Radiation toxicity to the bladder results in irritation or obstructive symptoms, with acute toxicity reported in 20–80% of patients [20]. Chronic cystitis can develop with bladder fibrosis and vascular derangements and is generally considered to be irreversible.

Pelvic radiation causes skeletal injury through a variety of mechanisms including vascular abnormalities, increased connective tissue, and impaired ability to handle physical or cellular stress [21]. Patients are often asymptomatic, with radiation-induced skeletal alterations diagnosed on routine surveillance imaging [22]. However, those presenting with pain may demonstrate signs of pelvic insufficiency fractures. Musculoskeletal pain from radiation osteitis is characterized by impaired osteoblast function resulting in bone matrix resorption. Additional mechanisms include bone marrow fibrosis, trabecular microfractures, and areas of focal necrosis [23]. Radiological evidence of radiation-induced osteitis may demonstrate patchy, mottled bone with coarse trabeculation. However, similar radiographic changes may occur with cancer recurrence, radiation-induced malignancy, and potential infection [22].

Late effects of pelvic radiation include femoral head and neck necrosis, acetabular necrosis, pelvic insufficiency, and subsequent stress fractures [19]. Radiation-induced bone changes typically occur on the iliac side of the sacroiliac joint and then progress to the joint itself. Among women treated with radiation for pelvic malignancies, the incidence of pelvic fractures was increased compared to those spared radiation, with an incidence ranging from 8% to 31% depending on the cancer site treated and generally at doses greater than 45 Gy [19, 24, 25]. Pelvic insufficiency fractures typically manifest with severe low back or pelvic pain, resulting in functional limitations and disability.

Radiation-Induced Neural Injury

Radiation-induced toxicity involving the nervous system includes neuropathies, myelopathies, and nerve entrapment. The evaluation of radiation-induced nerve injuries can be challenging, as they manifest with variable symptomatology and onset time, often further complicated by changes resulting from prior surgeries, chemotherapy, and hormonal therapy [26]. Several chronic pain syndromes have been described based on the involvement of particular nerve roots or trunks.

Radiation-induced peripheral neuropathies occur as a late manifestation of radiation toxicity. The mechanism of this neural injury is considered a combination of initial microvascular injury followed by radiation-induced fibrosis [27]. Radiation-induced nerve injury is initially asymptomatic with a pre-fibrotic phase marked by chronic inflammation. It gradually progresses to an organized fibrotic phase with increased extracellular matrix deposition, which is eventually followed by a late phase characterized by retractile fibrosis and poor vascularity (Fig. 6.2).

Cytokines such as transforming growth factor-β1 may play a central role in the initiation of radiation-induced fibrosis and the progression of fibroproliferation [28]. Radiation exposure to peripheral nerves also results in acute transient electrophysiological, biochemical, permeability alterations

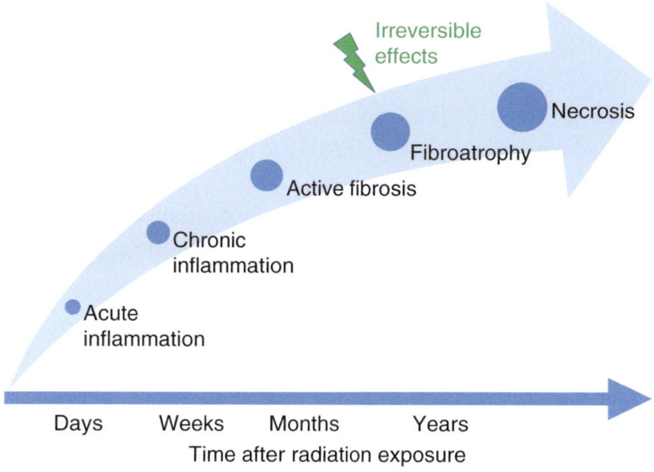

Fig. 6.2 Pathophysiology of radiation-induced fibrosis

compounding upon direct axonal injury, demyelination, and fibrosis. Radiation-specific risk factors include a large total dose (greater than 50 Gy to the plexus and greater than 60 Gy to cranial nerves) [29–31], a large dose per fraction (greater than or equal to 2.5 Gy) [30, 32], radiation therapy within a region of high nerve fiber density [33], heterogeneous high-dose distribution [34], and salvage radiation therapy to a previously irradiated area [35]. When combined with chemotherapy, the risk of developing neuropathies increases further. Additional risk factors include young or old age, obesity, and comorbidities such as diabetes, hypertension, dyslipidemias, and vasculopathies [27].

Radiation-Induced Brachial Plexopathy

Radiation-induced brachial plexopathy is most commonly seen following the treatment of breast cancer and less commonly after the treatment of lung cancer and lymphoma. As radiation therapies and fractionation schedules have refined over the past several decades, the incidence of radiation-induced brachial plexopathy has decreased. Recent estimates report the development of plexopathy in less than 1–2% of patients receiving plexus total doses of less than 55 Gy [36, 37]. The onset is delayed and ranges quite broadly from 6 months to up to 30 years posttreatment, with a peak seen at 2–4 years [36, 38, 39].

The clinical presentation of radiation-induced brachial plexopathy includes paresthesia or dysesthesia, which dissipates as hypoesthesia begins to develop. Neuropathic pain may be associated with brachial plexopathies, with approximately 18% of cases noting pain on presentation [40]. Painful neuropathy is typically moderate in severity, while predominant symptoms include progressive motor weakness with fasciculations and amyotrophy [27, 38, 41, 42]. Symptoms arise gradually and progress over months or years, commonly occurring first in the median nerve and spreading proximally to the forearm and upper arm. The diagnosis of brachial plexopathy includes an evaluation with magnetic resonance imaging (MRI) or positron emission tomography (PET), as well as electromyography (EMG) to help distinguish radiation-induced plexopathy from tumor recurrence [27]. Myokymic discharges (spontaneous fasciculations) on EMG may also suggest radiation-induced injury in the appropriate clinical scenario [41, 43].

Radiation-Induced Lumbosacral Radiculoplexopathy

Compared to radiation-induced brachial plexopathies, lumbosacral nerve radiation injuries are less common [27]. A majority of radiation-induced lumbosacral radiculoplexopathies are described following the treatment of gynecological malignancies. The onset following radiation exposure ranges from 1 to 30 years, with a median of approximately 5 years [44, 45]. Symptoms present gradually as with other neuropathies; however, in contrast to brachial plexopathies, neurological manifestations include predominately motor features with few or late-presenting sensory deficits or paresthesias [46].

Bilateral distal leg weakness is the most common presenting symptom. The presence of pain can be an important diagnostic feature, as acute onset pain with associated motor deficits may suggest plexopathy from tumor invasion, while delayed pain is more likely a radiation-induced plexopathy [45]. Additionally, pelvic malignancies treated with radiation may also be complicated by intestinal or urinary dysfunction as a result of peripheral neurogenic damage or pelvic fibrosis [44]. The use of MRI and PET scans is beneficial in ruling out malignancy recurrence in the setting of new neurological symptoms [33]. EMG will likely demonstrate abnormalities involving multiple nerve roots, with preserved sensory potentials, while the presence of myokymia may again suggest radiation-induced nerve injury [41, 44]. Table 6.2 summarizes factors useful for distinguishing radiation-induced plexopathy from tumor invasion or recurrence.

Table 6.2 Distinguishing factors of radiation-induced plexopathy versus plexopathy from tumor invasion [18, 45]

	Radiation-induced plexopathy	Tumor invasion
Onset	Delayed 1–10 years after RT	Shorter time of onset
Pain	Delayed	Present at onset
Edema	Present	Absent
MRI findings	Unremarkable	Signs of nerve enhancement
EMG	Presence of myokymia	Rare myokymia

Radiation-Induced Cranial Neuropathy

Intracranial, skull-based, and sinus tumors may receive radiation therapy in conjunction with surgical treatment, thus exposing cranial nerves to radiation-induced injury. The most common cranial neuropathy occurs with the optic nerve. Involvement of the optic nerve typically presents with sudden-onset, painless, and monocular visual loss occurring 3 months to 8 years postradiation exposure [47]. This is a progressive condition in which visual loss continues over a course of weeks. If the radiation injury is predominately in the anterior optic nerve, the clinical presentation will be that of acute loss of visual acuity [48]. In contrast, if the injury occurs in the posterior portion of the optic nerve, the loss of visual acuity is more gradual, occurring over 1–14 years postradiation.

The pathophysiology of radiation-induced optic neuropathy is thought to be related to cellular damage from the generation of ROS, primarily affecting white matter as noted by ischemic demyelination [47]. Radiation-induced optic neuropathy requires total doses greater than 50 Gy, and those cases occurring at a lower dose range may be due to concurrent chemotherapy administration. The second most common radiation-induced cranial neuropathy is hypoglossal palsy following the treatment of head and neck malignancies and typically presents 1–10 years after radiation treatment [49]. Symptoms include tongue hemiatrophy, fasciculations, and tongue deviation. Additional cranial neuropathies include facial paralysis from cranial nerve VII palsy resulting from parotid tumor radiation and trigeminal neuropathy following cavernous sinus tumor radiation [44].

Radiation-Induced Myelopathy

Ionizing radiation exposure to the spinal cord can result in neural injury and the destruction of white matter. The clinical constellation of symptoms varies with the location of spinal radiation exposure and the degree of injury. Radiation-induced myelopathy is a potential side effect of the treatment of primary or metastatic malignancies of the spine, spinal cord, head and neck, and lungs [50]. The implementation of stereotactic body radiotherapy (SBRT) has improved the ability to administer high-dose radiation with tremendous precision while simultaneously limiting exposure to surrounding structures. The incidence of permanent neurological injury is quite low, ranging from 0.03% to 0.2%, with total spinal cord doses less than 45–50 Gy in 1.8–2 Gy daily fractions [51, 52]. Important risk factors in the development of radiation-induced myelopathy include the total radiation dose, fractionation, and irradiated volume.

Patients with radiation-induced myelopathy may exhibit both acute and late manifestations. Acute symptoms include sensory deficits and motor weakness, which typically resolve [52, 53]. Patients with exposure to spinal radiation may also exhibit Lhermitte's syndrome, characterized by paresthesias in the back and extremities upon neck flexion occurring 2–4 months posttreatment [53, 54]. Lhermitte's syndrome is also self-limited, with full neurological recovery expected a few months after symptom onset. Delayed radiation-induced myelopathy typically presents after a latency period of 5–6 months, with a subtle onset of sensory and motor deficits, gait disturbances, incontinence, and occasionally pain [55, 56]. Compared to early radiation-induced myelopathy, late manifestations are generally not reversible and may progress to chronic neurological deficits. The pathophysiology of radiation-induced myelopathy is characterized by white matter necrosis, demyelination, and vascular dysfunction [55, 57]. Diagnostic imaging with MRI continues to be a central component in the evaluation of radiation-induced myelopathy.

Radiation-Induced Chest Wall Pain

Stereotactic body radiation therapy is used for the treatment of inoperable early stage non-small cell lung cancer and metastatic pulmonary and hepatic lesions [58–61]. SBRT may result in both acute and late chest wall toxicity marked by skin changes, rib fractures, and chest wall neuropathic pain [58, 59, 62]. The incidence of chest wall pain varies widely from 10% to 40%. Dermatological reactions typically occur 3–6 weeks posttreatment and include erythema, ulceration, and fibrosis [58, 63]. In most patients, radiation-induced chest wall pain is a temporary, mild reaction treated with nonsteroidal anti-inflammatory drugs; however, the pain may persist often requiring chronic opioid therapy [59]. The time course for chronic chest wall pain occurs at a median of 6 months posttreatment [58]. Studies evaluating the risk of postradiation chest wall pain have estimated a 30% risk of toxicity when 40 mL of tissue volume receives 30 Gy or 15 mL receives 40 Gy [60]. An absolute volume of chest wall tissue at a threshold of 30 cm^3 exposed to greater than or equal to 30 Gy has been implicated as a risk factor for the development of radiation-induced chest wall pain [62, 64].

Conclusion

As opposed to chemotherapy- and surgery-induced pain syndromes, pain associated with radiation may manifest in occult ways at variable time points. A thorough understanding of a cancer patient's radiation dosage and field of exposure is needed to understand the potential pain syndromes that may occur in the future. Exposure to radiation may lead to various bone and neuropathic pain symptoms that may be treated with pharmacologic and interventional pain options.

References

1. Van den Beuken-van Everdingen MH, De Rijke JM, Kessels AG, Schouten HC, Van Kleef M, Patijn J. Prevalence of pain in patients with cancer: a systematic review of the past 40 years. Ann Oncol. 2007;18(9):1437–49.
2. Delaney G, Jacob S, Featherstone C, Barton M. The role of radiotherapy in cancer treatment. Cancer. 2005;104(6):1129–37.
3. Siegel R, Naishadham D, Jemal A. Cancer statistics, 2012. CA Cancer J Clin. 2012;62(1):10–29.
4. Hubenak JR, Zhang Q, Branch CD, Kronowitz SJ. Mechanisms of injury to normal tissue after radiotherapy: a review. Plast Reconstr Surg. 2014;133(1):49e.
5. Zhao W, Diz DI, Robbins ME. Oxidative damage pathways in relation to normal tissue injury. Br J Radiology. 2007;80(1):23–31.
6. Rzeszowska-Wolny J, Przybyszewski WM, Widel M. Ionizing radiation-induced bystander effects, potential targets for modulation of radiotherapy. Eur J Pharmacol. 2009;625(1):156–64.
7. Begg AC. Can the severity of normal tissue damage after radiation therapy be predicted? PLoS Med. 2006;3(10):e440.
8. Wong PC, Dodd MJ, Miaskowski C, Paul SM, Bank KA, Shiba GH, Facione N. Mucositis pain induced by radiation therapy: prevalence, severity, and use of self-care behaviors. J Pain Symptom Manag. 2006;32(1):27–37.
9. Dirix P, Nuyts S, Van den Bogaert W. Radiation-induced xerostomia in patients with head and neck cancer. Cancer. 2006;107(11):2525–34.
10. Pico JL, Avila-Garavito A, Naccache P. Mucositis: its occurrence, consequences, and treatment in the oncology setting. Oncologist. 1998;3(6):446–51.
11. Cooper JS, Fu K, Marks J, Silverman S. Late effects of radiation therapy in the head and neck region. Int J Radiat Oncol Biol Phys. 1995;31(5):1141–64.
12. Scully C, Epstein J, Sonis S. Oral mucositis: a challenging complication of radiotherapy, chemotherapy, and radiochemotherapy: part 1, pathogenesis and prophylaxis of mucositis. Head Neck. 2003;25(12):1057–70.
13. Teng MS, Futran ND. Osteoradionecrosis of the mandible. Curr Opin Otolaryngol Head Neck Surg. 2005;13(4):217–21.
14. Yeoh A, Gibson R, Yeoh E, Bowen J, Stringer A, Giam K, Logan R, Keefe D. Radiation therapy-induced mucositis: relationships between fractionated radiation, NF-κB, COX-1, and COX-2. Cancer Treat Rev. 2006;32(8):645–51.
15. Classen J, Belka C, Paulsen F, Budach W, Hoffmann W, Bamberg M. Radiation-induced gastrointestinal toxicity. Pathophysiology, approaches to treatment and prophylaxis. Strahlenther Onkol. 1998;174:82–4.
16. Shadad AK, Sullivan FJ, Martin JD, Egan LJ. Gastrointestinal radiation injury: symptoms, risk factors and mechanisms. World J Gastroenterol. 2013;19(2):185–98.
17. Bye A, Tropé C, Loge JH, Hjermstad M, Kaasa S. Health-related quality of life and occurrence of intestinal side effects after pelvic radiotherapy: evaluation of long-term effects of diagnosis and treatment. Acta Oncol. 2000;39(2):173–80.
18. Brown MR, Ramirez JD, Farquhar-Smith P. Pain in cancer survivors. Br J Pain. 2014;8(4):139–53.
19. Levy MH, Chwistek M, Mehta RS. Management of chronic pain in cancer survivors. Cancer J. 2008;14(6):401–9.
20. Kolla SB, Dash A. Radiation cystitis: acute and chronic. In: Radiation therapy for pelvic malignancy and its consequences. New York: Springer; 2015. p. 111–8.
21. Parker RG, Berry HC. Late effects of therapeutic irradiation on the skeleton and bone marrow. Cancer. 1976;37(S2):1162–71.
22. Bluemke DA, Fishman EK, Scott WW Jr. Skeletal complications of radiation therapy. Radiographics. 1994;14(1):111–21.

23. Massin PH, Duparc JA. Total hip replacement in irradiated hips. A retrospective study of 71 cases. J Bone Joint Surg. 1995; 77(6):847–52.
24. Baxter NN, Habermann EB, Tepper JE, Durham SB, Virnig BA. Risk of pelvic fractures in older women following pelvic irradiation. JAMA. 2005;294(20):2587–93.
25. Reimer NB, Nystrom LM, Dean CW. Miscellaneous pelvic effects: pelvic/sacral insufficiency fractures. In: Radiation therapy for pelvic malignancy and its consequences. New York: Springer; 2015. p. 167–80.
26. Paice JA. Chronic treatment-related pain in cancer survivors. Pain. 2011;152(3):S84–9.
27. Delanian S, Lefaix JL. The radiation-induced fibroatrophic process: therapeutic perspective via the antioxidant pathway. Radiother Oncol. 2004;73(2):119–31.
28. Martin M, Lefaix JL, Delanian S. TGF-β1 and radiation fibrosis: a master switch and a specific therapeutic target? Int J Radiat Oncol Biol Phys. 2000 May 1;47(2):277–90.
29. Parsons JT, Bova FJ, Fitzgerald CR, Mendenhall WM, Million RR. Radiation optic neuropathy after megavoltage external-beam irradiation: analysis of time-dose factors. Int J Radiat Oncol Biol Phys. 1994;30(4):755–63.
30. Stoll BA, Andrews JT. Radiation-induced peripheral neuropathy. Br Med J. 1966;1(5491):834.
31. Maier JG, Perry RH, Saylor W, Sulak MH. Radiation myelitis of the dorsolumbar spinal cord. Radiology. 1969;93(1):153–60.
32. Johansson S, Svensson H, Denekamp J. Dose response and latency for radiation-induced fibrosis, edema, and neuropathy in breast cancer patients. Int J Radiat Oncol Biol Phys. 2002;52(5):1207–19.
33. Thomas JE, Cascino TL, Earle JD. Differential diagnosis between radiation and tumor plexopathy of the pelvis. Neurology. 1985;35(1):1.
34. Delanian S, Pradat PF. Posteriori conformal radiotherapy using three-dimensional dosimetric reconstitution in a survivor of adult-onset Hodgkin's disease for definitive diagnosis of lower motor neuron disease. J Clin Oncol. 2010;28(30):e599–601.
35. Ashenhurst EM, Quartey GR, Starreveld A. Lumbo-sacral radiculopathy induced by radiation. Can J Neurol Sci. 1977;4(04):259–63.
36. Powell S, Cooke J, Parsons C. Radiation-induced brachial plexus injury: follow-up of two different fractionation schedules. Radiother Oncol. 1990;18(3):213–20.
37. Rawlings G, Arriagada R, Fontaine F, Bouhnik H, Mouriesse H, Sarrazin D. Radiation-induced brachial plexopathy. Bull Cancer. 1983;70(2):77–83.
38. Kori SH, Foley KM, Posner JB. Brachial plexus lesions in patients with cancer= 100 cases. Neurology. 1981;31(1):45.
39. Bajrovic A, Rades D, Fehlauer F, Tribius S, Hoeller U, Rudat V, Jung H, Alberti W. Is there a life-long risk of brachial plexopathy after radiotherapy of supraclavicular lymph nodes in breast cancer patients? Radiother Oncol. 2004;71(3):297–301.
40. Kori SH. Diagnosis and management of brachial plexus lesions in cancer patients. Oncology (Williston Park, NY). 1995 Aug;9(8):756–760.
41. Delanian S, Lefaix JL, Pradat PF. Radiation-induced neuropathy in cancer survivors. Radiother Oncol. 2012;105(3):273–82.
42. Killer HE, Hess K. Natural history of radiation-induced brachial plexopathy compared with surgically treated patients. J Neurol. 1990;237(4):247–50.
43. Roth G, Magistris MR, Le Fort D, Desjacques P. Post-radiation brachial plexopathy. Persistent conduction block. Myokymic discharges and cramps. Rev Neurol. 1987;144(3):173–80.
44. Pradat PF, Delanian S. Late radiation injury to peripheral nerves. Handb Clin Neurol. 2012;115:743–58.
45. Merrell RT. Radiation-induced lumbosacral plexopathy. In: Radiation therapy for pelvic malignancy and its consequences. New York: Springer; 2015. p. 181–7.
46. Feistner H, Weissenborn K, Münte TF, Heinze HJ, Malin JP. Post-irradiation lesions of the caudal roots. Acta Neurol Scand. 1989;80(4):277–81.
47. Danesh-Meyer HV. Radiation-induced optic neuropathy. J Clin Neurosci. 2008;15(2):95–100.
48. Flickinger JC. Cranial nerves. In: Human radiation injury. Philadelphia: Lippincott Williams Wilkins; 2011. p. 210–6.
49. Berger PS, Bataini JP. Radiation-induced cranial nerve palsy. Cancer. 1977;40(1):152–5.
50. Wong CS, Fehlings MG, Sahgal A. Pathobiology of radiation myelopathy and strategies to mitigate injury. Spinal Cord. 2015;53(8):574–80.
51. Schultheiss TE. The radiation dose–response of the human spinal cord. Int J Radiat Oncol Biol Phys. 2008;71(5):1455–9.
52. Kirkpatrick JP, van der Kogel AJ, Schultheiss TE. Radiation dose–volume effects in the spinal cord. Int J Radiat Oncol Biol Phys. 2010;76(3):S42–9.
53. Gibbs IC, Patil C, Gerszten PC, Adler JR Jr, Burton SA. Delayed radiation-induced myelopathy after spinal radiosurgery. Neurosurgery. 2009;64(2):A67–72.
54. Wong CS, Van der Kogel AJ. Mechanisms of radiation injury to the central nervous system: implications for neuroprotection. Mol Interv. 2004;4(5):273.
55. New P. Radiation injury to the nervous system. Curr Opin Neurol. 2001;14(6):725–34.
56. Daly ME, Gibbs IC. Spinal radiosurgery: delayed radiation-induced myelopathy. In: Tumors of the central nervous system, vol. 6. Dordrecht: Springer Netherlands; 2012. p. 135–40.
57. Okada S, Okeda R. Pathology of radiation myelopathy. Neuropathology. 2001;21(4):247–65.
58. Stephans KL, Djemil T, Tendulkar RD, Robinson CG, Reddy CA, Videtic GM. Prediction of chest wall toxicity from lung stereotactic body radiotherapy (SBRT). Int J Radiat Oncol Biol Phys. 2012;82(2):974–80.
59. Din SU, Williams EL, Jackson A, Rosenzweig KE, Wu AJ, Foster A, Yorke ED, Rimner A. Impact of fractionation and dose in a multivariate model for radiation-induced chest wall pain. Int J Radiat Oncol Biol Phys. 2015;93(2):418–24.
60. Andolino DL, Forquer JA, Henderson MA, Barriger RB, Shapiro RH, Brabham JG, Johnstone PA, Cardenes HR, Fakiris AJ. Chest wall toxicity after stereotactic body radiotherapy for malignant lesions of the lung and liver. Int J Radiat Oncol Biol Phys. 2011;80(3):692–7.
61. Mutter RW, Liu F, Abreu A, Yorke E, Jackson A, Rosenzweig KE. Dose–volume parameters predict for the development of chest wall pain after stereotactic body radiation for lung cancer. Int J Radiat Oncol Biol Phys. 2012;82(5):1783–90.
62. Creach KM, El Naqa I, Bradley JD, Olsen JR, Parikh PJ, Drzymala RE, Bloch C, Robinson CG. Dosimetric predictors of chest wall pain after lung stereotactic body radiotherapy. Radiother Oncol. 2012;104(1):23–7.
63. Welsh J, Thomas J, Shah D, Allen PK, Wei X, Mitchell K, Gao S, Balter P, Komaki R, Chang JY. Obesity increases the risk of chest wall pain from thoracic stereotactic body radiation therapy. Int J Radiat Oncol Biol Phys. 2011;81(1):91–6.
64. Dunlap NE, Cai J, Biedermann GB, Yang W, Benedict SH, Sheng K, Schefter TE, Kavanagh BD, Larner JM. Chest wall volume receiving> 30 Gy predicts risk of severe pain and/or rib fracture after lung stereotactic body radiotherapy. Int J Radiat Oncol Biol Phys. 2010;76(3):796–801.

Part III

Paradigms in Cancer Pain Syndromes

General Pain Management Concepts

7

Dhanalakshmi Koyyalagunta, Maureen J. Simmonds, and Diane M. Novy

Introduction

As a result of significant advancements in early diagnosis and treatment, there are an estimated 13.7 million cancer survivors in the United States [1]. Almost 25% of these patients have ongoing pain that may last for years, depression, and fatigue that impacts their functioning and quality of life [2–6]. The classic chronic pain rehabilitation program that incorporated multiple disciplines was introduced by Drs. John Bonica and Wilburt Fordyce at the University of Washington Medical School and was designed to treat the complex symptom burden experienced by patients with chronic pain [7, 8]. With the growing costs of treating chronic pain over the last few decades, chronic pain rehabilitation programs (CPRPs) have been established with a focus on education, improving physical activity and functional restoration [9]. Indeed, a robust body of evidence now supports both general and specific health benefits of physical activity for individuals with acute and chronic disease for a range of physiological, physical, psychological, and social outcomes. Current evidence supports the efficacy of CPRPs for non-cancer pain [10, 11].

We elaborate the need for such rehabilitation programs in cancer survivors, adopting components from the CPRPs [12] and tailoring them to the needs of this population. The growing number of cancer survivors has created an overwhelming need for CPRPs for chronic cancer pain. CPRPs provide medical attention to pain management, physical and occupational therapy, psychological therapy using various modalities with a patient-centered approach, and goal-oriented treatment. In the chronic non-cancer pain population, when resolution of pain is not possible, treatment strategies may target different goals that address and ameliorate the impact of pain. These strategies include improving physical function, reducing non-beneficial health-care services, and increasing pain self-management.

Because behavioral, psychological, and social factors have shown reliably significant associations with pain severity, disability, work status, emotional distress, and health-care use among individuals with chronic pain, CPRPs incorporate methods to address these factors. Operant-behavioral therapy (OBT) and cognitive-behavioral therapy (CBT) for chronic pain have been the predominant psychological treatments used for the past 30 years, along with conservative medical treatment and physical rehabilitative interventions. CPRPs that include these approaches along with medical management, interventional therapies, and physical therapy are accessible to many patients with chronic pain. Studies of multidisciplinary treatment have shown that these treatments are useful in reducing pain, restoring lost function (including the ability to work), and reducing reliance on medical care.

Program Structure

CPRPs are most often multidisciplinary, with several disciplines working together at different facilities and providing coordinated care with varying degrees of communication. Interdisciplinary models may be more optimal, with multiple disciplines working together in a single facility with facilitated communication and well-coordinated care [9, 13]. The economic burden of these programs continues to be a barrier to more widespread use, even among the chronic pain patients, despite evidence supporting good outcomes.

D. Koyyalagunta (✉)
Department of Pain Medicine, UTMD Anderson Cancer Center, Houston, TX, USA
e-mail: dkoyyala@mdanderson.org

M. J. Simmonds
University of Texas, Physical Therapy Department, San Antonio, TX, USA
e-mail: simmondsm@uthscsa.edu

D. M. Novy
Department of Pain Medicine, The University of Texas MD Anderson Cancer Center, Houston, TX, USA
e-mail: dnovy@mdanderson.org

A. Gulati et al. (eds.), *Essentials of Interventional Cancer Pain Management*, https://doi.org/10.1007/978-3-319-99684-4_7

A cancer pain rehabilitation program must mirror what is available for chronic pain, along with some adaptation to the symptom cluster that is considered classic among patients with chronic cancer pain. The goal is "functional restoration" (mental and physical) using multiple modalities. The multidisciplinary team should include the physician, psychologist, physical/occupational therapist, and nursing staff (Table 7.1).

Assessment Process

Although some structural differences across CPRPs exist (e.g., duration of program, focus on opioid detoxification, facility resources for physical therapy) [9], most share common components. Determining the fit of the patient's medical condition and goals with those of the program is a first step. Assessing physical and mental impairments that lead to a poor HRQol is crucial so that a patient's rehabilitation needs can be tailored accordingly. The overarching purpose of the clinical interview is to gain an understanding of the patient's perspective of their history and treatment, especially as it relates to current symptoms and the impact of symptom burden on function, perceived barriers to improved function, previous physical therapy experiences, and their own treatment expectations and goals.

Barriers to improved function/activity may be impairment-based and due to pain, particularly pain related to activity, but they may also be due to muscle weakness, joint stiffness, edema, fatigue, nausea, and other causes. Barriers to activity may also be related to psychological issues, such as inadequate knowledge about exercise, anxieties related to physical activity, or inadequate social support for increasing activity.

Table 7.1 Health-care providers and respective role in interdisciplinary chronic pain management in cancer survivors

Health-care provider	Role
Physician	Evaluation of pain syndrome, anxiety, depression, fatigue, and other symptom cluster Treatment of pain syndromes with pharmacotherapy and interventions Treatment of comorbid medical and psychological issues Serve as liaison for coordinated care
Psychologist	Complete psychological evaluation Treatment with cognitive-behavioral techniques and biofeedback Provide psychological support to patient and family Coordinate care with other disciplines
Physical therapist	Evaluate limitation in function and cause Assess physical limitation at work Teach activity pacing Coordinate care with other disciplines

Adapted from Gatchel et al. [12]

The most commonly cited goals of physical therapy are to decrease pain and symptom burden and improve movement and function. In that sense, physical therapists work with the multidisciplinary team and the patient to ensure shared understanding, treatment aims, and short- and long-term management goals. Physicians, psychologists, and physical therapists assess the medical and rehabilitation potential of each patient. They evaluate everyone for symptoms of chronic pain, fatigue, cognitive dysfunction (chemotherapy-related or from other causes), alteration in sexual function, functional limitations, and other comorbidities.

Cancer-Related Pain Syndromes in Survivors

Surgery can produce chronic painful syndromes as well as distress from "disfigurement" and difficulty with mobility and swallowing. The overall incidence of pain is 33% in survivors [14], more than 60% among patients post-thoracotomy, 50–65% among patients post-mastectomy, 50–80% post-amputation, and more than 50% of patients post-neck dissection. Preoperative pain, anxiety, type of surgery, and uncontrolled postoperative pain are predictors of chronic pain after surgery [15]. Radiation to the affected area, as well as neurotoxic chemotherapeutic agents, may increase the incidence [16].

Certain chemotherapeutic agents (e.g., taxanes, platinum, thalidomide, bortezomib, and vincristine) can be associated with painful neuropathies [5, 17–19]. The onset of chemotherapy-induced peripheral neuropathy (CIPN) can present with the initial dose and escalate weeks to months after the last dose, known as "coasting." Advanced age, genetic polymorphisms, and pre-existing neuropathies are risk factors for CIPN [20]. Vinca alkaloids typically cause a sensorimotor neuropathy with autonomic features in up to 30%. Sensory or sensorimotor neuropathy is seen with platinum compounds, and ototoxicity may occur as well. Taxanes lead to classic distal sensory neuropathy, with rare motor involvement. Bortezomib can lead to debilitating dose-dependent neuropathy and "coasting" with motor and gait dysfunction and autonomic changes [16, 19].

Myalgias and arthralgias are commonly seen in breast, prostate, and gynecological cancer patients on maintenance hormonal therapy as well as those who have received systemic or oral steroids. Aromatase inhibitors (AI) lead to estrogen deprivation and associated osteopenia and osteoporosis. AI can cause joint stiffness, most often affecting the hands but can also involve the knees, ankles, and hips. It is usually worse in the morning with some improvement with movement. In one study, more than a third of patients on AI therapy reported these symptoms [21]. Previous hormonal therapy, obesity, chemotherapy, and treatment with anastrazole were risk factors to the development of arthralgias.

Radiation can lead to plexopathies, chronic pelvic pain, osteoradionecrosis, fractures, and secondary malignancies. Radiation-induced colitis and cystitis can lead to severe abdominal pain and/or other gastrointestinal or urinary symptoms, including incontinence. Neural injury after radiation (plexopathies) can lead to severe neuropathic pain, which can transform into a central pain syndrome. Very often these syndromes are much delayed in their occurrence and sometimes difficult to establish a causality.

Chronic graft vs. host disease (GVHD) affects multiple organs including the skin, gastrointestinal tract, oral mucosa, and eyes. It is seen in almost 30–80% of patients surviving for more than 6 months with a mortality rate of 40% at 5 years [22]. Patients have pain with involvement of the skin, mucosa, and eyes. There is atrophy and ulceration of skin and contracture of the joints, like scleroderma.

Physician Assessment

Chronic cancer pain is due to the cancer itself or treatment-related toxicities from chemotherapy, radiation, and/or surgery. It is different from chronic pain as identifiable tissue damage typically leads to the chronic cancer pain syndromes (Table 7.2). Pain can be somatic or visceral, nociceptive or neuropathic in nature, or sometimes a mixed pattern. Assessment includes a detailed history of the pain's intensity using the Brief Pain Inventory (BPI) [23] and the Edmonton Symptom Assessment Scale (ESAS) for collateral symptoms [24]. A thorough assessment and evaluation of the pain syndrome (somatic, visceral, and/or neuropathic) will determine the optimal pharmacotherapeutic agent or interventional therapies that would be optimal.

Table 7.2 Chronic cancer-related pain syndromes [22, 40, 41]

Cancer therapy	Pain syndrome
Chemotherapy	Chemotherapy-induced peripheral neuropathy
	Arthralgia/myalgia
	Muscle cramps
	Osteoporosis
Surgery	Post-mastectomy pain
	Post-thoracotomy pain
	Post-radical neck dissection
	Stump and phantom pain
	Chronic pelvic/abdominal pain
	Frozen shoulder
	Lymphedema
Corticosteroids	Avascular necrosis
	Vertebral compression fractures
	Myalgias, arthralgias
Hormonal therapy	Myalgias, arthralgias
	Muscle spasms
Radiation	Brachial plexopathy
	Lumbosacral plexopathy
	Radiation enteritis, cystitis
	Myelopathy
	Osteoradionecrosis
Bisphosphonates	Osteoradionecrosis
Post-stem cell transplantation (graft vs. host disease)	Abdominal/pelvic pain
	Myalgias
	Arthralgias
	Peripheral neuropathy
	Mucositis

Patients who experience post-thoracotomy pain syndrome usually complain of pain and or muscle spasms along the incision. They may also complain of ipsilateral shoulder pain and symptoms of frozen shoulder. Post-mastectomy pain patients usually have nociceptive or neuropathic pain at the incision site, phantom pain in the excised breast, neuralgia in the arm, and/or discomfort associated with lymphedema or frozen shoulder. More than half of patients experience pain after treatment for head and neck cancer. They have significant nociceptive pain associated with muscle atrophy and spasms as well as neuropathic pain. Phantom pain after amputations can be debilitating and difficult to treat. These patients also have stump pain related to neuromas or pressure from prosthetic devices.

Chemotherapy-induced peripheral neuropathy (CIPN) commonly presents as symmetrical distal sensory neuropathy in the "stocking-glove" distribution. Symptoms may vary from mild dysesthesia to severe allodynia and decreased sensation (hypesthesia). Patients experience significant neuropathic pain and are unable to remain active, leading to deconditioning and musculoskeletal pain. Evaluate for sensory, motor, and autonomic deficits.

Symptoms from radiation-induced neuralgias can range from mild hypesthesia to severe allodynia as well as motor deficits. In some cases, it can also transform to a central pain syndrome which may be difficult to treat. Examine for any sensory and motor deficits associated with plexopathies. EMG and NCV studies are done as indicated. The increase in pain or change in character of pain must trigger work-up to rule out cancer recurrence. GVHD can present with severe mucositis affecting various organs. Evaluate for oral and vaginal ulcerations that may lead to poor nutrition and Qol. These patients are immunocompromised and are prone to infections as well as bleeding secondary to thrombocytopenia. Evaluate for colonization of the open mucosal lesions with any organisms. Assess for pain and mobility associated with joint contractures.

Cancer survivors are at risk for insufficiency fractures and associated pain due to steroid-related osteoporosis or radiation-related osteitis. Vertebral compression fractures cause pain at the level with movement and can be reproduced with percussion over the involved level. Evaluate for any radicular symptoms and MRI to be done to determine the age of the fracture. An overall decrease in their immunity makes them prone to shingles and postherpetic neuralgia.

Fatigue can reduce physical functioning and lead to an inability to perform activities of daily living (ADLs). Evaluating whether these are due to physical deconditioning, treatment-related side effects (infection, anemia, malnutrition, diarrhea, anorexia, cardiomyopathy), and/or comorbid medical conditions will help to tailor the patient's rehabilitation treatment. Cognitive functioning can be assessed by interviewing the patient and his or her family members. Assess for medications (prescribed and/or over-the-counter) that may be related to a decline in function or in "chemo brain."

Physical Therapy Clinical Assessment

The standard physical therapy assessment includes a range of standardized patient-reported measures that evaluate, as appropriate, pain, fatigue, physical function, and activities of daily living and may include health-related quality of life. The physical therapy assessment includes measures of physical impairment of the affected body area, such as specific muscle strength, or joint range of motion (Table 7.3). In recent years, clinical assessment has emphasized measures of physical function [25] that have more relevance to patients' overall ability to function. Physical performance measures complement patient self-reports of their ability to function and are stronger predictors of outcome than are traditional impairment-based measures.

Within the clinical assessment, and because a major component of best-evidence physical therapy for cancer is physical activity, it is important for the physical therapist to understand the patient's attitudes toward physical activity. This understanding should include their activity preferences, willingness or readiness to engage in physical activity, and any perceived vulnerabilities they may have toward exercise and activity. For example, post-breast cancer and mastectomy, some individuals are concerned that strenuous arm exercise might increase lymphedema. Others, at some point during their care, may have been advised to "take it easy" but were never advised as to what that actually means.

The same issues may apply to family members who may be anxious and/or overly solicitous in relation to physical activity. Research on health literacy has revealed some remarkable gaps in knowledge among patients, caregivers, and providers [26]. Clearly, when patients or caregivers hold misbeliefs or unhelpful attitudes, it is important to correct and change those beliefs and attitudes in a sensitive manner. Reassurance and advice that appear dismissive or patronizing will not be helpful [27]. With regard to physical activity, misbeliefs and unhelpful attitudes may be attributable to a misunderstanding or a lack of understanding about basic physical activity and/or safe and effective exercise as part of rehabilitation. This is especially true when patients or caregivers are concerned that the presence of pain or discomfort during or after unaccustomed exercise may be an indication of cancer recurrence.

Table 7.3 Functional status assessment [25, 42]

	Examples of tests	Description	Psychometrics
Functional status Physical performance	Walking speed (timed 50-foot walk)	Patients walk 25 feet, turn around, and walk back as fast as they can. Walking time is recorded in seconds	Excellent inter- and intra-rater reliabilities and day-to-day stabilities $r > 0.98$ Construct, convergent, and discriminant validities established
	Distance walked in 2 or 6 min	Patients are instructed to walk as far and as fast as they can in the designated time, and total distance walked is recorded. (Subjects are allowed to use a walking aid but should do so consistently from test to test)	Excellent reliabilities $r = >0.9$. Construct, convergent, and discriminant validities established
	Chair rise time (2 or 5 reps)	From a seated position in a regular chair, patients are instructed to rise to standing and sit back down (×2 or 5) as fast but as safely as they can. After a brief rest, they repeat the task, and the average of the two times is used as the outcome	Excellent inter- and intra-rater reliabilities and day-to-day stabilities $r > 0.98$. Construct, convergent, and discriminant validities established

Psychological Assessment

The psychologist's primary role is to gather psychosocial information during a face-to-face interview with a patient and possibly from one or more of the patient's family members. Although a patient's demographic and clinical information is obtained from the medical record, the psychologist will ask about the pain experience and focus on treatments tried, useful coping strategies, and the impact of pain on the patient's life. Psychologists in a cancer setting also ask about the impact of cancer on the patient's life. The interview addresses current features of depression and anxiety as well as sources of stress and concern for the patient. A psychologist will also assess the risk of suicide, including any current passive or active thoughts regarding suicide and specifics about past attempts and other risk factors.

Questioning also focuses on any past psychological or psychiatric treatments, any perceptual distortions, and family history of psychological problems. Current and past substance use is also assessed. The questioning also focuses on current social support from family and friends and colleagues at work. Information about the patient's education, employment history, skills, and financial status are also sought. Finally, the patient is asked about his or her goals for treatment. Oftentimes patients will say that their hope is for "no pain." This is an opportunity to discuss the reality of that goal with the patient and the possibility of focusing on different and more attainable rehabilitation goals related to function and quality of life.

Different CPRPs may include self-report psychological questionnaires [28] to supplement information gathered by the team's assessment. Stanos' article outlines some of these differences [9]. In this article, the Mayo Clinic Pain Rehabilitation Center (Rochester, MN) implements a battery of questionnaires that assess the multidimensional pain experience, including depression and catastrophizing, whereas other centers use only a structured interview [9]. Currently, at MDACC, the psychologist employs a structured pain interview to gather information, make a diagnosis, and assess suitability for a treatment regimen consistent with the patient's health status and goals. We currently use the Edmonton Symptom Assessment Scale (ESAS) to capture ratings of fatigue, shortness of breath, poor appetite, depression, anxiety, drowsiness, difficulty in thinking clearly, insomnia, body appearance, body functioning, sexual functioning, spiritual pain, and financial difficulties. Currently, the risk of opioid misuse is assessed with the SOAPP (Screener and Opioid Assessment for Patients with Pain) [29–33]. Urine drug screens, pill counts, and prescription drug monitoring programs are useful in high-risk patients. No one tool by itself has been found to be reliable in terms of clinical outcomes [30, 34]. We have found that in patients with cancer pain, those with a high SOAPP score tend to be younger, endorse more pain, have a higher morphine equivalent daily dose (MEDD) requirement, and endorse more symptoms of depression and anxiety [35].

Treatment

CPRPs focus on optimizing medications, interventional therapies to minimize pain, physical reconditioning, occupational therapy, and group educational and psychological therapy. The treatment of chronic cancer pain should be based upon principles traditionally used with chronic pain but with modifications. The focus in chronic pain rehabilitation programs is opioid wean or holiday. This may be a challenge with chronic cancer pain patients because a significant number of these patients are on high-dose opioids initiated because of active cancer-related or treatment-related pain syndromes. It may be necessary to continue with opioids and adjuvants during initial rehabilitation and then wean as tolerated, unless patients have medication-related side effects of fatigue and/or cognitive impairment. Long-acting formulations may be better tolerated, with baseline pain control and breakthrough medications prescribed as necessary.

Choice and dose of opioid are based on patients' general condition, including renal and hepatic function and type of pain syndrome. Strong opioids include morphine, methadone, fentanyl, oxycodone, oxymorphone, and hydromorphone. Tapentadol is a μ agonist with norepinephrine reuptake inhibitor properties. Tramadol is a weak opioid with some tricyclic antidepressant (TCA)-like properties. In opioid-naïve patients, start with weak opioids, and titrate as tolerated as opioids have no ceiling effect. Common side effects of sedation, nausea, and constipation should be addressed as these may hinder rehabilitation. Morphine metabolites may accumulate in the presence of renal dysfunction and must be used with caution. EKG monitoring may be necessary with high-dose methadone or concomitant medications that can prolong QTc. In patients at risk for opioid misuse, wean opioids as tolerated, and add adjuvant therapies as indicated by pain syndromes.

Risk management strategies (risk assessment tools, urine drug screen (UDS), pill counts, and frequent follow-ups) are used in chronic pain patients [36]. NSAIDs, COX-2 inhibitors, duloxetine, and pregabalin are beneficial for patients with musculoskeletal pain. NSAIDs must be used with caution in patients with renal dysfunction, bleeding diathesis, and peptic ulcer disease. TCAs, selective serotonin reuptake inhibitors (SSRIs), and anti-epileptics can be added in the presence of a significant neuropathic component. Multiple topical creams are available with a combination of local anesthetics, neuropathic agents (gabapentin, ketamine), and NSAIDs. Treatment of depression and anxiety with pharmacological or psychological modalities is key to pain management. Methylphenidate or modafinil may be initiated to treat symptoms of fatigue. Pain can be optimized with procedural interventions (Table 7.4) as indicated. Neurolytic blocks should be used with caution in patients with no active cancer as permanent neurologic injuries are a concern [37].

Psychological Treatment

Psychological treatment is usually provided in group and individual format to patients participating in pain rehabilitation. Group therapy focuses on common elements of the pain experience, whereas individual therapy will be tailored to

Table 7.4 Interventions for chronic cancer pain syndromes

Pain syndrome	Interventional modalities
Chemotherapy-induced peripheral neuropathy	Spinal cord stimulator, intrathecal therapy
Post-mastectomy pain syndrome	Intercostal nerve blocks, intercostal nerve radio frequency or chemical ablation, spinal cord stimulator, intrathecal therapy
Post-thoracotomy pain syndrome	Intercostal nerve blocks, intercostal nerve radio frequency or chemical ablation, trigger-point injection, neuroma injection, spinal cord stimulator, intrathecal therapy
Phantom pain syndrome	Sympathetic blocks and ablation, neuroma injection, spinal cord stimulator, intrathecal therapy
Post-head and neck cancer treatment pain	Local trigger-point injection, botulinum toxin injection, peripheral nerve/neuroma injection, spinal cord stimulator, intrathecal therapy
Postradiation neuritis	Sympathetic blocks, peripheral somatic nerve blocks and neurolysis, spinal cord stimulator, intrathecal therapy
Abdominal/pelvic pain syndromes	Sympathetic blocks/neurolysis, spinal cord stimulator, intrathecal therapy
Vertebral compression fractures	Vertebroplasty, kyphoplasty, facet blocks

each patient. In the context of pain rehabilitation, apply psychological principles to change the overt behavior, thoughts, or feelings of people with chronic pain in order to help them experience less distress and to have more satisfying and productive daily lives. The goals of OBT (Operant Behavioral Therapy) and CBT (Cognitive Behavioral Therapy) are to replace maladaptive patient behaviors and cognitions with more adaptive ones.

Behavioral interventions include pacing and activity modulation, relaxation techniques, and biofeedback. Cognitive-behavioral interventions include coping skills in using cognitive or behavioral distraction, relaxation, pacing of activities, and the appropriate use of social support. Attention is paid to factors that increase or decrease pain, and these factors guide the application of pain-coping skills. Cognitive restructuring is used to challenge negative self-talk and catastrophizing; not necessarily positive thinking is emphasized. CBT is often short term and skill oriented. Group CBT has long been considered the mainstay of CPRP.

Two additional complementary therapies are gaining acceptance in the field of pain rehabilitation. Motivational interviewing (MI) has had a role in pain rehabilitation since the 1990s. It is a useful psychological approach that takes into account a patient's readiness to make proactive changes in his or her life (e.g., physical activity, healthful diet, relaxation practice or mindfulness, cessation of tobacco or other substance use) [38]. MI is particularly useful in helping patients taper off opioids to reassess their need for these medications. As part of this therapy, the psychologist solicits a patient's motivation and solutions for changing a target behavior.

A second therapy is acceptance and commitment therapy (ACT) and mindfulness for chronic pain [27]. Although aspects of this treatment fall within the family of CBT, they also extend this therapy in its approach to thoughts, feelings, experiences, and memories by not deeming them helpful or unhelpful based on their form, frequency, or appearance alone. Within ACT, two routes lead to healthy functioning: in one, certain methods can reduce the intensity or frequency of psychological experiences such as pain, fear, or sadness; these psychological experiences exert over behavior without necessarily reducing their intensity or frequency. Therapy is focused on improving psychological flexibility and helping patients accept the adversity in their lives. Another part of ACT is training in attention flexibility. Specifically, this training involves using breath as an anchor for guiding and taming one's attention. By doing so, attention is on the moment-to-moment experience of breathing, while competing thoughts and sensations (e.g., pain, fear, and sadness) are responded to in a nonjudgmental and accepting manner and purposely and gently overlooked in favor of attention on the breath. Through this process, patients learn to selectively "let go" and focus on the aspect of their experience that they want to place the most attention on [27, 39].

Physical Therapy Management

Physical therapy management focuses on working with the patient to improve movement and function and to overcome role limitations, with the goal of self-management. A clinical assessment in which the therapist is focused on listening (rather than talking) should help elicit information on the patient's primary barriers to improved function and to long-term self-management. Barriers may be primarily physiological, physical, and/or psychosocial. Actual or anticipated pain, muscle weakness, or joint stiffness, lack of knowledge or lack of access to an appropriate and engaging, and in some geographic areas (weather-proof) environment for pleasurable and preferred exercise e.g. swimming pool or indoor or outdoor walking trails—that will more likely be adhered to.

Lifestyle approaches to cancer survivors as well as other groups include an active lifestyle approach such as walking. General lifestyle approaches that address physical activity, good nutrition, and partners or family concerns are enhancing adherence and maintenance of an active and healthy survivorship. Exercise has been shown to have long-term benefits across a range of physical and psychosocial measures. However, no consensus exists regarding the differential effectiveness of specific exercises or activity regimens. A major difficulty is that for the benefits of exercise to accrue in terms of muscle strength, flexibility, or cardiovascular conditioning, the exercise must be performed consistently. In this regard, it seems to matter less whether the exercise is supervised or not but rather whether and to what extent the exercise is performed.

For individuals with minimal experience in exercising and in engaging in other physical activity—especially if they have concerns about activity—physical therapy supervision during exercise can help build the patient's self-confidence as well as his or her physical capacity as they move toward a self-managed exercise program. Participation in group exercise and the social and peer support provided by the interaction can be helpful for some individuals.

In general, an exercise program will include a series of exercises to enhance strength, flexibility, and endurance and thereby improve physical functioning. The exercises should be performed at least 3 to 4 days a week and should be challenging enough to provide a physiological training effect. The physical therapist should work with the individual patient to help him or her understand the importance of exercise and set progressive but achievable exercise goals in terms of increasing the intensity, duration, or frequency of exercises. These goals should be aligned with American College of Sports Medicine (ACSM) guidelines.

References

1. de Moor JS, Mariotto AB, Parry C, Alfano CM, Padgett L, Kent EE, Forsythe L, Scoppa S, Hachey M, Rowland JH. Cancer survivors in the United States: prevalence across the survivorship trajectory and implications for care. Cancer Epidemiol Biomark Prev. 2013;22:561–70.
2. Baker F, Denniston M, Haffer SC, Liberatos P. Change in health-related quality of life of newly diagnosed cancer patients, cancer survivors, and controls. Cancer. 2009;115:3024–33.
3. Levy MH, Chwistek M, Mehta RS. Management of chronic pain in cancer survivors. Cancer J. 2008;14:401–9.
4. Mishra SI, Scherer RW, Geigle PM, Berlanstein DR, Topaloglu O, Gotay CC, Snyder C. Exercise interventions on health-related quality of life for cancer survivors. Cochrane Database Syst Rev. 2012;8:Cd007566.
5. Burton AW, Fanciullo GJ, Beasley RD, Fisch MJ. Chronic pain in the cancer survivor: a new frontier. Pain Med. 2007;8:189–98.
6. Smith T, Stein KD, Mehta CC, Kaw C, Kepner JL, Buskirk T, Stafford J, Baker F. The rationale, design, and implementation of the American Cancer Society's studies of cancer survivors. Cancer. 2007;109:1–12.
7. Bonica JJ. Basic principles in managing chronic pain. Arch Surg. 1977;112:783–8.
8. Aronoff GM, Evans WO, Enders PL. A review of follow-up studies of multidisciplinary pain units. Pain. 1983;16:1–11.
9. Stanos S. Focused review of interdisciplinary pain rehabilitation programs for chronic pain management. Curr Pain Headache Rep. 2012;16:147–52.
10. Oslund S, Robinson RC, Clark TC, Garofalo JP, Behnk P, Walker B, Walker KE, Gatchel RJ, Mahaney M, Noe CE. Long-term effectiveness of a comprehensive pain management program: strengthening the case for interdisciplinary care. Proc (Baylor Univ Med Cent). 2009;22:211–4.
11. Chou R, Huffman LH. Nonpharmacologic therapies for acute and chronic low back pain: a review of the evidence for an American Pain Society/American College of Physicians clinical practice guideline. Ann Intern Med. 2007;147:492–504.
12. Gatchel RJ, McGeary DD, McGeary CA, Lippe B. Interdisciplinary chronic pain management: past, present, and future. Am Psychol. 2014;69:119–30.
13. Boon H, Verhoef M, O'Hara D, Findlay B. From parallel practice to integrative health care: a conceptual framework. BMC Health Serv Res. 2004;4:15.
14. van den Beuken-van Everdingen MH, de Rijke JM, Kessels AG, Schouten HC, van Kleef M, Patijn J. Prevalence of pain in patients with cancer: a systematic review of the past 40 years. Ann Oncol. 2007;18:1437–49.
15. Perkins FM, Kehlet H. Chronic pain as an outcome of surgery. A review of predictive factors. Anesthesiology. 2000;93:1123–33.
16. Glare PA, Davies PS, Finlay E, Gulati A, Lemanne D, Moryl N, Oeffinger KC, Paice JA, Stubblefield MD, Syrjala KL. Pain in cancer survivors. J Clin Oncol. 2014;32:1739.
17. Burton AW, Fine PG, Passik SD. Transformation of acute cancer pain to chronic cancer pain syndromes. J Support Oncol. 2012;10:89–95.
18. Windebank AJ, Grisold W. Chemotherapy-induced neuropathy. J Peripher Nerv Syst. 2008;13:27–46.
19. Grisold W, Cavaletti G, Windebank AJ. Peripheral neuropathies from chemotherapeutics and targeted agents: diagnosis, treatment, and prevention. Neuro-Oncology. 2012;14(Suppl 4):iv45–54.
20. Vincenzi B, Frezza AM, Schiavon G, Spoto C, Silvestris N, Addeo R, Catalano V, Graziano F, Santini D, Tonini G. Identification of clinical predictive factors of oxaliplatin-induced chronic peripheral neuropathy in colorectal cancer patients treated with adjuvant Folfox IV. Support Care Cancer. 2013;21:1313–9.
21. Sestak I, Cuzick J, Sapunar F, Eastell R, Forbes JF, Bianco AR, Buzdar AU. Risk factors for joint symptoms in patients enrolled in the ATAC trial: a retrospective, exploratory analysis. Lancet Oncol. 2008;9:866–72.
22. Paice JA. Chronic treatment-related pain in cancer survivors. Pain. 2011;152:S84–9.
23. Cleeland CS, Ryan KM. Pain assessment: global use of the Brief Pain Inventory. Ann Acad Med Singap. 1994;23:129–38.
24. Chang VT, Hwang SS, Feuerman M. Validation of the Edmonton Symptom Assessment Scale. Cancer. 2000;88:2164–71.
25. Simmonds MJ. Physical function in patients with cancer: psychometric characteristics and clinical usefulness of a physical performance test battery. J Pain Symptom Manag. 2002;24:404–14.
26. Institute of Medicine Committee on Advancing Pain Research CaE. The national academies collection: reports funded by National Institutes of Health. In: Relieving pain in America: a blueprint for transforming prevention, care, education, and research. Washington, DC: National Academies Press (US), National Academy of Sciences; 2011.
27. McCracken LM, Vowles KE. Acceptance and commitment therapy and mindfulness for chronic pain: model, process, and progress. Am Psychol. 2014;69:178–87.
28. Turk DC, Melzack R, editors. Handbook of pain assessment. 3rd ed. New York: The Guilford Press; 2010.
29. Chou R, Fanciullo GJ, Fine PG, Miaskowski C, Passik SD, Portenoy RK. Opioids for chronic noncancer pain: prediction and identification of aberrant drug-related behaviors: a review of the evidence for an American Pain Society and American Academy of Pain Medicine clinical practice guideline. In: *J Pain*. United States, 2009;10:131–146.
30. Solanki DR, Koyyalagunta D, Shah RV, Silverman SM, Manchikanti L. Monitoring opioid adherence in chronic pain patients: assessment of risk of substance misuse. Pain Physician. 2011;14:E119–31.
31. Butler SF, Budman SH, Fernandez KC, Houle B, Benoit C, Katz N, Jamison RN. Development and validation of the Current Opioid Misuse Measure. Pain. 2007;130:144–56.

32. Akbik H, Butler SF, Budman SH, Fernandez K, Katz NP, Jamison RN. Validation and clinical application of the Screener and Opioid Assessment for Patients with Pain (SOAPP). J Pain Symptom Manag. 2006;32:287–93.
33. Butler SF, Fernandez K, Benoit C, Budman SH, Jamison RN. Validation of the revised Screener and Opioid Assessment for Patients with Pain (SOAPP-R). J Pain. 2008;9:360–72.
34. Chou R, Ballantyne JC, Fanciullo GJ, Fine PG, Miaskowski C. Research gaps on use of opioids for chronic noncancer pain: findings from a review of the evidence for an American Pain Society and American Academy of Pain Medicine clinical practice guideline. J Pain. 2009;10:147–59.
35. Koyyalagunta D, Bruera E, Aigner C, Nusrat H, Driver L, Novy D. Risk stratification of opioid misuse among patients with cancer pain using the SOAPP-SF. Pain Med. 2013;14:667–75.
36. Koyyalagunta D, Burton AW, Toro MP, Driver L, Novy DM. Opioid abuse in cancer pain: report of two cases and presentation of an algorithm of multidisciplinary care. Pain Physician. 2011;14:E361–71.
37. Koyyalagunta D, Burton AW. The role of chemical neurolysis in cancer pain. Curr Pain Headache Rep. 2010;14:261–7.
38. Motivational interviewing: preparing people for change. New York, 2002.
39. Kabat-Zinn J, Hanh TN. Full catastrophe living (revised edition): using the wisdom of your body and mind to face stress, pain, and illness. New York: Random House Publishing Group; 2013.
40. Portenoy R, Conn M. Cancer pain syndromes. Cambridge: Press syndicate of the University of Cambridge; 2003.
41. Davies PS. Chronic pain management in the cancer survivor: tips for primary care providers. Nurse Pract. 2013;38:28–38; quiz 38-29.
42. Montoya M, Fossella F, Palmer JL, Kaur G, Pace EA, Yadav R, Simmonds M, Gillis T, Bruera E. Objective evaluation of physical function in patients with advanced lung cancer: a preliminary report. J Palliat Med. 2006;9:309–16.

8 Head and Neck Cancer Pain

Vinay Puttanniah and Elena V. Zininberg

Introduction

Cancers of the head and neck only account for approximately 3–5% of malignancies in the United States, but prevalence of pain syndromes associated with head and neck cancer has been reported as high as 86% and is considered among the worst symptoms of the cancer [1, 2]. Head and neck cancer (HNC) embodies a group of cancers arising in the head and neck region including the nasal cavity, oral cavity, pharynx, larynx, and associated structures including lips, sinuses, and salivary glands [3], with squamous cell cancer accounting for the most common histological type [4]. Understanding the underlying causes of head and neck cancer-related pain and awareness of treatment options is imperative in order to optimize the quality of life for patients suffering from these syndromes.

There are several ways to categorize pain caused by head and neck cancer. The pain can be nociceptive, including somatic and visceral pain syndromes resulting from damage to various tissue and organs, or neuropathic resulting from damage to components of the nervous system. Pain can result directly from the cancer such as mass effect from the tumor or malignant infiltration of nearby soft and bony structures as well as by neurological invasion and entrapment. Alternatively, pain can be the consequence of various cancer therapies including sequelae of various surgeries, radiation-induced tissue fibrosis, as well as mucositis and neuropathies resulting from both radiation and chemotherapy [5].

V. Puttanniah (✉)
Memorial Sloan Kettering Cancer Center, Anesthesiology and Critical Care Medicine, New York, NY, USA
e-mail: puttannv@mskcc.org

E. V. Zininberg
Weill Cornell School of Medicine, Department of Anesthesiology, New York, NY, USA

Department of Anesthesiology/Pain Management, Memorial Sloan Kettering, New York, NY, USA

Initial treatment of pain caused by head and neck cancer is typically based on the World Health Organization's cancer pain ladder which utilizes systemic analgesics in a stepwise fashion of increasingly potent opioids combined with non-opioid adjuncts and interventional techniques when they are available. In the following sections, we will focus on various interventional techniques that can be considered in the treatment of pain syndromes related to head and neck cancer.

Nociceptive Pain Syndromes

Nociceptive pain is caused by stimulation of the peripheral nociceptive nerves (A-delta and C-fibers) that are present in most tissues [6]. When considering pain resulting from head and neck cancer, nociceptive pain can be a direct effect of the tumor from expansion, inflammation, compression, ischemia, and destruction of surrounding tissue versus pain resulting from various cancer treatments such as surgery, radiation therapy, and chemotherapy. Pain location can vary enormously from dysphagia to pain in the face, occiput, and neck, myofascial pain, and articular pain at the cervical, scapular, and temporomandibular joints [7]. Nociceptive pain frequently responds to systemic analgesics which can help reduce the transmission of noxious stimuli, but various anatomic structures can also be targeted by interventional techniques to further accomplish pain relief [8].

Pain from Direct Tumor Involvement

Bone Invasion

Bone invasion is the leading cause of somatic pain in cancer [9]. Although the pathophysiologic mechanism is not fully understood, it is widely accepted that neurophysiologic changes related to malignancy sensitize peripheral nociceptors to mechanical and chemical stimuli. These receptors

A. Gulati et al. (eds.), *Essentials of Interventional Cancer Pain Management*, https://doi.org/10.1007/978-3-319-99684-4_8

are consequently activated by compression, ischemia, and release of local algesic factors [10]. Tumor-mediated imbalance between bone formation and resorption also plays an essential role in bone pain and predisposes to pathological fractures and nerve compression [11]. Pain secondary to bone involvement is typically well localized and constant, lasting days to weeks.

Nerve Compression and Invasion

Perineural tumor invasion is a well-reported phenomenon among patients with head and neck cancer. The primary tumor disseminates to noncontiguous regions along the endoneurium or perineurium causing nerve compression or infiltration [12]. Common nerves affected include the trigeminal nerve (V) and its branches, the facial nerve (VII), and the glossopharyngeal nerve (IX), though virtually any sensory nerves in the face, skull, neck, or shoulder can be involved [6]. Pain results in the anatomical distribution of the affected nerve(s).

Headache

Headache is a symptom frequently experienced with the presence of intracranial lesions, occurring in approximately 60% of patients presenting with primary brain tumors and in 35% of those with cerebral metastases [13]. Tumor-induced headaches are classically present on awakening, dull in nature, and intermittent, lasting up to several hours. Typically they are bifrontal and of mild to moderate intensity, but location can vary depending upon the location of the lesion [14].

Treatment-Associated Nociceptive Pain Syndromes

Chemotherapy or Radiation Therapy-Induced Oral Mucositis

Oral mucositis is a side effect of chemotherapy or radiation to the head and neck. Not only is it the most frequently reported pain syndrome in head and neck cancer, affecting up to 80% of patients, but patients report it is the most debilitating side effect of their therapy [15]. Ulceration leads to severe pain which interferes with speaking, eating, and drinking. This can be so incapacitating that cancer therapy may need to be interrupted or modified which may reduce survival [16]. Current pain regimens for oral mucositis rely primarily on the use of oral and intravenous analgesics, with the goal of managing pain in order to maximize patient swallowing efforts to prevent atrophy and fibrosis and optimize long-term swallow function [15]. Other commonly employed treatments include topical agents, usually in the form of mouthwash, to desensitize oral mucosa. Formulations commonly include local anesthetics such as lidocaine alone or as a mixture with morphine. Oral cryotherapy has also received attention as a preemptive measure employed to reduce the incidence and severity of mucositis in patients receiving certain types of chemotherapy [16].

Radiation-Induced Pain Syndromes

Radiation therapy is one of the most commonly employed treatment modalities in head and neck cancer. Although radiation targets the cancer as precisely as possible, sensitive organs within close proximity can be affected. Radiation to the head and neck can cause damage to the skin, mucosa, salivary glands, nerves, and bones. The diverse pathological effects include fibrosis, necrosis, tissue atrophy, and vascular damage [17].

Late xerostomia is one of the most common consequences of head and neck radiation primarily due to parotid gland damage. Besides simply causing the discomfort of dry mouth, xerostomia can cause difficulties with food intake and oral hygiene, significantly decreasing quality of life [18].

Skin and mucosa exposed to radiation often become friable and susceptible to recurrent painful ulceration.

Radiation-induced tissue fibrosis is another well-documented sequelae that can cause great pain and discomfort. It is a late manifestation of ionizing radiation which causes cellular damage by direct DNA damage as well as the creation of free radicals which lead to a localized inflammatory response. This inflammation ultimately leads to increased collagen deposition, poor vascularity, and scarring. Regional syndromes specific to radiation of the head and neck region can include trismus, dysphagia, aspiration, and localized pain [19].

Mandibular osteoradionecrosis is a relatively rare but devastating complication of radiation to the head and neck region. The incidence, which is relatively low at approximately 5–7%, depends largely on the amount of radiation delivered to the mandible and baseline oral hygiene. [18]

Postsurgical Pain

Many head and neck cancers including oropharyngeal, hypopharyngeal, and supraglottic laryngeal cancer result in nodal metastases to the neck requiring surgical treatment [20]. Neck and shoulder pain along with functional impairment are frequently reported complications after neck dissection surgery, with prevalence of shoulder complaints reaching up to 80% after lymph node dissection [21, 22]. Temporary or permanent denervation of the trapezius muscle secondary to spinal accessory nerve (CNXI) damage is the most common cause of shoulder pain and dysfunction. Multiple studies have shown that sparing the accessory nerve during neck dissection significantly decreases both acute and chronic postoperative shoulder pain and improves functional status [23]. Other surgeries such as mandibular resection and maxillectomy frequently result in sensory impairment causing allodynia, hyperalgesia, and persistent pain for years after surgery [24].

Neuropathic Pain Syndromes

It has been reported that up to 30% of HNC patients suffer from neuropathic pain because of cancer or its treatments [25]. Neuropathic pain is the result of a primary lesion or dysfunction involving the peripheral or central nervous system. Direct damage to peripheral pain neurons (C-fibers) causing abnormal regulation of sodium channels and signal transmission is one mechanism resulting in neuropathic pain. Alternatively, neuropathic pain can develop secondary to persistent, unrelieved nociceptive pain which can alter central pain pathways and lead to spinal cord hyperexcitability [26, 27]. Neuropathic pain usually manifests as abnormal numbness, burning, tingling, or shooting sensations and can include allodynia and/or hyperalgesia. In patients with head and neck cancer, neuropathic pain can be exacerbated by chewing, swallowing, and facial movements.

Neuropathic pain can be caused by a variety of mechanisms. Just as tumors can invade soft and bony tissues, malignancies can also invade and/or compress nervous structures resulting in abnormal transmission of pain signals. The distribution of abnormal sensation generally correlates to the specific nerve or plexus that is compressed or otherwise damaged. Alternatively, neuropathies can arise from various chemotherapies and/or prolonged radiation secondary to nerve damage. Finally, as described earlier, nerve damage can be caused during surgical dissection, leading to abnormal propagation of pain signals along the damaged nerves.

Interventional Pain Management

For patients who do not obtain satisfactory relief from oral analgesics, utilization of various interventional techniques may be indicated. Nerve blocks targeting central and peripheral nerves are often done diagnostically first, followed by longer-acting therapeutic injections. Other interventional options include neuromodulation, neural destructive techniques, and intraspinal drug delivery (see Fig. 8.1).

Nerve Blocks

Autonomic Nerve Blocks

Stellate Ganglion Block

Blockade of the stellate ganglion provides valuable diagnostic and therapeutic benefit in sympathetically mediated pain syndromes affecting the head, neck, and upper extremities. This type of block is traditionally used to alleviate upper extremity pain associated with complex regional pain syndrome. However, blockade of sympathetic fibers traveling to the head at either the C5 or C6 vertebra has been shown to produce more successful sympathetic blockade to the head and neck with less effect to the upper extremities [28]; this can prove useful in pain caused by head and neck cancer. There is anecdotal experience with short duration of efficacy with this procedure though it is not universally successful.

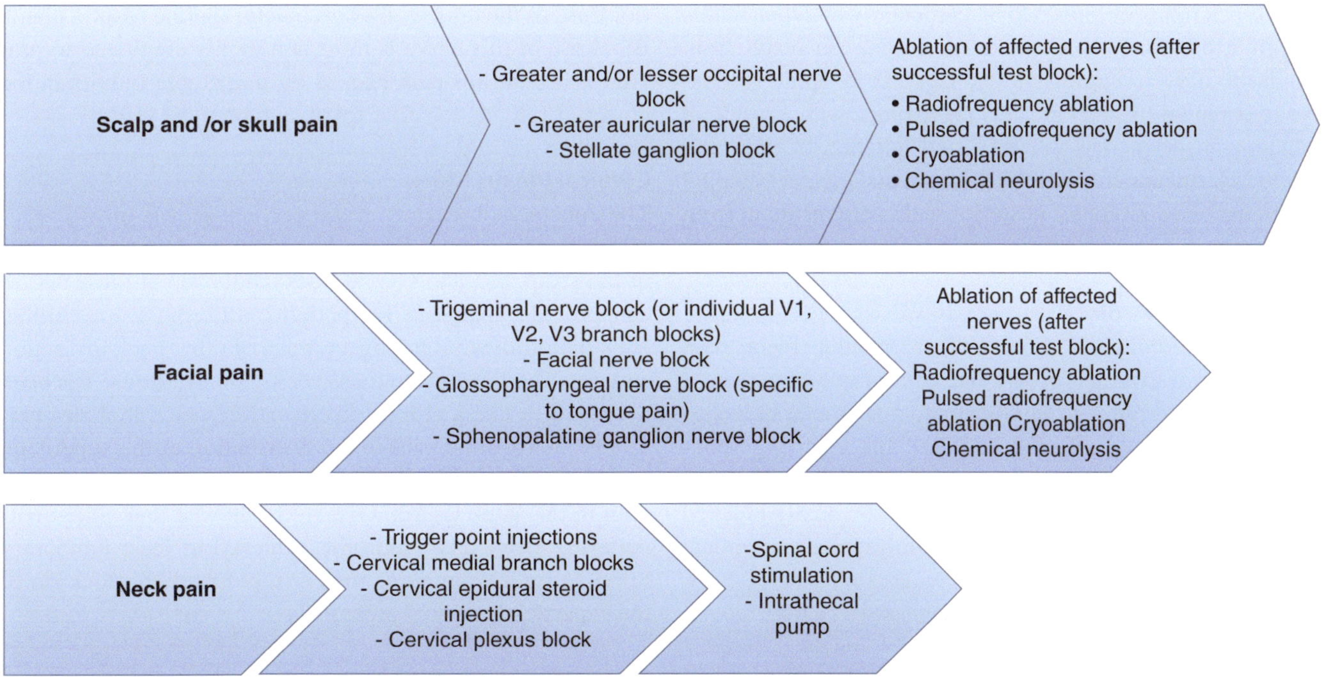

Fig. 8.1 Sequence of interventions for malignancy-associated head and neck pain syndromes by anatomic location. Suggested interventions after failed conservative management. Therapies may be used concurrently

Neurolysis of the ganglion that may rarely be indicated and theoretically may be considered for prolonged relief with the reconciliation of the risk for side effects, including prolonged Horner's syndrome.

Sphenopalatine Ganglion Block

The sphenopalatine ganglion is comprised of both sympathetic and parasympathetic fibers and has been implicated in the transmission of a variety of craniofacial pain syndromes. Blockade of the sphenopalatine ganglion has been proven to be an effective treatment for refractory facial pain due to a variety of causes including nerve compression secondary to neoplasm [29].

The evidence for this procedure is lacking; however, this target has anecdotal value in modulating oncologic facial pain. Consideration to anatomic changes secondary to tumor invasion, surgery, and radiation is important when performing this procedure, especially given the transmucosal or fluoroscopic guidance approaches rely on "normal" anatomy.

Somatic Nerve Blocks

Occipital Nerve Block

Occipital (third, lesser, and greater) nerve block can be used to treat several pain syndromes related to head and neck cancer. The conditions more commonly treated with occipital nerve block include cervicogenic headaches and occipital neuralgia. Cervicogenic headache is a general term used to describe headaches referred from a source in the neck and is quite common in head and neck cancer. Greater occipital nerve block has been shown to be particularly effective in this type of headache [30]. Occipital neuralgia can result from neoplastic nerve compression and can also be quite responsive to occipital (usually greater) nerve block with a resultant reduction in frequency, intensity, and duration of pain episodes [31]. Anecdotally, the third, lesser, and greater occipital nerves may be a target for posterior scalp pain resultant from craniotomy, tumor, or posterior scalp radiation treatments.

Trigeminal Nerve Block

Trigeminal neuralgia is a form of neuropathic facial pain resulting from irritation of any one or multiple branches of the trigeminal nerve. The maxillary and mandibular branches are most commonly affected with patients reporting spontaneous, severe facial pain in those distributions. Terminal divisions of the trigeminal nerve can be individually blocked for pain syndromes confined to a more precise anatomical location.

- V1: Ophthalmic nerve
- Blockade of the supraorbital and supratrochlear nerves, which are terminal divisions of the ophthalmic nerve, provides analgesia to the forehead area which is useful in pain resulting from tumors of the skull base, meningiomas, and neuromas of the trigeminal root [13].
- V2: Maxillary nerve
- Cancers of the upper jaw cause pain by a combination of stretching periosteal nociceptive fibers causing somatic pain and by putting pressure on the nerve itself resulting in maxillary neuralgia. Blockage of the maxillary nerve provides analgesia to the upper jaw and is useful in this setting.
- V3: Mandibular nerve
- Blockade of the mandibular nerve provides analgesia for pain in the distribution of the lower jaw, teeth, and floor of the mouth. Case reports have even described use of an indwelling mandibular catheter for intractable mandibular pain secondary to cancer [32].

Cervical Medial Branch Blocks

Neck pain secondary to direct tumor infiltration or nerve compression can be the cause of much patient discomfort. Blockade of the cervical medial branches, usually performed under fluoroscopic guidance, can provide analgesia to the head and neck area. Patients undergoing cervical neck surgery frequently suffer from persistent neck pain. Though there are only limited recommendations, one study suggests that early intervention with therapeutic medial branch blocks can be beneficial in these postsurgical patients [33].

Glossopharyngeal Nerve Block

The glossopharyngeal nerve provides sensation to the posterior third of the tongue, the soft palate, and the parotid gland. Blockade of this nerve is most commonly employed to provide analgesia for pain caused by inoperable tumors in the posterior tongue, tonsillar fossa, and pharynx [13].

Cervical Plexus Block

The cutaneous branches of the cervical plexus provide sensation to many areas of the head and neck including parts of the scalp, ear, and ventral neck. Blockade of these nerves can provide analgesia for patients suffering from chronic neck pain following laryngectomies or other neck dissection surgery. The term postradical neck pain syndrome has been used to describe a clinical presentation which includes persistent neuropathic pain in the distribution of the superficial cervical plexus which may be accompanied by myofascial pain in the same region. One study showed that all patients suffering from this syndrome achieved at least temporary relief or improvement of their symptoms with blockade of the superficial cervical plexus [34].

Trigger Point Injections

Myofascial pain in head and neck cancer can be the result of surgical intervention as described earlier in postradical neck dissection syndrome. Pain is most often in the distribution of the trapezius or sternocleidomastoid and may respond to trigger point injections similarly to myofascial pain affecting other parts of the body. Similarly, the use of botulinum toxin may be considered for the treatment of cervical dystonia, resulting from radiation fibrosis or surgery [35].

Neuromodulation

Transcutaneous Electrical Nerve Stimulation (TENS)

Transcutaneous electrical nerve stimulation is the application of various frequencies of electrical current through electrodes placed on the skin which achieves pain control by activating specific receptors in the spinal cord and brainstem [36]. TENS has most often been used to treat chronic neuropathic pain, including CRPS and diabetic neuropathy. More recently its use has become more widespread to include a plethora of chronic pain conditions as well as acute perioperative pain [37, 38]. This suggests that application of TENS could be beneficial in the perioperative period for patients undergoing radical neck dissections. Furthermore, several studies have demonstrated that extra-oral application of TENS during or postradiation therapy stimulates salivary flow, rendering it an effective adjunct in the treatment of radiation-induced xerostomia [39, 40].

Spinal Cord Stimulation (SCS)

Spinal cord stimulation is achieved by placing electrodes on the spinal cord which deliver impulses that may reduce pain. This technique is widely accepted for treatment of a variety of chronic pain conditions. Although there has not been enough evidence to establish its use in the treatment of cancer pain, it has become a topic of interest. In one study, Yakovlev et al. describe the successful implementation of SCS in the treatment of intractable cancer-related chest wall pain in a group of 14 patients [41]. While not necessarily for cancer-related pain, newer advances in neuromodulation for facial pain may one day be options for patients suffering from head and neck cancer-related pain [42].

Intrathecal Drug Delivery

Implantable intrathecal drug delivery systems work by delivering select medications directly into the cerebrospinal fluid for pain control. Studies suggest that use of intrathecal catheters for refractory cancer pain provides superior pain relief with fewer side effects when compared to traditional comprehensive medical management [43]. Appelgren et al. were one of the earliest studies investigating the safety and efficacy of continuous intracisternal and high cervical intrathecal bupivacaine infusion for the treatment of refractory head and neck cancer pain. Reportedly, the majority of the 13 patients in this study reported satisfactory pain relief and reduced opioid consumption [44]. More recently, Lundborg and colleagues reported on the use of high intrathecal bupivacaine for refractory pain involving the head and neck in a significantly larger group, consisting of 40 patients. They too concluded that most patients experienced complete pain relief with few side effects [45]. Placement of the catheter at the C1–C2 level appears to be superior for treating pain involving the head and neck, while placement at the C4–C5 is beneficial in treating shoulder and extremity pain [46].

Intraventricular Opiates

Several publications have described intraventricular morphine administration through an implanted catheter as an effective method of alleviating intractable cancer pain. The therapeutic effects of direct intraventricular administration of opiates are due to the high concentration of opioid receptors in the third ventricle and periaqueductal gray [46]. All studies, to our knowledge, have limited use of this therapy to patients with terminal head and neck cancer. In one study including 82 patients, Lazorthes et al. reported 80% of patients experienced good or excellent analgesia [47].

Neurodestructive Techniques

Radiofrequency Ablation

Radiofrequency ablation (RFA) is a technique that utilizes thermal ablation to achieve targeted cellular death. This technique is most often employed as a long-term method of analgesia after diagnostic blockade of a specific nerve or ganglion has proven beneficial. RFA for head and neck disease was first reported in 1975 for treatment of trigeminal neuralgia [48]. Several studies since have confirmed efficacy of trigeminal rhizotomy for trigeminal neuralgia, and more recently RFA has been employed in the treatment of several other head and neck pain syndromes. Various reports describe use of RFA targeting various nerves for treatment of refractory occipital neuralgia [49–51], chronic neck pain [52], and cervicogenic headache [53, 54].

Pulsed Radiofrequency

Pulsed radiofrequency (PRF) is an alternative technique developed in an attempt to limit the amount of tissue destruction when compared with traditional continuous radiofrequency ablation. This is particularly important in dealing with nerve targets that have motor function which would be compromised by thermal ablation. Although the mechanism of action of PRF is not entirely clear, studies attribute pain relief to changes in synaptic transmission along pain fibers [55]. Reported efficacy of PRF has been variable, but trials continue in similar applications as traditional RFA including treatment of trigeminal neuralgia [56, 57], occipital neuralgia

[58, 59], cervical radiculopathy [60], and cervicogenic head [61] and chronic shoulder pain [62].

Chemical Neurolysis

Chemical neurolysis, or denervation, refers to the use of chemical ablative agents in order to interrupt nerve signal transmission. Most commonly employed agents include alcohol, phenol, and botulinum toxin. This technique is older than RFA and PRF and has generally fallen out of favor, though its use has been well documented in ablation of the trigeminal ganglion, occipital nerves, and glossopharyngeal nerve [63]. The use of chemical neurolysis is generally accepted only in patients with intractable pain secondary to terminal cancer with a short life expectancy. The risks, including necrosis of the skin and nontarget tissue, neuritis, as well as the possibility of prolonged motor paralysis, are thought to outweigh the benefits in other patient populations [64].

Conclusions

The extremely high prevalence of pain syndromes associated with head and neck cancers is greatly detrimental to these patients' quality of life. Though medical management of head and neck cancer pain is generally effective, alternative interventional options must be considered to treat patients with intractable pain. A variety of peripheral, ganglionic, and axial nerve blocks exist that have had much success in treatment of various head and neck pain syndromes. More long-term solutions including radiofrequency ablation, chemical neurolysis, and pulsed radiofrequency can be employed once diagnostic blocks have been rendered useful. Both invasive and noninvasive neuromodulatory techniques have also been effective in alleviating various types of head and neck pain. Interventions should be selected based on individual symptoms, response to various techniques, and overall prognosis.

References

1. Chaplin JM, Morton RP. Prospective, longitudinal study of pain in head and neck cancer patients. Head Neck. 1999;21(6):531–7.
2. Breivik H, Cherny N, Collett B, de Conno F, Filbet M, Foubert AJ, Cohen R, Dow L. Cancer-related pain: a pan-European survey of prevalence, treatment, and patient attitudes. Ann Oncol. 2009;20(8):1420–33.
3. Davies L, Welch HG. Epidemiology of head and neck cancer in the United States. Otolaryngol Head Neck Surg. 2006;135(3):451–7.
4. Sanderson RJ, Ironside JA. Squamous cell carcinomas of the head and neck. BMJ. 2002;325(7368):822–7.
5. Caraceni A, Portenoy RK. An international survey of cancer pain characteristics and syndromes. IASP task force on cancer pain. International association for the study of pain. Pain. 1999;82(3):263–74.
6. Vecht CJ, Hoff AM, Kansen PJ, et al. Types and causes of pain in cancer of the head and neck. Cancer. 1992;70(1):178–84.
7. Trotter PB, et al. Pharmacological and other interventions for head and neck cancer pain: a systematic review. J Oral Maxillofac Res. 2012;3(4):e1.
8. Binczak M, et al. Management of somatic pain induced by head-and-neck cancer treatment: definition and assessment guidelines of the French Oto-Rhino-Laryngology- Head and Neck Surgery Society. Eur Ann Otorhinolaryngol Head Neck Dis. 2014;131(4):243–7.
9. Villaret D, Weymuller E. Pain caused by cancer of the head and neck. In: Loeser J, Butler S, Chapman R, editors. Bonica's management of pain. Philadelphia: Lippincott Williams & Wilkins; 2001. p. 948–65.
10. Foley KM. The treatment of cancer pain. N Engl J Med. 1985;313:84–95.
11. Roodman GD. Mechanisms of bone metastasis. N Engl J Med. 2004;350:1655–64.
12. Caldemeyer KS, Mathews VP, Righi PD, Smith RR. Imaging features and clinical significance of perineural spread or extension of head and neck tumours. Radiographics. 1998;18(1):97–110.
13. Mehio AK, Shah SK. Alleviating head and neck pain. Otolaryngol Clin N Am. 2009;42(1):143–59.
14. Alentorn A, et al. Presenting signs and symptoms in brain tumors. Handb Clin Neurol. 2016;134:19–26.
15. Mirabile A, et al. Pain management in head and neck cancer patients undergoing chemo-radiotherapy: clinical practical recommendations. Crit Rev Oncol Hematol. 2016;99:100–6.
16. Riley P, Glenny AM, Worthington HV, Littlewood A, Clarkson JE, McCabe MG. Interventions for preventing oral mucositis in patients with cancer receiving treatment: oral cryotherapy. Cochrane Database Syst Rev. 2015;(12). Art. No.: CD011552.
17. Pandya JA, et al. Post-radiation changes in oral tissues – an analysis of cancer irradiation cases. South Asian J Cancer. 2014;3(3):159–62.
18. Henriques de Figueiredo B, Grégoire V. How to minimize morbidity in radiotherapy of pharyngolaryngeal tumors? Curr Opin Otolaryngol Head Neck Surg. 2016;24(2):163–9.
19. Straub JM, et al. Radiation-induced fibrosis: mechanisms and implications for therapy. J Cancer Res Clin Oncol. 2015;141(11):1985–94.
20. Chan JY, et al. Shoulder dysfunction after selective neck dissection in recurrent nasopharyngeal carcinoma. Otolaryngol Head Neck Surg. 2015;153(3):379–84.
21. Lauchlan DT, McCaul JA, McCarron T. Neck dissection and the clinical appearance of post-operative shoulder disability: the post-operative role of physiotherapy. Eur J Cancer Care. 2008;17(6):542–8. [PubMed].
22. Rogers SN, Ferlito A, Pellitteri PK, Shaha AR, Rinaldo A. Quality of life following neck dissections. Acta Otolaryngol. 2004;124(3):231–6. [PubMed].
23. Terrell JE, et al. Pain, quality of life, and spinal accessory nerve status after neck dissection. Laryngoscope. 2000;110(4):620–6.
24. Epstein JB, Wilkie DJ, Fischer DJ, Kim Y-O, Villines D. Neuropathic and nociceptive pain in head and neck cancer patients receiving radiation therapy. Head Neck Oncol. 2009;1:26.
25. Grond S, et al. Validation of World Health Organization guidelines for pain relief in head and neck cancer. A prospective study. Ann Otol Rhinol Laryngol. 1993;102(5):342–8.
26. Coderre TJ, et al. Contribution of central neuroplasticity to pathological pain: review of clinical and experimental evidence. Pain. 1993;52(3):259–85.
27. Connolly I, et al. Management of severe neuropathic cancer pain: an illustrative case and review. Am J Hosp Palliat Care. 2013;30(1):83–90.
28. Mastsumoto S. Thermographic assessment of the sympathetic blockade by stellate ganglion block (20); Comparison between C7-SGB and C6-SGB in 20 healthy volunteers. Masui. 1991;40:692–701.

29. Prasanna A, Murthy PS. Sphenopalatine ganglion block and pain of cancer. J Pain Symptom Manag. 1993;8(3):125.
30. Levin M. Nerve blocks in the treatment of headache. Neurotherapeutics. 2010;7(2):197–203.
31. Dach F, et al. Nerve block for the treatment of headaches and cranial neuralgias – a practical approach. Headache. 2015;55(Suppl 1):59–71.
32. Kohase H, Umino M, Shibaji T, et al. Application of a mandibular nerve block using an indwelling catheter for intractable cancer pain. Acta Anaesthesiol Scand. 2004;48(3):382–3.
33. Klessinger S. The benefit of therapeutic medial branch blocks after cervical operations. Pain Physician. 2010;13(6):527–34.
34. Sist T, Miner M, Lema M. Characteristics of postradical neck pain syndrome: a report of 25 cases. J Pain Symptom Manage. 1999;18(2):95–102.
35. Stubblefield MD, Levine A, Custodio CM, Fitzpatrick T. The role of botulinum toxin type A in the radiation fibrosis syndrome: a preliminary report. Arch Phys Med Rehabil. 2008;89(3):417–21.
36. DeSantana JM, Walsh DM, Vance C, Rakel BA, Sluka KA. Effectiveness of transcutaneous electrical nerve stimulation for treatment of hyperalgesia and pain. Curr Rheumatol Rep. 2008;10(6):492–9.
37. DeSantana JM, Santana-Filho VJ, Guerra DR, et al. Hypoalgesic effect of the transcutaneous electrical nerve stimulation following inguinal herniorrhaphy: a randomized, controlled trial. J Pain. 2008;9:623–9.
38. Solak O, Turna A, Pekcolaklar A, et al. Transcutaneous electric nerve stimulation for the treatment of postthoracotomy pain: a randomized prospective study. Thorac Cardiovasc Surg. 2007;55:182–5.
39. Vijayan A, et al. Prospective phase II study of the efficacy of transcutaneous electrical nerve stimulation in post-radiation patients. Clin Oncol (R Coll Radiol). 2014;26(12):743–7.
40. Lakshman AR, et al. Evaluation of effect of transcutaneous electrical nerve stimulation on salivary flow rate in radiation induced xerostomia patients: a pilot study. J Cancer Res Ther. 2015;11(1):229–33.
41. Yakovlev AE, et al. Treatment of cancer-related chest wall pain using spinal cord stimulation. Am J Hosp Palliat Care. 2010;27(8):552–6.
42. Maniam R, Kaye AD, Vadivelu N, Urman RD. Facial pain update: advances in neurostimulation for the treatment of facial pain. Curr Pain Headache Rep. 2016;20(4):24.
43. Smith TJ, et al. Randomized clinical trial of an implantable drug delivery system compared with comprehensive medical management for refractory cancer pain: impact on pain, drug-related toxicity, and survival. J Clin Oncol. 2002;20(19):4040–9.
44. Appelgren L, Janson M, Nitescu P, Curelaru I. Continuous intracisternal and high cervical intrathecal bupivacaine analgesia in refractory head and neck pain. Anesthesiology. 1996;84(2):256–72.
45. Lundborg C, et al. High intrathecal bupivacaine for severe pain in the head and neck. Acta Anaesthesiol Scand. 2009;53(7):908–13.
46. Datta S, Pai UT. Interventional approaches to management of pain of oral cancer. Oral Maxillofac Surg Clin North Am. 2006;18(4):627–41.
47. Lazorthes YR, Sallerin BA, Verdié JC. Intracerebroventricular administration of morphine for control of irreducible cancer pain. Neurosurgery. 1995;37(3):422–8.
48. Onofrio BM. Radiofrequency percutaneous Gasserian ganglion lesions. Results in 140 patients with trigeminal pain. J Neurosurg. 1975;42(2):132–9.
49. Dubuisson D. Treatment of occipital neuralgia by partial posterior rhizotomy at C1–3. J Neurosurg. 1995;82(4):581–6.
50. Choi I, Jeon SR. Neuralgias of the head: occipital neuralgia. J Korean Med Sci. 2016;31(4):479–88.
51. Gande AV, et al. Long-term outcomes of intradural cervical dorsal root rhizotomy for refractory occipital neuralgia. J Neurosurg. 2015;18:1–9.
52. McDonald GJ, et al. Long-term follow-up of patients treated with cervical radiofrequency neurotomy for chronic neck pain. Neurosurgery. 1999;45(1):61–7.
53. Blume HG. Cervicogenic headaches: radiofrequency neurotomy and the cervical disc and fusion. Clin Exp Rheumatol. 2000;18(2):S53–8.
54. Lee JB, et al. Clinical efficacy of radiofrequency cervical zygapophyseal neurotomy in patients with chronic cervicogenic headache. J Korean Med Sci. 2007;22(2):326–9.
55. Cahana A, Zundert J, Macrea L, Kleef M, Sluijter M. Pulsed radiofrequency: current clinical and biological literature available. Pain Med. 2006;7(5):411–23.
56. Erdine S, Ozyalcin NS, Cimen A, Celik M, Talu GK, Disci R. Comparison of pulsed radiofrequency with conventional radiofrequency in the treatment of idiopathic trigeminal neuralgia. Eur J Pain. 2007;11(3):309–13.
57. Zundert J, Brabant S, Kelft E, Vercruyssen A, Buyten JP. Pulsed radiofrequency treatment of the Gasserian ganglion in patients with idiopathic trigeminal neuralgia. Pain. 2003;104(3):449–52.
58. Choi HJ, et al. Clinical outcomes of pulsed radiofrequency neuromodulation for the treatment of occipital neuralgia. J Korean Neurosurg Soc. 2012;51(5):281–5.
59. Vanelderen P, et al. Pulsed radiofrequency for the treatment of occipital neuralgia: a prospective study with 6 months of follow-up. Reg Anesth Pain Med. 2010;35(2):148–51.
60. Choi G-S, et al. Short-term effects of pulsed radiofrequency on chronic refractory cervical radicular pain. Ann Rehabil Med. 2011;35(6):826–32.
61. van Suijlekom JA, van Kleef M, Barendse G. Radio-frequency cervical zygapophyseal joint neurotomy for cervicogenic headache. A prospective study in 15 patients. Funct Neurol. 1998;13:297–303.
62. Liliang PC, et al. Pulsed radiofrequency lesioning of the suprascapular nerve for chronic shoulder pain: a preliminary report. Pain Med. 2009;10(1):70–5.
63. Koyyalagunta D, Burton AW. The role of chemical neurolysis in cancer pain. Curr Pain Headache Rep. 2010;14:261–7.
64. Joo YC1, Park JY, Kim KH. Comparison of alcohol ablation with repeated thermal radiofrequency ablation in medial branch neurotomy for the treatment of recurrent thoracolumbar facet joint pain. J Anesth. 2013;27(3):390–5.

Breast Cancer Pain: A Review of Pathology and Interventional Techniques

9

Ali Valimahomed, Jennifer Zocca, and Amitabh Gulati

Introduction

Breast cancer-related pain may be divided into three distinct categories: tumor-related pain, treatment-related pain, and debility or pain unrelated to cancer [1]. During active treatment and in advanced oncological disease, the tumor itself is typically the progenitor of breast cancer-related pain; however, in breast cancer survivors, pain is typically the sequela of the treatment itself – i.e., chemotherapy, radiation, hormonal therapy, etc. [2]. It is estimated that one-third of cancer patients experience chronic pain following curative treatment [3]. In a random self-reported sample survey of 2000 Denmark breast cancer survivors, 42% had chronic breast pain 5 years after their primary surgery [4]. A later study by Hofsø et al. [5] surveyed 188 Norwegian women with breast cancer for side effects following radiation therapy and found that 51% of patients complained of pain [5]. Van den Beuken-van Everdingen et al. [3] performed a meta-analysis of 7 studies and found the prevalence of pain in breast cancer patients to be 54% (44–64%) [3].

More aggressive breast cancer treatments, such as mastectomy, axillary lymph node dissection, and radiation therapy, are associated with increased shoulder pathology when compared to more conservative treatment such as lumpectomy, sentinel lymph node dissection, and less aggressive or no radiation therapy [6]. A review of recent literature surrounding breast cancer estimates that the prevalence of arm and shoulder pain following breast surgery is anywhere from 9% to 68% [7]. In patients with breast cancer who have had surgery, being younger than 40 years old, axillary dissection, and radiotherapy are associated with increased pain [8]. Oddly enough, the use of chemotherapy or the type of surgery (breast-conserving compared to mastectomy) does not influence the level of pain [8].

Breast cancer pain leads to a myriad of side effects including depression, insomnia, and decreased quality of life [2]. Cancer-related pain is underdiagnosed and undertreated [2]. According to a study by Von Roenn et al. [9], more than half (57–76%) of medical oncologists do not ask their patients about pain, and only half of these practitioners (51%) believe their patients' pain is well controlled [9]. A recent systematic review by van den Beuken et al. [3] found that in patients with cancer, pain was present in 64% of those with metastatic, advanced, or terminal disease, 59% of those undergoing cancer treatment, and 33% of those in remission [3]. This issue is clearly important, as reduced upper extremity function negatively influences a patient's ability return to work and to help care for family [10]. Unemployment rates are 1.37 times higher in cancer patients compared to their equivalent healthy counterparts [10, 11].

According to the Surveillance, Epidemiology, and End Results Program, there were an estimated 232,670 new cases of breast cancer in 2014, which represents 14% of all new cancer cases [12]. Data from 2009 to 2011 suggests that approximately 12.3% of all women in the United States will be diagnosed with cancer at some point during their lifetime [12]. 25.5% of breast cancer patients are between ages 55 and 64 at the time of diagnosis, and the median age at diagnosis is 61 years of age [12]. At the time of diagnosis, 61% will have localized disease confined to the primary site, 32% will have regional involvement or spread to regional lymph nodes, 5% will have metastases, and 2% is unknown or unstaged [12]. In 1980, the 5-year survival rate for breast cancer was 74.9%; however, in 2006 the 5-year survival rate for breast cancer had improved to 90.6% [12].

A. Valimahomed, M.D. (✉)
Department of Physical Medicine and Rehabilitation, New York-Presbyterian Hospital, Weill Cornell Medical College/Columbia University Vagelos College of Physicians and Surgeons, New York, NY, USA

J. Zocca, M.D.
Department of Anesthesiology, New York-Presbyterian Hospital, Weill Cornell Medical College, New York, NY, USA

A. Gulati, M.D.
Department of Anesthesiology and Critical Care, Memorial Sloan Kettering Cancer Center, New York, NY, USA

A. Gulati et al. (eds.), *Essentials of Interventional Cancer Pain Management*, https://doi.org/10.1007/978-3-319-99684-4_9

Innervation of the Breast

The thoracic dorsal root (sensory) and the ventral root (motor) combine in the intervertebral foramen and continue as the mixed spinal nerve. More distally, in the paravertebral space, the spinal nerve divides into the dorsal primary rami and the ventral primary rami. The dorsal primary rami course posteriorly to supply the zygapophyseal joints, midline muscles, and skin of the back. The ventral primary rami travels anteriorly in the thorax, inferior to costal groove, and is sheltered by the overlying ribs, in between the parietal pleura and the posterior intercostal membrane to form the intercostal nerve [13, 14].

The breast receives cutaneous innervation from the anterior and lateral cutaneous branches of intercostal nerves T1–T6 [15]. The lateral cutaneous branch arises at the midaxillary line (MAL) and splits into anterior and posterior branches to supply the skin of the lateral thoracic walls (from the scapular line to midclavicular line) [13, 16]. The anterior cutaneous branch of the intercostal nerve arises at the parasternal line and supplies the anterior portion of the thoracic wall [13, 16]. Collateral branches from the intercostal nerves supply motor innervation to the intercostal muscles and sensory innervation to the parietal pleura [14]. Each intercostal nerve innervates a characteristic band-like dermatomal distribution of the skin, with additional cross innervation between levels [17]. Of note, the first intercostal nerve is small; it does not have an anterior cutaneous branch, and a portion (equivalent to the lateral cutaneous branch) branches off to contribute to the brachial plexus [17].

The lateral branch of the second intercostal nerve does not divide into anterior and posterior portions, but instead forms the intercostobrachial nerve (occasionally there is contribution from the third intercostal nerve). The intercostobrachial nerve joins the medial brachial cutaneous nerve to provide sensation to the superior medial aspect of the arm and axilla [14, 18, 19].

The supraclavicular nerves, originating from C3 to C4 (primarily C4), also supply cutaneous innervation to the superior aspect of the chest and the shoulders [14, 16]. The medial pectoral nerve branches from the medial cord of the brachial plexus, derived from ventral rami of C8–T1, to innervate both the pectoralis minor and part of the pectoralis major. The lateral pectoral nerve branches from the lateral cord of the brachial plexus, derived from the ventral rami of C5–C7, and innervates the pectoralis major. The long thoracic nerve (LTN) is also derived from the ventral rami of C5–C7, traversing the anterolateral aspect of the first rib into the axilla to innervate the serratus anterior muscle. Damage to the LTN may occur during mastectomy and may result in a winged scapula [14] (Figs. 9.1, 9.2, and 9.3).

Pain relating to breast cancer may be conceptualized in several different ways. The pain syndromes can be thought of on a temporal spectrum, i.e., acute, subacute, and chronic. However, there can be significant variation and overlap when considering the time course of these various pain syndromes, and it is slightly easier to examine pain syndromes relating to breast cancer in an organ system-based approach. The primary organ systems affected in patients with breast cancer are the musculoskeletal, neurologic, lymphatic, and integumentary systems.

Musculoskeletal

Pain can arise from direct tumor burden affecting the muscles and bones, both from primary tumor burden and from metastases. Of note, surgical treatment itself can result in significant musculoskeletal pain, which will be discussed in

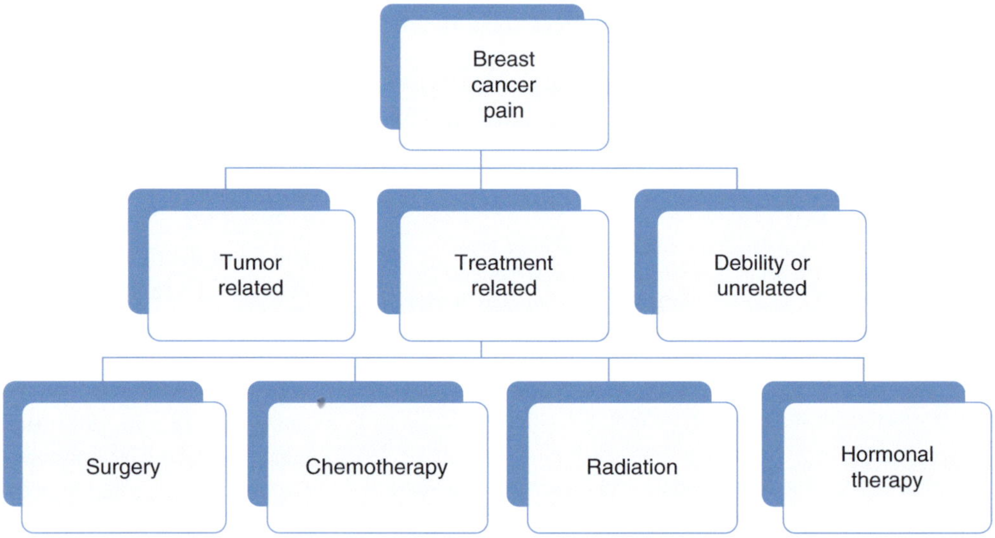

Fig. 9.1 Epidemiology of breast cancer pain

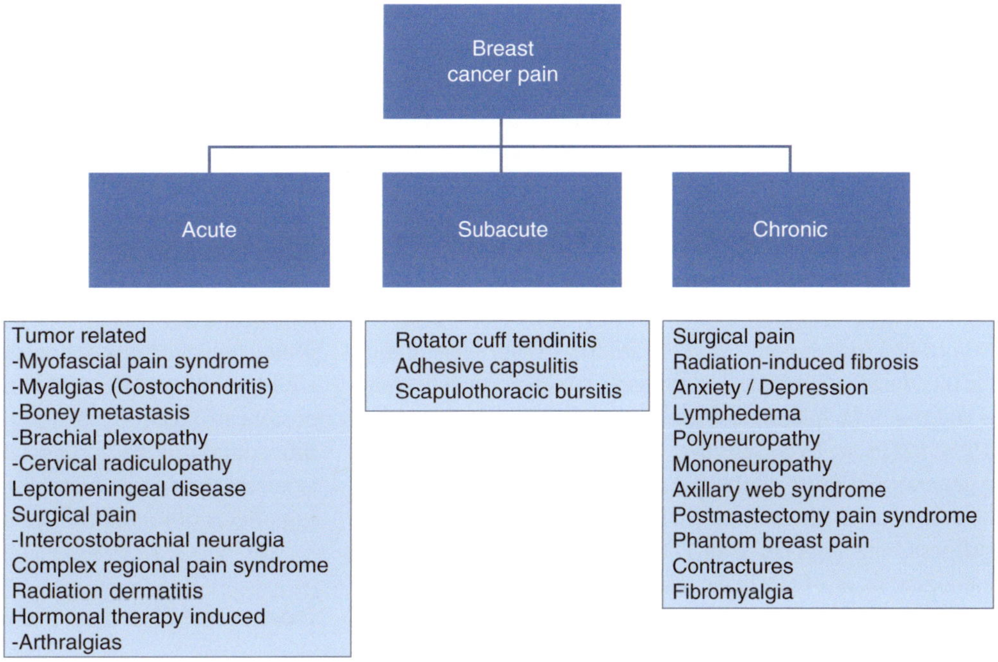

Fig. 9.2 Acute, subacute, and chronic pain disorders in breast cancer

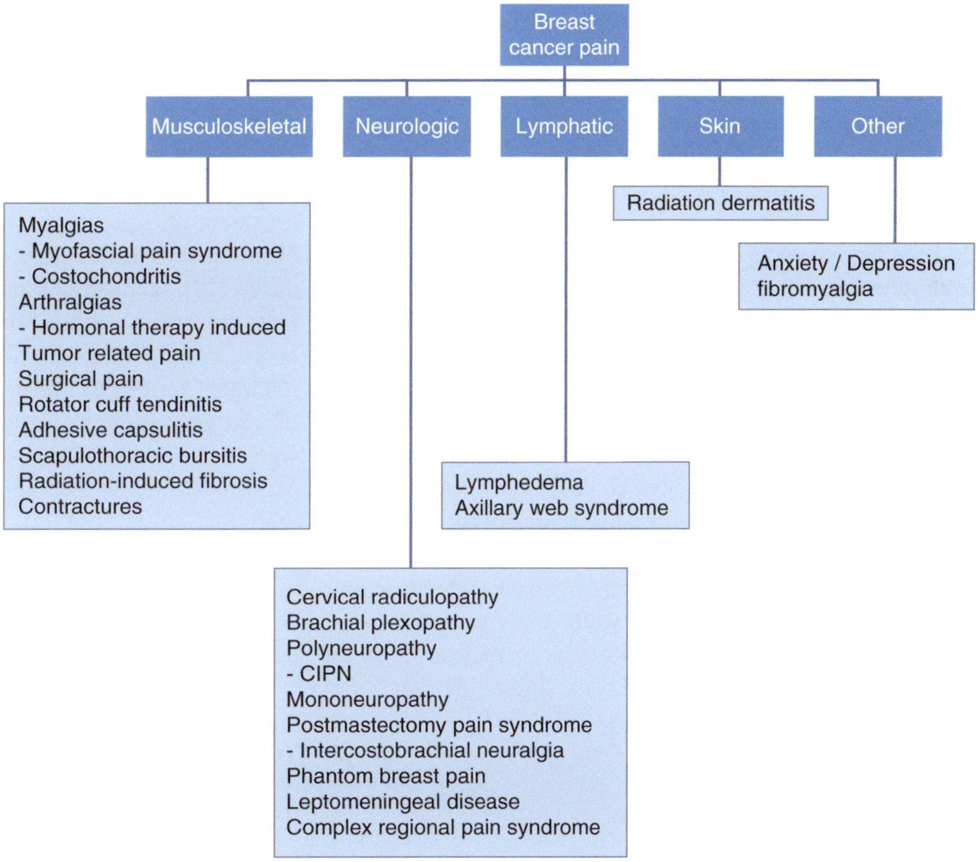

Fig. 9.3 Breast cancer pain by organ system

further detail. The shoulder can be affected by breast cancer and its treatment, and pain in this area can present as rotator cuff tendonitis, adhesive capsulitis, and scapulothoracic bursitis. It is also important to consider the role of radiation-induced fibrosis and contractures when evaluating pain syndromes relating to breast cancer.

Myofascial Pain Syndrome (MPS)

Myofascial trigger points (MTPs) are foci of taut skeletal muscle (i.e., localized muscle contractures), which occur at dysfunctional motor endplates, and lead to myofascial pain syndrome. These MTPs are hypersensitive, tender to palpation, and may be a generator of great discomfort and pain [20]. Symptoms may be associated with decreased range of motion, shoulder girdle stiffness, and regional pain [21]. It is hypothesized that the pathogenesis of MTPs is the result of noxious stimuli resulting in spontaneous discharges from the motor endplate, increased acetylcholine, leading to ischemia and subsequent inflammatory cascade (release of prostaglandin, bradykinin, capsaicin, serotonin, and histamine), causing peripheral and central sensitization [21, 22]. Continuous nociceptive stimuli may cause increased membrane excitability, reduced inhibition, and amplified signal at the spinal cord by deep afferent nociceptors connected to the dorsal horn, resulting in central sensitization. Patients with central sensitization complain of enhanced sensitivity, hyperalgesia, and allodynia [20, 23].

Breast cancer surgery leads to MPS through the ablation of the pectoral muscle and fascia, damage from intraoperative positioning, contractures from protective posturing, or fibrosis from radiation therapy and surgery [20, 21]. In a study of 116 women with breast cancer status post breast surgery, Lacomba et al. [20] found that 44.8% of these patients experienced MPS, primarily in the shoulder girdle (pectoralis major, serratus anterior, and upper trapezius). In patients with breast cancer, MPS typically occurs within the first 6 months following breast surgery [20]. Shin et al. [24] found that in breast cancer patients postmastectomy complaining of shoulder pain, ultrasound-guided trigger point injections of the subscapularis and/or pectoralis muscles were both diagnostic and efficacious in treatment of MTPs [24]. This study also found that treatment effects of trigger point injections were less in those patients where treatment was delayed, suggesting that early intervention may be beneficial [24].

Costochondritis

While the incidence of costochondritis and Tietze's syndrome is not well documented in breast cancer, it is something that is anecdotally observed in clinical practice. Costochondritis is characterized by inflammation at the costochondral junctions of ribs (typically ribs 2–5) or chondrosternal joints [25]. This process is typically self-limited, involves multiple rib levels, and is without swelling or erythema [25]. Symptoms include reproducible sharp, aching, pressure-like pain that is unilateral and aggravated by movement of the upper extremities and deep breathing [25]. Mainstay of treatment involves nonsteroidal anti-inflammatory drugs, heat, physical therapy, and local injection of corticosteroid plus local anesthetic for refractory cases [25]. Tietze's syndrome is a rarer pathology that also manifests as tenderness and pain at the parasternal joints; however, it is delineated from costochondritis by localized (second and third ribs) inflammation and swelling at the costal cartilage [26]. A study by Kamel and Kotob [26] found ultrasound-guided corticosteroid – local anesthetic injection is successful in the treatment of Tietze's syndrome, with lasting effects observed at 1 month [26].

Hormonal Therapy-Induced Arthralgias

In postmenopausal women with hormone-responsive breast cancer, aromatase inhibitors (anastrozole, letrozole, exemestane, etc.) are an effective class of medication for maintenance hormonal therapy [27]. Unfortunately, aromatase inhibitors are not without side effects; patients may suffer from arthralgias, osteoporosis, and fractures [27]. Among aromatase inhibitors, anastrozole appears to be associated with the highest rates of arthralgias, occurring in approximately 36% of patients, with an average onset of 14 months from initiation of treatment [27]. Interestingly, in those patients with previous chemotherapy, arthralgias present sooner and at a higher incidence [27]. One study found that in patients taking anastrozole, the mean onset until first painful arthralgic event is approximately 4 months [27]. It is postulated that aromatase inhibitors lead to painful arthralgias through the suppression of estrogen. Treatment of mild arthralgias typically involves weight loss, exercise, and lifestyle modifications [27]. Moderate to severe arthralgias are treated in a stepwise fashion with high-dose NSAIDs, co-codamol in instances where NSAIDs are contraindicated, NSAIDs plus codeine, or alternative endocrine breast cancer therapy (i.e., tamoxifen) [27]. Aromatase inhibitors also result in decreased bone mineral density, predisposing patients to fractures and pain [27].

Tumor-Related Pain

A full discussion of the ways in which direct tumor burden can affect the musculoskeletal system is outside the scope of this chapter; however, it is important to remember that the primary breast tumor itself and secondary metastases can directly impinge upon or infiltrate the muscles and bone, causing pain, instability, and loss of normal function [28–30].

The gold standard treatment for painful vertebral metastases is external beam radiation therapy [30, 31]. Although, other interventional pain procedures, such as local nerve blocks, radiofrequency ablation, and vertebroplasty, may also ameliorate pain [31, 32].

Surgical Pain

Insufficient acute postoperative pain management among breast surgery patients is one of the greatest predictors of chronic pain syndromes in this patient population [33, 34]. Surgical pain is likely influenced by the amount of tumor resection and surgical technique. Patients may be at lower risk for developing chronic pain following surgery if performed at a high-volume center as opposed to a low-volume center [35]. In the acute period of 1–3 years following breast cancer surgery, between 25% and 60% of patients experience pain, and between 20% and 80% experience sensory disturbances [8]. Interestingly, risk for chronic postoperative pain may also depend on whether or not breast reconstruction is performed. A survey by Wallace et al. [36] found that women who had breast reconstruction in addition to mastectomy experienced a higher incidence of pain at least 1 year postoperatively, as opposed to women who underwent mastectomy alone. In those who undergo breast augmentation, there does not appear to be a difference between the type of implant used, silicone versus saline, and pain [36].

Surgical therapy for breast cancer is typically divided into the mastectomy procedure and the lumpectomy procedure, also known as breast-conserving therapy. Radical mastectomy involves resection of the breast, skin and fat, pectoralis major and minor muscles, and all lymph nodes at the ipsilateral axilla [37]. The radical mastectomy has largely been replaced by the modified mastectomy. This procedure is identical to the radical mastectomy, except the pectoral muscles are spared [37]. Breast-conserving surgery or lumpectomy entails removal of the tumor with clear pathologic margins of normal tissue [37]. Variations of the lumpectomy include lumpectomy with axillary node dissection and lumpectomy with sentinel node biopsy [37]. The sentinel lymph node is the first node that receives lymphatic drainage from the breast. Dye or radio marker is injected into the tumor prior to surgery to identify this sentinel node, which is then removed and analyzed for pathology. Surgeons perform subsequent axillary dissection only in those patients with disease of the sentinel node as seen on pathologic analysis [37].

Many women choose to undergo breast reconstruction after initial surgical management of the disease. The process of breast reconstruction typically involves the placement of a tissue expander in the subpectoral space in order to create a potential space for implant placement [34]. Saline is injected through a port over the course of several weeks, and once the required volume is obtained, the temporary tissue expander is removed, and a permanent implant replaces it [34]. An autologous flap can also be used for reconstructive purposes in lieu of surgical implants [34]. Two of the more common flaps are the (1) transverse rectus abdominis myocutaneous flap (harvested from the anterior abdominal wall) and (2) latissimus dorsi myocutaneous flap (harvested from the back) [34]. During the later procedure, the harvested muscle flap is sutured to the inferomedial aspect of the detached pectoralis major muscle to ensure adequate coverage of the implant in order to prevent extrusion and potential complications [38].

The creation of a subpectoral cavity for breast implant placement during breast reconstruction surgery involves the separation of the serratus anterior muscle from its insertion on ribs 5–7 and dissection of the medial sternal border of the pectoralis major [34]. Local surgical trauma, stretching secondary to the expander, and spasms to the involved muscles (namely, the pectoralis major) are associated with nociceptive discomfort and pain in the acute phase following breast cancer surgery [34]. Nociceptive pain caused by local tissue damage is generally short-lived and resolves with the healing process [37]; however, this healing process may be delayed in the setting of chemotherapy and/or radiation therapy.

Rotator Cuff Tendonitis

Subacromial impingement syndrome, tendinitis, tendinosis, partial- and full-thickness tear of the rotator cuff, long-head biceps tendinitis/tendinosis, and subdeltoid bursitis are all diagnoses included under rotator cuff tendinopathy [39, 40]. Rotator cuff tendinopathy is an overuse condition that presents as pain around tendons of the shoulder [41]. The ability of the tendon to heal is limited by its avascular structure [39]. Failure to regenerate properly, i.e., tendon disorganization and thickening, leads to changes in physical properties, altered biomechanics, decreased tensile strength, diminished energy efficiency, and exacerbation of pain symptoms [41]. Interestingly, partial tears may be more painful than complete rotator cuff tears [42]. Similarly, bursal-side tears are often more painful than intratendinous tears [42].

The number of individuals that survive breast cancer continues to increase, and as this population rises, so does the prevalence of shoulder and arm pathology [6]. Prevalence of rotator cuff tendinopathy is estimated to be between 7.9% and 31% in the general population ages 40–69 years old; however, many of these cases are asymptomatic, as the incidence of rotator cuff disease increases with age [6, 43]. Breast cancer treatment places additional stress on the rotator cuff, likely increasing the number of symptomatic cases [6]. Incidence of rotator cuff tendinopathy in breast cancer is estimated to be between 6% and 30% [44].

Intrinsic factors leading to rotator cuff tendinopathy include degeneration, age, calcification, fibrovascular proliferation, overuse, and trauma [41]. Acutely, there can be hypovascularity of the rotator cuff tendons, leading to increased healing time [45]. Chronic rotator cuff tendinopathy is associated with neovascularization, which disrupts the extracellular matrix leading to weakness [45]. These changes in tendon morphology lead to increased shear forces and decreased elasticity, which contributes to rotator cuff tendinopathy [41].

Patients with rotator cuff tendinopathy complain of pain with overhead activities, particularly with the shoulder abducted greater than 90° [46]. On history and physical exam, patients demonstrate what is referred to as the "painful arc", or pain at the shoulder with abduction between 70° and 120°. Additional findings on history and physical exam include impaired shoulder function, weakness, pain, reduced range of motion, and stiffness [40, 41, 47, 48].

On imaging, excess fluid in the shoulder is indicative of a complete rupture of the rotator cuff and inconsistent with a partial tear [42]. Magnetic resonance imaging (MRI) and ultrasound (US) both have high accuracy in diagnosis of rotator cuff tears. A cadaveric study by Reilly et al. [50] found that the total prevalence of rotator cuff tears in asymptomatic patients to be 26% on MRI and 39% on US [50]. Treatment of breast cancer places further stressors on the already degenerated rotator cuff tendons, resulting in a higher incidence of symptomatic rotator cuff tendinopathy in the breast cancer population than would be expected for age [6].

Lymphedema, covered in further detail in the lymphatic system section, is present in more than 15% (and up to 56%) of breast cancer patients after treatment for breast cancer [51, 52]. Etiology of rotator cuff tendinopathy relating to lymphedema is thought to be secondary to a combination of factors including impingement of tendon fibers, functional overload, and intrinsic tendinopathy [53]. Lymphedema increases the limb weight, subsequently increasing the load placed upon the rotator cuff muscles and tendons, and potentially leading to excess stress and tendonitis [6, 53]. Studies have found atrophy and decreased muscle activity of the shoulder girdle muscles (i.e., pectoralis major, pectoralis minor, serratus anterior, upper trapezius, and rhomboid muscles) on the affected side of women with breast cancer, represented on CT and MRI as decreased muscle mass and on EMG as decreased muscle activity [54]. Weak rotator cuff and shoulder girdle musculature allows for abnormal glenohumeral movement, predisposes to rotator cuff impingement at the subacromial space, and causes subsequent pain [6]. In a similar mechanism, postsurgical pain can lead to learned disuse of the arm on the affected breast and protective posturing, resulting in shortening of the muscles of the anterior chest wall (namely, the pectorals), potentiating poor biomechanics, and pathology of the shoulder [6, 55].

Women with breast cancer demonstrate greater asymmetry of their resting shoulder girdle alignment as well as altered scapular motor patterns when compared to their aged-matched counterparts without breast cancer [56, 57]. Tightening of the anterior chest wall muscles, specifically the pectoralis major and minor, from surgery, protective posturing, postoperative pain, postoperative scar tissue formation, and fibrosis secondary to radiation results in a forward, depressed shoulder girdle [58]. Impaired resting alignment of the shoulder girdle creates an abnormal relationship between the humeral head and glenoid fossa. It also creates structural changes in the musculoskeletal tissues of the shoulder and decreased subacromial space, leading to altered shoulder girdle motion, degenerative changes, and subsequent pain and dysfunction of the rotator cuff muscles [59, 60]. A study comparing breast cancer survivors to healthy, matched controls by Harrington et al. [61] revealed that women with breast cancer have significantly decreased shoulder strength, decreased active and passive shoulder range of motion, and decreased shoulder function (as measured by the Disabilities of the Arm, Shoulder, and Hand (DASH) questionnaire and the Pennsylvania Shoulder Score (PSS)) [61].

Adhesive Capsulitis

In breast cancer patients, adhesive capsulitis is typically secondary to treatment effects, rotator cuff tendinopathy, and inflammatory changes [55, 62]. Treatment-related pain and fear of complications result in disuse and disincentive to move the affected shoulder [55]. A prospective cross-sectional study by Jeong et al. [63] analyzing shoulder pain in breast cancer patients with lymphedema discovered that adhesive capsulitis was present in 53% of patients [63].

The pathophysiology behind adhesive capsulitis is an inflammatory response leading to capsular fibrosis, contracture at the glenohumeral joint, reduction in the capsular volume, and resultant decreased glenohumeral movement [62]. Initial presentation of adhesive capsulitis is characterized as a painful shoulder accompanied by progressive loss of motion. The second phase of adhesive capsulitis is defined by decreased pain and marked stiffness. Treatment of adhesive capsulitis is performed in a stepwise manner with physiotherapy, steroid injections, manipulation under anesthesia (MUA), and arthroscopic capsular release [64].

In breast cancer patients with adhesive capsulitis, improvement of shoulder pain and range of motion is mainly dependent on the stage of cancer treatment [65]. Adhesive capsulitis is more prevalent in the acute and subacute phase following breast surgery. Patients are less likely to have adhesive capsulitis chronically as range of motion tends to improve as surgical pain dissipates [66]. Patients who have undergone mastectomy are at increased risk for developing adhesive capsulitis, and those who have undergone both mastectomy and reconstruction are at an even higher risk [67]. Radiation therapy may also be associated with the development of adhesive capsulitis, although more studies are needed to elucidate the dose at which this is more likely to occur [67]. A study by Hopwood et al. [68] found that approximately 20% of patients who had undergone radiation therapy after breast surgery experienced moderate to severe shoulder stiffness 5 years following breast surgery [68]. Multiple studies have found that radiation dose per fraction and duration of radiation treatment does not influence the extent of shoulder pain, stiffness, or range of motion in breast cancer patients with adhesive capsulitis [64, 68].

Scapulothoracic Bursitis

The scapulothoracic bursae lie between the scapula and the posterior aspect of ribs 2–7 and function to facilitate a smooth gliding movement throughout scapulothoracic articulation [69]. The two major or anatomic bursae are the infraserratus bursa (between the serratus anterior muscle and the chest wall) and the supraspinatus bursa (between the subscapularis and serratus anterior muscles). There are also four minor (or adventitial) bursa: two at the inferiormedial angle of the scapula, one at the inferior angle of the scapula, and the fourth at the trapezoid bursa, which may arise in response to abnormal biomechanics [69]. The precise mechanism through which scapulothoracic bursitis causes breast cancer pain is unknown, although it is hypothesized that it is due to abnormal scapular biomechanics resulting in inflammation of the scapulothoracic bursae and the adjacent T2–T7 intercostal nerves, which innervate the breast [70].

Symptoms include a history of overuse and a sense of fatigue before onset of symptoms. Physical exam may reveal crepitus, tenderness at the superior and medial aspect of the scapula between the second and seventh intercostal space, dyskinesis, decreased glenohumeral motion, scapular protrusion at the lateral border of the axilla, and enlarged bursa under ultrasound [69]. Focal muscle weakness or atrophy may also result in scapulothoracic bursitis from disuse or lesion of the long thoracic nerve resulting in scapular winging [69, 70]. A study by Boneti et al. [70] found that treatment of scapulothoracic bursitis with ultrasound-guided trigger point injections with local anesthetic and corticosteroid completely resolved pain symptoms within 15 minutes in the majority (86%) of patients [70]. Trigger point injections may be used for both diagnostic and short-term treatment of scapulothoracic bursitis [69].

Radiation-Induced Fibrosis

Radiation therapy results in acute tissue injury through DNA damage and the generation of reactive oxygen species, leading to cell damage, which induces an inflammatory response, followed by fibroblast recruitment and deposition of extracellular matrix [71]. Approximately 50% of patients with breast cancer undergo breast-conserving therapy; these individuals usually then obtain postoperative radiation treatment to the contralateral breast in addition to boost radiation at the lumpectomy site [72]. A study by Liss et al. [73] found that approximately 22% of women developed fair/poor cosmesis at a median follow-up of 2.5 years following breast irradiation [73]. Following radiation therapy, approximately 1/3 of breast cancer patients suffer from shoulder and arm pain at 5 years after treatment [68]; however, this statistic likely overestimates the incidence by encompassing other breast cancer-related pain.

The extent of radiation-induced fibrosis directly correlates with the total dose of radiotherapy, dose per fraction of radiotherapy (i.e., worse with hypofractionation), and increased field size [71]. A recent study by Bourgier et al. [74] revealed that although there is no statistical significant increase in the incidence of fibrosis between 40 Gy and 42 Gy divided in 10 twice-daily fractions, there is significantly more breast pain in the patients dosed with 42 Gy at 18 months [74]. Ataxia-telangiectasia mutated (ATM) gene has been found to be a genetic risk factor for radiation-induced fibrosis [75].

Radiation-induced fibrosis occurs between 4 and 12 months after radiation therapy and develops over years [71]. Typically radiation-induced fibrosis stabilizes after approximately 2 years [76]. Clinical signs and symptoms include skin induration and thickening, skin retraction, muscle shortening and atrophy, decreased tissue compliance, joint hypomobility, mucosal fibrosis, secondary functional limitation, and pain. More severe symptoms include lymphedema, ulceration, fistula, cervical plexopathy, brachial plexopathy, interstitial fibrosis, dyspnea, and decreased lung compliance [71, 72].

In patients with breast cancer complicated by radiation-induced fibrosis, pentoxifylline, an anti-inflammatory, and vitamin E, an antioxidant, have been shown to improve tissue compliance of the affected areas [77]. Physical therapy using the LPG Systems mechanical massage technique is shown to reduce pain symptoms and induce skin softening in cutaneous breast tissue of women with radiation-induced fibrosis [78]. Botulinum toxin injection may be effective at decreasing spasms and pain as a consequence of radiation-induced fibrosis, specifically in those with radiation-induced cervical dystonia [79]. Conservative treatment may be insufficient, and some patients require more aggressive management with surgical resection. Surgical resection is indicated for improved quality of life in patients with significant pain and functional limitations secondary to radiation-induced fibrosis refractory to conservative treatment [72].

Contractures

Once breast implants are placed, patients may suffer from a phenomenon known as post-augmentation breast pain [80]. The most common cause of post-augmentation breast pain is capsular contracture; thought to be an inflammatory reaction to foreign body, resulting in excess fibrosis [80]. While some fibrosis is desired to anchor the implant to the chest wall, too much fibrosis can be pathologic and potentially painful causing compression of the medial and lateral pectoral nerves posterior to the pectoral muscles [34, 80]. Level of contracture is described by the Baker classification scale I-IV, of which levels III-IV are clinically significant and symptomatic. Incidence of contracture is roughly 3–20% in the general population following breast augmentation [80]. Less commonly, the thoracodorsal nerve may become incidentally injured during latissimus dorsi flap harvesting for subpectoral implant, resulting in discomfort and spams of the latissimus dorsi muscle [38]. Possible treatments include intraoperative removal of the thoracodorsal nerve [38].

Chemodenervation via botulinum toxin (i.e., Botox) injection is a novel treatment that has been suggested in the treatment of acute pain associated with pectoral major spasms and contracture [81, 82]. In refractory cases, pectoral neurectomy has been shown to improve symptoms with variable success [38, 81]. Botox and neurectomy for treatment of breast cancer pain will be discussed later in the treatment sections.

Nervous System

Neurologic injury in breast cancer results from either direct tumor compression, lymphedema, cancer treatment (radiation-induced neuropathy and chemotherapy-induced neuropathy), paraneoplastic syndromes, and nerve damage or sacrifice during surgery [21]. Although rare, traction during surgery may result in brachial plexus injury [83]. While nociceptive pain typically resolves as damaged tissue heals, neuropathic pain may persist indefinitely. Treatment of a solid breast cancer tumor involving a nerve generally relies on radiation therapy and/or chemotherapy with or without addition of nerve-stabilizing agent (i.e., gabapentin) [21]. Primary tumor burden from breast cancer can directly impinge upon spinal cord, cervical nerve roots, brachial plexus, and peripheral nerves.

Cervical Radiculopathy

A study out of Rochester, Minnesota, found that the annual incidence rates of cervical radiculopathy per 100,000 people are reported to be 107.3 for men and 63.5 for women [84]. Anatomically, cervical radiculopathy results from dysfunction of the cervical nerve roots and commonly presents as neck pain, upper extremity pain, upper extremity paresthesias, and upper extremity weakness in patients with breast cancer [55]. Physical therapy, nonsteroidal anti-inflammatory medications, and anti-neuropathic medications (such as gabapentin) are used for conservative treatment, while epidural steroid injections via fluoroscopic guidance are typically reserved for those patients with more severe pain and weakness. Though similar treatments may work for patients with cervical radicular pain due to neoplasm (malignant radiculopathy), chemotherapy, radiation therapy, and surgery are the primary treatment modalities in order to reduce tumor size or remove compressive forces [55, 65].

Brachial Plexopathy

Brachial plexopathies are rare in the general population and less likely to present in the acute phase of breast cancer, unless the disease is advanced. In patients with breast cancer, brachial plexopathies are more likely the result of metastatic tumor involvement or breast cancer-related treatment (chemotherapy and radiation therapy) and present months to years from time of initial diagnosis/treatment [65]. Treatment of brachial plexopathies involves decreasing tumor mass effect through chemotherapy, radiation, and/or surgery. Symptoms are managed with a combination of physical therapy, NSAIDs, and nerve-stabilizing agents [65].

Horner's syndrome is another rare phenomenon that may occur in conjunction with a cervical radiculopathy due to injury of the sympathetic chain. Damage to the sympathetic chain is likely to be first order (central), lesions occur at the level of the cervical spinal cord between C8 and T2, or second-order (preganglionic) – lesions occur at the brachial plexus and neck. The classic triad of findings includes ipsilateral ptosis, anhidrosis, and miosis [85, 86].

Polyneuropathies

The most common classes of chemotherapy agents causing peripheral neuropathy are the platinum drugs (especially cisplatin and oxaliplatin), the taxanes (i.e., paclitaxel), vinca alkaloids, and bortezomib [87]. Taxanes and platinum-based drugs are more commonly used to treat breast cancer; however, these agents typically result in paresthesias and decreased sensation, not pain [87]. Preexisting neuropathies, such as diabetic neuropathy, place patients at increased risk for the development of neuropathic pain [88]. Pre-treatment with various agents has been suggested to mitigate the harsh neurotoxic effects of chemotherapy, e.g., magnesium, calcium, amifostine, vitamin E, glutathione, omega-3 fatty acids, cannabinoids, erythropoietin, and carbamazepine/oxcarbazepine. Unfortunately, randomized placebo-controlled, double-blinded clinical trials have not yielded significant results in favor of these agents [89–95].

Radiation-Induced Brachial Plexopathy

Radiation therapy is the standard of care following breast-conserving surgeries. Radiation-induced neuropathy is the result of ischemia secondary to microvascular damage, radiation-induced fibrosis, culminating in local nerve damage (direct axonal injury and demyelination) [96]. The incidence of radiation-induced brachial plexopathy (RIBP) is approximately <1–2% in patients receiving total doses <55 Gy at the plexus [96]. Large total radiation doses of >50 cGy to the plexus or large dose per fraction >2.5 cGy stereotactic radiosurgery are commonly associated with radiation-induced neuropathy [96].

Symptomatic progression of RIBP transitions from initial paresthesia or dysesthesia, which subsequently diminishes, to hypoesthesia followed by anesthesia [96]. Neuropathic pain, while more rare, does occur after failure of neurolysis [96]. Symptoms tend to start distally (emulating a carpal tunnel syndrome) and spread proximally. The majority of RIBP is known as a delayed progressive type; onset is insidious, occurring over months to years. Often symptoms are progressive and may lead to limb paralysis [96].

Diagnosis of radiation-induced neuropathy is based on clinical symptoms, namely, symptoms in the previous radiation field of numbness, tingling, burning or electrical sensations, weakness, atrophy, and fibrosis. Diagnosis can be further supported by electroneuromyography (EMG) and magnetic resonance imaging (MRI) [96]. EMG is instrumental in identifying the level of nerve injury at the root, plexus, or periphery [96]. Specifically, the presence of myokymic discharges on EMG is highly suggestive of radiation-induced nerve damage [96]. MRI is the primary diagnostic means to rule out a direct compressive neuropathy from tumor involvement and may also help further characterize fibrotic involvement.

Mononeuropathies

The most common upper extremity compression mononeuropathy is carpal tunnel syndrome (CTS), or entrapment of the median nerve at the level of the wrist [55, 97]. It has been suggested that lymphedema may lead to mononeuropathies, among them carpal tunnel syndrome (CTS); however, the data to support this claim is lacking [98]. Positive physical exam maneuvers in patients with CTS include Phalen's and Tinel's [99]. The current treatment guidelines from the European HANDGUIDE Study, established by therapists, physiatrists, and hand surgeons, suggest that splinting, corticosteroid injection, corticosteroid injections plus splinting, and surgery are all suitable treatment modalities for CTS [100].

Intercostobrachial Neuralgia (Postmastectomy Pain Syndrome)

During mastectomy the intercostobrachial nerve is often sacrificed, and it is often difficult to preserve the nerve during axillary dissection. A lesion to the intercostobrachial nerve may result in "hyposensitivity" and/or "hypersensitivity" [18]. Hyposensitivity is characterized as decreased nerve function, i.e., numbness, diminished sensation, or hypoesthesia, and hypersensitivity is characterized as pain, allodynia, dysesthesia, hyperesthesia, and paresthesias [18]. Intercostobrachial neuralgia (ICN) may present clinically as ipsilateral pain localized to the axilla, medial upper arm, and/or the anterior chest wall [37].

Neural blockade is instrumental in the diagnosis of specific nerves involved in neuropathic pain syndromes [19]; however, at this time, there is not a study specifically analyzing intercostobrachial nerve blocks with regard to ICN. Anticonvulsant medications such as gabapentin and pregabalin are efficacious in alleviating hyperalgesia and allodynia caused by neuropathic pain [7, 21]. Studies have shown that preoperative gabapentin results in a significant decrease in postoperative morphine consumption and movement-related pain [101].

Phantom Breast Pain

Phantom breast pain is the sensation of pain in the breast that is no longer there, not to be confused with a *non-painful* sensation of the breast that is no longer present [37]. It is often difficult for patients to quantify or describe symptoms of phantom breast pain [102]. Spatially it is difficult for patients to identify the location of the source of their pain [102], although the majority complain of pain at the entire breast [103]. An early study by Polinsky et al. [104] surveyed women after mastectomy for breast cancer and found that roughly 36% of women experienced phantom breast pain [104]. A prospective pilot study performed by Björkman et al. [102] followed 8 women status postmastectomy of which 50% experienced phantom breast pain. The study by Björkman et al. [102] also found that those with an absence of phantom breast pain in the initial month postoperatively were not likely to develop phantom breast pain in the coming months and years [102]. Later, Ahmed et al. [51] performed a larger prospective study of 80 patients undergoing modified radical mastectomy followed at 6 weeks, 6 months, and 12 months. The research found that phantom breast pain incidence increases from 5.4% to 13.6% at 6 weeks postoperatively as compared to 12 months postoperatively [103]. This most recent study suggests that phantom breast pain is less common than phantom limb pain, which has an incidence of approximately 59–85% [105].

Leptomeningeal Disease

Although leptomeningeal metastases (LM) may occur with any malignancy, it is most commonly seen in patients with breast cancer, with the incidence estimated between 1% and 8% [106]. Treatment of breast cancer LM is primarily focal radiotherapy to tumor burden or symptomatic areas [107]. Additional treatment options for breast cancer LM include intracerebrospinal fluid, intravenous, and oral chemotherapy [107]. Pain symptoms are primarily mitigated with radiotherapy, while chemotherapy is utilized to prolong survival [107, 108].

Complex Regional Pain Syndrome of the Breast

Complex regional pain syndrome (CRPS) of the breast is rare and has been reported only anecdotally as case reports in the literature. One case involved a 27-year-old woman who developed many symptoms consistent with CRPS after breast reduction, including breast swelling, burning pain, allodynia, temperature-related changes, skin changes, and reduced range of motion in her shoulder and upper arm. Of note, she had not been treated for breast cancer but, rather, had a modified radical mastectomy for macromastia [109]. She had symptomatic improvement with stellate ganglion block, which will be discussed below [109]. Another case series reported two women who had mastectomy for chronic mastalgia and subsequently developed CRPS of the upper extremity [110]. To our knowledge, only one case involving CRPS and breast cancer has been reported – that of a 24-year-old female who developed CRPS of her upper extremity after axillary node dissection [111]. She experienced dramatic improvement with physical therapy and stellate ganglion block [111].

Neuroma Pain

A traumatic neuroma is a reactive hyperplasia of nerve tissue. Traumatic neuromas can be divided into two groups: spindle neuromas and terminal neuromas. Spindle neuromas occur in intact nerves and are the result of repeated friction or irritation, and terminal neuromas occur in severed nerves and are located at the proximal end of said nerve [112]. Breast surgery, whether it is a mastectomy or lumpectomy, predisposes patients to scar tissue formation and thus neuromas and chronic pain [37]. Interestingly, studies have found that there is a lower incidence of neuromas in patients who undergo total mastectomy when compared to those treated with lumpectomy, axillary dissection, and radiotherapy [37]. Incidence of neuromas following breast cancer surgery is approximated to be anywhere from 23% to 49% [37]. Sensation to the breast and nipple is provided by the cutaneous branches of the anterior and lateral intercostal nerves [113]. The lateral zone of the breast accounts for nearly 80% of intercostal neuromas [37].

A thorough history reveals a pain localized to a specific point, sharp or stabbing in quality, occasionally associated with burning, paresthesias, and numbness. Physical exam is able to reproduce the pain localized over a point of maximal tenderness with (macroneuroma) or without (microneuroma) a palpable mass [37, 113, 114].

Ultrasound may be used to identify neuromas; they appear as a fusiform mass or enlargement, and terminal neuromas are distinct because of the presence of a bulbous end [115]. A local anesthetic peripheral nerve block with a 1:1 ratio of lidocaine 1% and 0.5% bupivacaine injection to the point of maximal tenderness with resolution of pain symptoms is diagnostic of a neuroma and suggests that a patient is a good surgical candidate for resection [113, 114]. Patients that fail conservative treatment have good outcomes with surgical intervention involving neuroma excision, nerve graft, and relocation of nerve to a more protected site buried beneath muscle to prevent reoccurrence and promote regeneration [113, 116].

In our practice, separating pain anatomically by location at the same times as making diagnostic decisions related to cause has allowed us to help guide treatments. Figure 9.4 below depicts some of the anatomical distribution of the pain syndromes.

Lymphatic System

Lymphedema

Lymphedema occurs when the transport capacity of the lymphatic system is unable to accommodate the lymphatic load [117]. Secondary lymphedema of breast cancer results from disease-related factors, such as disruption of lymphatic system from local tumor invasion and number of nodes involved, and treatment-related factors, such as surgery, chemotherapy, and/or radiotherapy [51]. As a result of the aforementioned factors, there is lymph stasis, the accumulation of proteins and cellular metabolites, thus raising the tissue colloid osmotic pressure and leading to accumulation of fluid in the interstitial space [51, 55]. Lymphedema effects roughly 15% of patients with breast cancer [52].

A leading risk factor for the development of lymphedema is surgery – specifically radical mastectomy (where the entire axillary lymph nodes are removed), modified radical mastectomy (only part of the axillary lymph nodes are removed), and lymph node dissection [117]. Another risk factor for developing lymphedema is radiation, which may result in fibrosis, impeding lymph transport, and interfering with

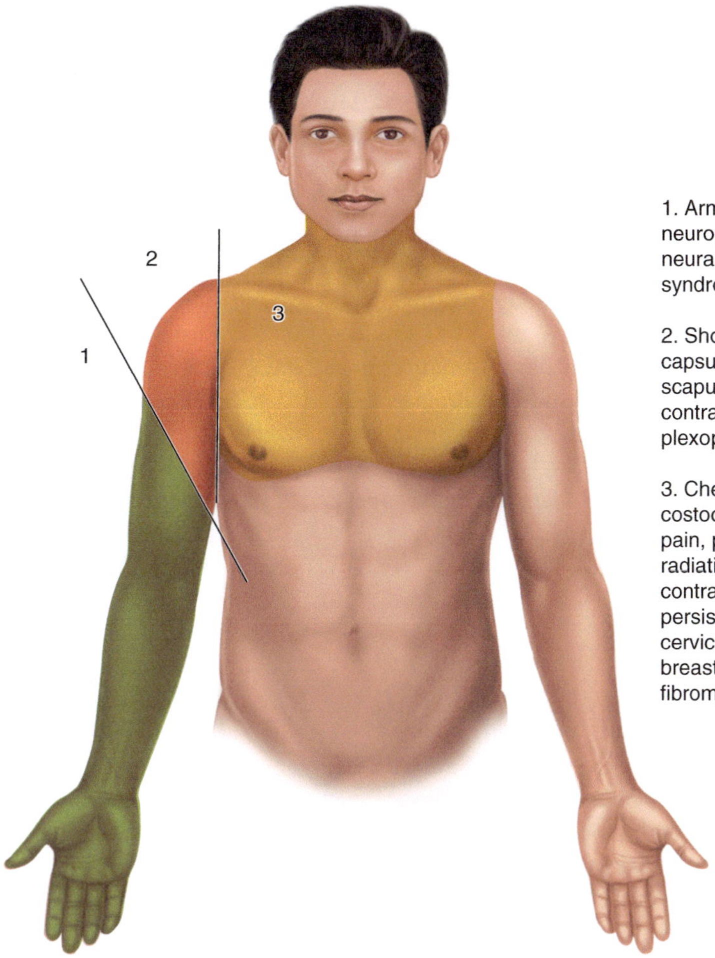

Fig. 9.4 Pain syndromes by anatomic location

lymph tissue regeneration [117]. It is hypothesized that radiation causes endothelial damage, dysregulation of the repair pathway (via TGF-β and endoglin), and macrophage infiltration all resulting in microvascular damage, tissue ischemia, and subsequent lymphatic damage [118].

Review of the literature defines lymphedema as a greater than 2 cm difference in circumference, greater than 200 ml difference in volume, or a greater than 3–10% difference in circumference or volume [52]. Physically, patients with lymphedema suffer from decreased functionality, specifically reduced elbow flexion and grip strength as well as decreased range of motion during shoulder abduction, resulting in impaired ability to complete activities of daily living (ADL) and independent activities of daily living (iADL) [51, 52]. As discussed earlier in this chapter, increased limb weight from lymphedema may result in subsequent abnormal biomechanics, leading to pathology, such as rotator cuff tendinopathy, shoulder impingement, adhesive capsulitis, etc. [6, 53].

Conservative treatment of lymphedema in breast cancer patients involves complete decongestive lymphatic therapy (DLT) with an "intense phase" – manual lymphatic drainage (MLD), compression dressings/gloves, and physical therapy to maximize functional ability and restore lymphatic circulation – and a "self-management phase" [117]. Intermittent pneumatic compression devices (PCDs) may also alleviate edema and symptoms; however, a recent meta-analysis performed in 2014 revealed that PCD as an adjunct to DLT is no more effective than DLT alone [119]. Oral pharmaceuticals are also used in lymphedema management; the most studied drugs are Cyclo-Fort, Daflon, 5–6 benzo-a-pyrone, and coumarin [120]. Low-level laser therapy (LLLT) is used for the treatment of secondary lymphedema in breast cancer patients; it is thought to work by decreasing fibrosis, stimulating lymphangiogenesis, and increasing overall lymphatic flow [121]. Surgical interventions such as lymphaticovenous anastomosis (LVA) and autologous lymph node transplantation (ALNT) are also available in the symptomatic treatment of lymphedema [122, 123].

Axillary Web Syndrome

Axillary web syndrome (AWS) is defined as a web of axillary skin overlying palpable cords of tissue, which are visible. Active range of motion of the shoulder into abduction results in tautening of this rope-like tissue and pain [124]. Symptoms of AWS are axillary pain radiating down the medial aspect of the arm to the elbow, occasionally extending along the ulnar aspect of the distal forearm and hand [125]. Associated symptoms include a subjective feeling of "tightness" and restricted range of motion at the shoulder [124]. The onset of AWS is typically within 3 months (mean 2 weeks) postoperatively following axillary surgery [125]. Treatment of AWS generally involves education, physiotherapy (myofascial release techniques, scar massage, manual lymphatic drainage), and pharmacologic agents (NSAIDs) [124].

Integumentary System

Radiation Dermatitis

The National Cancer Institute defines radiation-induced dermatitis (RID) as a "cutaneous inflammatory reaction occurring as a result of exposure to biologically effective levels of ionizing radiation" [126]. Irradiation of normal tissue may result in severe skin reactions, which may be painful and places the patient at increased risk for infection (e.g., *Staphylococcus aureus*) and fibrosis [127]. RID is influenced by the total dose, dose/fractionation, type and quality of the beam, volume, and total surface area exposed [128]. Overall RID may lead to significant discomfort, pain, and impaired quality of life. RID is one of the most common side effects of receiving radiotherapy, affecting up to 90% of patients [129, 130]. Acute changes are typically observed within 90 days from radiation exposure [128].

When referring to radiation-induced complications (tolerance of normal tissue to radiation therapy), tolerance doses (TDs) are utilized to calculate the risk of complication within a certain time frame [131]. For example, TD 5/5 refers to the probability of a 5% complication rate within 5 years from treatment, and TD 50/5 thus denotes the probability of 50% complication within 5 years [131]. Studies have found that radiation-induced complications are area dependent, and in the skin this is quantified in centimeters squared [131]. Skin necrosis in a 30 cm^2 field is seen at TD 3/5 of roughly 5700 cGy, and in a 10 cm^2 field, the TD 3/5 is about 6900 cGy [131]. Clinical myositis is seen at TD 1/5 of 5000 cGy with an incidence of roughly 1–5% [131].

Interestingly, the literature suggests that increased fraction size has a larger impact on late effects rather than acute effects (i.e., dermatitis) of radiotherapy [132]. Jagsi et al. found conventionally fractionated whole-breast radiotherapy had significantly higher incidence of grade ≥2 dermatitis, 62.6% vs. 27.4%, as well as a higher incidence of self-reported breast pain, moderate/severe pain, 41.1% vs. 24.2, compared to those treated with hypofractionation, 8–210 days post-radiotherapy [132]. A study by Shaitelman et al. found similar results when comparing conventionally fractionated whole-breast irradiation versus hypofractionated whole-breast irradiation, an increased incidence of acute dermatitis (36% vs. 69%) and breast pain (55% vs. 74%) [133].

Conservative management techniques for RID include the use of prophylactic in aqueous creams, natural topical agents (aloe vera and vitamin E), corticosteroid, topical acid (hyaluronic acid), and soap [134]. Bathing and washing with soap should be encouraged; studies suggest with varying results that patients who wash the irradiated skin sites may be less likely to experience erythema and desquamation [134]. Data does not support the use of topical corticosteroids for the treatment of pruritus and burning secondary to RID, and there is actually increased risk for potential thinning of the skin due to fat necrosis [134].

Treatment

The treatment options for pain relating to breast cancer may be conceptualized as conservative, namely, physical therapy and medical management, and interventional. Strategies for prevention of pain relating to breast cancer, particularly surrounding surgical interventions, are also being actively investigated and are briefly discussed below.

Conservative Treatment

Physical Therapy

Physical therapy as a treatment modality is grossly underutilized. A study by Cheville et al. [58] reported that among women with metastatic breast cancer, 90% would benefit from some form of therapy; however, only 30% receive said therapy [135]. Therapeutic ultrasound is commonly used in rehabilitation, however this modality should be avoided over areas of known or suspected malignancy, given potential risk for increased tumor burden or metastasis [136, 137].

Medication Management

The use of various medications for management of pain relating to breast cancer and its treatment has been a mainstay for many years. Multiple classes of medications have been utilized, including anti-epileptic medications such as gabapentin and pregabalin, sodium channel blockers like mexiletine, and antidepressant medications including venlafaxine and amitriptyline [35, 138, 139]. Ketamine and lidocaine infusions have also been utilized as preventative strategies and for treatment of chronic pain [138, 139]. Opioid medications continue to be frequently utilized for pain relating to malignancy, including breast cancer [140, 141].

Preventative Strategies

The utilization of a perioperative lidocaine infusion, administered initially as a bolus of 1.5 mg/kg and infused at 2 mg/kg/h until 2 h after arrival in the post-anesthesia care unit, has been shown to be associated with a 20-fold decrease in the incidence of chronic postsurgical pain in women undergoing mastectomy for breast cancer [142]. Additionally, the use of gabapentin or mexiletine in the perioperative period has been shown to be associated with a 50% decrease in the use of traditional analgesic medications in the first 10 days postoperatively and a reduction in the incidence of burning pain at 3 months postoperatively [143]. Venlafaxine, administered the evening before surgery and continued for 10 days, has been shown to be equipotent to gabapentin in reducing analgesic requirements post-surgery and significantly reduced the incidence of postmastectomy pain syndrome at 6 months post-surgery for breast cancer [144]. Multimodal analgesia using a combination of perioperative gabapentin, EMLA cream, and intraoperative irrigation of the brachial plexus and third, fourth, and fifth intercostal spaces with local anesthetic, significantly reduced analgesic consumption after surgery and the development of chronic pain at 3 months postsurgery for breast cancer [145].

Trigger Point Injections

Trigger point injection remains a commonly used technique for myofascial pain. Multiple different substances can be injected, including local anesthetics, botulinum toxin, sterile water, sterile saline, or dry needling [22]. A recent pilot study examining the use of ultrasound-guided trigger points in the subscapularis and pectoralis muscles in patients postmastectomy, found good immediate improvement in pain scores which lasted up to 3 months [24]. Although not specifically looking at patients with breast cancer, a recent meta-analysis found statistically significant improvement in pain scores in patients with myofascial pain treated with dry needling as compared to placebo in the short (immediate to 3 days) and medium term (9–28 days), but no effect in the long term (2–6 months) [146]. Data pooled from six studies found that wet needling, or trigger point injections with medication injected, was more effective than dry needling in the medium and long term for neck and shoulder pain [146].

Interventional Treatment Options

High-quality data assessing these interventions for the use of chronic pain posttreatment for breast cancer is, unfortunately, limited, and a recent systematic review found only seven studies assessing three targets: paravertebral blockade, stellate ganglion blockade, and intercostal neural blockade [19].

Suprascapular Nerve Block

It is estimated that the suprascapular nerve innervates 70% of the shoulder area, including the superior and posterior regions of the shoulder joint capsule and the acromioclavicular joint [147]. Suprascapular nerve blocks (SSNB) may be used for diagnostic and therapeutic pain relief of the shoulder with immediate onset and a relatively good safety profile [147–149]. SSNB is used to treat pain in several pathologies including adhesive capsulitis, rotator cuff tendinopathy, scapular fracture, and glenohumeral arthritis [17, 148, 150, 151]. When compared to intra-articular shoulder injections, SSNB have been found to provide significantly better pain relief at 12 weeks for the treatment of adhesive capsulitis [150]. When comparing the efficacy of physical therapy alone versus physical therapy plus prilocaine-triamcinolone SSNB, evidence suggests that there are both greater pain relief (measured using the Brief Pain Inventory-Short Form) and improved function (measured using the Constant Shoulder Scale) in SSNB treatment group [147]. Based on review of the literature, SSNB is a good short-term adjunct treatment option to facilitate painless range of motion during physical therapy.

Serratus Anterior Block

Another potential target for an interventional procedure for chronic pain after treatment for breast cancer is the serratus plane. The serratus plane block is a novel, ultrasound-guided nerve block which is able to anesthetize the hemithorax [152]. Anatomically, there are two different potential spaces, one superficial and one deep, which surround the serratus anterior muscle on the chest wall [152]. Local anesthetic and steroid may be deposited under ultrasound guidance into either of these spaces as treatment for chronic pain relating to breast cancer, although further high-quality studies investigating this technique are needed.

Paravertebral Blockade

A thoracic paravertebral block is a technique in which local anesthetic is targeted toward the thoracic spinal nerves as they emerge from the intervertebral foramen, in the paravertebral space. It is often conceptualized as a unilateral epidural anesthetic block in terms of the resulting ipsilateral somatic and sympathetic neural blockade. The paravertebral block can be performed either using landmarks or an ultrasound-guided technique [153, 154].

Paravertebral blockade has been shown to provide significant immediate postoperative analgesia after breast cancer surgery, with significantly less consumption of opioid medication [155]. Additionally, at 1-year follow-up, preoperative paravertebral blockade was associated with reduced prevalence and severity of pain symptoms [156]. Intruigingly, a retrospective, observational study suggests that there may be an association between lower frequency of breast cancer recurrence or metastases in those patients who receive preoperative paravertebral blockade prior to surgery for breast cancer [157]. A study by Kirvelä et al. [158] revealed that although initial pain relief from paravertebral blockade with 0.5% bupivacaine was very successful at 99% effective, only 12% had pain relief that lasted longer than 1 month. In this study, 20% of patients were pain-free after 5 months, but interpretation of this study is limited by inconsistent number of blocks per patient, lack of control, and insufficient blinding [158].

Stellate Ganglion Blockade

Cervical sympathetic blocks have typically been utilized for patients with complex regional pain syndrome of the upper extremities [159, 160]. This target has been investigated for the treatment of chronic pain relating to treatment for breast cancer. Of the two stellate ganglion blockade studies included in a recent systematic review of interventions for pain related to treatment for breast cancer, both showed statistically significant reduction in pain scores for up to 3 months after the procedure. However, in one study, gabapentin provided better pain relief in terms of numerical rating score as compared to the stellate ganglion block. These studies are relatively low quality and lack appropriate control groups or blinding of investigators [161, 162]. With regard to other chronic issues relating to treatment for breast cancer, a recent study investigating the use of stellate ganglion block for lymphedema found that 1 month after the last of three consecutive stellate ganglion blocks, forearm and upper arm circumferences were decreased significantly from baseline [163].

Intercostal Nerve Blockade

The intercostal nerve block procedure produces segmental anesthesia at the chosen levels in a band. Anatomically, the intercostal nerve lies inferiorly to the intercostal artery and vein on the inferior aspect of the rib. Cephalad-caudad spread of the anesthetic is much less common than with paravertebral blockade [164].

With regard to the utility of the intercostal nerve block for chronic pain relating to treatment for breast cancer, four intercostal nerve block studies performed in case series were included in a systematic review [19]. Fifty-three percent of patients had complete pain relief from local anesthetic blockade. All studies used this diagnostic block to aid the course of further treatment, either surgery or neurolysis. Unfortunately, none of these studies evaluated long-term effectiveness of the intercostal nerve block as a sole therapeutic option. Of note, surgical treatment was for resection of intercostal neuroma or relief of intercostal nerve entrapment [113, 165].

Pulsed Radiofrequency of Dorsal Root Ganglia

In consideration of the treatment of chronic pain relating to treatment of breast cancer, a retrospective study attempted to examine the utility of pulsed radiofrequency of the dorsal root ganglia. 49 patients were examined, 22.2% of whom had pain relating to mastectomy. This study also examined patients who had received pulsed radiofrequency therapy to the intercostal nerves. At 3 months, success, defined as greater than 50% pain relief, was significantly greater in the group of patients treated with radiofrequency to the dorsal root ganglion (53.8%) as compared to medication management alone or pulsed radiofrequency therapy to the intercostal nerves [166].

Pecs Block

These procedures include the "Pecs block" and the "modified Pecs block." Initially described by Blanco, the aim of the Pecs block is to place local anesthetic in the interfascial plane between the pectoralis major and minor muscles. His initial report of approximately 50 patients found minimal analgesic requirements postoperatively when this technique was used for breast surgery [167]. Blanco et al. later described a "modified Pecs block" also known as the "Pecs block type II." This procedure requires two needle approaches, the first to infiltrate between the pectoralis muscles and the second between the pectoralis minor and serratus anterior muscle. This approach attempts to block the axilla and intercostal nerves [168]. In a comparison of 60 patients undergoing breast surgery who either received a Pecs block or paravertebral block, the time for first request for morphine was significantly longer in the Pecs group, morphine consumption was lower at 24 h, and intensity of pain was lower in the first 12 h when compared to the paravertebral block group. However, pain intensity at 24 h was lower in the group of patients who received paravertebral block as compared to the Pecs block group [169].

Chemodenervation

Tumor resection for treatment of breast cancer, breast reconstruction therapy, and radiation therapy all may cause painful muscle spasms refractory to conservative measures and may require interventional treatment. Myospasms of the pectoralis major and minor muscles are frequently reported and may also be associated with cosmetic complications – i.e., high-riding implants. Studies have shown that intraoperative or postoperative botulinum toxin injection to the pectoral muscles is effective at decreasing muscle tone/spasms, resulting in decreased pain, while expediting recovery, and allowing for improved cosmetics [38, 82, 170, 171].

In order to inject into the pectoralis major, the needle is inserted into the anterior axillary fold. If the needle is advanced too dorsal, it will be in the coracobrachialis muscle, and if inserted too laterally, it will be in the biceps. EMG may be used to confirm needle placement in the pectoralis major muscles by asking the patient to perform horizontal adduction of the arm [172]. Insertion of the needle at the midclavicular line, deep to the pectoralis major, and anterior to the surface of the third rib provides ideal position for injection into the pectoralis minor. If the needle is superficial, injection will be into the pectoralis major. Ultrasound may also be used for safety to guide the needle to correct positioning [173]. Risks specific to this procedure include respiratory depression and pneumothorax given proximity to the pleural space [82].

In 2000, a case report by Senior and Fourie found that in patients developing tethering status post-breast augmentation, intraoperative injection of 100 units of Botox in a fanlike fashion to the muscle belly and tendon resulted in improved cosmetic appearance at 6 months [174]. In 2009, a study by Figus et al. found that 18.3% of patients who underwent breast reconstruction using latissimus dorsi flap plus subpectoral implants experienced discomfort secondary to involuntary contraction of the latissimus dorsi muscle and the visible contraction of the pectoral muscle [38]. Subsequent injection of botulinum toxin 100 units to the reconstructed breast resulted in significantly improved cosmetic appearance and reduced muscular tone, spasm, and pain, as soon as 14 days and as far out as 12 months [38]. A case study by Adkinson et al. [81] found that intraoperative injection of botulinum toxin 100 units resulted in relief of pain symptoms and improved cosmetic appearance immediately at 1 month post-procedurally with continued effects observed at 3 months [81]. A prospective, randomized, double-blinded controlled trial by Lo et al. in 2015 compared intraoperative injection of Botox 100 units to one pectoral muscle and normal saline on the contralateral side in patients undergoing breast reconstructive surgery following bilateral mastectomy [171]. This study concluded that there was no significant improvement in pain control with the use of Botox between 1 and 12 weeks postinjection [171].

Neuroma Injection

Cases of traumatic neuroma formation after surgery have been described in the literature [115]. In a review by Li et al., nodular masses may be viewed by ultrasound, presumed neuromas, which could be biopsied for confirmation. Neuroma formation tends to be at the area of scars and previous incisions. Neuromas may have a similar ultrasound structure (hyperechoic nodules) as tumors and lymphadenopathy; monitoring and further evaluation (including biopsy) should be considered. Treatments may include local anesthetic and steroid injection and ablative and surgical resections.

Spinal Cord Stimulation

Neurostimulation has been recognized as effective in the long term for nonmalignant painful conditions such as failed back syndrome [175]. There are some sporadic case series and cohorts of observational studies, not exclusively focusing on breast cancer, which have shown a marked reduction in pain intensity in patients experiencing pain relating to malignancy [176]. A systematic review in 2015 by the Cochrane Collaboration examined four before-and-after case series and found that current evidence was insufficient to establish the role of spinal cord stimulation in cancer pain, although the studies included did show improvement in pain relief and decrease in the use of analgesic medications [177]. There are no randomized controlled trials examining the use of neurostimulation for cancer pain in general or breast cancer specifically. More recent theories attribute pain relief to local effects at the spinal level with the release of GABA, acetylcholine, and serotonin as well as the inhibition of glutamate and aspartate – excitatory amino acids [178].

Intrathecal Pump Placement

As discussed in a recent review article, multiple studies have demonstrated the effectiveness of intrathecal pump drug delivery in the treatment of pain relating to cancer [179]. In fact, a study by Smith et al. showed not only improved pain control but also improved survival at 6 months [180]. This study included patients with breast cancer, but not exclusively. A retrospective review by Gulati et al. [181], examining interventional techniques for intractable chest wall pain in patients with cancer, did include patients with breast cancer and found that of the seven patients who underwent intrathecal pump placement, 100% had improvement (VAS improved >1) of pain relief [181]. Additionally, a cost-utilization analysis of intrathecal therapy for refractory cancer pain found that in select patients on high-cost opioid regimens, intrathecal pump placement becomes cost-beneficial within 6 months [182].

Fig. 9.5 Anatomical treatment paradigm

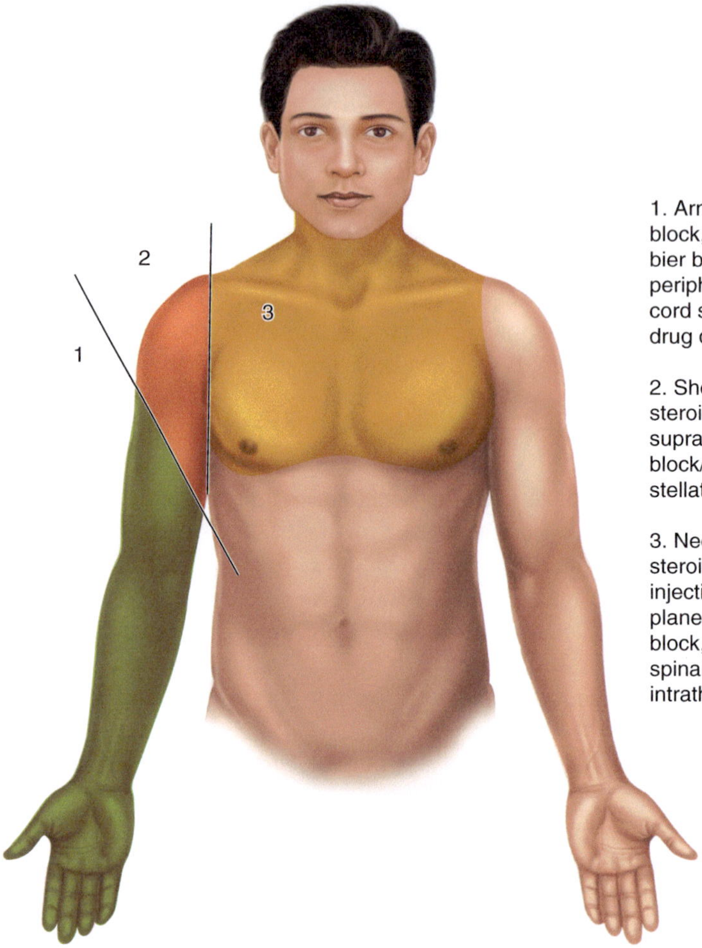

Interventional Treatment Paradigm

Pain related to breast cancer is often very complex and difficult to treat. As such, clinicians have been often moved away from intervention because of the difficulty with diagnostics. However, in our practice, we have often approached the previously discussed treatment options by considering both the cause and anatomical location of pain. Figure 9.5 depicts an anatomical approach to treatment of pain from breast cancer.

Conclusion

Pain relating to breast cancer is complex and multifactorial. It affects multiple organ systems in the acute, subacute, and chronic time frames. A deep understanding of the different mechanisms of pain relating to breast cancer and its treatment options, both conservative and interventional, is necessary in order to adequately treat women experiencing this type of pain.

References

1. Glare PA, Davies PS, Finlay E, et al. Pain in cancer survivors. J Clin Oncol. 2014;32(16):1739–47. https://doi.org/10.1200/JCO.2013.52.4629.
2. Pachman DR, Barton DL, Swetz KM, Loprinzi CL. Troublesome symptoms in cancer survivors: fatigue, insomnia, neuropathy, and pain. J Clin Oncol. 2012;30(30):3687–96. https://doi.org/10.1200/JCO.2012.41.7238.
3. van den Beuken-van Everdingen MHJ, de Rijke JM, Kessels AG, Schouten HC, van Kleef M, Patijn J. Prevalence of pain in patients with cancer: a systematic review of the past 40 years. Ann Oncol. 2007;18(9):1437–49. https://doi.org/10.1093/annonc/mdm056.
4. Peuckmann V, Ekholm O, Rasmussen NK, et al. Chronic pain and other sequelae in long-term breast cancer survivors: nationwide survey in Denmark. Eur J Pain. 2009;13(5):478–85. https://doi.org/10.1016/j.ejpain.2008.05.015.

5. Hofsø K, Rustøen T, Cooper BA, Bjordal K, Miaskowski C. Changes over time in occurrence, severity, and distress of common symptoms during and after radiation therapy for breast Cancer. J Pain Symptom Manag. 2013;45(6):980–1006. https://doi.org/10.1016/j.jpainsymman.2012.06.003.
6. Ebaugh D, Spinelli B, Schmitz KH. Shoulder impairments and their association with symptomatic rotator cuff disease in breast cancer survivors. Med Hypotheses. 2011;77(4):481–7. https://doi.org/10.1016/j.mehy.2011.06.015.
7. Ewertz M, Jensen AB. Late effects of breast cancer treatment and potentials for rehabilitation. Acta Oncol. 2011;50(2):187–93. https://doi.org/10.3109/0284186X.2010.533190.
8. Gärtner R, Jensen M-B, Nielsen J, Ewertz M, Kroman N, Kehlet H. Prevalence of and factors associated with persistent pain following breast cancer surgery. JAMA. 2009;302(18):1985–92. https://doi.org/10.1001/jama.2009.1568.
9. Von Roenn JH, Cleeland CS, Gonin R, Hatfield AK, Pandya KJ. Physician attitudes and practice in cancer pain management. A survey from the Eastern Cooperative Oncology Group. Ann Intern Med. 1993;119(2):121–6.
10. de Boer AGEM, Taskila T, Ojajärvi A, van Dijk FJH, Verbeek JHAM. Cancer survivors and unemployment: a meta-analysis and meta-regression. JAMA. 2009;301(7):753–62. https://doi.org/10.1001/jama.2009.187.
11. Tevaarwerk AJ, Lee JW, Sesto ME, et al. Employment outcomes among survivors of common cancers: the Symptom Outcomes and Practice Patterns (SOAPP) study. J Cancer Surviv. 2013;7(2):191–202. https://doi.org/10.1007/s11764-012-0258-2.
12. Howlader N, Noone AM, Krapcho M, et al. Surveillance, Epidemiology, and End Results (SEER) cancer statistics review. http://seer.cancer.gov/csr/1975_2012/. Published April 2015. Accessed 6 Nov 2015.
13. Netter FH. Atlas of human anatomy. Philadelphia: Elsevier Health Sciences; 2010.
14. Snell RS. Clinical anatomy by regions. Philadelphia: Lippincott Williams & Wilkins; 2011.
15. Moore KL, Dalley AF, Agur AMR. Clinically oriented anatomy. Philadelphia: Lippincott Williams & Wilkins; 2013.
16. Agur AMR, Dalley AF, Grant JCB. Grant's atlas of anatomy. Philadelphia: Lippincott Williams & Wilkins; 2013.
17. Deer TR, Leong MS, Gordin V. Treatment of chronic pain by medical approaches: the AMERICAN ACADEMY of PAIN MEDICINE textbook on patient management. New York: Springer; 2014.
18. Warrier S, Hwang S, Koh CE, et al. Preservation or division of the intercostobrachial nerve in axillary dissection for breast cancer: meta-analysis of randomised controlled trials. Breast. 2014;23(4):310–6. https://doi.org/10.1016/j.breast.2014.01.014.
19. Wijayasinghe N, Andersen KG, Kehlet H. Neural blockade for persistent pain after breast cancer surgery. Reg Anesth Pain Med. 2014;39(4):272–8. https://doi.org/10.1097/AAP.0000000000000101.
20. Torres Lacomba M, Mayoral del Moral O, Coperias Zazo JL, Gerwin RD, Goñí AZ. Incidence of myofascial pain syndrome in breast cancer surgery: a prospective study. Clin J Pain. 2010;26(4):320–5. https://doi.org/10.1097/AJP.0b013e3181c4904a.
21. Caban ME, Yadav R. Rehabilitation of breast cancer–related functional deficits. Crit Rev Phys Rehabil Med. 2008;20(1):1–23.
22. Lavelle ED, Lavelle W, Smith HS. Myofascial trigger points. Med Clin North Am. 2007;91(2):229–39. https://doi.org/10.1016/j.mcna.2006.12.004.
23. Latremoliere A, Woolf CJ. Central sensitization: a generator of pain hypersensitivity by central neural plasticity. J Pain. 2009;10(9):895–926. https://doi.org/10.1016/j.jpain.2009.06.012.
24. Shin HJ, Shin JC, Kim WS, Chang WH, Lee SC. Application of ultrasound-guided trigger point injection for myofascial trigger points in the subscapularis and pectoralis muscles to post-mastectomy patients: a pilot study. Yonsei Med J. 2014;55(3):792–8. https://doi.org/10.3349/ymj.2014.55.3.792.
25. Proulx AM, Zryd TW. Costochondritis: diagnosis and treatment. Am Fam Physician. 2009;80(6):617–20.
26. Kamel M, Kotob H. Ultrasonographic assessment of local steroid injection in Tietze's syndrome. Rheumatology. 1997;36(5):547–50. https://doi.org/10.1093/rheumatology/36.5.547.
27. Coleman RE, Bolten WW, Lansdown M, et al. Aromatase inhibitor-induced arthralgia: clinical experience and treatment recommendations. Cancer Treat Rev. 2008;34(3):275–82. https://doi.org/10.1016/j.ctrv.2007.10.004.
28. Coleman RE. Clinical features of metastatic bone disease and risk of skeletal morbidity. Clin Cancer Res. 2006;12(20 Pt 2):6243s–9s. https://doi.org/10.1158/1078-0432.CCR-06-0931.
29. Smith HS, Barkin RL. Painful boney metastases. Am J Ther. 2014;21(2):106–30. https://doi.org/10.1097/MJT.0b013e3182456dff.
30. Wallace AN, Robinson CG, Meyer J, et al. The metastatic spine disease multidisciplinary working group algorithms. Oncologist. 2015;20(10):1205–15. https://doi.org/10.1634/theoncologist.2015-0085.
31. Greenwood TJ, Wallace A, Friedman MV, Hillen TJ, Robinson CG, Jennings JW. Combined ablation and radiation therapy of spinal metastases: a novel multimodality treatment approach. Pain Physician. 2015;18(6):573–81.
32. Wallace AN, Tomasian A, Vaswani D, Vyhmeister R, Chang RO, Jennings JW. Radiographic local control of spinal metastases with percutaneous radiofrequency ablation and vertebral augmentation. AJNR Am J Neuroradiol. 2016;37(4):759–65. https://doi.org/10.3174/ajnr.A4595.
33. Tasmuth T, Smitten von K, Hietanen P, Kataja M, Kalso E. Pain and other symptoms after different treatment modalities of breast cancer. Ann Oncol. 1995;6(5):453–9.
34. Vadivelu N, Schreck M, Lopez J, Kodumudi G, Narayan D. Pain after mastectomy and breast reconstruction. Am Surg. 2008;74(4):285–96.
35. Tasmuth T, Blomqvist C, Kalso E. Chronic post-treatment symptoms in patients with breast cancer operated in different surgical units. Eur J Surg Oncol. 1999;25(1):38–43. https://doi.org/10.1053/ejso.1998.0597.
36. Wallace MS, Wallace AM, Lee J, Dobke MK. Pain after breast surgery: a survey of 282 women. Pain. 1996;66(2–3):195–205.
37. Jung BF, Ahrendt GM, Oaklander AL, Dworkin RH. Neuropathic pain following breast cancer surgery: proposed classification and research update. Pain. 2003;104(1):1–13. https://doi.org/10.1016/S0304-3959(03)00241-0.
38. Figus A, Mazzocchi M, Dessy LA, Curinga G, Scuderi N. Treatment of muscular contraction deformities with botulinum toxin type A after latissimus dorsi flap and sub-pectoral implant breast reconstruction. J Plast Reconstr Aesthet Surg. 2009;62(7):869–75. https://doi.org/10.1016/j.bjps.2007.07.025.
39. Ho JO, Sawadkar P, Mudera V. A review on the use of cell therapy in the treatment of tendon disease and injuries. J Tissue Eng. 2014;5(0):2041731414549678–18. https://doi.org/10.1177/2041731414549678.
40. Desmeules F, Boudreault J, Roy J-S, Dionne C, Frémont P, MacDermid JC. The efficacy of therapeutic ultrasound for rotator cuff tendinopathy: a systematic review and meta-analysis. Phys Ther Sport. 2015;16(3):1–9. https://doi.org/10.1016/j.ptsp.2014.09.004.
41. Factor D, Dale B. Current concepts of rotator cuff tendinopathy. Int J Sports Phys Ther. 2014;9(2):274–88.

42. Fukuda H. Partial-thickness rotator cuff tears: a modern view on Codman's classic. J Shoulder Elb Surg. 2000;9(2):163–8. https://doi.org/10.1067/mse.2000.101959.
43. Teunis T, Lubberts B, Reilly BT, Ring D. A systematic review and pooled analysis of the prevalence of rotator cuff disease with increasing age. J Shoulder Elb Surg. 2014;23(12):1913–21. https://doi.org/10.1016/j.jse.2014.08.001.
44. Petrek JA, Heelan MC. Incidence of breast carcinoma-related lymphedema. Cancer. 1998;83(12 Suppl American):2776–81.
45. Levy O, Relwani J, Zaman T, Even T, Venkateswaran B, Copeland S. Measurement of blood flow in the rotator cuff using laser Doppler flowmetry. J Bone Joint Surg Br. 2008;90(7):893–8. https://doi.org/10.1302/0301-620X.90B7.19918.
46. Brukner P, Khan K. Brukner & Khan's clinical sports medicine. Sydney: McGraw-Hill Education; 2011.
47. Lee TS, Kilbreath SL, Refshauge KM, Herbert RD, Beith JM. Prognosis of the upper limb following surgery and radiation for breast cancer. Breast Cancer Res Treat. 2007;110(1):19–37. https://doi.org/10.1007/s10549-007-9710-9.
48. Buckup K. Clinical tests for the musculoskeletal system. Stuttgart: Thieme; 2011.
49. Ardic F, Kahraman Y, Kacar M, Kahraman MC, Findikoglu G, Yorgancioglu ZR. Shoulder impingement syndrome: relationships between clinical, functional, and radiologic findings. Am J Phys Med Rehabil. 2006;85(1):53–60.
50. Reilly P, Macleod I, Macfarlane R, Windley J, Emery R. Dead men and radiologists don't lie: a review of cadaveric and radiological studies of rotator cuff tear prevalence. Ann R Coll Surg Engl. 2006;88(2):116–21. https://doi.org/10.1308/003588406X94968.
51. Ahmed RL, Prizment A, Lazovich D, Schmitz KH, Folsom AR. Lymphedema and quality of life in breast cancer survivors: the Iowa Women's Health Study. J Clin Oncol. 2008;26(35):5689–96. https://doi.org/10.1200/JCO.2008.16.4731.
52. Taghian NR, Miller CL, Jammallo LS, O'Toole J, Skolny MN. Lymphedema following breast cancer treatment and impact on quality of life: a review. Crit Rev Oncol Hematol. 2014;92(3):227–34. https://doi.org/10.1016/j.critrevonc.2014.06.004.
53. Herrera JE, Stubblefield MD. Rotator cuff tendonitis in lymphedema: a retrospective case series. Arch Phys Med Rehabil. 2004;85(12):1939–42. https://doi.org/10.1016/j.apmr.2004.06.065.
54. Shamley DR, Srinanaganathan R, Weatherall R, et al. Changes in shoulder muscle size and activity following treatment for breast cancer. Breast Cancer Res Treat. 2007;106(1):19–27. https://doi.org/10.1007/s10549-006-9466-7.
55. Stubblefield MD, Keole N. Upper body pain and functional disorders in patients with breast cancer. PMR. 2014;6(2):170–83. https://doi.org/10.1016/j.pmrj.2013.08.605.
56. Rostkowska E, Bak M, Samborski W. Body posture in women after mastectomy and its changes as a result of rehabilitation. Adv Med Sci. 2006;51:287–97.
57. Crosbie J, Kilbreath SL, Dylke E, et al. Effects of mastectomy on shoulder and spinal kinematics during bilateral upper-limb movement. Phys Ther. 2010;90(5):679–92. https://doi.org/10.2522/ptj.20090104.
58. Cheville AL, Tchou J. Barriers to rehabilitation following surgery for primary breast cancer. J Surg Oncol. 2007;95(5):409–18. https://doi.org/10.1002/jso.20782.
59. Borstad JD. Resting position variables at the shoulder: evidence to support a posture-impairment association. Phys Ther. 2006;86(4):549–57.
60. Levangie PK, Drouin J. Magnitude of late effects of breast cancer treatments on shoulder function: a systematic review. Breast Cancer Res Treat. 2008;116(1):1–15. https://doi.org/10.1007/s10549-008-0246-4.
61. Harrington S, Padua D, Battaglini C, et al. Comparison of shoulder flexibility, strength, and function between breast cancer survivors and healthy participants. J Cancer Surviv. 2011;5(2):167–74. https://doi.org/10.1007/s11764-010-0168-0.
62. Uppal HS. Frozen shoulder: a systematic review of therapeutic options. World J Orthod. 2015;6(2):263–7. https://doi.org/10.5312/wjo.v6.i2.263.
63. Jeong HJ, Sim Y-J, Hwang KH, Kim GC. Causes of shoulder pain in women with breast cancer-related lymphedema: a pilot study. Yonsei Med J. 2011;52(4):661–7. https://doi.org/10.3349/ymj.2011.52.4.661.
64. Leonidou A, Woods DA. A preliminary study of manipulation under anaesthesia for secondary frozen shoulder following breast cancer treatment. Ann R Coll Surg Engl. 2014;96(2):111–5. https://doi.org/10.1308/003588414X13824511649652.
65. Stubblefield MD, Custodio CM. Upper-extremity pain disorders in breast cancer. Arch Phys Med Rehabil. 2006;87(3 Suppl 1):S96–9; quiz S100-1. https://doi.org/10.1016/j.apmr.2005.12.017.
66. Leidenius M, Leivonen M, Vironen J, Smitten von K. The consequences of long-time arm morbidity in node-negative breast cancer patients with sentinel node biopsy or axillary clearance. J Surg Oncol. 2005;92(1):23–31. https://doi.org/10.1002/jso.20373.
67. Yang S, Park DH, Ahn SH, et al. Prevalence and risk factors of adhesive capsulitis of the shoulder after breast cancer treatment. Support Care Cancer. 2017;25(4):1317–22. https://doi.org/10.1007/s00520-016-3532-4.
68. Hopwood P, Haviland JS, Sumo G, et al. Comparison of patient-reported breast, arm, and shoulder symptoms and body image after radiotherapy for early breast cancer: 5-year follow-up in the randomised Standardisation of Breast Radiotherapy (START) trials. Lancet Oncol. 2010;11(3):231–40. https://doi.org/10.1016/S1470-2045(09)70382-1.
69. Conduah AH, Baker CL, Baker CL. Clinical management of scapulothoracic bursitis and the snapping scapula. Sports Health. 2010;2(2):147–55. https://doi.org/10.1177/1941738109338359.
70. Boneti C, Arentz C, Klimberg VS. Scapulothoracic bursitis as a significant cause of breast and chest wall pain: underrecognized and undertreated. Ann Surg Oncol. 2010;17(S3):321–4. https://doi.org/10.1245/s10434-010-1232-8.
71. Straub JM, New J, Hamilton CD, Lominska C, Shnayder Y, Thomas SM. Radiation-induced fibrosis: mechanisms and implications for therapy. J Cancer Res Clin Oncol. 2015;141(11):1–10. https://doi.org/10.1007/s00432-015-1974-6.
72. van Geel AN, Lans TE, Haen R, Tjong Joe Wai R, Menke-Pluijmers MBE. Partial mastectomy and m. latissimus dorsi reconstruction for radiation-induced fibrosis after breast-conserving cancer therapy. World J Surg. 2011;35(3):568–72. https://doi.org/10.1007/s00268-010-0911-8.
73. Liss AL, Ben-David MA, Jagsi R, et al. Decline of cosmetic outcomes following accelerated partial breast irradiation using intensity modulated radiation therapy: results of a single-institution prospective clinical trial. Int J Radiat Oncol Biol Phys. 2014;89(1):96–102. https://doi.org/10.1016/j.ijrobp.2014.01.005.
74. Bourgier C, Acevedo-Henao C, Dunant A, et al. Higher toxicity with 42 Gy in 10 fractions as a total dose for 3D-conformal accelerated partial breast irradiation: results from a dose escalation phase II trial. Radiat Oncol. 2012;7(1):141. https://doi.org/10.1186/1748-717X-7-141.
75. Edvardsen H, Tefre T, Jansen L, et al. Linkage disequilibrium pattern of the ATM gene in breast cancer patients and controls; association of SNPs and haplotypes to radio-sensitivity and post-lumpectomy local recurrence. Radiat Oncol. 2007;2(1):25–9. https://doi.org/10.1186/1748-717X-2-25.
76. Chen PY, Vicini FA, Benitez P, et al. Long-term cosmetic results and toxicity after accelerated partial-breast irradiation. Cancer. 2006;106(5):991–9. https://doi.org/10.1002/cncr.21681.
77. Jacobson G, Bhatia S, Smith BJ, Button AM, Bodeker K, Buatti J. Randomized trial of pentoxifylline and vitamin E vs standard

follow-up after breast irradiation to prevent breast fibrosis, evaluated by tissue compliance meter. Int J Radiat Oncol Biol Phys. 2013;85(3):604–8. https://doi.org/10.1016/j.ijrobp.2012.06.042.
78. Bourgeois JF, Gourgou S, Kramar A. A randomized, prospective study using the LPG® technique in treating radiation-induced skin fibrosis: clinical and profilometric analysis. Skin Res Technol. 2008. doi:https://doi.org/10.1111/j.1600-0846.2007.00263.x.
79. Stubblefield MD, Levine A, Custodio CM, Fitzpatrick T. The role of botulinum toxin type A in the radiation fibrosis syndrome: a preliminary report. Arch Phys Med Rehabil. 2008;89(3):417–21. https://doi.org/10.1016/j.apmr.2007.11.022.
80. Headon H, Kasem A, Mokbel K. Capsular contracture after breast augmentation: an update for clinical practice. Arch Plast Surg. 2015;42(5):532–12. https://doi.org/10.5999/aps.2015.42.5.532.
81. Adkinson JM, Miller NF, Murphy RX Jr. Neurectomy for breast reconstruction- related spasms of the pectoralis major muscle. Br J Plast Surg. 2014;67(2):257–9. https://doi.org/10.1016/j.bjps.2013.06.025.
82. O'Donnell CJ. Pectoral muscle spasms after mastectomy successfully treated with botulinum toxin injections. PMR. 2011;3(8):781–2. https://doi.org/10.1016/j.pmrj.2011.02.023.
83. Winfree CJ, Kline DG. Intraoperative positioning nerve injuries. Surg Neurol. 2005;63(1):5–18; discussion 18. https://doi.org/10.1016/j.surneu.2004.03.024.
84. Radhakrishnan K, Litchy WJ, O'Fallon WM, Kurland LT. Epidemiology of cervical radiculopathy. A population-based study from Rochester, Minnesota, 1976 through 1990. Brain. 1994;117(Pt 2):325–35.
85. Ma H, Kim I. Horner syndrome associated with a herniated cervical disc: a case report. Korean J Spine. 2012;9(2):108–10. https://doi.org/10.14245/kjs.2012.9.2.108.
86. Miller NR, Walsh FB, Hoyt WF. Walsh and Hoyt's clinical neuro-ophthalmology. Philadelphia: Lippincott Williams & Wilkins; 2005.
87. Carozzi VA, Canta A, Chiorazzi A. Chemotherapy-induced peripheral neuropathy: what do we know about mechanisms? Neurosci Lett. 2015;596:90–107. https://doi.org/10.1016/j.neulet.2014.10.014.
88. Chaudhry V, Chaudhry M, Crawford TO, Simmons-O'Brien E, Griffin JW. Toxic neuropathy in patients with pre-existing neuropathy. Neurology. 2003;60(2):337–40.
89. Albers JW, Chaudhry V, Cavaletti G, Donehower RC. Interventions for preventing neuropathy caused by cisplatin and related compounds. Albers JW, ed. Cochrane Database Syst Rev. 2014;3:CD005228. https://doi.org/10.1002/14651858.CD005228.pub4.
90. Piccolo J, Kolesar JM. Prevention and treatment of chemotherapy-induced peripheral neuropathy. Am J Health Syst Pharm. 2014;71(1):19–25. https://doi.org/10.2146/ajhp130126.
91. Verstappen CCP, Postma TJ, Geldof AA, Heimans JJ. Amifostine protects against chemotherapy-induced neurotoxicity: an in vitro investigation. Anticancer Res. 2004;24(4):2337–41.
92. Pachman DR, Barton DL, Watson JC, Loprinzi CL. Chemotherapy-induced peripheral neuropathy: prevention and treatment. Clin Pharmacol Ther. 2011;90(3):377–87. https://doi.org/10.1038/clpt.2011.115.
93. Gamelin L, Boisdron-Celle M, Delva R, et al. Prevention of oxaliplatin-related neurotoxicity by calcium and magnesium infusions: a retrospective study of 161 patients receiving oxaliplatin combined with 5-fluorouracil and leucovorin for advanced colorectal cancer. Clin Cancer Res. 2004;10(12 Pt 1):4055–61. https://doi.org/10.1158/1078-0432.CCR-03-0666.
94. Kottschade LA, Sloan JA, Mazurczak MA, et al. The use of vitamin E for the prevention of chemotherapy-induced peripheral neuropathy: results of a randomized phase III clinical trial. Support Care Cancer. 2011;19(11):1769–77. https://doi.org/10.1007/s00520-010-1018-3.
95. Amptoulach S, Tsavaris N. Neurotoxicity caused by the treatment with platinum analogues. Chemother Res Pract. 2011;2011(3):843019–5. https://doi.org/10.1155/2011/843019.
96. Delanian S, Lefaix J-L, Pradat P-F. Radiation-induced neuropathy in cancer survivors. Radiother Oncol. 2012;105(3):273–82. https://doi.org/10.1016/j.radonc.2012.10.012.
97. Burton CL, Chesterton LS, Chen Y, van der Windt DA. Clinical course and prognostic factors in conservatively managed carpal tunnel syndrome: a systematic review. Arch Phys Med Rehabil. 2015;97:836. https://doi.org/10.1016/j.apmr.2015.09.013.
98. Ganel A, Engel J, Sela M, Brooks M. Nerve entrapments associated with postmastectomy lymphedema. Cancer. 1979;44(6):2254–9.
99. Hansen JT. Netter's clinical anatomy. Philadelphia: Saunders; 2014.
100. Huisstede BM, Fridén J, Coert JH, Hoogvliet P, European HANDGUIDE Group. Carpal tunnel syndrome: hand surgeons, hand therapists, and physical medicine and rehabilitation physicians agree on a multidisciplinary treatment guideline – results from the European HANDGUIDE Study. Arch Phys Med Rehabil. 2014;95(12):2253–2263. https://doi.org/10.1016/j.apmr.2014.06.022.
101. Dirks J, Fredensborg BB, Christensen D, Fomsgaard JS, Flyger H, Dahl JB. A randomized study of the effects of single-dose gabapentin versus placebo on postoperative pain and morphine consumption after mastectomy. Anesthesiology. 2002;97(3):560–4.
102. Björkman B, Arnér S, Hydén L-C. Phantom breast and other syndromes after mastectomy: eight breast cancer patients describe their experiences over time: a 2-year follow-up study. J Pain. 2008;9(11):1018–25. https://doi.org/10.1016/j.jpain.2008.06.003.
103. Ahmed A, Bhatnagar S, Rana SPS, Ahmad SM, Joshi S, Mishra S. Prevalence of phantom breast pain and sensation among postmastectomy patients suffering from breast cancer: a prospective study. Pain Pract. 2013;14(2):E17–28. https://doi.org/10.1111/papr.12089.
104. Polinsky ML. Functional status of long-term breast cancer survivors: demonstrating chronicity. Health Soc Work. 1994;19(3):165–73.
105. Pohjolainen T. A clinical evaluation of stumps in lower limb amputees. Prosthetics Orthot Int. 1991;15(3):178–84.
106. Kak M, Nanda R, Ramsdale EE, Lukas RV. Treatment of leptomeningeal carcinomatosis: current challenges and future opportunities. J Clin Neurosci. 2015;22(4):632–7. https://doi.org/10.1016/j.jocn.2014.10.022.
107. Niwińska A, Rudnicka H, Murawska M. Breast cancer leptomeningeal metastasis: the & nbsp; results of combined treatment and the comparison of methotrexate and liposomal cytarabine as intra-cerebrospinal fluid chemotherapy. Clin Breast Cancer. 2015;15(1):66–72. https://doi.org/10.1016/j.clbc.2014.07.004.
108. Leal T, Chang JE, Mehta M, Robins HI. Leptomeningeal metastasis: challenges in diagnosis and treatment. Curr Cancer Ther Rev. 2011;7(4):319–27. https://doi.org/10.2174/157339411797642597.
109. Papay FA, Verghese A, Stanton-Hicks M, Zins J. Complex regional pain syndrome of the breast in a patient after breast reduction. Ann Plast Surg. 1997;39(4):347–52.
110. Graham LE, McGuigan C, Kerr S, Taggart AJ. Complex regional pain syndrome post mastectomy. Rheumatol Int. 2001;21(4):165–6. https://doi.org/10.1007/s00296-001-0152-0.
111. Khan F, Shaikh FM, Keane R, Conroy BP. Complex regional pain syndrome type I as a complication of axillary clearance. J Pain Symptom Manag. 2006;31(6):481–3. https://doi.org/10.1016/j.jpainsymman.2006.02.003.
112. Ashkar L, Omeroglu A, Halwani F, Alsharif S, Loutfi A, Mesurolle B. Post-traumatic neuroma following breast surgery. Breast J. 2013;19(6):671–2. https://doi.org/10.1111/tbj.12186.

113. Nguyen JT, Buchanan IA, Patel PP, Aljinovic N, Lee BT. Intercostal neuroma as a source of pain after aesthetic and reconstructive breast implant surgery. Br J Plast Surg. 2012;65(9):1199–203. https://doi.org/10.1016/j.bjps.2012.04.003.
114. Wong L. Intercostal neuromas: a treatable cause of postoperative breast surgery pain. Ann Plast Surg. 2001;46(5):481–4.
115. Li Q, Gao E-L, Yang Y-L, Hu H-Y, Hu X-Q. Traumatic neuroma in a patient with breast cancer after mastectomy: a case report and review of the literature. World J Surg Oncol. 2012;10(1):35. https://doi.org/10.1186/1477-7819-10-35.
116. Smith HS, Wu S-X. Persistent pain after breast cancer treatment. Ann Palliat Med. 2012;1(3):182–94. https://doi.org/10.3978/j.issn.2224-5820.2012.10.13.
117. Zuther JE, Norton S. Lymphedema management. New York: Thieme; 2012.
118. Russell NS, Floot B, van Werkhoven E, et al. Blood and lymphatic microvessel damage in irradiated human skin: the role of TGF-β, endoglin and macrophages. Radiother Oncol. 2015;116:455. https://doi.org/10.1016/j.radonc.2015.08.024.
119. Shao Y, Qi K, Zhou Q-H, Zhong D-S. Intermittent pneumatic compression pump for breast cancer-related lymphedema: a systematic review and meta-analysis of randomized controlled trials. Oncol Res Treat. 2014;37(4):170–4. https://doi.org/10.1159/000360786.
120. Moseley AL, Carati CJ, Piller NB. A systematic review of common conservative therapies for arm lymphoedema secondary to breast cancer treatment. Ann Oncol. 2007;18(4):639–46. https://doi.org/10.1093/annonc/mdl182.
121. E Lima MTBRM, E Lima JGM, de Andrade MFC, Bergmann A. Low-level laser therapy in secondary lymphedema after breast cancer: systematic review. Lasers Med Sci. 2014;29(3):1289–95. https://doi.org/10.1007/s10103-012-1240-y.
122. Mehrara BJ, Zampell JC, Suami H, Chang DW. Surgical management of lymphedema: past, present, and future. Lymphat Res Biol. 2011;9(3):159–67. https://doi.org/10.1089/lrb.2011.0011.
123. Travis EC, Shugg S, McEwan WM. Lymph node grafting in the treatment of upper limb lymphoedema: a clinical trial. ANZ J Surg. 2015;85(9):631–5. https://doi.org/10.1111/ans.13171.
124. Yeung WM, McPhail SM, Kuys SS. A systematic review of axillary web syndrome (AWS). J Cancer Surviv. 2015;9(4):576–98. https://doi.org/10.1007/s11764-015-0435-1.
125. Torres Lacomba M, Mayoral del Moral O, Coperias Zazo JL, Yuste Sánchez MJ, Ferrandez J-C, Zapico Goñi A. Axillary web syndrome after axillary dissection in breast cancer: a prospective study. Breast Cancer Res Treat. 2009;117(3):625–30. https://doi.org/10.1007/s10549-009-0371-8.
126. National Cancer Institute. Common terminology criteria for adverse events (CTCAE). NIH publication No. 09-5410. Bethesda: National Cancer Institute; 2010. Available at: https://www.eortc.be/services/doc/ctc/CTCAE_4.03_2010-06-14_QuickReference_5x7.pdf.
127. Chen M-F, Chen W-C, Lai C-H, Hung C-H, Liu K-C, Cheng Y-H. Predictive factors of radiation-induced skin toxicity in breast cancer patients. BMC Cancer. 2010;10(1):508–10. https://doi.org/10.1186/1471-2407-10-508.
128. Hymes SR, Strom EA, Fife C. Radiation dermatitis: clinical presentation, pathophysiology, and treatment 2006. J Am Acad Dermatol. 2006;54(1):28–46. https://doi.org/10.1016/j.jaad.2005.08.054.
129. Harper JL, Franklin LE, Jenrette JM, Aguero EG. Skin toxicity during breast irradiation: pathophysiology and management. South Med J. 2004;97(10):989–93. https://doi.org/10.1097/01.SMJ.0000140866.97278.87.
130. Chan RJ, Webster J, Chung B, Marquart L, Ahmed M, Garantziotis S. Prevention and treatment of acute radiation-induced skin reactions: a systematic review and meta-analysis of randomized controlled trials. BMC Cancer. 2014;14(1):53. https://doi.org/10.1186/1471-2407-14-53.
131. Emami B, Lyman J, Brown A, et al. Tolerance of normal tissue to therapeutic irradiation. Int J Radiat Oncol Biol Phys. 1991;21(1):109–22.
132. Jagsi R, Griffith KA, Boike TP, et al. Differences in the acute toxic effects of breast radiotherapy by fractionation schedule. JAMA Oncol. 2015;1(7):918–3. https://doi.org/10.1001/jamaoncol.2015.2590.
133. Shaitelman SF, Schlembach PJ, Arzu I, et al. Acute and short-term toxic effects of conventionally fractionated vs hypofractionated whole-breast irradiation. JAMA Oncol. 2015;1(7):931–11. https://doi.org/10.1001/jamaoncol.2015.2666.
134. Kumar S, Juresic E, Barton M, Shafiq J. Management of skin toxicity during radiation therapy: a review of the evidence. J Med Imaging Radiat Oncol. 2010;54(3):264–79. https://doi.org/10.1111/j.1754-9485.2010.02170.x.
135. Cheville AL, Troxel AB, Basford JR, Kornblith AB. Prevalence and treatment patterns of physical impairments in patients with metastatic breast cancer. J Clin Oncol. 2008;26(16):2621–9. https://doi.org/10.1200/JCO.2007.12.3075.
136. Carmeliet P, Jain RK. Angiogenesis in cancer and other diseases. Nature. 2000;407:249–57.
137. Maxwell L. Therapeutic ultrasound and tumour metastasis. Physiotherapy. 1995;81:272–5. https://doi.org/10.1016/S0031-9406(05)66822-8.
138. Humble SR, Dalton AJ, Li L. A systematic review of therapeutic interventions to reduce acute and chronic post-surgical pain after amputation, thoracotomy or mastectomy. Eur J Pain. 2015;19(4):451–65. https://doi.org/10.1002/ejp.567.
139. Mahran E, Hassan ME. Comparison of pregabalin versus ketamine in postoperative pain management in breast cancer surgery. Saudi J Anaesth. 2015;9(3):253–7. https://doi.org/10.4103/1658-354X.154697.
140. Kotlinska-Lemieszek A, Paulsen O, Kaasa S, Klepstad P. Polypharmacy in patients with advanced cancer and pain: a European cross-sectional study of 2282 patients. J Pain Symptom Manag. 2014;48(6):1145–59. https://doi.org/10.1016/j.jpainsymman.2014.03.008.
141. Portenoy RK, Ahmed E. Principles of opioid use in cancer pain. J Clin Oncol. 2014;32(16):1662–70. https://doi.org/10.1200/JCO.2013.52.5188.
142. Terkawi AS, Sharma S, Durieux ME, Thammishetti S, Brenin D, Tiouririne M. Perioperative lidocaine infusion reduces the incidence of post-mastectomy chronic pain: a double-blind, placebo-controlled randomized trial. Pain Physician. 2015;18(2):E139–46.
143. Fassoulaki A, Patris K, Sarantopoulos C, Hogan Q. The analgesic effect of gabapentin and mexiletine after breast surgery for cancer. Anesth Analg. 2002;95(4):985–91, table of contents.
144. Amr YM, Yousef AAA-M. Evaluation of efficacy of the perioperative administration of venlafaxine or gabapentin on acute and chronic postmastectomy pain. Clin J Pain. 2010;26(5):381–5. https://doi.org/10.1097/AJP.0b013e3181cb406e.
145. Fassoulaki A, Triga A, Melemeni A, Sarantopoulos C. Multimodal analgesia with gabapentin and local anesthetics prevents acute and chronic pain after breast surgery for cancer. Anesth Analg. 2005;101(5):1427–32. https://doi.org/10.1213/01.ANE.0000180200.11626.8E.
146. Liu L, Huang Q-M, Liu Q-G, et al. Effectiveness of dry needling for myofascial trigger points associated with neck and shoulder pain: a systematic review and meta-analysis. Arch Phys Med Rehabil. 2015;96(5):944–55. https://doi.org/10.1016/j.apmr.2014.12.015.
147. Klç Z, Filiz MB, Çakr T, Toraman NF. Addition of suprascapular nerve block to a physical therapy program produces an extra benefit to adhesive capsulitis: a randomized controlled trial. Am J Phys Med Rehabil. 2015;94(10 Suppl 1):912–20. https://doi.org/10.1097/PHM.0000000000000336.
148. Ozkan K, Ozcekic AN, Sarar S, Cift H, Ozkan FU, Unay K. Suprascapular nerve block for the treatment of fro-

zen shoulder. Saudi J Anaesth. 2012;6(1):52–5. https://doi.org/10.4103/1658-354X.93061.
149. Favejee MM, Huisstede BMA, Koes BW. Frozen shoulder: the effectiveness of conservative and surgical interventions – systematic review. Br J Sports Med. 2010;45(1):49–56. https://doi.org/10.1136/bjsm.2010.071431.
150. Jones DS, Chattopadhyay C. Suprascapular nerve block for the treatment of frozen shoulder in primary care: a randomized trial. Br J Gen Pract. 1999;49(438):39–41.
151. Dahan TH, Fortin L, Pelletier M, Petit M, Vadeboncoeur R, Suissa S. Double blind randomized clinical trial examining the efficacy of bupivacaine suprascapular nerve blocks in frozen shoulder. J Rheumatol. 2000;27(6):1464–9.
152. Blanco R, Parras T, McDonnell JG, Prats-Galino A. Serratus plane block: a novel ultrasound-guided thoracic wall nerve block. Anaesthesia. 2013;68(11):1107–13. https://doi.org/10.1111/anae.12344.
153. (null) NYSORA. Thoracic paravertebral block. http://www.nysora.com/techniques/neuraxial-and-perineuraxial-techniques/landmark-based/3077-thoracic-paravertebral-block.html. Published May 9, 2013. Accessed 8 Oct 2015.
154. Krediet AC, Moayeri N, van Geffen G-J, et al. Different approaches to ultrasound-guided thoracic paravertebral block: an illustrated review. Anesthesiology. 2015;123(2):459–74. https://doi.org/10.1097/ALN.0000000000000747.
155. Kairaluoma PM, Bachmann MS, Korpinen AK, Rosenberg PH, Pere PJ. Single-injection paravertebral block before general anesthesia enhances analgesia after breast cancer surgery with and without associated lymph node biopsy. Anesth Analg. 2004;99(6):1837–43, table of contents. https://doi.org/10.1213/01.ANE.0000136775.15566.87.
156. Kairaluoma PM, Bachmann MS, Rosenberg PH, Pere PJ. Preincisional paravertebral block reduces the prevalence of chronic pain after breast surgery. Anesth Analg. 2006;103(3):703–8. https://doi.org/10.1213/01.ane.0000230603.92574.4e.
157. Exadaktylos AK, Buggy DJ, Moriarty DC, Mascha E, Sessler DI. Can anesthetic technique for primary breast cancer surgery affect recurrence or metastasis? Anesthesiology. 2006;105(4):660–4.
158. Kirvelä O, Antila H. Thoracic paravertebral block in chronic postoperative pain. Reg Anesth. 1992;17(6):348–50.
159. Yucel I, Demiraran Y, Ozturan K, Degirmenci E. Complex regional pain syndrome type I: efficacy of stellate ganglion blockade. J Orthop Traumatol. 2009;10(4):179–83. https://doi.org/10.1007/s10195-009-0071-5.
160. Fishman S, Ballantyne J, Rathmell JP. Bonica's management of pain. In: Diagnostic and therapeutic nerve blocks. Philadelphia: Lippincott Williams & Wilkins; 2010. p. 1661.
161. Hoseinzade H, Mahmoodpoor A, Agamohammadi D, Sanaie S. Comparing the effect of stellate ganglion block and gabapentin on the post mastectomy pain syndrome. Rawal Med J. 2008;33(1):22–5. http://www.scopemed.org/?mno=7389
162. Nabil Abbas D, Abd El Ghafar EM, Ibrahim WA, Omran AF. Fluoroscopic stellate ganglion block for postmastectomy pain: a comparison of the classic anterior approach and the oblique approach. Clin J Pain. 2011;27(3):207–13. https://doi.org/10.1097/AJP.0b013e3181fb1ef1.
163. Park JH, Min Y-S, Chun SM, Seo KS. Effects of stellate ganglion block on breast cancer-related lymphedema: comparison of various injectates. Pain Physician. 2015;18(1):93–9.
164. New York School of Regional Anesthesia. Intercostal block. http://www.nysora.com/techniques/neuraxial-and-perineuraxial-techniques/landmark-based/3072-intercostal-block.html. Published March 9, 2013. Accessed 12 Oct 2015.
165. Ducic I, Larson EE. Outcomes of surgical treatment for chronic postoperative breast and abdominal pain attributed to the intercostal nerve. J Am Coll Surg. 2006;203(3):304–10. https://doi.org/10.1016/j.jamcollsurg.2006.05.018.
166. Cohen SP, Sireci A, Wu CL, Larkin TM, Williams KA, Hurley RW. Pulsed radiofrequency of the dorsal root ganglia is superior to pharmacotherapy or pulsed radiofrequency of the intercostal nerves in the treatment of chronic postsurgical thoracic pain. Pain Physician. 2006;9(3):227–35.
167. Blanco R. The "pecs block": a novel technique for providing analgesia after breast surgery. Anaesthesia. 2011;66(9):847–8. https://doi.org/10.1111/j.1365-2044.2011.06838.x.
168. Blanco R, Fajardo M, Parras Maldonado T. Ultrasound description of Pecs II (modified Pecs I): a novel approach to breast surgery. Rev Esp Anestesiol Reanim. 2012;59(9):470–5. https://doi.org/10.1016/j.redar.2012.07.003.
169. Wahba SS, Kamal SM. Thoracic paravertebral block versus pectoral nerve block for analgesia after breast surgery. Egypt J Anaesth. 2014;30(2):129–35. https://doi.org/10.1016/j.egja.2013.10.006.
170. Hoefflin SM. Botox alternatives. Plast Reconstr Surg. 1998;101(3):865.
171. Lo KK, Aycock JK. A blinded randomized controlled trial to evaluate the use of botulinum toxin for pain control in breast reconstruction with tissue expanders. Ann Plast Surg. 2015;74(3):281–3. https://doi.org/10.1097/SAP.0b013e31829be8d8.
172. Perotto A, Delagi EF. Anatomical guide for the electromyographer. Springfield: Charles C Thomas Publisher; 2005.
173. Doretti A, Gerevini S, Riccardi B, Gregorini F, Silani V, Maderna L. Flash posters. Eur J Neurol. 2015;22(S1):484–828. https://doi.org/10.1111/ene.12808.
174. Senior MA, Fourie LR. Botox and the management of pectoral spasm after subpectoral implant insertion. Plast Reconstr Surg. 2000;106(1):224–5.
175. Frey ME, Manchikanti L, Benyamin RM, Schultz DM, Smith HS, Cohen SP. Spinal cord stimulation for patients with failed back surgery syndrome: a systematic review. Pain Physician. 2009;12(2):379–97.
176. Yakovlev AE, Ellias Y. Spinal cord stimulation as a treatment option for intractable neuropathic cancer pain. Clin Med Res. 2008;6(3–4):103–6. https://doi.org/10.3121/cmr.2008.813.
177. Peng L, Min S, Zejun Z, Wei K, Bennett MI. Spinal cord stimulation for cancer-related pain in adults. Min S, ed. Cochrane Database Syst Rev. 2015;6(6):CD009389. https://doi.org/10.1002/14651858.CD009389.pub3.
178. Knotkova H, Rasche D. Textbook of neuromodulation. New York: Springer; 2014.
179. Christo PJ, Mazloomdoost D. Interventional pain treatments for cancer pain. Ann N Y Acad Sci. 2008;1138(1):299–328. https://doi.org/10.1196/annals.1414.034.
180. Smith TJ, Staats PS, Deer T, et al. Randomized clinical trial of an implantable drug delivery system compared with comprehensive medical management for refractory cancer pain: impact on pain, drug-related toxicity, and survival. J Clin Oncol. 2002;20(19):4040–9.
181. Gulati A, Shah R, Puttanniah V, Hung JC, Malhotra V. A retrospective review and treatment paradigm of interventional therapies for patients suffering from intractable thoracic chest wall pain in the oncologic population. Pain Med. 2015;16(4):802–10. https://doi.org/10.1111/pme.12558.
182. Brogan SE, Winter NB, Abiodun A, Safarpour R. A cost utilization analysis of intrathecal therapy for refractory cancer pain: identifying factors associated with cost benefit. Pain Med. 2013;14(4):478–86. https://doi.org/10.1111/pme.12060.

Thoracic Cancer Pain

10

Joseph C. Hung, Rajiv Shah, and Amitabh Gulati

Introduction

Lung cancer is the most common cancer in the world and the leading cause of cancer-related death worldwide [1]. By region, mortality rates are estimated to be the highest in Asian countries and lowest in Western Africa [2, 3]. Lung cancer mortality rates are closely related to smoking prevalence though secondhand tobacco smoke, indoor air pollution, outdoor air pollution, and occupational hazardous chemical exposure are also contributory [1]. It is fortunate that over time, lung cancer mortality has decreased in relation to the implementation of tobacco control policies – with higher socioeconomic groups in high-income countries becoming more likely to quit and less likely to begin using tobacco products [1].

Malignant pain from within the thoracic cavity may originate from primary or metastatic neoplasms involving the lungs, heart, esophagus, and neural structures such as the brachial plexus and intercostal nerves, osseous structures, or lymph nodes [4]. Pain most commonly arises from insult related to the underlying malignancy and usually affects multiple anatomic sites [5]. Examples include bony metastatic disease, tumor-induced mass effect on adjacent neural and soft tissue structures, and visceral or ischemic pain from organ parenchyma and lymph nodes [5]. Though lung cancer patients typically have highly variable cancer pain presentations, the chest and lumbar spine are the most frequently involved areas [5].

J. C. Hung
Memorial Sloan Kettering Cancer Center, Anesthesiology and Critical Care Medicine, New York, NY, USA
e-mail: jhung@alumni.upenn.edu

R. Shah
Washington University School of Medicine, Saint Louis, MO, USA

A. Gulati (✉)
Department of Anesthesiology and Critical Care, Memorial Sloan Kettering Cancer Center, New York, NY, USA

The thoracic cavity is also a common site for metastatic disease, including lesions from the lung, colon, and breast cancer [5]. Metastatic lung lesions are present in as many as 30% of patients with all cancer types [6]. Unfortunately, many of thoracic tumors are often incurable at the time of presentation, and treatment is targeted toward palliation of symptoms [7].

Thoracic Visceral Pain Syndromes

Lung Cancer

Pain is estimated to occur in up to 80% of patients with lung cancer and most often occurs unilaterally [8, 9]. Referred pain often occurs early in the course of disease to the ipsilateral shoulder and is commonly associated with cutaneous hypersensitivity of the T2–T5 dermatomes [9]. Upper lobe tumors more often cause referred visceral pain to the shoulder, while lower lobe tumors affect the lower chest [10]. Later in the course of disease, progressive involvement of pleural and neural structures often leads to poorly controlled and diffuse pain affecting the chest and shoulders [9].

Cardiac Tumors

Cardiac tumors are rare and for the most part benign [11]. Symptoms can vary widely and usually occur in an insidious fashion [11]. However, patients may present with severe findings including dizziness, dyspnea, palpitations, or even syncope from blood flow obstruction or disruption to the cardiac conduction system [11].

Thoracic visceral pain can refer to non-diseased areas, tends to be poorly localized, and can be hard to isolate [5]. It may be difficult to treat using targeted interventional pain management procedures and may be more responsive to either systemic pharmacotherapy or neuraxial-directed pain treatment options.

A. Gulati et al. (eds.), *Essentials of Interventional Cancer Pain Management*, https://doi.org/10.1007/978-3-319-99684-4_10

Thoracic Nociceptive Pain Syndromes

Primary Chest Wall Pain

Chest wall pain may result from malignant invasion of the ribs, intercostal spaces, adjacent soft tissue structures, or parietal pleura. It is most common with lung cancer and mesothelioma [12]. Primary chest wall tumors are rare and account for only 5% of all thoracic malignancies [13]. Primary bone tumors of the chest wall represent approximately only 8% of all primary bone tumor cases [13]. Most of these primary tumors present in the fifth and sixth decades of life and have an equal gender distribution [13].

Patients are often more comfortable at rest and commonly suffer from acute breakthrough pain with deep breathing or coughing. Those with lower rib fractures may have severe pain with contraction of the abdominal wall while twisting, sitting up, or laughing due to the attachment of the rectus muscles on the inner aspect of the lower ribs [14].

Pancoast Syndrome

Superior sulcus tumors involve the apical chest wall with resulting mass effect on adjacent structures including the lower part of the brachial plexus, upper ribs, vertebral bodies, subclavian vessels, or stellate ganglion. While over 95% of patients with Pancoast syndrome have either squamous cell or adenocarcinoma of the lung, small cell carcinoma, lymphoma, tuberculosis, or any other primary chest wall tumor can also be responsible [15].

Specific anatomic boundaries for the superior sulcus are lacking, but some authors have suggested using the cephalad portion of the costovertebral gutter extending from the first rib to the diaphragm or the subclavian artery as it crosses the top of the lung [15, 16]. Involvement of the chest wall below the level of the second rib or of only the visceral pleura is generally thought not to meet criteria for a Pancoast tumor [15].

Patients often present with severe and progressive ipsilateral shoulder pain, Horner syndrome, and upper extremity edema [16]. Pain may refer to the neck, axilla, or medial aspect of the arm. Further tumor growth may invade surrounding structures including the lower cervical or upper thoracic vertebrae, upper ribs, intervertebral foramen, spinal cord, superior vena cava, or recurrent laryngeal or phrenic nerves [10].

Tumor control using multimodal disciplinary oncologic management usually consisting induction chemoradiotherapy followed by surgery remains the best solution in terms of both pain management and also survival [15, 16]. Adverse prognostic factors are thought to include mediastinal lymph node metastasis, spine or subclavian vessel involvement, and limited resection [15]. Advancements in spine stabilization materials and multimodal surgical techniques incorporating complex spine reconstruction have increased the probability for complete resection of Pancoast tumors in recent years [15, 16].

Superior Vena Cava Obstruction

Obstruction of the superior vena cava can result from a mass in the middle or anterior mediastinum, intravascular devices such as stents, or even thrombosis without extrinsic compression [12, 17]. Patients can present with discomfort related to headache, increased swelling in the neck and arms, dyspnea, dysphagia, or even mental status changes secondary to cerebral edema [12, 17]. The severity of symptoms is related to the degree of vascular narrowing and the rapidity of onset [17]. Treatment usually consists of steroids, vascular stenting, or radiotherapy [12].

Skeletal Metastatic Disease

Breast and lung cancers are among the most frequent malignancies to spread to bone [18]. Among lung cancer patients, 30–40% will develop bony metastatic disease throughout their disease course with pain occurring as the initial presenting symptom 80% of the time [19]. Significant morbidity, quality of life reduction, and societal costs occur secondary to functional impairment and loss of independence in this patient population. After metastatic spread to bone, lung cancer patients are thought to have a 7-month median survival time [19].

The mechanism of malignant bone pain is thought to have components of neuropathic, inflammatory, and ischemic pain though osteoclastic bone resorption is thought to be a primary contributing mechanism [19, 20]. Compared to breakthrough pain, background pain is usually more responsive to analgesic therapy as incident pain episodes tend to occur rapidly and persist only for a short duration [20].

Bisphosphonates have long thought to be the standard of care for managing painful bony metastatic disease and reducing secondary complications as bone resorption inhibitors [21]. Even if pain is not present, all patients with malignant bone metastasis should be started on either bisphosphonate or denosumab therapy to prevent skeletal complications [22]. Compared to bisphosphonate therapy, denosumab, an antibody targeting receptor activator of nuclear factor kappa-B ligand (RANKL), has more recently thought to be superior in terms of time to skeletal-related events and time to pain onset in patients with bony mets [21, 22].

A large systemic review also found vertebral augmentation techniques to significantly reduce pain in cancer patients with metastatic spinal fractures unresponsive to conventional conservative and opioid therapies [23]. The same authors also noted efficacy regardless of cancer type and rare major complication rates and that the appropriate timing of vertebral augmentation techniques with regard to tumor control therapy has yet to be determined [23].

Radiotherapy and surgery should be rapidly considered as adjuvant therapies in the subset of patients with metastatic-related spinal cord compression or impending fracture [22].

C7-T1 Syndrome

Patients with metastatic pain to the vertebral bodies often complain of midline pain at the involved site [14]. Hematogenous spread of cancer from breast or bronchus malignancies often involve the C7 and T1 vertebral levels [14]. Referred pain from metastatic disease at these levels may additionally refer to between the shoulder blades [12]. Patients may complain of aching constant pain associated with unilateral radicular pain in a C7 or T1 distribution (medial aspect of the arm), triceps weakness, and sensory changes in the fourth and fifth digits [14]. Radiographic evaluation of the intrascapular area alone may miss the underlying pathology. Any patient with a known or suspected malignancy and progressive pain in this area should be evaluated for spine pathology.

Base of Skull Metastatic Disease

Malignant disease at the base of the skull often results in clinical symptoms secondary to compression of the exiting cranial nerves [24]. Metastatic spread from the nasopharynx is most frequently responsible though breast, bronchial, or prostate cancers are also causes [14].

Patients most often complain of headache with paresthesia and sensory changes in the distribution of one or more cranial nerves [14]. Involvement of the glossopharyngeal or accessory nerves exiting the jugular foramen results in the jugular foramen syndrome. Patients can develop pain in the ipsilateral neck, shoulder, or mastoid region associated with hoarseness, dysphagia, weakness of the palatal sternocleidomastoid, or trapezius muscles [24]. Compression of the vagus nerve can cause bradycardia or syncope. Disease in the area of the hypoglossal canal can cause dysarthria associated with paresis and atrophy of the ipsilateral tongue [14]. Symptoms can occur bilaterally with or without Horner's syndrome depending on involvement of the sympathetic nerves next to the jugular foramen [14].

Paraneoplastic Syndromes

Paraneoplastic syndromes are uncommon autoimmune disorders associated with certain types of cancers including small cell lung cancer, breast cancer, ovarian cancer, and thymoma [25]. Antibodies to markers found in tumor-related antigens and also physiologic neurologic tissue are thought to be responsible. Neurologic symptoms often manifest prior to an oncologic diagnosis and tend to be subacute with rapid progression [25]. They are highly heterogenous and are known to affect multiple different areas of the nervous system.

Mixed sensorimotor peripheral neuropathy is the most common pain causing pathology among paraneoplastic syndromes [26]. Pain, paresthesia, and nociceptive and proprioceptive loss accompanied with hyporeflexia or areflexia are common signs and symptoms [26]. Dorsal root ganglionitis and necrotizing myelopathy are also rare but painful paraneoplastic syndromes [26]. Patients afflicted with dorsal root ganglionitis initially present with sensory disturbances, sensory loss, ataxia, proprioceptive loss, and diminished dexterity [26]. Pathologic findings usually include T-cell-mediated inflammation around dorsal root ganglion cells and neural cell degeneration [26]. Necrotizing myelopathy usually starts in the cervical or upper thoracic region and causes a symmetric diffuse necrosis of both spinal cord white and gray matter [26]. Bladder and bowel incontinence are common presenting features in addition to radicular pain, progressive sensory loss, and paraplegia leading to what is usually a rapid death [26].

Various non-neuropathic mechanisms causing pain have also been described. Hypertrophic pulmonary osteoarthropathy presents as a rheumatoid-like polyarthritis affecting the knees, wrists, and ankles. The diagnosis can be confirmed by the radiographic presence of periostitis or positive bone scintigraphy at painful sites [12]. Paraneoplastic pemphigus produces widely disseminated mucocutaneous lesions compromising the face, conjunctiva, and genitalia and is seen with non-Hodgkin's lymphoma, leukemia, or thymoma [12]. Paraneoplastic gynecomastia typically associated with testicular, lung, gastric, or renal malignancies can produce breast enlargement and resulting discomfort [12]. Paraneoplastic Raynaud's phenomenon mimicking the nonmalignant disorder can cause peripheral arteriolar vasospasm leading to consequent pallor, cyanosis, and hyperemia [12]. It is most commonly linked with lung, ovarian, and testicular cancer [12].

Treatment usually consists of anti-neuropathic and analgesic systemic pharmacotherapy, but pain symptoms infrequently improve without successful antineoplastic therapy [26]. If eliminating the antineoplastic antigen source using either surgery, radiotherapy, or chemotherapy is not possible, some subsets of patients may benefit from immunomodulatory therapies such as corticosteroids, intravenous immunoglobulins, or plasma exchange [25]. In general, patients with paraneoplastic syndrome-induced peripheral nervous system derangements fare better than those with central nervous system pathology [25].

Malignancy-Associated Neuropathic Pain Syndromes

Intercostal Neuropathy

The most frequent causes of intercostal nerve damage are postherpetic neuralgia, thoracic surgery, and diabetes but also include lung malignancy, sarcoidosis, rib compression, and pleural mesothelioma [27]. Patients may present with neuropathic pain along the flank, cutaneous hypersensitivity, and dysesthesia in the distribution of the affected intercostal nerve(s) and altered touch discrimination also in the same distribution [27].

Brachial Plexopathy

Apical lung tumors, lymphadenopathy, radiation-induced fibrosis and inflammatory plexopathy, direct malignant invasion (often from lymphoma), and iatrogenic injury during surgery can all result in brachial plexus injury [12, 14]. Apical lung tumors that invade the lower aspect of the brachial plexus can cause neuropathic pain in the distribution of the lower cervical and upper thoracic nerve roots. Patients may present with neuropathic pain in the axilla, medial aspect of the arm, or distribution of the ulnar nerve associated with weakness and atrophy of the intrinsic hand muscles [16].

Continuous infusion of local anesthetic with or without opioid through a brachial plexus catheter placed using a classic interscalene approach or posterior paracervical technique may offer pain relief for brachial plexopathy-related neuropathic pain [28]. Ultrasound-guided diagnostic blockade of the C4–C7 nerve roots followed phenol percutaneous rhizotomy has also been successfully used to treat intractable neuropathic pain from Pancoast tumor [29].

Suprascapular Entrapment

The suprascapular nerve is a mixed peripheral nerve which supplies motor branches to the supraspinatus and infraspinatus muscles and sensory branches to the acromioclavicular and glenohumeral joints. Cachexia of the shoulder girdle musculature in cancer patients may cause winging of the scapula and resultant suprascapular nerve entrapment [14]. Upper extremity lymphedema, overuse of the accessory respiratory muscles, and corticosteroid-induced muscle atrophy can also cause suprascapular nerve entrapment in this population [30]. Out of the various steroid formulations, dexamethasone is known to cause more atrophy of the shoulder and hip muscles [30].

Pain is typically unilateral and worse with both upper extremity abduction and internal rotation [14]. Symptoms depend on the location of nerve entrapment [30]. Compression at the suprascapular notch usually results in abrupt shoulder pain affecting the posterolateral aspect of the shoulder, scapula, arm, or neck [30]. More distal compression at the spinoglenoid notch causes less pain but increased infraspinatus muscle atrophy [30]. Patients may present with weakness of the rotator cuff muscles and tenderness over the suprascapular fossa [14].

The diagnosis can be confirmed with pain relief following suprascapular nerve blockade. More definitive treatment consists of cryoablation, radiofrequency therapy, or peripheral neuromodulation. Though the suprascapular nerve has significant motor function, it is one of the few nerves that has been successfully treated with cryotherapy and thermal radiofrequency ablation without significant post-procedure impairment [30, 31]. As a last resort, surgical decompression can also be employed for those patients with significant pain or weakness despite more conservative non-operative therapy [30].

Facial Pain

Facial pain is common among lung cancer patients and can arise from one of several different mechanisms [32]. Metastatic disease to the cranium, meninges, or facial neural structures including the trigeminal ganglion may cause facial pain associated with neurologic deficits. In addition, various structures in the thorax including the pharynx, larynx, esophagus, and trachea may cause facial referred pain via the nerve of Arnold – a sensory branch of the vagus nerve [14, 32].

Spinal Cord Compression

The vertebral pedicle is a common site for the spread of metastatic disease, and disease progression may result in nerve root involvement or epidural extension [14]. Breast, lung, and prostate cancers are the most frequently implicated [12]. Compression tends to occur in the thoracic region in over two-thirds of cases with cervical compression occurring only about 10% of the time [14].

Patients often present initially with pain which may be somatic or neuropathic in origin. Any patient with a known malignancy that presents with neck or back pain should be monitored very closely for malignant neuraxial disease spread. Less than 50% of patients will have signs of neurologic dysfunction at presentation but may go on to develop impairment over weeks to months [12]. Many patients feel worse with lying flat [14]. Malignant radicular and funicular pain are often worse with increased intra-abdominal pressure (e.g., coughing or sneezing), spine flexion, or straight leg raise [14]. As stated above, urgent consultations for radiotherapy and surgical decompression should be initiated for these patients [22].

Treatment-Associated Pain Syndromes

Pain Related to Radiotherapy

Toxicity related to radiotherapy is thought to be most sensitive to the time duration over which treatment is delivered [33]. Prolonged courses of radiation may mitigate treatment-associated side effects but at the cost of less tumor control [33]. Cancer pain syndromes have been described with regard to radiotherapy delivered directly to or around the spine and brachial plexus [12].

Acute and transient brachial plexopathy has been known to occur either during or immediately following radiotherapy to the immediate area. Patients may present with neurologic symptoms including paresthesia, pain, and weakness affecting the ipsilateral upper extremity [12]. These symptoms tend to be self-limiting after several weeks [12]. Acute to subacute pain flares have also been described in association with radiotherapy targeting spinal metastatic disease [12]. Patients typically complain of shock-like pains (Lhermitte's sign) in the area of existing myelopathy [12]. Like radiation-associated transient plexopathy, these pains also tend to disappear after a period of weeks to months after cessation of radiotherapy [12].

It is clinically important to differentiate radiation-induced plexopathy from tumor-related plexopathy. Tumor-related insult often occurs earlier in the course disease and is associated with greater pain and Horner's syndrome [14]. Radiation-induced plexopathy tends not to cause significant pain, typically occurs 4–5 months after radiotherapy, and predominantly affects the upper cervical nerve roots (C5–C6 distribution) [5, 12]. An extremely late presentation of radiation-induced brachial plexopathy occurring several years after radiotherapy has also been described and is thought to have an incidence ranging from 14% to 73% [5]. In this variant, patients typically complain of sensory disturbances, weakness, and lymphedema more so than pain [5]. A radiation-damaged brachial plexus commonly has a diffusely thickened appearance in both T1- and T2-weighted magnetic resonance (MR) images [12]. The presence of myokymia during electrophysiologic testing can also confirm the diagnosis [12].

Radiotherapy-associated pain may also stem not only from neurologic structures but also the bone [34]. Osteoradionecrosis is a well-described pain syndrome thought secondary to radiation- induced bone hypoxia and deficient bone remodeling [34]. The mandible is frequently implicated as some of its portions have only a singular blood supply from the inferior alveolar artery [34]. The jaw may be included in radiation fields targeting the supraclavicular area, cervical spine, or chest in thoracic cancer patients.

Pain Related to Chemotherapeutic Agents

Many chemotherapeutic agents used to treat lung cancer may damage peripheral nerves [35]. Among the most frequently implicated include vinca alkaloids, taxane, and alkylating agents such as cisplatin [12, 26, 35]. Effects are typically dose dependent and can range from acute transitory paresthesia that subsides after treatment cessation to chronic intractable neuropathic pain [12].

Patients receiving 5-FU (5-fluorouracil) may also experience ischemic chest pain thought secondary to coronary vasospasm [10]. Those with coronary artery disease may be more susceptible.

Postsurgical Pain

Persistent postsurgical thoracic pain is relatively common and is seen in 5–65% of patients after thoracotomy and between 25% and 60% after mastectomy [36–38]. Numerous pathophysiologic mechanisms attributed to ribs, muscles, and nerves have been suggested in relation to the degree of surgical trauma, the need for chest tube insertion, or inadequate postoperative pain management [38, 39]. While minimally invasive surgical techniques may offer improved pulmonary function immediately following thoracotomy, the benefits for preventing chronic post-thoracotomy pain are less clear [38, 40]. The choice of acute pain management techniques including preoperative placement and usage of a thoracic epidural may have an important impact on the development of post-thoracotomy pain syndrome [41].

Interventional Pain Control Options

Many treatment options exist for patients with thoracic cancer pain. Most patients have their pain controlled with medications. In patients with intractable pain to medication management or side effects to medications, interventional techniques can provide better pain relief. Prior studies have shown that the location of the tumor within the thoracic cavity is crucial in choosing interventional techniques for pain control. Generally, the more peripheral the lesion, the more interventional treatment options are available for patients [42]. Interventional techniques can stop pain transmission by targeting the peripheral intercostal nerves, thoracic nerve roots, paravertebral space, epidural space, or intrathecal space.

Treatment Algorithm and Relevant Anatomy (Fig. 10.1)

To target pain from the anterior or lateral chest wall spanning only a few dermatomes – the initial procedure to perform is a diagnostic intercostal nerve blockade with local anesthetic and corticosteroid. In addition to providing analgesia, an intercostal nerve block can help differentiate between somatic (e.g., chest wall pain emanating from thoracic nerve roots and intercostal nerves) and visceral (e.g., visceral pleura innervated by the vagus nerve) sources of pain. Though a subset of patients may achieve prolonged pain relief with intercostal nerve blockade with steroid, information obtained from diagnostic intercostal blockade can help further guide which thoracic levels should be targeted if subsequent neurolysis is required [42]. The patient can also use diagnostic intercostal nerve blockade as a means to gauge the degree of expected motor and sensory impairment with ensuing neurolysis [43].

Targeted and Diagnostic Nerve Blockade

The intercostal nerves are the anterior rami from the T1–T11 spinal nerves. The anterior ramus from T12 traverses the anterior abdominal wall as the subcostal nerve. Each intercostal nerve typically provides four main branches: gray rami communicans postganglionic fibers that interface with the sympathetic chain, a posterior cutaneous branch, a lateral cutaneous branch, and an anterior cutaneous branch [43]. The lateral cutaneous branch of each intercostal nerve is given off near the anterior axillary line and further divides

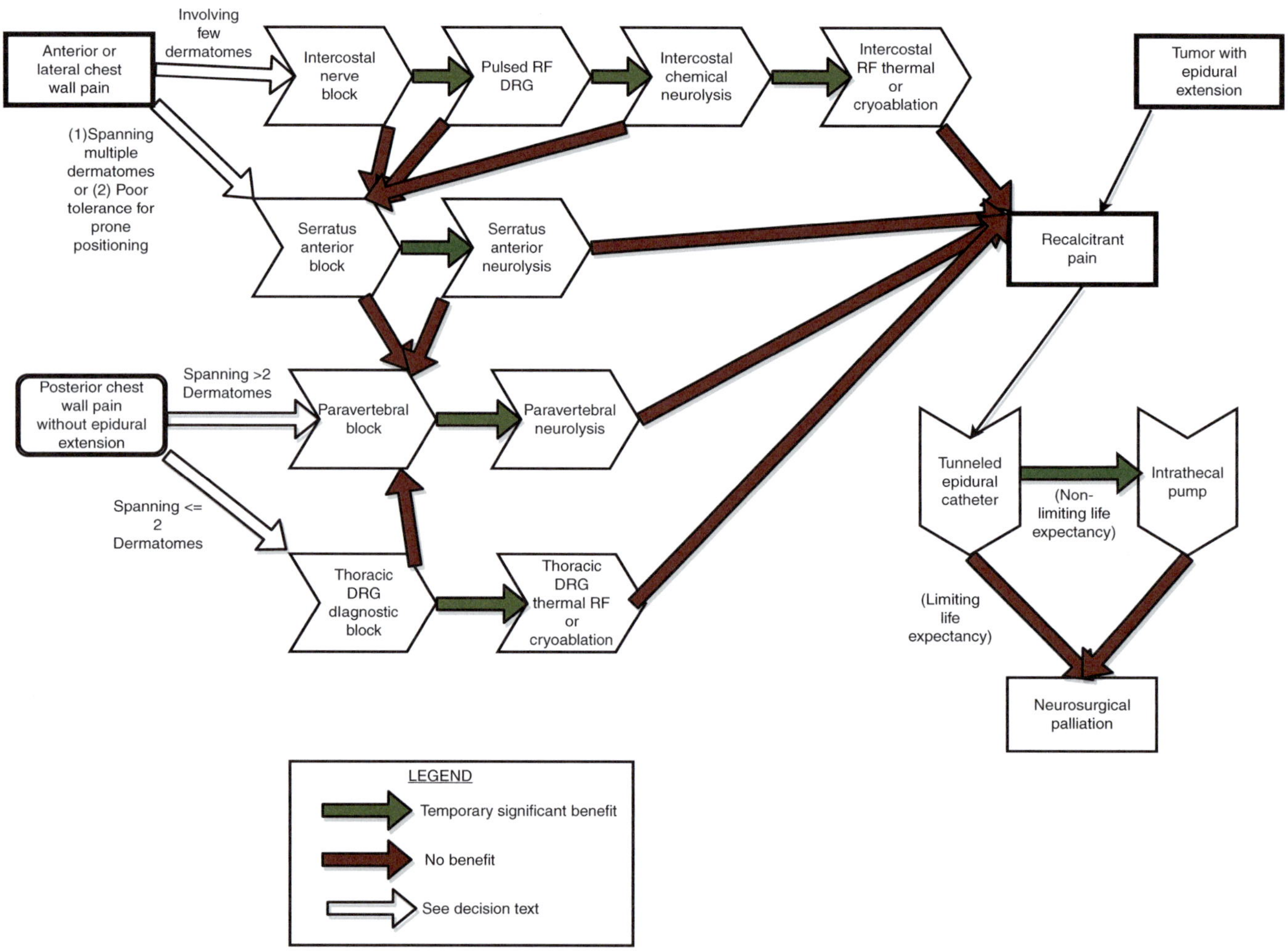

Fig. 10.1 Decision algorithm for chest wall pain

into anterior and posterior subbranches. It is these lateral cutaneous divisions that supply most of the sensation to the chest wall [43]. Each intercostal nerve terminates as an anterior cutaneous branch which supplies the anterior chest wall near midline. Sometimes these terminal divisions will cross midline and supply sensation to the contralateral chest wall [43]. Muscular subbranches supply the intercostal muscles, while pleural sensory and peritoneal sensory branches (from T7 to T11 only) innervate the parietal pleura and parietal peritoneum. The intercostal nerves are overall responsible for supplying sensation from the skin, parietal pleura, intercostal spaces, and chest wall musculature including the intercostal, levatores costarum, and serratus posterior muscles [44].

There is a higher chance of missing or incompletely blocking the posterior and lateral subdivisions of each intercostal nerve with more peripheral injection sites or with excessive movement during the procedure. This should be taken into consideration when treating cancer patients who have advanced disease, percutaneous tubes, or drains that may interfere with injection sites or cause great discomfort in the prone position for a prolonged period of time. Intercostal nerve blocks are limited in their ability to cover only a single dermatome with each needle placement. Large areas of pain that require multiple intercostal nerve blocks may cause significant procedure-related discomfort while increasing the chance for pneumothorax. For patients who are unable to tolerate lying in the prone position or those with thoracic pain spanning multiple dermatomes, a serratus plane block or paravertebral block may be a more suitable analgesic technique at the cost of being less precise than intercostal nerve blocks targeting specific dermatomes [45].

The serratus plane block is a newer ultrasound-guided pain management technique that is thought to provide anesthesia to the anterolateral hemithorax while having less risk and side effects compared to either paravertebral blockade or thoracic neuraxial anesthesia [46, 47]. Injection of anesthetic into the potential spaces above or below the serratus anterior muscle has been shown to provide long-lasting and predictable analgesia of the T2–T9 intercostal nerve branches that travel through these areas [46]. The long thoracic nerve and intercostobrachial nerve pierce the serratus anterior muscle and its fascia and are also consistently blocked with this technique [47]. Medication administration to the superficial serratus plane versus the deep plane has been theorized to be superior in terms of anesthetic spread, sensory distribution, and duration of analgesia [46, 47]. However, postsurgical scarring or postradiation fibrotic changes may interfere with medication spread more so in the superficial space [47].

The paravertebral block is another alternative that has traditionally been used in the perioperative period as a safe and effective alternative to thoracic epidural analgesia [48–50]. It is also a suitable technique for palliation of cancer-related thoracic pain, especially in those patients who develop tolerance or side effects to systemic analgesic therapies [42]. The paravertebral space is a triangular-shaped area bounded by the vertebral bodies and intervertebral discs medially, the parietal pleura and intercostal membrane anterolaterally, and thoracic vertebrae transverse processes, ribs, and superior costotransverse ligaments posteriorly [49, 51]. It contains the adipose tissue, the intercostal nerves, the sympathetic trunk, and the intercostal arteries and veins [51]. While the block can be performed without imaging guidance using a loss of resistance technique through the superior costotransverse ligament, a nerve stimulator or ultrasound guidance is often used to provide additional assistance [50]. A single-level paravertebral block at or slightly below the mid-dermatomal target level is usually capable of anesthetizing up to four dermatomes [49]. Multiple blocks are usually required to cover regions spanning greater than 3–4 ipsilateral dermatomes.

Neuromodulatory Techniques

For intractable cancer pain inadequately managed with intercostal nerve, paravertebral, or serratus plane blockade, neuromodulation or destructive techniques can be considered. Depending on factors including patient prognosis, risk tolerance, and preferences, an initial trial of pulsed radiofrequency ablation (PRF) or cryoablation of the thoracic nerve roots may provide adequate pain relief with less potential for serious neurologic complications compared to more aggressive neurolytic techniques [52–56]. It has been suggested that at least for post-thoracotomy pain, pulsed radiofrequency treatment of the thoracic dorsal root ganglion may be superior to both pulsed radiofrequency treatment directly to the intercostal nerves and also medical management with anticonvulsant/antidepressant therapy [57]. It should be noted that dorsal root ganglion pulsed radiofrequency therapy has yet to be studied for cancer-related thoracic pain [58].

Through our experience working at a large academic cancer treatment center, precise placement of the cryoprobe along the intercostal nerve can be difficult, and damage to the surrounding tissue is more prevalent [42]. Postradiation changes, tumor-induced soft tissue distortion, prior surgical manipulation, spinal spondylosis, and cervical torticollis may also obfuscate normal anatomic structures or interventional imaging guidance [29]. The efficacy of intercostal cryotherapy has also been questioned in terms of both pain relief and postoperative pulmonary function in the context of post-thoracotomy pain [59]. And furthermore, intercostal neuralgia lasting 2–4 weeks may develop in up to 20–30% of patients 6 weeks post-therapy [59].

Thermal radiofrequency ablation to the intercostal nerves for nonmalignant thoracic pain has also been described in the literature, but this technique shares similar technical-related concerns with cryoablation [60]. In general, thermal neurodestructive procedures are contraindicated for large myelinated nerves due to the possibility of developing post-treatment anesthesia dolorosa or neuromas [30]. However, these post-procedure complications may not apply to radiofrequency thermal lesioning of the thoracic dorsal root ganglion [61]. This technique has been used to treat intractable thoracic pain from bony pathology, intervertebral joint dislocations, intercostal neuropathy, or cancer [61]. In a study of 43 patients with thoracic pain resistant to conventional therapies, radiofrequency lesioning immediately adjacent to the thoracic dorsal root ganglion provided long-term (>36 weeks) pain relief in over half the treated group [61]. No major complications were reported though some patients reported having mild hypoesthesia and burning in the treated dermatomes [61]. All side effects resolved within 12 weeks without the need for intervention [61]. Of note, the same authors found significantly decreased efficacy of the thermal radiofrequency lesioning procedure for thoracic pain spanning greater than 2 dermatomes [61].

For those patients that desire more aggressive treatment or find it extremely difficult to tolerate going through multiple injections or procedures, commonly used neuroablative techniques include chemical neurolysis with alcohol or phenol. Neurolytic blocks applied to the intercostal nerves or paravertebral space are the most common in clinical practice. However, numerous case reports of neurologic injury including paraplegia have been reported with these techniques due to tracking of chemical neurolytic agents into the neuraxial space [62, 63]. The distribution of neurolytic agent after injection can be unpredictable. For example, thoracic paravertebral block injectate has been known to track to the contralateral side along the anterior aspect of the vertebral bodies [45]. Consequently, these procedures should be reserved for only those patients with intractable cancer-related pain and a poor prognosis [62]. Application of chemical neurolysis to the superficial serratus plane may be safer compared to neurolytic paravertebral blockade. However, ablation of the thoracodorsal and long thoracic nerves running through the same anatomic area may result in scapular winging after the procedure [47].

While follow-up neurolytic techniques can theoretically provide more sustained pain relief, they are often less effective compared to preceding diagnostic blocks targeting the same nerves [42]. The analgesic response to neurolytic blockade is influenced by various factors including concentration and volume of agent used in addition to rate of administration [14]. Other hypothesized reasons for decreased neurolytic efficacy include altered distribution of neurolytic agent in comparison to local anesthetic and steroid, increased patient discomfort and movement during neurolytic procedures, or variations between provider skills in performing neurolytic blocks [42].

Neuraxial Techniques

In patients with intractable pain despite the previous procedures, neuraxial-directed techniques provide at least equivocal pain control with fewer medication-related adverse side effects compared to systemic opioids [64–67].

Spinal cord stimulation (SCS) can be used to treat neuropathic and nociceptive pain. Though SCS has been typically indicated in patients suffering from nonmalignant conditions such as post-laminectomy pain syndrome and complex regional pain syndrome, it has also been reported as an effective technique in patients suffering from intractable cancer pain in smaller non-randomized clinical trials [68, 69]. Because evidence to support SCS for cancer-related pain from larger or high-level randomized controlled trials is still lacking, consideration for an epidural or intrathecal medication delivery device may be a more appropriate initial neuraxial pain treatment option [70].

A Cochrane review of uncontrolled studies reported excellent pain relief in 72% and 62% of cancer patients with the use of epidural and subarachnoid opioid infusions, respectively [71]. Other studies have found intrathecal drug delivery to be at least as effective as comprehensive medical management for refractory cancer pain with significantly less toxicity [65].

There are several important considerations when planning intrathecal medication delivery for malignant thoracic pain. When considering intrathecal medications, the use of only neuraxial opioids may incompletely control cancer-related pain, and addition of a local anesthetic drug is thought to enhance analgesia while reducing opioid requirements [72, 73]. While the addition of local anesthetic may cause additional adverse side effects including autonomic and neurologic dysfunction, orthostasis, and neurotoxicity, we still recommend a trial of combination of intrathecal medication as the initial first option.

More than 20 factors are thought to influence the spread of local anesthetic solutions in the cerebral spinal fluid after attainment of a pharmacologic steady state [74]. These influences include patient characteristics, injection technique, injection site, spinal fluid characteristics, and anesthetic solution characteristics [74]. Even hydrophilic compounds that undergo minimal spinal cord capillary losses are subject to a greater than 50% concentration loss along the length of the thoracic spinal cord when administered by slow intrathecal infusion [75].

Local anesthetics in the cerebrospinal fluid are thought to work by uptake into the nerve roots and into the spinal cord with the greatest uptake occurring where there is the highest concentration of medication [76]. When comparing the two processes, uptake of local anesthetic solution into the spinal cord is a slow process that preferentially occurs more so at the posterior and superficial regions [76]. Diffusion of local anesthetic deeper into the cord can also occur via the spaces of Virchow-Robin, but this is thought to be only a minor contributing mechanism [76]. Our experience with intrathecal pumps at a large academic cancer center also corroborates the primary mechanism of spinal anesthesia occurring more so at the thoracic nerve roots compared to spinal cord uptake. If spinal cord uptake were the primary mechanism of pain relief, patients should theoretically have enhanced analgesia everywhere caudal to the level of spinal cord blockade which we have not observed in patients with widely metastatic malignancies.

When infusing a local anesthetic and opioid combination, these significant considerations allude to the importance of aligning the final intrathecal catheter tip position to spinal nerve roots innervating the anatomic region causing the most distress. With this in mind, it is important to recall that spinal nerves originate at increasingly slanted angles in the cranial to caudal direction [77]. Spinal nerve roots in the thoracic region start descending approximately one vertebral level higher than their final vertebral column levels of exit [77, 78]. For those patients with a very limited life expectancy or with pain spanning a considerable region, placement of a tunneled epidural catheter may offer more superior pain relief compared to an intrathecal pump.

Neurosurgical Techniques

As a very last resort, neurosurgical palliative techniques including cordotomy can be considered. Precise sectioning of the spinothalamic tract results in contralateral loss of pain and temperature perception in up to several spinal segments below the incision level. It can be performed percutaneously or via open surgery. Several case studies have reported significant pain relief following cordotomy in up to 95% of treated patients with 75% maintaining pain control at 6 months [79, 80]. Postoperative neurologic issues are an obvious concern with this procedure, but several case series have reported only rare occurrences of motor weakness or incontinence following cordotomy [79, 81, 82]. It should be noted that bilateral cervical cordotomy confers a risk of sleep-associated apnea due to the presence of reticulospinal fibers responsible for spontaneous respiration traversing the area [79].

Summary

Pain syndromes related to thoracic malignancy are many and varied. Systemic analgesic therapy including opioids has the potential to provide significant pain relief in this population. However, some patients with gastrointestinal dysmotility or obstruction may have issues with conventional routes of medication administration. Others may fail to achieve meaningful pain relief or suffer from unbearable medication-related adverse side effects. In this subset of patients, interventional pain management techniques targeting the intercostal nerves, thoracic nerve roots, and/or neuroaxis can offer additional palliation when more conventional methods of pain control have failed.

References

1. Islami F, Torre LA, Jemal A. Global trends of lung cancer mortality and smoking prevalence. Transl Lung Cancer Res. 2015;4(4):327–38.
2. Fact Sheets by Cancer [Internet]. Available from: http://globocan.iarc.fr/Pages/fact_sheets_cancer.aspx.
3. Lung cancer mortality statistics|Cancer Research UK [Internet]. Available from: http://www.cancerresearchuk.org/health-professional/cancer-statistics/statistics-by-cancer-type/lung-cancer/mortality#heading-Five.
4. Al-Tariq QZ. Percutaneous strategies for the management of pulmonary parenchymal, chest wall, and pleural metastases. AJR Am J Roentgenol. 2014;203(4):709–16.
5. Mercadante S, Vitrano V. Pain in patients with lung cancer: pathophysiology and treatment. Lung Cancer. 2010;68(1):10–5.
6. Gough N, Miah AB, Linch M. Nonsurgical oncological management of cancer pain. Curr Opin Support Palliat Care. 2014;8(2):102–11.
7. Teunissen SCCM, Wesker W, Kruitwagen C, de Haes HCJM, Voest EE, de Graeff A. Symptom prevalence in patients with incurable cancer: a systematic review. J Pain Symptom Manag. 2007;34(1):94–104.
8. Marangoni C, Lacerenza M, Formaglio F, Smirne S, Marchettini P. Sensory disorder of the chest as presenting symptom of lung cancer. J Neurol Neurosurg Psychiatry. 1993;56(9):1033–4.
9. Marino C, Zoppi M, Morelli F, Buoncristiano U, Pagni E. Pain in early cancer of the lungs. Pain. 1986;27(1):57–62.
10. Fishman S, Ballantyne J, Rathmell JP, Bonica JJ, editors. Bonica's management of pain. 4th ed. Baltimore: Lippincott, Williams & Wilkins; 2010.
11. Yin L, He D, Shen H, et al. Surgical treatment of cardiac tumors: a 5-year experience from a single cardiac center. J Thorac Dis. 2016;8(5):911–9.
12. Bruera E, Portenoy RK, editors. Cancer pain: assessment and management. 2nd ed. Cambridge/New York: Cambridge University Press; 2010.
13. Hsu P-K, Hsu H-S, Lee H-C, et al. Management of primary chest wall tumors: 14 years' clinical experience. J Chin Med Assoc. 2006;69(8):377–82.
14. Rice ASC, editor. Clinical pain management. 2nd ed. London: Hodder Arnold; 2008.
15. Rusch VW. Management of Pancoast tumours. Lancet Oncol. 2006;7(12):997–1005.
16. Marulli G, Battistella L, Mammana M, Calabrese F, Rea F. Superior sulcus tumors (Pancoast tumors). Ann Translat Med. 2016;4(12):239.
17. Wilson LD, Detterbeck FC, Yahalom J. Clinical practice. Superior vena cava syndrome with malignant causes. N Engl J Med. 2007;356(18):1862–9.
18. Bone Metastasis: Which Cancers Cause It? [Internet]. Available from: http://www.webmd.com/cancer/common-cancers-that-metastasize-to-the-bones#1.

19. D'Antonio C, Passaro A, Gori B, et al. Bone and brain metastasis in lung cancer: recent advances in therapeutic strategies. Ther Adv Med Oncol. 2014;6(3):101–14.
20. Falk S, Dickenson AH. Pain and nociception: mechanisms of cancer-induced bone pain. J Clin Oncol. 2014;32(16):1647–54.
21. Sun L, Yu S. Efficacy and safety of denosumab versus zoledronic acid in patients with bone metastases: a systematic review and meta-analysis. Am J Clin Oncol. 2013;36(4):399–403.
22. Patrick DL, Cleeland CS, von Moos R, et al. Pain outcomes in patients with bone metastases from advanced cancer: assessment and management with bone-targeting agents. Support Care Cancer. 2015;23(4):1157–68.
23. Health Quality Ontario. Vertebral augmentation involving vertebroplasty or kyphoplasty for cancer-related vertebral compression fractures: a systematic review. Ont Health Technol Assess Ser. 2016;16(11):1–202.
24. Greenberg HS, Deck MD, Vikram B, Chu FC, Posner JB. Metastasis to the base of the skull: clinical findings in 43 patients. Neurology. 1981;31(5):530–7.
25. Storstein A, Vedeler CA. Paraneoplastic neurological syndromes and onconeural antibodies: clinical and immunological aspects. Adv Clin Chem. 2007;44:143–85.
26. Brady AM. Management of painful paraneoplastic syndromes. Hematol Oncol Clin North Am. 1996;10(4):801–9.
27. Trejo-Gabriel-Galan JM, Macarron-Vicente JL, Lázaro L, Rodriguez-Pascual L, Calvo I. Intercostal neuropathy and pain due to pleuritis. Pain Med. 2013;14(5):769–70.
28. Peláez R, Pascual G, Aguilar JL, Atanassoff PG. Paravertebral cervical nerve block in a patient suffering from a Pancoast tumor. Pain Med. 2010;11(12):1799–802.
29. Gofeld M, Bhatia A. Alleviation of Pancoast's tumor pain by ultrasound-guided percutaneous ablation of cervical nerve roots. Pain Pract. 2008;8(4):314–9.
30. Trescot, MD, ABIPP, FIPP, Andrea M, editor. Peripheral nerve entrapments [Internet]. Cham: Springer International Publishing; 2016 [cited 2016 Nov 20]. Available from: http://link.springer.com/10.1007/978-3-319-27482-9.
31. Simopoulos TT, Nagda J, Aner MM. Percutaneous radiofrequency lesioning of the suprascapular nerve for the management of chronic shoulder pain: a case series. J Pain Res. 2012;5:91–7.
32. Bindoff LA, Heseltine D. Unilateral facial pain in patients with lung cancer: a referred pain via the vagus? Lancet. 1988;1(8589):812–5.
33. Barnett GC, West CML, Dunning AM, et al. Normal tissue reactions to radiotherapy: towards tailoring treatment dose by genotype. Nat Rev Cancer. 2009;9(2):134–42.
34. Maesschalck TD, Dulguerov N, Caparrotti F, et al. Comparison of the incidence of osteoradionecrosis with conventional radiotherapy and intensity-modulated radiotherapy. Head Neck. 2016;38(11):1695–702.
35. Drugs Approved for Lung Cancer – National Cancer Institute [Internet]. Available from: https://www.cancer.gov/about-cancer/treatment/drugs/lung.
36. Meijuan Y, Zhiyou P, Yuwen T, Ying F, Xinzhong C. A retrospective study of postmastectomy pain syndrome: incidence, characteristics, risk factors, and influence on quality of life. Sci World J. 2013;2013:1–6.
37. Karmakar MK, Ho AMH. Postthoracotomy pain syndrome. Thorac Surg Clin. 2004;14(3):345–52.
38. Hopkins KG, Hoffman LA, Dabbs ADV, et al. Postthoracotomy pain syndrome following surgery for lung cancer: symptoms and impact on quality of life. J Adv Pract Oncol. 2015;6(2):121–32.
39. McGreevy K, Bottros MM, Raja SN. Preventing chronic pain following acute pain: risk factors, preventive strategies, and their efficacy. Eur J Pain Suppl. 2011;5(2):365–72.
40. Nagahiro I, Andou A, Aoe M, Sano Y, Date H, Shimizu N. Pulmonary function, postoperative pain, and serum cytokine level after lobectomy: a comparison of VATS and conventional procedure. Ann Thorac Surg. 2001;72(2):362–5.
41. Sentürk M, Ozcan PE, Talu GK, et al. The effects of three different analgesia techniques on long-term postthoracotomy pain. Anesth Analg. 2002;94(1):11–5, table of contents.
42. Gulati A, Shah R, Puttanniah V, Hung JC, Malhotra V. A retrospective review and treatment paradigm of interventional therapies for patients suffering from intractable thoracic chest wall pain in the oncologic population. Pain Med. 2015;16(4):802–10.
43. Waldman SD. Atlas of interventional pain management. 3rd ed. Philadelphia: Saunders/Elsevier; 2009.
44. Snell RS. Clinical anatomy by regions. Baltimore: Lippincott Williams & Wilkins; 2012.
45. Karmakar MK, Kwok WH, Kew J. Thoracic paravertebral block: radiological evidence of contralateral spread anterior to the vertebral bodies. Br J Anaesth. 2000;84(2):263–5.
46. Blanco R, Parras T, McDonnell JG, Prats-Galino A. Serratus plane block: a novel ultrasound-guided thoracic wall nerve block. Anaesthesia. 2013;68(11):1107–13.
47. Zocca JA, Chen GH, Puttanniah VG, Hung JC, Gulati A. Ultrasound-guided serratus plane block for treatment of postmastectomy pain syndromes in breast cancer patients: a case series. Pain Pract. 2017;17(1):141–6.
48. Grider JS, Mullet TW, Saha SP, Harned ME, Sloan PA. A randomized, double-blind trial comparing continuous thoracic epidural bupivacaine with and without opioid in contrast to a continuous paravertebral infusion of bupivacaine for post-thoracotomy pain. J Cardiothorac Vasc Anesth. 2012;26(1):83–9.
49. Tighe S, Greene MD, Rajadurai N. Paravertebral block. Contin Educ Anaesth Crit Care Pain. 2010;10(5):133–7.
50. Daly DJ, Myles PS. Update on the role of paravertebral blocks for thoracic surgery: are they worth it? Curr Opin Anaesthesiol. 2009;22(1):38–43.
51. Krediet AC, Moayeri N, van Geffen G-J, et al. Different approaches to ultrasound-guided thoracic paravertebral block: an illustrated review. Anesthesiology. 2015;123(2):459–74.
52. Connelly NR, Malik A, Madabushi L, Gibson C. Use of ultrasound-guided cryotherapy for the management of chronic pain states. J Clin Anesth. 2013;25(8):634–6.
53. Byas-Smith MG, Gulati A. Ultrasound-guided intercostal nerve cryoablation. Anesth Analg. 2006;103(4):1033–5.
54. Bogduk N. Pulsed radiofrequency. Pain Med. 2006;7(5):396–407.
55. Lord SM, Bogduk N. Radiofrequency procedures in chronic pain. Best Pract Res Clin Anaesthesiol. 2002;16(4):597–617.
56. Racz GB, Ruiz-Lopez R. Radiofrequency procedures. Pain Pract. 2006;6(1):46–50.
57. Cohen SP, Sireci A, Wu CL, Larkin TM, Williams KA, Hurley RW. Pulsed radiofrequency of the dorsal root ganglia is superior to pharmacotherapy or pulsed radiofrequency of the intercostal nerves in the treatment of chronic postsurgical thoracic pain. Pain Physician. 2006;9(3):227–35.
58. Facchini G, Spinnato P, Guglielmi G, Albisinni U, Bazzocchi A. A comprehensive review of pulsed radiofrequency in the treatment of pain associated with different spinal conditions. Br J Radiol. 2017;90:20150406.
59. Detterbeck FC. Efficacy of methods of intercostal nerve blockade for pain relief after thoracotomy. Ann Thorac Surg. 2005;80(4):1550–9.
60. Engel AJ. Utility of intercostal nerve conventional thermal radiofrequency ablations in the injured worker after blunt trauma. Pain Physician. 2012;15(5):E711–8.
61. van Kleef M, Barendse GA, Dingemans WA, et al. Effects of producing a radiofrequency lesion adjacent to the dorsal root ganglion in patients with thoracic segmental pain. Clin J Pain. 1995;11(4):325–32.
62. Malik T. Ultrasound-guided paravertebral neurolytic block: a report of two cases. Pain Pract. 2014;14(4):346–9.

63. Gollapalli L, Muppuri R. Paraplegia after intercostal neurolysis with phenol. J Pain Res. 2014;7:665–8.
64. McCartney CJL, Chambers WA. Central neuraxial techniques for cancer pain. Curr Anaesth Crit Care. 2000;11(3):166–72.
65. Smith TJ, Staats PS, Deer T, et al. Randomized clinical trial of an implantable drug delivery system compared with comprehensive medical management for refractory cancer pain: impact on pain, drug-related toxicity, and survival. J Clin Oncol. 2002;20(19):4040–9.
66. Brogan S, Junkins S. Interventional therapies for the management of cancer pain. J Support Oncol. 2010;8(2):52–9.
67. Mercadante S, Intravaia G, Villari P, et al. Intrathecal treatment in cancer patients unresponsive to multiple trials of systemic opioids. Clin J Pain. 2007;23(9):793–8.
68. Flagg A, McGreevy K, Williams K. Spinal cord stimulation in the treatment of cancer-related pain: "back to the origins". Curr Pain Headache Rep. 2012;16(4):343–9.
69. Yakovlev AE, Resch BE. Spinal cord stimulation for cancer-related low back pain. Am J Hosp Palliat Care. 2012;29(2):93–7.
70. Peng L, Min S, Zejun Z, Wei K, Bennett MI. Spinal cord stimulation for cancer-related pain in adults. Cochrane Database Syst Rev. 2015;6:CD009389.
71. Ballantyne JC, Carwood CM. Comparative efficacy of epidural, subarachnoid, and intracerebroventricular opioids in patients with pain due to cancer. Cochrane Database Syst Rev. 2005;1:CD005178.
72. Mercadante S. Neuraxial techniques for cancer pain: an opinion about unresolved therapeutic dilemmas. Reg Anesth Pain Med. 1999;24(1):74–83.
73. Farquhar-Smith P, Chapman S. Neuraxial (epidural and intrathecal) opioids for intractable pain. Br J Pain. 2012;6(1):25–35.
74. Greene NM. Distribution of local anesthetic solutions within the subarachnoid space. Anesth Analg. 1985;64(7):715–30.
75. Kroin JS, Ali A, York M, Penn RD. The distribution of medication along the spinal canal after chronic intrathecal administration. Neurosurgery. 1993;33(2):226–30; discussion 230.
76. NYSORA – The New York School of Regional Anesthesia – Spinal Anesthesia [Internet]. Available from: http://www.nysora.com/techniques/neuraxial-and-perineuraxial-techniques/landmark-based/3423-spinal-anesthesia.html.
77. Drake RL, Vogl W, Mitchell AWM, Gray H. Gray's anatomy for students. 3rd ed. Philadelphia: Churchill Livingstone/Elsevier; 2015.
78. Gosling JA. Human anatomy: color atlas and textbook. London: Mosby; 2008.
79. Atkin N, Jackson KA, Danks RA. Bilateral open thoracic cordotomy for refractory cancer pain: a neglected technique? J Pain Symptom Manag. 2010;39(5):924–9.
80. Kanpolat Y. The surgical treatment of chronic pain: destructive therapies in the spinal cord. Neurosurg Clin N Am. 2004;15(3):307–17.
81. Crul BJP, Blok LM, van Egmond J, van Dongen RTM. The present role of percutaneous cervical cordotomy for the treatment of cancer pain. J Headache Pain. 2005;6(1):24–9.
82. Raslan AM. Percutaneous computed tomography-guided radiofrequency ablation of upper spinal cord pain pathways for cancer-related pain. Neurosurgery. 2008;62(3 Suppl 1):226–33; discussion 233–4.

Gastrointestinal Cancer Pain

11

Daniel Pak and Joseph C. Hung

Introduction

The reported prevalence of pain syndromes associated with the most common gastrointestinal malignancies are 40–79% for colorectal cancer [1–5], 72–100% for pancreatic cancer [1, 3, 6], and 74–90% for gastric cancer.

In the sections below, we will focus on some techniques that may be considered for common pain syndromes associated with gastrointestinal malignancies (Table 11.1).

Gastrointestinal Visceral Pain Syndromes

As stated above, pain associated with noxious stimuli to abdominal organs tends to be diffuse, poorly localized, and dull in nature. These properties can be attributed to the low density of afferent nerve fibers located within viscera and also to the divergent nature of these inputs during central nervous system processing. Visceral pain secondary to tumors, both primary and metastatic, is most often due to organ distention or neural infiltration [7].

Pancreatic Cancer

Almost 90% of patients with tumors at the head of the pancreas experience pain, particularly if the growth is near the ampulla of Vater [8]. The pancreatic head is innervated by visceral afferent fibers that travel via the right thoracic splanchnic nerves. These arise from the thoracic sympathetic ganglia between the 6th and 12th vertebral bodies. Consequently, pain associated with the pancreatic head tends to be located near the epigastrium to the right of the midline. Tumors at the body of the pancreas also produce epigastric pain secondary to innervation from bilateral thoracic sympathetic ganglia and the right splenic nerves. Furthermore, tumors at the tail of the pancreas tend to produce left-sided epigastric pain secondary to innervation from the left splenic nerves and T6–L1 sympathetic ganglia.

Liver Cancer

Roughly 30% of patients with advanced hepatic cancers experience pain [8]. Potential pain generators in the hepatic region are numerous and include the liver capsule, hepatic

Table 11.1 Gastrointestinal malignancy pain syndromes

Gastrointestinal visceral pain syndromes
Pancreatic cancer
Liver cancer
Gastric cancer
Colorectal cancer
Retroperitoneal pain
Bowel obstruction
Peritoneal carcinomatosis
Ureteric obstruction
Gastrointestinal nociceptive pain syndromes
Malignant perineal pain
Anterior abdominal wall pain
Bone pain
Malignancy-associated neuropathic pain syndromes
Malignant radiculopathy
Malignant plexopathy
Malignant mononeuropathy
Treatment-associated pain syndromes
Chemotherapy-associated neuropathy
Postsurgical pain
Radiation-associated pain

D. Pak
Massachusetts General Hospital, Boston, MA, USA

J. C. Hung (✉)
Memorial Sloan Kettering Cancer Center, Anesthesiology and Critical Care Medicine, New York, NY, USA
e-mail: jhung@alumni.upenn.edu

A. Gulati et al. (eds.), *Essentials of Interventional Cancer Pain Management*, https://doi.org/10.1007/978-3-319-99684-4_11

vessels, and biliary tract. The liver parenchyma itself is innervated by the hepatic plexus, which is one of the largest derivatives of the celiac plexus.

The hepatic plexus carries both sympathetic fibers and parasympathetic fibers from the vagus nerve. Many of these nerves travel with divisions of the hepatic artery and bile ducts. The liver capsule also shares innervation from the lower intercostal nerves. As a result, liver malignancy pain is typically described as a dull right subcostal pain. Mass effect from hepatomegaly can result in distention of the liver capsule. In advanced disease this enlargement can be secondary to hemorrhage as well. Other potential sources of pain in the liver region include primary or secondary hepatic tumors and vessel distention as seen from portal obstruction. Any pressure on the diaphragm or biliary tract may result in referred pain transmitted via the phrenic nerve to the right supraclavicular region.

Pain from hepatic structures is frequently pleuritic and exacerbated with positional changes. On physical exam, patients may have hepatomegaly and tenderness to palpation at the right upper quadrant of the abdomen. A frictional rub may also be auscultated over this area.

Gastric Cancer

It is reported that 74–90% of patients with gastric cancer experience pain [1, 5]. The stomach receives innervation from presynaptic sympathetic fibers of the greater thoracic splanchnic nerves (T5–T9 segments) and parasympathetic innervation from the vagal trunk. These fibers synapse in the celiac ganglia. Patients with gastric visceral pain may present with dyspepsia and burning epigastric pain.

Colorectal Cancer

The small intestine and colon up to the splenic flexure receive parasympathetic innervation from the vagus nerve and sympathetic innervation from the greater (T5–T9) and lesser (T10–T11) thoracic splanchnic nerves. These nerves synapse via the celiac and superior mesenteric plexuses. The GI tract distal to the splenic flexure is innervated by sympathetic innervation from the lumbar splanchnic nerves (L1–L2) via the inferior mesenteric plexus.

Symptoms of colorectal cancers are dependent on the location of relevant pathology. Pain tends to be secondary to tumor growth into the intestinal lumen or nearby structures. In addition to weight loss, obstruction, melena, or hematochezia, patients can present with dull abdominal pain located roughly in the same area of tumor infiltration. Other sources of abdominal pain include distention secondary to obstruction, peritoneal metastasis, and/or intestinal perforation. Rectal or distal GI tract involvement can present with tenesmus and localized rectal pain that is worse with defecation.

Retroperitoneal Pain Syndrome

Tumor infiltration into the posterior abdominal wall, peritoneum, and neighboring neural structures can produce retroperitoneal pain syndrome. It is commonly experienced as a dull, aching pain in the epigastrium or mid-back that is exacerbated by lying down and relieved when sitting up. The most common causes are pancreatic cancer and retroperitoneal lymphadenopathy [9]. Pancreatic masses, in particular, can cause pain secondary to peritoneal invasion, compression of neighboring hepatic vessels, and/or spread to the liver.

Bowel Obstruction

Colorectal cancers as well as peritoneal carcinomatosis can cause intestinal bowel obstructions. This often presents with abdominal distention and pain. Small bowel obstructions tend to present with colicky discomfort located more at the mid-abdomen compared to large bowel obstructions where the pain is continuous and felt in the lower abdomen. Associated nausea, vomiting, and constipation are quite common. Bowel ischemia and perforation can also be seen with prolonged obstruction.

Peritoneal Carcinomatosis

The most common gastrointestinal malignancies causing peritoneal carcinomatosis are colorectal, gastric, and appendiceal cancers in addition to abdominal sarcomatosis [10]. Pain is inflammatory in nature and can subsequently lead to the development of both adhesions and ascites. Malignant bowel obstructions frequently occur. This pain syndrome is characterized by constant and diffuse abdominal pain that is tender with palpation.

Opiate analgesics have been found to be relatively ineffective [11]. Alternate analgesic options include control of disease using systemic and regional chemotherapy as well as operative cytoreduction in select patient populations.

Ureteric Obstruction

Obstructive uropathy is a structural hindrance of urine output that can lead to renal dysfunction and can be a recurrent issue when secondary to cancer. Colorectal cancer is a common cause [12]. Compression of the ureters causes unilateral flank pain that radiates to the ipsilateral inguinal region.

Pain is often described as colicky in nature and is associated with urination problems (e.g., anuria, polyuria). Treatment is often surgical in nature and often involves surgical decompression, percutaneous drainage, or stent placement.

Gastrointestinal Nociceptive Pain Syndromes

Malignant Perineal Pain

In addition to genitourinary malignancies, perineural invasion or infiltration of the pelvic musculature by colorectal tumors can cause a constant, dull pelvic pain that may be worsened by standing or sitting. Pain can be localized anteriorly or posteriorly or diffusely involve the perineal area. It may also be associated with bladder spasms or tenesmus. On physical exam, a digital rectal exam can demonstrate local tenderness or tumor.

Anterior Abdominal Wall Pain

Tumor cell seeding around port sites has been described as an unforeseen complication of laparoscopic surgery [13]. Abdominal wall metastases may arise from primary gastrointestinal malignancies – more commonly from those of hepatic and colorectal origin. Since abdominal wall metastasis is suggestive of widespread and/or advanced disease, differentiating abdominal wall pain from other malignant pain syndromes can be difficult. Presentation is varied, but palpable abdominal masses may be present and accompanied with localized pain.

Bone Pain

Bone metastasis is the most common cause of malignancy-associated chronic pain [7, 14]. Pain may be due to mass effect from large tumors or from metastatic infiltration into neural structures. Pathologic fractures may also cause pain, particularly with movement of the involved body part. Metastatic bone disease is a relatively uncommon occurrence in gastrointestinal malignancies, with most studies citing rates of less than 20% for pancreatic, gastric, and colorectal cancers [15–18].

Bone pain is classically a deep and aching pain that is continuous and exacerbated with movement. Patients may also experience mechanical allodynia. Vertebral body involvement causes axial back pain and associated tenderness on palpation. Infiltration of the epidural space may result in neurologic deficits and/or neuropathic pain. Two-thirds of the time, the thoracic spine is involved compared with cervical or lumbar regions [19]. The proximal femur is the most commonly affected peripheral site. Due to the role of the skeleton supporting the body, bony metastatic disease can be a major source of disability.

Opioid doses to effectively treat bone pain have been found to be higher than other pain syndromes of similar magnitude, thereby making it difficult to effectively manage with opiates alone [20, 21]. Therefore, adjuvant interventional techniques are frequently necessary for adequate pain control.

Malignancy-Associated Neuropathic Pain Syndromes

Tumor infiltration into neural structures can cause pain, sensory changes, and/or weakness in the distribution of the involved nerve root, plexus, or peripheral nerve.

Malignant Radiculopathy

Although not common with gastrointestinal malignancies, radicular pain may occur secondary to posterior extension of vertebral body metastatic disease. Involvement of the thoracic roots can cause flank pain described as a band around the chest or abdomen. It may also be accompanied with burning or electric shock-like sensations in the distribution of the involved nerve root. Focal neurologic deficits may be present. MR imaging is diagnostic and should be ordered to evaluate any oncologic patient presenting with neurologic dysfunction.

Malignant Plexopathy

Mass effect on nerve plexuses can cause severe discomfort and neurologic changes. Colorectal tumors may cause lumbar and/or sacral plexopathy. This condition tends to present with lower extremity pain, numbness, sensory changes, and/or weakness. Usually resulting from pressure on the psoas muscle, lumbar plexopathy affecting more cephalad nerve roots (L1–L4 distribution) causes pain in the anterolateral thigh, knee, and proximal leg. Cancers of the sigmoid colon and rectum may affect the lower lumbosacral plexus (L4–S1 distribution) and may manifest as pain in the buttocks, posterior leg, and foot. Patients with insult to the sacral plexus, usually from rectal tumors, tend to describe pain involving the buttocks, posterior legs, and perineum. Involvement of the coccygeal nerve can cause pain around the anus with associated sensory changes and also anal sphincter dysfunction. Symptoms are often worse with prolonged sitting and relieved with ambulation.

Any malignant plexopathy can also present with autonomic dysfunction [7]. Patients may complain of classic signs such as anhidrosis and vasodilation. This constellation of findings is often confused with complex regional pain syndrome (CRPS), which itself is also a potential complication secondary to malignant neuropathies. A diagnostic sympathetic nerve block may help to identify pain arising from a sympathetic origin [7].

Other plexopathies, for example, involving the cervical or brachial plexuses, are possible but rare with gastrointestinal malignancies.

Malignant Mononeuropathy

Compression or infiltration of a peripheral nerve can cause pain, dysesthesia, and/or neurologic deficits. Given the location of gastrointestinal malignancies away from most peripheral nerves, malignant mononeuropathy secondary to gastrointestinal cancer is relatively uncommon. When this syndrome does occur, examples include neuralgias involving the intercostal, lateral femoral cutaneous, hypogastric, or ilioinguinal nerves.

Treatment-Associated Pain Syndromes

Chemotherapy-Associated Neuropathies

Common chemotherapy agents used to treat gastrointestinal malignancies and can cause neuropathy include Taxol, docetaxel, oxaliplatin, cisplatin, and carboplatin [7, 22]. Nerves are damaged secondary to axonal atrophy and demyelination with resulting alteration of neural excitability. The degree of nerve damage is dependent on the type of drug, dose, duration of administration, and also pre-existing nerve damage.

In most cases, chemotherapy-induced neuropathy is acute and transient and appears within 24 h of initial administration [7]. Symptoms are usually reversible and resolve after stopping the agent or decreasing the dose. In some cases, symptoms appear or progress after cessation of therapy, which is a phenomenon known as "coasting." Less frequently, it persists as a chronic pain syndrome. Affected patients typically present with pain and dysesthesias affecting the distal extremities in a "stocking-glove" pattern. Other deficits such as weakness, loss of reflexes, and ataxia may also be present. Involvement of the autonomic nervous system results in orthostatic hypotension, constipation, paralytic ileus, urinary bladder dysfunction, and impotence.

Postsurgical Pain

Postsurgical pain is not uncommon within the oncologic population. The often extensive surgery that is necessary to remove cancerous tissue(s) can cause multiple acute and chronic pain symptoms. Given the anatomic location of gastrointestinal malignancies, chronic abdominal wall may stem from anterior cutaneous nerve entrapment. The pathophysiology underlying this condition is thought to be secondary to entrapment of the lower intercostal nerves at the lateral border of the rectus abdominis muscle from postsurgical scar tissue [23, 24]. Patients typically present with sharp and localized pain along the rectus abdominis muscle sheath. Carnett's sign, which is characterized by worsening pain with the Valsalva maneuver or with tensing the abdomen, may be indicative of this syndrome. Other pain syndromes resulting after abdominal surgery may arise from peripheral nerve injuries either from direct trauma or surgical positioning, adhesion formation, or bowel obstruction.

Radiation-Associated Pain

Radiation exposure typically causes tissue fibrosis, retraction of nerve trunks, direct nerve axon injury, and micro-infarction of nerves. The degree of neuronal damage depends primarily on the cumulative radiation dose and delivery technique [25]. However, advances within the field of radiation oncology, such as conformal radiation therapy, have improved upon tumor targeting techniques resulting in decreased radiation exposure to surrounding tissues. Lumbosacral plexopathy is most likely with abdominal radiation exposure. Afflicted patients are often seen with weakness, sensory changes, and burning, aching, and cramping pain in one or both legs. Symptoms may appear months to decades after completion of radiation therapy [26].

The incidence of radiation-induced enteritis is also high and results from tissue ischemia and its associated pathologic changes including mucosal friability, neovascularization, and fibrosis. Patients commonly experience colicky abdominal pain, bloating, loss of appetite, nausea, diarrhea, or fecal urgency during or shortly after a course of radiation therapy. Acute radiation-induced enteropathy is usually self-limited, often resolving within 3 months and requiring supportive measures such as fluid therapy, antidiarrheals, and cytoprotective agents (amifostine, sulfasalazine). Chronic enteropathy can develop several months to years after receiving radiation therapy [27]. Postprandial pain, acute or intermittent small bowel obstruction, nausea, anorexia, weight loss, diarrhea, and malabsorption are common.

Interventional Pain Control Options

Sympathetic Blocks for Visceral Pain

Given that the autonomic nervous system innervates much of the gastrointestinal tract, interventional techniques such as sympathetic nerve blocks can provide substantial pain relief for visceral pain syndromes.

Celiac Plexus Block

Afferent, sympathetic, and parasympathetic innervation of the abdominal viscera from the upper esophagus to the splenic flexure (including the pancreas, liver, biliary tract, gallbladder, spleen, adrenal glands, kidneys, mesentery, stomach, small and large bowels) are innervated by the celiac plexus, which is located in the retroperitoneum on the anterolateral surface of the aorta around the body of L1. Nearby structures include the celiac trunk and superior mesenteric artery (SMA). In addition to carrying visceral afferent fibers that transmit nociception, the celiac plexus also contains preganglionic sympathetic efferents from the splanchnic nerves as well as parasympathetic fibers from the vagus nerve.

Image-guided celiac plexus block can be performed for intractable pain originating from upper abdominal viscera. It is useful for treating pain secondary to primary/secondary tumors and also lymphadenopathy secondary to metastatic spread. In a meta-analysis retrospectively examining the effect of celiac plexus block on pancreatic cancer patients, this intervention provided partial to complete relief in 70–90% of patients at 3 months post-block and decreased overall analgesia consumption [28, 29]. Among other potential complications associated with celiac plexus blockade, the most common ones include back pain, transient diarrhea, hypotension, nerve injury, intravascular injection, bowel injury, and bleeding.

Splanchnic Nerve Block

The greater (T5–T9), lesser (T10–T11), and least (T12) splanchnic nerves provide afferent and sympathetic innervation to the abdominal viscera and travel through the celiac plexus. As an alternative to celiac plexus blockade via the transcrural needle approach, blockade of the splanchnic nerves can be performed in the retrocrural space. Advantages of this technique include enhanced medication spread and superior pain control when disease is located on or around the celiac axis (involving the body or tail of the pancreas) [30].

The choice of imaging modality for celiac/splanchnic nerve blockade is beyond the scope of this chapter. Ultrasound, fluoroscopic, and computed tomography (CT) guidance techniques have all been described. However, the use of CT has gained popularity for its ability to clearly visualize the procedure needle(s), avoid trauma to surrounding anatomy, and assess the spread of neurolytic agent.

Superior Hypogastric Plexus Block

The superior hypogastric plexus is situated on the anterior aspect of the L5–S1 vertebral bodies and branches into right and left trunks as it descends into the pelvis. It carries sympathetic and afferent nerve fibers from pelvic viscera as well as the bowel distal to the left colonic flexure. This block can provide effective pain relief for patients with abdominal pain from the descending colon, sigmoid colon, or rectum. Common complications include intravascular injection in the iliac vessels, discitis, and bladder or bowel incontinence.

Ganglion Impar Block

The two most caudal portions of the sympathetic ganglia fuse to form the ganglion impar, which lies anterior to the coccyx. The ganglion impair (or ganglion of Walther) provides sympathetic innervation for many of the structures in the pelvis, including the perineum, vulva, distal vagina, anus, distal rectum, and distal urethra. It can provide substantial relief for patients with pelvic pain syndromes, including anorectal and perineal pain. Ganglion impar blockade is typically facilitated with fluoroscopy or ultrasound. After diagnostic blockade, follow-up radiofrequency denervation or chemical neurolysis may be used for longer-term analgesia. The most common complications of this block include intravascular injection and transient bowel or bladder dysfunction.

Somatic Nerve Blocks

Thoracic Intercostal/Paravertebral Block

The abdominal wall is segmentally innervated by the intercostal nerves and can be organized by dermatomes. Nociceptive fibers from the liver, its surrounding capsule, portions of the diaphragm, and parietal pleura are known to travel with sympathetic fibers via the thoracic paravertebral ganglia as well as the greater and lesser splanchnic nerves. Analgesia involving the abdominal wall can be achieved by targeting individual intercostal nerves underneath each rib or by injecting anesthetic agents into the paravertebral space. Both techniques achieve ipsilateral somatic blockade in a dermatomal distribution. Compared with intercostal blocks, the paravertebral block has the added advantage of blocking the sympathetic chain as it travels through the paravertebral space and can be effective for blocking pain thought to be from the liver capsule.

The paravertebral space is wedge-shaped and bordered anterolaterally by the parietal pleura, posteriorly by the superior costotransverse ligament, and medially by the spine. Anesthetic agents introduced in this area can block spinal nerve roots before they form intercostal nerves in addition to the sympathetic chain which also travels through this location. Needle entry into the paravertebral space is normally facilitated using ultrasound guidance or anatomic landmarks. Several injections may be needed to adequately cover pain over many thoracic dermatomes. To cover liver capsule pain, the paravertebral blockade should be performed in the lower right-sided thoracic area in order to cover the lower thoracic sympathetic chain in addition to the exiting T10–T12 intercostal nerves.

Intercostal nerve blocks are easier to perform from a technical standpoint and are usually performed by placing a needle near the inferior border of the nearby rib so that the needle tip is in close proximity to the neurovascular bundle. These can be accomplished by either using anatomic landmarks or with image (most often fluoroscopic or ultrasound) guidance.

Compared with individual intercostal nerve blockade, the spread of anesthetic agent and resulting dermatomal coverage within the paravertebral space may be more unpredictable. This procedure is also more difficult to perform technically and carries a higher risk of pneumothorax. While easier to perform, intercostal nerve blocks are generally more time-consuming as each needle placement blocks only one thoracic dermatome. Other potential complications from the paravertebral block include vascular puncture or, rarely, trauma to nearby spinal structures. For both blocks, there is a risk of local anesthetic systemic toxicity due to close proximity of the intercostal vessels.

Transversus Abdominis and Subcostal Plane (TAP) Block

The transversus abdominis plane (TAP) and subcostal plane block is specifically used to block abdominal wall afferents, which are supplied by the lower six thoracic nerves and first lumbar nerve, by injection of local anesthetic into the region between the internal oblique and transversus abdominis muscles. With easily identifiable cutaneous nerve entrapments, surgical neurectomy or local nerve blocks are often suggested as first-line treatments compared to systemic analgesics. The TAP block has also traditionally been used for postoperative acute pain control following major abdominal and pelvic surgeries.

Malignant pain from the upper abdominal or chest walls from metastatic disease may also be treated using intercostal nerve block(s). Chemical neurolysis or radiofrequency denervation may be considered for longer-term relief. Both intercostal and TAP blocks target nerves carrying nociception from the abdominal or chest wall.

Neuraxial Pain Control Systems

Spinal Cord Stimulation

In patients with intractable visceral pain resistant to medical therapy and sympathetic blockade, spinal cord stimulation (SCS) may be a viable alternative. The theoretical mechanism of pain relief is that afferent pain inputs are modulated as they travel through the dorsal spinal column or the medial visceral tracts. SCS has been used to treat numerous pain syndromes including back pain, radicular pain, complex regional pain syndrome, and ischemic pain arising from vascular disease [31]. More recently, case reports have demonstrated success with using SCS for intractable visceral pain related to chronic pancreatitis [32–34]. The most common complications are electrode migration, hardware malfunction, infection, and subcutaneous hematoma.

Intrathecal, Epidural Drug Delivery Systems

Intrathecal pumps delivering local anesthetic or opioid in the intrathecal space are an effective long-term adjunct for the treatment of chronic refractory neuropathic or nociceptive pain syndromes. It reduces pain and opioid-related side effects from systemic delivery without interruption of motor or autonomic function.

Implantable intrathecal pump systems deliver anesthetic medications directly into the spinal fluid located in the intrathecal space. The pump itself is implanted in a small subcutaneous pocket usually created in the lower abdomen and connected to a tunneled intrathecal catheter. The tip of the catheter should be placed near the spinal level corresponding to the location of the patient's pain, which for visceral pain is around T5–T8.

Tunneled epidural catheter placement is another technique that allows for anesthetic medication delivery into the neuroaxis. Like intrathecal pumps, epidural catheters can be effective for treating refractory neuropathic or nociceptive cancer pain syndromes. Placement of the epidural catheter tip in the area of the spine corresponding to the location of pain is also necessary, usually T6 through T9. To reduce the potential for infection, the catheter can be completely tunneled ending with an injection port, which can be accessed percutaneously. Compared with intrathecal pumps, epidural catheters carry a higher risk of infection as portions of the drug delivery system are left outside the body and connected to an external reservoir. As such, tunneled epidural catheters are usually reserved for those patients with a limited life expectancy.

Infusion Therapies

Hyperalgesia as a result of recurrent noxious stimulus is thought to arise secondary to activation of N-methyl-D-aspartate (NMDA) receptors in the central nervous system [35]. The administration of NMDA receptor antagonists has been shown to limit the development of opioid tolerance while increasing pain tolerance thresholds resulting in improved analgesia [20, 36, 37]. Methadone and ketamine are commonly used NMDA antagonist agents used to treat pain syndromes.

Ketamine

Intravenous ketamine infusions have been found to substantially decrease pain scores in patients whose pain was not adequately controlled with traditional opiates [38, 39]. Because higher doses result in dysphoria, increased secretions, tachycardia, and hypnosis/sedation, reduced subanesthetic infusions are typically used for pain management. Most protocols involve an initial bolus dose ranging between 0.2 and 0.5 mg/kg followed by a repeated identical dose infused over 30 min to 1 h [40]. Duration of pain reduction can last up to several weeks [39]. If effective, repeat infusions may be necessary to maintain the analgesic effect.

Lidocaine

Lidocaine infusions have also been used for central or peripheral neuropathic pain, although they have not been found to be effective against plexopathies from tumor infiltration [40]. Analgesia is thought to result from blocking sodium channels in neuronal cell membranes that carry neuropathic and inflammatory pain signals. Doses of 1–5 mg/kg over 30 min to 2 h have demonstrated reduced pain scores in patients with intractable neuropathic pain [40]. Side effects are uncommon but can include seizures, confusion, numbness, nausea, and cardiac arrhythmias. Similar to the use of ketamine, pain reduction can last up to several weeks, and repeat infusions are often needed for continued relief.

Special Considerations for Specific Pain Syndromes

Neuropathic Pain

Primary malignancy- and treatment-associated neuropathic pain can be difficult to treat and frequently requires multimodal therapy. Typical regimens often include neuropathic agents (e.g., anticonvulsant and antidepressants) used with various opioid and non-opioid (e.g., acetaminophen and NSAID) analgesics. Because neuropathic pain syndromes often affect multiple extremities in a diffuse fashion (e.g., chemotherapy-induced neuropathy), systemic or neuraxial analgesic techniques are most often employed. Due to few side effects, infusion trials using either ketamine or lidocaine are reasonable initial steps. Systemic therapies can be augmented with lumbar sympathetic and/or stellate ganglion blocks depending on which extremities are affected. For refractory pain, more aggressive options such as spinal cord stimulation or implantation of an intrathecal delivery device may be warranted.

Lumbar sympathetic blocks may be attempted for generalized lower extremity neuropathic pain secondary to peripheral nerve or lumbosacral plexus pathology. Lumbar sympathetic blockade has been described to treat numerous conditions affecting the lower extremities including complex regional pain syndrome, phantom limb pain, vascular insufficiency, and postherpetic neuralgia [41].

The lumbar sympathetic chain is composed of three to five ganglia and is an extension of the thoracic sympathetic chain. It is located anterolaterally to the lumbar vertebral bodies, anterior to the psoas muscle, and posterior to the vena cava. Blockade of the lumbar sympathetic chain is most commonly performed at the anterolateral aspect of the L2 or L3 vertebral bodies and effectively interrupts sympathetic efferent flow to the ipsilateral lower extremity. Fluoroscopic guidance is usually used for this technique. Potential complications include accidental intravascular injection or blockade of the lumbosacral plexus within the psoas muscle.

Conclusion

Many varied pain treatment options exist for pain syndromes secondary to gastrointestinal malignancies and its associated treatments (Figs. 11.1, 11.2, and 11.3). Systemic therapy using the WHO analgesic ladder is a reasonable initial choice even for practitioners without special training in pain management. Unfortunately, many of these drugs are either insufficient when used as monotherapy or associated with intolerable medication-related adverse side effects. More aggressive or advanced pain therapy options should be pursued with the aid of an interventional pain management physician.

From a broad organizational standpoint, pain of visceral origin can be treated using celiac ganglion, hypogastric plexus, or ganglion of impar blockade, depending on the location within the linear gastrointestinal tract. In addition, right-sided paravertebral blockade can be considered for pain stemming from the hepatic capsule or nearby structures including the diaphragm or lower parietal pleura. Pain from the abdominal wall can be targeted using intercostal, paravertebral, or transversus abdominis plane blockade.

Neuropathic pain can be difficult to treat and often requires the use of multiple pain therapy options. Infusion therapies using lidocaine or ketamine are alternate systemic treatment options when opioids and neuropathic medications have failed. Pain in the distribution of an isolated peripheral nerve can be alleviated by blocking the involved peripheral nerve. However, extending the duration of pain relief beyond the initial diagnostic block can be challenging without causing additional disability to the patient.

The most aggressive therapies involve placement of analgesic devices near the spine for pain relief and should be considered only further downstream on potential pain treatment pathways. These options include spinal cord stimulation, which has traditionally been most effective for neuropathic pain affecting a single extremity, and intrathecal drug delivery systems.

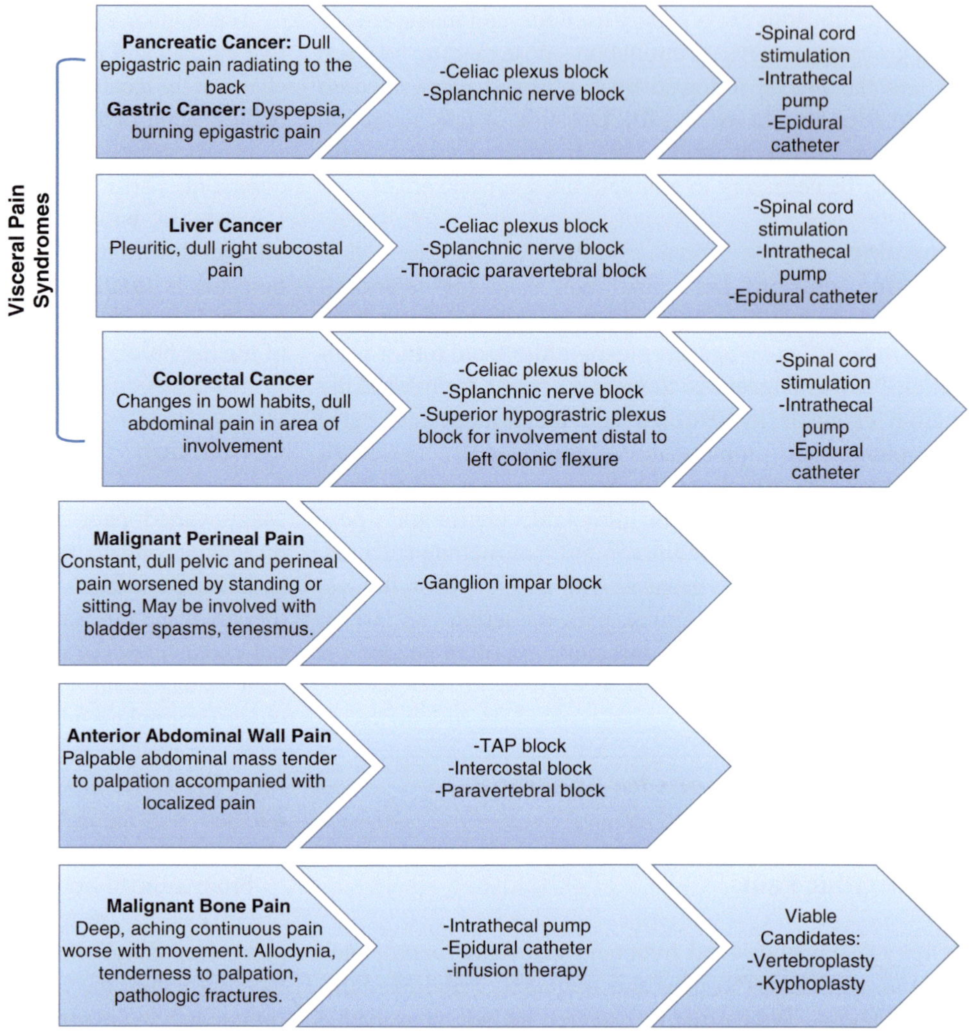

Fig. 11.1 Sequence of interventions for malignancy-associated visceral and nociceptive pain syndromes. Suggested interventions after failed conservative management. Therapies may be used concurrently

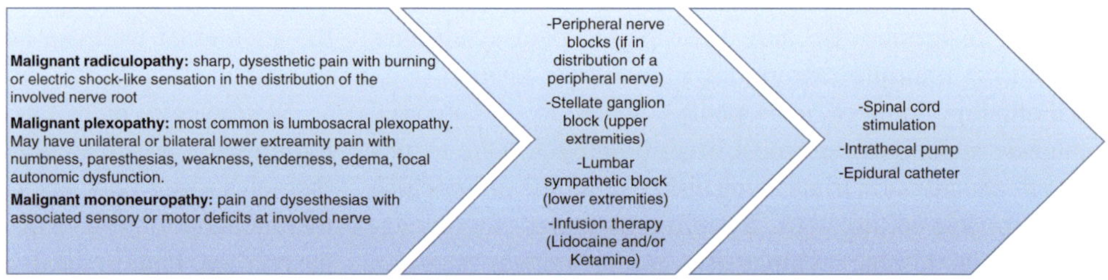

Fig. 11.2 Sequence of interventions for malignancy-associated neuropathic pain syndromes. Suggested interventions after failed conservative management. Therapies may be used concurrently

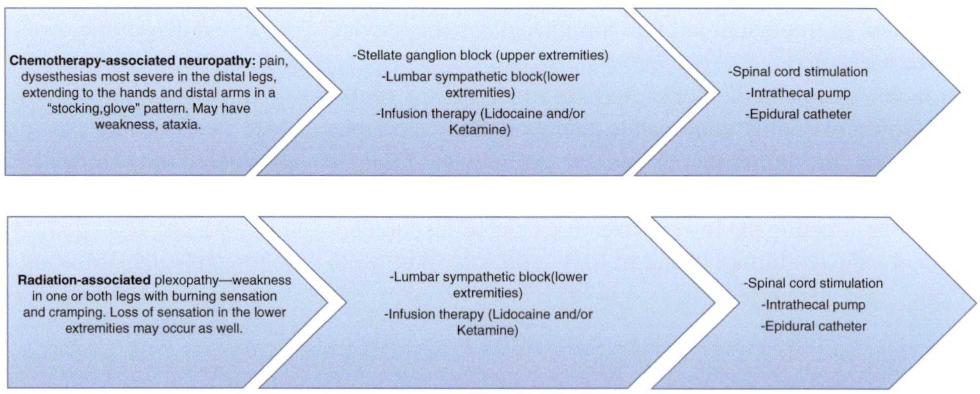

Fig. 11.3 Sequence of interventions for treatment-associated pain syndromes. Suggested interventions after failed conservative management. Therapies may be used concurrently

References

1. Chiu TY, Hu WY, Chen CY. Prevalence and severity of symptoms in terminal cancer patients: a study in Taiwan. Support Care Cancer Off J Multinatl Assoc Support Care Cancer. 2000;8:311–3.
2. Daut RL, Cleeland CS. The prevalence and severity of pain in cancer. Cancer. 1982;50:1913–8.
3. Donnelly S, Walsh D, Rybicki L. The symptoms of advanced cancer: identification of clinical and research priorities by assessment of prevalence and severity. J Palliat Care. 1995;11:27–32.
4. Portenoy RK, et al. Pain in ovarian cancer patients. Prevalence, characteristics, and associated symptoms. Cancer. 1994;74:907–15.
5. Vainio A, Auvinen A. Prevalence of symptoms among patients with advanced cancer: an international collaborative study. J Pain Symptom Manag. 1996;12:3–10.
6. Greenwald HP, Bonica JJ, Bergner M. The prevalence of pain in four cancers. Cancer. 1987;60:2563–9.
7. Bruera E, Portenoy R (eds.). Cancer pain assessment and management. Cambridge UK: Cambridge University Press; 2009. ISBN: 978-0521879279
8. Sykes N, Bennet M, Yuan C. Clinical pain management. 2nd Edition. Cancer Pain. Boca Raton, FL: CRC Press; 2008. ISBN: 978-0340940075.
9. Grahm AL, Andrén-Sandberg A. Prospective evaluation of pain in exocrine pancreatic cancer. Digestion. 1997;58:542–9.
10. Deraco M, Laterza B, Kusamura S, Baratti D. Updated treatment of peritoneal carcinomas: a reviewMinerva Chir. 2007;62:459–76.
11. Suzuki M, et al. Sensation of abdominal pain induced by peritoneal carcinomatosis is accompanied by changes in the expression of substance P and μ-opioid receptors in the spinal cord of mice. Anesthesiology. 2012;117:847–56.
12. Russo P. Urologic emergencies in the cancer patient. Semin Oncol. 2000;27:284–98.
13. Nduka CC, Monson JRT, Menzies-Gow N, Darzi A. Abdominal wall metastases following laparoscopy. Br J Surg. 1994;81:648–52.
14. Foley KM. Pain syndromes in patients with cancer. Med Clin North Am. 1987;71:169–84.
15. Borad MJ, et al. Skeletal metastases in pancreatic cancer: a retrospective study and review of the literature. Yale J Biol Med. 2009;82:1–6.
16. Ahn JB, Ha TK, Kwon SJ. Bone metastasis in gastric cancer patients. J Gastric Cancer. 2011;11:38–45.
17. Roth ES, et al. Does colon cancer ever metastasize to bone first? A temporal analysis of colorectal cancer progression. BMC Cancer. 2009;9:274.
18. Santini D, et al. Natural history of bone metastasis in colorectal cancer: final results of a large Italian bone metastases study. Ann Oncol Off J Eur Soc Med Oncol ESMO. 2012;23:2072–7.
19. Brihaye J, Ectors P, Lemort M, Van Houtte P. The management of spinal epidural metastases. Adv Tech Stand Neurosurg. 1988;16:121–76.
20. Mercadante S, Villari P, Ferrera P, Arcuri E, David F. Opioid switching and burst ketamine to improve the opioid response in patients with movement-related pain due to bone metastases. Clin J Pain. 2009;25:648–9.
21. Luger NM, et al. Efficacy of systemic morphine suggests a fundamental difference in the mechanisms that generate bone cancer vs inflammatory pain. Pain. 2002;99:397–406.
22. Quasthoff S, Hartung HP. Chemotherapy-induced peripheral neuropathy. J Neurol. 2002;249:9–17.
23. Boelens OB, Scheltinga MR, Houterman S, Roumen RM. Management of anterior cutaneous nerve entrapment syndrome in a cohort of 139 patients. Ann Surg. 2011;254:1054–8.
24. Akhnikh S, de Korte N, de Winter P. Anterior cutaneous nerve entrapment syndrome (ACNES): the forgotten diagnosis. Eur J Pediatr. 2014;173:445–9.
25. Kinsella TJ, et al. Threshold dose for peripheral neuropathy following intraoperative radiotherapy (IORT) in a large animal model. Int J Radiat Oncol. 1991;20:697–701.
26. Yi SK, et al. Development of a standardized method for contouring the lumbosacral plexus: a preliminary dosimetric analysis of this organ at risk among 15 patients treated with intensity-modulated radiotherapy for lower gastrointestinal cancers and the incidence of radiation-induced lumbosacral plexopathy. Int J Radiat Oncol Biol Phys. 2012;84:376–82.
27. Wj M. Surgical management of radiation enteropathy. Surg Clin North Am. 1991;71:977–90.
28. Eisenberg E, Carr DB, Chalmers TC. Neurolytic celiac plexus block for treatment of cancer pain: a meta-analysis. Anesth Analg. 1995;80:290–5.
29. Polati E, et al. Prospective randomized double-blind trial of neurolytic coeliac plexus block in patients with pancreatic cancer. Br J Surg. 1998;85:199–201.
30. Rykowski JJ, Hilgier M. Efficacy of neurolytic celiac plexus block in varying locations of pancreatic cancer: influence on pain relief. Anesthesiology. 2000;92:347–54.
31. Cameron T. Safety and efficacy of spinal cord stimulation for the treatment of chronic pain: a 20-year literature review. J Neurosurg Spine. 2004;100:254–67.
32. Kapural L, Rakic M. Spinal cord stimulation for chronic visceral pain secondary to chronic non-alcoholic pancreatitis. J Clin Gastroenterol. 2008;42:750–1.
33. Kim JK, Hong SH, Kim M-H, Lee J-K. Spinal cord stimulation for intractable visceral pain due to chronic pancreatitis. J Korean Neurosurg Soc. 2009;46:165.
34. Khan YN, Raza SS, Khan EA. Application of spinal cord stimulation for the treatment of abdominal visceral pain syndromes: case reports. Neuromodulation Technol Neural Interface. 2005;8:14–27.
35. Saito O, et al. Ketamine and N-acetylaspartylglutamate peptidase inhibitor exert analgesia in bone cancer pain. Can J Anaesth J Can Anesth. 2006;53:891–8.
36. Jackson K, et al. Burst' ketamine for refractory cancer pain: an open-label audit of 39 patients. J Pain Symptom Manag. 2001;22:834–42.
37. Mercadante S, Villari P, Ferrera P. Burst ketamine to reverse opioid tolerance in cancer pain. J Pain Symptom Manag. 2003;25:302–5.
38. Mercadante S, Arcuri E, Tirelli W, Casuccio A. Analgesic effect of intravenous ketamine in cancer patients on morphine therapy: a randomized, controlled, double-blind, crossover, double-dose study. J Pain Symptom Manage. 2000;20:246–52.
39. Patil S, Anitescu M. Efficacy of outpatient ketamine infusions in refractory chronic pain syndromes: a 5-year retrospective analysis. Pain Med Malden Mass. 2012;13:263–9.
40. Kosharskyy B, Almonte W, Shaparin N, Pappagallo M, Smith H. Intravenous infusions in chronic pain management. Pain Physician. 2013;16:231–49.
41. Day M. Sympathetic blocks: the evidence. Pain Pract Off J World Inst Pain. 2008;8:98–109.

Genitourinary Cancer Pain Syndromes

12

Ilan Margulis and Amitabh Gulati

Introduction

It is essential to characterize the underlying pathophysiology of your patient's pain to aid in diagnosis and subsequent targeted therapy. Pain can be described as either nociceptive pain, which can be further subdivided into somatic and visceral pain, or neuropathic pain. Somatic pain arises from injury to the skin, soft tissue, and bone and is mediated by somatic afferent A-delta and C fibers. It is often described as being sharp and well localized. Visceral pain arises from noxious stimuli involving the visceral organs and is mediated by nociceptive afferent fibers. Visceral pain is described as being dull and diffuse. Neuropathic pain arises from injury to some component of the nervous system and is described as burning, shooting, or electric-shock-like. These differences in patients' pain syndromes guide physicians as to how to best approach their patients' pain and provide them with an armamentarium of different treatment options.

Genitourinary Visceral Pain Syndromes

Visceral pain is the result of noxious stimuli or injury to the visceral organs and often presents with diffuse, dull, and poorly localized pain. It is mediated by visceral nociceptive afferent fibers that travel with sympathetic fibers, which is important when considering therapeutic approaches.

These syndromes may present as a result of the primary tumor, metastases, neural infiltration, or a combination of these events.

I. Margulis
Department of Anesthesiology, New York-Presbyterian Hospital/Weill Cornell Medicine, New York, NY, USA

A. Gulati (✉)
Department of Anesthesiology and Critical Care, Memorial Sloan Kettering Cancer Center, New York, NY, USA

Prostate Cancer

Prostate cancer is an increasing health concern in the aging population. It is estimated that 27% of men diagnosed with cancer in 2012 were diagnosed with prostate cancer [1]. When looking at deaths from cancer in the last years, approximately 10% of patients died from prostate cancer [1]. These disparate statistics highlight the fact that patients are living with prostate cancer for many years. Despite aggressive treatment, we are seeing more cases of progressed disease with associated symptomatology.

Pain can occur in each stage of prostate cancer, both early and late in the disease course. It is estimated that 30–50% of prostate cancer patients experience chronic pain, which increases to up to 90% of patients as they enter the terminal phase of the disease [1, 2]. The pain may be due to tumor infiltration of other organs, soft tissue, nerves, or bones. Almost 77% of patients with prostate cancer experience pain directly because of their pathology, and 19% experience pain as a result of their cancer treatment [1, 2]. Prostate cancer pain may also present with rectal pain, perineal pain, and tenesmus. Regardless of the cause of their pain, majority of prostate cancer patients experience pain at some point in the course of their disease [3–7].

Renal Cell Carcinoma

Renal cell carcinoma has non-specific symptoms and is often diagnosed late in the disease course. Patients may ultimately present with hematuria, flank pain, and weight loss. It commonly metastasizes to the lymphatic system, lungs, liver, adrenal glands, and bone. Initial treatment is often partial or total nephrectomy.

The kidneys are widely innervated by sympathetic, parasympathetic, and afferent sensory fibers. Sympathetic fibers originating in T10–L1 form the renal plexus via synapses in aorticorenal ganglia, celiac ganglia, and lesser splanchnic

A. Gulati et al. (eds.), *Essentials of Interventional Cancer Pain Management*, https://doi.org/10.1007/978-3-319-99684-4_12

nerves. All of which can be targeted when treating pain associated with this disease process [3].

Testicular Cancer

Testicular cancer is the most common solid organ cancer in younger males, despite being seen in only 1% of the male population [1]. Patients typically present with a testicular lump, which is often painless. Presenting with pain is uncommon and is said to occur in only 30% of patients [2]. Majority of patients present with stage 1 disease and do well with treatment. Fifteen percent of patients who present with stage 1 disease relapse and require more extensive therapy [2]. Pain seen in patients with testicular cancer is commonly seen in late and progressive disease as well because of treatment.

Another consideration in this patient population is pain after orchiectomy. Phantom testis syndrome is now being described in patients who underwent orchiectomy. One study estimated the incidence of phantom testis syndrome to be 25% [2].

Bladder Cancer

Bladder cancer is seen in both sexes, though it is more common in males. It is estimated that 7% of the patients diagnosed with cancer in the last years were diagnosed with bladder cancer [1, 2]. Patients often present with hematuria. Pain is not commonly the presenting symptoms and is often seen secondary to treatment of this cancer, including postoperative pain and post-radiation pain. It is often noninvasive and tends to recur.

Due to the relapsing nature of this disease process as well as the increase in the elderly population, we often see progressive disease. Progressive disease, including muscle invasive and distant disease, must be treated with surgical intervention, systemic therapy, and, possibly, radiotherapy. Bladder spasms because of cancer or its treatment have been described and potential treatments include sympathetic blockade [8].

Ovarian Cancer

Ovarian cancer typically has a prolonged course marked with varied symptomatology. Patients often get treated with a combination of surgical debulking and chemotherapeutic therapy. Given the prolonged nature of the disease, patients commonly present with pain as either the result of the cancer or its therapy. Patients typically complain of abdominal or pelvic pain associated with pressure and cramping. Pain often precedes recurrence and is seen in approximately 40% of patients, markedly impacting functionality [1, 2]. In one study, 62% of patients recalled experiencing pain before being diagnosed [1, 2]. Interestingly, in many of these patients, the pain dissipated after receiving systemic chemotherapy likely due to reduced tumor size [9].

Many of the commonly used therapeutic agents also cause specific pain syndromes. Certain drugs are directly related to the development of peripheral neuropathy, which is an unfortunate, yet, well-documented event. This is further discussed in other chapters.

Uterine Cancer

Uterine cancer typically presents in postmenopausal women. Symptoms commonly appear early in the disease course, leading to diagnosis in the earlier stages of the disease process. Women most commonly present with vaginal bleeding, prompting testing, and diagnosis. The two main types of uterine cancers are uterine sarcomas and endometrial carcinomas. Majority of uterine cancers are endometrial. Uterine sarcomas involve the myometrium or surrounding connective tissues. Often, patients will present with low abdominal and pelvic pain which is commonly visceral in origin. Postsurgical pain may result in pelvic floor dysfunction in distinction to visceral pain [10].

Cervical Cancer

Cervical cancer commonly presents late in the disease course. Early in the disease course, symptoms may be absent or non-specific. As the disease progresses, patients may present with many different symptoms including vaginal bleeding, mass, weight loss, and severe pelvic pain.

In patients with cervical cancer, their source of pain can be varied. It may be due to tumor bulk and infiltration of other sites and neural structures. It may also be due secondary to radiation or surgical resection. Often, it is due to a combination of factors and treatment must be approached accordingly. Primarily pelvic pain or pain due to compression of psoas (lumbar plexus pain) or sacral nerve roots (sciatic pain) occasionally pudendal nerve and finally visceral pain from the lower pelvis are described below.

Genitourinary Somatic Pain Syndromes

Bone Pain

Bone metastasis is an unfortunate, yet common, phenomenon seen in patients with cancer. It is a common cause of chronic pain in patients with various solid organ cancers.

Tumors may infiltrate bone and neural structures leading to severe pain. Metastases to bone also weaken the bone and make patients prone to developing pathologic fractures. The pathophysiology of metastatic bone disease can involve either osteolysis or bone sclerosis depending on the primary cancer. Prostate cancer has been described to metastasize to bone in approximately 65–75% of patients with advanced disease, more frequently than any other cancer [1, 2].

Bone pain tends to be severe and difficult to treat with one medication alone [11]. Often multimodal treatment is necessary, as opiates are commonly not sufficient [11]. Opioids, adjuvant medications, radiotherapy, and interventional procedures can be all employed to treat bone pain [11, 12]. Bisphosphonates have been shown to be very helpful in metastatic bone pain. An essential component to bone pain is osteolytic activity which is inhibited by bisphosphonates [11, 12]. Many studies have shown decreased pain scores in patients with metastatic bone pain after starting bisphosphonates [13]. Radiotherapy has been shown to be very effective in palliating metastatic bone disease. Single and fractionated doses have both been found to be effective in treating metastatic bone pain [11, 12].

Medial branch blocks and lateral branch blocks can be performed to treat certain cases of bone pain involving the zygophysial joints. Medial branch nerves supply zygophysial joints and can be targeted in cases of facet arthropathy and metastatic bone disease [14]. If diagnostic blocks are successful, ablative or neurolytic procedures can be performed for longer-lasting pain relief [14]. These procedures are more selective for C and A-delta fibers, mediating pain, secondary to their lack of myelinization and small diameter which allows motor and sensory fiber function to be preserved. Furthermore, disease affecting the lateral sacrum or posterior ileum may be targeted by sacroiliac joint injections [15].

Commonly metastasis of the prostate cancer may progress to the lumbar spine and sacroiliac space. While anecdotally epidural steroid injections and neuroaxial devices, such as the intrathecal drug delivery system, have been performed, paradigms have also been developed to treat pain of tumors near the sacroiliac joint [15].

Neuropathic Pain Syndromes

Malignant Radiculopathy/Plexopathy

Malignant radiculopathy and plexopathy are conditions seen in patients having pathology involving different neural structures. Pathology involving the proximal nerve root, seen with cancer involving the neural foramina or spinal canal, often leads to radiculopathy. Radiculopathy often presents with poorly defined sensory and motor symptoms and often has no autonomic symptoms since autonomic fibers join more distally [16]. A plexopathy is seen when pathology involves the plexus itself or the distal nerve roots. It often presents with poorly defined neurologic symptoms. However, unlike a radiculopathy, a plexopathy often presents with autonomic symptoms such as changes in skin color or loss of perspiration [16].

Pathology involving the lumbar and sacral nerve roots, the lumbosacral plexus, or the peripheral nerves given off by the plexus is referred to as lumbosacral plexopathy.

The lumbosacral trunk consists of a lumbar and sacral component; the lumbar component is formed by fibers of L4 and L5 which connect with the sacral plexus, consisting of fibers derived from S1 to S4 [16]. Malignant radiculopathy and plexopathy are seen when primary masses or metastases invade or compress neural structures. Treatment options include a multimodal medical approach, radiotherapy, and/or interventional (e.g., sympathetic blocks) blocks. One may consider neuraxial devices for pain management in patients with uncontrolled pain.

Interventional Pain Treatments

Sympathetic Blocks

The afferent nerve fibers that mediate visceral pain follow the autonomic nervous system; thus autonomic ganglia are frequently targeted when treating visceral pain [17]. Local anesthetic blockade of sympathetic ganglia allows practitioners to diagnose and treat pain mediated by the sympathetic nervous system. If successful, neurolysis can be performed for more permanent analgesia [17].

Lumbar Splanchnic Nerve Block

Lumbar splanchnic nerve blockade may be appropriate in some instances of lower abdominal and pelvic visceral pain. At times, this may be an easier target than the superior hypogastric plexus. The lumbar splanchnic ganglion and nerves are located on the anterolateral surface of lumbar vertebral bodies and are the target of this block. These are usually at the levels of L2–L5 though L3 and L4 may be the best targets. Treatment of lymphedema from gynecologic cancer with repetitive sympathetic blocks has been described in the literature [18]. Essentially, sympathetically mediated pain signals are interrupted by injection of local anesthetic or neurolytic medication [17, 19].

Superior Hypogastric Plexus Block

The superior hypogastric plexus block is often utilized when treating genitourinary and gastrointestinal cancer pain (especially of organs which originate embryonically from the hindgut). The superior hypogastric plexus lies in the retroperitoneal space, usually around the aortic and IVC bifurcations, and is located at the level of the L5 vertebral body and extending to the first sacral vertebral body [20, 21]. The superior hypogastric plexus is formed by visceral afferent and efferent sympathetic nerves from branches of the aortic plexus as well as by the splanchnic nerves [20, 21]. However, there is evidence that parasympathetic branches may join from the sacral plexus [22]. The plexus branches and descends into the pelvis innervating the uterus, bladder, prostate, testes, urethra, rectum and descending colon. Sympathetic lumbar and thoracic fibers communicate visceral impulses from pelvic structures to the dorsal horn through this plexus. This structure is often targeted when treating pain associated with these organs. This procedure can be performed under CT or fluoroscopic guidance. More recently, an ultrasound-guided approach has been reported [23]. Complications associated with this block include neuraxial injection, intravascular injection, infection, retroperitoneal bleeding, and damage to neurovascular structures.

Ganglion of Impar/Walther's Ganglion

The impar ganglion is the termination of the paravertebral sympathetic chains, where they converge and form a single ganglion located anterior to the coccyx [24]. The ganglion impar provides primarily sympathetic innervation for many retroperitoneal pelvic structures and can thus be targeted in patients with pelvic pain syndromes [24]. Blockade of this ganglion will relieve pain originating from the bladder, rectum, distal vagina, distal urethra, anus, and cervix [24]. Case reports have documented the successful use of this block in treating post-radiation proctitis in prostate cancer patients who underwent radiotherapy. Furthermore, many studies have documented the successful use of ganglion impar blocks to decrease pain scores in patients with both malignant and nonmalignant pain. Complications include perforation of the rectum, infection, and bowel/bladder/sexual dysfunction [24].

Pudendal Nerve

The pudendal nerve is involved with sensation from the external genitalia and skin around both the anus and perineum. The nerve can be injured because of local tumor involvement, most commonly in prostate cancer, and also as a result of radiation. Radiation in the pelvis has been associated with pudendal nerve entrapment [25]. In practice, pudendal nerve blocks can be performed under CT, fluoroscopy, ultrasound, or using a blind technique, and blocks can be performed for diagnostic or therapeutic purposes. In advanced cancer and refractory disease, neurolysis of the nerve has been performed using cytoablative techniques [26].

Neuroablative Procedures

Intrathecal Neurolysis

Though rarely used in pain clinics, refractory cancer pain may be managed with intrathecal neurolysis. Chemicals considered include phenol and alcohol, each with advantages and disadvantages [27]. Indications in the genitourinary population include tumors presenting with sacral (low pelvic and perineal pain). The conus of the spinal cord may be targeted, causing saddle anesthesia [27]. While posterior rootlets of the lumbar nerve roots may be targeted (and perhaps sacral nerve roots through the caudal space), the pain relief may be incomplete and further may result in unforeseen side effects [27]. Thus, these procedures are considered in the late stage of cancer diagnosis for patients.

Punctate Midline Myelotomy

This neuroablative procedure interrupts the midline of the dorsal column and has been shown to be very effective in treating intractable pain refractory to other treatments [28]. It has been postulated that a midline posterior column visceral pain pathway exists in the spinal cord. The dorsal columns contain this pathway and may be integral in transmitting the visceral pain signals than the spinothalamic tract [28, 29]. Studies have looked at the efficacy of targeting these structures in relieving refractory pain. A study revealed that a punctate midline myelotomy of the posterior columns in six patients with refractory visceral cancer pain yielded lower pain scores and lessened opiate use [29]. The midline lesions provided widespread pain relief and spared sensory and proprioception.

Neuraxial Pain Techniques

Severe refractory pain is often treated with high-dose opioids and other analgesics. These methods typically fail in treating pain secondary to the unwanted side effects and drug toxicities associated with the dosage required to treat pain adequately. Finding ways to treat pain and avoid systemic effects has been an area of focus in pain medicine.

Spinal Cord Stimulation

If medical therapy and sympathetic blockade fails in adequately controlling visceral pain, spinal cord stimulation may be considered. It is thought that spinal cord stimulation modulates afferent input as it travels through the dorsal columns of the spinal cord [30]. Electrodes are placed in the epidural space on the dorsal surface of the spinal cord. It is postulated that the impulses generated activate large myelinated fibers which inhibit the transmission of painful stimuli mediated by A-delta and C fibers. Many studies have documented improved pain scores, functionality, and patient satisfaction in patients who underwent SCS implantation as compared to medical management. A 20-year literature review evaluating the rate of complications in patients with SCS found the overall complication rate to be 34% with the most common complication being lead migration and lead fracture [31]. While this has not been described in the oncologic population to our knowledge, evidence is present in the chronic abdominal pain population [32].

Intrathecal and Epidural Drug Delivery Systems

Chronic refractory pain can be successfully treated using drug delivery systems. Intrathecal pumps deliver a desired drug to the intrathecal space, which maximizes drug effect while minimizing systemic side effects and maintaining motor and autonomic function. Intrathecal pumps deliver opiate, local anesthetic, or a combination to the intrathecal space.

A pump is implanted in a small subcutaneous pocket and the intrathecal catheter is tunneled and connected to it. Although many patients do very well with this treatment option, they are at risk for a unique complication. Granulomas may form at the intrathecal catheter tip which may cause spinal cord compression and neurological deficits, often associated with higher concentrations of infused drugs [33]. The decision of whether to use an intrathecal or epidural drug delivery system is complex and involves many considerations. Epidural drug delivery systems increase the likelihood of developing infection and are usually reserved for patients with limited life expectancy [33]. We recommend the use of intrathecal drug delivery if conservative medical management and neurolytic techniques are unsuccessful in managing a patient's pain in this population [34].

We describe a paradigm approach to management of patients suffering from intractable cancer pain in the genitourinary population (Fig. 12.1).

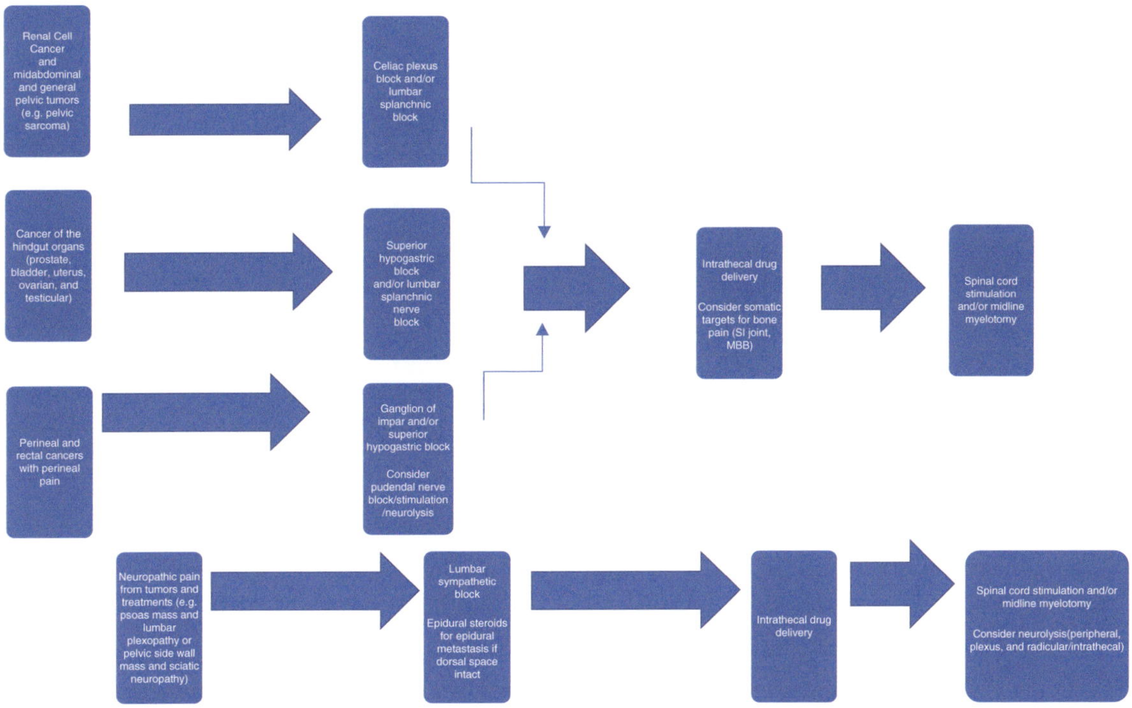

Fig. 12.1 A paradigm approach to interventional pain therapies for patients suffering from pain syndromes related to genitourinary cancers

References

1. Office for National Statistics Cancer statistics registrations: registrations of cancer diagnosed in 2002 England. Series MB1 no. 33. London: Office for National Statistics, 2005.
2. Siegel R, et al. Cancer statistics, 2014. CA Cancer J Clin. 2014;64(1):9–29.
3. Ali M, et al. Anatomy of the pelvic plexus and innervation of the prostate gland. Clin Anat. 2004;17(2):123–9.
4. Eman A, Serbülent G, Gürcü ME. Pain management in prostate cancer. Open J Urol. 2012;2(3):164.
5. Bader P, et al. Prostate cancer pain management: EAU guidelines on pain management. World J Urol. 2012;30(5):677–86.
6. Autio KA, et al. Prevalence of pain and analgesic use in men with metastatic prostate cancer using a patient-reported outcome measure. J Oncol Pract. 2013;9(5):223–9.
7. Khosla A, Adeyefa O, Nasir S. Successful treatment of radiation-induced proctitis pain by blockade of the ganglion impar in an elderly patient with prostate cancer: a case report. Pain Med. 2013;14:662–6. https://doi.org/10.1111/pme.12065.
8. Gulati A, Khelemsky Y, Loh J, Puttanniah V, Malhotra V, Cubert K. The use of lumbar sympathetic blockade at L4 for management of malignancy-related bladder spasms. Pain Physician. 2011; 14(3):305–10.
9. Portenoy RK, et al. Pain in ovarian cancer patients. Prevalence, characteristics, and associated symptoms. Cancer. 1994;74(3):907–15.
10. Noronha AF, Mello de Figueiredo E, Rossi de Figueiredo Franco TM, Cândido EB, Silva-Filho AL. Treatments for invasive carcinoma of the cervix: what are their impacts on the pelvic floor functions? Int Braz J Urol. 2013;39(1):46–54.
11. Coleman RE. Metastatic bone disease: clinical features, pathophysiology and treatment strategies. Cancer Treat Rev. 2001;27(3):165–76.
12. Serafini AN. Therapy of metastatic bone pain. J Nucl Med. 2001;42(6):895–906.
13. Buga S, Sarria JE. The management of pain in metastatic bone disease. Cancer Control. 2012;19(2):154–66.
14. Birthi P, Sloan P. Interventional treatment of refractory cancer pain. Cancer J. 2013;19(5):390–6.
15. Hutson N, Hung JC, Puttanniah V, Lis E, Laufer I, Gulati A. Interventional pain management for sacroiliac tumors in the oncologic population: a case series and paradigm approach. Pain Med. 2017;18(5):959–68.
16. Brejt N, et al. Pelvic radiculopathies, lumbosacral plexopathies, and neuropathies in oncologic disease: a multidisciplinary approach to a diagnostic challenge. Cancer Imaging. 2013;13(4):591.
17. Amr YM, Makharita MY. Neurolytic sympathectomy in the management of cancer pain – time effect: a prospective, randomized multicenter study. J Pain Symptom Manag. 2014;48(5):944–56.
18. Woo JH, Park HS, Kim SC, Kim YH. The effect of lumbar sympathetic ganglion block on gynecologic cancer-related lymphedema. Pain Physician. 2013;16(4):345–52.
19. de Oliveira R, dos Reis MP, Prado WA. The effects of early or late neurolytic sympathetic plexus block on the management of abdominal or pelvic cancer pain. Pain. 2004;110(1):400–8.
20. Ahmed DG, Mohamad MF, Mohamed SA-E. Superior hypogastric plexus combined with ganglion impar neurolytic blocks for pelvic and/or perineal cancer pain relief. Pain Physician. 2015;18(1):E49–56.
21. Stogicza A, et al. Inferior hypogastric plexus block affects sacral nerves and the superior hypogastric plexus. ISRN Anesthesiology. 2012;2012:1–5.
22. Saito T, Den S, Tanuma K, Tanuma Y, Carney E, Carlsson C. Anatomical bases for paravertebral anesthetic block: fluid communication between the thoracic and lumbar paravertebral regions. Surg Radiol Anat. 1999;21(6):359–63.
23. Mishra S, Bhatnagar S, Rana SP, Khurana D, Thulkar S. Efficacy of the anterior ultrasound-guided superior hypogastric plexus neurolysis in pelvic cancer pain in advanced gynecological cancer patients. Pain Med. 2013;14(6):837–42.
24. Eker HE, Cok OY, Kocum A, Acil M, Turkoz A. Transsacrococcygeal approach to ganglion impar for pelvic cancer pain: a report of 3 cases. Reg Anesth Pain Med. 2008;33(4):381–2.
25. Elahi, et al. Pudendal entrapment neuropathy: a rare complication of pelvic radiation therapy. Pain Physician. 2013;16:E793–7.
26. Prologo JD, et al. Percutaneous CT-guided cryoablation for the treatment of refractory pudendal neurologia. Skelet Radiol. 2015;44:709–14.
27. Candido K, Stevens RA. Intrathecal neurolytic blocks for the relief of cancer pain. Best Pract Res Clin Anaesthesiol. 2003;17(3):407–28. Becker R, Sure U, Bertalanffy H. Punctate midline myelotomy a new approach in the management of visceral pain. Acta Neurochir 1999;141(8): 881–883.
28. Becker R1, Gatscher S, Sure U, Bertalanffy H. The punctate midline myelotomy concept for visceral cancer pain control-case report and review of the literature. Acta Neurochir Suppl. 2002;79:77–8.
29. Nauta HJW, et al. Punctate midline myelotomy for the relief of visceral cancer pain. J Neurosurg Spine. 2000;92(2):125–30.
30. Flagg II, Artemus, McGreevy K, Williams K. Spinal cord stimulation in the treatment of cancer-related pain:"back to the origins". Curr Pain Headache Rep. 2012;16(4):343–9.
31. Cameron T. Safety and efficacy of spinal cord stimulation for the treatment of chronic pain: a 20-year literature review. J Neurosurg Spine. 2004;100(3):254–67.
32. Baranidharan G, Simpson KH, Dhandapani K. Spinal cord stimulation for visceral pain – a novel approach. Neuromodulation. 2014;17(8):753–8.
33. Deer TR, et al. Comprehensive consensus based guidelines on intrathecal drug delivery systems in the treatment of pain caused by cancer pain. Pain Physician. 2011;14(3):E283–312.
34. Bruel BM, Burton AW. Intrathecal therapy for cancer-related pain. Pain Med. 2016;17(12):2404–21.

Pediatric Cancer Pain Management

13

Stephen L. Long and Anurag K. Agrawal

Introduction

Pain in pediatric oncology patients can be secondary to the underlying tumor, due to treatment-related effects of chemotherapy and radiation therapy, or procedure-related. Utilizing appropriate pain intensity assessment tools and the World Health Organization analgesic ladder, most pediatric oncology patients can be appropriately treated without the need for interventional pain management. Collins et al. [1] identified 6% of pediatric oncology patients who required extraordinary measures including massive opioid infusions as well as epidural or subarachnoid infusions or palliative sedation. The need for interventional measures was found specifically in patients with solid tumors with metastases to the spinal nerve roots, nerve plexus, or large peripheral nerves with possible spinal cord compression [1]. Geeta et al. [2] showed that pediatric patients with leukemia in general did not require interventional therapies although those with bone pain and neuropathic pain required strong opioids and referral to a pain specialist service.

In a review of pediatric cancer pain and palliation, Lebel [3] notes that terminal symptoms, especially pain, and treatment-related pain remain inadequately controlled due to multiple factors including persistent misconceptions about pediatric pain, challenges in pain assessment due to variable cognitive and developmental stage, lack of pediatric pharmacokinetic data, lack of access to pediatric pain and palliation specialists, and, finally, limited training in palliation among pediatric oncologists. Additional misconceptions that have been discredited in the medical literature include neonatal hypoalgesia and the potential of opioid addiction although parent misperception about these issues must be adequately addressed by the healthcare team [3–5]. Here we discuss developmental aspects in the assessment and management of pediatric cancer pain, causes of treatment-related pain, and management strategies for refractory pain that is not well-controlled with high-dose opioid therapy both during treatment and for end-stage disease.

S. L. Long
Department of Anesthesiology, UCSF Benioff Children's Hospital Oakland, Oakland, CA, USA
e-mail: llong@mail.cho.org

A. K. Agrawal (✉)
Department of Hematology/Oncology, UCSF Benioff Children's Hospital Oakland, Oakland, CA, USA
aagrawal@mail.cho.org

Developmental Issues in Pediatric Pain Management

Unlike adult patients, multiple developmental issues must be considered to provide effective pain management in pediatric oncology patients. Pathways conducting nociceptive stimuli to the thalamus and cortex are fully myelinated in the newborn infant, while many neuromodulators and neurotransmitters are present in the fetus [3]. Afferent excitatory pathways develop prior to the maturation of descending inhibitory pathways [3, 4]. Undertreatment of pain in young children is known to have short-term physiologic effects and may influence later pain behaviors including those children with newly diagnosed cancer [3, 4]. Development must be considered in the assessment of pain; children under 3 years of age and those with developmental delay must have pain intensity measured by behavioral observation scales, while older children (e.g., >8 years) can utilize adult scales [4]. Multiple physiologic aspects can affect the pharmacokinetics and pharmacodynamics of analgesic drug delivery dependent on developmental stage and include reduced hepatic and possibly renal clearance in neonates, possible increased drug effect in neonates due to decreased protein-binding, increased water ratio in neonates increasing duration of action of water-soluble drugs, increased potential for sedation from hypoventilation in infants, and increased drug clearance in young children as compared to adults due to a larger proportional liver mass [4].

A. Gulati et al. (eds.), *Essentials of Interventional Cancer Pain Management*, https://doi.org/10.1007/978-3-319-99684-4_13

Assessment of Pediatric Oncology Pain

Multiple pain assessment tools are available in the medical literature although none has specifically been validated for pediatric oncology patients [3, 5–11]. Duhn and Medves [6] reviewed 35 infant pain assessment tools, while Stinson et al. [9] analyzed 34 pediatric pain assessment tools; none were felt to be ideal. Linder [7] specifically examined instruments measuring physical symptoms in children and adolescents with cancer; none were found to be explicit for the measurement of cancer-related pain in these patients. In the 2007 National Comprehensive Cancer Network Pediatric Cancer Pain Guidelines, Anghelescu et al. [12] utilize the Wong-Baker FACES® Pain Rating Scale (WBFPRS) for self-report and the FLACC (face, legs, activity, crying, consolability) scale for preverbal children although other sources feel that additional scales may be equal or better than these [13]. In a review of faces scales, Tomlinson et al. [14] found that the Faces Pain Scale, Faces Pain Scale-Revised, Oucher pain scale, and the WBFPRS all were well supported although children preferred the WBFPRS. Additionally, Wood et al. [15] showed a strong correlation between electronic and paper versions of a Faces Pain Scale with many children preferring the electronic version. Little data are available on the use of such scales in children between 3 and 5 years of age [14]. Pain assessment in infants with cancer is especially difficult and further research is required on optimal means [16]. Huguet et al. [17] recently published findings on the development of a scale to score pain-related fear in children and adolescents, an important area that deserves more research and consideration in pediatric oncology patients.

Behavioral and psychological assessment is a necessity in young, nonverbal children with the understanding that self-report is the best indicator of pain in all verbal patient populations (i.e., usually children ≥3 years) [13]. Additionally, it is usually the ability to see an improvement in the pain intensity rating with treatment that is more vital than the original number reported by the child [14]. More active involvement of the patient and family in pain assessment likely would improve quality of care, but this is not yet evidence-based [16, 18].

Authorized Agent Controlled Analgesia

Children >5–6 years with normal cognition are generally felt able to utilize patient-controlled analgesia (PCA), while those under this age or with developmental delay should utilize authorized agent controlled analgesia (AACA), as compared to unauthorized agent usage or, PCA by proxy [4, 19]. AACA can include either nurse-controlled or caregiver-controlled analgesia if the caregiver is consistently available, competent, and properly educated and the authorized agent is designated in the medical order [19]. AACA should not be used in conjunction with PCA for those patients competent and able to utilize the system independently, and there should be only one authorized agent at a given time [19]. Monitto et al. [20] prospectively evaluated 240 occasions of AACA usage over a 1-year period in children of an average 2.3 years of age and found 4 instances of naloxone treatment for apnea or desaturation; however, no historical side effect frequency could be found as a comparison in a like-aged patient population utilizing as needed opioid dosing Angheslescu et al. [21]. Anghelescu et al. similarly found one episode of naloxone requirement in 576 days of AACA usage in a pediatric oncology cohort with a lower overall complication rate as compared to a standard PCA group. A follow-up study by Anghelescu et al. [22] showed that AACA by either a parent or nurse was as safe as PCA in pediatric oncology patients. Important hypothesized factors in a low complication rate included the presence of institutional standards and guidelines, caregiver education materials, and frequent nursing bedside assessment [22].

Procedural Cancer Pain Management

The necessity for policies in the management of pain and anxiety with pediatric oncology procedures including lumbar puncture, bone marrow aspirate and biopsy, intravenous access, and intramuscular injection was first noted in 1990 by the American Academy of Pediatrics with the recommendation for pharmacologic and behavioral approaches [23]. Vital components from this protocol remain valid today including the necessity of parental education and preparation, developmentally appropriate preparation for the child, and ability to provide optimal analgesia and sedation when needed [24]. Child life specialists and cognitive-behavioral interventions such as distraction are especially valuable in preparing the child and allowing for effective coping and adjustment [24–26]. Proper parental communication is also critical in positively influencing the distress of the child with normalization and supportive communication styles, in addition to aiding in the utilization of cognitive-behavioral interventions, being most beneficial before and during the procedure [27]. Sedation should be utilized for bone marrow procedures and lumbar puncture in many pediatric cases after discussion with the family [23, 24]. Interestingly, Hedén et al. [28] showed no benefit with the addition of 0.25 mg/kg oral morphine to topical analgesia in decreasing fear, distress, or pain in children prior to needle insertion in a subcutaneously implanted intravenous port. Institutional guidelines are vital to ensure that children are comfortable especially during procedures that will be repeated multiple times during the course of cancer treatment [23, 24].

Treatment-Related Pain

Unlike adult oncology patients whose most frequent cause of pain is often secondary to the underlying disease, treatment-related pain is the most common cause in pediatric oncology patients and may be severe enough to require interdisciplinary care [29]. Neuropathic pain in children is often secondary to chemotherapeutic side effects and is likely under-recognized due to the inability of young children to describe the quality of neurologic symptoms [29]. Similarly, pain and neurologic symptoms after limb-salvage procedures and amputation are poorly described in pediatric patients and are likely underreported [30]. Evidence for the management of these syndromes in the pediatric literature is sparse.

Neuropathic Cancer Pain

Neuropathic cancer pain in pediatric oncology patients is poorly quantified as compared to nociceptive pain as well as neuropathic pain in adults. Neuropathic pain can be secondary to tumor invasion of the spinal cord or nerve roots, limb-sparing surgery, amputation, chemotherapy, radiation therapy, or hematopoietic stem cell transplantation [29, 31]. Anghelescu et al. [31] found that neuropathic pain occurred in 17% of pain referrals and was more common with solid tumors and after limb-sparing surgery. Neuropathic pain also appeared more difficult to treat, requiring more visits per patient and longer follow-up as compared to nociceptive pain referrals as well as complex pharmacological management [31]. Patients received a combination of opioids, anticonvulsants (e.g., gabapentin), tricyclic antidepressants (e.g., amitriptyline), as well as psychological interventions and physical therapy; regional anesthesia was not included as a management in the study [31]. Systematic evidence on the use of such adjuvant agents in pediatric oncology patients is lacking [29, 31]. Dougherty and DeBaun [32] note that opioid and benzodiazepine usage was statistically much higher at the end of life in a pediatric oncology cohort with neuropathic pain as compared to a group without, implying poor pain management that could be benefited by additional therapies; they suggest benefit with opioid rotation to methadone although further study in pediatric oncology patients is required. Interventional management strategies due to tumor invasion of the spinal cord or nerve roots are discussed in Section 11.5.2.

Pain After Limb-Salvage Procedures

Very limited evidence is available in the medical literature regarding the prevalence and management of pain after limb-salvage procedures in pediatric cancer patients. Anghelescu et al. [33] report a significant rate of long-term pain after limb-salvage of the long bones requiring increasingly complex multimodal therapy including standard pharmacologic agents as well as adjuvants for neuropathic pain, local anesthetic wound catheters, postoperative continuous epidural infusion, and continuous peripheral nerve block catheters [33]. Appropriate interdisciplinary pharmacologic, behavioral, and rehabilitative management (including early mobilization) likely improves postoperative outcomes and decreases the incidence of chronic pain in this patient population although further evidence is required [33].

Phantom Pain After Limb Amputation

As with neuropathic pain in general, phantom pain after limb amputation in pediatric oncology patients is poorly quantified and likely underreported [30]. Similar to myths about neonatal hypoalgesia, it was previously believed that young children did not experience phantom pain sensations [30]. Previous reports have described neurologic symptoms which have lasted months to years after amputation and more likely to occur in patients who experienced pre-amputation pain [30, 34, 35]. Burgoyne et al. [35] theorize that peri-amputation pain strategies including gabapentin as well as epidural analgesia and continuous peripheral nerve block may limit the long-term incidence of phantom limb pain. Sufficient pediatric evidence to support this conclusion is lacking, but the benefit of regional anesthesia in such cases should be considered.

Beyond Opioids in the Management of Pediatric Cancer Pain

Practitioners must be aware of additional options including anesthetic agents, interventional procedures, complementary and alternative therapies, and end-of-life measures including palliative radiation and sedation for which there is an evidence basis in pediatric oncology patients. Although these areas are far less studied as compared to adult oncology, pediatric patients whose pain is refractory to opioid therapy should be given the opportunity to have their pain relieved by such additional modalities through the utilization of an interdisciplinary team. End-stage cancer pain especially may require the consideration of such treatment options. Evidence for neuroablation and neurostimulation in refractory pediatric cancer pain is lacking.

Anesthetic Agents

High opioid doses for intractable cancer pain may ultimately be both ineffective and lead to untoward side effects, especially sedation, constipation, and respiratory depression, as well as possibly hyperalgesia, allodynia, myotonia, and seizures [36]. Intravenous anesthetic agents including ketamine, propofol, and lidocaine have all been reported effective in pediatric oncology patients. White et al. [37] reported on the use of ketamine in addition to morphine PCA for 24 of 92 patients with oral mucositis and rapidly increasing morphine doses. The addition of ketamine was effective in decreasing pain scores and morphine consumption with minimal side effects; no psychomimetic effects were noted [37]. Ketamine was conveniently mixed with morphine in a 1:1 ratio in a normal saline solution with similar PCA dosing as with morphine alone except for an increased initial 4 h maximum dose [37]. Patients who required the addition of ketamine tended to be older and more likely female [37]. Finkel et al. [36] similarly utilized subanesthetic doses of ketamine in 11 children with uncontrolled cancer pain on high opioid doses. Eight of the 11 children had improved pain control, decreased opioid usage, and increased ability to interact with their families on doses of 0.1–1.0 mg/kg/h with concomitant lorazepam 0.025 mg/kg every 12 h to prevent any psychomimetic effects [36]. The authors note that as an *N*-methyl-D-aspartate (NMDA) receptor antagonist, ketamine may have beneficial effect on opioid tolerance and hyperalgesia [36]. Additional pediatric case reports have similarly shown benefit of low-dose intravenous ketamine in treatment of end-stage cancer and neuropathic pain [38–42].

Low-dose propofol and lidocaine intravenous infusions have also been noted to be beneficial for end-stage pediatric cancer pain not well-controlled with opioids and benzodiazepines [42–45]. Hooke et al. [43] reported on the use of propofol in nine pediatric patients receiving palliation for pain from nerve compression, organ metastases, organ capsule expansion, and increased intracranial pressure with continued use until death in eight of the nine with relative stabilization of the opioid dose in seven of the nine patients. Patients were able to have periods of wakefulness and meaningful interaction while receiving low-dose propofol at an initial median dose of 0.6 mg/kg/h until terminal coma with final median doses of 3.2 mg/kg/h; adverse effects were not uncommon and included agitation in five, hallucinations in two, and twitching in one, all controllable with benzodiazepines and none requiring medication discontinuation [43]. One patient had severe tetany resulting in the need for temporary discontinuation of the propofol infusion which was later restarted at a lower dose without adverse effect. Propofol may also have beneficial antiemetic properties in such patients [43, 44]. Two case reports describe the benefit of intravenous lidocaine in end-stage cancer pain with opioid tolerance at dose ranges of 9–63 mcg/kg/min although the patient in the study by Kajiume et al. [42] was also receiving intravenous ketamine [45]. Lidocaine is thought to work by blocking voltage-gated sodium channels, and potential side effects due to this inhibition, especially cardiac dysrhythmias, must be considered although were not seen in the two reported patients and are more likely at doses higher than that administered [42, 45].

Regional Anesthesia Interventional Procedures

Patients who fail therapy with high-dose opioids and potentially adjuvant anesthetic agents, develop intolerable side effects, or have severe but localized pain should be considered for regional anesthesia interventional procedures. In a survey of pediatric oncology patients over an approximate 8-year period, Collins et al. [46] found that about 3% of children dying from malignancy required epidural or subarachnoid infusions, mainly in those with solid tumors. Anghelscu et al. [47] reported that approximately 5% of pediatric oncology pain service consultations ultimately required regional anesthesia. Pediatric evidence for regional anesthesia was reviewed by Rork et al. [48] and found to be limited to case reports and case series such that only provisional recommendations can be made; yet, for those patients with refractory pain not responding to other modalities, regional analgesia must be considered under consultation with palliative and pain management services (Fig. 13.1).

Interventional procedures are likely underutilized due to a lack of exposure to such procedures as well as an absence of local pain specialty services at many centers [3, 49]. Pediatric guidelines outlining regional anesthesia techniques for peripheral nerve and plexus blocks or infusions, neurolytic blocks, central neuraxial infusions, and implanted intrathecal ports are derived from the adult literature, and therefore many of the techniques outlined in this book can and should be applied to pediatric patients [48]. Fear of complications or affecting the desired place of death should not preclude the investigation of such modalities; Anghelscu et al. [47] showed in a small cohort of pediatric oncology patients that such interventions could be done with little risk of complication without compromising the desired place of death.

Because interventional regional anesthesia procedures often result in reduced opioid consumption, these techniques are especially important for patients experiencing intolerable opioid-related side effects or opioid tachyphylaxis [50]. Broadly speaking, interventional regional anesthesia

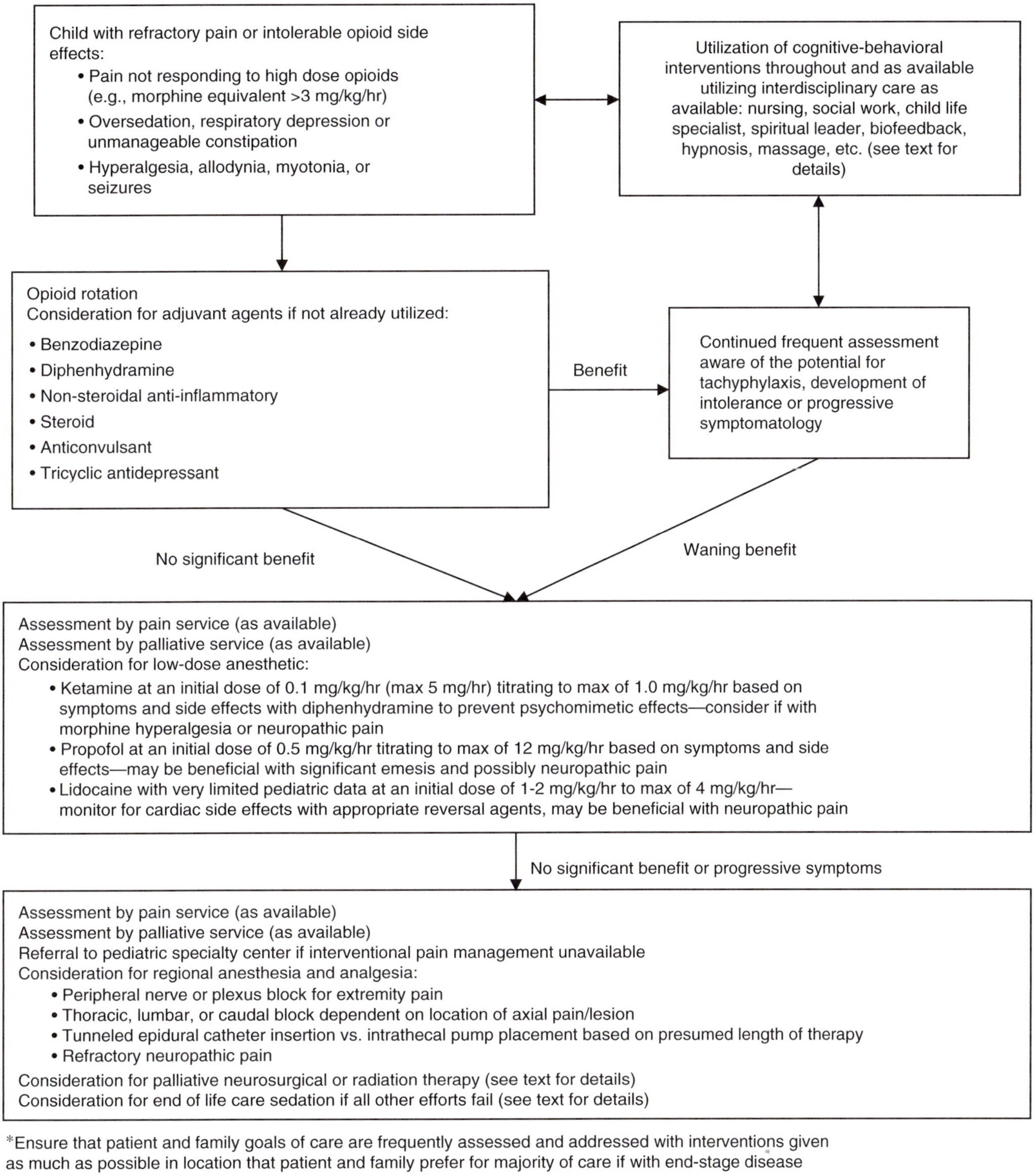

Fig. 13.1 Algorithm for the utilization of interventional pain services in pediatric oncology*

procedures in children can be divided into two categories: *neuraxial* nerve blocks and *peripheral* nerve blocks. Neuraxial nerve blocks target the spinal cord and the spinal cord nerve roots. These techniques involve administering medications directly into the intrathecal or epidural spaces, often via catheters. Because neural conduction is blocked at the level of the spinal cord nerve roots, the resultant analgesia typically encompasses a large area of the body (i.e., several dermatomes bilaterally). Peripheral nerve blocks, on the other hand, provide analgesia for a single peripheral nerve (e.g., femoral nerve) or group of nerves (e.g., transversus abdominis plane block). Peripheral nerve blocks are ideal for well-localized pain and, as described below, have a better safety profile than neuraxial nerve blocks. However, for larger areas of pain involving multiple nerves, neuraxial blocks are superior.

In general, many interventional regional anesthesia procedures performed on adults can be successfully performed on children. However, age-related differences in anatomy, pharmacokinetics, and pharmacodynamics can affect the regional technique or imaging modality used or the drug administered. For example, the conus medullaris of neonates terminates further caudad than that of older children and adults, potentially affecting the placement of lumbar epidural catheters in this age group [51]. Increasingly, ultrasonography is used to identify anatomic differences and facilitate regional procedures, especially peripheral nerve blocks; however, fluoroscopy, which is commonly used to facilitate neuraxial procedures in adults, may be less appropriate in children due to concerns for cumulative radiation exposure [52, 53]. In addition, well-known pharmacokinetic differences between children and adults, such as the effect of age on the free fraction of local anesthetics in the blood, may drastically change the dosing of these drugs for regional techniques in neonatal patients [54]. Moreover, preclinical data suggest the developing neonatal nervous system, including the spinal cord, may be vulnerable to neuraxial drug-related toxicity [55]. Taken together, anatomical and pharmacological considerations inform the practice of interventional regional anesthesia in children, with emphasis in the neonatal population.

As with any procedure, the risk/benefit calculus for interventional regional anesthesia is addressed first and foremost; and with this comes the question, how safe are the procedures in children? Our current understanding of the risk of neuraxial and peripheral nerve blocks comes from nearly 50,000 pediatric patients taken from two separate datasets [56, 57]. Overall the risk of serious complications from neuraxial and peripheral nerve blocks was low, on the order of 1–2 serious complications (e.g., cardiac toxicity, dural puncture, nerve injury, visceral puncture, infection) per 1000 blocks [56, 57]. The majority of the complications arose from neuraxial procedures and all complication-related morbidity resolved within 1 year. Although severe permanent neurologic complications were not seen in these two datasets, catastrophic complications from neuraxial procedures have been reported elsewhere [58].

Risk of bleeding secondary to thrombocytopenia and risk of infection secondary to neutropenia must be considered prior to an interventional procedure; Anghelscu et al. [47] suggest a platelet count $\geq 100 \times 10^9$/L prior to epidural catheter placement. Potential contraindications to regional anesthesia and the necessity to reduce suffering in an end-stage patient must be balanced through interdisciplinary discussion [48]. In a review of long-term epidural catheter placement for adult chronic pain, Strafford et al. [59] note a 2.4% incidence of infection. No similar data are available in the pediatric literature, but practitioners should be cognizant of infection risk. As with adult patients, a combination of an opioid, a local anesthetic (e.g., bupivacaine), and an α_2 adrenergic agonist (e.g., clonidine) is utilized in pediatric regional anesthesia [48, 49]. Tachyphylaxis to the local anesthetic agent as well as systemic toxicity can occur [48, 60]. In adult studies, use of an opioid in combination with a local anesthetic has been shown to reduce overall opioid consumption and clonidine has been noted effective for neuropathic pain; pediatric data are lacking [49]. Motor blockade, loss of bowel and bladder function, and respiratory depression depending on the level of spinal anesthesia as well as hemodynamic compromise secondary to sympathetic blockade are potential serious side effects that must be considered in pediatric patients as well as adults [48, 60].

Most interventional regional anesthesia procedures in children occur in the perioperative setting. However, the demand to treat acute or chronic nonsurgical pain with interventional techniques is growing [61]. The utility of neuraxial or peripheral nerve blocks for nonsurgical pain (e.g., pathologic pain, traumatic pain, neuropathies) has been well-demonstrated for adults, but the present literature for children, while promising, is mostly restricted to smaller studies and case reports [62–65]. Nonetheless, the application of interventional regional anesthesia is potentially far-reaching and includes pediatric palliative care [47, 48].

Decision to utilize a peripheral nerve block versus a neuraxial infusion should be based on the location of the tumor and subsequent pain [47]. Anghelscu et al. [47] do not recommend intrathecal ports over tunneled epidural catheters in end-stage pediatric oncology patients due to their shortened life expectancy; on the other hand, Rork et al. [48] note that intrathecal ports more conveniently allow for medication refill. Though not utilized commonly, neurolysis of the celiac plexus has been noted to be beneficial in two case reports of pediatric abdominal tumors [66, 67].

In summary, excellent pain relief with interventional regional anesthesia procedures is well-documented in children in the perioperative setting. Few serious complications from these procedures are observed, especially with respect to peripheral nerve blocks. When performing these procedures, age-related considerations are especially important for neonatal patients. The utility of neuraxial and peripheral nerve blocks outside of the operating room is increasingly reported in the literature, with benefits seen for nonsurgical pathologic and traumatic pain, neuropathies, and palliation.

Complementary Therapies

Cognitive behavioral interventions and complementary therapies should not be overlooked as potentially important ways to improve pain and quality of life for pediatric oncology patients both during disease treatment and at the end of life. Areas that have a limited evidence basis for pediatric patients include massage, hypnosis, acupuncture, music therapy, virtual reality, yoga, as well as biofeedback and relaxation techniques. Many of the reports are in relation to procedure-related pain but can likely be applied to treatment-related pain, pain from the underlying disease, and pain at the end of life.

A recent Cochrane Collaboration review of non-pharmacologic management of procedure-related pain in young children was mixed, showing no conclusively beneficial treatments in young infants although neonates were shown to benefit from sucking-related interventions as well as rocking and holding [68]. A similar review for children and adolescents undergoing needle-related procedures showed potential benefit for distraction, hypnosis, and combined cognitive behavioral interventions [69]. Specifically for pediatric oncology patients, Landier et al. [70] concluded in a systematic review that hypnosis, distraction, and imagery may be helpful for procedure-related pain. Wild et al. [71] and Richardson et al. [72] noted similar results when specifically reviewing hypnosis for procedural pain and distress in children with cancer although also noted that further evidence is required before hypnosis can be recommended routinely. A Cochrane Collaboration review of music therapy in oncology patients determined that there may be a beneficial impact on pain although many studies had a high risk of bias [73]. Nguyen et al. [74] specifically analyzed the benefit of music therapy on pain and anxiety with lumbar puncture in pediatric oncology patients and found that music decreased both procedural pain and fear.

Shockey et al. [75] conducted a feasibility study on the utilization of relaxation and biofeedback to minimize preprocedural distress in pediatric oncology patients and found that such therapy could be beneficial to patients at risk although further study is required. Distraction through virtual reality prior to needle-related procedures may also be beneficial in children with cancer [76]. Systematic reviews of acupuncture, yoga, and massage therapy have all shown potential benefit in reducing pain and anxiety in pediatric oncology patients [77–81]. Adams et al. [82] analyzed the risk of adverse events from acupuncture and found an acceptable rate of risk although disease-specific risk of infection and bleeding must be considered in pediatric oncology patients. Excluding acupuncture, complementary therapies come with little risk in children with cancer and may provide some pain relief; therefore, resources for exploration of such modalities should be routinely provided to patients and their families both during treatment of disease and at the end of life.

Palliative Radiation Therapy

Although palliative radiation therapy (PRT) is a routine part of adult oncology care, the usage of this treatment modality for end-stage pediatric cancer pain is likely underutilized and should be considered in patients with pain from soft tissue masses and metastases to the bone, brain, and liver [83]. In a survey of Canadian pediatric oncologists, Tucker et al. [83] reported many obstacles for utilization of PRT including a lack of education and training, poor communication with patients, families and interdisciplinary teams, poor healthcare coordination, and a lack of treatment guidelines. The evidence in the medical literature for palliative radiotherapy in pediatric cancer patients is limited, with reports of benefit in relapsed and metastatic Wilms tumor, neuroblastoma, Ewing sarcoma, and osteosarcoma [84–87]. These studies commonly showed an improvement in pain for the majority of patients receiving PRT, with some having a durable response until death [84–87].

Palliative Sedation Therapy

Practitioners should be aware that pain control is often suboptimal in the last days of life [88]. In a review of palliative sedation therapy (PST), Kiman et al. [89] note that such a strategy should be utilized as a last resort in terminally ill patients with severe symptoms that persist despite the intensive efforts of an interdisciplinary team, decreasing patient awareness to the necessary level to relieve the burden of intractable suffering in a manner ethically acceptable to the patient, family, and healthcare providers. Due to a lack of evidence-based research, an international panel of 29 palliative care experts made the following recommendations for adults which can be extrapolated for pediatric oncology patients: (1) the decision to utilize PST should arrive through interdisciplinary discussion with the healthcare team, family, and patient if developmentally appropriate; (2) sedative drugs should be titrated to the cessation of refractory symptoms; (3) in the case of continuous deep PST, disease should be irreversible with death expected in hours to days; (4) midazolam should be considered first-line sedative therapy; and (5) phenobarbital and propofol are reasonable second-line therapies [90]. Pediatric data are lacking although Anghelescu et al. [91] reported on the use of propofol for PST in three pediatric oncology patients at the end of life.

Integration of Pain Services into Pediatric Oncology

A recent survey of participating institutions in the Children's Oncology Group (COG) showed that although a pain service was available in 90%, a median of two patients per institution with newly diagnosed cancer and one patient per institution with relapsed cancer was referred to the service [92]. It is unclear why underutilization of the service occurs but is likely multifactorial with a lack of health provider education and exposure being potential easy areas for improvement [3, 49]. Meyer [93] describes a successful model for the integration of anesthesiology services into pediatric oncology through the development of acute pain, chronic pain, palliative care, and procedure management sections. Key personnel include pain management physicians, nurse practitioners, clinical nurse specialists, as well as psychology faculty. Ultimately the recognition of the necessity for interdisciplinary expertise and the desire for active interdisciplinary communication and participation are required to manage complex refractory pain in pediatric oncology patients.

Summary

Pain in pediatric oncology patients can be managed utilizing both nonopioid and opioid medications. Developmental and cognitive status must be considered in the appropriate assessment of pediatric cancer pain. A small fraction of patients, especially those noted to have solid tumors with metastases to the spinal nerve roots, nerve plexus, or large peripheral nerves may develop refractory pain requiring regional anesthesia interventional procedures. The literature regarding such procedures in pediatric patients is sparse, and therefore treatment guidelines must be based on adult evidence. The pediatric literature regarding palliative radiation therapy and sedation for pain are even more limited. Complementary therapies must be considered in pediatric patients, especially for procedure-related pain and pain at the end of life. The integration of pain and palliative care services with pediatric oncology is required to provide the appropriate level of interdisciplinary management in complex patients with refractory pain during treatment for cancer and for those with end-stage disease.

References

1. Collins JJ, Grier HE, Kinney HC, et al. Control of severe pain in children with terminal malignancy. J Pediatr. 1995;126:653–7.
2. Geeta MG, Geetha P, Ajithkumar VT, et al. Management of pain in leukemic children using the WHO analgesic ladder. India J Pediatr. 2010;77:665–8.
3. Lebel A. Cancer pain and palliative care in children. Tech Reg Anesth Pain Manage. 2005;9:145–51.
4. Berde CB, Sethna NF. Analgesics for the treatment of pain in children. N Engl J Med. 2002;347:1094–103.
5. Anand KJ, International Evidence-Based Group for Neonatal Pain. Consensus statement for the prevention and management of pain in the newborn. Arch Pediatr Adolesc Med. 2001;155:173–80.
6. Duhn LJ, Medves JM. A systematic integrative review of infant pain assessment tools. Adv Neonatal Care. 2004;4:126–40.
7. Linder LA. Measuring physical symptoms in children and adolescents with cancer. Cancer Nurs. 2005;28:16–26.
8. Hummel P, van Dijk M. Pain assessment: current status and challenges. Semin Fetal Neonatal Med. 2006;11:237–45.
9. Stinson JN, Kavanagh T, Yamada J, et al. Systematic review of the psychometric properties, interpretability and feasibility of self-report pain intensity measures for use in clinical trials in children and adolescents. Pain. 2006;125:143–57.
10. von Baeyer CL, Spagrud LJ. Systematic review of observational (behavioral) measures of pain for children and adolescents aged 3 to 18 years. Pain. 2007;127:140–50.
11. Cohen LL, Lemanek K, Blount RL, et al. Evidence-based assessment of pediatric pain. J Pediatr Psychol. 2008;33:939–55.
12. Anghelescu DL, Berde C, Cohen KJ, et al. NCCN clinical practice guidelines in oncology: pediatric cancer pain v1. 2007. Accessed from www.nccn.org.
13. Huguet A, Stinson JN, McGrath PJ. Measurement of self-reported pain intensity in children and adolescents. J Psychosom Res. 2010;68:329–36.
14. Tomlinson D, von Baeyer CL, Stinson JN, et al. A systematic review of faces scales for the self-report of pain intensity in children. Pediatrics. 2010;126:e1168–98.
15. Wood C, von Baeyer CL, Falinower S, et al. Electronic and paper versions of a faces pain intensity scale: concordance and preference in hospitalized children. BMC Pediatr. 2011;11:87.
16. Stevens B. Pain assessment and management in infants with cancer. Pediatr Blood Cancer. 2007;49:1097–101.
17. Huguet A, McGrath PJ, Pardos J. Development and preliminary testing of a scale to assess pain-related fear in children and adolescents. J Pain. 2011;12:840–8.
18. Franck LS, Allen A, Oulton K. Making pain assessment more accessible to children and parents: can greater involvement improve the quality of care? Clin J Pain. 2007;23:331–8.
19. Wuhrman E, Cooney MF, Dunwoody CJ. Authorized and unauthorized ("PCA by proxy") dosing of analgesic infusion pumps: position statement with clinical practice recommendations. Pain Manage Nurs. 2007;8:4–11.
20. Monitto CL, Greenberg RS, Kost-Byerly S, et al. The safety and efficacy of parent−/nurse-controlled analgesia in patients less than six years of age. Anesth Analg. 2000;91:573–9.
21. Anghelescu DL, Burgoyne LL, Oakes LL, et al. The safety of patient-controlled analgesia by proxy in pediatric oncology patients. Anesth Analg. 2005;101:1623–7.
22. Anghelescu DL, Faughnan LG, Oakes LL, et al. Parent-controlled PCA for pain management in pediatric oncology: is it safe? J Pediatr Hematol Oncol. 2012;34:416–20.
23. Zeltzer LK, Altman A, Cohen D, et al. Report of the subcommittee on the management of pain associated with procedures in children with cancer. Pediatrics. 1990;86:826–31.
24. Hockenberry MJ, McCarthy K, Taylor O, et al. Managing painful procedures in children with cancer. J Pediatr Hematol Oncol. 2011;33:119–27.
25. Hedén L, von Essen L, Ljungman G. Randomized interventions for needle procedures in children with cancer. Eur J Cancer. 2009;18:358–63.
26. Sadeghi T, Mohammadi N, Shamshiri M, et al. Effect of distraction on children's pain during intravenous catheter insertion. J Spec Pediatr Nurs. 2013;18:109–14.
27. Cline RJ, Harper FW, Penner LA, et al. Parent communication and child pain and distress during painful pediatric cancer treatments. Soc Sci Med. 2006;63:883–98.
28. Hedén LE, von Essen L, Ljungman G. Effect of morphine in needle procedures in children with cancer. Eur J Pain. 2011;15:1056–60.

29. Jacob E. Neuropathic pain in children with cancer. J Pediatr Nurs. 2004;21:350–7.
30. Weinstein SM. Phantom limb pain and related disorders. Neurol Clin. 1998;16:919–35.
31. Anghelescu DL, Faughman LG, Popenhagen MP, et al. Neuropathic pain referrals to a multidisciplinary pediatric cancer pain service. Pain Manage Nurs. 2014;15:126–31.
32. Dougherty M, DeBaun MR. Rapid increase of morphine and benzodiazepine usage in the last three days of life in children with cancer is related to neuropathic pain. J Pediatr. 2003;142:373–6.
33. Anghelescu DL, Oakes LL, Hankins GM. Treatment of pain in children after limb-sparing surgery: an institution's 26-year experience. Pain Manage Nurs. 2011;12:82–94.
34. Krane EJ, Heller LB. The prevalence of phantom sensation and pain in pediatric amputees. J Pain Symptom Manag. 1995;10:21–9.
35. Burgoyne LL, Billups CA, Jirón JL Jr, et al. Phantom limb pain in young cancer-related amputees: recent experience at St Jude children's research hospital. Clin J Pain. 2012;28:222–5.
36. Finkel JC, Pestieau SR, Quezado ZM. Ketamine as an adjuvant for treatment of cancer pain in children and adolescents. J Pain. 2007;8:515–21.
37. White MC, Hommers C, Parry S, et al. Pain management in 100 episodes of severe mucositis in children. Paediatr Anaesth. 2011;21:411–6.
38. Klepstad P, Borchgrevink P, Hval B, et al. Long-term treatment with ketamine in a 12-year-old girl with severe neuropathic pain caused by a cervical spinal tumor. J Pediatr Hematol Oncol. 2001;23:616–9.
39. Tsui BC, Davies D, Desai S, et al. Intravenous ketamine infusion as an adjuvant to morphine in a 2-year-old with severe cancer pain from metastatic neuroblastoma. J Pediatr Hematol Oncol. 2004;26:678–80.
40. Conway M, White N, St. Jean C, et al. Use of continuous intravenous ketamine for end-stage cancer pain in children. J Pediatr Oncol Nurs. 2009;26:100–6.
41. Fine PG. Low-dose ketamine in the management of opioid nonresponsive terminal cancer pain. J Pain Symptom Manag. 1999;17:296–300.
42. Kajiume T, Sera Y, Nakanuno R, et al. Continuous intravenous infusion of ketamine and lidocaine as adjuvant analgesics in a 5-year-old patient with neuropathic cancer pain. J Palliat Med. 2012;15:719–22.
43. Hooke MC, Grund E, Quammen H, et al. Propofol use in pediatric patients with severe cancer pain at the end of life. J Pediatr Oncol Nurs. 2007;24:29–34.
44. Glover ML, Kodish E, Reed MD. Continuous propofol infusion for the relief of treatment-resistant discomfort in a terminally ill pediatric patient with cancer. J Pediatr Hematol Oncol. 1996;18:377–80.
45. Massey GV, Pedigo S, Dunn NL, et al. Continuous lidocaine infusion for the relief of refractory malignant pain in a terminally ill pediatric cancer patient. J Pediatr Hematol Oncol. 2002;24:566–8.
46. Collins JJ, Grier HE, Sethna NF, et al. Regional anesthesia for pain associated with terminal pediatric malignancy. Pain. 1996;65:63–9.
47. Anghelescu DL, Faughnan LG, Baker JN, et al. Use of epidural and peripheral nerve blocks at the end of life in children and young adults with cancer: the collaboration between a pain service and a palliative care service. Paediatr Anaesth. 2010;20:1070–7.
48. Rork JF, Berde CB, Goldstein RD. Regional anesthesia approaches to pain management in pediatric palliative care: a review of current knowledge. J Pain Symptom Manag. 2013;46:859–73.
49. Saroyan JM, Schechter WS, Tresgallo ME, et al. Role of intraspinal analgesia in terminal pediatric malignancy. J Clin Oncol. 2005;23:1318–21.
50. Morton NS, Errera A. APA national audit of pediatric opioid infusions. Paediatr Anaesth. 2010;20:119–25.
51. Van Schoor AN, Bosman MC, Bosenberg AT. Descriptive study of the differences in the level of conus medullaris in four different age groups. Clin Anat. 2015;28:638–44.
52. Reinoso-Barbero F, Saavedra B, Segura-Grau E, et al. Anatomical comparison of sciatic nerves between adults and newborns: clinical implications for ultrasound guided block. J Anat. 2014;224:108–12.
53. Hernanz-Schulman M, Ahlswede E, Bercha IH, et al. Pause and pulse: image gently in fluoroscopy. Image gently. The alliance for radiation in pediatric imaging. Web http://www.imagegently.org/Procedures/Fluoroscopy#1931727-what-is-fluoroscopy. 13 Jan 2016.
54. Lerman J, Strong HA, LeDez KM, et al. Effects of age on the serum concentration of alpha 1-acid glycoprotein and the binding of lidocaine in pediatric patients. Clin Pharmacol Ther. 1989;46:219–25.
55. Walker SM, Yaksh TL. Neuraxial analgesia in neonates and infants: a review of clinical and preclinical strategies for the development of safety and efficacy data. Anesth Analg. 2012;115:638–62.
56. Polaner DM, Taenzer AH, Walker BJ, et al. Pediatric Regional Anesthesia Network (PRAN): a multi-institutional study of the use and incidence of complications of pediatric regional anesthesia. Anesth Analg. 2012;115:1353–64.
57. Ecoffey C, Lacroix F, Giaufré E, et al. Epidemiology and morbidity of regional anesthesia in children: a follow-up one-year prospective survey of the French-language Society of Paediatric Anaesthesiologists (ADARPEF). Paediatr Anaesth. 2010;20:1061–9.
58. Meyer MJ, Krane EJ, Goldschneider KR, et al. Case report: neurological complications associated with epidural analgesia in children: a report of 4 cases of ambiguous etiologies. Anesth Analg. 2012;115:1365–70.
59. Strafford MA, Wilder RT, Berde CB. The risk of infection from epidural analgesia in children: a review of 1620 cases. Anesth Analg. 1995;80:234–8.
60. Tobias JD. Applications of intrathecal catheters in children. Paediatr Anaesth. 2000;10:367–75.
61. Dadure C, Marec P, Veyckemans F, et al. [Chronic pain and regional anesthesia in children] [French]. Arch Pediatr. 2013;20:1149–57.
62. Martin DP, Bhalla T, Rehman S, et al. Successive multisite peripheral nerve catheters for treatment of complex regional pain syndrome type I. Pediatrics. 2013;131:e323–6.
63. Cucchiaro G, Craig K, Marks K, et al. Diffuse complex regional pain syndrome in an adolescent: a novel treatment approach. Clin J Pain. 2013;29:e42–5.
64. Frenkel O, Mansour K, Fischer JW. Ultrasound-guided femoral nerve block for pain control in an infant with a femur fracture due to nonaccidental trauma. Pediatr Emerg Care. 2012;28:183–4.
65. Dubrovsky AS, Friedman D, Kocilowicz H. Pediatric post-traumatic headaches and peripheral nerve blocks of the scalp: a case series and patient satisfaction survey. Headache. 2014;54:878–87.
66. Berde CB, Sethna NF, Fisher DE, et al. Celiac plexus blockade for a 3-year-old body with hepatoblastoma and refractory pain. Pediatrics. 1990;86:779–81.
67. Staats PS, Kost-Byerly S. Celiac plexus blockade in a 7-year-old child with neuroblastoma. J Pain Symptom Manage. 1995;10:321–4.
68. Pillai Riddell RR, Racine NM, Turcotte K, et al. Non-pharmacological management of infant and young child procedural pain. Cochrane Syst Rev. 2011;10:CD006275.
69. Uman LS, Chambers CT, McGrath PJ, et al. Psychological interventions for needle-related procedural pain and distress in children and adolescents. Cochrane Syst Rev. 2006;4:CD005179.
70. Landier W, Tse AM. Use of complementary and alternative medical interventions for the management of procedure-related pain, anxiety, and distress in pediatric oncology: an integrative review. J Pediatr Nurs. 2010;25:566–79.

71. Wild MR, Espie CA. The efficacy of hypnosis in the reduction of procedural pain and distress in pediatric oncology: a systematic review. J Dev Behav Pediatr. 2004;25:207–13.
72. Richardson J, Smith JE, McCall G, et al. Hypnosis for procedure-related pain and distress in pediatric cancer patients: a systematic review of effectiveness and methodology related to hypnosis interventions. J Pain Symptom Manag. 2006;31:70–84.
73. Bradt J, Dileo C, Grocke D, et al. Music interventions for improving psychological and physical outcomes in cancer patients. Cochrane Syst Rev. 2011;8:CD006911.
74. Nguyen TN, Nilsson S, Hellström AL, et al. Music therapy to reduce pain and anxiety in children with cancer undergoing lumbar puncture: a randomized clinical trial. J Pediatr Oncol Nurs. 2010;27:146–55.
75. Shockey DP, Menzies V, Glick DF, et al. Preprocedural distress in children with cancer: an intervention using biofeedback and relaxation. J Pediatr Oncol Nurs. 2013;30:129–38.
76. Nilsson S, Finnström B, Kokinsky E, et al. The use of virtual reality for needle-related procedural pain and distress in children and adolescents in a paediatric oncology unit. Eur J Oncol Nurs. 2009;13:102–9.
77. Kundu A, Berman B. Acupuncture for pediatric pain and symptom management. Pediatr Clin N Am. 2007;54:885–99.
78. Jindal V, Ge A, Mansky PJ. Safety and efficacy of acupuncture in children: a review of the evidence. J Pediatr Hematol Oncol. 2008;30:431–42.
79. Moody K, Daswani D, Abrahams B, et al. Yoga for pain and anxiety in pediatric hematology-oncology patients: case series and review of the literature. J Soc Integr Oncol. 2010;8:95–105.
80. Beider S, Mahrer NE, Gold JI. Pediatric massage therapy: an overview for clinicians. Pediatr Clin N Am. 2007;54:1025–41.
81. Hughes D, Ladas E, Rooney D, et al. Massage therapy as a supportive care intervention for children with cancer. Oncol Nurs Forum. 2008;35:431–42.
82. Adams D, Cheng F, Jou H, et al. The safety of pediatric acupuncture: a systematic review. Pediatrics. 2011;128:e1575–87.
83. Tucker TL, Samant RS, Fitzgibbon EJ. Knowledge and utilization of palliative radiotherapy by pediatric oncologists. Curr Oncol. 2008;17:48–55.
84. Paulino AC. Relapsed Wilms tumor: is there a role for radiation therapy? Am J Clin Oncol. 2001;24:408–13.
85. Paulino AC. Palliative radiotherapy in children with neuroblastoma. Pediatr Hematol Oncol. 2003;20:111–7.
86. Deutsch M, Tersak JM. Radiotherapy for symptomatic metastases to bone in children. Am J Clin Oncol. 2004;27:128–31.
87. Koontz BF, Clough RW, Halperin EC. Palliative radiation therapy for metastatic Ewing sarcoma. Cancer. 2006;106:1790–3.
88. Friedrichsdorf SJ, Kang TI. The management of pain in children with life-limiting illnesses. Pediatr Clin N Am. 2007;54:645–72.
89. Kiman R, Wuiloud AC, Requena ML. End of life care sedation for children. Curr Opin Support Palliat Care. 2011;5:285–90.
90. de Graeff A, Dean M. Palliative sedation therapy in the last weeks of life: a literature review and recommendations for standards. J Palliat Med. 2007;10:67–85.
91. Anghelescu DL, Hamilton H, Faughnan LG, et al. Pediatric palliative sedation therapy with propofol: recommendations based on experience in children with terminal cancer. J Palliat Med. 2012;15:1082–90.
92. Johnston DL, Nogel K, Friedman DL, et al. Availability and use of palliative care and end-of-life services for pediatric oncology patients. J Clin Oncol. 2008;26:4646–50.
93. Meyer MJ. Integration of pain services into pediatric oncology. Int Anesthesiol Clin. 2006;44:95–107.

14 Pain in Hematologic Malignancies

Kanu Sharan

Introduction

Many pain syndromes can be associated with HTM [1, 2]. Bone pain due to osteolytic lesions is a very common debilitating symptom with myeloma. Diffuse bone pain can be due to involvement of bone marrow with acute leukemia and aggressive lymphomas, and these patients describe this as a dull or throbbing deep pain. Pain due to cord compression can be seen in myeloma and aggressive lymphomas. Neuropathic pain can be disease related such as plasma cell disorders, amyloid, or monoclonal gammopathy of undetermined significance. This can be infection related due to herpes zoster in patients immunosuppressed with chemotherapy and post hematopoietic stem cell transplant.

Other important causes of neuropathic pain are involvement of vertebral bodies with extradural compression of spinal cord, generally seen with myeloma and lymphoma as well as infiltration or compression by cervical, axillary, para-aortic, or retroperitoneal lymph nodes of adjacent nerve plexus. In addition, neuropathic pain can be iatrogenic due to chemotherapeutic agents like vinca alkaloids, platinum agents, etc. Headaches can be disease related or iatrogenic. CNS involvement with aggressive lymphomas and leukemias can present with headaches and visual difficulties. Lumbar puncture, intrathecal chemotherapy, and chemotherapy agents can precipitate headaches. Other disease-related pain scenarios can be visceral (lymphomas/leukemias), cutaneous (mycosis fungoides), and mucus membrane tumor involvement, space-occupying masses, bulky lymph nodes, and organ enlargement such as hepatosplenomegaly. Patients with BRC are also highly susceptible to painful infections, such as pneumonia, urinary tract infections, cellulitis, oral and gastrointestinal mucositis, esophagitis with candida, herpes zoster, and postherpetic neuralgia.

K. Sharan (✉)
MD Anderson Cancer Center at Cooper, Department of Hematology/Oncology, Camden, NJ, USA
e-mail: sharan-kanu@CooperHealth.edu

General Approach to Pain in BRC

Disease-related management is guided by two principles: treatment of the underlying condition by tumor-directed therapies, radiotherapy, orthopedic devices or surgery, and analgesic strategies to relieve pain irrespective of cause. Induction chemotherapy is considered causal measure as it not only reduces malignant bone pain but also relieves the pain due to disease burden. Corticosteroids may be a causal measure, especially for those with lymphomas. Corticosteroids are effective not only in ameliorating bone pain but also significantly improve pain due to neural infiltration or compression of neural structures as seen in patients with spinal cord compression.

Analgesic drugs can be administered with chemotherapy, radiotherapy, and adjuvant agents. Since HTM can be associated with severe neutropenia, thrombocytopenia, and coagulopathies, appropriate analgesic should be carefully selected. Non-steroidal anti-inflammatory drugs (NSAIDs) should be avoided in these patients because of their effects on renal blood flow and need caution for use in patients who are at risk for bleeding due to thrombocytopenia or coagulopathy. These can be replaced with acetaminophen or tramadol. However, these agents may mask fever and therefore an underlying septic condition, which can be of serious concern in the management of neutropenic patients. The safety of COX-2 inhibitor-specific NSAIDs needs to be specifically studied in this setting. These agents could be considered suitable alternatives in patients with BRC, as they exert no effect on the hemostatic system.

Opioids are the mainstay of analgesic therapy in patients with HTM [1, 2]. The opioid of choice is morphine in both immediate and sustained release preparations. Intravenous route is the fastest way to achieve effective analgesia in patients with rapidly escalating or uncontrolled pain. Fentanyl can be a reasonable option and is available for transdermal, buccal, submucosal, and intranasal routes. Transdermal route is optimal in patients with stably maintained analgesia and is not indicated when urgent pain relief or fast titration is required.

A. Gulati et al. (eds.), *Essentials of Interventional Cancer Pain Management*, https://doi.org/10.1007/978-3-319-99684-4_14

Adjuvant drugs such as antidepressants, antiepileptics, and membrane-stabilizing agents (gabapentin, pregabalin) can be useful adjuncts to opiate therapy as they not only enhance the efficacy of opioids but also exert an independent analgesic effect in neuropathic pain. In addition, psychological support, cognitive behavioral interventions, coping strategies, physical therapies, rehabilitation, and biomechanical interventions should be also factored in the comprehensive management of pain in these patients.

Specific Pain Syndromes in BRC

Bone Pain

The most important disease-related pain experienced by patients with BRC is bone pain. The two most common pathophysiologies resulting in bone pain include pain due to lytic bone lesions and infiltration of bone marrow by malignant cells [2]. A common iatrogenic cause of bone pain is administration of growth factors such as pegfilgrastim.

Bone Lesions

Bone lesions occur rarely in patients with hematologic malignancies; however, they are quite common in patients with multiple myeloma and adult T-cell leukemia/lymphoma (ATL) associated with the human T-cell leukemia/lymphoma virus-1 (HTLV-1) virus. Bone lesions may occur in some lymphoproliferative disorders such as Waldenstrom's macroglobulinemia disease or in myeloproliferative disorders [3]. The primary mechanism for bone destruction in patients with myeloma and lymphoma is increased osteoclastic bone resorption.

Multiple myeloma (MM) is a relatively common hematologic malignancy. Bone involvement is the hallmark of MM, characterized by presence of lytic bone lesions. These lesions are associated with bone pain, pathological fractures, spinal cord compression, or hypercalcemia. Sixty percent of patients present with bone pain, and 60% develop a pathological fracture during their disease, thereby affecting the quality of life. These lytic lesions are the result of excessive bone resorption due to increased osteoclast formation and activity as well as inhibition of new bone formation by osteoblasts. Many chemokines and cytokines have been identified as the osteoclast-activating factors (OAF). These OAFs, produced by both myeloma cells and bone marrow stromal cells, can stimulate osteoclast formation, differentiation, and activity. These also suppress osteoblast activity.

Treatment for pain due to myeloma-related lytic bone lesions will include both symptomatic and disease-specific management. Opioids will be initiated with both short-acting and long-acting medications. This will likely be a combination of morphine or oxycodone or fentanyl patch.

Approximately 20% of myeloma patients will require radiation. Local radiation can be started simultaneously as this can reduce pain significantly. Single fraction radiation treatment has proven to be an efficient and cost-effective alternative to traditional multi-fractionated radiotherapy. If pain control is the exclusive goal, a single dose or a short course fractionation will be ideal, especially in patients with decreased performance status and short life expectancy. However, in the majority of multiple myeloma patients with long life expectancy in whom recalcification is the most important goal, a more fractionated schedule is recommended.

Bisphosphonates are also mainstay for treatment of such painful lytic lesions in myeloma. They inhibit osteoclast recruitment and maturation, prevent the development of monocytes into osteoclast, induce osteoclast apoptosis, and interrupt their attachment to the bone [4]. Several clinical trials of zoledronic acid or pamidronate have shown to be beneficial, both in terms of anti-myeloma effect and for bone strengthening. These agents will usually be administered monthly for up to 2 years. A large phase III randomized, double-blind trial confirmed that zoledronic acid and pamidronate had similar efficacy in reducing the risk of skeletal-related events in myeloma patients. However, ease of administration is more with zoledronic acid as this is infused over 15 min, while pamidronate requires to be infused over 3 h. Denosumab, a monoclonal antibody, functioning as a RANK ligand inhibitor, is now FDA approved for the prevention of skeletal-related events (SREs) in patients with multiple myeloma. Denosumab demonstrated noninferiority to zoledronic acid at delaying the time to the first SRE in patients with multiple myeloma. It can be administered easily as a subcutaneous injection once a month.

Osteonecrosis of the jawbone with extensive dental work is a potential rare side effect of bisphosphonates and Denosumab, which results in a difficult to treat painful condition. Prevention is key, and patients are required to have a dental evaluation and clearance prior to start of these agents. In addition, if they require dental work while they are no these agents, then it will be prudent to temporarily hold the drugs and to be restarted when complete healing has occurred.

Patients with large lytic lesions in weight-bearing bones may require orthopedic procedures and surgery for pain control and as prophylaxis against fractures. Vertebral augmentation has become increasingly common treatment for pain caused by vertebral compression fractures. Randomized controlled trials of patients with osteoporosis and solid metastatic neoplasms have shown that vertebroplasty and kyphoplasty reduce pain, decrease use of analgesic drugs, increase vertebral height, and improve functional ability. Even though these procedures are increasingly used to palliate vertebral lesions in myeloma, data for these procedures is limited to small experiential case series [5].

Khan et al. [5] performed a systematic literature review of 23 published case series with the aim to analyze data on vertebral augmentation procedures in myeloma. Even though this review had many intrinsic limitations, their analysis demonstrated that spinal augmentation in patients with myeloma is effective, with decreased postoperative pain and decreased analgesic drug use. The benefit was immediate and sustained, with associated complications rates being low.

Bone Pain Due to Pegfilgrastim

The clinical consequences of chemotherapy-induced neutropenia are often severe and can be potentially life threatening. Patients who develop febrile neutropenia often need to be hospitalized, reducing their quality of life and increasing costs. Neutropenia can also compromise the ability to deliver chemotherapy at the full dose and on schedule. To help prevent the occurrence of neutropenia, patients with high risk of developing chemotherapy-related infections may be given prophylactic colony-stimulating factors, such as filgrastim.

Bone pain is a common side effect of treatment with filgrastim. Pegfilgrastim is a pegylated long-acting analogue of filgrastim that is administered once per chemotherapy cycle [6].

Pegfilgrastim is a white blood cell growth factor and works by stimulating the bone marrow to produce new granulocytes. This stimulation of the bone marrow often leads to some degree of bone pain, typically lasting for a few days after the growth factor injection. Pain is generally reported in the pelvis and femur, as the greatest marrow reserves are in these regions.

Pawloski et al. [7] reported that pegfilgrastim-associated bone pain occurred in 19% and loratadine was the most common medication used to treat it. Potential risk factors for bone pain in patients receiving myelosuppressive chemotherapy and primary prophylactic pegfilgrastim identified in one study were younger age and history of bone pain [8].

Traditionally, this has been managed with NSAIDs for mild pain and opioids for moderate to severe pain. But these often fall short in controlling the pain, requiring reduction in the dose of pegfilgrastim. A phase III randomized placebo-controlled clinical trial demonstrated that naproxen at a dose of 500 mg twice per day is effective in reducing the incidence and severity of pegfilgrastim-induced bone pain [9]. Based on anecdotal reports, there has been increasing use of loratadine for this in the outpatient oncology setting.

A recent phase II study showed that administration of prophylactic loratadine does not decrease the incidence of severe bone pain or improve quality of life in high-risk patient population receiving chemotherapy [10].

Headaches

Headache is a commonly encountered and often non-specific symptom in patients with hematologic malignancies. While primary headaches are a potential cause, consideration must be given to unique disease-related and treatment-related etiologies in this patient population. Disease-related causes include central nervous system involvement, cerebrospinal fluid obstruction, intracranial hemorrhage, anemia, venous thrombosis, and hyperviscosity syndromes. Headaches may also be post-procedural (after lumbar puncture) or therapy related (aseptic meningitis from intrathecal chemotherapy or IVIG, all-trans-retinoic acid-induced intracranial hypertension).

ATRA-Induced Headaches

Acute promyelocytic leukemia (APL) is a distinct clinico-pathologic disorder that accounts for 10–15% of cases of acute myeloid leukemia (AML). All-trans-retinoic acid (ATRA), a derivative of vitamin A, is an essential component in the treatment of acute promyelocytic leukemia (APL). ATRA has been associated with pseudotumor cerebri (PC), seen predominantly in pediatric patients. However, several incidences have been reported in adults with a slight preponderance in overweight young females of childbearing age. These signs and symptoms of PC usually develop 2 weeks after initiation of ATRA [11].

All patients on ATRA who develop PC report headaches and 50% of them report diplopia. Less common complaints are nausea, vomiting, and blurred vision. Treatment options have been analgesics, withdrawal of ATRA, antiemetics, acetazolamide, and therapeutic lumbar puncture.

A literature review of 23 cases of ATRA-induced intracranial hypertension looked at the treatments used and time to resolution of symptoms [12]. The primary treatment used was withdrawal of ATRA. Lumbar punctures and acetazolamide were used alone or in combination with withdrawal of ATRA to reduce cerebrospinal fluid pressure. Acetazolamide treatment showed to be ineffective in one case for which ultimately therapeutic lumbar puncture in addition to ATRA withdrawal achieved relief of the symptoms [13]. Therapeutic lumbar punctures have shown to provide symptoms resolution anywhere from immediate relief to after 3 weeks of repeated procedures [14, 15].

Procedure-Related Headaches

CNS involvement can occur with certain HTM such as aggressive NHL (Burkitt's and diffuse large B-cell lymphoma) and acute lymphoblastic leukemia. Intrathecal chemotherapy, both prophylactic and therapeutic, has been an integral part of management of these HTM and has led to significant improvement in outcomes of these patients. Headache is a common adverse event in patients who receive intrathecal chemotherapy, with one study reporting 39% of patients [16]. In less severe cases, these were attributed to lumbar puncture itself and were responsive to supportive care measures, such as mild analgesics and prolonged supine position. Other more serious cases are due to the chemotherapy itself. Liposomal cytarabine has been associated with papilledema, increased intracranial pressure, and encephalitis [16]. There have been deaths reported due to encephalitis from liposomal cytarabine [16]. Four studies that reviewed acute lymphoblastic lymphoma and Burkitt's lymphoma patients receiving hyper-CVAD chemotherapy suggested <1% of cases with the severe toxicity of papilledema, pseudotumor cerebri, and encephalitis from standard intrathecal chemotherapy of cytarabine alternating with methotrexate [17–20]. Other studies have shown that 7% to 15% of cases with aseptic meningitis symptoms are from liposomal cytarabine [21]. Treatments used for headache related to intrathecal treatment include conservative measurements like, bed rest, fluids, caffeine, and oral analgesics. In some patients, additional measures like steroids and intravenous opioids may be required [16, 21]. Rarely IV caffeine and epidural blood patch may be required in select patients if headaches do not improve by above interventions.

Pain Due to Peripheral Neuropathy

Peripheral neuropathy is defined as a disease or degenerative state of the peripheral nerves in which motor, sensory, or vasomotor nerve fibers are affected. The condition appears clinically as muscle weakness and atrophy, pain, and numbness. Peripheral neuropathy (PN) and associated pain in BRC can occur from disease-related conditions, chemotherapy/treatment induced, and infections such as postherpetic neuralgia. HTM such as multiple myeloma, Waldenstrom's macroglobulinemia, POEMS syndrome, and light chain amyloidosis generate paraproteins, which are immunoglobulins produced in excess by an abnormal clonal proliferation of B-lymphocytes or plasma cells. These frequently present with peripheral neuropathy resulting in pain. In addition, myeloma, non-Hodgkin lymphomas, and leukemias can cause neuropathy by compression or invasion of extra-/intradural space. Chemotherapy-induced peripheral neuropathy (CiPN) has been consistently reported with platinum compounds, vinca alkaloids, proteasome inhibitors, and immunomodulatory drugs with different and often specific clinical characteristics. Increased collaboration between hematologists and neurologists is required in differentiation, early recognition and treatment of these painful neuropathies [22].

Paraproteinemic Neuropathy

Baseline paraproteinemic PN (PPN) may be observed in nearly 50% of newly diagnosed patients with plasma cell dyscrasias [23]. This may be due to the presence of monoclonal protein or compression of nerve roots. PPN may be caused by interaction of antibodies with specific antigenic targets on peripheral nerves or by deposition of immunoglobulins or amyloid. IgM monoclonal protein could bind to the myelin-associated glycoprotein, thereby causing damage to the nerves. The association and pathogenesis of IgA or IgG monoclonal gammopathy with polyneuropathy is less clear. Small fiber neuropathy is often seen in amyloidosis and may be a result of pro-inflammatory cytokines and vasoactive peptides. IgM paraprotein-related neuropathy is more commonly seen with MGUS and Waldenstrom's macroglobulinemia, whereas IgA/IgG is more commonly associated with myeloma.

Typically manifested neurologically as a length-dependent axonal loss sensorimotor polyneuropathy, PPN affects some or all sensory modalities causing allodynia, hyperpathia, cramps, or mild distal weakness (rarely it can be associated with more profound motor symptoms). Electrodiagnostic studies show mixed demyelinating and axonal features and often may be indistinguishable from findings in chronic inflammatory demyelinating polyneuropathy.

Definitive therapy with chemotherapy or immunomodulatory agents will need to be initiated quickly. However, these can inherently be associated with risks of neuropathy.

Plasmapheresis and IVIG can be used as initial treatment along with definitive therapy to rapidly decrease the amount of paraprotein; response is generally being short term [24].

Corticosteroids, when given in conjunction with other therapies, produce a response in about half of the patients with high anti-MAG IgM but are seldom effective as a single therapy. However, long-term use of corticosteroids is prohibitive as it can suppress pituitary-adrenal axis and increases patient susceptibility for infection.

After IVIG and corticosteroids, azathioprine and rituximab may be considered as alternative immunosuppressive agents. These agents are less commonly used since definitive therapy for the HTM is far more essential.

Symptomatic treatment of the neuropathy itself usually involves membrane stabilizers, tricyclic antidepressants, and/or serotonin-norepinephrine reuptake inhibitors with or without opioids based on severity and chronicity of symptoms.

Chemotherapy-Induced Peripheral Neuropathy (CIPN)

CiPN is caused by damage to nerve fibers, more specifically the axon and dorsal root ganglion (DRG). Although this is generally associated with distal symmetrical sensory neuropathy, motor and/or autonomic nerve fibers may be affected.

Platinum compounds such as cisplatin is used as a salvage regimen in lymphomas. Platinum-induced neuropathy occurs in about 30% of patients and is related to total cumulative dose [22]. DRG is the main target.

Vinca alkaloids (vincristine/vinblastine) are used in regimens for lymphomas, leukemia, and rarely plasma dorsal root ganglion (DRG) cell dyscrasias. Neurotoxicity has been reported in 30–40% of patients and is total cumulative dose related. These agents inhibit microtubule formation for their antineoplastic effect and affect neuronal function this way. A significant proportion of patients on vinca alkaloids also develop autonomic symptoms, like orthostatic hypotension, gastrointestinal dysmotility, urinary retention, or erectile dysfunction.

Proteasome inhibitors such as bortezomib and carfilzomib are standard therapies for myeloma. Bortezomib preferentially causes painful sensory neuropathy in approximately 30% of patients as compared to that reported in 15% of patients with carfilzomib. These agents induce PN by blocking transcription of nerve growth factor by inhibiting nuclear factor kB but also induce mitochondrial mediated apoptosis. Bortezomib-induced PN can be reversible.

Immunomodulatory agents, such as thalidomide, preferentially cause mixed sensory-motor type of neuropathy with a reported prevalence of 10–55%. Pathogenesis of thalidomide-induced PN is poorly understood but could be related to its anti-angiogenic and immunomodulatory effects, resulting in partially irreversible damage to the distal axons and DRG neurons. Currently lenalidomide is used for myeloma and myelodysplasia more commonly than thalidomide, and this has been reported to cause less PN.

Early detection of treatment-related PN is essential for timely and appropriate intervention. Patients with pre-existing PN should be monitored closely for signs of deterioration. Implementation of patient-focused tools for screening and grading of neuropathy and symptom evaluation and a focused clinical neurological examination including the evaluation of sensation, distal muscle strength, ankle reflexes, and supine versus upright blood pressure should be performed. Nerve conduction studies and needle electromyography can help to quantify the severity of neuropathy and to differentiate treatment-related (mostly primarily axonal neuropathies) from disease-related (often demyelinating) PN and from non-neurological problems.

One of the most widely used grading systems for assessing CiPN in hematology clinical practice is the NCI CTC criteria version 4.0 (Table 14.1).

Dose reduction or dose modification of these drugs is the first step in the management of CiPN, as this can prevent more serious and potentially irreversible neurologic damage. Discontinuation of drugs may have to be considered, in case of severe symptoms. Clinical studies have shown that dose reduction of bortezomib or change from twice weekly to weekly dosing can improve and prevent progress of PN. In addition, subcutaneous dosing of bortezomib resulted in much less incidence of PN as compared to intravenous administration.

First-line treatment of pain from CiPN includes drugs like gabapentin and pregabalin, with titration to a tolerable dose with maximal benefit. Alternative medications can be tricyclic antidepressants, serotonin reuptake inhibitors, and antiepileptics. Opioid analgesics and tramadol are generally considered second-line treatment for neuropathic pain but can be initiated simultaneously with gabapentin and pregabalin. Local application of lidocaine or menthol cream may temporarily alleviate symptoms. Transcutaneous electrical nerve stimulation is safe and may be help for symptom relief. The evidence of supplements such as vitamin B complex and/or alpha lipoic acid in myeloma and other HTM remains anecdotal, and their use is based on extrapolation from trials with other neurotoxic drugs in different diseases such as diabetic neuropathy. A complementary role of these supplements has been suggested and therefore at times used in HTM.

Table 14.1 CTCAE v5.0 – November 27, 2017: peripheral neuropathy

Nervous system disorders					
CTCAE term	Grade 1	Grade 2	Grade 3	Grade 4	Grade 5
Peripheral sensory neuropathy	Asymptomatic	Moderate symptoms; limiting instrumental ADL	Severe symptoms; limiting self-care ADL	Life-threatening consequences; urgent intervention indicated	-

Definition: A disorder characterized by damage or dysfunction of the peripheral sensory nerves
Navigational note: -

Herpes Zoster and Postherpetic Neuralgia

Herpes zoster (HZ) or shingles is due to viral reactivation of latent VZV. HTM patients with HZ tend to have more HZ-relatedcomplications, as they are more immunosuppressed than patients with solid tumor malignancies and have a tendency to recur [25]. The incidence of varicella-zoster infection ranges from 2% among patients with chronic myeloid leukemia (CML) receiving imatinib mesylate to 10–15% in patients with chronic lymphocytic leukemia (CLL) receiving fludarabine or alemtuzumab, to 25% of patients with Hodgkin lymphoma or autologous stem cell transplant recipients, and to 45–60% among allogeneic stem cell transplant recipients. Postherpetic neuralgia is a complication of shingles, which is caused herpes zoster virus. Postherpetic neuralgia affects nerve fibers and the skin, causing burning pain that lasts long after the rash and blisters of shingles disappear. Severe pain can continue for more than 1–3 months in the same place that the shingles occurred, which can be very debilitating for these patients [26].

Treatment of VZV disease should include the early institution of antiviral therapy (valacyclovir, acyclovir, or famciclovir). There is no evidence that intravenous immunoglobulin or corticosteroids add benefit in the treatment of VZV disease in immunocompromised patients. Opioids, tramadol, and gabapentin are used as adjunct for symptomatic relief. Lidocaine or capsaicin patch may provide local symptom relief.

Prevention of VZV reactivation among patients with hematologic malignancy remains controversial. Acyclovir and valacyclovir are highly effective. Despite its efficacy in preventing VZV disease, antiviral prophylaxis is not routinely recommended by many clinical care guidelines. The reluctance to recommend routine prophylaxis appears to be based on observations that VZV disease may still occur after the discontinuation of VZV prophylaxis. However, antiviral prophylaxis with valacyclovir (500 mg BID) is routinely prescribed for the first year after stem cell transplantation and for patients who receive intensive therapy or alemtuzumab [26].

The Food and Drug Administration has approved the use of the varicella-zoster vaccine (Zostavax) for adults' age 50 and older. The shingles vaccine doesn't guarantee complete prevention of shingles but will likely reduce the course and severity of the disease and reduce the risk of postherpetic neuralgia.

The shingles vaccine is used only as a prevention strategy. It's not intended to treat people who currently have the disease. The vaccine contains live virus and is therefore not given to patients with HTM, who are immunosuppressed.

Oral Mucositis

Whether under active treatment or in advanced phase of the disease, oral mucositis is one of the most painful complications that patients with hematologic malignancies experience [1]. This can cause considerable impact on their quality of life due to pain, poor food intake, and increased risk of local infections. Treatment-induced mucositis is a pathological process which is characterized by mucosal damage, ranging from mild inflammation to deep ulcerations and affecting one or more parts of the alimentary tract. The incidence of oral mucositis-related pain syndromes is 40–70% among patients treated with chemotherapy, 100% in those who received radiation for head and neck tumors, and 60–80% in the setting of allogeneic SCT, with significant pain lasting from the 4th to the 11th day after transplantation [27].

Pain symptoms can range from a sense of burning in the initial phases up to severe forms and are caused by a mixture of different types of pain. The main component is nociceptive pain, mediated by C fibers and relievable by opioids. The second component is incidental pain, caused by movement and contact with the mucosal surface, mediated by the fast-conducting A-δ fibers. This latter component is insensitive to analgesics and the only effective pain treatment is the functional exclusion of the anatomic parts involved until the resolution of the ulcers and full recovery of the mouth's functionality. The symptoms of GIM are visceral pain (ranging from mild pain to projected abdominal wall pain) and hypermobility with diarrhea, starting from the 3rd day after the beginning of the treatment and resolving by the 7th day, coinciding with the full clinical flare of the OM.

NCI CTC version 4.0 also has a system of grading for mucositis, which is common in hematology practice (Table 14.2).

Table 14.2 CTCAE v5.0 – November 27, 2017: oral mucositis

Gastrointestinal disorders					
CTCAE term	Grade 1	Grade 2	Grade 3	Grade 4	Grade 5
Mucositis oral	Asymptomatic or mild symptoms; intervention not indicated	Moderate pain or ulcer that does not interfere with oral intake; modified diet indicated	Severe pain; interfering with oral intake	Life-threatening consequences; urgent intervention indicated	Death

Definition: A disorder characterized by ulceration or inflammation of the oral mucosal
Navigational note: -

Currently, no standard therapy prevents or treats severe oral mucositis. Good oral hygiene, dietary adjustments, topical agents, application of local anesthetic, cryotherapy, antibiotics, and opioids as systemic analgesics currently remain the cornerstones of mucositis care. Analgesic therapy can allow the resumption of feeding. The mainstay of analgesic therapy is the parenteral administration of opioids. Tramadol can be used for mild to moderate pain.

Palifermin, a human recombinant keratinocyte growth factor, is the most promising agent. Palifermin has been shown to significantly and consistently reduce the duration and incidence of oral mucositis after intensive chemotherapy, radiotherapy, and autologous hematopoietic stem cell transplantation. Particularly, it markedly reduced the incidence of oral mucositis of WHO grade 4 (20%, as compared with 62% in the placebo group; $P < 0.001$), the most debilitating form of oral mucositis, in which oral alimentation is impossible [28]. This agent and two human fibroblast growth factors could become the targeted therapy for prevention of mucositis in future.

Procedure-Related Pain

Bone marrow biopsy and lumbar puncture are indicated for diagnosis in hematologic malignancies. In addition, venous access with a port or PICC is integral for administration of chemotherapy and other supportive therapies. These pain scenarios are generally acute and transient [1]. Careful needle selection, appropriate practice, correct technique and local anesthetic may decrease the painful complications.

Light sedation with benzodiazepines can further enhance the comfort of the patient. At times, a brief unconscious sedation, in close collaboration with anesthetists, may be recommended for painful diagnostic procedures in children and in selected adult patients [1].

Back Pain from Cord Compression

Aggressive lymphomas such as Burkitt's and diffuse large B-cell lymphoma and plasmacytomas can present with spinal involvement resulting in cord compression. Clinically, these patients can present with pain and neurologic deficits. Surgery is indicated in patients with spinal cord compression syndrome. Early diagnosis is associated with better prognosis. Recommended treatment can include acute surgical decompression and systemic and intrathecal chemotherapy adapted to the histological sub-type of each tumor. In selected cases, radiotherapy can also be utilized. Consensus does not exist regarding the degree of neurologic deficit and the timing of surgery versus radiotherapy. Corticosteroid use is an initial treatment and often is immediately started when neurologic symptoms are confirmed from spinal cord compression. Corticosteroids both serve to stabilize neural membranes, treat spinal vasogenic cord edema, and serve as part of a chemotherapeutic regimen. In addition, corticosteroids can preserve neurologic function and improve overall outcome after specific therapy. One of the most common regimens used is dexamethasone. High doses of dexamethasone can also result in sudden pain relief.

Bone Marrow Transplant

Pain is a common symptom in patients undergoing hematopoietic stem cell transplant (HSCT) for HTM, and a multitude of pain scenarios can be seen in transplant recipients. HSCTs can be autologous which means stem cells from patient to himself or allogeneic SCT, which is from another individual to patient.

The major cause of pain in HSCT recipients is a result of injury to mucosal tissues induced by the conditioning regimen, infections, and acute and chronic GVHD (graft vs. host disease) [29]. Apart from the recipients, donors can experience deep somatic pain from growth factors such as filgrastim and pegfilgrastim used for stem cell mobilization and collection. Bone pain has generally been reported in about 60% and headaches in 25% of growth factor-stimulated patients.

Hematopoietic stem cells are collected more commonly from peripheral blood and less often by bone marrow harvest. In the setting of marrow harvest, incidence of pain was reported in 30%.

Another common scenario is superficial somatic pain from oral mucositis. The severity of oral mucositis is closely related to the conditioning regimen. It has been reported to be as high as 75% in lymphoma patients undergoing autologous SCT and almost all patients with allogeneic SCT, grade 3 or 4 in 60%. With the conditioning regimen used in myeloma, oral mucositis has been reported in 30–35%. In addition, gastrointestinal mucositis is frequently associated with visceral pain.

Acute visceral pain occurs in allogeneic SCT patients due to hepatic veno-occlusive disease. This has been attributed to cytotoxic drug-induced damage to the endothelium of hepatic sinusoids. Patients present with right upper quadrant pain due to distension of Glisson's capsule.

Other cases of visceral pain in patients who have undergone allogeneic SCT include mucosal damage induced by GVHD and intestinal dysmotility due to neuropathy. Drugs used for GVHD prophylaxis, such as calcineurin inhibitors, may induce neurotoxicity and neuropathic pain. Lastly another cause of visceral pain can be urinary bladder irritation and /or hemorrhagic cystitis, generally in those who have been conditioned with total body irradiation and cyclophosphamide-based regimens.

Another unique pain syndrome reported in recipients of allogeneic SCT is bone marrow necrosis. This is a rare but very painful complication in patients undergoing allogeneic SCT following GCSF administration or due to acute GVHD.

In general, pain should be routinely assessed in all HSCT patients together with the assessment of other vital signs. Opioids are the mainstay of pain management in HSCT patients. Partial mixed opiate receptor agonists and mild opioids, such as hydrocodone, codeine, and tramadol, are beneficial for relieving moderate pain. However, the pure μ-opiate receptor agonists or strong opioids, such as morphine or fentanyl, are the drugs of choice for treating severe pain. Adjuvant pain therapy can be added to the analgesic regimen. NSAIDs should not be administered to HSCT patients as they are at high risk because of coexisting renal dysfunction, gastropathy, or hemostatic defects.

Conclusion

The control of pain is therefore essential in the complete management of patients with active BRC as well as long-term survivors. A multidisciplinary approach is the need for appropriate pain management of these patients. The WHO analgesic ladder for cancer pain is effective in most cases. However, targeted measures, adjuvant agents, and non-pharmacological interventions also play a significant role in relieving pain in certain circumstances. A rational treatment strategy should be based on causal interventions along with analgesic measures.

References

1. Niscola P, et al. Pain syndromes in hematologic malignancies: an overview. Hematol J. 2004;5:293–303.
2. Niscola P, et al. Pain in blood cancers. Indian J Palliat Care. 2011;17(3):175–83.
3. Roodman, GD. Mechanisms of bone lesions in myeloma and lymphoma. Cancer. 1997;80(8):1557–63.
4. Pathogenesis and Management of Myeloma Bone Disease. Christoulas, et al. Expert Rev Hematol. 2009;2(4):385–98.
5. Khan OA, et al. Vertebral augmentation in patients with multiple myeloma: a pooled analysis of published case series. Am J Neuroradiol. 2014;35:207–10.
6. Kubista E, Glaspy J, Holmes FA, Green MD, Hackett J, Neumann T, Pegfilgrastim Study Group. Bone pain associated with once-per-cycle pegfilgrastim is similar to daily filgrastim in patients with breast cancer. Clin Breast Cancer. 2003;3(6):391–8.
7. Pawloski PA, Larsen M, Thoresen A, Giordana MD. Pegfilgrastim use and bone pain: a cohort study of community-based cancer patients. J Oncol Pharm Pract. 2015 May 7. pii: 1078155215585188. [Epub ahead of print].
8. Xu H, Gong Q, Vogl FD, Reiner M, Page JH. Risk factors for bone pain among patients with cancer receiving myelosuppressive chemotherapy and pegfilgrastim. Support Care Cancer. 2016;24(2):723–30. https://doi.org/10.1007/s00520-015-2834-2. Epub 2015 Jul 11.
9. Kirshner JJ, Heckler CE, Janelsins MC, Dakhil SR, Hopkins JO, Coles C, Morrow GR. Prevention of pegfilgrastim-induced bone pain: a phase iii double-blind placebo-controlled randomized clinical trial of the university of rochester cancer center clinical commun oncol program research base. J Clin Oncol. 2012;30(16):1974–9. https://doi.org/10.1200/JCO.2011.37.8364. Epub 2012 Apr 16.
10. Moukharskaya J, Abrams DM, Ashikaga T, Khan F, Schwartz J, Wilson K, Verschraegen C, Openshaw T, Valentine J, Eneman J, Unger P, Ades S. Randomized phase II study of loratadine for the prevention of bone pain caused by pegfilgrastim. Support Care Cancer. 2016 Feb 19. [Epub ahead of print].
11. Visani G, Bontempo G, Manfroi S, Pazzaglia A, D'Alessandro R, Tura S. All-trans-retinoic acid and pseudotumor cerebri in a young adult with acute promyelocytic leukemia: a possible disease association. Haematologica. 1996;81(2):152–4. Review.
12. Visani G, Bontempo G, Manfroi S, Pazzaglia A, D'Alessandro R, Tura S. All-trans-retinoic acid and pseudotumor cerebri in a young adult with acute promyelocytic leukemia: a possible disease association. Haematologica. 1996;81(2):152–4.
13. Guirgis MF, Lueder GT. Intracranial hypertension secondary to all-trans retinoic acid treatment for leukemia: diagnosis and management. J AAPOS. 2003;7(6):432–4.
14. Decaudin D, Adams D, Naccache P, Castagna L, Munck JN. Maintained all-trans retinoic acid therapy in a patient with pseudotumour cerebri despite aggravated symptoms. Leuk Lymphoma. 1997;27(3–4):373–4.
15. Jabbour E, O'Brien S, Kantarjian H, Garcia-Manero G, Ferrajoli A, Ravandi F, Cabanillas M, Thomas DA. Neurologic complications associated with intrathecal liposomal cytarabine given prophylactically in combination with high-dose methotrexate and cytarabine to patients with acute lymphocytic leukemia. Blood. 2007;109(8):3214–8. Epub 2007 Jan 5.
16. Kantarjian HM, O'Brien S, Smith TL, et al. Results of treatment with hyper-CVAD, a dose-intensive regimen, in adult acute lymphocytic leukemia. J Clin Oncol. 2000;18:547–61.
17. Kantarjian H, Thomas D, O'Brien S, et al. Long-term follow-up results of hyperfractionated cyclophosphamide, vincristine, doxorubicin, and dexamethasone (hyper-CVAD), a dose-intensive regimen, in adult acute lymphocytic leukemia. Cancer. 2004;101:2788–801.
18. Thomas DA, O'Brien S, Cortes J, et al. Outcome with the hyper-CVAD regimens in lymphoblastic lymphoma. Blood. 2004;104:1624–30.
19. Thomas DA, Faderl S, O'Brien S, et al. Chemoimmunotherapy with hyper-CVAD plus rituximab for the treatment of adult Burkitt and Burkitt-type lymphoma or acute lymphoblastic leukemia. Cancer. 2006;106:1569–80.
20. Scott BJ, van Vugt VA, Rush T, Brown T, Chen CC, Carter BS, Schwab R, Fanta P, Helsten T, Bazhenova L, Parker B, Pingle S, Saria MG, Brown BD, Piccioni DE, Kesari S. Concurrent intrathecal methotrexate and liposomal cytarabine for leptomeningeal metastasis from solid tumors: a retrospective cohort study. J Neuro Oncol. 2014 Jun 19. [Epub ahead of print].
21. Chamberlain MC. Neurotoxicity of intra-CSF liposomal cytarabine (DepoCyt) administered for the treatment of leptomeningeal metastases: a retrospective case series. J Neuro-Oncol. 2012;109(1):143–8. https://doi.org/10.1007/s11060-012-0880-x. Epub 2012 Apr 27.
22. JLM J, et al. Chemotherapy induced peripheral neuropathies in hematological malignancies. J Neuro-Oncol. 2015;121(2):229–37.

23. Sonneveld P, et al. Dealing with neuropathy in plasma-cell dyscrasias. ASH Education Book. 2010;2010(1):423–30.
24. Rison RA, et al. Paraproteinemic neuropathy: a practical review. BMC Neurol. 2016;16:13.
25. Tran TN, et al. Complications of herpes zoster in cancer patients. Scand J Infect Dis. 2014;46(7):528–32.
26. Wade J. Viral infections in patients with hematological malignancies. ASH Education Book. 2006;2006(1):368–74.
27. Niscola P, et al. Mucositis in patients with hematologic malignancies: an overview. Haematologica. 2007;92(2):222–31.
28. Spielberger R, et al. Palifermin for oral mucositis after intensive therapy for hematologic cancers. N Engl J Med. 2004;351(25):2590–8.
29. Niscola P, et al. Pain syndromes in the setting of haematopoietic stem cell transplantation for haematological malignancies. Bone Marrow Transplant. 2008;41:757–64.

15 Dermatologic Cancer Pain Syndromes

Katerina Svigos, Viswanath Reddy Belum, and Mario E. Lacouture

Abbreviations

APC	Antigen-presenting cell
DPD	Dihydropyrimidine dehydrogenase
HFS	Hand-foot syndrome
HFSR	Hand-foot skin reaction
HZ	Herpes zoster
MHC	Major histocompatibility complex
NSAID	Nonsteroidal anti-inflammatory drug
PHN	Postherpetic Neuralgia
PPES	Palmar-Plantar Erythrodysesthesia Syndrome
TS	Thymidylate synthase
UV	Ultraviolet
VZV	Varicella-zoster virus

Introduction

Along with burning, pruritus, and skin irritation, pain is one of the most common symptoms treated in dermatology clinics. Pain in the oncologic population may result from iatrogenic interventions (e.g., medications and procedures) or an underlying malignancy (e.g., immunocompromised status). Many dermatologic symptoms are preventable and/or easily managed. In this chapter, we provide an overview of the anatomy and physiology of skin, followed by a discussion of common painful skin conditions and their management.

K. Svigos (✉)
New York University School of Medicine, New York, NY, USA
e-mail: katerina.svigos@nyumc.org

V. R. Belum · M. E. Lacouture
Department of Medicine, Memorial Sloan Kettering Cancer Center, New York, NY, USA
e-mail: belumv@mskcc.org; lacoutum@mskcc.org

Anatomy and Physiology of Skin

The epidermis is the outermost layer of the skin and renews itself approximately every 28 days. It varies in thickness, ranging between 0.05 mm and 1.5 mm, and is comprised of four layers of keratinocytes (skin cells): stratum basale, stratum spinosum, stratum granulosum, and the stratum corneum. The stratum basale is the lowermost layer of the epidermis and is attached to the underlying basement membrane by hemidesmosomes. It is comprised of mitotically active cells, which terminally differentiate into anucleate keratinized corneocytes as they transition through the overlying (four) layers of the skin. The stratum spinosum and the stratum granulosum are the middle layers of the epidermis. These layers are comprised of keratinocytes that are tightly bound together by intercalated desmosomes or adhesion proteins held together by intermediate filaments. The outermost layer of the skin, the stratum corneum, is a compact, tight layer of corneocytes, interwoven with proteins and lipids that together serve as a barrier and maintain moisture within the body.

Besides keratinocytes, major cell types in the epidermis include melanocytes and Langerhans cells. The melanocytes are dendritic cells that release melanin, a pigment primarily responsible for skin color. The Langerhans cells are antigen-presenting cells (APCs) that play a critical role in mounting immune responses against various microbial antigens (including tumor cells). The function of the epidermis is to provide a protective barrier to the skin by retaining moisture, assist in thermoregulation, and provide protection from UV rays. It also aids in regulating desquamation and immunological surveillance, prevents permeation of toxins, and activates anti-microbial responses.

The dermis is the intermediate layer of the skin, which, like the epidermis, varies in its thickness and ranges from 0.3 mm to 3.0 mm. It is organized in two layers: the upper papillary dermis and the lower reticular dermis. The upper papillary dermis is comprised of collagen fibers connected to proteins of the epidermal-dermal junction. The reticular dermis is composed

A. Gulati et al. (eds.), *Essentials of Interventional Cancer Pain Management*, https://doi.org/10.1007/978-3-319-99684-4_15

of proteoglycans, glycoproteins, and tightly interwoven collagen fibrils, which render elasticity and tensile strength to the skin. It is also a site of immune response activity to pathogens by antibodies, fibroblasts, macrophages, mast cells, and circulating cells.

Macrophages carry out a variety of functions such as phagocytosis of foreign bodies and presentation of antigens on extracellular major histocompatibility complexes (MHCs). Mast cells are skin cells that release several pro-inflammatory mediators including histamine (from secretory granules), in response to microbial pathogens. Histamine aids in blood vessel dilation and permeation, allowing immune cells to access the site of infection. Within the dermis, blood vessels branch into arterioles and further into arterial and venous capillary beds, to provide the most effective mode of oxygen and nutrient delivery to tissues. This branching also allows for efficient transportation of immune cells to the infected areas of the dermis [1].

The skin contains a variety of receptors that respond to different stimuli (e.g., mechanical, chemical, thermal). Nociceptors are small, excitatory neurons that transmit signals from the dermis along nerve fibers to the spinal cord (dorsal root ganglion) and brain and are most involved with the sensation of pain. One such example is the trigeminal nerve, which has nerve endings that are sensitive to pain, pruritus, and temperature.

Other types of sensory receptors include the Pacinian corpuscles, Merkel cells, Ruffini cells, and Meissner's corpuscle, which are innervated by low threshold A-fibers (or sensory neurons). C-fibers are responsible for heat sensation, while A-fibers are mostly responsible for heat and mechanosensation [2]. Pacinian corpuscles are large encapsulated endings that are highly concentrated in the palm of hands and fingertips and serve to detect large, deep vibrations and pressure. Merkel cells are sensory mechanoreceptors in the epidermis (around the hair follicles) that mediate sensations of gentle touch pressure. The Ruffini cells are slow-adapting receptors, located in the deep subcutaneous tissue of the skin and are sensitive to sustained pressure. Meissner's corpuscles are rapidly adapting receptors, located throughout the body, but concentrated in thick, hairless skin such as finger pads and lips. They are sensitive to pressure and vibration. In general, these receptors work to transmit a signal to the brain by the firing of electrical action potentials. This signal occurs at a rapid rate and begins in an afferent nerve that synapses in the spinal cord on another neuron that eventually terminates in the brain to give the individual a sensory experience [3].

Pain Syndromes and Management

Injection Site Reactions

Central and peripheral venous access (IV) are commonly required in cancer patients. Peripheral venous access permits infusion of medications, hydration fluids, blood products, and nutritional supplements. In most cases, IV placement is a safe procedure and poses little serious risk. In cancer patients however, central venous access is often required for the administration of chemotherapeutic drugs, to minimize patient discomfort (since they are frequently administered in cycles) and because of the smaller caliber of a peripheral vein.

A common complication of injections at peripheral and central venous site is phlebitis, i.e., inflammation of the veins, which often manifests with erythema, pain, tenderness, and induration around the injection site (Fig. 15.1). Thrombophlebitis occurs in up to 15% of patients with

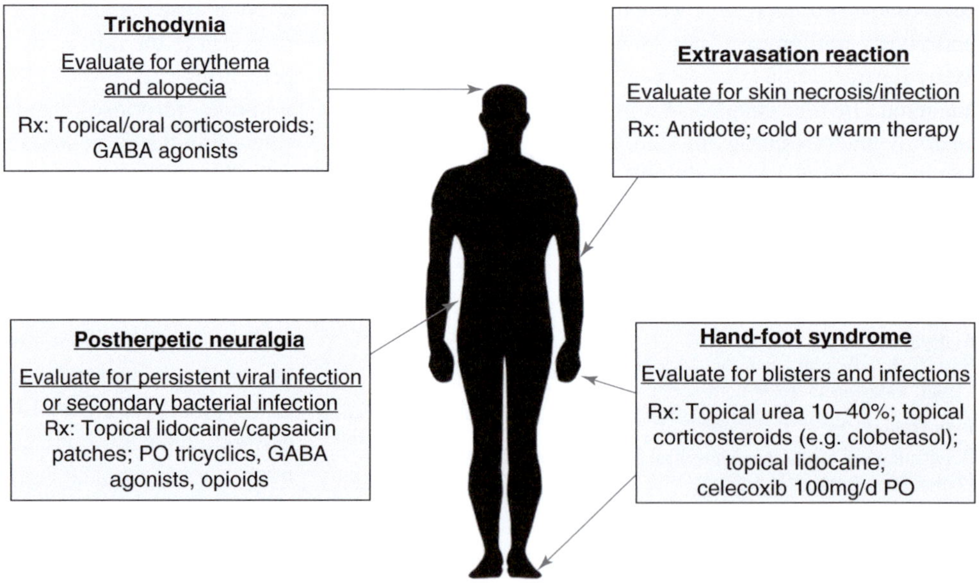

Fig. 15.1 Dermatologic cancer pain syndromes

peripheral venous catheters [4]. It occurs more commonly in immunocompromised patients, as in the case of cancer patients, and can at times lead to bloodstream infections (e.g., sepsis) [5].

Prophylaxis of phlebitis involves maintaining adequate circulation and reducing the risk of blood clots. Measures include avoidance of IV catheter placement in the lower extremities, minimizing catheter mobility, placing catheters of the smallest caliber, and removing the catheter as soon as possible [6, 7]. First-line treatment of phlebitis includes discontinuing IV infusion and removing the catheter. Pain may be further alleviated by extremity elevation, warm or cool compresses, and oral nonsteroidal anti-inflammatory drugs (NSAIDs). For patients with superficial thrombophlebitis involving an extremity, anticoagulation medications are recommended to reduce blood clotting. In patients experiencing persistent pain, suppurative phlebitis or vein inflammation due to infection should be suspected, and treatment with an antibiotic should be instituted.

Another common injection site complication is extravasation, or the unintended leakage of drugs into the extravascular space. The frequency of extravasation is between 0.1% and 6% in peripheral injections and lower in central lines [8]. Extravasation reactions can cause severe tissue damage and result in lasting injury. Anthracyclines have been reported to cause more serious reactions such as tissue necrosis with skin ulceration and thinning of skin. Local inflammatory reactions such as burning, tightness, pain, and phlebitis, accompanied by erythema and tenderness, are commonly reported issues with other chemotherapeutic agents.

Risk factors for extravasation from peripheral venous sites include small/ fragile veins, obesity (obscures veins from view and palpation), multiple previous venipunctures, and disseminated skin disease such as eczema or psoriasis. Additionally, patient movement during IV placement and sensory deficits that impair the patient's ability to detect sensory changes at the site of IV infusion may also lead to peripheral extravasation [9–11]. Risk factors specific to extravasation from central venous catheters include difficulty encountered during the insertion of the device, misplacement of the device when a catheter tip is placed outside of the vein, and gradual catheter migration from the vein out into the tissue. The risk of extravasation from central venous access is also increased with long dwell times of 6 or more months, presence of fibrin sheath or thrombus at catheter tip (which causes chemotherapy to backtrack along the catheter and leak from the vein), and a deeply implanted port [12, 13].

Symptoms of extravasation are usually experienced immediately but may be delayed for days to weeks. The initial clinical manifestations include local burning or tingling, mild erythema, pruritus, and swelling. After about 3 days, patients commonly experience increasing erythema, pain, brawny discoloration, induration, dry desquamation, and/or blistering at the site [14]. In more serious cases, patients may develop necrosis, eschar formation, and ulceration with raised, red, painful edges and a yellow necrotic base.

Avoidance of extravasation includes administering drugs only through IVs placed within large, intact, and patent veins. The patency of the IV should first be checked by flushing. To reduce the risk of extravasation, veins should be inspected and accessed in the following order: the forearm, the dorsum of the hand, the wrist, and the antecubital fossae. Veins should be inspected prior to administering any medication and checked daily. Sites with sclerosis, thrombosis, scar formation, or previously irradiated areas should be avoided, and patency of the IV should first be confirmed by flushing. Patients should also be instructed to notify their clinician immediately if they experience any pain, leakage, or changes in sensation [15, 16].

Pain due to extravasation may be managed by discontinuing the infusion and elevation of the affected extremity. The catheter should not be removed, but rather left in place to aspirate the fluid. Topical application of ice is also helpful for minimizing pain, except when vinca alkaloids (e.g., vincristine, vinblastine, vinorelbine) or epipodophyllotoxins (e.g., etoposide) are being administered. Several medications, depending on the causative agent, have also been shown to be effective in the prevention of necrosis and ulceration. Dexrazoxane is particularly effective as it provides protection against extravasated anthracyclines [17]. Other medications include sodium thiosulfate following mechlorethamine, dacarbazine, or cisplatin, DMSO following mitomycin, or hyaluronidase following vinca alkaloids, paclitaxel, epipodophyllotoxins, and ifosfamide. In the event of a nonhealing ulcer, patients will require debridement and skin grafting [15, 16, 18, 19].

Postherpetic Neuralgia

Postherpetic neuralgia (PHN) is defined by the persistence of pain beyond 4 months, from the initial onset of rash of herpes zoster (HZ) [20]. The latter occurs due to the reactivation of varicella-zoster virus (VZV), which normally remains dormant for years in the dorsal root ganglia of cranial or spinal nerves, after resolution of the initial infection. The risk of reactivation of VZV, however, increases with impairment of the immune system, which could be idiopathic or secondary to physical/ psychosocial stress. When cellular immunity wanes, VZV is transported along the peripheral nerves, producing an acute neuritis that is characterized by hemorrhagic inflammation and eventually fibrosis, upon resolution.

Approximately, 600,000 to 1 million people are newly infected with VZV [21] per year, while the incidence of HZ is around 3/1000 patients per year [22]. It is noteworthy, however, that the incidence of HZ is 2–4 times higher in cancer patients, as opposed to the general population. For example, in patients with Hodgkin's lymphoma, it has been estimated that around 48 patients per thousand develop HZ [23]. The type of chemotherapy and/or the dose of corticosteroid play an important role in altering the immune function, therefore increasing the risk in this subset of patients.

Since at least 90% of adults show evidence of VZV, they are potentially at risk for PHN [24]. PHN is also common in patients with HIV infection or cancer, with lymphomas and leukemias posing the greatest risk among the latter. Around 47% of HZ patients with hematologic cancers and 41% of patients with solid tumors develop PHN [23]. These numbers are much higher as opposed to the incidence (25%) in the general population [25]. In general, VZV is strongly associated with the presence of an active tumor at the time of infection [26].

Clinically, patients commonly complain of a "burning" pain, and 90% have allodynia (pain evoked by normally nonpainful stimuli, e.g., light touch). It is likely secondary to inflammation related to the movement of viral particles from sensory nerves to skin and subcutaneous tissues, as well as secondary to damage to the nerve structures [27–29]. This pain may be significant enough to interfere with appetite, sleep, or sexual function [30, 31]. Patients also often also demonstrate areas of anesthesia such as deficits of thermal, tactile, pinprick, and vibration sensations, within the affected areas [32] (Fig. 15.1).

Initiation of treatment for HZ within the first 5 days of onset decreases the risk of PHN. The VZV vaccine reduces the risk of developing HZ and PHN by 51% and 67%, respectively [33]. First-line treatment for PHN is tricyclic antidepressants such as amitriptyline, nortriptyline, and desipramine, which work by inhibiting the reuptake of norepinephrine and serotonin in the central nervous system and increasing the inhibition of nociceptive signals from the periphery. Their benefit is limited because of the anticholinergic side effects such as sedation and dry mouth. Other forms of treatment include neuromodulators such as gabapentin, pregabalin, and valproic acid, which are commonly used for neuropathic pain. Opioids, while effective, are considered second- or third-line drugs, given their high risk of physical dependence, tolerance, addiction, and risk for overdosing. Topical treatment with lidocaine or capsaicin patches temporarily alleviates the pain and results in minimal systemic absorption and fewer adverse events. Several studies have shown that lidocaine is effective in providing pain relief as well [34], although skin irritation at the site of the patch is frequently reported [35]. With capsaicin, burning, stinging, and erythema of the skin are common; however, repeated applications can result in desensitization of unmyelinated epidermal nerve cells [36].

Patients experiencing PHN affecting nerves other than the trigeminal nerve may be offered intrathecal glucocorticoids, although there is insufficient data supporting its efficacy, and besides, serious adverse events may occur (e.g., aseptic meningitis, transverse myelitis, cauda equina syndrome, lumbar radiculitis, headache, urinary retention, and arachnoiditis). NMDA receptor antagonists such as ketamine and dextromethorphan can relieve neuropathic pain in humans; however, these antagonists may cause sedation, dysphoria, and dissociative episodes as well. Cryotherapy is another modality of treatment, which involves ablation of the affected nerve, but like many of these forms of treatments, the results are inconsistent. Patients who fail all conservative treatments may be suitable candidates for surgery. Possible procedures include electrical stimulation of thalamus, anterolateral cordotomy, and electrocoagulation of the dorsal root. However, there are substantial risks of permanent neurologic deficits with surgery, and no consistent benefit has been reported.

Palmar-Plantar Erythrodysesthesia

Palmar-plantar erythrodysesthesia (PPE) is a drug-induced pain syndrome, which encompasses two distinct conditions with overlapping symptomatology—the hand-foot syndrome (HFS) and hand-foot skin reaction (HFSR). It is a common occurrence among cancer patients receiving systemic cytotoxic and targeted anticancer treatments [37]. The former includes drugs such as cytarabine, capecitabine, doxorubicin (including pegylated liposomal), or 5-fluorouracil [38–40], all of which can cause HFS. Among the targeted therapies, multitargeted tyrosine-kinase inhibitors (e.g., all-grade HFSR—regorafenib, 60.5%; cabozantinib, 35.3%; sorafenib, 33.8%; axitinib, 29.2%; sunitinib, 18.9%) are most commonly associated with HFSR [38, 41]. Of note, some of these medications appear to cause PPE in patients who are genetically predisposed. One example is capecitabine-induced HFS, which is associated with genetic polymorphisms of dihydropyrimidine dehydrogenase (DPYD) and thymidylate synthase (TYMS)—two enzymes that are involved in metabolism of the drug [42]. In general, the patient's risk of developing PPE depends on the drug's dose, formulation, and administration schedule, and sustained serum levels of cytotoxic agents lead to HFS more frequently.

PPE occurs on the distal aspects of the hands and feet, and patients initially present with complaints of a tingling sensation on the palms and/or soles followed by edema and tender, symmetrical erythema over the fat pads of the distal phalanges (Fig. 15.1). HFS and HFSR symptoms present primarily on the surfaces of the palms and soles. However, HFS is associated with diffuse pain, edema erythema, and desquamation, while HFSR tends to be dose-dependent and affects pressure/friction-prone regions (e.g., heels) and often results in callus formation and blistering of the affected area. The pain accompanying PPE may limit daily activities such as walking and grasping objects and can lead to the loss of fingerprints over time.

Large-scale trials investigating the treatment of PPE are lacking, although small case studies have noted improvement in the symptoms with topical dimethyl sulfoxide, nicotine patch, oral vitamin E, and amifostine. However, the most efficient interventions are dose modification and symptom management. The latter includes high-potency topical corticosteroids and topical keratolytics [38]. General prophylactic measures include urea-based creams, avoidance of hot water, and activities that contribute to the development of blisters during treatment (e.g., excessive walking and handling of heavy objects). It is important to document the baseline status of susceptible areas before initiating anticancer treatment with PPE-inducing drugs. After administration of the first dose, patients should be monitored often, and after the first two doses, they should be inspected every 1–2 weeks. If symptoms appear, physicians must first aim to rule out other conditions such as fungal infections, persisting sensory neuropathy following cytotoxic chemotherapy, and even erythema multiforme [41].

Trichodynia

Trichodynia is a condition characterized by the occurrence of a painful or abnormal sensation on the scalp [43] (Fig. 15.1). It may be accompanied by hair loss or may be a warning sign of impending hair fall and is commonly noted with various types of hair loss such as telogen effluvium, androgenetic alopecia/female pattern androgenetic alopecia, alopecia areata, and folliculitis decalvans [44]. Although the exact prevalence is not known, studies have reported rates ranging from 14.3% to 73.6% in patients with alopecia. It is more common in women [45], and in patients with telogen effluvium [46–48].

Clinically patients complain of a burning or painful sensation of either the entire scalp or patchy areas of the scalp [43]. The severity may vary, and in some cases, it may be severe enough to cause insomnia and behavioral problems. This is associated with increased hair loss from primarily the painful areas of the scalp [44]. Some practitioners believe that trichodynia is associated with anxiety and depression and may be considered an equivalent of glossodynia or vulvodynia [49]. Although the pathogenesis of trichodynia remains unclear, it is thought that inflammation of the hair follicle may be the primary underlying process. A close interplay between substance P (pro-inflammatory) and mast cells via the neurokinin-1 (NK-1) receptor may together initiate and perpetuate neurogenic inflammation around the hair follicle [50], which explains its concurrent occurrence with other scalp inflammatory conditions that cause alopecia.

There is no well-defined treatment for this condition and with most interventions being empirical. Corticosteroids are used to treat some types of alopecia and may lead to resolution of trichodynia. Other drugs that have been tried are L-cysteine preparations, antidepressant and antianxiety medications, and cannabinoids [49, 51, 52].

Conclusion

Cancer patients commonly experience painful skin conditions. In addition to cancer-related pain, dermatologic conditions such as injection site reactions, postherpetic neuralgia, PPE, and trichodynia are other important causes of pain in cancer patients (Fig. 15.1). Although the conditions have been extensively studied and documented in dermatology and oncology literature, the underlying pathophysiology remains elusive. Therefore, it is important to recognize these conditions early on and understand their management as treatment continues to be nonstandardized, to maintain consistent dosing and satisfactory patients' health-related quality of life.

References

1. Lacouture ME. 3/structure and function of the intergumentary system and the dermatology lexicon. Dermatologic principles and practice in oncology: conditions of the skin, hair, and nails in cancer patients. Hoboken: Wiley Blackwell; 2014. 95+. Print.
2. Dubin AE, Patapoutian A. Nociceptors: the sensors of the pain pathway. J Clin Invest. 2010;120(11):3760–72.
3. Purves D. Mechanoreceptors specialized to receive tactile information. Neuroscience. 2nd ed. U.S. National Library of Medicine, 1 Jan 1970. Web. 12 Apr 2017.
4. Monreal M, Oller B, Rodriguez N, Vega J, Torres T, Valero P, Mach G, Ruiz AE, Roca J. Infusion phlebitis in post-operative patients: when and why. Haemostasis. 1999;29(5):247–54.
5. Otten TR, Stein PD, Patel KC, Mustafa S, Silbergleit A. Thromboembolic disease involving the superior vena cava and brachiocephalic veins. Chest J. 2003;123(3):809–12.
6. Haddad FG, Waked CH, Zein EF. Peripheral venous catheter-related inflammation. A randomized prospective trial. J Med Liban. 2006;54(3):139–45.
7. Singh R, Bhandary S, Pun KD. Peripheral intravenous catheter related phlebitis and its contributing factors among adult population at KU Teaching Hospital. Kathmandu Univ Med J (KUMJ). 2008;6(24):443–7.
8. Scjrijvers DL. Extravasation: a dreaded complication of chemotherapy. Ann Oncol. 2003;14(3):26–30.
9. Goolsby TV, Lombardo FA. Extravasation of chemotherapeutic agents: prevention and treatment. Semin Oncol. 2006;33(1):139–43.
10. Schulmeister L. Extravasation management: clinical update. Semin Oncol Nurs. 2011;27(1):82–90.
11. Doellman D, Hadaway L, Bowe-Geddes LA, Franklin M, LeDonne J, Papke-O'Donnell L, Pettit J, Schulmeister L, Stranz M. Infiltration and extravasation: update on prevention and management. J Infus Nurs. 2009;32(4):203–11.
12. Sauerland C, Engelking C, Wickham R, Corbi D. Vesicant extravasation part I: mechanisms, pathogenesis, and nursing care to reduce risk. Oncol Nurs Forum. 2006;33(6):1134–41.

13. Schulmeister L, Camp-Sorrell D. Chemotherapy extravasation from implanted ports. Oncol Nurs Forum. 2000;27(3):531–8.
14. Loth TS, Eversmann WW Jr. Treatment methods for extravasations of chemotherapeutic agents: a comparative study. J Hand Surg Am. 1986;11(3):388–96.
15. Polovich M, Whitford JM, Olsen M. Chemotherapy and biotherapy guidelines and recommendations for practice. 3rd ed. ONS News. 2009;Section V:105. Available online: http://www.ons.org/about/FAQ/Clinical/#extravasation
16. Perez Fidalgo JA, Garcia Fabregat L, Cervantes A, Margulies A, Vidall C, Roila F, ESMO Working Group. Management of chemotherapy extravasation: ESMO-EONS clinical practice guidelines. Ann Oncol. 2012;23(7 Suppl):vii167–73.
17. Jensen JN, Lock-Anderson J, Langer SW, Mejer J. Dexrazoxane – a promising antidote in the treatment of accidental extravasation of antracyclines. Scand J Plast Resconstr Surg Hand Surg. 2003;37:174–5.
18. Cox K, Stuart-Harris R, Abdini G, Grygiel J, Raghavan D. The management of cytotoxic-drug extravasation: guide-lines drawn up by a working party for the Clinical Oncological Society of Australia. Med J Aust. 1988;148(4):185–9.
19. Albanell J, Baselga J. Systemic therapy emergencies. Semin Oncol. 2000;27(3):347–61.
20. Dworkin RH, Portenoy RK. Pain and its persistence in herpes zoster. Pain. 1996;67(2–3):241–51.
21. Quan D, Cohrs R, Mahalingam R, Gilden DH. Prevention of shingles: safety and efficacy of live zoster vaccine. Ther Clin Risk Manag. 2007;3(4):633–9.
22. Sampathkumar P, Drage LA, Martin DP. Herpes zoster (shingles) and postherpetic neuralgia. Mayo Clin Proc. 2009;84(3):274–80.
23. Yenikomishian MA, Guignard AP, Haguinet F, LaCasce AS, Skarin AT, Trahey A, Karner P, Duh MS. The epidemiology of herpes zoster and its complications in Medicare cancer patients. BMC Infect Dis. 2015;15(106):1–10.
24. Gnann JW, Whitley RJ. Herpes Zoster. N Engl J Med. 2002;347:340–6.
25. Johnson RW. Herpes zoster and postherpetic neuralgia. Multispecialty. 2010;9(3s):21–6.
26. Rusthoven JJ, Ahlgren P, Elhakim T, Pinfold P, Reid J, Stewart L, Feld R. Varicella-zoster infection in adult cancer patients. A population study. Arch Intern Med. 1988;148(7):1561–6.
27. Watson CP, Morshead C, Van der Kooy D, Deck J, Evans RJ. Post-herpetic neuralgia: post-mortem analysis of a case. Pain. 1988;34(2):129.
28. LaMotte RH, Shain CN, Simone DA, Tsai EF. Neurogenic hyperalgesia: psychophysical studies of underlying mechanisms. J Neurophysiol. 1991;66(1):190.
29. Simone DA, Baumann TK, LaMotte RH. Dose-dependent pain and mechanical hyperalgesia in humans after intradermal injection of capsaicin. Pain. 1989;38(1):99.
30. Drolet M, Brisson M, Schmader KE, Levin MJ, Johnson R, Oxman MN, Patrick D, Blanchette C, Mansi JA. The impact of herpes zoster and postherpetic neuralgia on health-related quality of life: a prospective study. CMAJ. 2010;182(16):1731–6.
31. Johnson RW, Bouhassira D, Kassianos G, Leplège A, Schmader KE, Weinke T. The impact of herpes zoster and post-herpetic neuralgia on quality-of-life. BMC Med. 2010;8:37.
32. Bowsher D. Pathophysiology of postherpetic neuralgia: towards a rational treatment. Neurology. 1995;45(12 Suppl 8):S56–7.
33. Tseng HF, Smith N, Harpaz R, Bialek SR, Sy LS, Jacobsen SJ. Herpes zoster vaccine in older adults and the risk of subsequent herpes zoster disease. JAMA. 2011;305(2):160–6.
34. Comer AM, Lamb HM. Lidocaine patch 5%. Drugs. 2000 Feb;59(2):245–9.
35. Meier T, Wasner G, Faust M, Kuntzer T, Ochsner F, Hueppe M, Bogousslavsky J, Baron R. Efficacy of lidocaine patch 5% in the treatment of focal peripheral neuropathic pain syndromesL a randomized, double-blind, placebo-controlled study. Pain. 2003;106(1–2):151–8.
36. Nolano M, Simone DA, Wendelschafer-Crabb G, Johnson T, Hazen E, Kennedy WR. Total capsaicin in humans: parallel loss of epidermal nerve fibers and pain sensation. Pain. 1999;81(1–2):135–45.
37. Gomez P, Lacouture ME. Clinical presentation and management of hand-foot skin reaction associated with Sorafenib in combination with cytotoxic chemotherapy: experience in breast cancer. Oncologist. 2011;16(11):1508–19.
38. Miller KK, Gorcey L, McLellan BN. Chemotherapy-induced hand-foot syndrome and nail changes: a review of clinical presentation, etiology, pathogenesis, and management. J Am Acad Dermatol. 2014;71(4):787.
39. Hoff PM, Valero V, Ibrahim N, Willey J, Hortobagyi GN. Hand-foot syndrome following prolonged infusion of high doses of vinorelbine. Cancer. 1998;82(5):965.
40. Eich D, Scharffetter-Kochanek K, Eich HT, Tantcheva-Poor I, Krieg T. Acral erythrodysesthesia syndrome caused by intravenous infusion of docetaxel in breast cancer. Am J Clin Oncol. 2002;25(6):599.
41. McLellan B, Ciardiello F, Lacouture M, Segaert S, Van Cutsem E. Regorafenib-associated hand-foot skin reaction: practical advise on diagnosis, prevention, and management. Ann Oncol. 2015;26(8):2017.
42. Rosmarin D, Palles C, Church D, Domingo E, Jones A, Johnstone E, Wang H, Love S, Julier P, Scudder C, Nicholson G, Gonzalez-Neira A, Martin M, Sargent D, Green E, McLeod H, Zanger UM, Schwab M, Braun M, Seymour M, Thompson L, Lacas B, Boige V, Ribelles N, Afzal S, Enghusen H, Jensen SA, Etienne-Grimaldi MC, Milano G, Wadelius M, Glimelius B, Garmo H, Gusella M, Lecomte T, Laurent-Puig P, Martinez-Balibrea E, Sharma R, Garcia-Foncillas J, Kleibl Z, Morel A, Pignon JP, Midgley R, Kerr D, Oncol TIJC. Genetic markers of toxicity from capecitabine and other fluorouracil-based regimens: investigation in the QUASAR2 study, systematic review, and meta-analysis. J Clin Oncol. 2014;32(10):1031–9. Epub 2014 Mar 3.
43. Sulzberger MB, Witten VH, Kopf AW. Diffuse alopecia in women: its unexplained apparent increase in incidence. AMA Arch Derm. 1960;81(4):556–660.
44. Baldari M, Montinari M, Guarrera M, Rebora A. Trichodynia is a distinguishing symptom of telogen effluvium. J Eur Acad Dermatol Venereol. 2009;23:733–4.
45. Willimann B, Trüeb RM. Hair pain (trichodynia): frequency and relationship to hair loss and patient gender. Dermatology. 2002;205:374–7.
46. Grimalt R, Ferrando J, Grimalt F. Trichodynia. Dermatology (Basel, Switzerland). 1998;196(3):374.
47. Kivanç-Altunay İ, Savaş C, Gökdemir G, Köşlü A, Ayaydin EB. The presence of trichodynia in patients with telogen effluvium and androgenetic alopecia. Int J Dermatol. 2003;42:691–3.
48. Durusoy C, Ozenli Y, Adiguzel A, Budakoglu IY, Tugal O, Arikan S, Uslu A, Gulec AT. The role of psychological factors and serum zinc, folate and vitamin B_{12} levels in the aetiology of trichodynia: a case–control study. Clin Exp Dermatol. 2009;34:789–92.
49. Hoss D, Segal S. Scalp dysesthesia. Arch Dermatol. 1998;134(3):327–30.
50. O'Connor TM, et al. The role of substance P in inflammatory disease. J Cell Physiol. 2004;201(2):167–80.
51. Trüeb RM. Trichodynie. Hautarzt. 1997;48(12):877–80.
52. Wu M, Ma D. Total syntheses of (±)-Spiroquinazoline,(−)-Alantryphenone,(+)-Lapatin a, and (−)-Quinadoline B. Angewandte Chemie. 2013;125(37):9941–4.

Part IV

Percutaneous Pain Techniques and Anatomy

Ablative Techniques

16

Simon Guo and Jack W. Lam

Diagnostic Versus Therapeutic Blocks

When performing any type of procedure, it is important to first narrow the field of diagnosis. Therefore, when considering a more definitive analgesic treatment, it is crucial that one considers performing diagnostic injections first. This will allow the clinician to gain valuable information regarding possible targets for therapeutic intervention. Diagnostic injections with local anesthetics and often with particulate steroids may provide both diagnostic information and therapeutic treatment. Practitioners can then use information related to target localization, degree of pain relief, and duration of pain relief to further determine potential benefits of neuroablation.

It is often wise to have at least one or more diagnostic injections before proceeding with an ablative procedure to confirm that a specific nerve is the source of pain. The patient should also understand the extent of pain relief possible from a neuroablative procedure and be comfortable with the associated risks. Neuroablative procedures generally take longer to perform and are often associated with more intra- and post-procedural pain related to the type of lesioning. Because of the increased duration and procedure-related discomfort, patients may require a degree of sedation in order to comfortably complete the procedure. In addition, neuroablative techniques can be associated with a significant risk to adjacent tissues. All of these risks are specific to the target site and mechanism of ablation chosen. As neuroablative procedures for cancer are entirely elective procedures, it is very important to fully educate the patient and family regarding risks before proceeding.

S. Guo
Northport Veterans Affairs Medical Center, Department of Anesthesia, Northport, NY, USA

J. W. Lam (✉)
Rex Hospital, Wake Med Cary Hospital, Duke Raleigh Hospital, Department of Anesthesia, Raleigh, NC, USA

Radiofrequency Ablation

Continuous Thermal Radiofrequency Ablation

The first lesions in neural tissue were used in the nineteenth century by applying electrical direct currents on the body [1]. A thermal radiofrequency ablation involves a high-frequency current that is applied to the surrounding tissues. A voltage is generated between the tip of a needle and a dispersion pad with the patient acting to close the circuit. This generates an electric field that causes the ions within the surrounding tissue to rapidly move back and forth to generate heat. This heat is then absorbed by the electrode which registers the temperature reading typically ranging between 60 °C and 80 °C. The resultant lesion that is created depends on electric field size, temperature, and duration of heat creation [2]. During the procedure, prior to ablation, both sensory and motor stimulation is often conducted if the target involves anatomy close to valuable nerve fibers.

Thermal radiofrequency may have many advantages. One is that the lesions tend to be smooth and well-circumscribed. The lesion sizes can be reproducible and quantified using temperature monitoring at the tip of the lesion electrode. Adverse effects such as boiling, charring, and sticking can be avoided by temperature monitoring. The target localization and stability of the radiofrequency electrode positioning can be better accomplished because of the easy application of stimulation, impedance monitoring, and the adaptation to stereotactic or fixation devices. Finally, the electrodes are robust and easily made in different configurations to suit a specific anatomical usage [1].

Cooled Radiofrequency Ablation

Cooled radiofrequency ablation is a newer technique that functions much like the conventional thermal process.

A. Gulati et al. (eds.), *Essentials of Interventional Cancer Pain Management*, https://doi.org/10.1007/978-3-319-99684-4_16

However, the lesion created is larger due to its mechanics. In thermal radiofrequency ablation, the highest temperature of a lesion is at the tissue and probe interface. The tissue immediately surrounding the probe heats up very quickly. If the tissue gets too hot (90–95 °C), the tissue becomes vaporized and/or carbonized. When this occurs, it acts like an insulator and prevents tissue distal to it from being heated (i.e., reduced current density) and subsequently ablated. Therefore, the lesion size is limited near the tissue and probe interface. Cooling allows the removal of heat from the hottest area of the lesion, therefore decreasing the carbonization of the surrounding tissue. The tissue temperature immediately adjacent to the probe is maintained at 60 °C, while the surrounding target tissue is heated to 75 °C. This will provide a lesion of approximately 8–10 mm and also allows lesioning at the tip of the probe.

Pulsed Radiofrequency Treatment

Pulsed radiofrequency treatment is a form of neuromodulation whereby radiofrequency currents are usually delivered in short (20 ms), high-voltage bursts with periods of 480 ms (at 2 Hz but can also be 5 Hz and 50 ms pulses) to allow heat dissipation. This gives it unique features of pain control without the complete tissue destruction and sometimes, painful sequelae of continuous thermal radiofrequency ablation. The mechanism of action is not entirely clear, but may involve temperature-independent effects which modulate neural structures and neural behavior by applying rapidly changing electric field [3]. In contrast to traditional thermal radiofrequency ablation, the temperature around the probe tip is kept around 40 °C during a typical lesioning cycle ranging from 2 to 8 min. According to Sluijter et al., pulsed radiofrequency ablation is advantageous compared to traditional thermal radiofrequency ablation as it tends to be painless, there is lack of actual nerve tissue destruction, and it may be applied to a broad range of neuropathic pain conditions where heat generation is not recommended, such as in a very narrow intervertebral foramen [4].

Chemical Neurolysis

Neurolysis via chemical destruction can also be achieved through the application of alcohol, phenol, or glycerol. Analgesia is obtained by interruption of pain pathways through chemical induced neural destruction. As mentioned previously, it is typically performed only after a trial of diagnostic block has proven successful.

Ethyl Alcohol Neurolysis

Ethyl alcohol is typically available in 1 or 5 ml hypobaric aliquots at high concentrations which must subsequently be diluted. It is often recommended to inject local anesthetic prior to injecting ethyl alcohol as it can cause a burning sensation along the neural distribution when given [5]. Nerve tissue destruction is thought to occur via dehydration, mucoprotein precipitation, and extraction of vital biochemical components including cholesterol, cerebrosides, and phospholipids [6]. The end result is destruction of the myelin sheath and nerve fibers leading ultimately to Wallerian degeneration. An approximate concentration of at least 50% is needed to have satisfactory results. When compared to glycerin and phenol, ethyl alcohol typically requires more volume due to its rapid spread from site of injection. One of the drawbacks is unwanted spread to nearby tissues. Other side effects should be kept in mind such as arterial vasospasm, deafferentation pain, post procedure neuritis, and a temporary rise in blood alcohol concentration. If injected intravascularly, alcohol can cause thrombosis. The analgesic effects occur as early as 12 h after treatment and may last for weeks to months before neural regeneration may take place.

Phenol Neurolysis

The use of phenol was first described by Doppler in Germany in 1925. By 1950, it was established as a commonly used neurolytic agent for relief of chronic pain. Phenol or carbolic acid is a benzene ring with one hydroxyl group substituted for a hydrogen ion [7]. Compared to alcohol, phenol causes similar neural tissue destruction and is hyperbaric when compared to cerebrospinal fluid. It also exhibits a local anesthetic like effects which results in less procedural related pain. As it is not commercially available, phenol is typically custom made by local compounding pharmacies. It is commonly mixed with viscous glycerin which may result in limiting the spread within the injection site. This partially explains the shorter duration and less intense analgesia seen with phenol compared to alcohol. Wide ranges of concentrations used in clinical practice have been described ranging from 2% to 10%. Many practitioners choose the middle of this range (5%) and believe this to be the optimal concentration to cause indiscriminate damage to afferent and efferent nerve fibers [8]. In a review article, Wood (1978), a wide range of neurolysis dose (2–10%) had been studied without definite recommendation on the specific dose to use [7]. Neural destruction is thought to occur from protein coagulation and necrosis associated with axonal degeneration and Wallerian degeneration. If injected intravascularly, one may see convulsions due to an increase in acetylcholine within the central nervous system and cardiovascular collapse. Lower amounts of intravascular uptake can present with local anesthetic toxicity with side effects of tinnitus and flushing [7].

Glycerol

Hakanson accidentally discovered glycerol after it was injected into the trigeminal ganglion for treatment of trigeminal neuralgia [9]. Propane-1,2,3-triol or glycerol is structurally similar to alcohol as both contain an active hydroxyl group. The high viscosity and poor miscibility of glycerol in water offer advantages over ethanol such as diffusing slower than ethanol, allowing for better positional control of spread of the chemical agent. However, compared to phenol and alcohol, glycerol is the weakest of the neurolytic agents. Glycerol is thought to cause myelin disintegration, axonolysis, and Wallerian degeneration when applied to peripheral nerves [10]. Nerve destruction is also through Wallerian degeneration [11].

Cryoneurolysis

Denny-Brown et al. first reported the use of extreme cold to cause peripheral nerve injury and found larger nerves to be more susceptible [12]. Since then, cryoneurolysis has been refined to cause ischemic necrosis to neural tissue through the formation of ice crystals below −20 °C. The quality of lesioning is thought to rely upon the rate of freezing and thawing [13]. Cryoablation is typically accomplished by using a hollow tube containing a smaller inner tube. The smaller inner tube releases pressurized gas (usually argon, nitrogena, or nitrous oxide) which subsequently leads to gas expansion and heat extraction from the probe tip. Surrounding vascular injury and edema results from diapedesis of polymorphonuclear cells through vessel walls and ultimately Wallerian degeneration [14]. Once the formation of ice crystals begins, patients may experience a burning sensation lasting for approximately 30 s. A typical treatment cycle consists of 1–3 min of freezing followed by 30 s of thawing time, performed two or three times in succession on a single target.

High-Intensity Focused Ultrasound (HIFU)

HIFU is a newer ablative technique which utilizes high-intensity ultrasound energy focused upon a specific target area. The resulting heat causes tissue destruction which is proportional to the duration of treatment and rate of temperature increase. A main drawback of HIFU is that cavitation can result. During this process, tiny bubbles can form within the target area and impede ongoing acoustic wave delivery. These bubbles can inadvertently serve as conduits for unintentional thermal energy delivery should they burst. On the other hand, acoustic cavitation may lead to desired effects of neural destruction if tissue is properly targeted. Gulati et al. have been leading ongoing research on this promising treatment modality using swine models [15].

References

1. Cosman ER, Nashold BS, Ovelmann-Levitt J. Theorectical aspects of radiofrequency lesions in the dorsal root entry zone. Neurosurgery. 1984;15:945–50.
2. Cosman E, Cosman B. Methods of making nervous system lesion. In: Wilkens R, Rengachary SS, editors. Neurosurgery. New York: McGraw-Hill; 1984. p. 2490–9.
3. Cosman EJ, Cosman ES. Electric and thermal field effects in tissue around radiofrequency electrodes. Pain Med. 2005;6:405–24.
4. Sluijeter ME, Cosman ER, Rittman WB III, et al. The effects of pulsed radiofrequency firelds applied to the dorsal root ganglion-a preliminary report. Pain Clin. 1998;11:109–17.
5. Raj PP, Patt RB, Neurolysis P. In: Raj PP, editor. Pain medicine: a comprehensive review. St. Louis: Mosby; 1996. p. 288–96.
6. Rumbsy MG, Finean JB. The action of organic solvents on the myelin sheath of peripheral nerve tissue: II. Short-chain aliphatic alcohols. J Neurochem. 1966;13:1509.
7. Wood KM. The use of phenol as a neurolytic agent: a review. Pain. 1978;5:205–29.
8. de Leon-Casasola OA, Ditonto E. Drugs commonly used for nerve blocking: neurolytic agents. In: Raj PP, editor. practical management of pain. 3rd ed. St. Louis: Mosby; 2000. p. 575–8.
9. Håkanson S. Trigeminal neuralgia treated by the injection of glycerol into the trigeminal cistern. Neurosurgery. 1981;9:638–46.
10. Rengachary SS, Watanabe IS, Singer P, et al. Effect of glycerol on peripheral nerve: an experimental study. Neurosurgery. 1983;13:681–8.
11. de Leon-Casasola OA, Ditonto E. Drugs commonly used for nerve blocking: neurolytic agents. In: Raj PP, editor. Practical management of pain. 3rd ed. St. Louis: Mosby; 2000. p. 575–8.
12. Denny-Brown D, Adams RD, Brenner C, et al. The pathology of injury to nerve induced by cold. J Neuropathol Exp Neurol. 1945;4:305–23.
13. Mazur P. Rand RW, editor. Physical and chemical factors underlying cell injury in cryosurgical freezing, Cryosurgery. Springfield: Charles C. Thomas. p. 1968.
14. Meyers RR, Katz J. Neural pathology of neurolytic and semidestructive agents. In: Cousins MJ, Bridenbaugh PO, editors. Neural blockade in clinical anesthesia and management of pain. Lippincott Williams & Wilkens, Philadelphia PA USA. 1988.
15. Gulati A, et al. Novel use of noninvasive high intensity focused ultrasonography for intercostal nerve neurolysis in a swine mondel. Reg Anesth Pain Med. 2014;39:26–30.

Sympathetic Nervous System Blocks for the Treatment of Cancer Pain

17

Nadya M. Dhanani, Wilson A. Almonte, and Mitchell P. Engle

Introduction

The anatomist Galen first described the sympathetic nervous system (SNS) in the second century AD. However, a more complete anatomical description of the iconic paravertebral chains would be delineated by the Oxford scholar Thomas Willis in his remarkable book *De Cerebri Anatome* (1664 AD). Experimentally, the French scientist Francois Pourfour du Petit (1664–1741 AD) is credited with transecting the superior cervical chain in a dog which resulted in what would later be known as Horner's triad [1]. This experiment appears to be the first purposeful SNS block that would be easily understood by the modern physician. In 1948, Dargent published the first major case series assessing the role of the SNS in cancer pain by evaluating percutaneous cocaine sympathetic blocks and surgical sympathectomies [2].

The autonomic nervous system is comprised of the sympathetic nervous system, parasympathetic nervous system, and enteric nervous system. Anatomically, the SNS is composed of both pre- and postganglionic neurons. The soma of preganglionic sympathetic neurons is located in the intermediolateral column of the spinal cord from T1 to L2. These neurons then leave the spinal canal as myelinated neurons on the ventral nerve root and travel to the thoracic paravertebral ganglia. These are paired ganglia on the anterolateral surface of the vertebrae. Embryologically, paired ganglia are formed for every vertebral level, but during development sequential ganglia can fuse, particularly in the cervical region. Preganglionic neurons can synapse at the same paravertebral ganglion level that they enter, or they can ascend or descend before synapsing. Postganglionic neurons with their soma in the paravertebral ganglia then track toward their target organs (Fig. 17.1). Alternatively, some presynaptic neurons pass through the paravertebral ganglia forming splanchnic nerves. These nerves synapse in prevertebral ganglia which unlike the paravertebral ganglion are not paired. Postganglionic neurons with their soma in the prevertebral ganglia then track toward their target organs (Fig. 17.1).

Thoracic, abdominal, and pelvic sympathetic nerves are generally paired with visceral afferent nerves which both track along visceral vascular supplies. The visceral afferent nerves, like somatic afferent nerves, have their soma in the dorsal root ganglia (DRG) with synaptic connections in lamina I, II outer, V, and X of the spinal cord dorsal horn. In addition, synaptic connections are also made in the intermediolateral column and on ventral motor neurons for coordination of complex visceral reflexes. Ascending spinal pathways for this lamina are principally contained in the anterolateral pathways and in the dorsal columns [3].

The role of the sympathetic nervous system in pain has a relatively recent history. Several conditions, most notably being complex regional pain syndrome, can have strong sympathetic components in the initiation and maintenance of the pain. The diagnosis of sympathetically mediated pain is generally made by associating pain with other signs of sympathetic dysregulation such as vasomotor changes, edema, tremor, and trophic changes of the affected body region [4, 5].

It is likely that several mechanisms underlie the development and maintenance of sympathetically mediated pain. Following nerve injury, nociceptors in the periphery become sensitized to direct norepinephrine application or sympathetic stimulation [6] providing a peripheral mechanism for efferent-afferent coupling. Peripheral nerve injury also triggers sympathetic efferents to sprout into the DRG and form

N. M. Dhanani
Memorial Hermann Hospital/Mischer Neuroscience Institute, Department of Pain Management/Neurosurgery, Houston, TX, USA
e-mail: Nadya.m.dhanani@uth.tmc.edu

W. A. Almonte
Victoria Pain and Rehabilitation Center, Victoria, TX, USA

M. P. Engle (✉)
Institute of Precision Pain Medicine, Corpus Christi, TX, USA
e-mail: mpengle@mdanderson.org

A. Gulati et al. (eds.), *Essentials of Interventional Cancer Pain Management*, https://doi.org/10.1007/978-3-319-99684-4_17

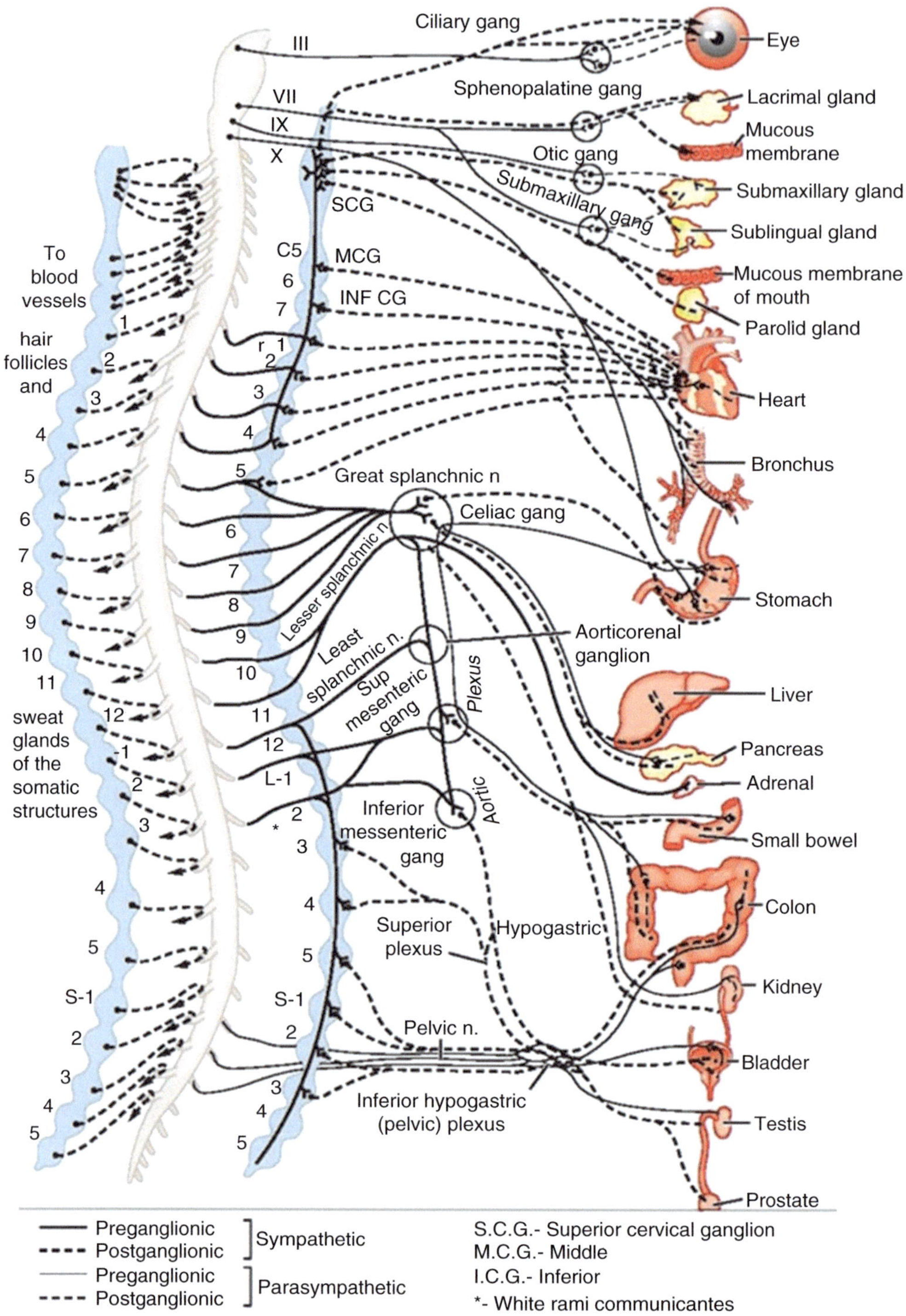

Fig. 17.1 Schematic of the peripheral sympathetic nervous system. Sympathetic fibers exit the spinal cord from T1 to L2 and enter the paravertebral chain (blue column to the right of the spinal cord). These fibers can either synapse at the same level or ascend along the paravertebral chain before synapsing at a higher level. Alternatively, some fibers pass through the paravertebral ganglia and form the splanchnic nerves before synapsing in the prevertebral ganglia. Target organs of post-sympathetic efferents are indicated on the right side of the figure. (Adapted from Griffin et al. [75] with permission from Wolters Kluwer)

"baskets" around large diameter afferent neuron providing a DRG mechanism for efferent-afferent coupling [7]. Finally, much work has also occurred in recent years regarding the role of nerve growth factor (NGF) in animal models of cancer pain. These studies have shown that NGF released by inflammatory cells near an osseous tumor can sensitize primary afferent neurons and lead to sprouting and neuroma formation of both sensory afferent and sympathetic efferent fibers [8] providing a neuroanatomical underpinning for how the sympathetic nervous system may be involved in osseous cancer pain.

The SNS can be blocked at the level of the ganglia or anywhere along a sympathetic pathway. This chapter will concentrate on the seven major sympathetic blocks commonly performed in clinical practice for the treatment of cancer pain.

Sphenopalatine Ganglion Block

Anatomy

The sphenopalatine ganglion (SPG) also known as the pterygopalatine ganglion is the most cephalad sympathetic pathway for which diagnostic and therapeutic blocks are commonly performed. The ganglion is also the largest group of neurons outside the cranial cavity. It is primarily a parasympathetic ganglion that also contains sensory and sympathetic fibers. The postganglionic sympathetic fibers that course through the sphenopalatine ganglion originate in the superior cervical ganglia. These nerves initially travel through the carotid artery plexus and then through the deep petrosal and vidian nerves before reaching the sphenopalatine ganglion in the pterygopalatine fossa. These postganglionic fibers provide sympathetic innervation to the lacrimal glands as well as nasal and palatine mucosa. Importantly, sensory afferent fibers from the maxillary nerve also pass through the sphenopalatine ganglia [9, 10].

Indications

The primary indications for the sphenopalatine block are sphenopalatine neuralgia, trigeminal neuralgia, headache (migraine and cluster), and atypical facial pain. In addition, publications have documented the effect of the block for cancer pain involving the tongue and floor of the mouth [9–11].

Evidence

The evidence for the effectiveness of the sphenopalatine ganglion block is derived from multiple case series that mainly emphasized headache, sphenopalatine neuralgia, and atypical facial pain. For example, Sanders and colleagues studied 56 patients with episodic and 10 patients with chronic cluster headaches. They all underwent radiofrequency ablation of the sphenopalatine ganglion, and 60% of the episodic and 30% of the chronic patients had total pain relief at a mean follow-up of 29 months [12]. Additionally, Narouze and colleagues performed infrazygomatic SPG radiofrequency ablation (RFA) on 15 people with chronic cluster headache and showed a significant reduction in mean attack intensity and frequency [13]. Puig and colleagues performed repeated chemical neurolysis of the SPG on eight patients with sphenopalatine neuralgia. The patients reported on average 90% pain relief with an average duration of pain relief of 9.5 months [14]. Finally, a study by Bayer and colleagues followed 30 patients with chronic face and head pain. The patients were evaluated 4–52 months after radiofrequency ablation of the SPG, resulting in 21% of patients reporting complete pain relief and 65% reporting mild to moderate relief [15].

The evidence for the SPG block in the treatment of cancer pain is specifically limited to a few small case series. Prasanna and colleagues reported ten patients with cancer of the tongue or floor of the mouth that reported significant pain relief with repeated transnasal SPG blocks [16]. In addition, another case report documented excellent pain relief in a patient with buccal mucosa cancer with significant extension into the maxilla and mandible following both diagnostic and neurolytic transnasal SPG blocks [17].

Intranasal Technique

The patient is placed supine on the procedure table. Long cotton tip applicators are then soaked in local anesthetic (commonly 4% viscous lidocaine). These applicators are then inserted through the nares and are slowly advanced to the back of the nasal pharynx. A second applicator is then advanced through the same nare, and the tip is seated immediately superior and lateral to the first applicator. These applicators are left in place for 30–60 min. The sphenopalatine ganglion is near the lateral nasal mucosa and can be blocked by diffusion of the local anesthetic through the mucosa. If additional local anesthetic is necessary, newly soaked applicators can replace the initial applicators, or local anesthetic can be trickled down the shafts of the initial applicators [9–11].

Infrazygomatic Fluoroscopic Technique

This technique can be used for diagnostic blockade and should be employed prior to SPG neurolysis. One should consider obtaining intravenous access since the patient may require sedation for successful completion of this procedure. The patient is placed supine with the head slightly turned away from the physician. Then, lateral fluoroscopic guidance is used to align the ipsilateral and contralateral mandibles. The pterygopalatine fossa is a vase-shaped structure that can be visualized under the ipsilateral zygomatic arch and posterior to the maxillary sinus. Cephalad tilt of the C-arm frequently helps visualization. Next, anesthetize the skin and subcutaneous tissues over the fossa but anterior to the mandibular rami using a 25-gauge 1.5-inch needle. Then, insert a 22-gauge 3.5-inch spinal needle under the zygoma and in the coronoid notch, and advance toward the middle of the pterygopalatine fossa. This will likely be in a medial, cephalad, and slightly posterior trajectory. Alternate between anteroposterior and lateral views as the spinal needle is advanced toward the middle turbinate on AP view. Note that the sinus bones are exceptionally thin and easily penetrated by a needle. A reasonable argument can be made for use of blunt needles for this reason. The final position is determined in the AP view with the needle tip adjacent to the nasal mucosa. After negative aspiration, inject 0.5 ml of contrast solution to verify appropriate needle position in the fossa and to ensure that there is no vascular or intranasal spread of contrast. Then, 2 ml of 0.25% bupivacaine should be injected into the fossa. The needle can then be removed [9, 10, 18] (Fig. 17.2).

Neurolysis of the ganglia can be performed following a positive diagnostic block using either radiofrequency ablation or chemical neurolysis. For radiofrequency ablation, a 10-cm needle with a 5-mm active tip is inserted using the infrazygomatic approach as previously described. Use sensory stimulation at 50–100 Hz and 0.1–1 V to elicit paresthesia at the root of the nose. If paresthesia is felt in the upper teeth, the needle needs to be redirected inferior and medial [9]. Following appropriate needle position confirmation, inject 1–2 ml of local anesthetic. Radiofrequency ablation can be performed at 80 °C for 90 s. Alternatively, pulsed radiofrequency modulation can be performed at 42 °C for 120 s. When considering chemical neurolysis, it is critically important to inject contrast to evaluate for vascular uptake and to identify the extent of neurolytic solution spread [9–11].

Side Effects and Complications

The sphenopalatine block and neurolysis is a relatively advanced procedure that should only be performed by physicians well trained in the technical aspects of the block and potential complications. Blocking the ganglion will commonly result in ipsilateral tearing due to unopposed parasympathetic activity. Infection is possible if sterile technique is compromised or if the nasal mucosa is breeched by penetrating the lateral aspect of the nasal wall. Bleeding and hematoma are certainly considerations given the maxillary artery and vascular plexus is near the ganglion. Dysesthesia of the palate, maxilla, and oropharynx has been reported following radiofrequency ablation. Damage to the globe is possible if the needle is advanced through the inferior orbital fissure. Finally, a bradycardic reflex can occur during RFA that occasionally requires pharmacologic therapy during the procedure [9, 10, 18].

Stellate Ganglion Block

Anatomy

The stellate ganglion is commonly formed by the fusion of the inferior cervical and first thoracic sympathetic ganglia. The structure is anatomically located anterior to the neck of the first rib and C7 transverse process. The sympathetic chain proceeding through this critical structure supplies the

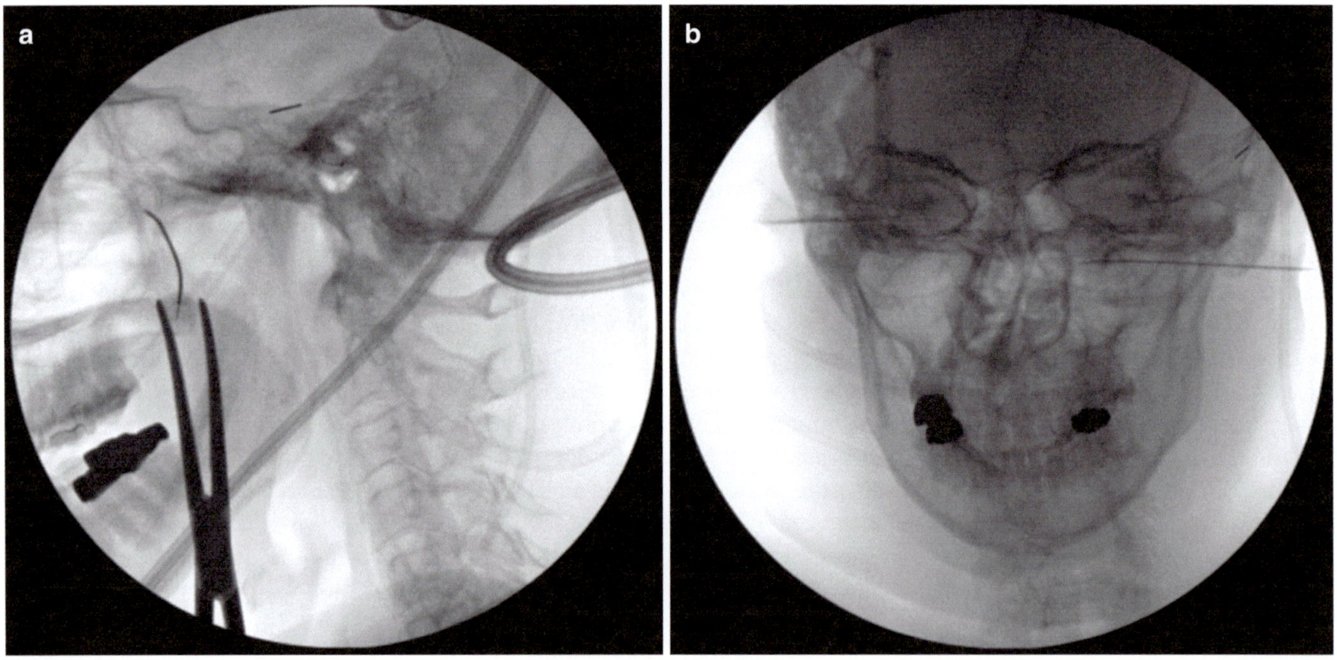

Fig. 17.2 Infrazygomatic sphenopalatine block. (a) Lateral view demonstrating the needle tip in the sphenopalatine foramen which is shaped like a vase. (b) AP view demonstrating the needle tip is immediately lateral to the lateral wall of the maxillary sinus

sympathetic innervation to the ipsilateral head, neck, and upper extremity. The stellate ganglion block is frequently performed at the C6 vertebral level, although some practitioners perform it at C7 or T1 levels. The C6 location is rostral to the actual ganglion but helps avoid inadvertent contact with both the apex of the lung and unprotected portion of the vertebral artery as it travels through the transverse foramen of the cervical vertebrae. At the level of C6, the cervical sympathetic chain is posterior to the carotid artery and jugular vein, anterior to the C6 transverse process and longus colli muscle, lateral to the thyroid and esophagus, and medial to the anterior scalene muscle and vertebral artery.

Indications

The three most commonly recognized indications for the stellate ganglion block (SGB) are vascular insufficiency, hyperhidrosis, and sympathetically mediated pain (SMP) syndromes affecting the face or upper extremity. As mentioned previously, SGB can be used to diagnose and treat a variety of sympathetically mediated pain disorders affecting the head, neck, or upper extremity. These include CRPS and herpetic neuralgia. In terms of cancer-related pain, SGB may be effective for regional pain associated with a solid tumor, upper extremity pain due to superior sulcus lung tumors, postmastectomy pain syndrome, brachial plexopathy, and postradiation neuritis. The SGB has also been described for treating post-traumatic stress disorder in addition to hot flashes and nighttime awakenings frequently present in breast cancer survivors.

Evidence

Studies investigating the efficacy of the SGB have predominantly focused on patients with CRPS and acute herpetic neuralgia. When used to treat CRPS, SGB is thought to be more effective when performed closer to onset of symptoms [19, 20]. In 2013, Kastler and colleagues reported on a series of patients with type I CRPS that underwent CT-guided radiofrequency neurolysis or block. Patients who underwent neurolysis were more likely to have greater than 50% pain relief at 2 years than patients who underwent block alone (68% versus 21%) [21]. A cadaver study examining the ideal volume compared 5, 10, and 20 ml injections and found the most favorable spread with 5 ml [22]. Although not performed at our center, chemical neurolysis of the stellate ganglion has also been described in the literature. Arter and colleagues reported no serious complications in a series of over 150 SGB with 3% phenol [23].

Several studies have evaluated the effectiveness of the SGB on trigeminal and cervical acute herpetic neuralgia [24]. In 2012, Makharita and colleagues reported a randomized, placebo-controlled study investigating the effect of early stellate ganglion blockade for facial pain from acute herpes zoster on the subsequent development of postherpetic neuralgia. They concluded that early SGB performed within 2 weeks of rash onset can rapidly relieve acute pain from herpes zoster with a possible reduction in the incidence of postherpetic neuralgia [25].

The SGB has been utilized for the treatment of several cancer-associated pain syndromes. In 2002, Noguchi and colleagues reported that SGB relieved trigeminal neuralgia caused by a cerebellopontine angle tumor [26]. Lipov and colleagues reported a prospective pilot study of 13 breast cancer survivors who underwent SGB for the treatment of hot flashes and night awakenings. They found that one or two SGB very effectively reduced the incidence of hot flashes and night awakenings for up to a year. Interestingly, the authors noted the projection of stellate ganglion efferents to the hypothalamus, a critical center in thermoregulation [27, 28].

In 2004, an oblique fluoroscopic technique was published by Abdi and colleagues [29]. Subsequently, a prospective study compared the classical anterior and oblique block techniques in 50 patients with postmastectomy pain syndrome. They found that both block procedures decreased pain scores, daily morphine consumption, areas of allodynia, and patient satisfaction for up to 3 months after the last block. However, the authors reported higher incidence of side effects with the classic anterior approach than with the oblique approach [30].

Anterior Paratracheal Fluoroscopic Technique

Always obtain verified intravenous access prior to performing this procedure due to risks of hemodynamic and neurological complications. Heart rate, blood pressure, and pulse oximetry monitors should be applied. The patient is positioned supine on the fluoroscopic table with the neck slightly extended and the head slightly turned away from the physician. Use PA fluoroscopic imaging to identify the uncinate process of the C6 vertebral body. Slight caudal tilt may enhance visualization. Anesthetize skin over the uncinate process using a 25-gauge 1.5-inch needle. Next, laterally retract the ipsilateral carotid artery to prevent inadvertent vascular puncture. A 25-gauge spinal needle is then inserted through the skin and advanced toward the C6 transverse process immediately inferior to the uncinate process. This process should be performed while maintaining lateral retraction on the carotid artery, and needle advancement should be performed using coaxial technique. After the needle contacts the C6 transverse process, the needle should be withdrawn several millimeters to prevent injection into the longus colli muscle. Following negative aspiration, 1–2 ml of contrast should be injected under live fluoroscopic imaging to demonstrate the lack intravascular injection and to ensure appropriate spread of contrast along the muscle. Next, slowly inject 0.5 ml of 0.25% bupivacaine and wait at least 1 min to ensure lack of vascular injection. Then slowly inject an additional 4.5 ml of 0.25% bupivacaine. The needle is removed. In our practice, we commonly add 25 mcg of clonidine to the injection mixture.

Neurolysis of the stellate ganglion has been reported following positive diagnostic blockade using both radiofrequency ablation and chemical neurolysis. In our clinical practice, we do not perform neurolysis of this ganglion due to the proximity to critical vascular and neurological structures. Several reports have documented stellate ganglion radiofrequency ablation using the technique previously described. Sensory stimulation for paresthesias should be undertaken at 50–100 Hz and 0.1–1.5 V. Motor testing to identify the phrenic nerve and recurrent laryngeal nerve should be carried out at 2 Hz and 0.1–1.5 V. A small volume of local anesthetic and particulate (or non-particulate depending on a practitioner's concern of vascular uptake in the cervical region) steroid is injected after negative aspiration. Radiofrequency ablation is then typically performed at 60 °C for 60 s.

Oblique Fluoroscopic Technique

An alternative technique uses an oblique approach to avoid the major vascular structures of the neck. Again, IV access and cardiorespiratory monitors should be used while performing the block. With the patient in the supine position, the C6 vertebrae are visualized using PA fluoroscopy. The fluoroscope is then tilted obliquely until the neuroforamen are visualized. The skin overlying the junction of the C6 uncinate and transverse process is anesthetized with local anesthetic using a 25-gauge 1.5-inch needle. A 25-gauge spinal needle is then inserted through the skin and advanced toward the junction between the C6 uncinate and transverse processes. After appropriate needle placement, the procedure is like the standard PA procedure (Fig. 17.3).

Ultrasound-Guided Technique

Ultrasound has gained considerable standing in the past decade for the performance of blocks. Ultrasound-guided SGB has the unique advantage of allowing the physician to directly visualize and avoid critical vascular and neural structures in the neck. Prior to beginning the block, intravenous access and cardiorespiratory monitors are applied, and the patient is placed supine on the procedure table with the neck slightly extended and head turned away from the physician. The cricoid cartilage is then palpated to identify the C6 vertebral level. Using sterile technique, a high-frequency linear ultrasound probe is placed in the transverse position at the level of the cricoid cartilage. The neck is then scanned medial to lateral to identify the trachea, esophagus, thyroid, carotid artery, jugular vein, C6 transverse process, longus colli muscle, anterior scalene, brachial plexus, and middle scalene muscles. The sympathetic chain usually lies posterior (deep) to the carotid artery and anterior to the longus colli muscle. The block is performed using an in-plane needle placement technique from either the medial or lateral aspect of the probe. The lateral approach is preferred at our institution. For this technique, the skin lateral to the probe is anesthetized with local anesthetic using a 25-gauge 1.5-inch needle. Using an in-plane technique, an echogenic needle is inserted through the skin immediately superior to the brachial plexus. The needle is then advanced toward the sympathetic chain being careful not to contact the brachial plexus, jugular vein, or carotid artery. The final needle position should be posterior to the carotid artery and superior to the longus colli muscle. Following negative aspiration, 0.5 ml of 0.25% bupivacaine is injected. After 1 min with no neurological symptoms, the remaining 4.5 ml of 0.25% bupivacaine can be injected. The needle can then be removed. Unlike the fluoroscopic technique, no contrast is utilized during the ultrasound procedure because the vascular structures can be directly visualized and avoided (Fig. 17.4).

Side Effects and Complications

The stellate ganglion block is an advanced procedure regardless of technique utilized and should only be performed by physicians appropriately trained in the technique and potential complications. Following the block, ipsilateral Horner's syndrome with ptosis, miosis, and occasionally enophthalmos and conjunctival injection is expected and indicative of a successful block. This block should be avoided in patients with significant pulmonary disease, since phrenic nerve block is a frequent side effect. In addition, patients should be instructed not to eat or drink anything for several hours after the block since recurrent laryngeal nerve block is also a common side effect. Rarely, branches of the brachial plexus will inadvertently be blocked due to proximity of the plexus. This block is also associated with several significant complications such as pneumothorax, vascular injury, epidural or intrathecal injections, cardiovascular collapse due to sudden loss of sympathetic tone, seizure related to arterial injection of local anesthetic, and disruption of the vertebral artery causing thrombus, dissection, or infarction. Inadvertent puncture of the cervical esophagus is possible when performing the procedure, particularly on the left side. A rare delayed complication is retropharyngeal hematoma which can cause complete airway obstruction [31]. These complications highlight the necessity of appropriate intravenous access, cardiopulmonary monitoring, and rapidly available ACLS support.

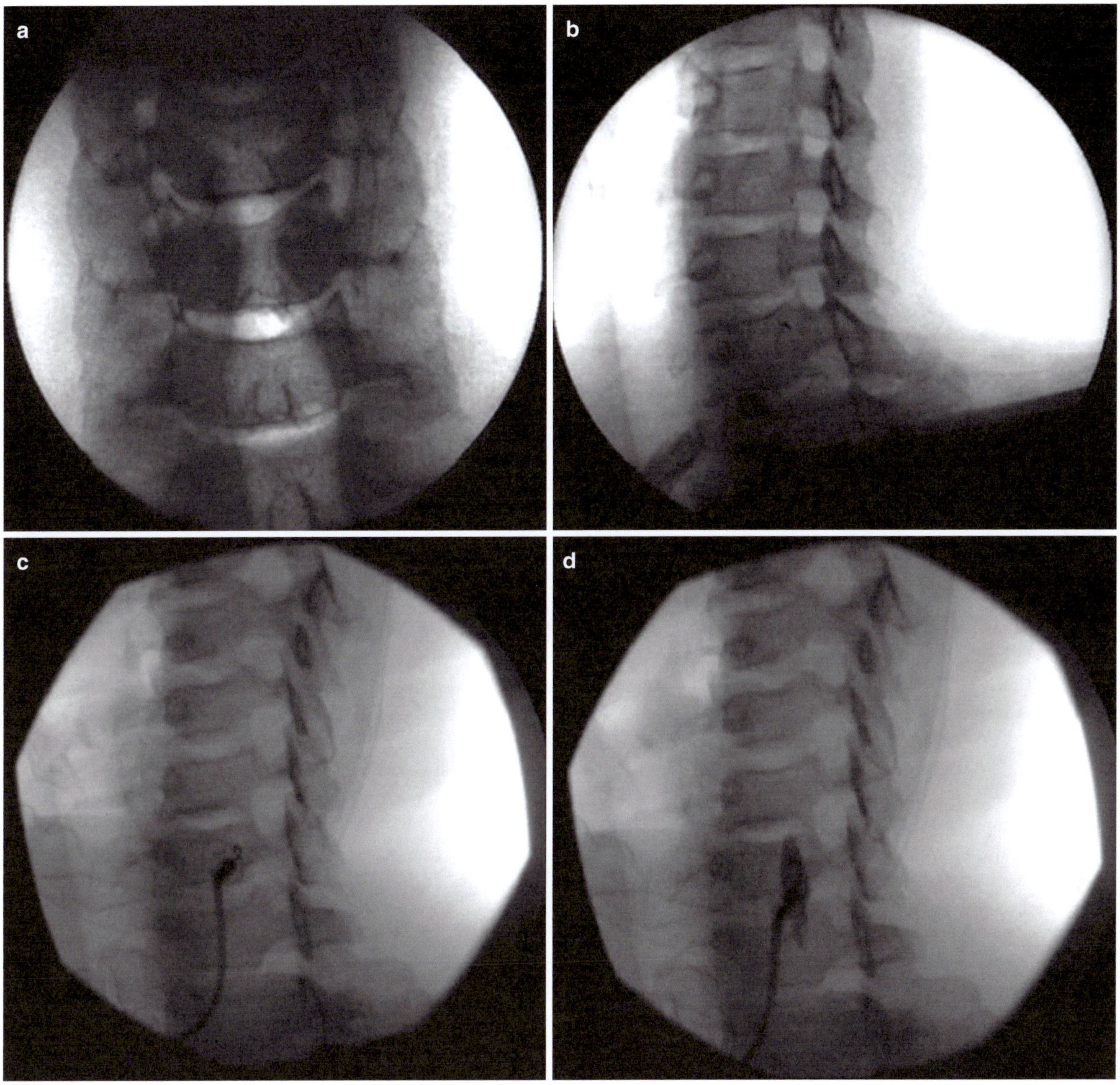

Fig. 17.3 Oblique stellate ganglion block. (**a**) AP fluoroscopic view with caudal tilt to square the end plates. (**b**) Oblique view demonstrating a clear view of the neuroforamen. (**c**) The needle is placed at the base of the uncinate process. (**d**) Appropriate contrast spread. (Adapted from Abdi et al. [29] with permission from the American Society of International Pain Physicians)

Thoracic Sympathetic Ganglion Blocks

Anatomy

The thoracic sympathetic ganglia provide sympathetic innervation to the upper extremities, chest wall, and upper abdominal wall. The superior thoracic sympathetic ganglia often fuse with the inferior cervical ganglia to form the stellate ganglia. Although these ganglia do provide passage for the majority of the upper extremity sympathetic fibers, at least 20% of people have significant contributions from the T2 and T3 thoracic sympathetic ganglia. The fibers from these ganglia are commonly referred to as Kuntz nerves. Failure to block these fibers may lead to lack of success with the SGB when targeting sympathetic fibers to the upper extremity. Since preganglionic neurons of the upper extremity typically

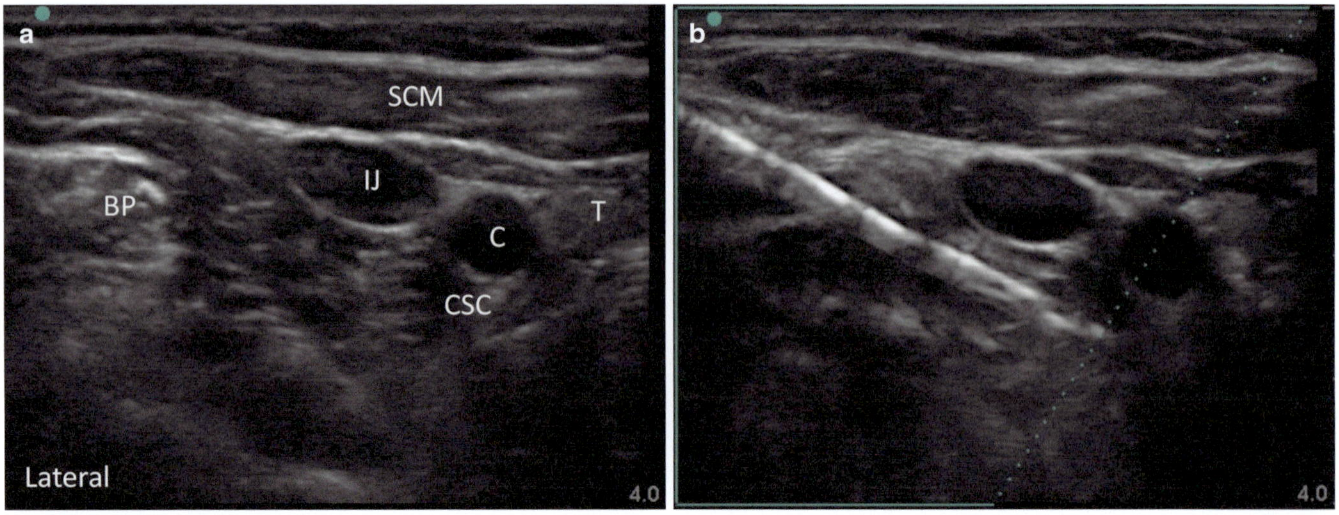

Fig. 17.4 Ultrasound-guided stellate ganglion block (lateral approach). (**a**) Transverse ultrasound view at the level of the cricoid cartilage demonstrating the brachial plexus (BP), sternocleidomastoid (SCM), thyroid (T), internal jugular (IJ) vein, carotid artery (C), and cervical sympathetic chain (CSC). (**b**) Similar image after lateral in-plane needle placement above the brachial plexus with the final needle tip position at cervical sympathetic chain deep to the carotid artery

originate from T2 to T8 and ascend to the T3, T2, stellate, and middle cervical ganglia, blockade of the upper thoracic ganglia should ensure complete blockade of the sympathetic innervation to the upper extremity [32].

The T2 and T3 sympathetic ganglia lie on the lateral aspect of their respective vertebral bodies approximately halfway between the anterior and posterior longitudinal lines. The ganglia are several millimeters superior to the cranio-caudal midpoint of the vertebrae as well. Of note, the ganglia are in relatively close approximation to the parietal pleura and intercostal nerves [33].

Indications

The indications for the upper thoracic sympathetic ganglia block are similar to those for the stellate ganglion block. These indications are vascular insufficiency, hyperhidrosis, and SMP syndromes. The most common of the sympathetically mediated pain syndromes is complex regional pain syndrome of the upper extremity. This technique has also been reported for the diagnosis and treatment of phantom breast pain, acute herpes zoster, angina pectoris, and refractory polymorphic tachycardia [34].

Evidence

Few studies have investigated the effectiveness of thoracic sympathetic ganglion blockade or ablation. A retrospective analysis of CT-guided interventions in 293 patients with intractable neuropathic pain reported that continuous infusion of ropivacaine or chemical neurolysis produced significant reductions in patient reported pain [35]. Another study reported sustained relief of sympathetically mediated pain for greater than 1 year following thoracic sympathetic ganglia thermal radiofrequency ablation [36]. In general, it has been reported that thoracic sympathetic blocks are more likely to be effective if performed within 1 year of pain onset [34].

Fluoroscopic T2–T3 Technique

Always obtain verified intravenous access prior to performing this procedure due to risks of hemodynamic and neurological complications. Cardiopulmonary monitors should be applied. The patient is positioned prone on a fluoroscopic table. AP fluoroscopy is used to identify the T2 vertebral body, and the end plates are squared. Oblique the C-arm approximately 20° to the ipsilateral side. Anesthetize the skin immediately lateral to the T2 vertebral body just caudal to the second rib. Using coaxial technique, a 22-gauge spinal needle is then inserted through the skin immediately lateral to the T2 vertebral body. The needle is advanced using frequent oblique and lateral imaging. The needle should closely approximate the T2 vertebral body during the entire procedure. The final needle position is halfway between the anterior and posterior longitudinal lines for the vertebrae and slightly superior to the cranial caudal axis of the vertebrae. Inject 2 ml of contrast solution to verify appropriate ventral spread along the sympathetic chain. If the contrast follows the dome of the lung, this indicates that the parietal pleura has been breached and the needle should be redirected medially. For a diagnostic block, 6–8 ml of 0.25% bupivacaine is injected. The needle is then withdrawn, and the patient is taken to the recovery room where a chest X-ray is obtained to evaluate for pneumothorax [32].

Chemical neurolysis is not commonly performed by many physicians due to the proximity of the thoracic nerve roots. Instead, radiofrequency ablation is more commonly used. The neuroablation procedure is usually technically similar to diagnostic blockade except that an additional needle is placed at the T3 vertebral level to completely capture sympathetic fibers from T2 and T3. Applying thermal energy also requires the use of specialized curved thermal RF cannulas (usually with 10 mm active lesioning tips). It is important to perform both sensory (50 Hz up to 1 V) and motor testing (2 Hz up to 2 V) to ensure that the lesion area will not encompass the thoracic nerve root. Prior to lesioning, a small volume of local anesthetic is injected. The lesion is typically performed at 80 °C for 90 s (Fig. 17.5) [32].

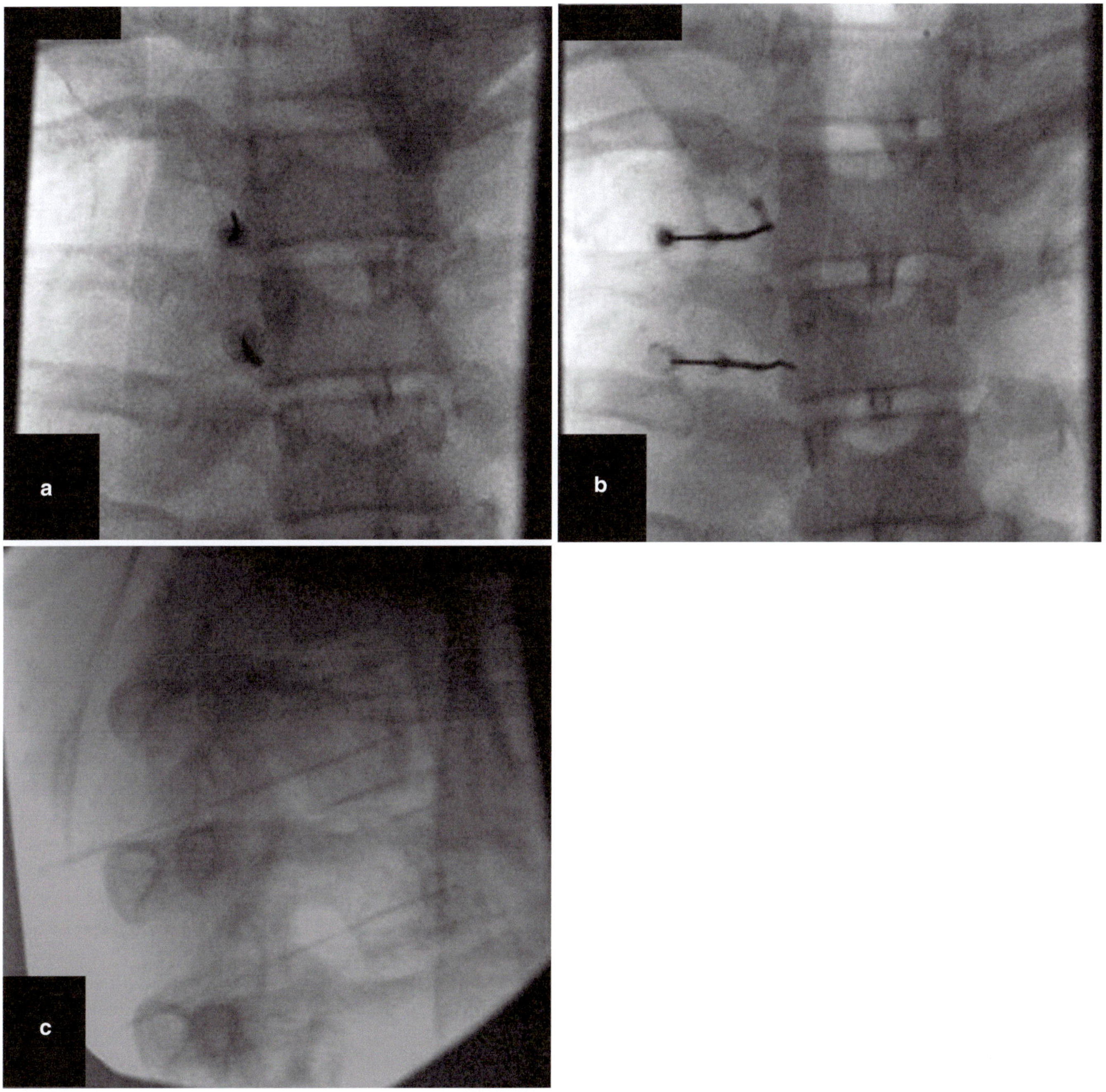

Fig. 17.5 Thoracic sympathetic ganglion block. (**a**) Using a 20° ipsilateral oblique view, the needles are placed and advanced immediately inferior to the transverse process along the vertebral body. Final needle placement in the AP (**b**) and lateral (**c**) views. (Images courtesy of Miles Day, M.D., Department of Anesthesiology and Pain Management, Texas Tech University Health Sciences Center, Lubbock, Texas)

Side Effects and Complications

The thoracic sympathetic block is an advanced procedure and should only be performed by physicians appropriately trained in the technique and potential complications. Similar to the stellate ganglion block, ipsilateral Horner's syndrome is an expected side effect. Rarely, branches of the brachial plexus will inadvertently be blocked due to variable contribution of the intercostal nerves to the brachial plexus. The most common complication is pneumothorax which is documented to occur in 1.8–2.4% of cases performed by experienced practitioners [32, 36]. This complication highlights the importance of the post-procedural chest X-ray to evaluate for pneumothorax and the need to inform patients of the possible delayed development of a pneumothorax. Less common complications include sudden cardiovascular collapse due to blockade of cardiac sympathetic fibers, epidural or intrathecal injection, intercostal nerve injury, and local anesthetic toxicity. These complications again highlight the necessity of appropriate intravenous access, cardiopulmonary monitoring, and rapidly available ACLS support.

Celiac Plexus and Splanchnic Nerve Block

Anatomy

Although many presynaptic sympathetic neurons synapse in the paravertebral ganglia, a portion of them bypass the ganglia as splanchnic nerves. Instead, these presynaptic sympathetic fibers synapse at unique prevertebral ganglia that typically lie anterior to the aorta. The greater splanchnic nerve is derived from the medial branches of the fifth through ninth thoracic sympathetic ganglia. These nerves descend obliquely, perforating the diaphragm before terminating in the celiac ganglion [37]. The lesser splanchnic nerves are formed from the ninth and tenth thoracic ganglia and terminate in the aorticorenal ganglion. The least splanchnic nerve is highly variable and generally originates from the 11th and 12th thoracic ganglia and synapses in the renal plexus [37].

The celiac plexus is the best known of the prevertebral ganglia, and it surrounds the celiac artery which is usually located at the L1 vertebral level. The plexus is an important pathway for sympathetic efferent and visceral afferent nerves innervating the pancreas, liver, gallbladder, spleen, distal esophagus, stomach, adrenals, kidneys, small intestine, and large intestine to the splenic flexure.

Indications

The celiac plexus block is one of the oldest sympathetic blocks having been first described in 1914 by Max Kappis for the management of abdominal pain [38]. Today the block is used most commonly for the treatment of intra-abdominal cancer pain, most commonly pain associated with pancreatic cancer. The technique is commonly carried out using a neurolytic technique with alcohol or phenol solutions. The procedure has been described using many different techniques including anatomical landmark, fluoroscopy, CT guidance (posterior or anterior), abdominal ultrasound, and endoscopic ultrasound-guided approaches. The selection of technique frequently depends on locally available technology and physician expertise.

The terms neurolytic celiac plexus block (NCPB) and neurolytic splanchnic nerve block are commonly and inappropriately used as synonyms. The NCPB is a transcrural technique that targets the prevertebral synaptic ganglion. Conversely, the neurolytic splanchnic nerve block is a retrocrural technique that specifically targets the splanchnic nerves before they pierce the diaphragm and synapse in the celiac ganglion. Some practitioners choose the splanchnic nerve neurolysis over a true celiac plexus neurolysis because it avoids penetration of the diaphragm and its clinical success is less likely to be influenced by intra-abdominal tumor burden around the prevertebral celiac plexus.

Evidence

The first high-quality double-blind randomized controlled trial was performed by Lillemoe and colleagues in 1993. This study evaluated intraoperative chemical splanchnicectomy with 50% alcohol ($N = 65$) versus a placebo injection of saline ($N = 72$) in patients with histologically proven unresectable pancreatic cancer. The chemical splanchnicectomy group reported decreased pain scores for up to 6 months. Interestingly, the chemical splanchnicectomy group had improved survival compared to the saline group [39].

Mercadante performed a prospective randomized controlled trial on 20 patients with pancreatic cancer comparing the effectiveness of neurolytic celiac plexus block (NCPB) versus oral analgesics. Though the study did not find statistically significant differences in pain scores between the two groups, the NCPB group consumed significantly less opioids [40]. In addition, Kawamata and colleagues conducted a randomized prospective study to evaluate the effectiveness of NCPB versus NSAID and morphine treatment in 21 pancreatic cancer patients. They reported lower pain scores for the first 4 weeks in the NCPB group with reduced morphine consumption to 7 weeks [41].

Polati and colleagues conducted a double-blind randomized controlled trialed comparing neurolytic celiac plexus blocks ($N = 12$) with pharmacologic therapy ($N = 12$). Short-term pain relief was superior in the neurolytic celiac plexus block group, although long-term relief was not different between the groups. Opioid consumption was also noted to be lower in the neurolytic celiac plexus block group [42]. Similarly, Zhang and colleagues in an unblinded randomized controlled study investigated the efficacy of CT-guided NCPB compared with pharmacological therapy in 56 patients. The authors demonstrated a significant decrease in pain score for 2 weeks and a decreased in opioid consumption for 90 days in the NCPB group [43].

In 2004, Wong and colleagues performed a prospective double-blind randomized controlled trial that examined the effect of NCPB versus a sham injection on pain relief, quality of life, and survival in 100 patients with unresectable pancreatic cancer. The patients were followed weekly for at least 1 year or until death. Neurolytic celiac plexus block produced superior analgesia to the sham procedure, although both groups reported significant pain reduction out to 24 weeks. Despite changes in pain, the NCPB showed no effect on opioid consumption, quality of life, or survival [44].

Wyse and colleagues in a prospective double-blind randomized controlled trial studied the effect of endoscopic ultrasound-guided celiac plexus neurolysis for newly diagnosed inoperable pancreatic cancer. This study determined that the endoscopic technique also resulted in decreased pain burden and possibly decreased morphine consumption over 3 months [45].

In 2011, Arcidiacono and colleagues published a meta-analysis at the Cochrane Collaboration evaluating the effectiveness of NCPB on pain reduction and opioid utilization. The analysis used many of the studies already described in this section and reported a significant and highly homogenous reduction in pain at 4 weeks. This effect was not maintained at 8 weeks with a significant increase in heterogeneity. Opioid utilization was significantly decreased at both 4 and 8 weeks [46].

Since the clinical effectiveness of NCPB tends to wane with time, repeat NCPB are occasionally performed. McGreevy and colleagues reported that repeat NCPB have a lower chance of achieving 50% pain relief than the initial block (67% vs. 29%) and that the mean duration of pain relief is decreased for the second block (3.4 months vs. 1.6 months) [47]. In addition, anatomical distortions caused by adenopathy or tumor around the frontal plane quadrants of the celiac axis can have significant impact on the effectiveness of the NCPB. De Cicco and colleagues published two reports evaluating the effect of anatomic distortions on contrast spread and pain relief. When contrast spreads to all four quadrants around the celiac axis, the chance of prolonged pain relief is quite high. However, when two or fewer quadrants demonstrate contrast spread, the chance of prolonged pain relief is very low [48, 49].

Fluoroscopic Celiac Plexus or Splanchnic Nerve Block

Always obtain verified intravenous access prior to performing this procedure due to high likelihood of significant hemodynamic changes. If appropriate, infuse 500–1000 ml of crystalloid prior to the procedure to increase cardiac preload. Cardiopulmonary monitors should be applied. The patient is positioned prone on a fluoroscopic table. The patient may require sedation to lie on their abdomen for an extended period. Visualize the T12 and L1 vertebral body in an AP fluoroscopic view and square the end plates. Next, oblique the C-arm approximately 20–30° ipsilateral until the T12 transverse process is encompassed within the lateral border of the vertebral body. Anesthetize the skin and subcutaneous tissues immediately lateral to the vertebral body and inferior to the rib head in this view with 1% lidocaine using a 25-gauge 1.5-inch needle. For the splanchnic nerve block, the needle insertion site is immediately superior to the 12th rib and just lateral to the vertebral body. For the celiac plexus block, the needle insertion site is at the superolateral border of the L1 vertebrae in the oblique view. Curved tip 5–7-inch 22-gauge spinal needles are commonly used for this procedure. For the splanchnic nerve block, the needle trajectory has a slight angulation toward the T12 vertebral body. In either case, alternate between oblique and lateral views as the spinal needle is advanced. Once periosteum is contacted, the spinal needle is then "walked" along the lateral edge of the vertebra. For the splanchnic nerve block, final needle position is at the anterior edge of the T12 vertebral body in the lateral view (Fig. 17.6).

For the celiac plexus block, the needle trajectory is truly coaxial along the lateral border of the L1 vertebral body. The left side needle should be placed at the location of the aorta, which can be mapped from a prior CT scan of the patient's abdomen. Alternate between oblique and lateral views every few centimeters as the spinal needle is advanced. After the anterior edge of the vertebral body is reached in the lateral view, it is advanced under constant aspiration. If blood is aspirated, a transaortic technique can be performed by advancing until blood can no longer be aspirated. The final needle position is 2–3 cm anterior to the vertebral body in the lateral view and medial to the pedicle in the AP view. This should allow for injection of contrast and neurolytic anterior to the aorta.

After determination of the final needle position, inject 0.5–1 ml of contrast solution through each needle to verify appropriate anterolateral spread along the vertebral body for the splanchnic nerve block and preaortic spread for the celiac plexus block. Then, after negative aspiration for blood, inject 10 ml of 0.25% bupivacaine through each needle. The needles are then removed.

For chemical neurolysis, after contrast spread is verified, 10 ml of 1% lidocaine (or 2% chloroprocaine) is injected through each needle. After 10–12 min, hip flexion motor testing is then performed to verify that the local anesthetic did not track posterior to the nerve roots or spinal cord. If motor function remains intact, 6–10 ml (usually higher volumes are chosen for the transcrural

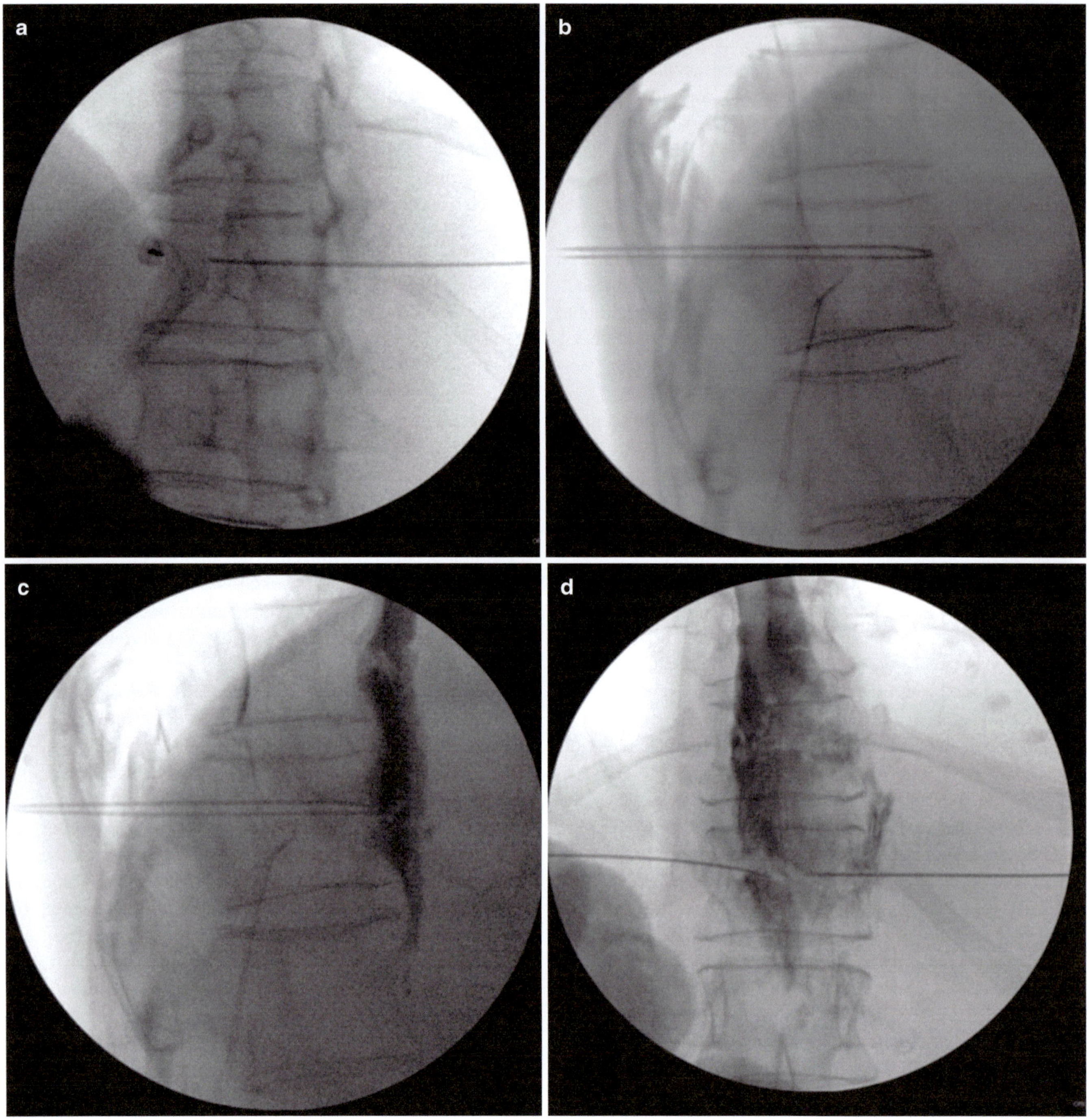

Fig. 17.6 Splanchnic nerve block. (**a**) In an oblique view, the needle is placed superior to the head of the 12th rib immediately lateral to the vertebral body (a similar contralateral needle was already placed). (**b**) Final needle position at the anterior border of the T12 vertebral body. Appropriate prevertebral contrast spread in the lateral (**c**) and AP (**d**) views

approach) of 98% alcohol or 6–10% phenol per side is then injected slowly in 1 ml increments over the course of 5–10 min. The spinal needles should be flushed with saline or local anesthetic solution prior to removal to prevent posterior tracking of alcohol. Many practitioners also inject non-particulate steroid during the flush procedure to reduce the chance of chemical neuritis (Fig. 17.6).

Computed Tomography (CT)-Guided Celiac Plexus and Splanchnic Nerve Block: Posterior Approach

Following placement of verified intravenous access and cardiopulmonary monitors similar to the fluoroscopic approach, the patient is positioned prone on the CT scanner table.

Sequential 5 mm slices are then obtained from T11-L1 to locate the celiac artery and other vasculature in relationship to the lung and soft tissue structures. Planned pathways to the retrocrural space using two needles or the transcrural space using one or two needles are commonly mapped prior to needle placement using the CT image viewer tools. A radiopaque measurement grid taped to the patient or a sterile ruler can be further used to identify specific needle entry sites in the axial and sagittal planes. Typical entry points are no greater than 7 cm from midline. After anesthetizing all entry sites with local anesthetic, 5- or 7-inch 22-g spinal needles are then directed using intermittent CT guidance toward their respective targets. The needles should pass medial to the kidneys and either anterior to the aorta for the transcrural (celiac plexus block) technique or lateral to the aorta and behind the diaphragm when utilizing the retrocrural (splanchnic nerve block) technique. Repeat imaging should be obtained every 1–2 cm while attempting to keep the needle shaft in the current CT axial plane. Following negative aspiration, a small volume of contrast is injected. The contrast should spread bilaterally around the anterior surface of the aorta using the transcrural approach and through the retrocrural space when using the retrocrural approach. If adequate spread of contrast along both sides of the aorta is not appreciable when targeting the transcrural space, an identically placed needle should be placed on the contralateral side. Two needles are almost always required for the retrocrural technique in that the aorta typically prevents spread of injected material to the contralateral side. But in general, lower volumes are typically required for the retrocrural approach given that the splanchnic nerves lie within this confined space. Following confirmation of bilateral contrast spread, 10–30 ml of 0.25% bupivacaine divided among one or two needles can be injected when performing a diagnostic block. When planning neurolysis, 5 ml of 1% lidocaine is first injected through each needle. After performing a neurological test and waiting 10–12 min, 5–15 ml of 50–100% alcohol is subsequently slowly injected through each needle when using a two-needle technique. If a single-needle transcrural approach is utilized, up to 20–40 ml of neurolytic agent can be given in total. The needles are then flushed and removed similar to the fluoroscopic approach (Fig. 17.7).

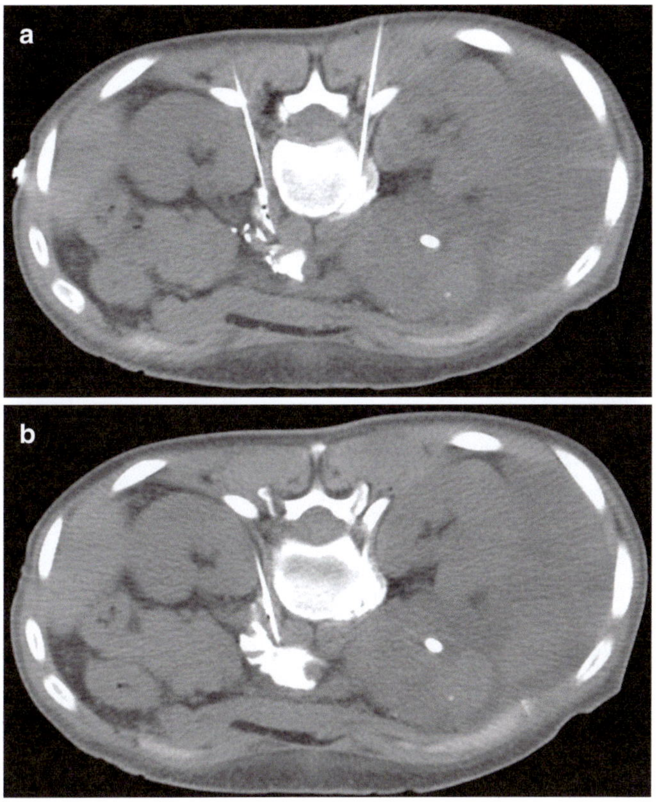

Fig. 17.7 Celiac plexus block (CT guided). (**a**) In a prone position, the right needle tip is placed at the anterolateral aspect of the L1 vertebral body with appropriate contrast spread. (**b**) The left needle tip is placed near the celiac artery branch point from the abdominal aorta. Contrast shows an appropriate preaortic spread. (Images courtesy of Vinay Puttanniah, M.D., Department of Anesthesiology and Critical Care Medicine, Memorial Sloan Kettering Cancer Center, New York, New York)

Side Effects and Complications

Hypotension is a common side effect following CPB and may be symptomatic. This effect is due to vasodilation and pooling of blood within the splanchnic vasculature and is generally responsive to the infusion of crystalloid. The patient should be monitored after the procedure with vital signs obtained at regular intervals. Orthostatic hypotension is generally transient but has been reported up to 1 week [43]. Diarrhea is another common side effect due to the unopposed parasympathetic tone with the blockade of the sympathetic fibers. For this reason, this procedure should not be performed in patients with known or suspected bowel obstruction due to the risk of bowel perforation. The most common significant complication is pneumothorax due to the inadvertent puncture of the parietal pleura during needle placement. The reported incidence of pneumothorax is 1–2% [50–52]. The risk for this complication increases with more cephalad needle placements. As such, immediate ACLS should be available whenever this procedure is performed. Additional reported side effects include hemorrhage due to patient coagulopathy or aortic puncture, aortic wall dissection [53], hematuria from renal puncture, and hemorrhagic gastritis [54]. The most feared complications of this procedure are neurological, ranging from local chemical neuritis to paralysis. Although less severe, hip flexor paresis or paralysis can occur from unintentional lumbar plexus neurolysis in the psoas compartment. Spinal paralysis can be caused by posterior tracking of the neurolytic agent toward spinal cord or vasospasm of the anterior spinal vasculature. In a large retrospective series of 2730 NCPB procedures performed in the late 1980s under radiographic guidance, 4 events of paralysis were reported for an incidence of 1:683 [55].

Lumbar Sympathetic Block

Anatomy

The lumbar sympathetic chain is a series of paired ganglia anterolateral to the L2-L4 vertebral bodies. The preganglionic neurons that synapse in these ganglia arise from the T11-L2 region of the spinal cord [56]. These ganglia are responsible for the majority of the sympathetic innervation to the lower extremities.

Indications

The lumbar sympathetic block (LSB) is used for both diagnostic and therapeutic purposes. It is primarily indicated for sympathetically mediated pain involving the lower extremities. Pain conditions that have been treated by lumbar sympathetic block include complex regional pain syndrome, peripheral vascular disease, postherpetic neuralgia, diabetic neuropathy, phantom limb pain, and groin and testicular pain. Cancer-specific diagnoses for which this block has been utilized include tumor-related lumbosacral neuropathy, postradiation plexopathy [5], and tumor-related bladder spasms [57].

Evidence

Most of the evidence demonstrating the efficacy of lumbar sympathetic blockade is from patients with CRPS. In 1994, Cameron and colleagues studied 29 patients with CRPS involving the lower extremity following total knee replacement. They found 45% of the patients had complete pain relief with the intervention [58]. Another study by Rocco and colleagues assessed the effectiveness of lumbar sympathetic chain radiofrequency ablation in 20 patients with CRPS. Of the 18 patients who completed treatment, 14 demonstrated some degree of response, with 5 patients reporting complete resolution of pain [59]. More recently, Manjunath and colleagues conducted a randomized controlled trial of 20 patients comparing radiofrequency ablation versus phenol for CRPS involving the lower extremities. The study found no significant difference between the two methods of neurolysis [60]. Finally, Carroll and colleagues reported the use of botulinum toxin A along with bupivacaine in LSB for the treatment of CRPS. They found that the addition of botulinum toxin A significantly increased the duration of effect of the block from 10 to 71 days [61].

The utilization of LSB for cancer-related pain has not been widely published. In 2011, Gulati and colleagues reported the use of an LSB at L4 for the treatment of malignancy-related bladder spasms. The three patients reported had bladder spasms caused by local tumor progression, metastatic tumor infiltration, and/or intravesicular chemotherapy. All three patients had significant pain reduction following the procedure [57].

Fluoroscopic Lumbar Sympathetic Block

Consider obtaining intravenous access before proceeding. It is possible for patients to become hypotensive after during the procedure. Cardiopulmonary monitors are applied. The patient is placed in the prone position. A pillow may be placed underneath the patient's abdomen to reduce lumbar lordosis. Identify the L2 vertebral body using AP fluoroscopy, and square the end plates using a caudal tilt of the C-arm. This block can be performed anywhere from the inferior aspect of L2 to the superior aspect of L4. Oblique the C-arm approximately 20–30° ipsilateral until the lateral tip of the transverse process is encompassed within the L2 vertebral body. Anesthetize the skin and subcutaneous tissues over the inferior portion of the lateral border of the L2 vertebral body using a 25-gauge 1.5-inch needle. A 22-gauge spinal needle is then inserted through the skin slightly lateral to the lateral border of the L2 body. Using coaxial technique, the needle is advanced toward the lateral border of the vertebral body. The lateral border of the vertebral body should then be contacted, and the needle is "walked off" the body using lateral fluoroscopic imaging. The final needle position should lie within the anterior 1/3 of the vertebral body in the lateral fluoroscopic view. After negative aspiration, inject 0.5–1 ml of contrast solution to verify appropriate ventral spread along the anterolateral aspect of vertebral body and not in the psoas muscle. Blockade is then typically achieved using 10 ml of 0.25% bupivacaine injected in 2 ml increments through each needle (Fig. 17.8).

Lumbar sympathetic chain neurolysis can be accomplished using either radiofrequency ablation (RFA) or chemical neurolysis. For chemical neurolysis, needles are placed at the L2, L3, and L4 spinal levels like the technique described for the L2 needle placement. Following negative aspiration for blood and appropriate contrast spread, 2 ml of 2% chloroprocaine is injected slowly through each needle. After waiting approximately 10 min, perform a hip flexion motor testing to ensure the local anesthetic did not spread to the motor nerves. If motor strength is still intact, then slowly inject 2 ml of 50–98% alcohol or 6% phenol through each needle.

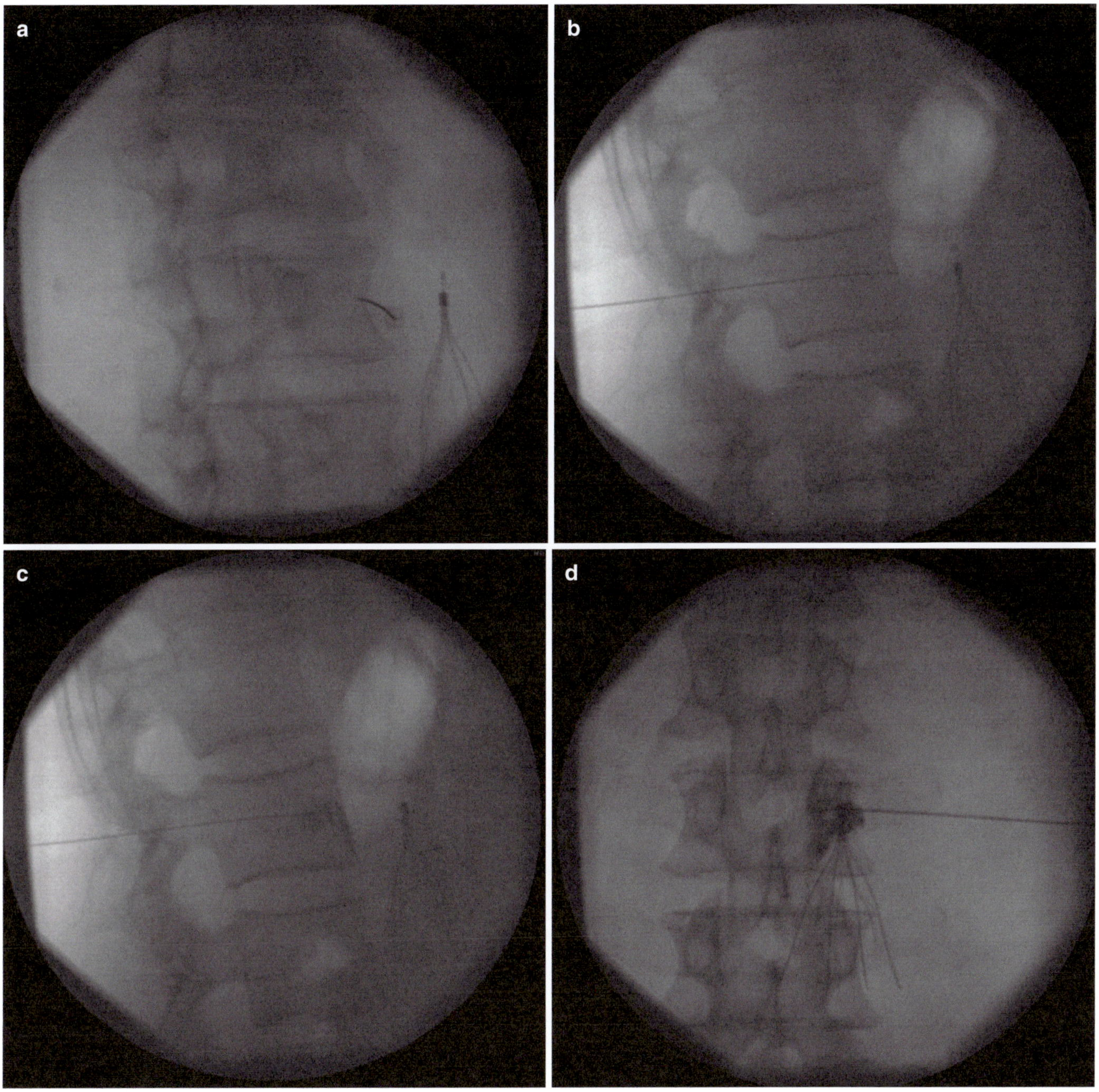

Fig. 17.8 Lumbar sympathetic block. (**a**) The needle is placed and advanced immediately lateral to the L2 vertebral body in an oblique view. (**b**) Final needle position at the anterior border of the L2 vertebral body. Appropriate prevertebral contrast spread in the lateral (**c**) and AP (**d**) views

For RFA, 15-cm RFA needles with 10-mm active tips are placed over the anterolateral aspect of the L2, L3, and L4 vertebral bodies. Sensory testing should be conducted and generally results in difficult to localize back and abdominal pain. Motor testing should also be performed with 2 Hz up to 3 V to ensure the needle tip is an appropriate distance from critical motor structures. No lower extremity movement is expected with motor testing at this site. 1 ml of 2% lidocaine is then injected followed by lesioning at 80 °C for 90 s. Non-particulate steroids are frequently injected following RFA prior to needle removal.

Side Effects and Complications

The most common side effect for this procedure is hypotension. Patients should be monitored carefully post-procedure with vital signs obtained at regular intervals. In addition, the temperature of the lower extremity on the ipsilateral side of the performed block may increase secondary to increased blood flow. Some practitioners use a temperature increase of 2 °C as an indication of a successful block. Genitofemoral neuralgia can occur from direct mechanical injury to the genitofemoral nerve which presents as pain in the groin and anterior thigh. A recent publication also reported permanent lesioning of the lateral femoral cutaneous nerve after low-volume chemical neurolysis with alcohol [62]. Hemorrhage is always possible given proximity to major vascular structures. Hematuria can occur from placement of the needle through the kidney and is normally self-limited. Finally, neuroablative procedures carry the added possible complications of chemical neuritis, femoral nerve neurolysis, and paralysis with mechanisms like those described in the neurolytic celiac plexus block section.

Superior Hypogastric Plexus Block

Anatomy

The superior hypogastric plexus is a collection of retroperitoneal sympathetic fibers that are anterior to the L5 and S1 vertebral bodies. These fibers then continue to the inferior hypogastric plexus at the S2 to S4 levels where they receive additional parasympathetic inputs. Visceral afferent and sympathetic efferent nerves in the superior hypogastric plexus innervate the prostate, bladder, uterus, ovaries, proximal vagina, and rectum.

Indications

Indications for the superior hypogastric plexus block (SHPB) include pain originating from the pelvic viscera, gynecologic disorders, endometriosis, adhesions, interstitial cystitis, irritable bowel syndrome, and malignancies in the pelvic viscera. Diagnostic blocks may be effective in determining the pelvic pain generator. Neurolytic blocks are frequently used for pelvic tumor-related pain.

Evidence

Numerous reports exist regarding the effectiveness of SHPB for the management of pelvic pain associated with cancer. Plancarte and colleagues reported a significant decrease in pain scores after SHPB for patients with cervical, prostate, and bladder cancer pain [63]. De Leon and colleagues reported that 69% of patients had significant pain reduction with superior hypogastric plexus neurolysis for pelvic pain arising from gynecologic, colorectal, or urinary cancer [64]. Plancarte and colleagues later reported the largest cohort of superior hypogastric neurolysis in 227 patients with gynecological, colorectal, or genitourinary cancer. The neurolytic procedure reduced pain by 50% for greater than 1 month in 72% of patients who responded to a diagnostic block and 51% of all patients that enrolled in the study. In addition, mean opioid use decreased by 40% [65]. Predictors of successful pain reduction following superior hypogastric plexus neurolysis included increased age and bladder cancer [66].

The transdiscal approach is an alternative to the classical paravertebral superior SHPB. Erdine and colleagues performed the transdiscal block on 20 patients with pelvic pain due to cancer. Sixty percent had significant pain relief and decreased daily analgesic requirements for up to 3 months [67]. A formal comparison of the two block techniques demonstrated equivalence in pain reduction, with decreased time to perform the transdiscal approach [68]. The transdiscal approach may be particularly helpful as a rescue technique if the classical approach is not possible due to anatomic limitations such as large transverse processes or iliac crests [69].

Fluoroscopic Technique

The patient is placed prone on the fluoroscopy table. Place a pillow underneath the patient's iliac crest to decrease lumbar lordosis. Locate the S1 sacral segment and square the superior end plate using cranial tilt. Turn oblique approximately 20–30 ipsilateral to the side of needle placement. The ideal trajectory will be inferior to the L5 transverse process, medial to the iliac crest, and lateral to the lateral aspect of the vertebral body in this view. It is frequently necessary to adjust the degree of oblique tilt to obtain the clearest view. Anesthetize the skin and soft tissues over the proposed trajectory. Insert a curved tip 5- or 7-inch 22-gauge spinal needle immediately lateral to the lateral border of the L5 vertebral body. Advance the needle along this path using a slight medial deviation. Once the vertebral body is contacted, turn to a lateral view, and slowly walk the needle to the anterior portion of the L5 vertebral body. The ideal position is along the inferior aspect of the L5 or superior aspect of the S1 body on lateral imaging. This technique frequently requires bilateral needle placement. Inject 1–2 ml of contrast solution to verify appropriate prevertebral along the sacral promontory in both AP and lateral images.

A transdiscal approach can also be used for this block and frequently only requires one needle placement. We frequently provide prophylactic antibiotics prior to a transdiscal procedure. This approach uses a similar initial fluoroscopic view with careful attention to "squaring" off the superior S1 end plate. The fluoroscope is then turned oblique 15–25°. The needle entry point is like L5-S1 discography, immediately lateral to the sacral ala over the disc. A 22-gauge 7-cm spinal needle is inserted through the skin and advanced through the disc. Once in the disc, use lateral guidance to advance the needle until the needle tip has exited the disc. Inject 3 ml of contrast solution to verify appropriate prevertebral along the sacral promontory in both AP and lateral images (Fig. 17.9).

After appropriate contrast spread and negative aspiration for blood, 8–10 ml of 0.25% bupivacaine is slowly injected through each needle for the block. For neurolysis, first inject 8 ml of 1% lidocaine (or 2% chloroprocaine) through each needle. We routinely wait 10–12 min and repeat motor testing (ankle plantar and dorsiflexion). If motor function is intact, slowly inject 5–8 ml of 98% alcohol or 6% phenol in 1 ml aliquots over 5 min. The needles are then flushed with

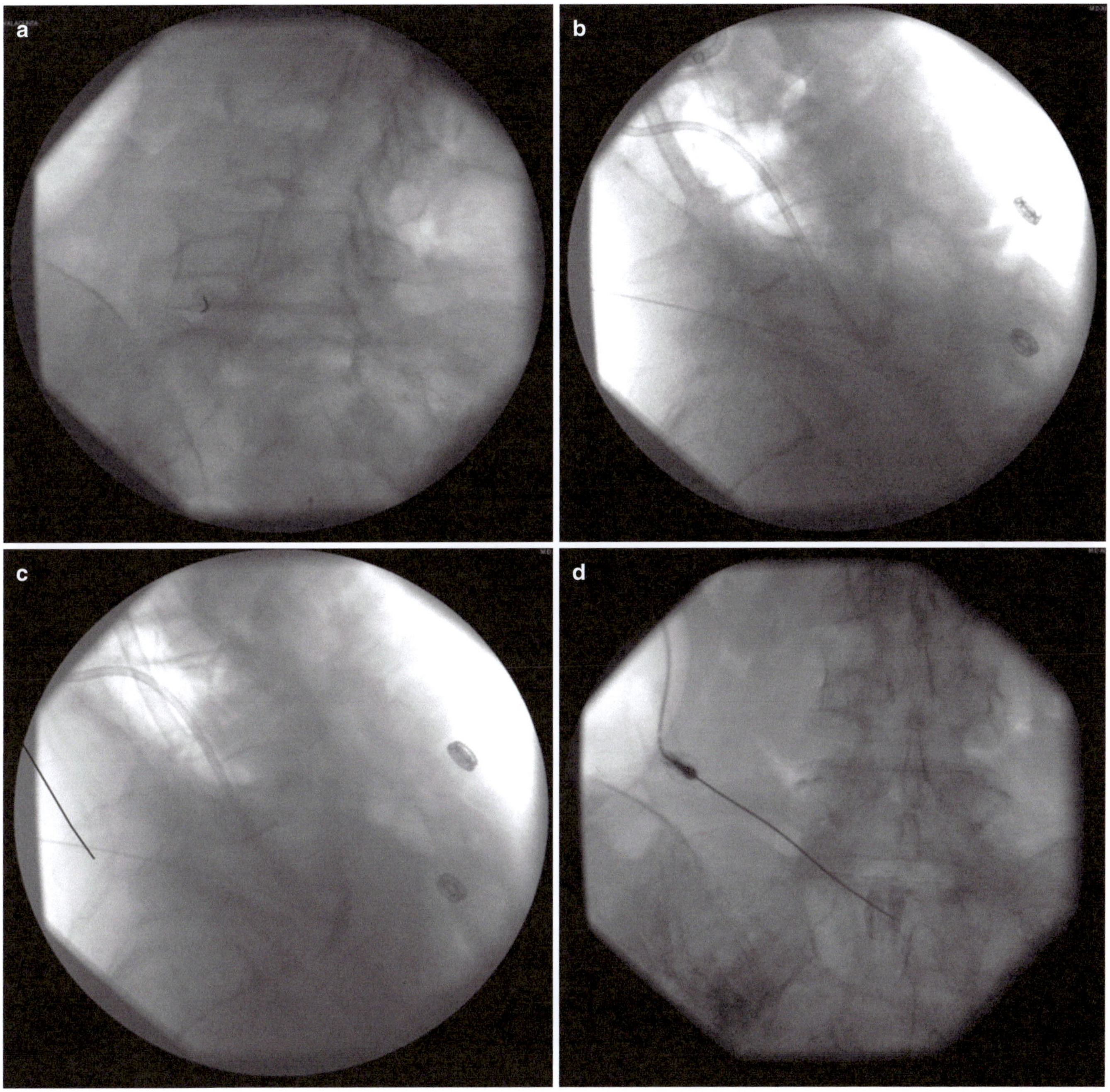

Fig. 17.9 Superior hypogastric plexus block (transdiscal approach). Cranial tilt is used to visualize the L5-S1 intervertebral disc. (**a**) Following 20–30° of oblique angulation, the needle is placed and advanced immediately lateral to the sacral ala through the L5-S1 disc. (**b**) Final needle position immediately anterior the disc. Appropriate contrast spread over the sacral promontory in the lateral (**c**) and AP (**d**) views

local anesthetic and steroid and are then removed. Care must be taken to flush the needles prior to removing them because the path of the needle is near the L5 spinal nerve.

Side Effects and Complications

Due to the plexus location directly posterior to the iliac vessel bifurcation, inadvertent intravascular injection of medications with resultant systemic toxicity is possible. Additionally, strict sterile technique should be used when performing the transdiscal technique in conjunction with intravenous prophylactic antibiotics (such as cefazolin) to help prevent the development of discitis. Since the L5 nerve root is commonly in the path of needle placement for this block, the patient should be awake while the needle is advanced past the neuroforamen. Needle repositioning is frequently needed during the procedure to avoid contacting the L5 spinal nerve. Finally, rare painful sacral neuritis has been observed in our clinical practice and is thought to be related to tracking of neurolytic agent along the sacral nerve roots.

Ganglion Impar Block

Anatomy

The ganglion impar (ganglion of Walther) is the most caudal ganglion of the sympathetic chain. It is a solitary midline ganglion formed from the union of bilateral paravertebral ganglia. The structure is located anterior to the inferior sacral or superior coccygeal segments in the retrorectal space. The ganglion contains sympathetic, parasympathetic, and visceral afferent fibers innervating the distal rectum, anus, perineum, vulva, distal vagina, and distal urethra.

Indications

The ganglion impar block is usually performed in patients with pelvic and perineal pain from the rectum, anus, vagina, and vulva. For tumor-related pain, neurolysis of this ganglion is a commonly employed practice. Local anesthetic blockade and radiofrequency ablation have also been used to relieve chronic pain from coccydynia.

Evidence

Several small case reports have been published evaluating the role of the procedure in treating pelvic and perineal pain due to cancer. The original technique for blocking the impar ganglion was published in abstract form by Plancarte and colleagues in 1990 [70]. In the study, 16 patients underwent the block and over half reported having complete relief of previous pain symptoms. Similar pain reduction has been reported in other small case series [71, 72].

The commonly used transarticular approach was described in 1998 by Swafford and colleagues [73]. In this report, 20 patients with perineal pain all reported at least 50% pain relief, with 5 patients reporting complete relief. A more recent prospective study from 2005 by Reig and colleagues looked at radiofrequency ablation for noncancer-related perineal pain. The group found that all 13 patients receiving the treatment had an average decrease in their pain score by 50% [74].

Fluoroscopic Technique

The patient is placed prone on the fluoroscopic table. Lateral fluoroscopic imaging is used to identify the interspace between the last sacral segment and the first coccygeal segment using a metallic pointer. Holding the pointer in place, an AP image is then obtained ensuring the entry point is midline on the sacrum. The site is then anesthetized with local anesthetic. A 22- or 25-gauge 2-inch spinal needle is inserted through the skin and advanced through the sacrococcygeal ligament in the lateral view. The needle tip is advanced several millimeters past the anterior border of the sacrum. Following negative aspiration for blood, 0.5 ml of contrast solution is injected to verify presacral spread in the lateral view. AP imaging is used to confirm midline spread of the contrast. For the block 5 ml of 0.25% bupivacaine is injected and the needle is withdrawn. For chemical neurolysis, 3–4 ml of 1% lidocaine is injected, and after 7–10 min, 3–4 ml of 50–98% alcohol or 6% phenol is then injected. The needle is then flushed and removed. Many practitioners inject a small amount of steroid to help prevent neuritis. For radiofrequency ablation, a 5-mm active tip RFA needle is placed as described above with only the active tip anterior to the sacrum. Motor and sensory testing are typically performed. Radiofrequency ablation is then performed at 80 °C for 90 s (Fig. 17.10).

Side Effects and Complications

Significant complications from this block are relatively rare. Inadvertent puncture of the rectum with the needle can occur. The risk for this complication increases as the size of a pelvic tumor increases. In neutropenic patients, this can result in a presacral abscess. In addition, rectal fistula formation is possible. Finally, the injectate can track anterior to the sacrum and adversely affect the sacral nerve roots and parasympathetic nerves.

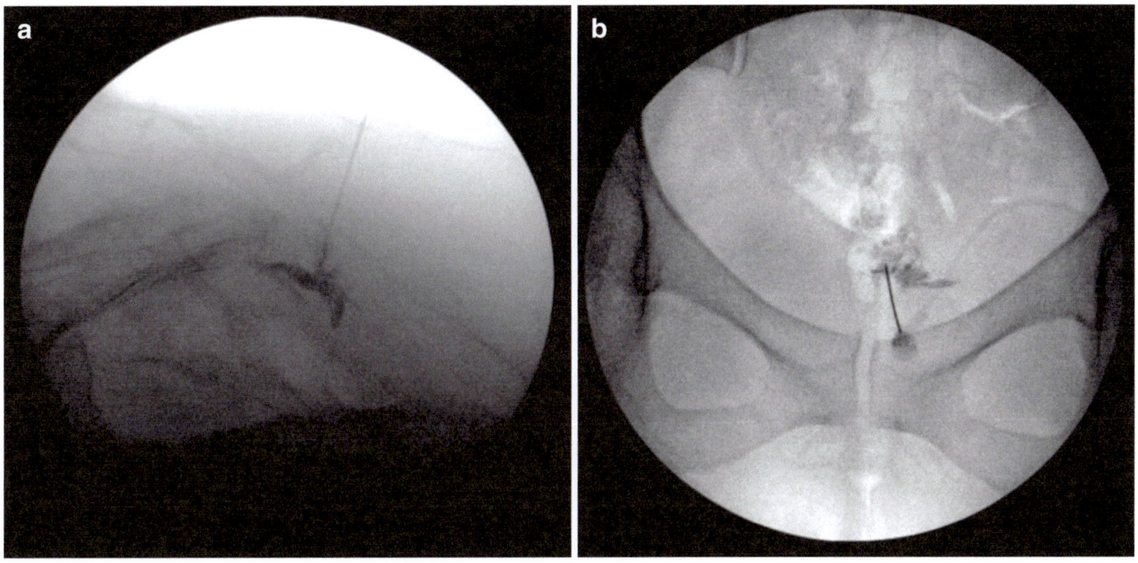

Fig. 17.10 Impar ganglion block. Initial approach in the lateral view between coccygeal segments. The final needle position is immediately anterior to the segments. Appropriate pre-coccygeal contrast spread in the lateral (**a**) and AP (**b**) views

Fig. 17.11 Potential sympathetic blocks based on the anatomical site of lesion or injury

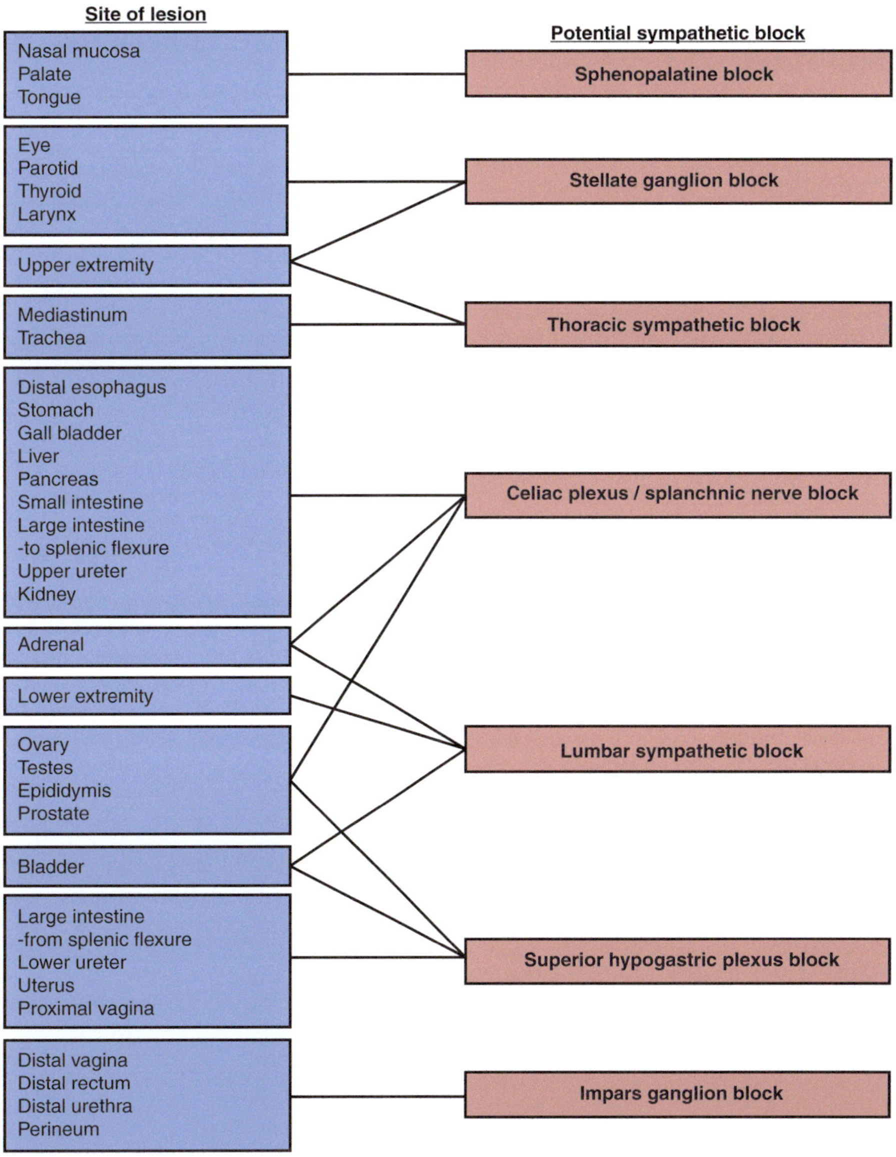

Conclusion

Blocks of the sympathetic nervous system are some of the oldest and most reported interventional pain techniques. These blocks have been shown to be effective in treating sympathetically mediated pain syndromes in addition to malignant visceral pain. Determination of the appropriate sympathetic block can be challenging due to the diffuse nature of both sympathetic and visceral innervations. Figure 17.11 was constructed to assist interventional pain physicians in choosing the most appropriate sympathetic block based on the anatomical location of the tumor or cancer treatment.

Although several randomized controlled trials have been conducted for the celiac plexus block, few high-quality studies have been performed for the other techniques outlined in this chapter. Future directions for the field of interventional cancer pain medicine should aim to include more high-quality prospective studies examining the benefit of these procedures in the context of cancer-related pain.

References

1. Ackerknecht EH. The history of the discovery of the vegetative (autonomic) nervous system. Med Hist. 1974;18:1–8.
2. Dargent M. Role of sympathetic nerve in cancerous pain; an inquiry on 300 cases. Br Med J. 1948;1:440–2.
3. Gebhart GF, Bielefeldt K. Visceral pain. In: Basbaum AI, Masland RH, editors. The senses: a comprehensive reference. Amsterdam: Elsevier; 2008. p. 543–62.
4. Martin LA, Hagen NA. Neuropathic pain in cancer patients: mechanisms, syndromes, and clinical controversies. J Pain Symptom Manag. 1997;14:99–117.
5. Wilsey B, Teicheira D, Caneris OA, Fishman SM. A review of sympathetically maintained pain syndromes in the cancer pain population: the spectrum of ambiguous entities of RSD, CRPS, SMP and other pain states related to the sympathetic nervous system. Pain Pract. 2001;1:307–23.
6. Sato J, Perl ER. Adrenergic excitation of cutaneous pain receptors induced by peripheral nerve injury. Science. 1991;251:1608–10.
7. McLachlan EM, Janig W, Devor M, Michaelis M. Peripheral nerve injury triggers noradrenergic sprouting within dorsal root ganglia. Nature. 1993;363:543–6.
8. Mantyh PW, Koltzenburg M, Mendell LM, Tive L, Shelton DL. Antagonism of nerve growth factor-TrkA signaling and the relief of pain. Anesthesiology. 2011;115:189–204.
9. Day M. Neurolysis of the trigeminal and sphenopalatine ganglions. Pain Pract. 2001;1:171–82.
10. Piagkou M, Demesticha T, Troupis T, Vlasis K, Skandalakis P, Makri A, et al. The pterygopalatine ganglion and its role in various pain syndromes: from anatomy to clinical practice. Pain Pract. 2012;12:399–412.
11. Leong MS, Gjolaj MP, Gaeta RR. Sphenopalatine ganglion block. New York: Springer. 2013.
12. Sanders M, Zuurmond WW. Efficacy of sphenopalatine ganglion blockade in 66 patients suffering from cluster headache: a 12- to 70-month follow-up evaluation. J Neurosurg. 1997;87:876–80.
13. Narouze S, Kapural L, Casanova J, Mekhail N. Sphenopalatine ganglion radiofrequency ablation for the management of chronic cluster headache. Headache. 2009;49:571–7.
14. Puig CM, Driscoll CL, Kern EB. Sluder's sphenopalatine ganglion neuralgia – treatment with 88% phenol. Am J Rhinol. 1998;12:113–8.
15. Bayer E, Racz GB, Miles D, Heavner J. Sphenopalatine ganglion pulsed radiofrequency treatment in 30 patients suffering from chronic face and head pain. Pain Pract. 2005;5:223–7.
16. Prasanna A, Murthy PS. Sphenopalatine ganglion block and pain of cancer. J Pain Symptom Manag. 1993;8:125.
17. Varghese BT, Cherian Koshy R, Sebastian P, Joseph E. Combined sphenopalatine ganglion and mandibular nerve, neurolytic block for pain due to advanced head and neck cancer. Palliat Med. 2002;16:447–8.
18. Syed MI, Shaikh A. Radiology of non-spinal pain procedures: a guide for the interventionalist. New York: Springer. 2013.
19. Yucel I, Demiraran Y, Ozturan K, Degirmenci E. Complex regional pain syndrome type I: efficacy of stellate ganglion blockade. J Orthop Traumatol. 2009;10:179–83.
20. Ackerman WE, Zhang JM. Efficacy of stellate ganglion blockade for the management of type 1 complex regional pain syndrome. South Med J. 2006;99:1084–8.
21. Kastler A, Aubry S, Sailley N, Michalakis D, Siliman G, Gory G, et al. CT-guided stellate ganglion blockade vs. radiofrequency neurolysis in the management of refractory type I complex regional pain syndrome of the upper limb. Eur Radiol. 2013;23:1316–22.
22. Feigl GC, Rosmarin W, Stelzl A, Weninger B, Likar R. Comparison of different injectate volumes for stellate ganglion block: an anatomic and radiologic study. Reg Anesth Pain Med. 2007;32:203–8.
23. Arter OE, Racz GB. Pain management of the oncologic patient. Semin Surg Oncol. 1990;6:162–72.
24. Higa K, Hori K, Harasawa I, Hirata K, Dan K. High thoracic epidural block relieves acute herpetic pain involving the trigeminal and cervical regions: comparison with effects of stellate ganglion block. Reg Anesth Pain Med. 1998;23:25–9.
25. Makharita MY, Amr YM, El-Bayoumy Y. Effect of early stellate ganglion blockade for facial pain from acute herpes zoster and incidence of postherpetic neuralgia. Pain Physician. 2012;15:467–74.
26. Noguchi I, Hasegawa J, Kobayashi K, Takahashi H. Pain relief by stellate ganglion block in a case with trigeminal neuralgia caused by a cerebellopontine angle tumor. Anesth Prog. 2002;49:88–91.
27. Lipov EG, Joshi JR, Xie H, Slavin KV. Updated findings on the effects of stellate-ganglion block on hot flushes and night awakenings. Lancet Oncol. 2008;9:819–20.
28. Lipov EG, Joshi JR, Sanders S, Wilcox K, Lipov S, Xie H, et al. Effects of stellate-ganglion block on hot flushes and night awakenings in survivors of breast cancer: a pilot study. Lancet Oncol. 2008;9:523–32.
29. Abdi S, Zhou Y, Patel N, Saini B, Nelson J. A new and easy technique to block the stellate ganglion. Pain Physician. 2004;7:327–31.
30. Nabil Abbas D, Abd El Ghafar EM, Ibrahim WA, Omran AF. Fluoroscopic stellate ganglion block for postmastectomy pain: a comparison of the classic anterior approach and the oblique approach. Clin J Pain. 2011;27:207–13.
31. Higa K, Hirata K, Hirota K, Nitahara K, Shono S. Retropharyngeal hematoma after stellate ganglion block: analysis of 27 patients reported in the literature. Anesthesiology. 2006;105:1238–45; discussion 5A-6A.
32. Skaebuland C, Racz G. Indications and technique of thoracic(2) and thoracic(3) neurolysis. Curr Rev Pain. 1999;3:400–5.
33. Yarzebski JL, Wilkinson HA. T2 and T3 sympathetic ganglia in the adult human: a cadaver and clinical-radiographic study and its clinical application. Neurosurgery. 1987;21:339–42.
34. Yoo HS, Nahm FS, Lee PB, Lee CJ. Early thoracic sympathetic block improves the treatment effect for upper extremity neuropathic pain. Anesth Analg. 2011;113:605–9.
35. Agarwal-Kozlowski K, Lorke DE, Habermann CR, Schulte am Esch J, Beck H. Interventional management of intractable sympathetically mediated pain by computed tomography-guided catheter implantation for block and neuroablation of the thoracic sympathetic chain: technical approach and review of 322 procedures. Anaesthesia. 2011;66:699–708.

36. Wilkinson HA. Percutaneous radiofrequency upper thoracic sympathectomy. Neurosurgery. 1996;38:715–25.
37. Loukas M, Klaassen Z, Merbs W, Tubbs RS, Gielecki J, Zurada A. A review of the thoracic splanchnic nerves and celiac ganglia. Clin Anat. 2010;23:512–22.
38. Kappis M. Erfahrungen mit local anasthesie bie bauchoperationen. Verh Dtsch Gesellsch Chir. 1914;43:87–9.
39. Lillemoe KD, Cameron JL, Kaufman HS, Yeo CJ, Pitt HA, Sauter PK. Chemical splanchnicectomy in patients with unresectable pancreatic cancer. A prospective randomized trial. Ann Surg. 1993;217:447–55. discussion 56-7
40. Mercadante S. Celiac plexus block versus analgesics in pancreatic cancer pain. Pain. 1993;52:187–92.
41. Kawamata M, Ishitani K, Ishikawa K, Sasaki H, Ota K, Omote K, et al. Comparison between celiac plexus block and morphine treatment on quality of life in patients with pancreatic cancer pain. Pain. 1996;64:597–602.
42. Polati E, Finco G, Gottin L, Bassi C, Pederzoli P, Ischia S. Prospective randomized double-blind trial of neurolytic coeliac plexus block in patients with pancreatic cancer. Br J Surg. 1998;85:199–201.
43. Zhang CL, Zhang TJ, Guo YN, Yang LQ, He MW, Shi JZ, et al. Effect of neurolytic celiac plexus block guided by computerized tomography on pancreatic cancer pain. Dig Dis Sci. 2008;53:856–60.
44. Wong GY, Schroeder DR, Carns PE, Wilson JL, Martin DP, Kinney MO, et al. Effect of neurolytic celiac plexus block on pain relief, quality of life, and survival in patients with unresectable pancreatic cancer: a randomized controlled trial. JAMA. 2004;291:1092–9.
45. Wyse JM, Carone M, Paquin SC, Usatii M, Sahai AV. Randomized, double-blind, controlled trial of early endoscopic ultrasound-guided celiac plexus neurolysis to prevent pain progression in patients with newly diagnosed, painful, inoperable pancreatic cancer. J Clin Oncol. 2011;29:3541–6.
46. Arcidiacono PG, Calori G, Carrara S, McNicol ED, Testoni PA. Celiac plexus block for pancreatic cancer pain in adults. Cochrane Database Syst Rev. 2011;3:CD007519.
47. McGreevy K, Hurley RW, Erdek MA, Aner MM, Li S, Cohen SP. The effectiveness of repeat celiac plexus neurolysis for pancreatic cancer: a pilot study. Pain Pract. 2013;13:89–95.
48. De Cicco M, Matovic M, Balestreri L, Fracasso A, Morassut S, Testa V. Single-needle celiac plexus block: is needle tip position critical in patients with no regional anatomic distortions? Anesthesiology. 1997;87:1301–8.
49. De Cicco M, Matovic M, Bortolussi R, Coran F, Fantin D, Fabiani F, et al. Celiac plexus block: injectate spread and pain relief in patients with regional anatomic distortions. Anesthesiology. 2001;94:561–5.
50. Brown DL, Bulley CK, Quiel EL. Neurolytic celiac plexus block for pancreatic cancer pain. Anesth Analg. 1987;66:869–73.
51. Brown DL, Moore DC. The use of neurolytic celiac plexus block for pancreatic cancer: anatomy and technique. J Pain Symptom Manag. 1988;3:206–9.
52. Brown DL. A retrospective analysis of neurolytic celiac plexus block for nonpancreatic intra-abdominal cancer pain. Reg Anesth. 1989;14:63–5.
53. Kaplan R, Schiff-Keren B, Alt E. Aortic dissection as a complication of celiac plexus block. Anesthesiology. 1995;83:632–5.
54. Pello S, Miller A, Ku T, Wang D. Hemorrhagic gastritis and duodenitis following celiac plexus neurolysis. Pain Physician. 2009;12:1001–3.
55. Davies DD. Incidence of major complications of neurolytic coeliac plexus block. J R Soc Med. 1993;86:264–6.
56. Rathmell JP. Atlas of image-guided intervention in regional anesthesia and pain medicine: Wolters Kluwer Health; 2012.
57. Gulati A, Khelemsky Y, Loh J, Puttanniah V, Malhotra V, Cubert K. The use of lumbar sympathetic blockade at L4 for management of malignancy-related bladder spasms. Pain Physician. 2011;14:305–10.
58. Cameron HU, Park YS, Krestow M. Reflex sympathetic dystrophy following total knee replacement. Contemp Orthop. 1994;29:279–81.
59. Rocco AG. Radiofrequency lumbar sympatholysis. The evolution of a technique for managing sympathetically maintained pain. Reg Anesth. 1995;20:3–12.
60. Manjunath PS, Jayalakshmi TS, Dureja GP, Prevost AT. Management of lower limb complex regional pain syndrome type 1: an evaluation of percutaneous radiofrequency thermal lumbar sympathectomy versus phenol lumbar sympathetic neurolysis – a pilot study. Anesth Analg. 2008;106:647–9. table of contents
61. Carroll I, Clark JD, Mackey S. Sympathetic block with botulinum toxin to treat complex regional pain syndrome. Ann Neurol. 2009;65:348–51.
62. Pennekamp W, Krumova EK, Feigl GP, Frombach E, Nicolas V, Schwarzer A, et al. Permanent lesion of the lateral femoral cutaneous nerve after low-volume ethanol 96% application on the lumbar sympathetic chain. Pain Physician. 2013;16:391–7.
63. Plancarte R, Amescua C, Patt RB, Aldrete JA. Superior hypogastric plexus block for pelvic cancer pain. Anesthesiology. 1990;73:236–9.
64. de Leon-Casasola OA, Kent E, Lema MJ. Neurolytic superior hypogastric plexus block for chronic pelvic pain associated with cancer. Pain. 1993;54:145–51.
65. Plancarte R, de Leon-Casasola OA, El-Helaly M, Allende S, Lema MJ. Neurolytic superior hypogastric plexus block for chronic pelvic pain associated with cancer. Reg Anesth. 1997;22:562–8.
66. Kroll CE, Schartz B, Gonzalez-Fernandez M, Gordon AH, Babade M, Erdek MA, et al. Factors associated with outcome after superior hypogastric plexus neurolysis in cancer patients. Clin J Pain. 2014;30:55–62.
67. Erdine S. Transdiscal approach for hypogastric plexus block. Reg Anesth Pain Med. 2003;28:304–8.
68. Gamal G, Helaly M, Labib YM. Superior hypogastric block: transdiscal versus classic posterior approach in pelvic cancer pain. Clin J Pain. 2006;22:544–7.
69. Nabil D, Eissa AA. Evaluation of posteromedial transdiscal superior hypogastric block after failure of the classic approach. Clin J Pain. 2010;26:694–7.
70. Plancarte R, Amescua C, Patt RB. Presacral blockade of the ganglion impar (ganglion of Walther). Anesthesiology. 1990. (Abstract;73:A751.
71. Eker HE, Cok OY, Kocum A, Acil M, Turkoz A. Transsacrococcygeal approach to ganglion impar for pelvic cancer pain: a report of 3 cases. Reg Anesth Pain Med. 2008;33:381–2.
72. Bhatnagar S, Khanna S, Roshni S, Goyal GN, Mishra S, Rana SP, et al. Early ultrasound-guided neurolysis for pain management in gastrointestinal and pelvic malignancies: an observational study in a tertiary care center of urban India. Pain Pract. 2012;12:23–32.
73. Swofford JB, Ratzman DM. A transarticular approach to blockade of the ganglion impar (ganglion of walther). Reg Anesth Pain Med. 1998;23:25.
74. Reig E, Abejon D, del Pozo C, Insausti J, Contreras R. Thermocoagulation of the ganglion impar or ganglion of Walther: description of a modified approach. Preliminary results in chronic, nononcological pain. Pain Pract. 2005;5:103–10.
75. Griffin R, Fink E, Brenner GJ. Bonica's management of pain. In: Fishman S, Ballantyne J, Rathmell JP, Bonica JJ, editors. Baltimore: Lippincott, Williams & Wilkins; 2010. p. 98–119.

18 Peripheral Nerve Blocks

Nantthasorn Zinboonyahgoon, Christopher R. Abrecht, and Sanjeet Narang

Introduction

Cancer-related pain is often multifactorial in etiology and taxonomy. Tumor invasion and associated oncologic therapies such as chemotherapy, radiotherapy, and surgery have all been known to cause a myriad of pain syndromes that have nociceptive, neuropathic, and visceral components. Somatic and peripheral nerve blockade for malignant pain control is often delayed until goals of care have become palliative in nature. However, these oncologic pain interventions have been proven effective for treating cancer-related pain even early in the disease course.

No panacea exists for malignant pain management; combinations of blocks are often indicated and required. A patient with invasive rectal cancer, for instance, might require a combination of somatic and autonomic blocks such as bilateral S3 blocks targeting the pudendal nerve plus a ganglion of impar block. Another possibility for such a patient might be a block plus an intrathecal opioid trial.

Corticosteroid may enhance the therapeutic duration of peripheral nerve blocks on the order of weeks. If destructive neurolytic chemicals are employed, analgesia has the potential to last several months before regeneration of nerve tissue. Local anesthetic peripheral nerve blockade often provides immediate gratification which may instill patient confidence and provide opportunity for further treatment. Practitioners who may not have access to guidance by ultrasound or other forms of imaging may rely on classical surface anatomy-based techniques.

N. Zinboonyahgoon (✉)
Department of Anesthesiology, Faculty of Medicine Siriraj Hospital, Mahidol University, Bangkok, Thailand

Department of Anesthesiology, Perioperative and Pain Medicine, Brigham and Women's Hospital, Harvard Medical School, Boston, MA, USA

C. R. Abrecht
Department of Anesthesiology, Perioperative and Pain Medicine, Brigham and Women's Hospital, Harvard Medical School, Boston, MA, USA

S. Narang
Department of Anesthesiology, Perioperative and Pain Medicine, The Pain Management Center at Brigham and Women's Hospital, Harvard Medical School, Chestnut Hill, MA, USA

Pharmacology

Non-neurolytic Block Agents

Local anesthetics and corticosteroids are among the more commonly used non-neurolytic agents. Local anesthetics inhibit sodium channels needed for nerve conduction and have the potential to provide immediate pain relief. They also provide sensory information which is useful in determining the distribution and quality of the block. Local corticosteroids in nerve blocks work by a mechanism not completely understood. Potential mechanisms of effect include direct inhibition of inflammation caused by an invasive tumor, suppression of spontaneous ectopic discharge and injured nerves, and inhibition of painful transmission through afferent nociceptive fibers [1]. Furthermore, many patients even experience analgesia beyond the longevity of large particle depot steroid formulations suggesting that interruption of central sensitization may serve as an additional mechanism of action. Often an inflammatory component exists in many cancer pain syndromes. Invasive tumors may cause inflammation via mass effect or tissue destruction. In addition, the body may treat cancer cells as a hostile presence by mounting a natural inflammatory response against this threat [2].

Systemic toxicity and unwanted side effects occur frequently with local anesthetic administration. Systemic toxicity can be mitigated by careful aspiration, incremental injection, and contrast usage to minimize the risk of intravascular injection.

Corticosteroids, through their physiologic effects, have been known to cause adrenal suppression, glaucoma, edema,

A. Gulati et al. (eds.), *Essentials of Interventional Cancer Pain Management*, https://doi.org/10.1007/978-3-319-99684-4_18

hypertension, psychotropic derangements, weight gain, and hyperglycemia. These adverse side effects are more likely to occur with higher doses and more frequent administration. As there is not sufficient data regarding the "safe" dose of particulate steroid injection for nerve blocks, methylprednisolone 40–80 mg (or its equivalent) is commonly used. A total dose of 120 mg on any one occasion is normally not exceeded at our institution.

Neurolytic Block Agents

Alcohol and phenol are among the available neurolytic agents used to provide irreversible conduction block and destroy nerve bundles. Other methods of neurolysis include cryotherapy or radio-frequency ablation. None of these blocks are, however, truly permanent because nerve fibers regenerate; pain may return in 3–6 months.

Neurolytic blocks are a widely used and evidence-based intervention for sympathetic blocks. For somatic blocks, however, the application is quite limited because somatic nerves carry both sensory and motor fibers. Therefore, patients who receive neurolytic block may develop peripheral neuritis, deafferentation pain, and analgesia dolorosa, as well as motor deficits. For these reasons, neurolytic blocks for somatic nerves are usually reserved as last resort for refractory malignant pain with expected short life span. The patient should have successful pain control and accept the sense of numbness and motor deficit experienced with the diagnostic block before proceeding to neurolytic block.

Ethyl alcohol provides immediate neurolytic effect and is administered as a 98% solution alone or as a 60–80% solution when diluted with contrast or local anesthetics. At these high concentrations, it is rapidly absorbed into blood stream and may cause sedation or a disulfiram-like reaction. It also causes burning pain on injection, so stronger local anesthetic should be administered prior to the injection of ethyl alcohol [3].

Phenol provides delayed neurolysis (i.e., 15 min) and is administered in 4–10% solutions that are not commercially available and must be compounded individually by a hospital or commercial pharmacist. When prepared with glycerin, phenol spread is confined and well localized; however, it is very difficult to inject through narrower bore needles; hence, it may be mixed in sterile water instead. Regardless of the preparation, phenol has weak local anesthetic properties and is associated with non-painful warmth and local anesthetic action. Compared to ethyl alcohol, nerve regeneration occurs faster [3].

Somatic Nerve Blocks

Somatic blocks used in the management of cancer pain can be diagnostic, prognostic, or therapeutic. Somatic blocks can be used diagnostically to confirm or exclude a suspected pain generator. For example, a transversus abdominis block will provide analgesia for pathology affecting the abdominal wall but not the underlying visceral organs. Similarly, a pudendal nerve block done for pelvic pain may aid in the differentiation of pudendal neuralgia from visceral pelvic pain. They are prognostic in that a successful somatic block would suggest a higher rate of benefit from subsequent neurolysis or ablation. And the aim is always for oncologic interventions to therapeutically improve patient quality of life.

In general, the principles of peripheral nerve block for the management of patients with non-cancer pain can be applied to patients with malignant pain. All nerves that are accessible to neural blockade are legitimate targets. Clarity of anatomic location of pain is key for successful block of the appropriate nerve or groups of nerves. A thorough history and physical are essential. Practitioners are urged to meticulously record the pain history and examination with the aim of finally visualizing the pain as a three-dimensional physical entity, occupying the relevant area of the patient's body. Nuances of precipitating and aggravating factors will help determine etiology and therefore alter the targets to be blocked.

Procedure-related factors pertaining to the oncologic patient present additional challenges. For instance, anatomic distortion from tumor compression, surgery, or radiotherapy may increase the technical difficulty of any procedures. Multiple comorbidities and a decreased functional capacity may also prevent the patient from assuming certain positions required for performing the block (e.g., the prone position). Moreover, many cancer patients are coagulopathic either through cytotoxic cancer therapy or secondary to poor nutritional status. A significant portion of this population may also be receiving oncologic therapies that increase the risk of bleeding (bevacizumab) or on anticoagulant therapy given the prothrombotic nature of malignancy.

Clinicians as well as these patients may, however, be willing to accept an elevated risk of bleeding, even if in a noncompressible space, if there is possibility for significant pain relief in the context of a terminal illness. Elevated risk of infection is also a concern in oncology patients. In addition, many patients may have chronic non-healing wounds requiring long-term prophylactic antibiotic therapy. Carefully avoiding infected areas and adherence to strict aseptic technique will tilt the balance in favor of avoiding infectious complications. In such cases where there is intense pain but a limited life expectancy, diagnostic and therapeutic blocks may be performed during the same procedure session (e.g., an intercostal nerve block resulting in intense pain relief could be followed immediately with a neurolytic block). Similarly, it is also common practice to perform multiple procedures (e.g., a pudendal nerve block and a ganglion of impar block in one session).

Somatic nerve blocks are most commonly guided by anatomic landmarks, fluoroscopy, computed tomography, ultrasound, or a combination of these. The ultrasound-guided technique has gained popularity because it provides real-time needle guidance and visualization of neurovascular structures. Ultrasound has the potential to increase success rate, decrease time until onset of sensory block, reduce the number of needle attempts, lower the minimum anesthetic dose used, and aid in the detection of intraneural and intravascular injection. These benefits are especially useful in an anatomically challenging situation, as is often the case in the oncologic population. Ultrasound technology has become portable, not associated with radiation exposure, and has no known absolute contraindications [4].

However, ultrasound is not without limitations. For example, it has limited depth and cannot penetrate through certainstructures such as the bone. Target sites that are deep or encased within bone may be reached easier using other imaging modalities such as fluoroscopy. Depth of target tissue may also be a factor in choosing fluoroscopy over ultrasound. In all cases, though, the choice of the technique depends in large part on the experience and comfort level of the interventionist.

Truncal Blocks

Thoracic Paravertebral Block (TPVB)

TPVB provides unilateral somatic and sympathetic block in multiple contiguous thoracic dermatomes. Given the ability to block several adjacent dermatomes with a single injection, the TPVB is effective for treating acute and chronic pain affecting the thorax and upper abdomen. Unfortunately, mastectomy and thoracotomy are frequently performed surgeries in the oncologic population that are associated with a high subsequent incidence of chronic pain [5]. Rates are thought to range from 20 to 40% for mastectomy and as high as 50% for thoracotomy [6, 7]. The TPVB can be utilized for both perioperative pain control and also to treat the subsequent development of chronic postmastectomy or post-thoracotomy pain. Case series of neurolytic TPVB have also been reported in patients with chest wall and rib metastasis [8].

Anatomy The thoracic paravertebral space is a triangular space located at anterolateral side of thoracic vertebra and contains adipose tissue, intercostal neurovasculature, and the sympathetic trunk. Boundaries are the parietal pleura (anterolateral), superior costotransverse ligament (posterior), and vertebral body/intervertebral foramen (medial). The thoracic paravertebral space connects with epidural space medially and with the intercostal space laterally (Fig. 18.1). Because the TPVS is contiguous in the rostral and caudal directions, a large-volume single injection may cover multiple dermatome levels.

Technique The patient may be in the sitting, lateral decubitus, or prone position. For persistent postmastectomy pain, the goal is to cover the T2–T6 dermatomes, often with 0.25% bupivacaine 15–20 mL with or without additives such as corticosteroids via a single injection at T4. This single injection of 15–20 mL usually spreads 3–4 dermatomes and sufficiently covers the painful territory. In all cases, injection should only follow anaspiration negative for blood, air, and CSF.

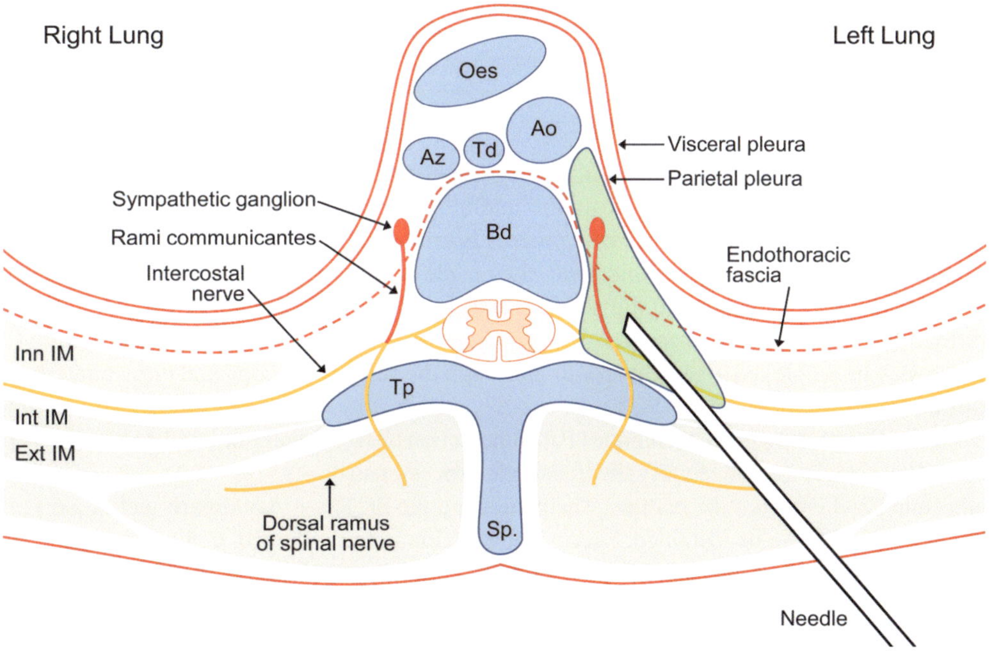

Fig. 18.1 Anatomy of thethoracic paravertebral space (triangle). *Tp* transverse process, *Sp* spinous process, *Bd* vertebral body, *Oes* esophagus, *Ao* aorta

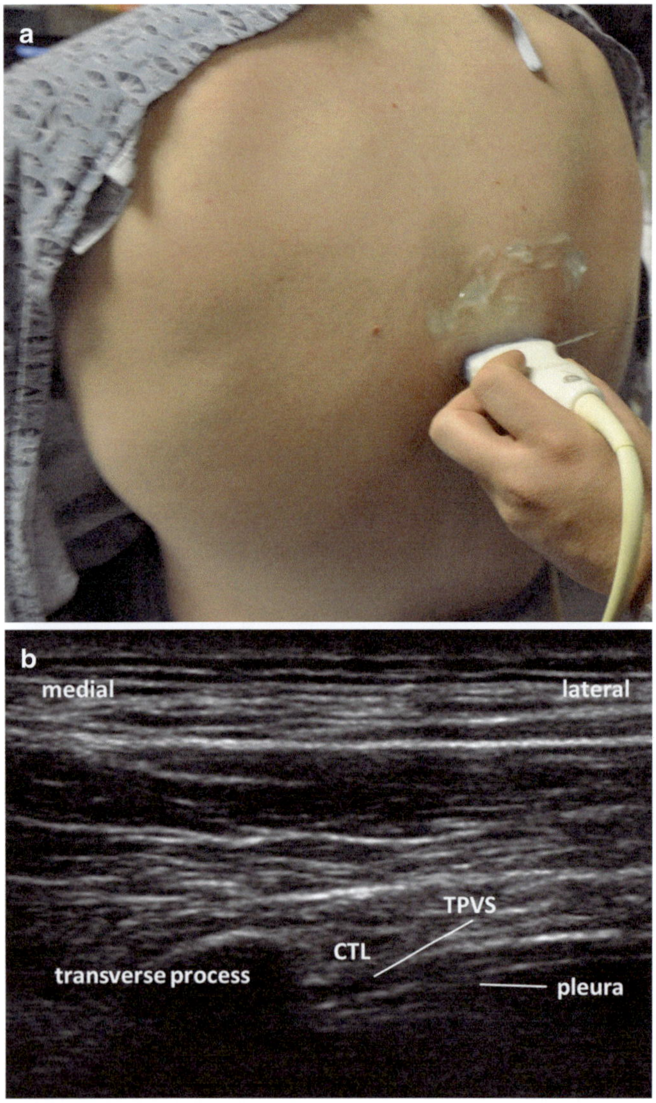

Fig. 18.2 (**a**) Transverse scan for TPVB (left). (**b**) Sonographic image shows the thoracic paravertebral space (TPVS) and related structures; *CTL* costotransverse ligament (right)

In the landmark technique, a 21G, 10 cm spinal or epidural needle is advanced 2–3 cm from the midline, perpendicular to the skin, until the transverse process is contacted, usually at about 3–6 cm [9]. At this point, the needle is redirected cephalad or caudad until the needle advances slightly further past the transverse process. A loss of resistance technique may be employed to indicate passing through the superior costotransverse ligament (SCT).

In the ultrasound-guided technique [10], either a transverse or sagittal scan is used to identify the transverse process, usually found 2–3 cm from the midline. The pleura and the SCT ligament should also be identified. Successful injection in the TPVS should displace the pleura (Figs. 18.2 and 18.3).

Benefit Kirvelä et al. demonstrated in a case series of 281 TPVBs that successful pain relief for persistent postmastectomy and post-thoracotomy was achieved using PVB with bupivacaine without steroid. In this study, most patients had pain relief lasting at least 4 weeks and, in some cases, more than 5 months. For unclear reasons, benefit appeared to be superior in post-thoracotomy patients in terms of duration compared to the postmastectomy group [7].

Complications and Side Effects Pneumothorax, intravascular injection, epidural or spinal spread, hypotension, Horner's syndrome (when performed at the upper thoracic levels), pleural puncture, pneumothorax, vascular puncture, hematoma, unintentional neuraxial spread, and infection are all potential risks associated with these blocks.

Intercostal Block

Intercostal block provides a unilateral dermatomal blockade at the targeted thoracic level which it is performed. Malignant chest wall invasion and rib metastases causing somatic pain are common indications for this block. Given that breast and lung cancer often metastasizes to the ribs, the intercostal block may be especially useful in this population [11]. Compared to paravertebral blockade, intercostal blocks have a theoretical decreased chance of injectate tracking into the neuroaxis. This increased control comes at the disadvantage of only covering one segmental dermatome per injection.

Anatomy The thoracic nerve roots originate from T1–T12, exit the spine through their respective intervertebral foramina as spinal nerves, and then divide into the dorsal and ventral rami. The dorsal rami run posteriorly to supply the paraspinal region. The ventral rami run laterally and then anteriorly, becoming the intercostal nerves. At the angle of the rib, the intercostal nerve lies next to the innermost of the internal intercostal muscles in the subcostal groove just inferior to the intercostal vessels at the inferior border of the corresponding rib. At the midaxillary line, the intercostal nerve divides into the lateral branch, which supplies the lateral trunk, and into the anterior branch, which supplies the anterior trunk (Fig. 18.4).

Technique The patient position can be sitting, lateral decubitus, or prone. The procedure may be done by anatomic landmarks with or without imaging guidance such as fluoroscopy and ultrasound. In all cases, after an aspiration negative for blood or air, an injection of 2–3 mL of neurolytic agent or local anesthetic is performed at each level.

Landmark technique [12]: Start at the inferior border of the rib, 6–8 cm from the midline (i.e., the spinous process). Point the needle 20° cephalad until contact is made with the

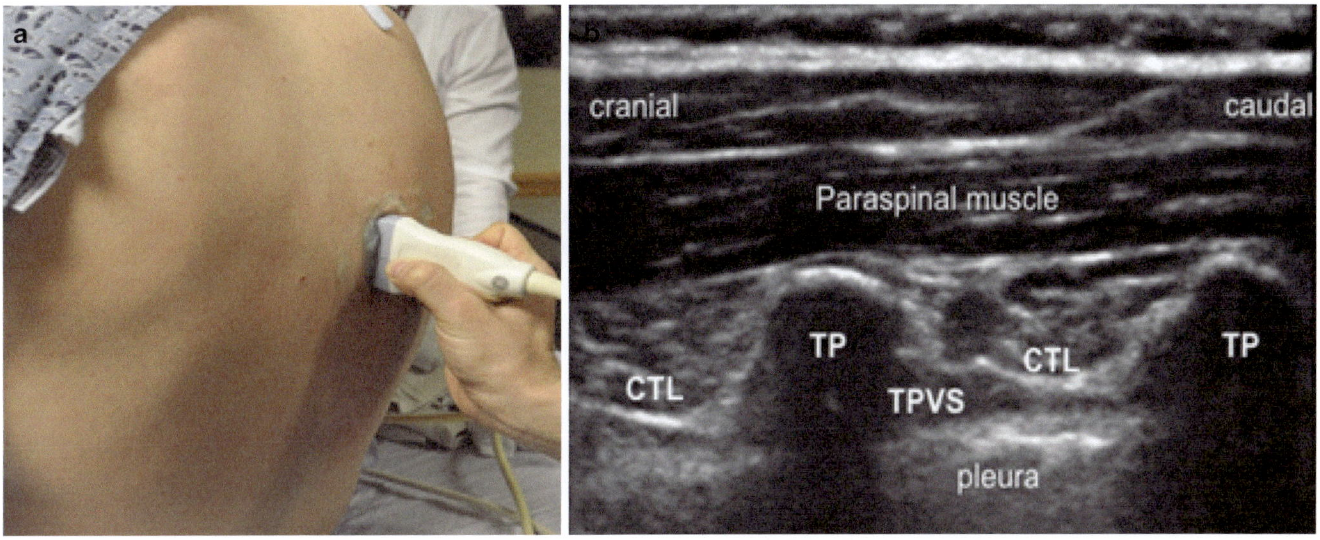

Fig. 18.3 (**a**) Sagittal paramedian scan for TPVB (left). (**b**) Sonographic image shows the thoracic paravertebral space (TPVS) and related structures; *TP* transverse process (right)

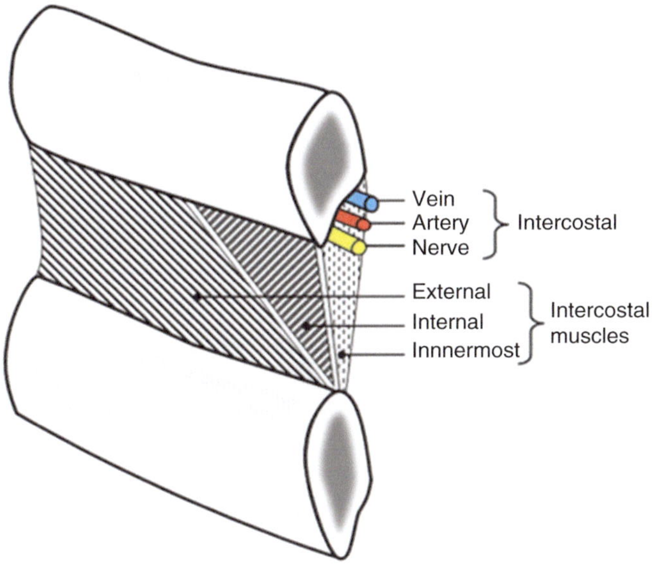

Fig. 18.4 Anatomy of intercostal nerve

rib, then maintain a cephalad angle, and pull the skin inferiorly as the needle is walked off the inferior border of the rib and into subcostal groove. Once the inferior margin has been passed, the needle is slightly advanced, and the injectate is administered after negative aspiration.

Ultrasound guided [13]: Ultrasound is usually performed with the probe in the sagittal plane. Start by scanning transversely 6–8 cm from the midline and identify the desired rib space as well as the pleura. Rib spaces can be identified and counted usually from the caudal or cephalad direction. A spinal needle is commonly used and advanced in-plane just deep to or at the internal intercostal muscle. The pleura should be visualized to minimize the risk of inadvertent puncture. Successful injection will spread in the intercostal space (Fig. 18.5).

Benefit Case series by Wong et al. showed successful pain relief from rib metastasis in terminal-stage cancer patients following neurolytic intercostal block. Ninety-six percent of the patients experienced immediate pain relief following diagnostic blockade. Over 80% still had significant analgesia with subsequent neurolysis which lasted anywhere from 5 to 158 days [14]. In this case series, patients on high-dose opioids with severe and intractable pain symptoms demonstrated the most benefit.

Complications Pneumothorax, intravascular injection, hematoma, infection, and neuraxial spread are all possible complications. Paraplegia after neurolytic block is also possible and thought to result from medial spread of agent through the intervertebral foramen [3].

Transversus Abdominis Plane Block (TAP Block)

TAP block provides somatic block of the unilateral abdominal wall in multiple dermatomes with a single injection. It can be applied for diagnostic or therapeutic purposes. As a diagnostic block, it can distinguish abdominal wall pain from visceral. As a therapeutic block, it has been employed for perioperative pain control during and after abdominal surgery. In addition, local anesthetic and neurolytic blocks have been utilized for malignant pain related to tumor invasion of the abdominal wall.

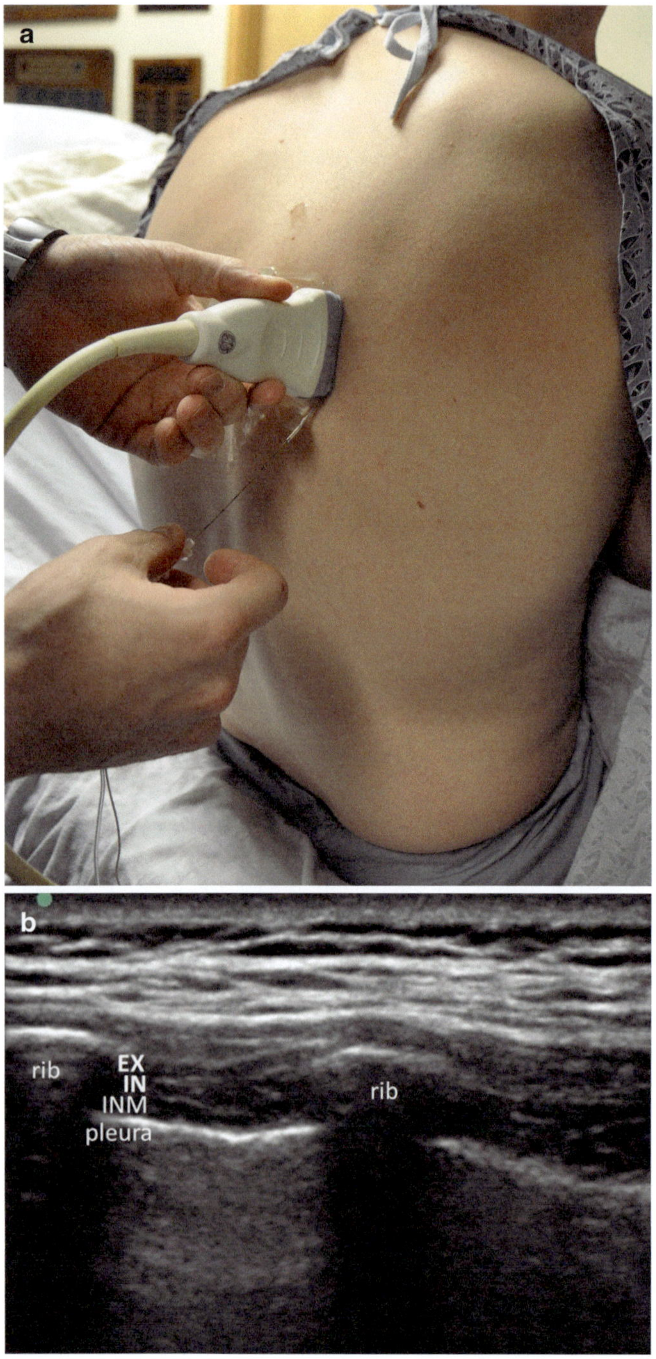

Fig. 18.5 (**a**) Sagittal paramedian scan of ribs (left). (**b**) Sonographic image shows the intercostal space and layers of intercostal muscle; *INM* innermost, *IN* internal, *EX* external (right)

Anatomy The anterior rami of T7–L1 travel from the intercostal space toward midline. In the abdominal wall, they pass through the plane between internal abdominal oblique and transversus abdominis muscles before terminating as the cutaneous branches (Fig. 18.6).

Technique [15] The original description of TAP block was a landmark-based technique; however, ultrasound has gained increasing favor to better visualize the appropriate target plane in addition to surrounding soft tissue structures. The TAP block can be done by two approaches: the classic approach at midaxillary line which better covers the lower abdomen (below umbilicus) and the subcostal approach, which is superior for pain arising from the upper abdomen. Hebbard [16] described the subcostal oblique hydrodissection approach which can cover both the unilateral upper and lower abdomen in a single injection but requires a higher volume of injectate. For diffuse abdominal pain suspected to be from the abdominal wall, both the midaxillary and subcostal approachescan be utilized.

For the ultrasound approach, the patient is in supine position and the ultrasound probe applied to abdominal wall. For the traditional approach, the probe is placed along the lateral abdominal wall between the inferior costal margin anterior crest. For the subcostal approach, it is common to scan along the inferior costal margin (Fig. 18.5). The goal is to deposit the injectate (usually 10–20 ml) between the internal oblique and transversus abdominis muscle planes. In terms of identification, the internal oblique tends to be the thickest and the transversus abdominis the thinnest among the abdominal wall muscle layers. For intractable malignant pain, subsequent neurolytic agent (6% phenol or 60–100% alcohol) can be used for longer-lasting pain relief. After the operator is satisfied with the spread, inject 10–20 ml of 6% phenol or 60–98% alcohol for neurolysis (author suggestion).

Benefit There are case series [17] and reports [18–20] that demonstrate significant pain relief and decreased opioid consumption following TAP blockade in the oncologic population suffering from abdominal wall tumor invasion. Some patients may need both the classic and the subcostal approaches to cover all painful areas.

Complications As it targets peripheral anatomic areas away from most critical structures, bleeding sequelae are less concerning with this technique. However, local anesthetic toxicity, visceral organ puncture, and infection are still possible complications.

Peripheral Nerve Block

Brachial Plexus Block

Indication The brachial plexus block provides sensory and motor block in the territory of the brachial plexus. Malignant invasion of the brachial plexus is uncommon, occurring in less than 3% of patients of lung and breast cancer, but it accounts for one-third of intractable pain in patients with lung and breast cancer [21–23]. Non-neurolytic brachial

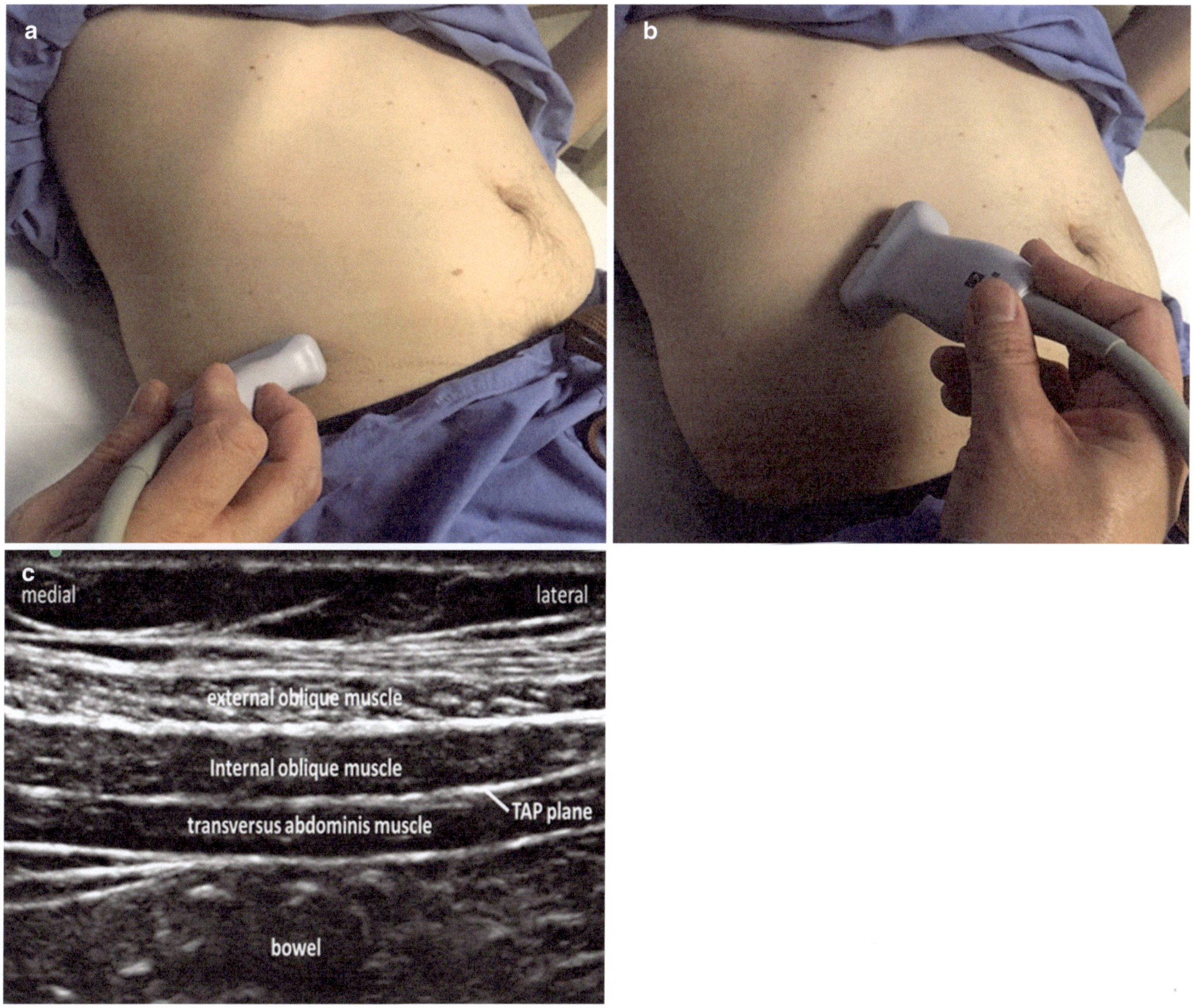

Fig. 18.6 Location for ultrasound probe application for Transversus Abdominis Plane (TAP) block; (**a**) midaxillary approach (left), (**b**) subcostal approach (middle). (**c**) Image from ultrasound guided TAP block (right)

plexus block may be prognostic, predicting a response to neurolytic block or nerve root ablation. It may also act a therapeutic bridge prior to radiation therapy.

Anatomy The brachial plexus originates from the ventral rami of C5–T1 and then travels inferiorly and laterally to form three trunks between the anterior and middle scalen-emuscles, where it may be targeted via the interscalene approach. The trunks then separate into the anterior and posterior divisions at the first rib lateral to the subclavian artery. This spot is the target for the supraclavicular approach. The divisions then travel under the clavicle to the axilla and form three cords surrounding the axillary artery, at which point they may be targeted via the infraclavicular approach. Finally, the cords give rise to the terminal branches at the axilla.

Technique [24] The block should be performed proximal to the site generating pain. For tumors invading the lung apex, the interscalene or supraclavicular approaches are often chosen. As with previous interventional techniques in this chapter, ultrasound has gained popularity over using anatomic landmarks solely. Nerve stimulation is, however, still a useful adjunct to ultrasound to identify and confirm the nerve bundle.

The patient is supine with the head turned to the opposi-tesite. Next, an echogenic needle is advanced, in-plane or out-of-plane, toward the target. After negative aspiration of blood or air, volumes of 10–20 ml of local anesthetic with or

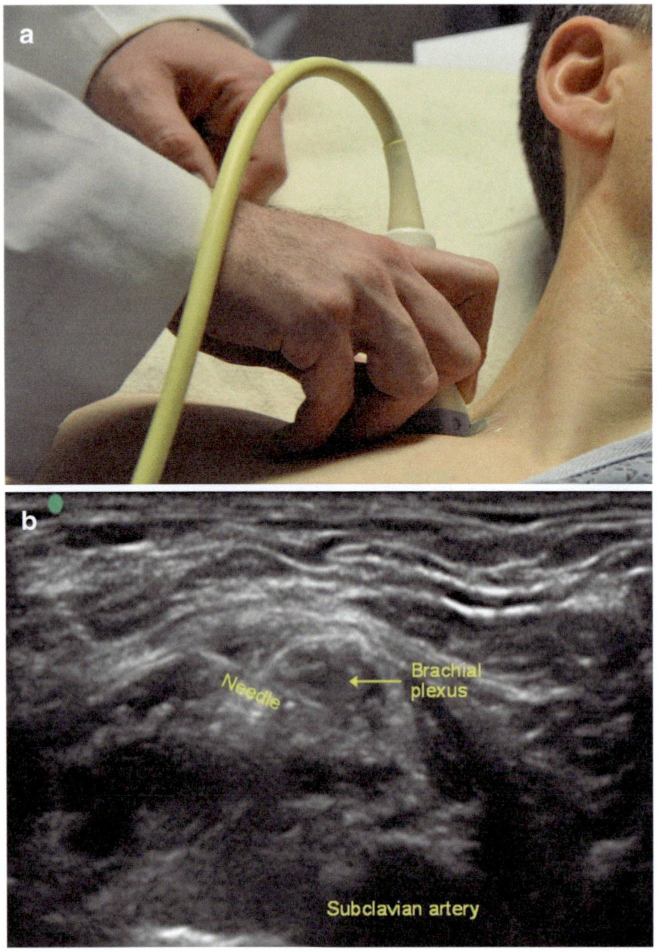

Fig. 18.7 (**a**) A transverse scan at supraclavicular fossa (left). (**b**) Sonographic image of the brachial plexus block for a patient with pancoast tumor at the supraclavicular level

without steroid are administered around the targeted neural structures [25].

Supraclavicular Approach To perform this block, scan transversely in the supraclavicular fossa at the mid-clavicle, and tilt the probe to identify subclavian artery beneath the clavicle. The brachial plexus at this level will appear as a mix of hypoechoic and hyperechoic round structures superior and lateral to the subclavian artery (Fig. 18.7).

Interscalene Approach The trunks of the brachial plexus can be identified by scanning lateral at the level of the cricoid cartilage to identify the anterior and middle scalene muscles. The three hypoechoic round structures between these two muscles will be the trunks of the brachial plexus. If visualization is difficult, the brachial plexus can be traced cephalad from the supraclavicular view (Fig. 18.8).

Benefit The senior author of this chapter presented a case series of single shot brachial plexus block with local anesthetic and corticosteroid to treat intractable pain from neoplastic brachial plexopathy [25]. The procedures were not associated with any immediate complications and in some cases provided pain relief for 4–8 weeks. This technique can be used as an analgesic bridge before the often-delayed pain relief expected following tumor shrinkage chemoradiation therapies. It can also be a bridge before the end-of-life palliative pain control, as well as a predictor for responsiveness to other interventions such as continuous blockade via an indwelling perineural catheter or nerve root ablation. Vranken et al. demonstrated that continuous brachial plexus block not only dramatically decreased pain scores and opioid

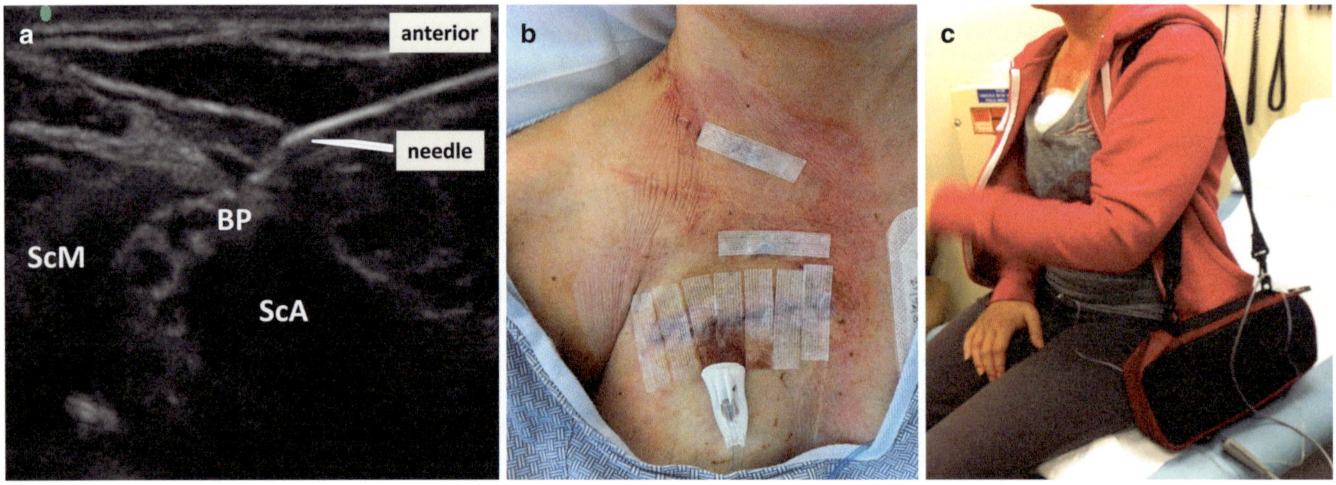

Fig. 18.8 (**a**) Sonographic image of an interscalene brachial plexus block with a catheter (left) (**b**) Port-a-Cath™ on patient's chest attached to the interscalene catheter (middle). (**c**) Ambulatory patient with interscalene catheter wearing a travel case containing bupivacaine reservoir (right)

consumption but also improved performance scores and quality of life in patients with intractable pain from neoplastic brachial plexopathy [26].

Complications Pneumothorax, local anesthetic systemic toxicity, intravascular injection, nerve injuries, diaphragmatic paralysis, Horner's syndrome, hematoma, and infection are all possible complications. For obvious reasons, neurolytic brachial plexus block may be associated with sensory and motor deficit and should therefore be preserved for terminal cancer patients.

Other Peripheral Nerve Blocks Case series and case reports also describe the use of other peripheral nerve blocks in selected cancer patients. For instance, the pudendal nerve block may be a diagnostic or therapeutic intervention for the treatment of pelvic pain. Like TAP block, pudendal nerve block done for pelvic pain may aid in the differentiation of pudendal neuralgia from visceral pelvic pain [27]. Pudendal nerve block may be performed at the ischial spine or the sacral nerve roots [28]. In the therapeutic context, the pudendal nerve block also often combined with the ganglion of impar block to cover both somatic and visceral pain.

Other case reports have also demonstrated significant pain relief following lumbar plexus neurolysis to treat metastatic disease to the hip [29]. Others have reported improvement of femoral bony metastatic pain with continuous femoral peripheral nerve blockade using a catheter tunneled to a subcutaneous injection port [30].

Cranial Nerve Block

Gasserian Ganglion Block

The Gasserian ganglion block may be used to treat malignant facial pain, as might occur from invasion of tumor into the orbit, maxillary sinus, or mandible. The Gasserian ganglion (trigeminal nerve ganglion) is located within Meckel's cave near the petrous part of the temporal bone and contains both sensory and motor from all three divisions of trigeminal nerve: ophthalmic, maxillary, and mandibular. The ganglion lies near vital structures including surrounding dura mater. Neurolytic procedures have been associated with significant adverse consequences including unintended injection of agent into CSF, deafness, and temporal fossa hemorrhage. Radio-frequency ablation or peripheral branch neurolysis (of the supraorbital, infraorbital, or mandibular nerves [31]) may be alternative options for the interventionist. The senior author of this chapter presented a case series of single shot Gasserian ganglion block with local anesthetic and corticosteroid to treat intractable pain from head and neck cancer with trigeminal nerve invasion. The procedures were not associated with any immediate complications and provided-pain relief for 2–6 weeks (Fig. 18.9) [32].

Other Cranial Nerve Blocks

Blocks for cancer-related pain include Kohase et al. reported mandibular nerve block used to treat tongue cancer invading the mandible and ultrasound neurolytic glossopharyngeal nerve block used to treat invasive squamous cell carcinoma at the base of the tongue [31, 33].

Nerve Root Block

Selective nerve root blockade with subsequent neurolysis [34] or epidural steroid injections [35] have been utilized to treat cancer-related pain. Engle et al. presented a case series of epidural steroid injections for the treatment of tumor-related radicular pain [35]. Quinn et al. reported case series of CT-guided nerve root ablation with alcohol in cancer-related pain [34]. Thoracic dermatomes have simpler anatomic patterns, and nerve roots in this region are not associated with significant motor function and thus may be safer to neurolyze.

In contrast, cervical and lumbosacral may be associated with motor deficits due to the complex innervation and major motor function. Gofeld and Bhatia reported significant success using cervical nerve root ablation as an alternative to brachial plexus blockade for pain related to Pancoast tumor [36]. Cok et al. reported benefit using sacral nerve root blockade as an alternative to pudendal nerve block. [28].

Autonomic Nerve Blocks

Stellate Ganglion Block

Malignant pain in the upper extremity, neck, and head may respond to stellate ganglion block. Common indications are ischemic neuropathies, shingles, and radiation-induced neuritis [37]. While the combined landmark and fluoroscopic technique is most commonly used today, the incorporation of ultrasound is gaining traction, in part given the multiple delicate structures in the neck not visualized on fluoroscopy (Fig. 18.10).

Evidence of a successful stellate ganglion block is synonymous with evidence of sympathetic blockade: a Horner's syndrome, anhidrosis, nasal congestion, as well as venodilation and a temperature increase by at least 1 °C in the affected upper extremities. Multiple complications are possible from wayward spread of the injected agent. If, for instance, local anesthetic spreads to the nearby recurrent laryngeal nerve, hoarseness or dyspnea may result.

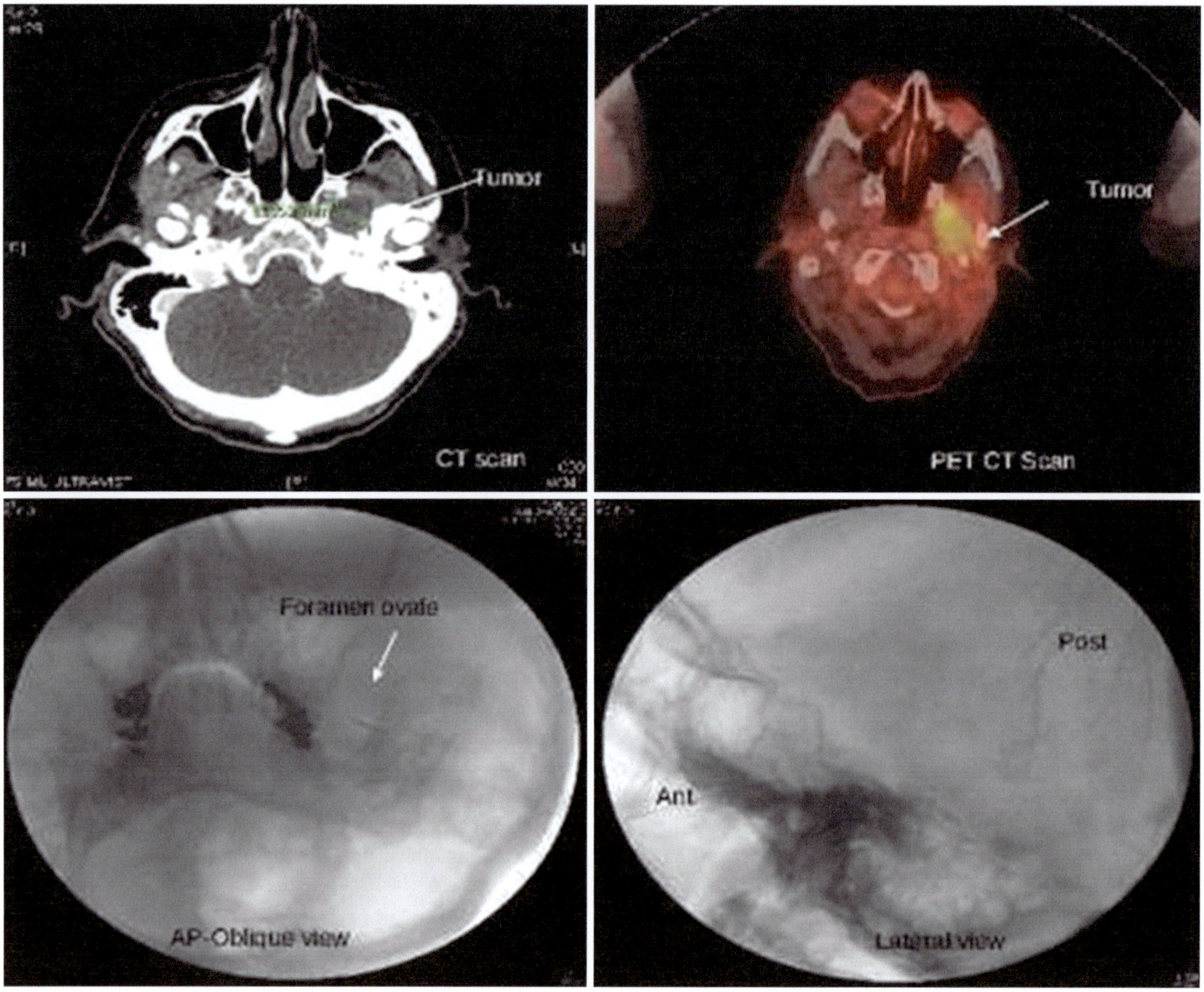

Fig. 18.9 Gasserian ganglion block for patient with facial pain from squamous cell carcinoma with trigeminal nerve invasion: CT scan and PET scan (upper left and right), fluoroscopic image of skull AP and lateral, focus at target of block, foramen ovale (lower left and right)

For this reason, stellate ganglion blocks should not be performed on both sides simultaneously and should be performed in caution with patients with known contralateral recurrent laryngeal nerve damage. Another common and related complication is spread of the agent to the phrenic nerve, resulting in unilateral diaphragmatic paresis. In a related vein, spread of the agent toward the brachial plexus may cause upper extremity sensory or motor deficits, requiring that the patient go home with an arm sling. More dire complications include unintended epidural or spinal blockade, usually the result of a too-lateral entry point combined with medial angulation of the needle. Of note, an epidural injection of a long-lasting local anesthetic may not result in evidence of an intended neuraxial blockade for 15 min or more; all patients undergoing this procedure should therefore be monitored closely for at least 30 min post-procedure. Finally, intravascular injection is always a concern. In the advent of injection into the vertebral artery, or, less likely, the carotid artery, a generalized seizure may occur [38].

Celiac Plexus Block

Malignant pain in abdominal viscera may be amenable to treatment with a celiac plexus block. Targeted structures include the pancreas, liver, gallbladder, omentum, mesentery, and alimentary tract from the stomach to the transverse colon. The most common indication for celiac plexus block is pain from pancreatic cancer and other intra-abdominal malignancies [39] given the strong evidence that this technique results in at least equal analgesia compared to medical

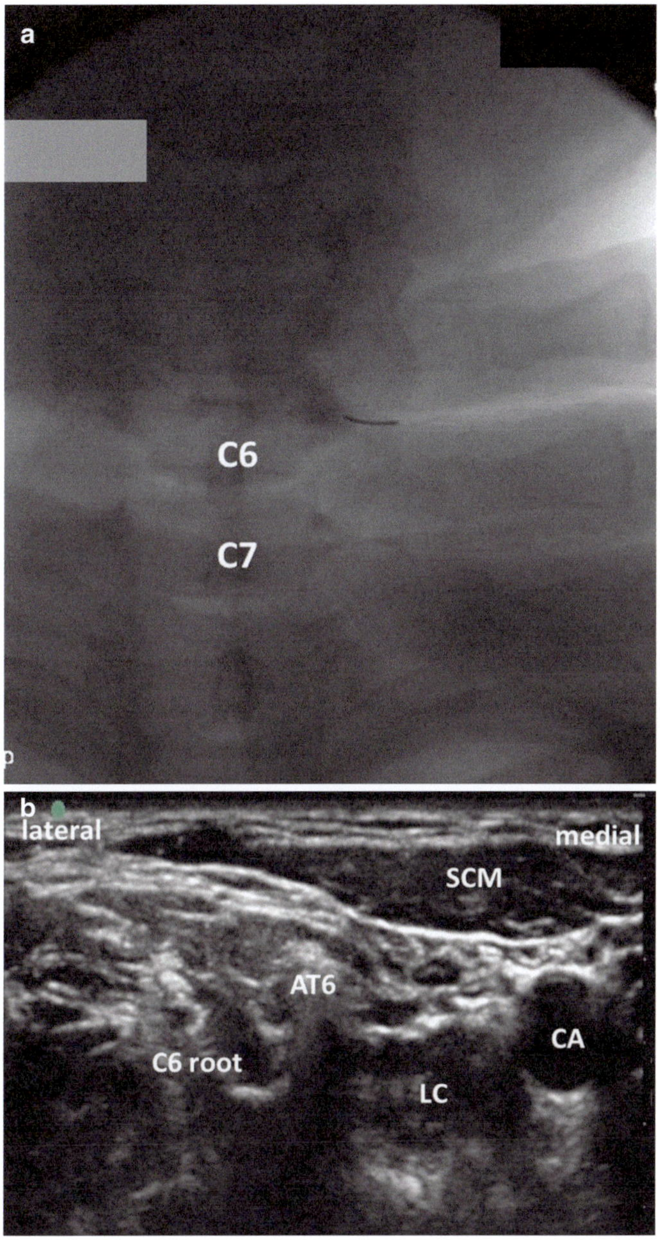

Fig. 18.10 (**a**) Fluoroscopic-guided stellate ganglion block (left), (**b**) Ultrasound imaging for a right stellate ganglion block. *SCM* sternocleidomastoid muscle, *AT6* anterior tubercle of C6 (Chassaignac's tubercle), *C6 root* C6 nerve root, *LC* longus coli muscle, *CA* carotid artery (right). Target for ultrasound-guided stellate ganglion block is a potential space between prevertebral fascia and longus coli muscle

therapy but has many fewer troubling adverse effects (e.g., the constipation, sedation from opioids) [40]. Prospective studies of patients with intra-abdominal malignancies have even shown that celiac sympathectomy results in improved pain control and higher quality of life before Step 2 of the WHO analgesic ladder [41].

The myriad techniques available to achieve celiac plexus block include guidance by fluoroscopy, CT, or ultrasound as well as direct surgical visualization. The classic technique is percutaneous, guided by fluoroscopy, with the patient in the prone position (Fig. 18.11).

An expected side effect of a celiac plexus block is diarrhea and cramping due to unopposed parasympathetic activity in the gastrointestinal tract as well as hypotension due to splanchnic vasodilation. The diarrhea and cramping are usually transient, resolving within a week; the hypotension usually responds to intravenous hydration. Complications include errant needles causing pneumothorax, retroperitoneal bleed, or perforation of other visceral organs. Most of the complications associated with this block, however, relate to intravascular injection into the aorta, celiac trunk, or artery of Adamkiewicz. Alcohol intoxication may occur with intravascular injection of ethanol; seizures and cardiovascular collapse, like the presentation of local anesthetic toxicity, may occur with the intravascular injection of phenol. The most feared complication, however, involves the artery of Adamkiewicz, which originates in most patients on the left side at around T12–L1 and supplies the anterior two-thirds of the spinal cord in the lumbar region. In the event of injection of neurolytic or particulate steroid into this vessel, paraplegia may result.

Superior Hypogastric Plexus Block

Malignant pain in the pelvic viscera may be treated with superior hypogastric plexus block. The applicable organs include the bladder, uterus, rectum, vagina, and prostate. While there are no randomized controlled trials assessing a superior hypogastric plexus neurolysis compared to medical management alone, prospective studies have shown that this technique results in a significant reduction of pain and opioid analgesic use in patients with pelvic malignancies [42].

The superior hypogastric plexus consists of sympathetic and parasympathetic fibers innervating the pelvic viscera and is located anterior to the L5 vertebral body, immediately below the aortic bifurcation (Fig. 18.12). As was the case in the celiac plexus, visceral pelvic afferents travel with the autonomic fibers and are therefore blocked at the superior hypogastric plexus [43].

Few large studies have examined the complications associated with superior hypogastric plexus block, but the most common would likely be intravascular injection into the iliac vessels, bladder puncture, or lumbar plexus injury given the proximity of these structures to the superior hypogastric plexus.

Ganglion of Impar Block

Malignant pain in the territory of the perineum, distal rectum, anus, distal third of the vagina, and vulva is among the targets of the ganglion of impar block. Small case series have demonstrated patients with pelvic pain receiving significant

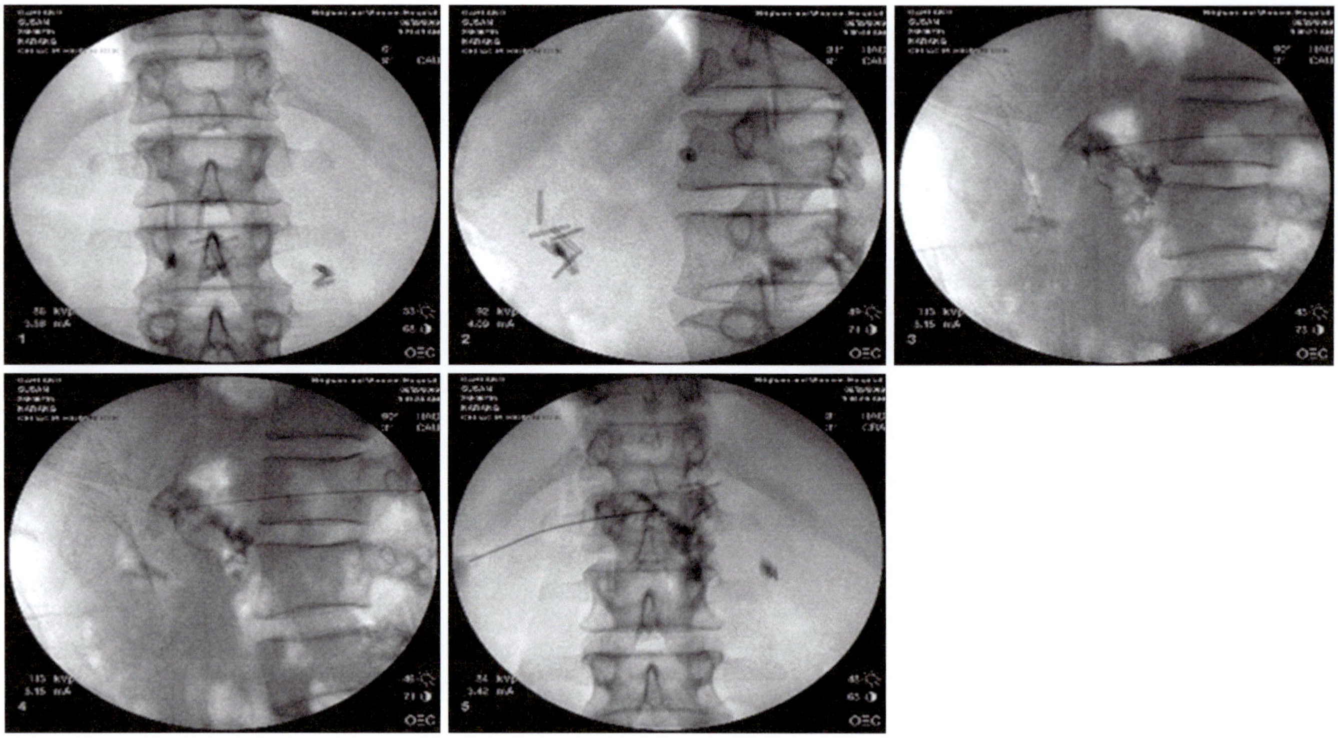

Fig. 18.11 Fluoroscopic-guided trans-aortic celiac plexus block

pain relief with the ganglion of impar block or neurolysis [44]. Other common indications include nonmalignant coccygodynia and chronic pelvic pain.

The ganglion of impar is the termination of the sympathetic chain, typically located anterior to the sacrococcygeal junction, though it has been observed in case reports to stray as far from this classic location as below the midpoint of the coccyx (Fig. 18.13).

There is little published data on the frequency of complications following this block. According to case reports and consideration of nearby anatomic structures, however, possible complications include retroperitoneal bleeding and damage to visceral organs. The original technique, for instance, via the ano-coccygeal ligament using a bent spinal needle, may have an increased risk of rectal perforation.

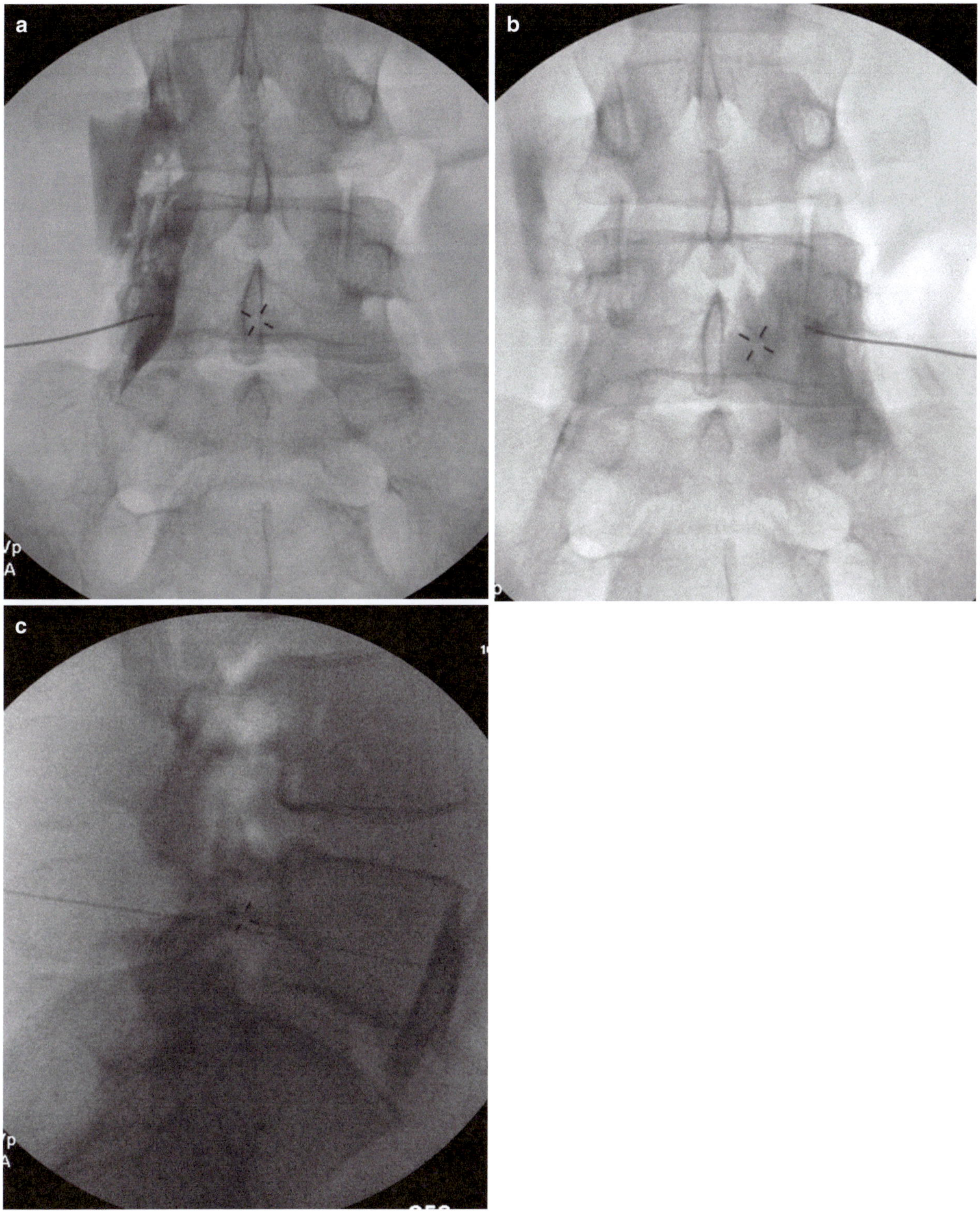

Fig. 18.12 (**a-c**) Fluoroscopic-guided hypogastric plexusblock

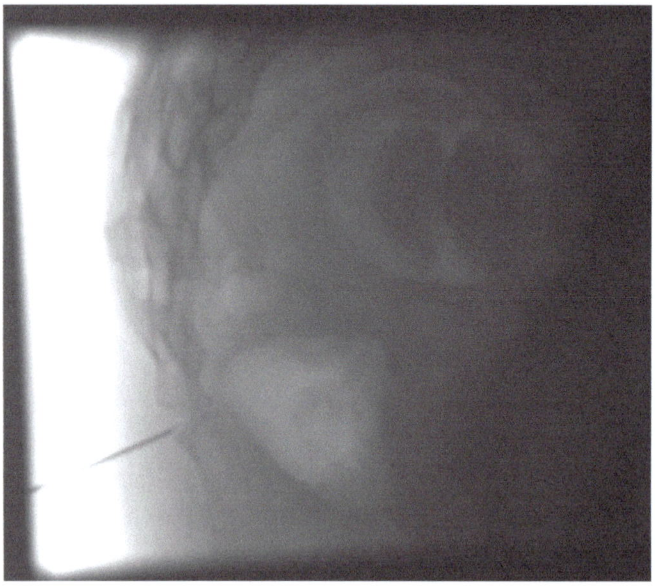

Fig. 18.13 Fluoroscopic-guided ganglion impar block

Conclusion

Knowledge in anatomy and regional anesthesia techniques used for the non-cancer patient can be applied for cancer-related pain. However, this specific population may present unique challenges in terms of distorted anatomy and frail physiology. Diagnostic and neurolytic nerve blocks can be widely applied in the oncologic population in those who have survived cancer as well as those with unfortunate terminal-stage disease. As cancer-related pain is usually multifactorial, multiple techniques may be required to control pain. The evidence suggests that nerve blocks are not only effectively alleviate pain, but some blocks may also be associated with improved quality of life, enhanced functional status, and even prolonged survival in cancer patients.

References

1. Anitescu M, Benzon H, Variakojis R. Pharmacology for the interventional pain physician. In: Benzon H, Rathmell J, Wu C, Turk D, Argoff C, Hurley R, editors. Practical management of pain. 5th ed. Philadelphia: Elsevier; 2014. p. 596–614.
2. Hotchkiss RS, Moldawer LL. Parallels between cancer and infectious disease. N Engl J Med. 2014;371(4):380–3.
3. Adams M, Benzon H, Hurley R. Chemical neurolysis blocks. In: Benzon H, Rathmell J, Wu C, Turk D, Argoff C, Hurley R, editors. Practical management of pain. 5th ed. Philadelphia: Elsevier; 2014. p. 784–93.
4. Collins A, Gray A. Peripheral nerve blocks. In: Miller R, Pardo M, editors. Basic of Anesthesia. 6th ed. Philadelphia: Elsevier; 2011. p. 284–99.
5. Schreiber KL, Martel MO, Shnol H, et al. Persistent pain in postmastectomy patients: comparison of psychophysical, medical, surgical, and psychosocial characteristics between patients with and without pain. Pain. 2013;154(5):660–8.
6. Klepstad P, Kurita GP, Mercadante S, Sjøgren P. The evidence of peripheral nerve blocks for cancer-related pain: a systematic review. Minerva Anestesiol. 2015;81(7):789–93.
7. Kirvelä O, Antila H. Thoracic paravertebral block in chronic postoperative pain. Reg Anesth. 1992;17(6):348–50.
8. Malik T. Ultrasound-guided paravertebral neurolytic block: a report of two cases. Pain Pract. 2014;14(4):346–9.
9. Hadzic A. Thoracic paravertebral block. In: Hadzic A, editor. Hadzic's peripheral nerve blocks and anatomy for ultrasound-guided regional anesthesia. New York: McGrawHill Medical; 2012. p. 291–302.
10. Karmakar M. Ultrasound-guided thoracic paravertebral block. In: Narouze S, editor. Atlas of ultrasound-guided procedures in interventional pain management. New York: Springer; 2010. p. 133–47.
11. Kakhki VR, Anvari K, Sadeghi R, Mahmoudian AS, Torabian-Kakhki M. Pattern and distribution of bone metastases in common malignant tumors. Nucl Med Rev Cent East Eur. 2013;16(2):66–9.
12. Hadzic A. Intercostal block. In: Hadzic A, editor. Hadzic's peripheral nerve blocks and anatomy for ultrasound-guided regional anesthesia. New York: McGrawHill Medical; 2012. p. 304–10.
13. Bhatia A, Peng P. Ultrasound-guided peripheral nerve blockade in chronic pain management. In: Narouze S, editor. Atlas of ultrasound-guided procedures in interventional pain management. New York: Springer; 2010. p. 279–92.
14. Wong FC, Lee TW, Yuen KK, Lo SH, Sze WK, Tung SY. Intercostal nerve blockade for cancer pain: effectiveness and selection of patients. Hong Kong Med J. 2007;13(4):266–70.
15. Narouze S. Ultrasound-Guided Transversus Abdominis Plane (TAP) block. In: Narouze S, editor. Atlas of ultrasound-guided procedures in interventional pain management. New York: Springer; 2010. p. 193–8.
16. Hebbard PD, Barrington MJ, Vasey C. Ultrasound-guided continuous oblique subcostal transversus abdominis plane blockade: description of anatomy and clinical technique. Reg Anesth Pain Med. 2010;35(5):436–41.
17. Hung JC, Azam N, Puttanniah V, Malhotra V, Gulati A. Neurolytic transversus abdominal plane block with alcohol for long-term malignancy related pain control. Pain Physician. 2014;17(6):E755–60.
18. Gebhardt R, Wu K. Transversus abdominis plane neurolysis with phenol in abdominal wall cancer pain palliation. Pain Physician. 2013;16(3):E325–30.
19. Restrepo-Garces CE, Asenjo JF, Gomez CM, et al. Subcostal transversus abdominis plane phenol injection for abdominal wall cancer pain. Pain Pract. 2014;14(3):278–82.
20. Sakamoto B, Kuber S, Gwirtz K, Elsahy A, Stennis M. Neurolytic transversus abdominis plane block in the palliative treatment of intractable abdominal wall pain. J Clin Anesth. 2012;24(1):58–61.
21. Davis G, Knight S. Pancoast tumors. Neurosurg Clin N Am. 2008;19(4):545–57.
22. Watson P, Evans R. Intractable pain with lung cancer. Pain. 1987;29(2):163–73.
23. Wood J, Gawler J, Whittle RJ, Staunton MD. Brachial plexopathy in breast carcinoma-an unsolved problem. Eur J Surg Oncol. 1991;17:265–9.
24. Hadzic A. Ultrasound-guided interscalene brachial plexus block. In: Hadzic A, editor. Hadzic's peripheral nerve blocks and anatomy for ultrasound-guided regional anesthesia. New York: McGrawHill Medical; 2012. p. 353–60.
25. Zinboonyahgoon N, Vlassakov K, Abrecht CR, Srinivasan S, Narang S. Brachial plexus block for Cancer-related pain: a case series. Pain Physician. 2015;18(5):E917–24.
26. Vranken J, van der Vegt M, Zuurmond W, Pijl AJ, Dzoljic M. Continuous brachial plexus block at the cervical level using a

posterior approach in the management of neuropathic cancer pain. Reg Anesth Pain Med. 2001;26(6):572–5.
27. Elahi F, Callahan D, Greenlee J, Dann TL. Pudendal entrapment neuropathy: a rare complication of pelvic radiation therapy. Pain Physician. 2013;16(6):E793–7.
28. Cok OY, Eker HE, Cok T, Akin S, Aribogan A, Arslan G. Transsacral S2–S4 nerve block for vaginal pain due to pudendal neuralgia. J Minim Invasive Gynecol. 2011;18(3):401–4.
29. Kaki AM, Lewis GW. Inguinal paravascular (lumbar plexus) neurolytic block – description of a catheter technique: case report. Reg Anesth Pain Med. 1998;23(2):214–8.
30. Khor KE, Ditton JN. Femoral nerve blockade in the multidisciplinary management of intractable localized pain due to metastatic tumor: a case report. J Pain Symptom Manag. 1996;11(1):57–6.
31. Kohase H, Umino M, Shibaji T, Suzuki N. Application of a mandibular nerve block using an indwelling catheter for intractable cancer pain. Acta Anaesthesiol Scand. 2004;48(3):382–3.
32. Srinivasan S, Issa M, Narang S. The use of gasserian ganglion block in neoplastic trigeminal neuralgia – a case series. Poster presented at ASRA annual meeting; 11/2013: Phoenix, AZ.
33. Bedder MD, Lindsay D. Glossopharyngeal nerve block using ultrasound guidance: a case report of a new technique. Reg Anesth. 1989;14(6):304–7.
34. Quinn SF, Murtagh FR, Chatfield R, Kori SH. CT-guided nerve root block and ablation. AJR Am J Roentgenol. 1988;151(6):1213–6.
35. Shah K, Novy D, Koyyalakunta D, Chai T, Bruel B, Yu J, Dong W, Engle M. The effectiveness and safety of epidural steroid injections for the tumor related radicular pain. Oral presentation at the third annual meeting cancer pain research consortium. Phoenix; 4/2017.
36. Gofeld M, Bhatia A. Alleviation of Pancoast's tumor pain by ultrasound-guided percutaneous ablation of cervical nerve roots. Pain Pract. 2008;8(4):314–9.
37. Keel JC, Bodas AV. Chapter 147: interventional pain management I: epidural, ganglion, and nerve blocks. In: Vacanta CA, Sikka PK, Urman RD, Segal BS, editors. Essential clinical anesthesia. 1st ed. Cambridge: Cambridge University Press; 2011. p. 907–18.
38. Rathmell JP. Chapter 10: stellate ganglion block. In: Rathmell JP, editor. Atlas of image-guided intervention in regional anesthesia and pain medicine. 2nd ed. Philadelphia: Lippincott Williams & Wilkins; 2011. p. 115–21.
39. Srinivasan S, Zinboonyahgoon N, Narang N. Celiac plexus block for non-pancreatic intra-abdominal malignancies – results and outcomes. Poster presented at NYOSRA annual meeting; 2014: New York, NY.
40. Arcidiacono PG, Calori G, Carrara S, et al. Celiac plexus block for pancreatic cancer pain in adults. Cochrane Database Syst Rev. 2011;16(3):CD007519.
41. Amr YM, Makharita MY. Neurolytic sympathectomy in the management of cancer pain-time effect: a prospective, randomized multicenter study. J Pain Symptom Manag. 2014;48(5):944.
42. Plancarte R, de Leon-Casasola OA, El-Helaly M, Allende S, Lema MJ. Neurolytic superior hypogastric plexus block for chronic pelvic pain associated with cancer. Reg Anesth. 1997;22(6):562.
43. Rathmell JP. Chapter 13: superior hypogastric block and neurolysis. In: Rathmell JP, editor. Atlas of image-guided intervention in regional anesthesia and pain medicine. 2nd ed. Philadelphia: Lippincott Williams & Wilkins; 2011. p. 143–9.
44. Scott-Warren JT, Hill V, Rajasekaran A. Ganglion impar blockade: a review. Curr Pain Headache Rep. 2013;17:306.

19 Cranial Nerve Targets

Jill E. Sindt

Introduction

Cancers of the head and neck account for less than 5% of cancers diagnosed in the United States, with approximately 75,000 new cases each year [1]. However cancer-associated pain occurs in 70–85% of these patients and is rated among the worst symptoms of the cancer [2, 3]. Patients rate pain control just behind achieving a cure and living as long as possible as their priorities after diagnosis [4]. Pain is associated with decreased quality of life for patients and increases in prevalence and intensity as the cancer progresses [5, 6].

Head and neck cancers are a heterogeneous group of diagnoses that affect a variety of anatomic locations and tissue types. Cancers of the thyroid, larynx, oropharynx, tongue, and soft tissue account for the majority of cases, but cancer can also occur in the salivary gland, nose and nasopharynx, lip, bone, and larynx [1]. More than 90% of tumors in the head and neck are squamous cell carcinomas [7].

Pain from head and neck cancer can result from several different mechanisms. It can be nociceptive, neuropathic, or referred in character. Pain can result from direct tumor invasion of nearby soft tissue, mucosa, and bone as well as involvement in nervous system structures. It can also occur as a consequence of treatment. Surgery can result in chronic infection, difficulties with wound healing, and nerve damage. Radiation can cause tissue fibrosis and plexopathy, and both radiation and chemotherapy can lead to neuropathy and mucositis [8].

Treatment of cancer-associated head and neck pain is based on the World Health Organization's Cancer Pain Relief Ladder emphasizing a stepwise method utilizing increasingly potent opioids in combination with non-opioid adjunct medications. In addition to medication management, many patients benefit from interventional techniques addressing specific underlying sources of pain. Targets for intervention discussed below and summarized in Table 19.1 include cranial nerve as well as peripheral nerves.

Cranial Nerve Targets

Trigeminal Nerve: Anatomy and Innervation

The trigeminal nerve is the fifth cranial nerve and is responsible for sensation over much of the face as well as motor function of the muscles of mastication. It arises from the brainstem at the level of the pons. It then joins the gasserian or trigeminal ganglion in the middle cranial fossa in a region known as Meckel's cave, an invagination of the dura in a depression in the petrous apex. The trigeminal nerve then divides into its three primary branches: the ophthalmic nerve (V1), the maxillary nerve (V2), and the mandibular nerve (V3). These branches exit the skull through the superior orbital fissure, foramen rotundum, and foramen ovale, respectively.

The ophthalmic nerve is a pure sensory nerve and innervates the skin of the scalp, forehead, upper eyelid, and tip of the nose as well as the conjunctiva, cornea, and frontal sinuses. It branches into frontal, lacrimal, and nasociliary nerves. The frontal nerve further divides into its terminal branches, the supraorbital and supratrochlear nerves, both of which are amenable to procedural intervention.

The maxillary nerve is also a sensory nerve and provides sensory innervation to the skin of the cheek, lower eyelid, nares, and upper lip as well as the upper teeth and gums, the palate and roof of the pharynx and the nasal mucosa and maxillary, and ethmoid and sphenoid sinuses. Shortly after leaving the trigeminal ganglion, the zygomatic and superior alveolar nerves branch off, and it continues on as the infraorbital nerve.

The mandibular nerve has both motor and sensory functions. It supplies sensory innervation to the chin, jaw, lower

J. E. Sindt, MD (✉)
University of Utah, Department of Anesthesiology, Salt Lake City, UT, USA
e-mail: jill.sindt@hsc.utah.edu

A. Gulati et al. (eds.), *Essentials of Interventional Cancer Pain Management*, https://doi.org/10.1007/978-3-319-99684-4_19

Table 19.1 Summary of head and neck interventional targets

Nerve	Innervation/Function	Interventional techniques
Trigeminal ganglion	Sensory innervation to skin of face and motor innervation to muscles of mastication	Nerve block Chemical neurolysis Pulsed radiofrequency ablation Balloon compression Cryoablation
Maxillary nerve	Sensory innervation of middle 1/3 of face	Nerve block Chemical neurolysis Pulsed radiofrequency ablation Cryoablation
Mandibular nerve	Sensory innervation of lower 1/3 of the face Motor innervation of the muscles of mastication	Nerve block Chemical Neurolysis Pulsed radiofrequency ablation Cryoablation
Supraorbital nerve	Sensory innervation of forehead, upper eyelid, and anterior scalp	Nerve block Pulsed radiofrequency ablation Peripheral nerve stimulation Cryoablation
Supratrochlear nerve	Sensory innervation of medial forehead, bridge of nose, medial upper eyelid	Nerve block Pulsed radiofrequency ablation Peripheral nerve stimulation Cryoablation
Infraorbital nerve	Sensory innervation of lower eyelid, medial cheek, lateral naris, upper lip	Nerve block Chemical neurolysis Pulsed radiofrequency ablation Cryoablation
Mental nerve	Sensory innervation of lower lip and chin	Nerve block Chemical neurolysis Pulsed radiofrequency ablation Cryoablation
Glossopharyngeal nerve	Sensory innervation of the external ear, posterior pharynx and tongue, and carotid body and sinus Parasympathetic innervation to the parotid gland Motor innervation to the stylopharyngeus muscle	Nerve block Chemical neurolysis Pulsed radiofrequency ablation
Vagus nerve	Sensory innervation of the external auditory meatus and mucosa of the larynx and vocal cords Motor innervation of the pharyngeal and laryngeal muscles Parasympathetic innervation to intrathoracic and abdominal organs	Nerve block Chemical neurolysis Pulsed radiofrequency ablation
Sphenopalatine ganglion	Sensory innervation of the nasal and palatine mucosa, soft palate, pharynx and lacrimal gland	Nerve block Chemical neurolysis Thermal radiofrequency ablation Pulsed radiofrequency ablation
Temporomandibular joint	Rotational and translational movement of the jaw, including mastication and opening of the jaw	Intraarticular joint injection
Greater and lesser occipital nerve	Sensory innervation to the posterior scalp	Nerve block Thermal radiofrequency ablation Pulsed radiofrequency ablation Cryoablation Peripheral nerve stimulation
Superficial cervical plexus	Sensory innervation of the lower mandible, anterolateral neck and supraclavicular fossa	Nerve block
Deep cervical plexus	Sensory innervation of the lower mandible, anterolateral neck, and supraclavicular fossa Motor innervation of the paravertebral and deep muscles of the neck. Provides motor fibers to phrenic and spinal accessory nerves	Nerve block

lip, external ear, lower teeth, and gums via the auriculotemporal, lingual, buccal, inferior alveolar, and mental nerves. Its branches also innervate the muscles of mastication including the temporal, masseter, lateral pterygoid, and medial pterygoid muscles [9]. (Fig. 19.1).

Trigeminal Nerve: Procedural Interventions

The trigeminal nerve and its branches can be targeted at multiple sites depending on the pain location and reason for pain as summarized in Table 19.2.

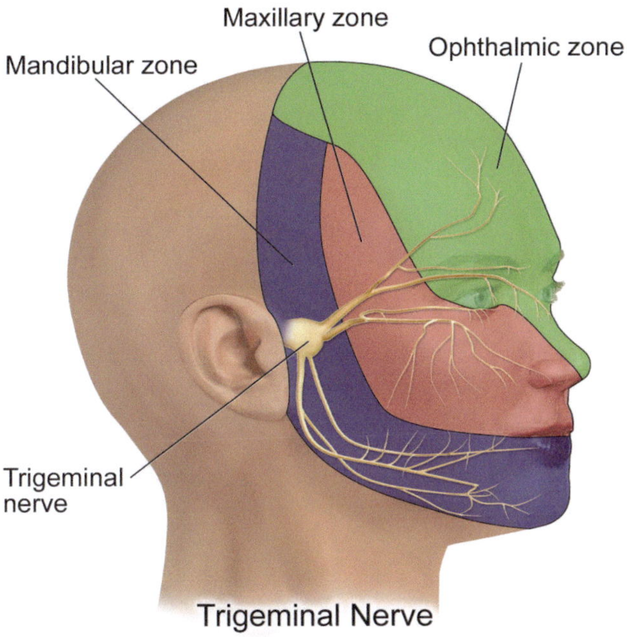

Fig. 19.1 Trigeminal nerve distribution Madhero88 (https://commons.wikimedia.org/wiki/File:Trig_innervation.svg), "Trig innervation," https://creativecommons.org/licenses/by/3.0/legalcode

Table 19.2 Summary of trigeminal nerve targets

Anatomic target	Innervation
Trigeminal ganglion	Sensory innervation of the face Motor innervation of muscles of mastication
Maxillary nerve	Sensory innervation of middle 1/3 of the face
Mandibular nerve	Sensory innervation of lower 1/3 of the face Motor innervation of muscles of mastication
Supraorbital nerve	Sensory innervation of forehead, upper eyelid, and anterior scalp
Supratrochlear nerve	Sensory innervation of medial forehead, bridge of nose, medial upper eyelid
Infraorbital nerve	Sensory innervation of lower eyelid, medial cheek, lateral naris, upper lip
Mental nerve	Sensory innervation of lower lip and chin

Trigeminal (Gasserian) Ganglion Neurolysis

Clinical Indications Trigeminal ganglion neurolysis is most commonly used as a treatment for trigeminal neuralgia; however it has been used successfully for cancer patients with pain that is located in areas supplied by the trigeminal nerve. Pain amenable to this approach is often described as a burning or lancing pain in the midface with extension into the forehead or mandible area. It is best performed early in the course of head and neck cancer before significant anatomic distortion is present. Pain relief typically lasts months and the procedure can berepeated if necessary.

Anatomic Considerations The trigeminal ganglion is accessed via the foramen ovale. It is bound medially by the cavernous sinus, superiorly by the temporal bone, and posteriorly by the dura and brainstem. In addition the area is highly vascular, and the middle meningeal and carotid arteries lie in the vicinity of the ganglion. Fluoroscopic guidance should be used to minimize the risks of encountering these structures, and care must also be taken to avoid penetration of the oral cavity during needle advancement [10]. While the success rate for trigeminal neurolysis for cancer-related pain is unknown, pain relief is reported in 80–90% of patients with trigeminal neuralgia who undergo the procedure, though recurrence of pain occurs in 20–50% of these patients within 1–2 years [11].

Procedure Description The patient is placed supine on the fluoroscopy table with the cervical spine slightly extended. Moderate sedation is used. Skin entry should be approximately 2.5 cm lateral to the corner of mouth. C-arm is used to identify the foramen ovale using an approximately 30 ° caudal angulation and 20 ° lateral oblique rotation. In this view the foramen will appear as an oval-shaped area just inferior to the orbit and lateral to the ethmoid sinuses (see Fig. 19.2). The needle is advanced toward the foramen ovale under fluoroscopic guidance. The trajectory of the needle should be in line with the pupil of the eye and cephalad toward the external auditory meatus at an angle of 30–45 ° at the skin (see Fig. 19.3). The foramen ovale is sometimes difficult to identify with fluoroscopy, in particular if the anatomy has been altered by tumor or cancer treatment. In these cases initial advancement of the needle using the skin site and trajectory described above may help to more clearly identify the foramen ovale.

The needle is advanced until lateral view shows appropriate placement in the foramen ovale, directly inferior to the sella turcica (see Fig. 19.4). Often contact with bone is made first, at which point the needle should be "walked off" the bone usually posteriorly until it enters the foramen. Patients may experience a paresthesia in the distribution of the mandibular nerve as the needle enters the foramen.

After negative aspiration for blood and CSF, contrast administration (0.1–0.5 mL) should be used to verify correct placement of the needle in the foramen. Local anesthetic blockade can be performed at this time with 0.1–0.5 mL of local anesthetic for an "on the table" trial if desired. Neurolysis can then be completed. Volumes of 0.3–0.5 mL are usually adequate and should not exceed 1 mL to avoid-spread to other structures. Absolute alcohol, 6–10% phenol, and sterile glycerol have all been used successfully. Phenol has the advantage of painless application, near-immediate onset, and less spread to other structures due to its viscosity.

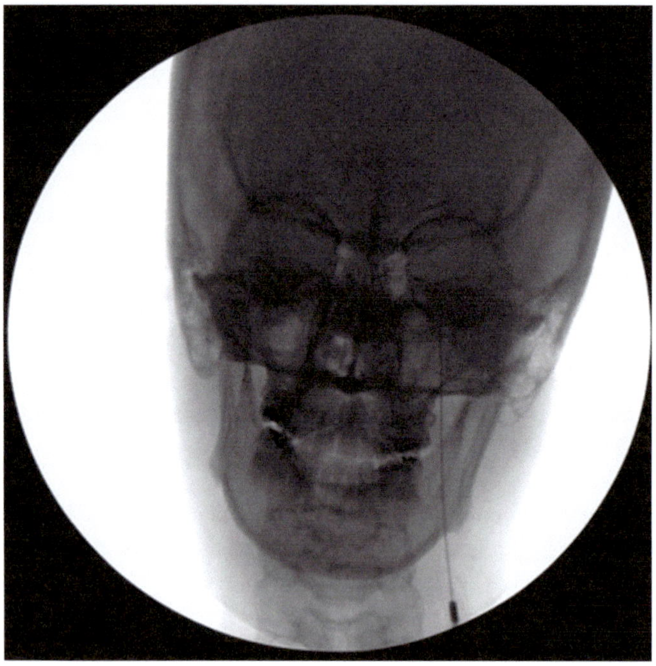

Fig. 19.2 Fluoroscopic view of the foramen ovale with needle in place – AP view

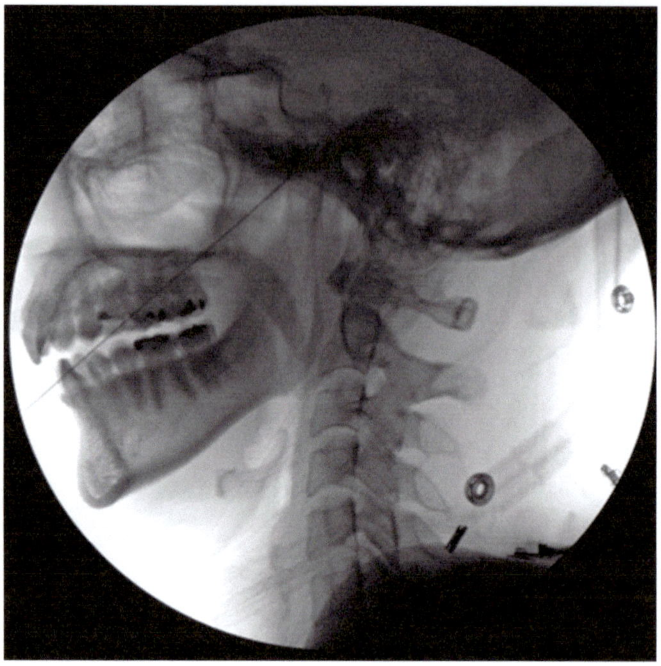

Fig. 19.4 Fluoroscopic view of the foramen ovale with needle in place – lateral view

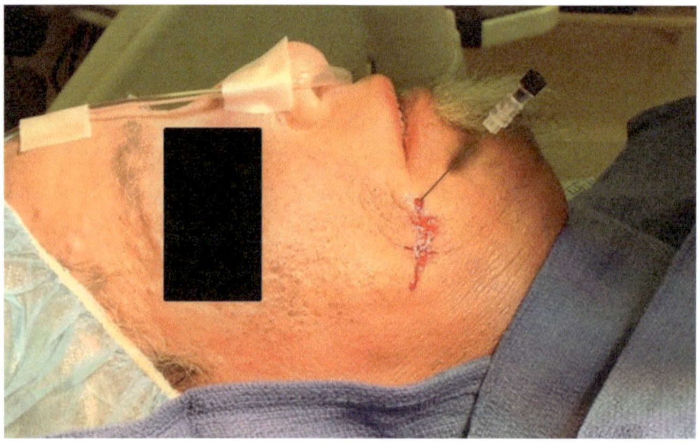

Fig. 19.3 Skin insertion site for trigeminal ganglion block

Glycerol may not produce analgesia for 6–10 days but may result in a longer duration and is the most commonly used agent for trigeminal ganglion neurolysis [12]. If glycerol is used, the patient should be moved to the sitting position with the head tipped downward prior to injection and should remain in this position for 2 h after the procedure to avoid unwanted spread to other areas.

If CSF is encountered with advancement of the needle, the tip can be slowly withdrawn until CSF is no longer aspirated and neurolysis can proceed as above, with any medication administered in aliquots of 0.1 mL and careful observation due to the risks of high spinal or spread of the neurolytic agent to the brainstem. Alternatively the needle can be left in place, and a retrogasserian approach can be employed by injecting up to 0.5 mL of glycerol in aliquots of 0.1 mL. The patient is moved to the sitting position with head tipped downward prior to injection and remains in this position for 2 h after the procedure to prevent glycerol spread to the brainstem. This technique is well described and safe when performed correctly and may permit more selective destruction of maxillary and mandibular distributions due to glycerol's hyperbaricity [13] (Figs. 19.2, 19.3, and 19.4).

Side Effects/Complications Due to the vascular nature of the area, subscleral and facial hematoma may occur. Numbness of the face also occurs commonly, and patients should be warned about facial asymmetry and weakness of the muscles of mastication, though this is rarely clinically relevant. Trigeminal ganglion neurolysis can lead to reactivation of herpes labialis or herpes zoster in a significant percentage of patients. Neurolysis of the ophthalmic division may produce impairment of the corneal reflex and corneal anesthesia, which in severe cases can lead to keratitis and vision impairment. Dysesthesia has been reported in 6–44% of subjects, and anesthesia dolorosa is a rare but potential complication of trigeminal neurolysis [14].

Trigeminal (Gasserian) Ganglion Radiofrequency Ablation

Clinical Indications Trigeminal ganglion radiofrequency lesioning is performed for the same clinical indications as trigeminal ganglion neurolysis as above. It is done most frequently for trigeminal neuralgia, but it has been used successfully for cancer-associated pain [15]. Radiofrequency ablation may allow for more selective destruction of one trigeminal division and eliminates the risks of spread of neurolytic agents to nearby structures [10]. It also may result in longer duration of analgesia as compared tochemical neurolysis [13].

Anatomic Considerations Trigeminal ganglion radiofrequency ablation is performed using the same trans-foramen ovale approach as trigeminal ganglion chemical neurolysis; thus anatomic considerations are identical to those previously described.

Procedure Description The foramen ovale is accessed in the same method as described above for trigeminal ganglion chemical neurolysis. Once the cannula is appropriately positioned by fluoroscopic guidance and aspiration is negative for CSF or blood sensory stimulation at 50 Hz with 0.1–0.5 V should be performed to confirm placement, and the patient should note sensation in the appropriate division. Next motor stimulation at 2 Hz with 0.5–1.5 V should be performed. If the needle is in proximity to the mandibular division, contraction of the ipsilateral muscles of the lower mandible will be observed. If the needle is in proximity to the ophthalmic or maxillary division, no motor response will be observed [16].

Thermal radiofrequency ablation is the most common method of RF used for trigeminal ablation. Lesioning is delivered in 60- to 90-s cycles at 60–90 C until the patient develops hypoalgesia, as evidenced by perception of sharp pinprick as light touch in the corresponding area. Facial flushing in the corresponding division(s) may also occur. Up to 1 mL of lidocaine in divided doses should be injected prior to lesioning to ease the pain of thermal ablation with careful monitoring for intravascular and intrathecal injection.

Pulsed radiofrequency ablation has also been described using 2–3 cycles of lesioning at 42 °C for 120 s. Pulsed radiofrequency ablation is postulated to result in a lower incidence of dysesthesia following the procedure, but less data is available on efficacy or complications as compared to thermal radiofrequency ablation [11]. Administration of local anesthetic prior to lesioning is not required due to the lower temperature used in pulsed radiofrequency.

Side Effects/Complications Similar complications occur with radiofrequency ablation of the trigeminal ganglion as chemical neurolysis, though without risks of neurolytic agent spreading to unwanted areas. There have been reports of hematoma, facial numbness, weakness of the muscles of mastication, reactivation of herpes infections, and corneal anesthesia as complications. However the incidence of dysesthesia and anesthesia dolorosa may be lower than chemical neurolysis [17, 18]. In addition stimulation or lesioning of the trigeminal ganglion may result in acute bradycardia; atropine and cardiopulmonary resuscitation equipment should be immediately available.

Trigeminal (Gasserian) Ganglion Balloon Compression

Clinical Indications Trigeminal ganglion balloon compression is performed for the same clinical indications as trigeminal ganglion neurolysis and radiofrequency ablation as above. Success rate when performed for trigeminal neuralgia is above 90%, and recurrence may be lower with balloon compression as compared with other methods of trigeminal ganglion procedures [19].

Anatomic Considerations Similar to those for trigeminal ganglion radiofrequency ablation.

Procedure Description Balloon compression is usually completed under general anesthesia. The foramen ovale is accessed in a similar method as described above for trigeminal ganglion chemical neurolysis, though the needle is placed so that just the tip of the needle engages in the foramen ovale. This is often accompanied by significant bradycardia, and atropine and cardiopulmonary resuscitation equipment should be immediately available. A Fogarty catheter is the placed through the needle into Meckel's cave and inflated with contrast medium under fluoroscopic visualization until a pear-shaped image is observed with the stem end facing posteriorly, indicating that the balloon is occupying the entire cave and adequate compression is occurring. Compression times of 2–7 min have been used. The catheter and needle are then removed.

Side Effects/Complications Similar complications occur with radiofrequency ablation of the trigeminal ganglion as radiofrequency ablation, though studies indicate lower rates of complications, in particular dysesthesia and anesthesia dolorosa, as compared to other trigeminal ganglion procedures [20].

Selective Maxillary Nerve Block and Radiofrequency Ablation

Clinical Indications For patients suffering from pain limited to the maxillary nerve distribution of the trigeminal nerve, the maxillary nerve can be selectively blocked using a lateral coronoid approach. Anestheticnerve block can be used for diagnostic purposes, and steroid is often added to local anesthetic for therapeutic benefit. Pulsed radiofrequency ablation has also been reported with successful treatment of trigeminal neuralgia in the maxillary distribution [21].

Anatomic Considerations The maxillary nerve exits the middle cranial fossa via the foramen rotundum and then traverses the pterygopalatine fossa. The nerve can be selectively blocked in the anterior portion of the pterygopalatine fossa before it passes through the inferior orbital fissure and emerges onto the surface of the face through the infraorbital foramen. A lateral approach via the coronoid notch is used (see Fig. 19.5) [22].

Procedure Description The patient is placed supine on the fluoroscopy table with a neutral neck position, and the patient is asked to slightly open their jaw into a "slack jaw" position to facilitate identification of the coronoid notch just anterior to the external auditory meatus and inferior to the zygomatic arch. A lateral fluoroscopic view is used to identify the pterygopalatine fossa as a V-shaped structure superior to the upper molars and inferior to the orbit. Side-to-side rotation of the head may be used to help identify the fossa and align it fluoroscopically with the pterygopalatine fossa on the contralateral side of the head for appropriate positioning.

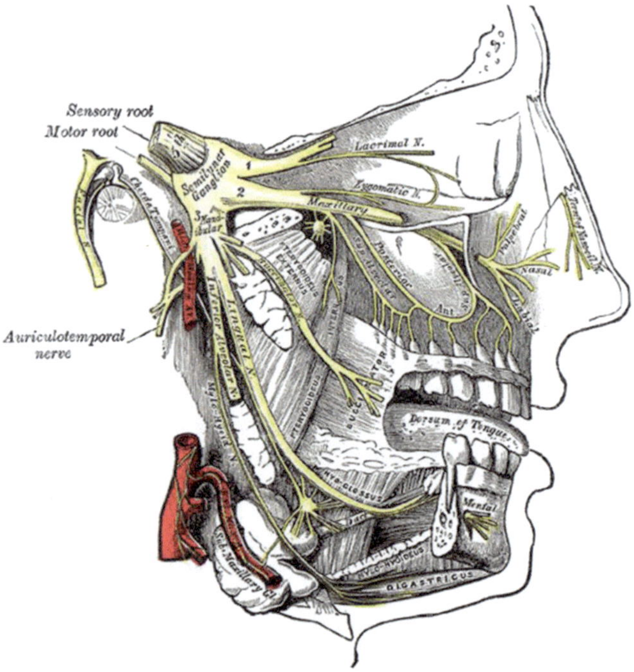

Fig. 19.5 Anatomic course of the maxillary nerve. (From Henry Gray (1918) *Anatomy of the Human Body* via Wikipedia Commons. https://commons.wikimedia.org/wiki/Trigeminal_nerve#/media/File:Gray778.png. In public domain)

The needle is inserted in the coronoid notch and directed in a plane perpendicular to the skull toward the pterygopalatine fossa, usually 4–5 cm. Often the lateral pterygopalatine plate is encountered, and the needle should then be redirected anteriorly and superiorly and advanced approximately 0.5–1 cm to enter the pterygopalatine fossa. Maxillary nerve paresthesia often occurs with this advancement. The needle should be directed to the superior anterior part of the pterygopalatine fossa (see Fig. 19.6). On AP fluoroscopic view, the needle should be lateral to the middle nasal turbinate (see Fig. 19.7) Contrast can be used to confirm appropriate placement.

If anesthetic blockade is desired, 3 to 5 mL of local anesthetic is injected in divided doses with patient monitoring. Steroid, such as depot methylprednisolone 40–80 mg, is often added to the local anesthetic. Chemical neurolysis for palliation of severe cancer pain has been reported anecdotally using phenol or alcohol by some practitioners, but no case reports or studies have been published.

If pulsed radiofrequency ablation isused, sensory stimulation at 50 Hz with 0.1–1 V should be performed, and the patient should experience the stimulation in the upper teeth and/or over the skin of the midface. Lesioning is then performed at 42 °C for 90 s. Two to three rounds of lesioning are often performed for improved efficacy.

Side Effects/Complications Due to thevascular nature of the area, facial hematoma is a common side effect. Dysesthesia may occur, and anesthesia dolorosa is possible, though it has not been reported in the literature.

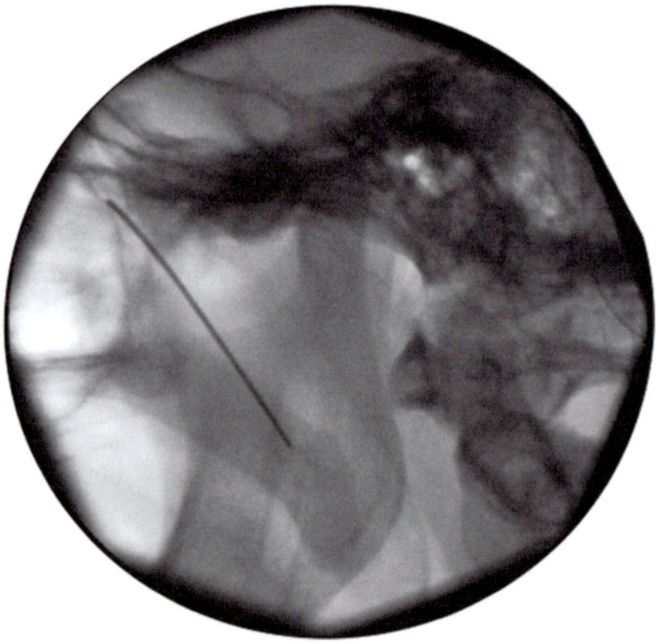

Fig. 19.6 Lateral view of maxillary nerve block with needle in the superior anterior part of the pterygopalatine fossa

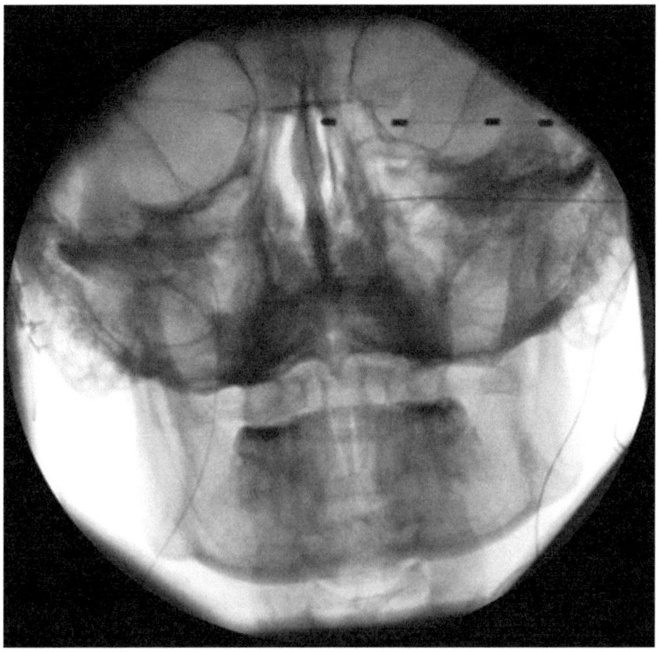

Fig. 19.7 AP view of maxillary nerve block

Selective Mandibular Nerve Block and Radiofrequency Ablation

Clinical Indications For patients suffering from pain limited to the mandibular nerve distribution of the trigeminal nerve, the mandibular nerve can be selectively blocked also using a lateral coronoid approach. Anesthetic nerve block can be used for diagnostic purposes, and steroid can be added to local anesthetic for therapeutic benefit [23]. Chemical neurolysis with 0.4–1 mL of alcohol or phenol has been used successfully for trigeminal neuralgia and cancer-associated pain, as has an indwelling continuous local anesthetic infusion via catheter and pulsed radiofrequency ablation [24–26].

Anatomic Considerations The mandibular nerve is composed of a large sensory root and smaller motor root. These roots combine shortly after exiting the middle cranial fossa via the foramen ovale to form the mandibular nerve. It then descends inferior to the lateral pterygoid plate, at which point it can be blocked beforedividing into its terminal branches. A lateral approach via the coronoid notch is used.

Procedure Description The patient is placed supine on the fluoroscopy table with a neutral neck position, and the patient is asked to slightly open their jaw into a "slack jaw" position to facilitate identification of the coronoid notch just anterior to the external auditory meatus and inferior to the mandible. An AP fluoroscopic view is usedto guide needle placement.

The needle is inserted in the coronoid notch and directed in a plane perpendicular to the skull until the lateral pterygopalatine plate is encountered. The needle is then redirected posteriorly and inferiorly advanced approximately 0.5–1 cm to slip past the inferior edge of the lateral pterygoid plate. Mandibular nerve paresthesia is often encountered and used to confirm appropriate positioning of the needle. Local anesthetic blockade can be accomplished with 3–5 mL of local anesthetic with or without depot steroid. Pulsed radiofrequency lesioning can be performed following sensory stimulation at 50 Hz with 0.1–1 V confirming appropriate mandibular distribution of stimulation and motor stimulation at 2 Hz with 0.5–1.5 V, which should result in contraction of the ipsilateral muscles of the lower mandible. Lesioning using two to three rounds at 42 °C for 90 s is then performed. For end of life care, a cannula can be inserted through the needle and left in place for continuous local anesthetic infusion or later chemical neurolytic block.

Side Effects/Complications Due to the vascular nature of the area, facial hematoma is a common side effect. Dysesthesia may occur, and anesthesia dolorosa is possible, though it has not been reported in the literature. Neurolysis or radiofrequency ablation may result in motor dysfunction and facial asymmetry due to weakness of the muscles of mastication, though this is usually not clinically relevant.

Supraorbital and Supratrochlear Nerves: Local Anesthetic Block and Pulsed Radiofrequency Ablation

Clinical Indications The supraorbital and supratrochlear nerves are terminal nerve branches of the ophthalmic nerve. The supraorbital nerve provides sensory innervation to the skin of the forehead, upper eyelid, and anterior scalp, while the supratrochlear nerve provides sensory innervation to the medial upper eyelid and forehead and bridge of the nose. Pain in this area is most commonly due to trauma or idiopathic supraorbital neuralgia though treatment techniques have been expanded to treat cancer-associated pain in this area.

Anatomic Considerations The supraorbital nerve exits the skull at the supraorbital foramen in the supraorbital rim, and the supratrochlear nerve exits the skull more medially at the supratrochlear notch, just lateral to the junction of the supraorbital rim and the bridge of the nose.

Procedure Description: Supraorbital Nerve The patient is positioned supine with the head in a neutral position. The supraorbital notch along the supraorbital ridge is palpated, or fluoroscopy can be used to identity the notch. A needle is advanced toward the notch in a slight medial direction until bone is contacted. Care should be taken not to enter the foramen itself. The needle should be withdrawn slightly from the periosteum, and 1–3 mL of local anesthetic, with or without depot steroid, should be deposited in the area being careful to avoid spillage into the eye (see Fig. 19.8). The patient may experience a paresthesia in the distribution of the supraorbital nerve. If pulsed radiofrequency ablation is desired, two 5 cm radiofrequency cannulas should be inserted, one with a final needle tip position overlying the superior margin of the supraorbital notch and one with a final needle tip position overlying the middle or inferior aspect of the notch. Skin sites for cannulas insertion should be 1–2 cm medial or lateral to the foramen to allow the needle tip to be perpendicular to the nerve in its final position. Sensory stimulation should be performed at 50 Hz with 0.1–1 V confirming appropriate supraorbital distribution of stimulation, and then lesioning with 2 to 3 cycles of 42 °C for 90 s should be completed [28]. Conventional thermal radiofrequency ablation should not be used due to the risk of thermal damage to the skin and eyebrow.

Procedure Description: Supratrochlear Nerve The patient is positioned supine with the head in a neutral position. The supratrochlear notch along the medial aspect of the supraorbital ridge just lateral to the junction of the supraorbital ridge and the bridge of the nose is palpated or fluoroscopically identified. A needle is advanced toward the notch until bone is contacted. The needle should be withdrawn slightly, and 1–3 mL of local anesthetic, with or without depot steroid, is deposited in the area in a fanlike distribution, being careful to avoid spillage into the eye. If pulsed radiofrequency ablation is desired, a 5 cm radiofrequency cannula should be inserted with final needle tip position in the supratrochlear notch. Sensory stimulation should be performed confirming appropriate supratrochlear distribution of stimulation, and then lesioning with 2 to 3 cycles of 42 °C for 90 s should be completed [28]. Conventional thermal radiofrequency ablation should notbe used due to the risk of thermal damage to the skin and eyebrow.

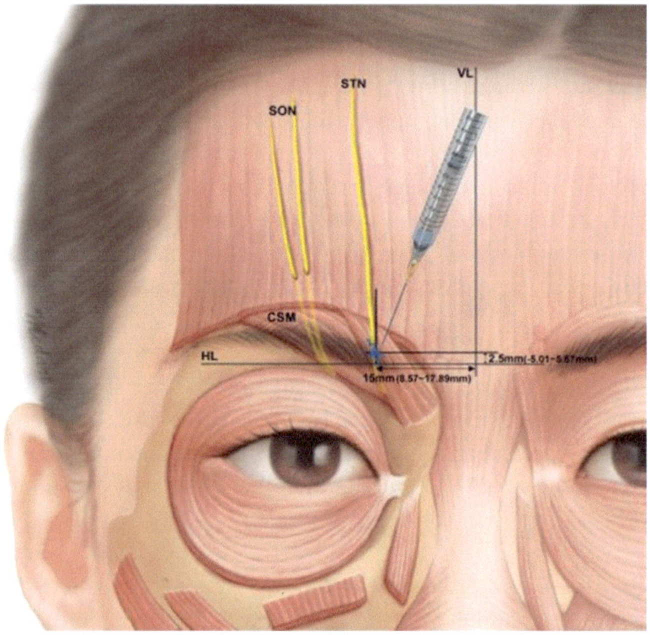

Fig. 19.8 Supraorbital and supratrochlear nerve block (*SON* supraorbital nerve, *STN* supratrochlear nerve, *CSM* corrugator supercilii muscle, *VL* vertical reference line, *HL* horizontal reference line). (Lee et al. [27])

Side Effects/Complications Given the vascular nature of the area, periorbital ecchymosis and hematoma formation may occur. With repeated injections using depot steroid, subcutaneous fat atrophy and skin discoloration may occur. Radiofrequency lesioning has the potential to lead to dysesthesias though this has been infrequently reported.

Supraorbital and Supratrochlear Peripheral Nerve Stimulation

Clinical Indications The supraorbital nerve provides sensory innervation to the skin of the forehead, upper eyelid, and anterior scalp, while the supratrochlear nerve provides sensory innervation to the medial upper eyelid and forehead and bridge of the nose. For patients with longer life expectancy who have responded well to diagnostic supraorbital and supratrochlear nerve blocks, peripheral nerve stimulation may provide long-lasting pain control.

Anatomic Considerations The supraorbital and supratrochlear nerves exit the skull at the supraorbital and supratrochlear foramen, respectively, and then travel over the forehead superiorly. Peripheral nerve stimulator leads can be positioned to overly these nerves as they cross the forehead above the eyebrow. As positioning of these peripheral stimulator leads requires traversing the temporal nerve and artery, this should be done by experienced practitioners only or in coordination with a neurosurgeon to avoid damage to the temporal artery or nerve. Permanent implantation is generally performed by neurosurgeons or plastic surgeons due to the need to tunnel the stimulator leads through the neck into the infraclavicular area where the generator is implanted. Thus only the placement of trial spinal cord stimulator leads is described here.

Procedure Description The patient ispositioned supine with the head in a neutral position and moderate sedation is used. A small area just posterior and superior to the top of the ear is shaved and the skin cleansed. Sterile prep, drapes, gloves, and gowns should be used. A small incision is made, and the stimulator lead is inserted, often with the help of a flexible blunt tunneling device. The stimulator lead is slowly advanced under AP fluoroscopic guidance with constant tactile contact with the tip of the lead through the skin and with great care taken to avoid the temporal artery and nerve. The lead is advanced until the lead contacts are just superior to both the supraorbital and supratrochlear foramens (see Fig. 19.9). On-the-table stimulation and programming should be done to ensure coverage of both the supraorbital and supratrochlear nerves. The lead is then sutured to the skin at its entry site, and copious tape is used to secure the lead to the skin behind the ear before connecting to a temporary generator. The patient should be advised to minimize movement of their head to prevent dislodging the trial lead. Some practitioners place patients in a soft cervical collar to protect against head movement during the duration of the trial, which lasts 2–7 days. The procedure is repeated on the contralateral side in the event of bilateral symptoms [29].

Side Effects/Complications The most dangerous complication of peripheral nerve stimulator trial is damage to the temporal nerve and artery. Thus this procedure should only be performed by experienced practitioners or in coordination with a neurosurgeon to avoid damage to these structures. Given the vascular nature of the scalp, bleeding and hematoma may occur. Infection is a rare complication, but care should be taken to use sterile technique throughout the procedure, in particular because trial leads may remain in place for several days. Complications of permanent implantation of peripheral stimulator leads include bleeding, infection, lead erosion through the skin, lead migration, damage to vascular and nervous system structures in the neck and supraclavicular area during tunneling, and generator placement and generator malfunction [30].

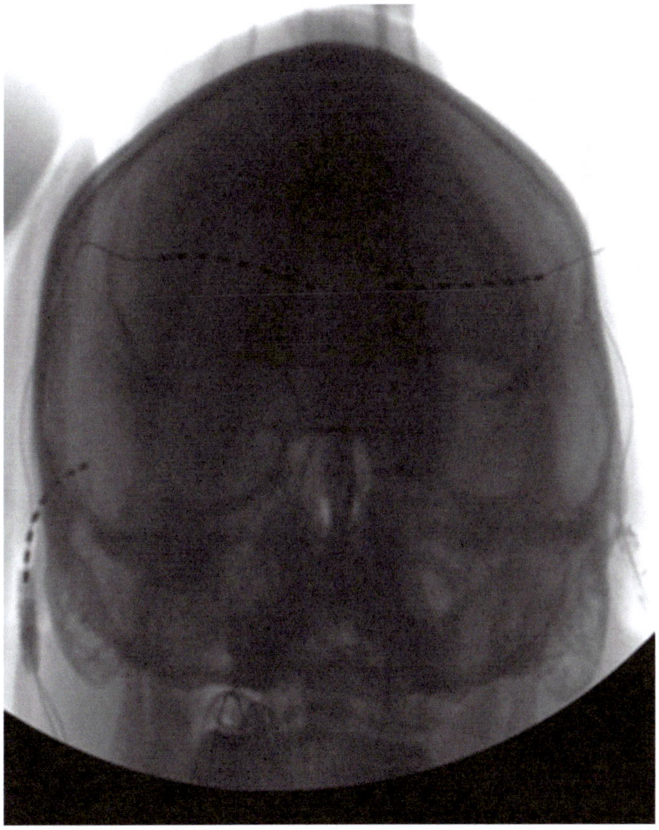

Fig. 19.9 Fluoroscopic view of supraorbital/supratrochlear peripheral nerve stimulator leads

Infraorbital Nerve Block, Neurolysis, and Pulsed Radiofrequency Ablation

Clinical Indications The infraorbital nerve is a terminal nerve branch of the maxillary nerve. It provides sensory innervation to the lower eyelid, medial cheek, and lateral nares and upper lip and can be damaged by direct tumor invasions or surgical intervention.

Anatomic Considerations The infraorbital nerve arises from the maxillary nerve shortly after it exits the middle cranial fossa at the foramen rotundum. It then passes along the floor of the orbit in the infraorbital groove and canal and exits the skull via the infraorbital foramen, approximately 2.5 cm lateral of midline and 1 cm inferior to the orbit. Needle trajectory should be superior and lateral for appropriate placement [31].

Procedure Description The patient is positioned supine with the head in a neutral position. The infraorbital notch is identified using AP fluoroscopy. A needle is inserted 1 cm below and 1 cm lateral to the foramen directed in an upward lateral trajectory toward the foramen. For local anesthetic blockade, the needle should be advanced until it contacts the periosteum but should not enter the foramen to prevent compression neuropathy. Three milliliters of local anesthetic, with or without depot steroid, is deposited in a fanlike distribution. Neurolysis with 0.5 mL of glycerol using this approach has also been described [32].

For radiofrequency ablation the needle tip should enter the infraorbital foramen slightly, which may elicit a paresthesia. Sensory stimulation should be performed at 50 Hz, and then pulsed radiofrequency lesioning with 2 to 3 cycles of 42 °C for 90 s and conventional thermal radiofrequency ablation with 30-s cycles at 75–80 C until anesthesia in the infraorbital area is obtained have both been described. However, care must be taken to avoid thermal damage to the skin and subcutaneous tissue if thermal ablation is used.

Side Effects/Complications Given the vascular nature of the area, ecchymosis and hematoma formation may occur. With repeated injections using depot steroid, subcutaneous fat atrophy and skin discoloration may occur. Radiofrequency lesioning has the potential to lead to dysesthesias though this has been infrequently reported.

Mental Nerve Block, Neurolysis, and Pulsed Radiofrequency Ablation

Clinical Indications The mental nerve is a terminal nerve branch of the mandibular nerve. Mental neuralgia most often occurs not as a result of head and neck cancer but rather as a site of metastatic disease from breast cancer or lymphomas. While mental neuralgia often presents with painless hypoesthesia or numbness of the chin, painful varieties occur as well [33].

Anatomic Considerations The mental nerveis a branch of the inferior alveolar nerve. It exits the mandible via the mental foramen in the chin and courses superiorly toward the lower lip. It supplies sensory information to the chin, lower lip, and buccal gingival.

Procedure Description The patient is placed in a supine position and the mental foramen is palpated. A needle is directed toward the foramen with in a slightly medial direction until bone is contacted. Entry into the foramen should be avoided to prevent compression neuropathy. Fluoroscopic guidance can also be used. After negative aspiration 2–3 mL of local anesthetic, with or without depot steroid, is injected in a fanlike distribution. Neurolysis using this approach with 1 mL glycerol has been described as well [32]. Pulsed radiofrequency ablation of the mental nerve requires placement of the needle tip just inside the mental foramen and can be accomplished with 2–3 cycles at standard lesioning parameters after appropriate sensory stimulation [34].

Side Effects/Complications Ecchymosis and hematoma formation may occur. With chemical neurolysis or repeated injections using depot steroid, subcutaneous fat atrophy and skin discoloration may occur. Radiofrequency lesioning has the potential to lead to dysesthesias thoughthis has not been reported.

Cryoablation of the Trigeminal Nerve and Its Branches

Cryoablation of the above nerve targets has been reported in the literature, though minimal data regarding efficacy, specific complications, and comparison to other methods of neural blockade has been published. Cryoablation can be performed by placing a large-bore catheter, such as a 14-gauge intravenous catheter, in the appropriate location and using a nerve stimulator to identify concordant sensory distribution. Local anesthetic block is then undertaken prior inserting a 1.4 mm cryoablation probe. Generally, 2–3 2-minute cycles are adequate [35].

Glossopharyngeal Nerve: Anatomy and Innervation

The glossopharyngeal nerve is the ninth cranial nerve. It arises from the brainstem at the level of the medulla and exits the skull through the jugular foramen. The glossopharyngeal nerve is a mixed nerve with motor, sensory, and parasympathetic functions. It provides sensory innervation of the external ear, posterior pharynx, posterior one-third of the tongue (including taste sensation), carotid body, and sinus. It also provides parasympathetic innervation to the parotid gland and motor innervation to the stylopharyngeus muscle, which is responsible for pharyngeal dilation during swallowing (see Fig. 19.10).

Glossopharyngeal Nerve Block, Chemical Neurolysis, and Pulsed Radiofrequency Ablation

Clinical Indications Glossopharyngeal neuralgia is a rare clinical syndrome characterized by lancing, often episodic pain in the tonsillar area with radiation to the ear. The nearby vagus nerve can also be involved in a minority of patients leading to bradycardia and syncope [36]. While most cases are idiopathic in nature, secondary glossopharyngeal neuralgia may occur as a result of invasive cancer or as a result of

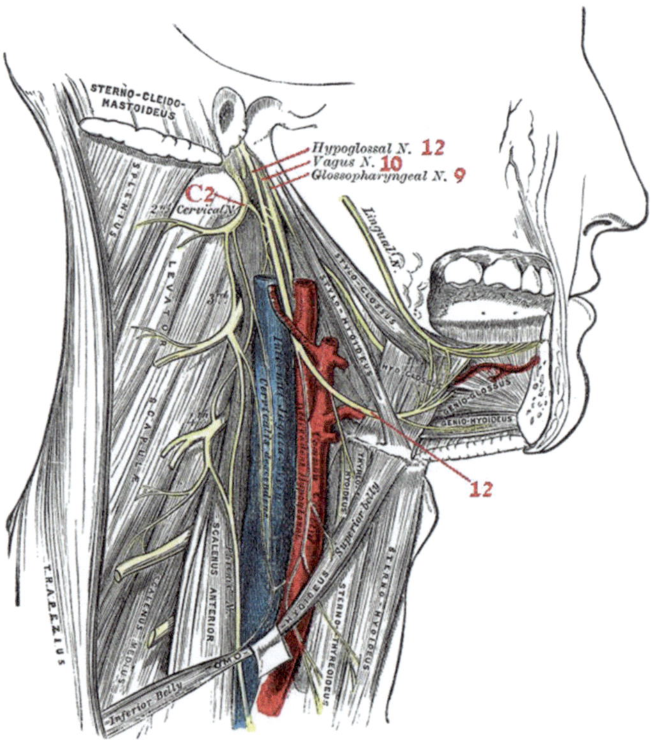

Fig. 19.10 Glossopharyngeal and vagus nerve anatomy. (From Henry Gray (1918) *Anatomy of the Human Body* via Wikipedia Commons https://commons.wikimedia.org/wiki/File:Gray794A.png. In public domain)

radiation therapy [37]. Nerve blocks, chemical neurolysis, and pulsed radiofrequency have all been described.

Anatomic Considerations After leaving thejugular foramen, the glossopharyngeal nerve descends in front of the internal carotid artery and passes below the styloid process before running along the pharyngeal muscles and eventually terminating in palatine tonsil and base of the tongue. The nerve can be accessed percutaneously where it contacts the styloid process using fluoroscopic guidance or via an intraoral approach in the tonsillar pillars.

Procedure Description: Percutaneous Approach The patient is placed supine with neck in a neutral position. Lateral fluoroscopy is used to identify the styloid process posterior and superior to the angle of the mandible, approximately. A needle is inserted from a lateral approach approximately 1.5–3 cm until contact with the styloid process is made. After contact with the styloid process is made, the needle should be redirected posteriorly and advanced another 0.5–1.5 cm. The glossopharyngeal nerve lies in close proximity to the internal and external carotid arteries, and intermittent AP and lateral fluoroscopy should be used to guide needle placement. After negative aspiration contrast should be used to verify lack of vascular uptake. Nerve block can be accomplished with 2–3 mL of local anesthetic in divided doses with close observation, with or without depot steroid. Pulsed radiofrequency ablation has also been described using this approach. Sensory stimulation should produce symptoms at the base of the tongue, pharynx, and ipsilateral tonsils, whereas motor stimulation should produce local pharyngeal muscle contraction and the absence of diaphragmatic and trapezius muscle action. Due to the nearby vagus nerve, the patient should be monitored for bradycardia and hypotension during stimulation. Lesioning with 2–3 cycles of 120 s at 42 °C is then completed [38]. Thermal radiofrequency ablation has also been reported but carries an increased risk of neuritis and damage to the nearby vagal nerve.

Procedure Description: Intraoral Approach The patient is placed supine with neck in neutral position. Topical lidocaine spray is used to anesthetize the tonsil and posterior pharynx. A needle is then inserted into the lateral portion of the anterior tonsillar pillar approximately 0.5 cm lateral to the base of the tongue. Additional lidocaine can be deposited here for nerve block, or chemical neurolysis can be accomplished with injection of 0.3–1 mL of glycerol in the upper and lower portions of the lateral anterior tonsillar pillar.

Side Effects/Complications Given the proximity of the internal and external carotid arteries, care should be taken to avoid vascular injury to prevent hematoma. In addition the risk of intravascular injection is significant. The vagal nerve also lies posterior and lateral to the glossopharyngeal nerve, and stimulation in this area may result in vagal response with bradycardia and hypotension. Inadvertent blockade of the hypoglossal and spinal accessory nerves will result in weakness of the tongue and trapezius muscles.

Vagus Nerve: Anatomy and Innervation

The vagus nerve is the tenth cranial nerve. It arises from the medulla and exits the skull through the jugularforamen along with the glossopharyngeal nerve. It then descends in the carotid sheath between the internal carotid artery and internal jugular vein before continuing on through the neck, thorax, and abdomen. The vagus nerve is a mixed nerve with motor and sensory functions. It provides motor innervation to the majority of the pharyngeal and laryngeal muscles and sensory innervation to the posterior external auditory meatus, inferior tympanic membrane, and mucosa of the larynx and vocal cords. It also provides parasympathetic innervation to most intrathoracic and abdominal organs (see Fig. 19.11).

Vagus Nerve Block, Chemical Neurolysis, and Pulsed Radiofrequency Ablation

Clinical Indications Pain attributable to the vagus nerve is a diagnosis of exclusion given its rarity. It is similar to glossopharyngeal neuralgia in that patients experience shocking,

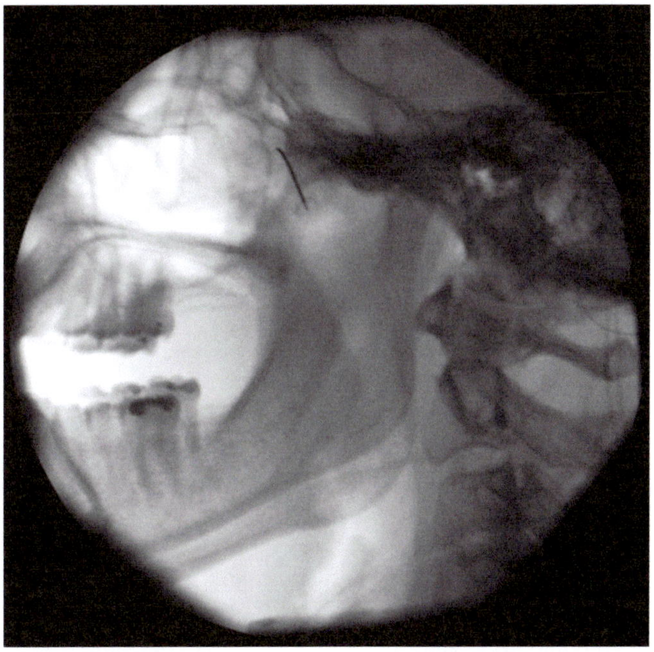

Fig. 19.11 Fluoroscopic image of sphenopalatine ganglion block with needle in middle anterior portion of the pterygoid fossa – lateral view

episodic pain in the posterior pharynx, though vagal neuralgia often also causes pain in the thyroid area with radiation to the upper chest and/or jaw. Nerve blocks, chemical neurolysis, and pulsed radiofrequency ablation of the vagus nerve have all been described [39]. Given the risks of this procedure, it should only be performed when more conservative treatments have failed and in the hands of experienced practitioners.

Anatomic Considerations The vagus nerve can be blocked at the level of the styloid process where it lies posterior to the glossopharyngeal, accessory, and hypoglossal nerves and superficial to the internal jugular vein. Fluoroscopic guidance is used to identify the styloid process to guide appropriate placement via a percutaneous approach.

Procedure Description The patient isplaced supine with neck in a neutral position. Lateral fluoroscopy is used to identify the styloid process posterior and superior to the angle of the mandible. A needle is inserted from a lateral approach until contact with the styloid process is made, approximately 1.5–3 cm. After contact with the styloid process, the needle is redirected posteriorly and inferiorly and advanced another 0.5 cm. Intermittent fluoroscopy should be used to guide needle placement. After negative aspiration contrast should be used to verify lack of vascular uptake. Nerve block can be accomplished with 3–5 mL of local anesthetic in divided doses with close observation, with or without depot steroid. Chemical neurolysis with small quantities of alcohol, phenol, or glycerol and radiofrequency ablation have been described [39].

Side Effects/Complications Given the proximity of the internal and external carotid arteries, care should be taken to avoid vascular injury to prevent hematoma. In addition the risk of intravascular injection is significant. Stimulation in this area may result in vagal response with bradycardia and hypotension. Inadvertent blockade of the hypoglossal and spinal accessory nerves will result in weakness of the tongue and trapezius muscles.

Other Head and Neck Nerve Targets

Sphenopalatine Ganglion: Anatomy and Innervation

The sphenopalatine ganglion is a complex network of neural connections. It lies in the pterygopalatine fossa posterior to the middle turbinate of the nose just deep to the lateral nasal mucosa. It has motor, sensory, and autonomic functions and sends connections to multiple other important facial structures including the trigeminal ganglion, carotid plexus, facial nerve, and superior cervical ganglion. Sensory, motor, parasympathetic, and sympathetic nerve fibers pass through or synapse in the ganglion and are dispersed to the nasal membranes, lacrimal glands, soft palate, and pharynx [40].

Sphenopalatine Ganglion Nerve Block, Chemical Neurolysis, Pulsed Radiofrequency Ablation, and Thermal Radiofrequency Ablation

Clinical Indications Sphenopalatine ganglion blocks for the treatment of headaches have been used for decades, in particular headaches with autonomic features such as lacrimation and nasal congestion. It has also been helpful for cancer patients, in particular with cancers of the tongue and floor of the mouth [41]. Patients who describe midface pain, pain behind the nose or inferior forehead, and frontal headache may benefit from sphenopalatine intervention [42].

Anatomic Considerations The sphenopalatine ganglion lies in the pterygopalatine fossa just deep to the middle nasal turbinate. A thin layer of connective tissues separates the ganglion and the superior aspect of the middle nasal turbinate. Sphenopalatine ganglion blockade with local anesthetic can be performed from a transnasal approach or via a lateral approach through the coronoid notch, similar to maxillary nerve blockade. However chemical neurolysis or radiofrequency ablation should be performed only from a lateral approach to more specifically localize the ganglion and reduce risk of damage to nearby structures.

Procedure Description: Transnasal Approach The patient is placed in a supine position with cervical extension in a "sniffing" position. Lidocaine nasal spray is used for topical anesthesia. A cotton-tipped applicator soaked in local anesthetic is advanced posteriorly along the superior aspect of the middle nasal turbinate until resistance is met at the posterior aspect of the nasal pharynx. The applicator is left in place for 15–20 min. Additional local anesthetic can be delivered by allowing it to "trickle down" the applicator to the cotton-tipped end.

Procedure Description: Lateral Approach The patient is placed supine on the fluoroscopy table with a neutral neck position, and the patient is asked to slightly open their jaw into a "slack jaw" position to facilitate identification of the coronoid notch just anterior to the external auditory meatus and inferior to the zygomatic arch. A lateral fluoroscopic view is used to identify the pterygopalatine fossa as a V-shaped structure superior to the upper molars and inferior to theorbit. Side-to-side rotation of the head may be used to help identify the fossa and align it fluoroscopically with the pterygopalatine fossa on the contralateral side of the head for appropriate positioning.

The needle is inserted in the coronoid notch and directed in a plane perpendicular to the skull toward the pterygopalatine fossa, usually 4–5 cm. Often the lateral pterygopalatine plate is encountered, and the needle should then be redirected anteriorly and superiorly and advanced approximately 0.5–1 cm to enter the pterygopalatine fossa. Maxillary nerve paresthesia may occur with this advancement. The needle should be directed to the middle anterior part of the pterygopalatine fossa so that the needle tip rests inferior to the maxillary nerve (see Fig. 19.11). On AP fluoroscopic view, the needle should be just lateral to the middle nasal turbinate. Contrast can be used to confirm appropriate placement.

If anesthetic blockade is desired, 2 mL of local anesthetic is injected in divided doses with patient monitoring with or without depot steroid. Chemical neurolysis for palliation of severe cancer pain has been reported using glycerol, phenol, or alcohol with volumes of 0.3–0.5 mL.

If radiofrequency ablation is used, sensory stimulation at 50 Hz with 0.1–1 V should be performed, and the patient should experience the stimulation at the base of the nose. Pulsed radiofrequency lesioning is then performed at 42 °C for 90 s. Two to three rounds of lesioning are often performed for improved efficacy [43]. Thermal radiofrequency ablation has been performed using temperatures ranging from 60 to 90C for 60–90 s, though risk of damage to nearby structures increases with this method [11].

Side Effects/Complications Due to the vascular nature of the area, facial hematoma is a common side effect. Dysesthesia may occur and anesthesia dolorosa is possible, though it has not been reported in the literature. Some patients may experience orthostatic hypotension after sphenopalatine ganglion blockade.

Temporomandibular Joint: Anatomy and Innervation

The temporomandibular joint, commonly referred to as TMJ, is a synovial articulation between the temporal bone and the mandible. It is composed of an articular disc between the two bones and encompassed by a dense, fibrous joint capsule lined by a synovial membrane. It is involved in both rotational and translational movements of the jaw, including mastication and opening of the jaw. The joint can be directly invaded by tumor and damaged with surgical intervention or develop an inflammatory arthropathy due to chemotherapy or radiation therapy [44].

Clinical Indications Patients with temporomandibular joint pain describe a dull, aching pain over the area that radiates into the ear, temporaland periorbital region, mandible, and posterior neck. Movement of the mandible exacerbates pain, and patients frequently describe a "locking" of their jaw in either the closed or open position prohibiting normal jaw movement. There is limited range of motion of the jaw and often a "clicking" sound with jaw movement. Panoramic radiographs or CT imaging can be used to help confirm the diagnosis [45].

Anatomic Considerations The temporomandibular joint lies approximately 1 cm anterior to the tragus and 2 mm inferior to the tragal-canthal line. It lies in close proximity to the facial nerveas well as the superficial temporal artery and nerve.

Procedure Description The patient is placed in the supine position with the cervical spine and the jaw in a neutral position. A point 1 cm anterior to the tragus and 2 mm below the tragal-canthal line is the insertion point. The needle is advanced approximately 0.5–0.75 cm in a plan perpendicular to the skull until a "pop" is felt as the needle enters the joint space. Afternegative aspiration 1 mL of local anesthetic, with or without depot steroid, is injected [46, 47].

Risks/Complications Hematoma and ecchymosis are not uncommon. If the facial nerve is inadvertently damaged or anesthetized, facial weakness can occur and corneal lubrication and patching is necessary. While the procedure may be repeated every 5–7 days as needed for end-of-life palliative care, repeated injections can result in joint necrosis over time.

Greater and Lesser Occipital Nerves: Procedural Intervention

Anatomy and Innervation

The greater occipital nerve arises from the dorsal rami of the C2 and C3cervical nerves. They ascend in the posterior neck and pierces the fascia just below the nuchal ridge medial to the occipital artery. The lesser occipital nerve arises from the ventral rami of the C2 and C3 cervical nerves and ascends more laterally and superficially in the posterior neck on top of the sternocleidomastoid muscle before dividing into cutaneous branches above the nuchal ridge. Together these nerves provide sensory innervation to the posterior head and scalp [48].

Greater Occipital and Lesser Occipital Nerve Blocks, Radiofrequency Ablation, and Cryoablation

Clinical Indications Occipital neuralgia is a syndrome of paroxysms of pain or dysesthesia in the distribution of these nerves with tenderness over the area. Clinically it may be accompanied by headache in the occipital region. While occipital neuralgia may be the presenting symptom of cancer in rare instances, more often patients develop pain in this region following resectionof intracranial masses [49].

Anatomic Considerations The greater and lesser occipital nerves can be accessed at the level of the nuchal ridge where they both lie just superficial to the periosteum. If a line is drawn between the external occipital protuberance and the mastoid process, the greater occipital nerve is located at approximately the 1/3 mark, and the lesser occipital nerve is located at approximately the 2/3 mark along this line. The occipital artery is located just lateral to the greater occipital nerve and is an important landmark. Neural blockade has been described using landmark technique, fluoroscopy, and ultrasound guidance. In addition to local anesthetic block with or without steroid, cryoablation and pulsed radiofrequency ablation have been described [50] [35].

Procedure Description The patient is positioned in a chair and the posterior scalp is cleansed with alcohol. For greater occipital nerve block, the occipital artery is palpated at the level of the superior nuchal ridge. A needle is inserted just medial to the artery in a plan perpendicular to the skull until periosteum is contacted. The needle is withdrawn slightly and directed superiorly, and 3–5 mL of local anesthetic, with or without depot steroid, is injected in a fanlike distribution after negative aspiration. For lesser occipital nerve block, a line is imagined between the external occipital protuberance and the mastoid process. At a point 2/3 along this line, a needle is inserted perpendicular to the scalp until bone is contacted. The needle is withdrawn, and 3–5 mL of local anesthetic, with or without depot steroid, is injected in a fanlike distribution. Fluoroscopic guidance is sometimes employed to clearly identify the aforementioned bony landmarks in the case of anatomic distortion. Ultrasound guidance can also be used by placing the ultrasound transducer parallel to the superior nuchal ridge just below the inion and scanning laterally along the nuchal ridge until the nerve is seen. Doppler ultrasound can be used to identify the occipital artery just lateral to the nerve (see Figs. 19.12 and 19.13) [51, 52].

Thermal radiofrequency ablation at90 °C for 90–120 s and pulsed radiofrequency ablation at 42 °C for 2–3 cycles of 120 s have been described [50]. Appropriate concordant sensory stimulation prior to lesioning is important as the nerve can be difficult to locate. Cryoablation of the GON under ultrasound guidance has also been described using temperatures of negative 60–70 ° for 2–3 min [53]. Ablative techniques have not been described for the lesser occipital nerve given its less dependable anatomic position.

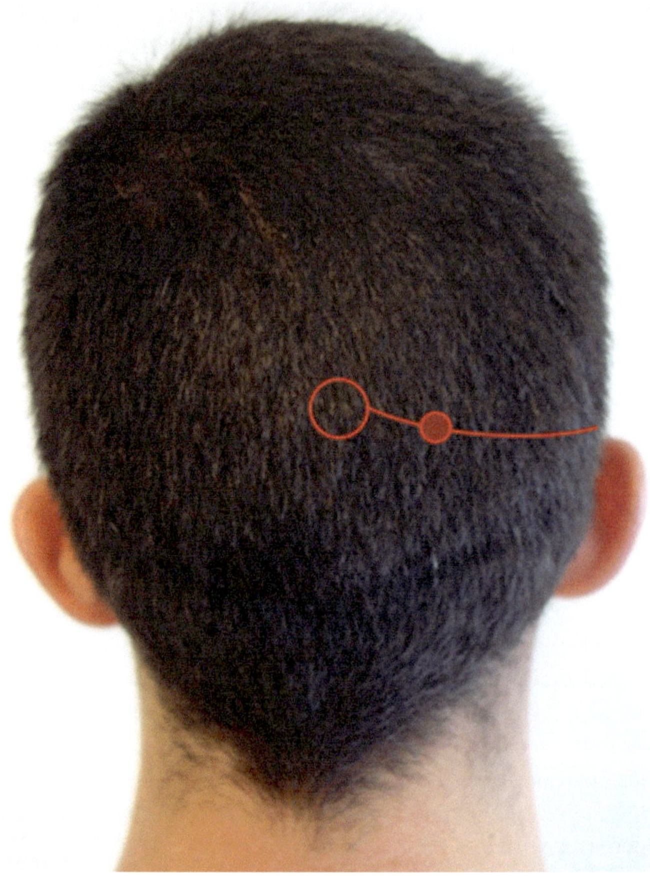

Fig. 19.12 Greater and lesser occipital nerve block. Line indicates the superior nuchal ridge. Open circle indicates occipital protuberance, and closed circle indicates approximate needle entry point just medial to the occipital artery

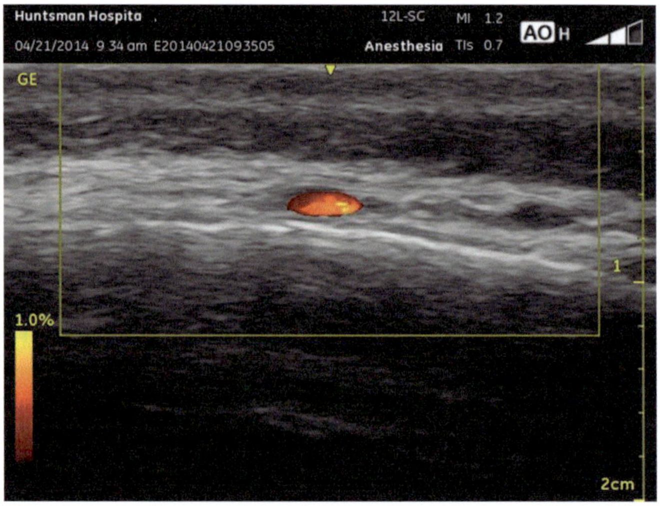

Fig. 19.13 Ultrasound image of greater occipital nerve – the occipital artery is identified, and the neural target lies just medial

Risks/Complications Given the vascular nature and the scalp and the proximity to the occipital artery, bleeding and hematoma may occur. In addition care should be taken not to insert the needle into the nearby foramen magnum due to the risks of administering local anesthetic in the subarachnoid space and developing a total spinal. Ablative procedures also carry the risk of neuritis or dysesthesia following the procedure.

Greater and Lesser Occipital Nerve Peripheral Nerve Stimulation

Clinical Indications Occipital nerve peripheral nerve stimulation is performed for the same indications as greater and lesser occipital nerve block above [49]. Following successful diagnostic nerve blocks, implanted peripheral nerve stimulation may be used to provide long-lasting pain relief.

Anatomic Considerations The greater andlesser occipital nerves can be accessed at the level of the nuchal ridge where they both lie just superficial to the periosteum. If a line is drawn between the external occipital protuberance and the mastoid process, the greater occipital nerve is located at approximately the 1/3 mark, and the lesser occipital nerve is located at approximately the 2/3 mark along this line. Thus it is important to place the stimulator leads in a position to cover both these landmarks. Placement of trial peripheral nerve stimulator leads is described below; implantation of permanent leads is often performed by neurosurgeons given the need for tunneling in the neck and thorax for generator implantation.

Procedure Description The patient is positioned prone with slight cervical flexion and the posterior scalp is shaved and cleansed. Sterile prep, drapes, gloves, and gowns should be used. Fluoroscopic guidance is used to identify anatomic midline and the dens of C2. A 1 cm incision in the posterior scalp is made just superior to the dens after skin localization. The peripheral nerve stimulator lead is inserted through a Tuohy needle or with the help of a flexible introducer device. The lead is advanced under live fluoroscopic guidance with a slightly cranial trajectory in a fascial plane below the skin but superficial to the muscle until the lead contacts cover the anticipated locations of the greater and lesser occipital nerves (see Fig. 19.14). On-the-table stimulation and programming should be done to ensure coverage of both the greater occipital and lesser occipital nerves. The lead is then sutured to the skin at its entry site at the scalp, and copious tape is used to secure the lead to the skin of the neck before connecting to a temporary generator. The patient should be advised to minimize movement of their head to prevent dislodging the trial lead. Some practitioners place patients in a soft cervical collar to protect against head movement during the duration of the trial, which lasts 2–7 days. The procedure is repeated on the contralateral side in the event of bilateral symptoms. The procedure has also been described using a lateral to medial trajectory of the leads with the scalp incision placed just behind the ear [54].

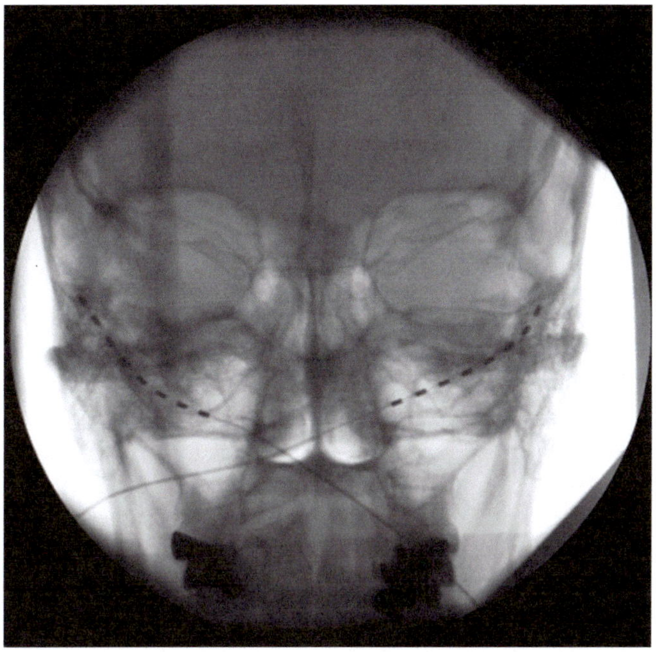

Fig. 19.14 Fluoroscopic view of occipital nerve stimulator leads

Risks/Complications Given the vascular nature and the scalp and the proximity to the occipital artery, bleeding and hematoma may occur. Infection is an uncommon complication, but care should be taken to use sterile technique throughout the procedure, in particular because trial leads may remain in place for several days. Complications of permanent implantation of peripheral stimulator leads include bleeding, infection in up to 20% of implanted devices, lead erosion through the skin, lead migration, damage to vascular and nervous system structures in the neck during tunneling, and generator placement and generator malfunction [55].

Cervical Plexus: Procedural Intervention

Anatomy and Innervation

The cervical plexus is made up of fibers from the ventral rami of the C1–C4 cervical nerves. These nerves travel from the intervertebral foramina to the lateral aspect of the corresponding transverse processes just behind the sternocleidomastoid muscle. From here cutaneous branches emerge from the posterior aspect of the sternocleidomastoid at its midpoint. These branches, the superficial cervical plexus, provide cutaneous sensory innervation to the lower mandible, anterolateral neck, supraclavicular fossa, and pre- and retroauricular area. Muscular branches of the cervical plexus remain deep in the deep cervical plexus and provide motor fibers to the phrenic nerve to control diaphragmatic movement, the spinal accessory nerve which innervates the trapezius and sternocleidomastoid muscles, as well as direct motor innervation of the paravertebral and deep muscles of the neck.

Cervical Plexus Nerve Block

Clinical Indications Cervical plexus block can be useful in patients who have acute, uncontrolled pain arising from superficial or deep structures in the neck [56]. Blockade of both the deep and superficial cervical plexus will provide cutaneous analgesia to the lower mandible, anterolateral neck, supraclavicular fossa, and preauricular and retroauricular area. Deep cervical plexus block will also result in blockade of the diaphragm via the phrenic nerve, the trapezius, and sternocleidomastoid muscles via the spinal accessory nerve, as well as the paravertebral and deep muscles of the neck. Superficial and deep cervical plexus blocks are most commonly done via landmark guidance.

Anatomic Considerations The superficial cervical plexus can be blocked at the posterior margin of the sternocleidomastoid muscle, whereas the deep cervical plexus is blocked near the transverse processes. The deep cervical plexus lies in close proximity to the vertebral artery, the epidural space, and the subarachnoid space, and care must to be taken to avoid these structures.

Procedure Description: Superficial Cervical Plexus The patient is placed supine with the neck slightly extended and turned away from the side of interest. The posterior sternocleidomastoid muscle is palpated, and the midpoint of the muscle is identified. In the event of difficult palpation, the midpoint of a line between the mastoid process and the insertion of the sternocleidomastoid muscle on the clavicle can be used. After cleansing the skin, a needle is inserted, and 5 mL of local anesthetic, with our without depot steroid, is deposited along the posterior edge of the sternocleidomastoid muscle subcutaneously and superficial and deep to the fascia of the muscle at a depth of approximately 0.5–1.5 cm in an average patient. The needle is directed cranial and caudal, and an additional 5–10 mL is deposited in a fanlike distribution (see Fig. 19.15) [57]. For continuous superficial plexus blockade, a catheter can be left in the area [58].

Procedure Description: Deep Cervical Plexus The patient isplaced supine with the neck slightly extended and turned away from the side of interest. The mastoid process and the C6 transverse process (Chassaignac's tubercle) are palpated, and a line is drawn on the skin between the two structures. Needle insertion sites are then marked on the skin along this line at 2 cm, 4 cm, and 6 cm caudal to the mastoid process, corresponding to the C2, C3, and C4 transverse processes. After the skin along the line is anesthetized, a needle is inserted at each site perpendicular to the skin with a slight caudal tilt. The needle is advanced until it contacts the transverse process. It is thenwithdrawn slightly, and 3–5 mL of local anesthetic, with our without depot steroid, is injected slowly after negative aspiration (see Fig. 19.16). If the transverse process is not contacted within 2 cm of the skin, the needle should be withdrawn

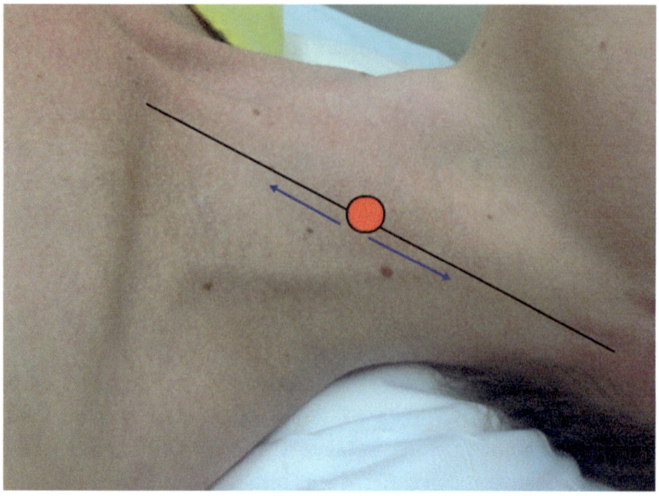

Fig. 19.15 Superficial cervical plexus block. Black line delineates the posterior border of the sternocleidomastoid muscle. Red circle shows initial needle placement, and blue arrows indicate redirection of needle caudal and cranial to initial placement

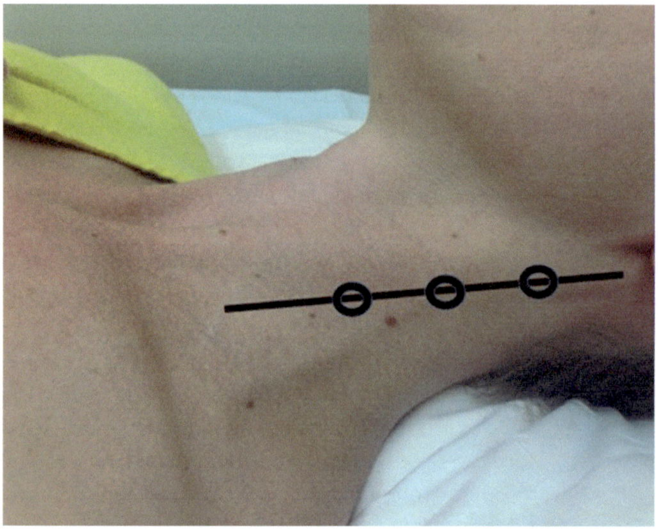

Fig. 19.16 Deep cervical plexus block. Line connects mastoid process and C6 tubercle. Hatches identify needle placements

and redirected. The process is then repeated at the other two levels. A catheter can be left in the area for continuous analgesia [58].

Risks/Complications Hematoma and bleeding may occur as the superficial cervical plexus in close proximity to the external jugular vein, whereas the deep cervical plexus lies close to the vertebral artery. Care should be taken to avoid intravascular injection. The deep cervical plexus also lies close to the neuraxial structures, and significant motor weakness or high spinal may result from inadvertent injection in these locations. The phrenic nerve is always blocked with deep cervical plexus block and may be blocked with superficial cervical plexus block, and patients with respiratory compromise should be monitored carefully. Bilateral deep cervical plexus block should be undertaken only in rare circumstances due to risk bilateral phrenic blockade [59].

References

1. Davies L, Welch HG. Epidemiology of head and neck cancer in the United States. Otolaryngol Head Neck Surg. 2006;135(3):451–7.
2. Breivik H, Cherny N, Collett B, De Conno F, Filbet M, Foubert AJ, et al. Cancer-related pain: a pan-European survey of prevalence, treatment, and patient attitudes. Ann Oncol. 2009;20(8):1420–33.
3. van den Beuken-van Everdingen MHJ, de Rijke JM, Kessels AG, Schouten HC, van Kleef M, Patijn J. Prevalence of pain in patients with cancer: a systematic review of the past 40 years. Ann Oncol. 2007;18(9):1437–49.
4. List MA, Stracks J, Colangelo L, Butler P, Ganzenko N, Lundy D, et al. How do head and neck cancer patients prioritize treatment outcomes before initiating treatment? J Clin Oncol. 2000;18(4):877–84.
5. Hammerlid E, Bjordal K, Ahlner-Elmqvist M, Boysen M, Evensen JF, Biörklund A, et al. A prospective study of quality of life in head and neck cancer patients. Part I: at diagnosis. Laryngoscope. 2001;111(4 Pt 1):669–80.
6. Bjordal K, Elmqvist MA, Hammerlid E. A prospective study of quality of life in head and neck cancer patients. Part II: longitudinal data. Laryngoscope. 2001;111:1440–52.
7. Sanderson RJ, Ironside J. Squamous cell carcinomas of the head and neck. BMJ. 2002;325:822–7.
8. Caraceni A, Portenoy RK. An international survey of cancer pain characteristics and syndromes. IASP task force on Cancer pain. International Association for the Study of Pain. Pain. 1999;82(3):263–74.
9. Hickey AH, Scrivani SS, Bajwa ZH. Cranial Neuralgias. In: Fishman SM, Ballantyne JC, Rathmell JP, editors. Bonica's Management of Pain. 4th ed. Baltimore: Lippincott Williams and Wilkins; 2010. p. 953–71.
10. Erdine S. Interventional treatment of cancer pain. Eur J Cancer Supp. 2005;3(3):97–106.
11. Day M. Neurolysis of the trigeminal and sphenopalatine ganglions. Pain Pract. 2001;1(2):171–82.
12. Saini SS. Reterogasserian anhydrous glycerol injection therapy in trigeminal neuralgia: observations in 552 patients. J Neurol Neurosurg Psychiatry. 1987;50(11):1536–8.
13. Peters G, Nurmikko TJ. Peripheral and gasserian ganglion-level procedures for the treatment of trigeminal neuralgia. Clin J Pain. 2002;18(1):28–34.
14. Ischia S, Luzzania A, Polati E. Retrogasserian glycerol injections: a retrospective study of 112 patients. Clin J Pain. 1990;6(4):291–6.
15. Mendelsohn D, Ranjan M, Hawley P, Honey CR. Percutaneous trigeminal rhizotomy for facial pain secondary to head and neck malignancy. Clin J Pain. 2013;29(10):e4–5.
16. Waldman SD. Gasserian ganglion block radiofrequency lesioning. In: Waldman SD, editor. Atlas of interventional pain management. 3rd ed. Philadelphia: Saunders Elsevier; 2009. p. 38–44.
17. Spincemaille GH, Dingemans W, Lodder J. Percutaneous radiofrequency Gasserian ganglion coagulation in the treatment of trigeminal neuralgia. Clin Neurol Neurosurg. 1985;87(2):91–4.
18. Kanpolat Y, Savas A, Bekar A, Berk C. Percutaneous controlled radiofrequency trigeminal rhizotomy for the treatment of idiopathic trigeminal neuralgia: 25-year experience with 1,600 patients. Neurosurgery. 2001;48(3). 524–32–discussion 532–4
19. Fraioli B, Esposito V, Guidetti B, Cruccu G, Manfredi M. Treatment of trigeminal neuralgia by Thermocoagulation, Glycerolization, and percutaneous compression of the gasserian ganglion and/or retrogasserian rootlets: long-term results and therapeutic protocol. Neurosurgery. 1989;24(2):239.
20. Skirving DJ, Dan NG. A 20-year review of percutaneous balloon compression of the trigeminal ganglion. J Neurosurg. 2001;94(6):913–7.
21. Nguyen M, Wilkes D. Pulsed radiofrequency V2 treatment and intranasal sphenopalatine ganglion block: a combination therapy for atypical trigeminal neuralgia. Pain Pract. 2010;10(4):370–4.
22. Singh B, Srivastava SK, Dang R. Anatomic considerations in relation to the maxillary nerve block. Reg Anesth Pain Med. 2001;26(6):507–11.
23. Kohase H, Umino M, Shibaji T, Suzuki N. Application of a mandibular nerve block using an indwelling catheter for intractable cancer pain. Acta Anaesthesiol Scand. 2004;48(3):382–3.
24. Takemura H, Masuda Y, Yatsushir R. Mandibular nerve block treatment for trismus associated with hypoxic-ischemic encephalopathy. Reg Anesth Pain Med. 2002;27(3):313–5.
25. Wells J. The use of nerve destruction for relief of pain in cancer: a review. Palliat Med. 1989;3(4):239–47.
26. Wilkinson HA. Trigeminal nerve peripheral branch phenol/glycerol injections for tic douloureux. J Neurosurg. 1999;90(5):828–32.
27. Lee HJ, Choi KS, Won SY, et al. Topographic Relationship between the Supratrochlear Nerve and Corrugator Supercilii Muscle—Can This Anatomical Knowledge Improve the Response to Botulinum Toxin Injections in Chronic Migraine? Toxins. 2015;7:2629–38.
28. Koyyalagunta D, Mazloomdoost D. Radiofrequency and cryoablation for cancer pain. Tech Reg Anesth Pain Med. 2010;14:3–9.
29. Osenbach R. Neurostimulation for the treatment of intractable facial pain. Pain Med. 2006;7(S1):S126–36.
30. Vaisman J, Markley H, Ordia J. The treatment of medically intractable trigeminal autonomic cephalalgia with supraorbital/supratrochlear stimulation: a retrospective case series. Neuromodulation. 2012;15:374–80.
31. Rahman M, Richter EO, Osawa S, Rhoton AL. Anatomic study of the infraorbital foramen for radiofrequency neurotomy of the infraorbital nerve. Neurosurgery. 2009;64(5 Suppl 2):423–7.
32. Erdem E, Alkan A. Peripheral glycerol injections in the treatment of idiopathic trigeminal neuralgia: retrospective analysis of 157 cases. J Oral Maxillofac Surg. 2001;59(10):1176–80.
33. Faltas B, Phatak P, Sham R. Mental nerve neuropathy: frequently overlooked clinical sign of hematologic malignancies. Am J Med. 2011;124(1):e1–2.
34. Park HG, Park PG, Kim WJ, Park YH, Kang H, Baek CW, et al. Ultrasound-assisted mental nerve block and pulsed radiofrequency treatment for intractable postherpetic neuralgia: three case studies. Korean J Pain. 2014;27(1):81–5.
35. Trescot AM. Cryoanalgesia in interventional pain management. Pain Physician. 2003;6(3):345–60.

36. Kandan SR, Khan S, Jeyaretna DS, Lhatoo S, Patel NK, Coakham HB. Neuralgia of the glossopharyngeal and vagal nerves: long-term outcome following surgical treatment and literature review. Br J Neurosurg. 2010;24(4):441–6.
37. Shin HY, Park HJ, Choi Y-C, Kim SM. Clinical and electromyographic features of radiation-induced lower cranial neuropathy. Clin Neurophysiol. 2013;124(3):598–602.
38. Shah RV, Racz GB. Pulsed mode radiofrequency lesioning to treat chronic post-tonsillectomy pain (secondary glossopharyngeal neuralgia). Pain Pract. 2003;3(3):232–7.
39. Waldman SD. Vagus nerve block. In: Waldman SD, editor. Atlas of interventional pain management. 3rd ed. Philadelphia: Saunders Elsevier; 2009. p. 104–7.
40. Windsor RE, Jahnke S. Sphenopalatine ganglion blockade: a review and proposed modification of the transnasal technique. Pain Physician. 2004;7(2):283–6.
41. Varghese BT, Koshy RC, Sebastian P, Joseph E. Combined sphenopalatine ganglion and mandibular nerve, neurolytic block for pain due to advanced head and neck cancer. Palliat Med. 2002;16(5):447–8.
42. Day M. Sympathetic blocks: the evidence. Pain Pract. 2008;8(2):98–109.
43. Bayer E, Racz GB, Miles D, Heavner J. Sphenopalatine ganglion pulsed radiofrequency treatment in 30 patients suffering from chronic face and head pain. Pain Pract. 2005;5(3):223–7.
44. Kim M-J, Ye Y-M, Park H-S, Suh C-H. Chemotherapy-related arthropathy. J Rheumatol. 2006;33(7):1364–8.
45. Scrivani SJ, Keith DA, Kaban LB. Temporomandibular disorders. N Engl J Med. 2008;359(25):2693–705.
46. Guarda-Nardini L, Stifano M, Brombin C, Salmaso L, Manfredini D. A one-year case series of arthrocentesis with hyaluronic acid injections for temporomandibular joint osteoarthritis. Oral Surg Oral Med Oral Pathol Oral Radiol Endod. 2007;103(6):e14–22.
47. Waldman SD. Temporomandibular joint injection. In: Waldman SD, editor. Atlas of pain injection techniques. 3rd ed. Philadelphia: Saunders Elsevier; 2013. Ch 1.
48. Ward JB. Greater occipital nerve block. Semin Neurol. 2003;23(1):59–62.
49. Ducic I, Felder JM, Endara M. Postoperative headache following acoustic neuroma resection: occipital nerve injuries are associated with a treatable occipital neuralgia. Headache. 2012;52(7):1136–45.
50. Navani A, Mahajan G, Kreis P, Fishman SM. A case of pulsed radiofrequency lesioning for occipital neuralgia. Pain Med. 2006;7(5):453–6.
51. Shim JH, Ko SY, Bang MR, Jeon WJ, Cho SY, Yeom JH, et al. Ultrasound-guided greater occipital nerve block for patients with occipital headache and short term follow up. Korean J Anesthesiol. 2011;61(1):50–4.
52. Skaribas I, Aló K. Ultrasound imaging and occipital nerve stimulation. Neuromodulation. 2010;13(2):126–30.
53. Fredriksen TA. Cervicogenic headache: invasive procedures. Cephalalgia. 2008;28(s1):39–40.
54. Slavin KV, Colpan ME, Munawar N, Wess C. Trigeminal and occipital peripheral nerve stimulation for craniofacial pain: a single-institution experience and review of the literature. Neurosurg Focus. 2006;15:374–80.
55. Hong J, Ball PA, Fanciullo GJ. Neurostimulation for neck pain and headache. Headache. 2014;54(3):430–44.
56. Sist T, Miner M, Lema M. Characteristics of postradical neck pain syndrome: a report of 25 cases. J Pain Symp. 1999;18:95.
57. Pandit JJ, Bree S, Dillon P, Elcock D. A comparison of superficial versus combined (superficial and deep) cervical plexus block for carotid endarterectomy: a prospective, randomized study. Anest Analg. 2009;91:781–6.
58. Arnér S. The role of nerve blocks in the treatment of cancer pain. Acta Anaesthesiol Scand. 1982;74(S):104–8.
59. Pandit JJ, Dutta D, Morris JF. Spread of injectate with superficial cervical plexus block in humans: an anatomical study. Brit J of Anaesth. 2003;91(5):733–5.

Vertebroplasty, Kyphoplasty, and Sacroplasty

20

Dawood Sayed and Shervin Razavian

Introduction

First described by Galibert and colleagues in 1984 to treat a C2 hemangioma, the original vertebroplasty procedure has undergone many different technical revisions and has been used to treat a myriad of different cancer-related and non-cancer-related conditions that cause painful vertebral body compression fractures [1]. During this time period, several variant procedures including kyphoplasty and sacroplasty have been introduced as well, with the aim of providing relief to those afflicted by painful injuries of the vertebral column through a minimally invasive approach. Overall, vertebroplasty has seen a rise in popularity. As reported by Weinstein, the number of vertebroplasty procedures performed for all indications more than doubled from 0.43 to 0.89 per 1000 Medicare enrollees during the time period 2001–2006 [2]. This chapter aims to provide greater insight into the procedures of vertebroplasty, kyphoplasty, and sacroplasty. As mentioned previously, these procedures may be used for several different conditions that cause painful fractures of the spinal column. Given the scope of this textbook, however, we will focus on the use of these procedures for cancer-related vertebral body compression fractures.

The incidence of vertebral compression fracture in cancer patients is relatively high as shown in Table 20.1 [3]. The median survival for patients with lung cancer and bone metastasis is 6 months; the median survival for patients with breast cancer and bone metastasis is 24 months; and multiple myeloma patients with metastatic bone disease have shown a median survival of 8 months [4, 5]. These procedures have the ability to profoundly impact the lives of those afflicted by painful vertebral body fractures secondary to malignancy, and their use for treatment of these conditions must be strongly considered [6].

Pathophysiology of Cancer Bone Pain

Painful and debilitating vertebral metastases are a common complication of solid malignancies, most commonly prostate, breast, lung, thyroid, and genitourinary cancers. The musculoskeletal system is the third most common site of metastasis by a solid tumor, with the spinal column being the most common site of skeletal metastasis [7]. The specific incidence of vertebral metastasis ranges from 30 to 95% of patients with cancers of the aforementioned and other primary origins. Many patients with multiple myeloma also have osteolytic lesions or generalized osteoporosis during the course of their disease [4]. 10% of all cancer patients will present with symptoms related to vertebral metastasis and of these patients; 40–70% will have involvement at multiple levels of the spinal column [8]. Patients with bone cancer pain must often deal with a poor quality of life. Skeletal complications as a sequela of metastatic disease manifest in approximately 70% of advanced breast, prostate, and lung carcinomas, and skeletal metastases are discovered in >90% of patients who die of these conditions [4] (Fig. 20.1). Bone-related cancer pain secondary to spinal metastasis can make even the most basic of bodily functions including coughing, turning in bed, and modest limb use result in severe pain. The back pain encountered by cancer patients afflicted with spine metastasis is related to two primary factors: tumor-related bone pain and mechanical pain. Tumor-related bone pain is primarily nocturnal or occurs in the early morning. Typically, tumor-related bone pain improves with activity during the day. The neurochemical and cellular characteristics of bone cancer pain are unique when compared to inflammatory or neuropathic pain. The bone contains a highly concentrated mosaic of primary sensory afferent and sympathetic nerve fiber innervation embedded in both the periosteum

D. Sayed (✉)
University of Kansas Medical Center, Department of Anesthesiology and Pain Medicine, Kansas City, KS, USA

S. Razavian
Anesthesia Associates of Kansas City, Overland Park, KS, USA

A. Gulati et al. (eds.), *Essentials of Interventional Cancer Pain Management*, https://doi.org/10.1007/978-3-319-99684-4_20

and the intramedullary space of the bone. The mediators of bone cancer pain cause reorganization and sensitization of the central dorsal horn of the spinal cord. This is manifested by several different neurochemical and cellular processes, including increased expression of the prohyperalgesic peptide dynorphin, enhanced neuronal activity monitored by increased c-Fos expression, and profound astrocytosis. Further, while bone cancer pain does not produce significant expression of substance P and CGRP in the dorsal horn of the spinal cord or GAL and NPY protein in the primary afferent neurons, it does increase the expression of glial fibrillary acidic protein markedly [9]. Mechanical cancer-related bone pain results from structural destruction of the spine that results in instability. This pain is movement related and is exacerbated by increasing the axial load on the spine. In patients with malignancy, the infiltrating tumor destroys the integrity of the vertebrae, which is followed by vertebral collapse, thereby leading to the severe pain with movement. Multiple myeloma is characterized by the accumulation of malignant plasma cells in the bone marrow leading to impaired hematopoiesis and bone disease including lytic lesions, pathological fractures, hypocalcemia, and osteoporosis (Fig. 20.2). Specifically, myeloma bone disease is a result of increased osteoclast activity without a concurrent increase in osteoblast activity, ultimately leading to bone resorption. Cytokine mediators including IL-6, M-CSF, TNF, RANK, and RANKL are all thought to play a role in this osteoclast activation. Cancer pain is typically managed with a combination of medical and/or surgical therapy. Medical treatment options for cancer bone pain include monotherapy with

Table 20.1 Incidence of compression fracture in cancer patients

Cancer (%)	Incidence (%)
Multiple myeloma	24
Breast	14
Prostate	6
Lung	8

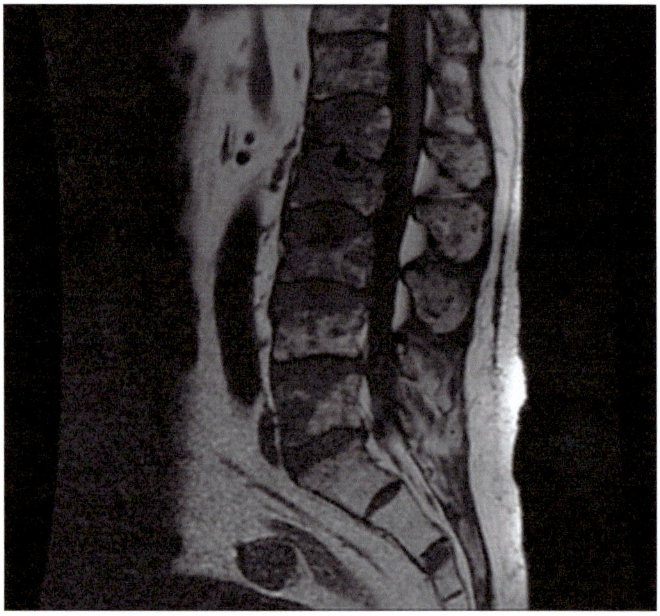

Fig. 20.2 MRI of patient with multiple myeloma of the spine and multilevel pathological compression fractures

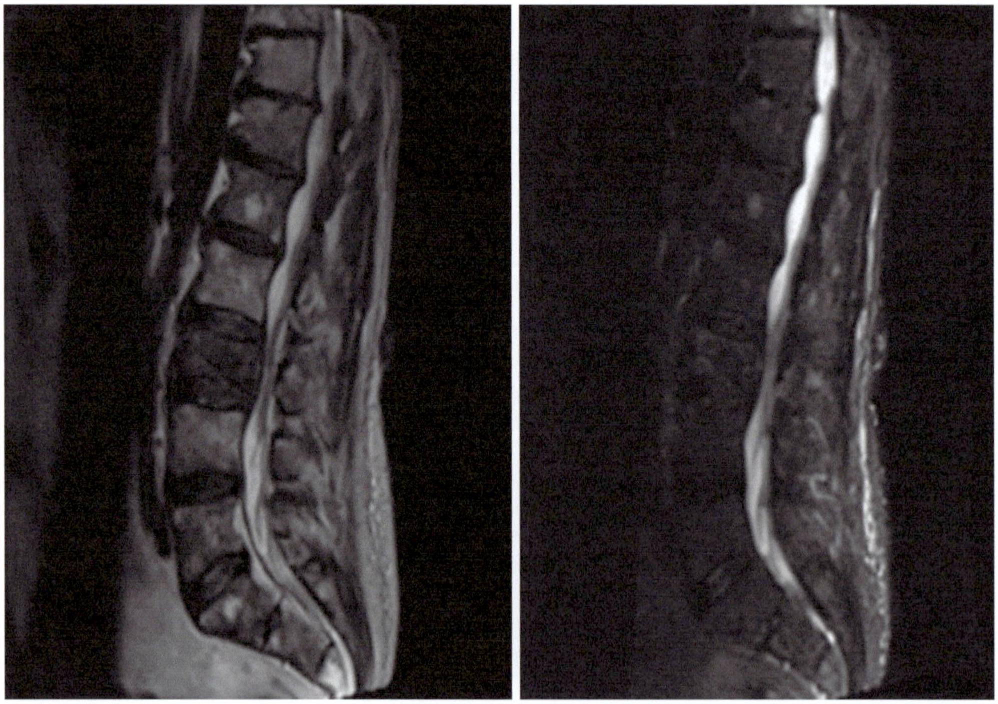

Fig. 20.1 Sagittal MRI of patient with metastatic lung cancer and diffuse spinal vertebral metastasis with L3 pathological fracture

a combination of NSAIDs, COX-2 inhibitors, chemotherapy, radiation, bisphosphonates, and opioids. Typically NSAIDs or COX-2 inhibitors are considered first-line treatment and provide a source of pain relief by inhibiting peripheral sources of pain. The advantage of COX-2 inhibitors compared to NSAIDS is that the former has less of a gastrointestinal side effect profile compared to the later. Chemotherapy may eradicate the tumor; however, it does not address the issue of mechanical pain relief. External beam radiation is highly effective in alleviating tumor-induced bone pain, with greater than 90% of patients receiving some pain relief and 50% of patients having complete pain relief. This relief is not without several consequences. First, it was reported that more than 50% of patients who undergo radiation treatment and experience pain relief will acquire a relapse of pain equivalent to pretreatment levels [10]. In addition, there are reports of radiation therapy, especially radiosurgery, contributing to osteonecrosis [11]. Radiotherapy also has the potential for damaging nearby normal tissue, resulting in fibrosclerosis and excessive extracellular matrix and collagen deposition, which may manifest as fibrosis and/or vascular or other tissue damage [12]. Further, other serious reported adverse effects include the development of a second primary tumor due to toxicity to nearby normal tissue, as well as hematologic toxicity that may limit the use of chemotherapy [13, 14]. Spinal metastatic disease from renal cell cancer is also known to be very radioresistant (Fig. 20.3). Bisphosphonates produce a direct inhibition of osteoclasts and osteoclast precursor cells, thereby inhibiting bone resorption and allowing for mechanical stabilization.

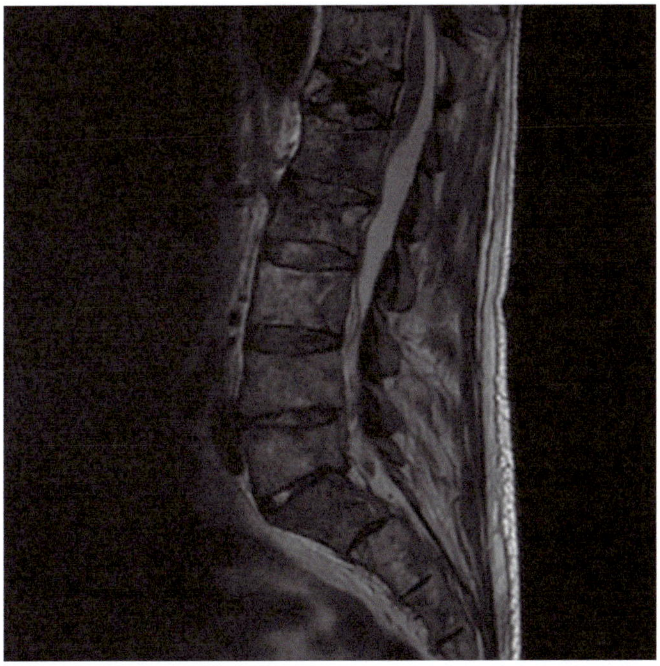

Fig. 20.3 Post vertebroplasty MRI of patient with pathological compression fracture of L2 secondary to metastatic renal cell cancer

Bisphosphonate use entails several side effects as well, osteonecrosis of the jaw being chief among them. Either concurrently or when all of the aforementioned treatment options fail, cancer-related bone pain is often treated with strong opioid pain medications. Unfortunately, given the intense pain often experienced due to cancer bone pain, high-dose opioids are needed. This leads to several undesired consequences, including confusion, constipation, respiratory depression, and somnolence. One study examined patients receiving opioid therapy for moderate to severe cancer-related pain. Within 4 weeks of seeing their physician, 73% of terminally ill patients reported that their pain was still moderate to severe, and 40% of those patients who rated their pain as severe requested an increase in opioid treatment [15].

Often, medical treatment for cancer itself may be a source of cancer-related bone destruction and pain. Aromatase inhibitors for breast cancer and antiandrogens for prostate cancer, as well as the metabolic burden placed on the bone by solid tumors themselves, can all lead to generalized bone loss and the possibility of painful vertebral compression fractures. Surgical therapy for cancer-related bone pain is typically palliative, and the aims include providing pain control and maintaining neurologic function as well as spinal stability. There are, however, a significant number of complications associated with performing surgery on patients with metastatic tumor(s) to the spinal column, making the procedure a high-risk endeavor. Studies have shown that laminectomy either alone or with adjunct radiation therapy yield poor results [16]. Specifically, laminectomy often does not provide exposure to resect lateral and anterior vertebral body tumors. Further, resection of the posterior element often leads to kyphosis and an increased number of neurologic deficits. Tseng et al. reported that upon a review of the literature, surgery for metastatic spinal tumors has been demonstrated to yield an overall complication rate of 10–52% [16]. Specific complications of surgery for skeletal column metastasis include deep venous thrombosis, myocardial ischemia and infarction, and bronchopulmonary pneumonia. Further complications of these procedures also include failed fixation requiring revision and postoperative hematoma, in addition to the universal surgical risks of infection and wound dehiscence. There are instances, however, where surgical intervention is not only warranted but imperative. Such cases include unclear diagnosis of a spinal lesion, neurologic compromise with concurrent or impending decline, and compression from an epidural tumor or bone fragments, among others [16].

Clinical Evaluation

Patients presenting for a possible vertebral augmentation procedure will often do so in excruciating pain. Despite this, it is important to obtain a detailed history and physical examination, including any events or potentially traumatic injuries that may have occurred prior to the onset of the patient's pain. Other causes of back pain including muscle spasm, disc herniation, spinal stenosis, osteoarthritis, ankylosing spondylitis, and infection should be actively investigated and eliminated. Imaging studies, including any available MRI studies, should be thoroughly reviewed. Often, but not always, the patient will present with pain and tenderness that will correlate with the spinal level(s) seen to be affected on MRI. There are several MRI findings that are very consistent with the diagnosis of a tumor-related vertebral compression fracture. Abnormal signal(s) in the posterior element, expansion of the contour of the vertebral body or posterior elements, along with an associated epidural or extravertebral soft-tissue mass favor this diagnosis. Only a few lab tests are necessary; specifically, the PTT, PT, and platelet count should be normal. There are several absolute and relative contraindications to performing vertebroplasty or its related procedures. Absolute contraindications include epidural abscess, systemic sepsis, osteomyelitis, discitis, a bone that is too sclerotic for the procedure, and uncorrectable coagulopathy. Several patient and institutional factors may also serve as absolute contraindications including severe, active, and non-optimized cardiopulmonary disease, patient's inability to tolerate conscious sedation or general anesthesia, and lack of patient monitoring facilities in the event of an unanticipated complication of the procedure. Relative contraindications to vertebroplasty and related procedures include radiculopathy and severe vertebral body collapse/vertebra plana, and destruction of posterior cortex. As mentioned previously, the presence of an epidural tumor or bone fragments in the epidural space along with a resultant neurologic compromise should be viewed as an absolute contraindication, and immediate surgical consultation should be considered. Radiculopathy is considered a relative contraindication because of the potential for exacerbating nerve root compression by polymethylmethacrylate (PMMA) cement extrusion into the neural foramen. Severe vertebral body collapse is also considered a relative contraindication as there is likely to be difficulty in passing the trocars through the pedicle without entering the spinal canal. It is certainly possible to perform the procedure on patients with severe vertebral body collapse; however, the trocars should be placed as laterally as possible in the pedicle. This will obviously make the kyphoplasty technique almost impossible to perform. Careful attention must also be paid to the viscosity of the cement that is to be injected. Specifically, it should be of an appropriate viscosity that prevents the entrance of PMMA cement into the epidural space. The number of levels that may be performed at once has been a topic of contention, as well, mainly because of the potential for PMMA toxicity. Peters et al. suggested no more than two levels be corrected at once [17]. Hentschel et al., as well as other authors, have demonstrated the ability to perform the procedure on three levels safely [18]. A couple of authors have reported correcting four levels at once [19]. The decision to augment multiple levels must be determined based on history, exam, and imaging globally, not solely on imaging. Hentschel did identify a statistically significant increase in the incidence of PMMA cement extrusion in patients undergoing a vertebroplasty with the aforementioned contraindications; however, all but one were asymptomatic (and the one exception resulted in transient radicular pain) [18].

Vertebroplasty

As mentioned previously, vertebroplasty was first described by Galibert in 1984 to treat a C2 hemangioma [1]. While it is still used to treat painful vertebral hemangiomas, the procedure has been also used to treat a variety of different benign and pathological conditions including osteoporotic vertebral compression fractures, vertebral metastasis of solid tumors or multiple myeloma, and Kümmel's spondylitis. Vertebroplasty targets the vertebral body. The transpedicular approach is preferred in the thoracic and lumbar regions. The pedicles, which form the lateral aspects of the spinal canal, offer a safe and effective route to the pathologic site in the lumbar and thoracic regions. If one is to perform the procedure on the cervical region of the spine, the anterolateral approach is preferred as the pedicles are too small to accommodate the needles needed for the vertebroplasty procedure. Because of this, the posterolateral approach also carries a significant chance of injuring the associated vertebral artery. One must also be conscientious of the venous anatomy of the spine. Specifically, the epidural venous plexus is located in the anterior epidural space with longitudinal sinuses that extend around the circumference of the spinal canal. This plexus communicates with a basivertebral vein in the central aspect of the vertebral body and with intervertebral and lumbar veins that drain laterally. All of these veins eventually drain into either the inferior vena cava or azygous system. Once appropriate patient selection and anatomic considerations have taken place, the patient should be brought to the operatory suite with the minimum appropriate monitoring consisting of EKG and pulse oximetry, and a noninvasive blood pressure measurement device should be placed on the patient. An intravenous line is placed for procedural sedation as well as for administration of an antibiotic against common skin flora. The following is a summary of the "classic approach" for the thoracic and lumbar regions followed by the authors of this text, as well as which has been previously described by Fenton and Czervionke [20]. The patient is placed in the prone position. Patient positioning is variable by institution; however, proper positioning that allows easy access to the vertebra with concurrent patient comfort is imperative. While positioning, careful attention must also be paid to not cause any additional fractures in this patient population that is at risk for additional fractures. The patient's back is then prepared in a sterile fashion and draped. A wide area of the back should be prepped to allow for various angles of approach if necessary. The initial placement of the needle is a crucial step in the procedure. In the classic approach, the vertebral body is aligned in the straight anteroposterior (AP) and lateral projections. The superior and inferior end plates are aligned to a single line on the AP view with both pedicles visible and the spinous process in the midline. The ribs, pedicles, neural arches, and posterior aspects of contiguous vertebral bodies are aligned on the lateral view. This positioning typically allows for a good view of both sides of the vertebral body for needle placement. Other approaches have been described with good efficacy, and the reader is encouraged to consider all approaches available for this procedure. Once alignment has been confirmed and an entry point has been chosen, local anesthesia with 1% lidocaine or a similar local anesthetic agent is injected subcutaneously. The tract of the needle should be infiltrated to the pedicle, and a generous amount of local anesthetic should be applied to the pedicle. This step can be performed by a 22–25-gauge spinal needle and is also an optimal way to judge the trajectory of the working cannula. A small skin incision is then made with a scalpel, and the larger-caliber vertebroplasty needle is then placed in the mid to upper outer third of the pedicle into the vertebral body. Optimal needle placement involves positioning the tip of the outer needle cannula at the junction of the middle and anterior thirds of the vertebral body as close to the center as possible (Fig. 20.4). If necessary, needle path adjustments should be made with the needle still in the pedicle. With the assistance of fluoroscopic guidance, the needle should be visualized to be lateral to the medial cortical edge of the pedicle until it has passed anteriorly into the vertebral body (Fig. 20.5). This point cannot be understated. If this medial cortex of the pedicle is violated, trauma to the thecal sac or spinal cord with possible tearing of the epidural veins may occur. With mild vertebral body collapse, the needle may be placed on the involved side. If the collapse is severe, it may be necessary to place the needle on the side with more residual vertebral body. If there is severe collapse involving the central portion, bilateral needle placement will likely be required, as a single pedicle approach will likely not result in PMMA distribution across the midline (Fig. 20.6). Once past the posterior edge of the vertebral body, with visualization in the lateral plane, the needle can be advanced more rapidly under continuous fluoroscopy. Patients will move during this procedure, and the fluoroscopic image may not reflect a true lateral position. If the needle is advanced too far anteriorly, an off-midline needle tip could perforate the ventral cortex of the vertebral body. This has the potential for perforating the

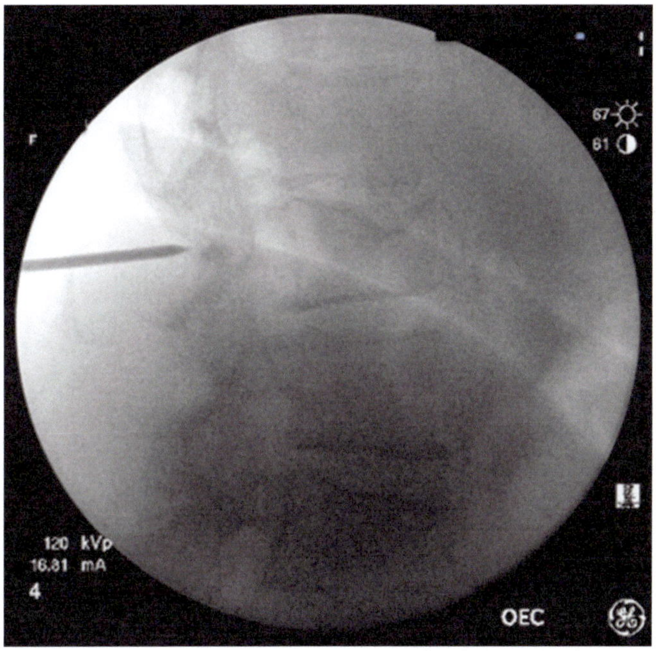

Fig. 20.4 Lateral fluoroscopic image of working cannula access of L2 pedicle

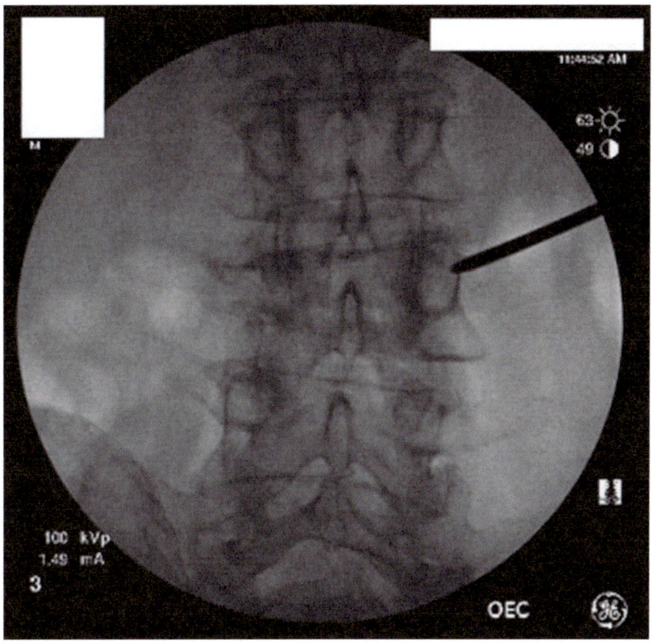

Fig. 20.5 AP fluoroscopic image of lumbar pedicle access with working cannula

aorta and inferior vena cava, which lie just anterior to the vertebral column in the thoracic and upper lumbar spine. When needle placement has been completed, a vertebral biopsy may be performed if the etiology behind the compression fracture is equivocal; otherwise, venography may be performed through the needle. Three to five milliliters of

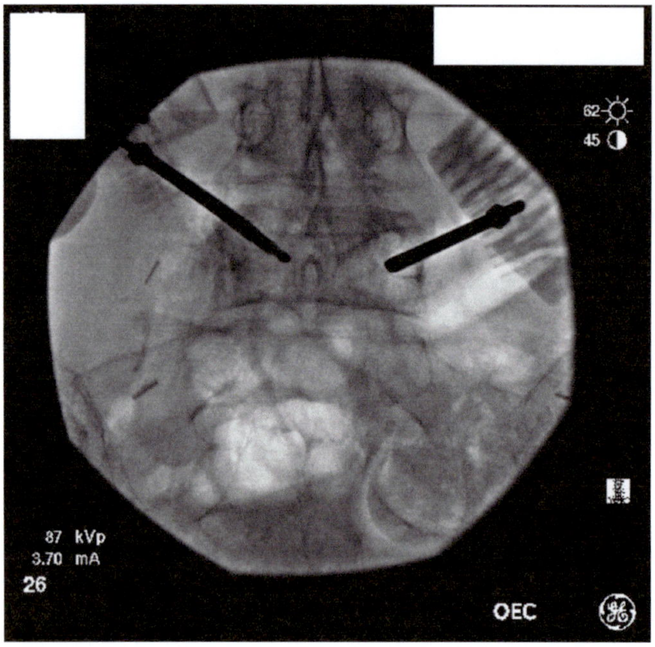

Fig. 20.6 AP fluoroscopic image of bilateral transpedicle access of L5 vertebrae

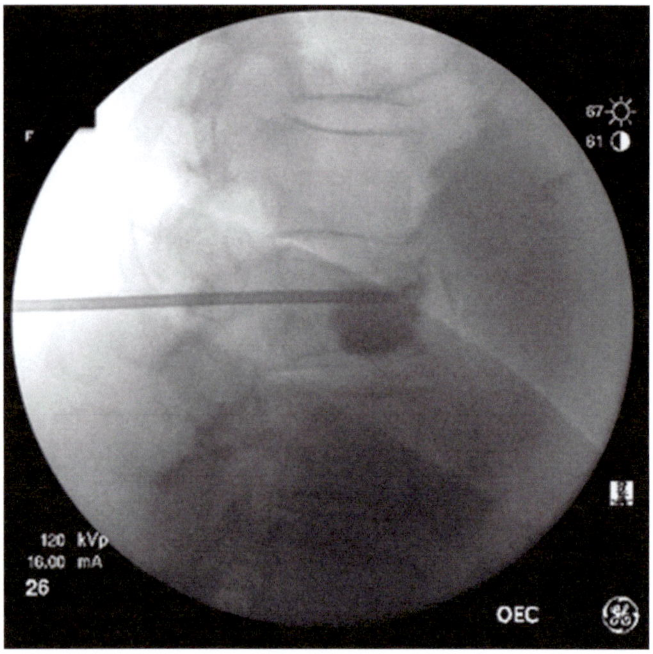

Fig. 20.7 Lateral fluoroscopic image of PMMA fill of pathological fracture during vertebroplasty procedure

half-strength contrast agent is injected to determine whether the needle is in or immediately adjacent to the basivertebral vein or another large draining vein or whether it is within a fissure continuous with paraspinal structures or adjacent disc spaces. This step reduces the likelihood of injection of PMMA cement into a vascular structure. The PMMA cement

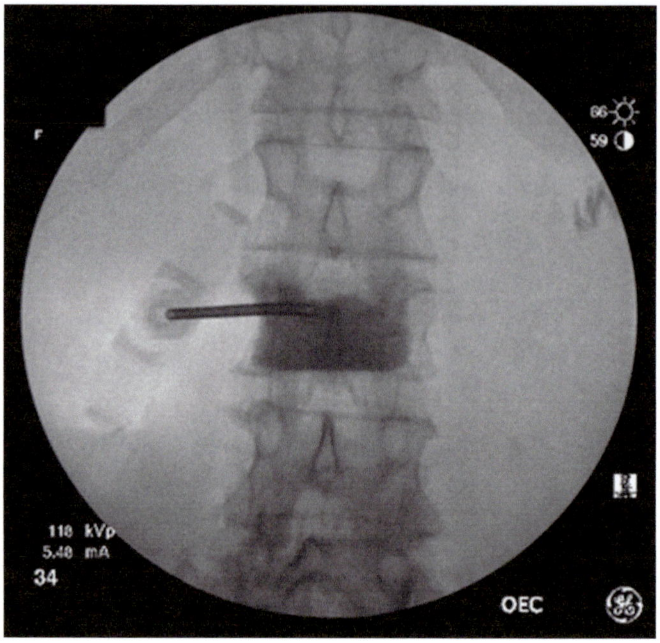

Fig. 20.8 AP fluoroscopic view of L2 vertebrae after PMMA injection. Note bilateral spread using unipedicular approach

is then prepared, and delivery of the mixture is accomplished under direct fluoroscopic visualization. This process should be viewed in a true lateral projection with particular attention to ensure no extravasation of PMMA into the basivertebral vein or through a fissure into the epidural space. The end point of injection varies; however, it is essential to avoid the deposition of cement at the posterior aspect of the vertebral body, which may lead to potential neurovascular compromise. Little clinical outcome is gained from filling the entire vertebral body. Needles should then be withdrawn, and AP and lateral final control photographs are taken (Figs. 20.7, 20.8, 20.9, and 20.10). Adhesive strips and sterile dressing are then applied to the skin. The patient is gently turned supine and transferred to the recovery area. Unlike surgical approaches, vertebroplasty provides immediate anterior stabilization of the vertebral column (Fig. 20.11).

Although there have been conflicting reports on the long-term efficacy of vertebroplasty for osteoporotic compression fractures, the evidence is much stronger for malignant fractures. Buchbinder et al. found that vertebroplasty did not result in a significant advantage in any measured outcome at any time point for the treatment of osteoporotic vertebral compression fractures; however, Gangi found favorable outcomes in 83% of patients presenting for vertebroplasty secondary to vertebral body factures due to malignant lesions [21, 22]. Similarly, Lee et al. found that following vertebroplasty for vertebral compression fractures secondary to malignant lesions, 84% of patients described a benefit with regard to pain relief within 24–48 h [8]. Overall, when Chen et al. reviewed recent literature on spinal metastases treated

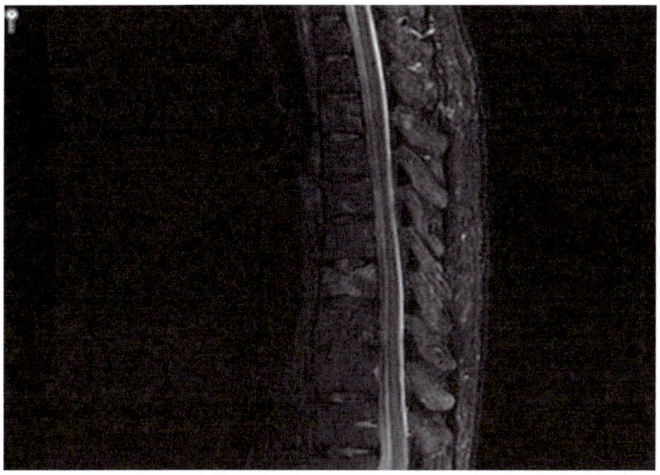

Fig. 20.9 Sagittal MRI noting T8 pathological compression fracture

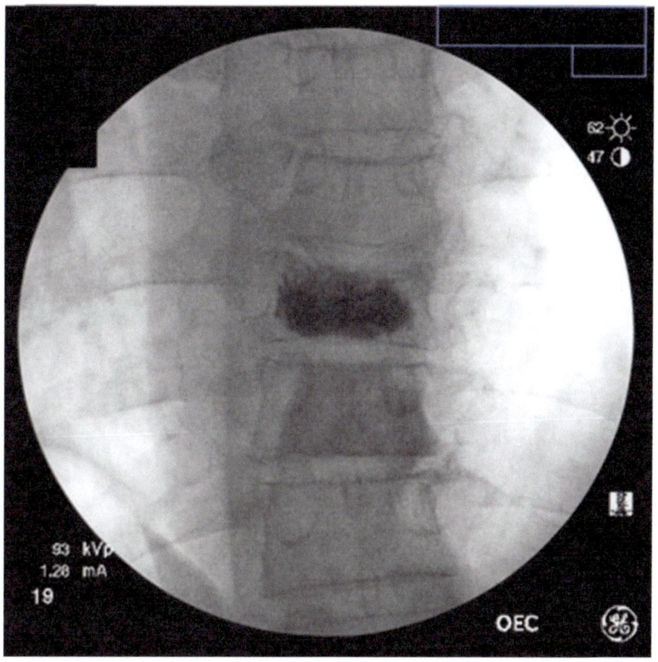

Fig. 20.10 AP fluoroscopic view of the same vertebrae from Fig. 20.9 after satisfactory vertebral augmentation

with vertebroplasty, they found that complete or partial pain relief was achieved in 75–89% of patients [23]. In the aforementioned review, there were no significant differences found in the pain relief of men versus women. The mechanisms by which vertebroplasty provides pain relief are likely due to several factors. Local tumoricidal effects around the area where cement was injected were noted in a postmortem study of six individuals [24]. An immediate analgesic effect that has been reported may be explained by in situ immobilization of the vertebral body fracture. Specifically, this internal stabilization prevents micromotion, and the subsequent related pain, as well as providing for an environment of healing [16].

Kyphoplasty

Balloon kyphoplasty was first described in 1998 [25] and has also seen a rise in its use since its inception [25]. A variant procedure of the previously described vertebroplasty, kyphoplasty is a method for treating compression fractures of the spine in which a balloon is placed coaxially through a needle into the vertebral body to reduce the fracture. This is then followed by cement augmentation in an approach similar to the one described above. Notable differences include the fact that kyphoplasty requires larger needles and a bipedicular approach. Because of this, kyphoplasty may only be attempted on the midthoracic and lumbar spinal levels (Fig. 20.12). In addition, the PMMA viscosity must be very low, and it must be injected under very low pressure. The main reported advantage of kyphoplasty over vertebroplasty is a restoration of height within the vertebral body, thereby potentially improving the biomechanics of the spine and possibly improving kyphosis. For this reason, kyphoplasty tends to be favored when the patient's kyphosis is greater than 20°. The nature of the procedure allows for more controlled delivery of bone cement, and so it is also favored when disruption of the posterior vertebral cortex is present. Further, in patients with severe vertebral collapse, kyphoplasty is preferred to restore height unless the collapse is too severe to permit insertion of balloon [26]. Results regarding pain relief in patients with cancer-related bone pain tend to be similar to those seen with vertebroplasty. Fourney et al. found that 86% of patients who underwent vertebroplasty for vertebral body fracture secondary to cancer reported improved or complete pain relief, compared to 80% of patients who underwent kyphoplasty. Only 9% of the patients who underwent either procedure reported no pain relief. In a more recent study, Berenson found that among patients with cancer and vertebral compression fractures who were treated with kyphoplasty, the patients who underwent kyphoplasty had a superior functional outcome at 1 month, showed a marked reduction in back pain, and showed improved quality of life, with fewer patients using pain medications, compared with those who were treated with conservative medical management [3]. As an advantage of kyphoplasty over vertebroplasty, Hentschel and Fourney found there to be less risk of PMMA cement extrusion with kyphoplasty compared to vertebroplasty [18, 26]. Unfortunately, kyphoplasty entails greater cost than vertebroplasty and usually requires a longer procedure time.

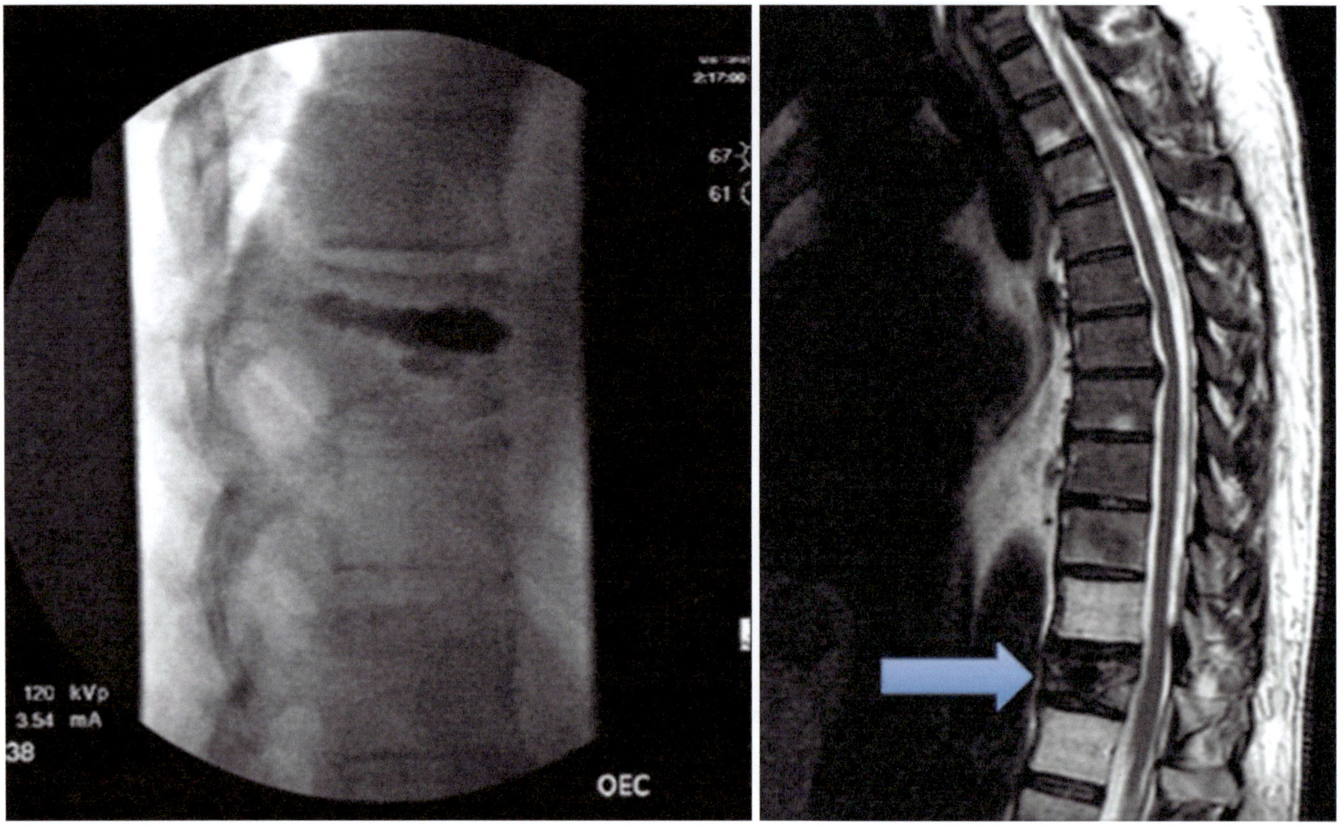

Fig. 20.11 Lateral fluoroscopic view after T11 vertebral augmentation procedure. Note 4-week post-procedure MRI that demonstrates anterior stabilization of vertebral body after vertebral augmentation

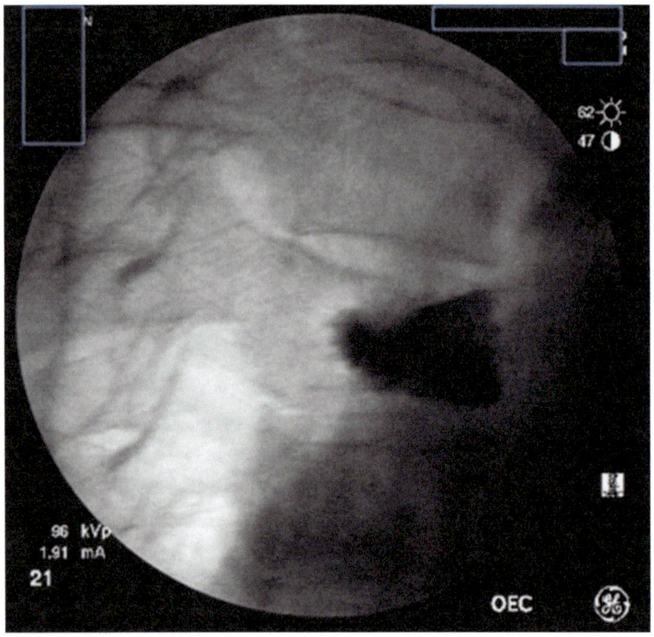

Fig. 20.12 Lateral fluoroscopic view after satisfactory kyphoplasty procedure

Sacroplasty

Spinal metastatic lesions most commonly occur in the thoracic spinal area followed by the lumbar spinal areas. However, sacral metastasis of a solid tumor or malignancy and spread of a primary pelvic lesion are well-described clinical entities. Spread is typically by hematologic dissemination with the exception of extension of primary pelvic lesions. Unfortunately, sacral lesions are often diagnosed in the advanced stages of the tumor and are often surrounding sacral nerves, vasculature, and nearby organs. X-ray films are typically not accurate, and, thus, the diagnosis is most often made with three-phase bone scintigraphy, CT scanning, MRI, or a combination of these. Based upon a review of several sources, Furman report that the 1-year mortality rate of patients with pelvic insufficiency fractures is 14.3% and 50% of affected patients will not return to their previous level of functioning [27]. Traditional therapy has consisted of extended bed rest with analgesics. However, this has several potentially fatal consequences including deep venous thrombosis, pulmonary embolism, muscle atrophy, cardiac deconditioning, decubitus ulcers, bone demineralization, and psychological changes, among other complications. Other treatment options include chemotherapy, radiotherapy, radiofrequency thermocoagulation, and surgical excision. By its nature, chemotherapy has several undesirable systemic consequences. Radiotherapy has the potential to damage collateral structures. Radiofrequency thermocoagulation palliates pain, however, not as quickly as sacroplasty. Goetz et al. found that radiofrequency thermocoagulation results in a three to four point drop in the numerical pain scores. However, this occurs over a 4–12-week period, and this time frame is often not acceptable to patients who present with cancer-induced sacral pain [28]. Surgical sacral intervention has many serious potential complications including massive bleeding, CSF leakage, neurologic defects, bowel and bladder dysfunction, and spinal and/or pelvic instability. All of these complications lead to an overall morbidity of 19–48% for sacral surgery [29]. For these reasons, sacral vertebroplasty and sacral kyphoplasty are becoming increasingly popular treatment options for patients presenting with sacral metastatic lesions.

Description of Procedure

The following is an abbreviated description of a short-axis fluoroscopic approach to sacral vertebroplasty. Prior to the procedure, standard monitoring equipment including EKG, pulse oximetry, and blood pressure cuff is applied. An intravenous line is established for preoperative antibiotic and procedural sedation. The patient is positioned prone, and the fluoroscope is obliqued contralaterally from the side being treated until the physician can superimpose the medial and lateral aspects of the sacroiliac joint. An 18-gauge needle is used to penetrate the skin, and a mallet is used to gently tap a 13- or 11-gauge trocar into the periosteum. A lateral view is used to confirm that the needle tip is located within the S1 and S2 vertebral segments and not ventral to them. The physician then returns to the AP view to properly visualize the sacral foramen and to confirm needle tip placement. Some physicians may consider placing contrast at the S1 nerve root for proper visualization of the nerve, and the same process may be repeated at S2. Depending on the extent of the fracture, the aforementioned process may need to be repeated at S3 and S4. When injecting the cement, it should be injected slowly with the use of the AP imaging to watch for medial spread of the cement toward the nerve roots. The majority of the S1 and S2 segments should be filled, as that is where most of the weight-bearing occurs, and approximately 5–8 ml of cement is placed in each sacral ala. Sacral kyphoplasty is a variation upon the procedure described above and incorporates the use of a tamping balloon similar to the variation upon spinal column vertebroplasty, as described above. This procedure may be performed either with fluoroscopy alone or with a combination of fluoroscopy and CT image guidance (Zhang 2008). The use of fluoroscopic guidance alone, however, may be problematic as reported by Zhang et al. [30]. The use of fluoroscopic guidance alone may lead to difficulty in visualizing the sacral foramina. CT guidance may give better definition of the spatial relationships, which aids in preventing injury to nearby vascular, neurologic, and visceral structures. Overall, sacroplasty, including both sacral vertebroplasty and sacral kyphoplasty, has been shown to be effective as a means of reducing pain and restoring functional ability to patients presenting with sacral metastases and sacral insufficiency fractures. Citing several previous case reports, as well as their own patients, Shah et al. found that sacroplasty patients demonstrated early, rapid, and durable pain relief (sustained at a 1-year time interval), functional improvement, and decreased opioid consumption [29].

Complications

Although these are procedures with an overall excellent safety profile, there are several possible complications of vertebroplasty, kyphoplasty, and sacroplasty. Leakage of PMMA cement is a known complication given the nature of the procedure, and this leakage, specifically through cortical defects with subsequent epidural compression of the neural elements, is of concern. In a case series by Cotten et al., it was found that cement leakage occurred in up to 73% of all procedures for cancer pain and myeloma [31]. The vast majority of these were found to be asymptomatic. This finding has been substantiated by more recent literature as well [18, 26]. Cement extrusion into the disc space and anterior spinal space (with the exception of the venous plexus) is typically of little significance (Fig. 20.13). Extrusion of cement into the nerve root foramen is likely to be of some clinical significance, as leakage into the relatively small space will typically result in a radiculopathy. Lee et al. found that this occurs in <0.5% of cases. In the literature, when this has been reported, it has been noted to be transient and will often respond well to corticosteroids [8, 18]. Injecting smaller volumes of PMMA cement likely reduces the incidence of cement extrusion, and, importantly, it has been demonstrated that the volume of cement injected is unrelated to patient outcome with respect to pain control [31]. Infiltration of PMMA cement into small veins while this substance is still in a liquid state could occur, thereby leading to the embolization of fat secondary to entrainment of this substance into the paravertebral vasculature. Based on other studies, Lee et al. reported that the overall risk of infection from vertebroplasty for all types of patients is at 0.5% [8].

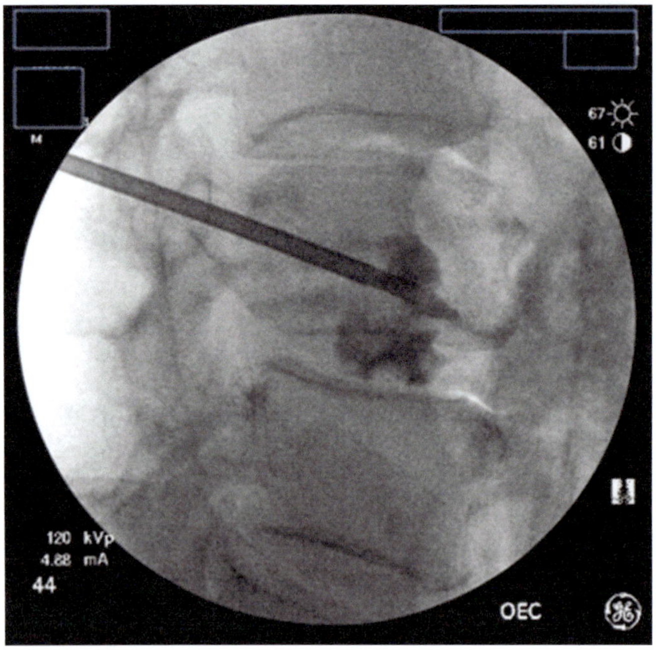

Fig. 20.13 Lateral fluoroscopic image of lumbar vertebroplasty with inferior endplate extravasation of PMMA into the lumbar disc

Additionally, there has been noted to be an association between vertebroplasty and new-onset fractures. Specifically, it has been shown that after vertebroplasty patients are at an increased risk of new-onset adjacent-level fractures and when they occur, they occur sooner than nonadjacent level fractures [32]. Trout et al. found a relative risk of 4.62 for fracture of vertebrae adjacent to treated levels versus fractures not adjacent to treated levels. The investigators hypothesized that this is potentially due to biomechanics in the treated area of the spine. Specifically, cement in an augmented vertebral body acts as a pillar that both reduces the normal inward bulge of the treated end plate and increases the stiffness of both the intervertebral joint and the whole motion segment. The pressure in the adjacent intervertebral disk increases significantly, resulting in higher loading forces on the adjacent vertebral bodies as well as increased deflection of the adjacent end plate. This can potentially lead to failure of adjacent vertebral bodies, especially in lower spinal loads [32]. Contrary to this, Taylor et al. found a reduction in incident fractures in 12 months following kyphoplasty for osteoporotic vertebral fractures compared to patients receiving conventional treatment [33]. Rare complications have been reported to occur as well, including cement extension into IVC, aortic puncture, local hematoma, cement pulmonary emboli, and loss of sensation at the dermatome of the vertebral body being worked upon. Sacroplasty carries with it the possible complication of bowel perforation, in addition to the aforementioned. Upon a review of the literature, Chew et al. state that a serious complication rate of around 2% has been observed in vertebroplasty being performed for malignant disease, compared to 1.5% in osteoporosis [5]. This slightly higher rate of complication may be related to a higher volume of cement that is often necessary to be used for vertebral compression fractures resulting from metastatic disease. Finally, citing other sources as well as their own findings, Lee et al. found that vertebroplasty is an overall safe procedure, with an overall risk of complications noted to be between 5% and 10% in metastatic disease [8].

Conclusion

Since being first described in the early 1980s, the vertebroplasty procedure has seen many variations in the technique and approach to the procedure, as well as several variant procedures that have allowed it to be used for an increasing number of different causes of malignant and nonmalignant vertebral body compression fractures. While clinically uncommon, transient, and serious complications have all been described as a consequence of performing vertebroplasty or one of the variant procedures, the success rates cited above certainly warrant its use as a treatment modality for those suffering from pain related to malignancy-induced vertebral compression fractures. Important topics for further research include the time frame at which vertebroplasty and its variant procedures are offered to patients and the maximal number of vertebral segments that can be treated at once. In the present, however, vertebroplasty and its related procedures should be viewed as an overall safe and effective treatment option for patients suffering from cancer pain secondary to malignancy-related vertebral compression fractures.

References

1. Galibert P, Deramond H, Rosat P, Le Gars D. Preliminary note on the treatment of vertebral angioma by percutaneous acrylic vertebroplasty. Neurochirurgie. 1987;33(2):166–8.
2. Weinstein JN. Balancing science and informed choice in decisions about vertebroplasty. N Engl J Med. 2009;361(6):619–21.
3. Berenson J, Pflugmacher R, Jarzem P, Zonder J, Schechtman K, Tillman JB, et al. Balloon kyphoplasty versus non-surgical fracture management for treatment of painful vertebral body compression fractures in patients with cancer: a multicentre randomised controlled trial. Lancet Oncol. 2011;12(3):225–35.
4. Coleman RE. Skeletal complications of malignancy. Cancer. 1997;80(8 Suppl):1588–94.
5. Chew C, Craig L, Edwards R, Moss J, O'Dwyer PJ. Safety and efficacy of percutaneous vertebroplasty in malignancy: a systematic review. Clin Radiol. 2011;66(1):63–72.
6. Chew C, Ritchie M, O'Dwyer PJ, Edwards R. A prospective study of vertebroplasty in patients with myeloma and spinal metastasis. Clin Radiol. 2011;66(12):1193–6.
7. Aaron AD. The management of cancer metastatic to bone. J Am Med Assoc. 1994;272(15):1206–9.

8. Lee B, Franklin I, Lewis JS, Coombes RC, Leonard R, Gishen P, et al. The efficacy of percutaneous vertebroplasty for vertebral metastasis associated with solid malignancies. Eur J Cancer. 2009;45(9):1597–602.
9. Goblirsch MJ, Zwolak PP, Clohisy DR. Biology of bone cancer pain. Clin Cancer Res. 2006;12(20 Pt 2):6231s–5s.
10. Tong D, Gillick L, Hendrickson FR. The palliation of symptomatic osseous metastases: final results of the study by the radiation therapy oncology group. Cancer. 2. Allan JM, Travis LB. Mechanisms of therapy related carcinogenesis. Nat Rev Cancer 2005;5(12):943–955. r 1982;50(5):893–899.
11. Rose PS, Laufer I, Boland PJ, Hanover A, Bilsky MH, Yamada J, et al. Risk of fracture after single fraction image-guided intensity-modulated radiation therapy to spinal metastasis. J Clin Oncol. 2009;27(30):5075–9.
12. Bentzen SM. Preventing or reducing late side effects of radiation therapy: radiobiology meets molecular pathology. Nat Rev Cancer. 2006;6(9):703–13.
13. Allan JM, Travis LB. Mechanisms of therapy related carcinogenesis. Nat Rev Cancer. 2005;5(12):943–55.
14. Jefferies S, Rajan B, Ashley S, Traish D, Brada M. Haematological toxicity of cranio-spinal irradiation. Radiother Oncol. 1998;48(1):23–7.
15. Coyle N, Adelhardt J, Foley KM, Portenoy RK. Character of terminal illness in the advanced cancer patient: pain and other symptoms during the last four weeks of life. J Pain Symptom Manag. 1990;5(2):83–93.
16. Tseng YY, Lo YL, Chen LH, Lai PL, Yang ST. Percutaneous polymethylmethacrylate vertebroplasty in the treatment of pain induced by metastatic spinal tumor. Surg Neurol. 2008;70(Suppl 1):S1 78–83.
17. Peters KR, Guiot BH, Martin PA, Fessler RG. Vertebroplasty for osteoporotic compression fractures: current practice and evolving techniques. Neurosurgery. 2002;51(5 Suppl):S96–103.
18. Hentschel SJ, Burton AW, Fourney DR, Rhines LD, Mendel E. Percutaneous vertebroplasty and kyphoplasty performed at a cancer center: refuting proposed contraindications. J Neurosurg Spine. 2005;2(4):436–40.
19. Amar AP, Larsen DW, Teitelbaum GP. Percutaneous carotid angioplasty and stenting with the use of gadolinium in lieu of iodinated contrast medium: technical case report and review of the literature. Neurosurgery. 2001;49(5):1262–6.
20. Fenton DS, Czervionke LF. Image-guided spine intervention. Philadelphia: Saunders; 2003.
21. Buchbinder R, Osborne RH, Ebeling PR, Wark JD, Mitchell P, Wriedt C, et al. A randomized trial of vertebroplasty for painful osteoporotic vertebral fractures. N Engl J Med. 2009;361(6):557–68.
22. Gangi A, Guth S, Imbert JP, Marin H, Dietemann JL. Percutaneous vertebroplasty: indications, technique, and results. Radiographics. 2003;23(2). https://doi.org/10.1148/rg.e10.
23. Chen KY, Ma HI, Chiang YH. Percutaneous transpedicular vertebroplasty with polymethyl methacrylate for pathological fracture of the spine. J Clin Neurosci. 2009;16(10):1300–4.
24. San Millan Ruiz D, Burkhardt K, Jean B, Muster M, Martin JB, Bouvier J, et al. Pathology findings with acrylic implants. Bone. 1999;25(2 Suppl):85s–90s.
25. Garfin SR, Yuan HA, Reiley MA. New technologies in spine: kyphoplasty and vertebroplasty for the treatment of painful osteoporotic compression fractures. Spine. 2001;26(14):1511–5.
26. Fourney DR, Schomer DF, Nader R, Chlan-Fourney J, Suki D, Ahrar K, et al. Percutaneous vertebroplasty and kyphoplasty for painful vertebral body fractures in cancer patients. J Neurosurg. 2003;98(1 Suppl):21–30.
27. Furman MB, Lee TS, Berkwitz L. Atlas of image-guided spinal procedures. Philadelphia: Saunders; 2012.
28. Goetz MP, Callstrom MR, Charboneau JW, Farrell MA, Maus TP, Welch TJ. Percutaneous image-guided radiofrequency ablation of painful metastasis involving bone: a multicenter study. J Clin Oncol. 2004;22(2):300–6.
29. Shah RV. Sacral kyphoplasty for the treatment of painful sacral insufficiency fractures and metastases. Spine J. 2012;12(2):113–20.
30. Zhang J, Wu CG, Gu YF, Li MH. Percutaneous sacroplasty for sacral metastatic tumors under fluoroscopic guidance only. Korean J Radiol. 2008;9(6):572–6.
31. Cotten A, Dewatre F, Cortet B, Assaker R, Leblond D, Duquesnov B, et al. Percutaneous vertebroplasty for osteolytic metastases and myeloma: effects of the percentage of lesion filling and the leakage of methyl methacrylate at clinical follow-up. Radiology. 1996;200(2):525–30.
32. Trout AT, Kallmes DF, Kaufmann TJ. New fractures after vertebroplasty: adjacent fractures occur significantly sooner. Am J Neuroradiol. 2006;27(1):217–23.
33. Taylor RS, Fritzell P, Taylor RJ. Balloon kyphoplasty in the management of vertebral compression fractures: an updated systematic review and meta-analysis. Eur Spine J. 2006;16(8):1085–100.

Treatment Considerations for Cancer Pain Syndromes

21

Devin Peck and Gendai J. Echezona

Concurrent Chemotherapy

While no formal recommendations have been made regarding interventions in patients undergoing chemotherapy, consensus statements address the implantation of intrathecal pumps in such patients. We can apply these recommendations to the use of other invasive pain therapies. A multi-institutional statement published in 2011 stated that a white blood cell count > 2 × 10^9/L and/or an absolute neutrophil count > 1000/μL is preferred. To optimize safety, interventions can be planned for cell count recovery periods in between cytotoxic oncologic treatments [1]. Close coordination and frequent communication with the oncologic team are strongly advised.

Platelet count levels mirror those of white blood cells with respect to effects of chemotherapeutic administration. In general, platelet counts of 100,000/μL are preferred for spinal interventions. Prior to any procedures, discussions regarding risk versus benefit should involve the pain physician, oncologist, palliative care team, and patient [2]. Additional consideration should be given to any concurrent chemotherapeutic regimens. As an example, bevacizumab is known to increase bleeding risk for up to a month following administration [3].

Coagulopathy and Anticoagulation

Anticoagulation is common in oncologic patients due to the pro-thrombotic physiologic changes caused by malignancy. Venous thromboembolism is a leading cause of morbidity and mortality in this population [4]. While the overall incidence of neuraxial hematoma is low (incidence rates of 1: 220,000 and 1: 150,000 for intrathecal and epidural interventions, respectively [1]), more recent epidemiological surveys suggest that certain groups or situations may be at additional risk. The risk of bleeding complications is increased in the geriatric population, in those with spinal abnormalities, or in the case of difficult needle placement. The American Society of Regional Anesthesia and Pain Medicine has reviewed various anticoagulants, antiplatelet agents, and thrombolytics to develop recommendations regarding their management in the setting of planned interventions [5].

Pain as a Result of Therapy

Chemotherapy-Induced Peripheral Neuropathy

Peripheral neuropathy is a commonly known side effect of chemotherapeutic agents. It may present as pain in the form of paresthesia or myalgias typically affecting the hands and feet. Symptoms may be explained by injury to axons, myelin sheaths, neural cell bodies, and glial structures, although the mechanism of nerve injury is not fully understood [6]. Pain may present shortly after the initiation of therapy or well after the medication has been discontinued. Agents commonly known to cause peripheral neuropathy include vinca alkaloids, taxols, platinum compounds, and suramin. The degree of nerve damage correlates with the type of agent, duration of treatment, and cumulative dose received [7, 8].

The nervous system has a remarkable ability to regenerate, which patients may perceive as an improvement in painful symptoms. For regeneration to occur, the cell bodies must be intact and further exposure to offending agents avoided. Unfortunately, regeneration may be incomplete and damage irreversible.

Medications used for the treatment of peripheral neuropathy include analgesics such as opioids and nonsteroidal anti-inflammatory agents, in addition to nerve stabilization agents

D. Peck
Physician, Austin Interventional Pain, Austin, TX, USA

G. J. Echezona (✉)
Eagle Consulting Services, White Plains, NY, USA
e-mail: Gendai.echezona@wchn.org

A. Gulati et al. (eds.), *Essentials of Interventional Cancer Pain Management*, https://doi.org/10.1007/978-3-319-99684-4_21

consisting of antidepressants or antiepileptics. Interventional techniques used for the treatment of peripheral neuropathy include transcutaneous electrical nerve stimulation (TENS) and spinal cord stimulation. Emerging therapies include neurosurgical intervention, peripheral nerve blocks, and peripheral nerve stimulation.

Transcutaneous electrical nerve stimulation alters pain perception through activation of sensory A-beta nerve fibers, which may then inhibit transmission of nociceptive A-delta or C fibers [9]. This mechanism of action is based on the "gate control" theory. Application of TENS over intact skin in a neurotome distribution typically causes non-noxious paresthesia. This can act to alleviate neuropathic pain. TENS can be self-administered by the patient following an in-office training session. It is generally well-tolerated and results in few adverse effects.

Spinal cord stimulation involves the implantation of electronic leads in the epidural space to transmit pulsed energy to the dorsal columns of the spinal cord or nerve roots [10]. Spinal cord stimulation has been used to treat failed back syndrome, radicular pain, complex regional pain syndrome, and peripheral neuropathies (including diabetic neuropathy and chemotherapy-induced neuropathy). The proposed mechanism of action for pain relief is based in part on the gate control theory. In addition, it has been proposed that activation of dorsal column fibers by electrical stimulation inhibits the hyperexcitability of wide-dynamic-range neurons that are sensitized by peripheral nerve injury [4].

Until recently, the use of spinal cord stimulation was limited in the cancer population due to MRI incompatibility as many oncologic patients may require scans in the future to assess disease progression, metastasis, or recurrence. The introduction of newer MRI compatible devices has allowed patients with implanted spinal cord stimulators to receive full-body MRI scans safely when certain restrictions are maintained [11]. Patients suffering from chemotherapy-induced neuropathy may now benefit from spinal cord stimulation without precluding future MRI.

Surgical decompression of affected nerves is an emerging treatment for chemotherapy-induced peripheral neuropathy. The ideal candidate for this therapy should meet certain criteria including having paresthesia, numbness, or burning pain in a symmetrical stocking distribution, a positive Tinel sign at the target nerve, developing symptoms after the initiation of chemotherapy. Efficacy of this technique is based on the "double-crush" theory of nerve injury. This theory states that repeated damage to the nervous system has an additive effect and that painful neuropathy may occur even when these traumatic steps are relatively minor and may not individually manifest as symptoms. In the context of oncologic neuropathic pain, the initial insult often occurs because of neurotoxic chemotherapeutic administration. This results in nerves which are more susceptible to further injury by compression at common susceptible anatomic sites [12].

Radiation Therapy-Induced Pain

Oral Mucositis

Oral mucositis is characterized by the presence of erythematous or ulcerative lesions involving the oral mucosa and is commonly associated with patients receiving chemotherapy or radiation treatment for cancers of the head and neck. Mucositis often causes a great deal of pain and other problems such as dysphagia, malnutrition, and infection. Severe oral mucositis has been reported in up to 60% of patients receiving standard radiation therapy and in 100% of those receiving hyperfractionation or accelerated hyperfractionation regimens [13]. Treatment risk factors include volume of mucosal exposure to radiation, cumulative radiation dose, dose schedule, and the use of concurrent chemotherapy [14].

Management of mucositis-related pain frequently requires opioid medications. Patients generally have difficulty swallowing and may require topical, transdermal, or intravenous medication delivery routes. For temporary relief of pain, topical anesthetics and mouthwashes are commonly used. Viscous lidocaine is a regularly used and effective temporary treatment. "Magic mouthwash," which is a combination of antacid, diphenhydramine, lidocaine, and the antifungal nystatin, is another often used topical therapy for symptomatic relief. Other swish and spit therapies may include coating agents such as sucralfate and antibiotics.

Osteonecrosis of the Jaw

Patients undergoing head and neck radiation therapy, chemotherapy, corticosteroid treatment, or bisphosphonate treatment are at risk for osteonecrosis of the jaw. A history of previous dental procedures is thought to also increase risk [15]. The incidence of radiation therapy-induced osteonecrosis ranges from 0.4% to 8.2% and varies depending on the dose, field, and fraction of radiation therapy [7]. While the underlying pathogenesis is not completely understood, radiation-induced osteonecrosis of the jaw is characterized by destruction of osteocytes and radiation-induced ischemic necrosis with the absence of new bone development [16].

Treatment may include saline irrigation, antibiotics to treat recurrent infections, hyperbaric oxygen, and surgical debridement of loose and exposed bone. Peripheral nerve blocks may be attempted for pain relief depending on the distribution of pain. More specifically, affected regions of the jaw supplied by the maxillary (V2) or mandibular (V3) branches of the trigeminal nerve are suitable targets. For mandibular pain, a mandibular nerve block, inferior alveolar nerve block, or mental nerve block with or without additive corticosteroid may be effective. For pain in the upper jaw, a maxillary nerve block may be performed. Patients may also present with painful osteonecrosis in multiple areas. This type of diffuse involvement may require Gasserian ganglion blockade, with consideration of further neurolysis for prolonged relief [17, 18].

Special considerations must be taken before performing a nerve block for osteonecrosis of the jaw as patients with this condition frequently have intraoral infections. Most interventional pain physicians perform these blocks percutaneously, while dentists often favor intraoral techniques. It is important to explore details and history related to infectious risk including antibiotic treatment prior to performing injections. In terms of obtaining confirmed consent, it is important to relay the possibility of numbness in the face or anterior tongue with any of the above interventions. And while the branches of the trigeminal nerve are largely sensory, the mandibular nerve does have a motor component that plays a role in mastication.

Cervical Dystonia

Patients receiving radiation to the head and neck are at risk for developing radiation-induced fibrosis and resulting cervical dystonia. The latter is characterized by painful spasms and contractures of the neck musculature causing abnormal posturing of the head. Commonly affected muscles include the sternocleidomastoid, scalene, and trapezius muscles. Abnormal nerve activity in the spinal accessory nerve, cervical nerve roots, and cervical plexus may additionally contribute to contracture and spasm of these muscles [19].

The primary treatment for cervical dystonia includes early physical therapy with the goal of maintaining range of motion of the head and neck. Additional treatment may be provided using neuropathic agents, muscle relaxants, or opioids on a case-by-case basis. Interventional approaches include trigger point injections, superficial cervical plexus blocks, and administration of botulinum toxin.

Trigger Point Injections

Trigger point injections into taut muscle bands may be used to treat painful cervical muscle spasms. A 25-gauge, 1–1.5 inch needle is usually sufficient to inject the relatively superficial muscles in the cervical region. The muscle of interest is identified, prepped with alcohol, and held firmly with the non-dominant hand, while the other hand inserts a sterile needle into the muscle belly usually in the direction of the muscle fibers. With or without dry needling, 0.5–1 ml of a local anesthetic solution, typically a mixture of 1% lidocaine and 0.25% bupivacaine, is injected. An ultrasound probe may be substituted in the non-dominant hand and helpful for identifying appropriate needle depth, specific facial muscles, and nerves.

Superficial Cervical Plexus Block

The superficial cervical plexus supplies cutaneous sensation to the neck and blockade may be beneficial for treating painful cervical dystonia. With the patient in the supine position and the head turned in the contralateral direction, the posterior border of the sternocleidomastoid muscle is identified. Chassaignac's tubercle – corresponding to the transverse process of C6 – can then be identified at the level of the cricoid cartilage. A 25–27-gauge, 1.5–2 inch needle is inserted at this level along the posterior edge of the sternocleidomastoid and advanced in a cephalad direction toward the mastoid process. Approximately 2.5–5 ml of local anesthetic and steroid mixture is injected. The needle is then redirected caudad in line with the posterior border of the muscle and another 2.5–5 ml of local anesthetic with or without corticosteroid is injected.

Botulinum Toxin

In 2000, the Food and Drug Administration approved botulinum toxins A and B for the treatment of cervical dystonia. These proteins are composed of a heavy chain and a light chain joined by a disulfide bond. Injection of botulinum toxin into target tissues results in binding of the heavy chain to glycoproteins found in muscle and exocrine gland cholinergic nerve terminals. Once internalized into the presynaptic cell, the light chain binds to and cleaves the transport protein responsible for acetylcholine release by the motor endplate (SNARE protein receptor complex) [20]. Flaccid paralysis results because of blocking acetylcholine release.

Botulinum toxin has also been postulated to inhibit neural pro-inflammatory substances in addition to pain signaling mediators including substance P, calcitonin gene-related peptide, and glutamate.

Botulinum toxins A and B differ in pharmacologic targets and properties, with each serotype having a specific binding site at presynaptic nerve terminals. Botulinum toxin A is more commonly used due to the lower incidence of adverse effects. It cleaves synaptosomal-associated protein of 25kD (SNAP-25) which ultimately inhibits pain neurotransmitter release [21].

Prior to injection of botulinum toxin, it is important to identify painful or dystonic muscle groups. This can be done clinically or with the use of EMG. Commonly injected muscles include the sternocleidomastoid, trapezius, and splenius capitis. The number of injections and total dose will vary with the muscle size. In general, patients should receive the minimal dose necessary to avoid adverse effects and immune resistance while still providing satisfactory relief. While large high-quality prospective trials have not examined the use of botulinum for the treatment of cervical dystonia, preliminary clinical results have been encouraging [21].

Radiation Proctitis

Patients undergoing radiation treatment to the pelvis for gynecologic, urologic, or anorectal cancers may develop radiation proctitis. Radiation proctitis is defined as injury to the rectum from radiation therapy and usually presents as diarrhea, mucus discharge, cramping, bloating, tenesmus, incontinence, rectal bleeding, or anal pain [22]. There are multiple interventional techniques which may help in the management of painful proctitis. These include caudal epidural injections, ganglion of impar blockade, and spinal cord stimulation.

Caudal Epidural Injection

Caudal epidural injections target the sacral spinal nerves with local anesthetic and corticosteroid, thereby reducing inflammation and pain transmission by afferent nociceptors. With the patient placed in the prone position, the sacral hiatus is identified by palpation of the sacral cornua and confirmed with fluoroscopy. After anesthetizing the skin, a Tuohy needle or spinal needle is advanced through the skin and sacral membrane. Once the caudal spinal canal is entered, the angle of the needle is decreased to lie in a closer plane to the sacrum. The needle can then be advanced another 1–2 cm. Placement of the needle is confirmed using radiographic contrast (Fig. 21.1). A solution of steroid and preservative-free saline or local anesthetic is injected.

Ganglion of Impar block

The ganglion of impar is a sympathetic ganglion located anterior to the sacrococcygeal junction. It is readily blocked using fluoroscopic guidance. The sacrococcygeal junction is identified in the lateral fluoroscopic view. After anesthetizing the skin, a 22–25-gauge needle is advanced through the sacrococcygeal ligament until the needle tip lies just anterior to the sacrum. Great care must be taken not to violate the posterior wall of the rectum. Needle placement is confirmed using radiographic contrast. A characteristic "reverse comma" appearance should result from the spread of the contrast (Fig. 21.2). A solution of local anesthetic with or without steroid is injected. If pain relief is significant but only transient, further chemical neurolysis of the ganglion of impar can be accomplished using dehydrated alcohol. Pulsed or thermal radiofrequency ablation treatments have also been described.

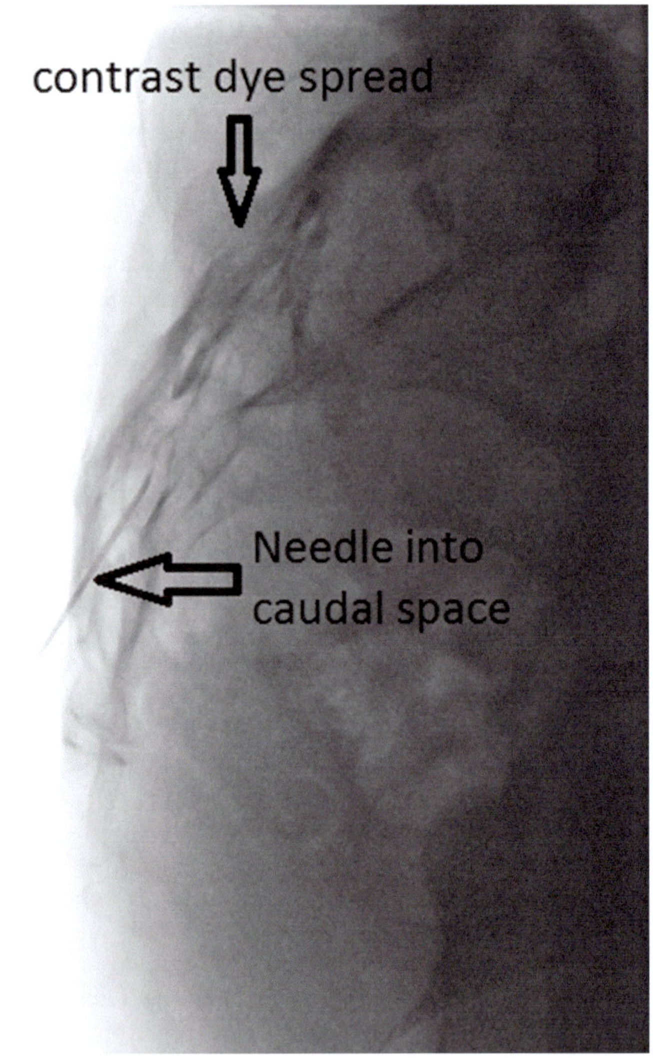

Fig. 21.1 Caudal injection in lateral view under fluoroscopy. Depicted is the needle showing dye spread into the epidural space

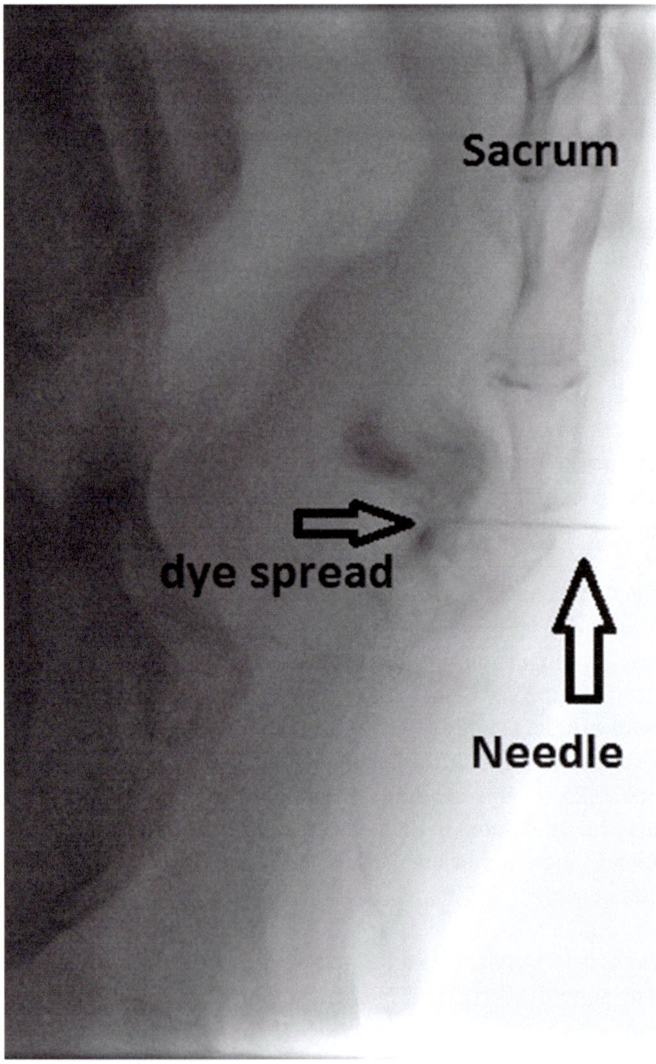

Fig. 21.2 Ganglion of impar block in lateral view under fluoroscopic guidance. Depicted is the needle placed to the anterior surface of the sacrum with appropriate anterior dye spread

Spinal Cord Stimulation

Spinal cord stimulation may be used to treat radiation proctitis pain refractory more conservative measures. The goal of traditional spinal cord stimulation is to produce paresthesia in areas of chronic pain. Proposed mechanisms of action include the gate control theory, conduction blockade of spinothalamic tracts, activation of supraspinal mechanisms, blockade of sympathetic activity, and release of neuromodulators [23].

Lead placement can be accomplished via a retrograde approach or via the sacral hiatus to cover the upper sacral nerve roots on both sides [24]. Other potential targets for lead placement include the conus medullaris (typically T12-L1) and the mid-thoracic (T6 or T7) levels where sensory afferent fibers from the caudad body segments travel more medially [25].

Radiation-Induced Neuropathy

Radiation-induced neuropathy is a rare and late complication of radiation therapy in long-term cancer survivors. Mechanisms of injury to the nerve are complex and multifactorial. Potential causes include nerve compression via adjacent radiation-induced fibrotic tissues, direct nerve injury resulting in axonal damage or demyelination, or vascular damage producing ischemic nerve injury [26]. Treatment risk factors include high total dose and high dose-per-fraction radiotherapy, short source-to-skin distance, salvage therapy of previously treated areas, and the use of certain chemotherapeutic agents known to be independently neurotoxic [27].

Interventional approaches to pain management include selective nerve blocks of affected peripheral nerves. Patients with trigeminal neuropathy after radiation for head and neck cancer may benefit from blockade of the Gasserian ganglion or one of its major divisions (see descriptions above). Spinal cord or peripheral nerve stimulation can also be effective.

Insufficiency Fractures

Many components of cancer therapy increase the risk of osteoporosis. These include systemic glucocorticoid therapy, androgen deprivation, the use of aromatase inhibitors, and gonadotropin-releasing hormone agonist therapy. A history of oophorectomy or chemotherapy-induced ovarian failure also confers additional risk. Radiation therapy can lead to osteonecrosis and eventually vertebral compression fractures [28–30]. Common fracture sites include the femoral neck, radius, pelvis, and spine. Interventional pain treatment options include kyphoplasty, vertebroplasty, and sacroplasty which are described in greater detail in Chap. 20.

Kyphoplasty and Vertebroplasty

Vertebroplasty involves the percutaneous instillation of cement – often polymethylmethacrylate (PMMA) – into the vertebral body of a spinal fracture. Kyphoplasty is a similar procedure in which a balloon is first inflated within the vertebral body prior to instillation of PMMA. We will primarily discuss kyphoplasty as this is the technique most utilized by interventionalists [31–33].

Sacroplasty

While sacral insufficiency fractures are less common than vertebral fractures, their diagnosis is increasing as is awareness of these fractures as part of the differential for acute low back pain. Pelvic MRI is the most sensitive and specific modality for diagnosis. Fracture lines can be seen longitudinally between the sacroiliac joints and neural foramina, either unilaterally or bilaterally. There may also be a horizontal fracture line, often located between the S1 and S2 levels. Pain due to sacral fractures is often localized to the sacral or buttock area although may be referred to the groin or hips. The pain is typically worsened with weight-bearing and improved with a supine position [34].

Conservative treatment involves medication management to reverse and prevent further osteoporosis and to treat pain and encourage weight-bearing. The latter can help stimulate osteoblast activity and new bone formation and repair [34]. When these measures fail, percutaneous repair with sacroplasty can be considered.

Sacral Kyphoplasty

Sacral kyphoplasty is a modification of the sacroplasty procedure. This procedure involves creating a bone void with a distensible balloon and then delivering cement to the defect. This procedure may be done under CT, CT fluoroscopy, or fluoroscopy. A PACS imaging system may be ideal for planning trocar trajectories. A retrospective case series report published in 2012 demonstrated early and rapid pain reduction which was sustained for almost 1 year [35].

Postsurgical Pain

Chronic pain because of surgery is not uncommon in the cancer survivor. There are many factors that may contribute to the development of chronic pain after surgery including preoperative pain, anatomic location of surgery, iatrogenic nerve injury, previous chemotherapy, or radiation therapy, in addition to patient factors such as depression or personality disorders

[36]. Some of the most implicated types of surgery include radical neck dissection, mastectomy, and thoracotomy.

Post Radical Neck Dissection Pain

The incidence of chronic pain in head and neck cancer patients is about 40% at 1 year and 15% at 5 years [36]. Surgery, radiation, and chemotherapy can all cause chronic pain in the oral cavity, neck, face, and shoulders. Neuropathic pain may arise from injury to the superficial cervical plexus or spinal accessory nerve. Interventional pain treatment options include trigger point injections, scar injections, and superficial cervical plexus blocks.

Scar Injections

Postsurgical scar formation in areas of high tension such as the neck may result in pruritus, pain, or contractures. Injections containing local and corticosteroid into the scar may provide pain relief while facilitating physical therapy and therapeutic myofascial release.

Postmastectomy Pain

About 50% of women will suffer chronic pain after mastectomy. The incidence is thought to be related to the intensity of acute postoperative pain, type of operation, involvement of lymph nodes, and radiation therapy [36]. Postmastectomy pain includes a spectrum of pain syndromes including phantom breast pain, intercostobrachial neuralgia, and neuroma pain. Pain may present in the breast, chest wall, neck, arm, or shoulder. Paresthesia, hyperalgesia, and dysesthesia, in addition to allodynia, are also common. Of note, late onset of pain or swelling postmastectomy are red flags which may indicate cellulitis, deep venous thrombosis, recurrence of tumor, or lymphedema [37].

Sensations or pain coming from the amputated breast is referred to as phantom breast pain. This pain is intermittent and can occur in the first months to years after mastectomy. Treatment includes physical therapy, skin desensitization, and myofascial release [37].

Neuroma Injections

Neuroma formation following surgery may cause significant discomfort. Histologically, a neuroma represents disorganized hyperplasia following injury or entrapment of nerve tissue. While diagnosis is primarily clinical, imaging studies such as MRI or ultrasound can be useful in characterizing the size, morphology, and location of a neuroma [38].

Surgical excision may not reliably provide pain relief. Infiltration with local anesthetic and corticosteroid with or without ultrasound guidance is a less invasive potential treatment option. Neuromas are usually seen under ultrasound as hypoechoic nodules surrounded by fibrous tissue. Serial injections may be required to provide adequate relief.

Neurolysis can also be utilized to obtain more prolonged relief. Available modalities include chemical neurolysis, radiofrequency ablation, pulsed radiofrequency ablation, and cryoneurolysis [38, 39]. Extracorporeal shockwave lithotripsy has also been described in the podiatric literature as a potential treatment for interdigital neuromas.

Intercostobrachial Nerve Block

The breast is innervated by the intercostal nerves from T2 through T6. The lateral cutaneous branch of the second intercostal nerve is called the intercostobrachial nerve. Intercostobrachial nerve damage during surgery is a common cause of postmastectomy pain syndrome and is more likely to occur when axillary lymph node dissection is performed [36]. Damage to this nerve presents as neuropathic pain involving the medial aspect of the upper arm.

An intercostobrachial nerve block may provide at least temporary pain relief. To perform this block, the arm is abducted and externally rotated. A field block is then performed using local anesthetic in a linear fashion starting at the deltoid prominence and ending inferiorly at the medial arm. This nerve can also be blocked at the T2 thoracic nerve root level or paravertebral block, since most of the innervation of the nerve is from the T2 thoracic nerve root.

Post-thoracotomy Pain Syndrome

The incidence of chronic pain following thoracotomy may be as high as 50% [36]. It is common for patients to have severe postoperative discomfort that gradually improves over months to years. Intercostal nerve injury, rib injury, and inflammation of the chest wall muscles are often contributory. Possible treatment modalities include intercostal nerve blocks, paravertebral blocks, TENS, lidocaine, and ketamine infusions, in addition to spinal cord or peripheral nerve stimulation.

The intercostal and paravertebral nerve blocks are described in greater detail in Chap. 18.

Intercostal Nerve Block

The intercostal nerve lies inferior to the intercostal vein and artery at the caudal border of each rib between the internal and innermost intercostal muscles. The nerve is best targeted at the angle of the rib as this is the region where the lateral cutaneous branches split off. These branches are responsible for supplying sensation from the anterolateral chest and abdominal wall [40].

Ultrasound guidance is advantageous for identifying the pleura and neurovascular structures in real time. Either the transverse or longitudinal orientation with respect to the rib can be used.

For the longitudinal technique, the patient is placed in a prone or lateral position, and the ribs are identified in a longitudinal plane. The three muscle layers are then identified just caudal to the rib of interest as the external, internal, and innermost intercostal muscles.

In the more commonly used transverse technique, the ribs are identified as hypoechoic oval structures with a bright hyperechoic cortex. The depth should be adjusted to adequately visualize the underlying pleura. The needle is inserted caudal to the ultrasound probe and advanced in-plane to the caudal surface of the rib. The medication is then deposited at this surface (Fig. 21.3).

It is worth noting that a cadaver study indicated that the nerve is located subcostally only 17% of the time and is more frequently found in the midcostal region [41]. This may reinforce the importance of targeting the proper muscle plane which is more easily appreciated in the longitudinal view.

Follow-up neurolytic or ablative techniques may be used if patients have adequate pain relief from diagnostic local anesthetic blocks. Dehydrated alcohol or 10% phenol is commonly used and injected under fluoroscopic guidance or ultrasound guidance using the techniques described above. Care must be taken to avoid intravascular uptake.

Cryoablation and pulsed radiofrequency of the intercostal nerve using image guidance are other options that may also provide long-term pain relief [42].

Paravertebral Block

The paravertebral block is another option to provide thoracic nerve blockade. The thoracic paravertebral space is a wedge-shaped space located on bilateral sides of the vertebral column. It is bordered by the parietal pleura anterolaterally and the superior costotransverse ligament posteriorly [43]. The paravertebral space communicates with the epidural space medially and the intercostal space laterally which accounts for its mechanism of action. The paravertebral block can be done using ultrasound guidance with a similar approach as the intercostal nerve block.

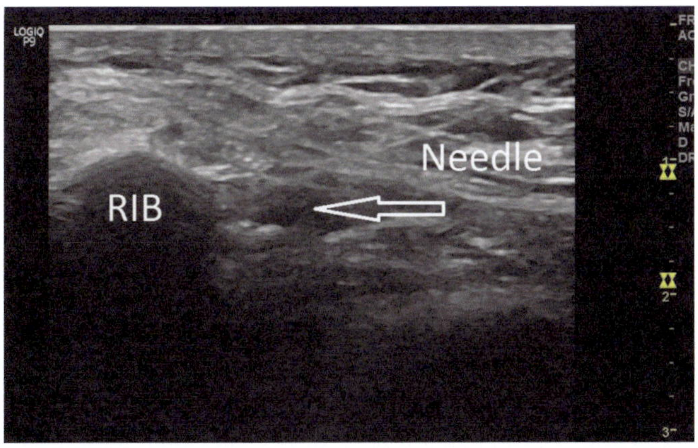

Fig. 21.3 Intercostal nerve block under ultrasound guidance. Depicted is needle placement at the inferior border of the rib with local anesthetic spread (arrow) in the internal intercostal muscle

TENS

Transcutaneous electrical nerve stimulation is a potentially effective and low-risk treatment option for post-thoracotomy pain [44]. The electrodes can be applied to the chest wall in a neurotomal distribution.

Intravenous Infusions

Neuropathic pain is a major component of post-thoracotomy pain syndrome. Patients with chronic neuropathic pain syndromes may benefit from intravenous infusions of lidocaine or ketamine.

Lidocaine is an amide local anesthetic that inhibits pain by blocking peripheral and central sodium channels. Lidocaine inhibits aberrant electrical discharges at sub-anesthetic doses and thus can be used to treat a broad spectrum of neuropathic pain syndromes [45]. Historically, lidocaine infusions have been given on a monthly basis. The dose is generally 1–3 mg/kg intravenously over 20–30 min. After this period, pain scores are assessed. If pain scores significantly decline over the bolus period, then an infusion of 1–3 mg/kg/h is initiated [46]. It is very important to monitor for signs of local anesthetic toxicity during this process. Systemic toxicity usually begins with perioral numbness or metallic taste but can progress to dizziness, disorientation, seizures, and cardiovascular collapse. Though toxicity is generally easily reversible by reducing or discontinuing the infusion, ACLS equipment, seizure-abortive therapies such as benzodiazepines, and Intralipid should be immediately available.

Ketamine is a dissociative anesthetic that blocks the N-methyl-D-aspartate (NMDA) receptor, a ligand-gated calcium channel activated by glutamate [47]. Activation of this channel contributes to the "windup" phenomenon which leads to central sensitization [47]. As it can potentially inhibit this process, ketamine has been used to treat numerous chronic neuropathic pain states. Intravenous ketamine infusions can be performed inpatient or outpatient setting, often with co-administration of a benzodiazepine and clonidine to mitigate its well-known psychotropic side effects. Other potential side effects include hypertension, tachycardia, and excess salivation. It should be used with caution in patients with known increased intracranial pressure or cardiovascular disease including hypertension, stroke, and ischemic heart disease.

Spinal Cord Stimulation

A few published case reports have described partial or complete resolution of chronic post-thoracotomy pain with the use of spinal cord stimulation. One case report from the

Western Pennsylvania Hospital for Pain Management reported complete resolution of post-thoracotomy pain symptoms after implantation of a spinal cord stimulator at the T3 superior endplate [48]. Another case report, presented at the annual meeting of the North American Neuromodulation Society in 2009, demonstrated greater than 75% improvement after implantation of a spinal cord stimulator at the T6–T7 level [49]; while these case reports have shown promising results, large-scale prospective studies are needed to further evaluate the effectiveness of spinal cord stimulation for post-thoracotomy pain syndrome.

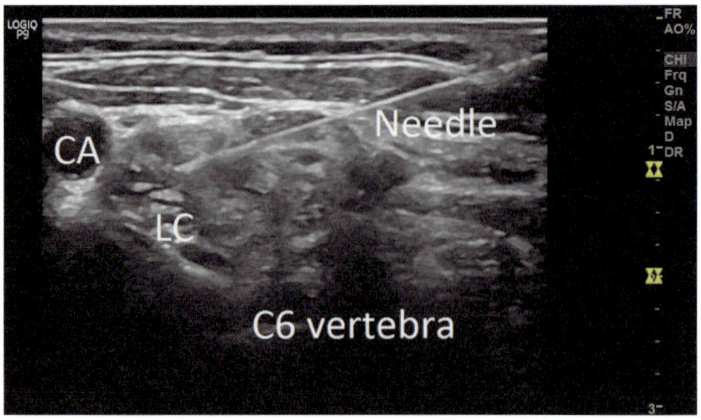

Fig. 21.4 Stellate ganglion block under ultrasound guidance. Depicted is the needle placement in the pre cervical fascia between the carotid artery (CA) and anterior to the longus colli muscle (LC). This is commonly done at the level of the C6 vertebrae above the level of the stellate ganglion, which is typically located at the C7 or T1 vertebrae

Phantom Limb Pain and Stump Pain

Phantom sensation, phantom pain, and stump pain maker after limb amputation [50]. Phantom sensation is defined as any non-painful sensation perceived from the amputated extremity as if it is still attached. Phantom pain is an intense sensation experienced as discomfort in the amputated extremity. Stump pain is a painful sensation that is localized to the stump. The incidence of phantom limb pain may be as high as 72% [36]. Predisposing factors are thought to include pre-amputation pain, female gender, severe postoperative pain, proximal amputations, poorly fitting prostheses, and the use of chemotherapy. Two thirds of patients with phantom limb pain may also suffer from stump pain [36].

Treatment options for phantom limb pain include sympathetic blockade, peripheral nerve blockade, botulinum toxin injections, and spinal cord stimulation. Treatment options for stump pain include scar or neuroma injections, peripheral nerve blocks, and botulinum toxin administration.

Sympathetic Nerve Blocks

Phantom limb pain may be difficult to treat as the mechanism of pain is often multifactorial. Peripheral, spinal, and supraspinal mechanisms of pain may all be responsible for phantom limb pain and stump pain. Dysfunction of the autonomic nervous system is often involved in many chronic pain syndromes. Pain that is categorized as sympathetically mediated may be characterized by increased responsiveness of injured sensory nerves to catecholamines, increased expression of alpha-1 adrenoreceptors on primary afferent nociceptors and hyperalgesic skin, central sensitization, and enhanced sympathetic discharge [51]. Sympathetic nerve blockade may be part of a multimodal treatment approach with stellate ganglion blocks used for upper extremity pain and lumbar sympathetic blocks used for lower extremity pain.

A stellate ganglion block can be performed on the ipsilateral side of the amputated limb using ultrasound guidance. With the patient supine and the neck extended, a linear probe is used to obtain a cross-sectional image of the neck anatomy at the level of C6. The level can be confirmed by identifying Chassaignac's tubercle. The carotid artery, internal jugular vein, thyroid gland, trachea, esophagus, longus colli muscle, C6 nerve root, and transverse process of C6 are visualized (Fig. 21.4).

When ultrasound guidance is used, this block can also be performed at the C7 level. This may offer superior coverage of the upper extremity. Since the vertebral artery will not be protected by Chassaignac's tubercle, great care must be taken to identify and avoid this structure.

For treatment of lower extremity phantom limb pain, a lumbar sympathetic block can be performed on the ipsilateral side of the amputated limb under fluoroscopic guidance. With the patient in the prone position, after adequate local anesthesia to the skin and subcutaneous tissue, a 22-gauge 5 inch needle is inserted in a coaxial plane to the anterolateral aspect of the lumbar vertebral body using oblique and lateral images. After negative aspiration, a 10 ml mixture of local anesthetic and steroid is injected.

Peripheral Nerve Blocks

Injury to peripheral nerves may occur during limb amputation. Subsequent changes in the brain and spinal cord may produce central sensitization, allodynia, and hyperalgesia in the affected limb.

Peripheral nerve blocks inhibit transmission of painful stimuli and offer at least a temporary means to alleviate phantom limb pain. Unfortunately, local anesthetics may have an analgesic effect of only a few hours. One small study published by a team at the University of California, San Diego, demonstrated prolonged pain relief after termination of a continuous nerve block. This suggests that continuous peripheral nerve blocks lasting days rather than hours may better reorganize cortical pain mapping [52]. In this context, a continuous catheter may be inserted at the brachial plexus to treat chronic upper extremity phantom limb pain. For lower extremity phantom limb pain, femoral and popliteal continuous nerve catheters may be used.

Scar Injection

Postsurgical scar and neuroma formation may result in pain or contractures in the affected limb. Like the technique described above for chronic head and neck oncologic pain, a mixture of local anesthetic with or without corticosteroid may be helpful for treating stump pain. A more prolonged response may be achieved with chemical ablation is appropriate cryoablation, or thermal radiofrequency ablation.

Botulinum Toxin Injections

Botulinum toxin administration to scars or areas of known neuroma formation may also be used to treat stump pain. Analgesia is thought to occur secondary to acetylcholine synaptic transmission inhibition at motor endplates and muscle spindles. Botulinum toxin is also thought to exhibit a direct influence on nociceptive transmitters. Some studies have demonstrated decreased opioid use, increased ability to participate in physical therapy, and better tolerance of prosthetics following treatments [53].

There have even been several case studies reporting efficacy with delivery of botulinum toxin into the muscle or subcutaneous tissues of painful limbs [36]. A randomized double-blinded pilot study found that injection of botulinum toxin A into stump tender points resulted in 6-month pain relief among amputees with chronic pain that already failed more conventional treatments [54]. The authors used 50 units of botulinum toxin at each tender point for a total of 250–300 units.

Spinal Cord Stimulation

The use of spinal cord stimulation for phantom limb pain has been described in case series as early as 1975 [55]. These documented significant pain relief using subdural dorsal cord stimulation for both upper and lower extremity phantom limb pain. Since the 1970s, spinal cord stimulation technology has evolved significantly and has been used increasingly for the treatment of medication refractory chronic neuropathic pain states. More recent publications have since corroborated the effectiveness of spinal cord stimulation for phantom limb pain in selected patients failing to obtain adequate pain relief with more traditional medical management [56].

Conclusion

Oncologic pain syndromes in patients with active disease and survivors represent a true challenge to the interventional pain physician. Not only does this patient population tend to be frail, but multiple causes of complex pain from a wide variety of potential sources often present simultaneously. Through this process, it is vital that clinicians remain in close communication with the primary oncology team and vigilant with regard to potential recurrence of disease.

Reference

1. Deer TR, et al. Comprehensive consensus based guidelines on intrathecal drug delivery systems in the treatment of pain caused by cancer pain. Pain Physician. 2011;14:E283–312.
2. Lin Y, Foltz LM. Proposed guidelines for platelet transfusion Issue. BCMJ. 2005;47(5):245–8.
3. Boehm S, Rothermundt C, Hess D, Joerger M. Antiangiogenic drugs in oncology: a focus on drug safety and the elderly – a mini-review. Gerontology. 2010;56:303–9.
4. Streiff MB. Diagnosis and initial treatment of venous thromboembolism in patients with cancer. J Clin Oncol. 2009;27:4889–94.
5. Terese T, Horlocker MD, et al. Regional anesthesia in the patient receiving antithrombotic or thrombolytic therapy-American Society of Regional Anesthesia and Pain Medicine Evidence-Based Guidelines (Fourth Edition). Reg Anesth Pain Med. 2018;43(2):263–309.
6. Malik B, Stillman M. Chemotherapy-induced peripheral neuropathy. Curr Neurol Neurosci Rep. 2008;8(1):56–65.
7. Quasthoff S, Hartung HP. Chemotherapy-induced peripheral neuropathy. J Neurol. 2002;249(1):9–17.
8. Chaudhry V, Eisenberger MA, Sinibaldi VJ, Sheikh K, Griffin JW, Cornblath DR. A prospective study of suramin-induced peripheral neuropathy. Brain. 1996;119(Pt 6):2039–52.
9. Loh J, Gulati A. The use of transcutaneous electrical nerve stimulation (TENS) in a major cancer center for the treatment of severe cancer-related pain and associated disability. Pain Med. 2013;16(6):1204–10.
10. Cata JP, Cordella JV, Burton AW, Hassenbusch SJ, Weng HR, Dougherty PM. Spinal cord stimulation relieves chemotherapy-induced pain: a clinical case report. J Pain Symptom Manag. 2004;27(1):72–8.
11. Medtronic, Inc. *MRI guidelines for Medtronic neurostimulation systems for chronic pain*. Minneapolis: Medtronic, Inc; 2013.
12. Dellon AL, Swier P, Maloney CT Jr, Livengood MS, Werter S. Chemotherapy-induced neuropathy: treatment by decompression of peripheral nerves. Plast Reconstr Surg. 2004;114(2):478–83.
13. Vera Llonch M, Oster G, Hagiwara M, Sonis S. Oral mucositis in patients undergoing radiation treatment for head and neck carcinoma. *Cancer*. 2006;*106*(2):329–36.
14. Rosenthal DI, Trotti A. Strategies for managing radiation-induced mucositis in head and neck cancer. In: Seminars in radiation oncology (Vol. 19, No. 1, pp. 29–34). WB Saunders; 2009.
15. Ruggiero S, Gralow J, Marx RE, Hoff AO, Schubert MM, Huryn JM, et al. Practical guidelines for the prevention, diagnosis, and treatment of osteonecrosis of the jaw in patients with cancer. J Oncol Pract. 2006;2(1):7–14.
16. Jereczek-Fossa BA, Orecchia R. Radiotherapy-induced mandibular bone complications. Cancer Treat Rev. 2002;28(1):65–74.
17. Erdine S, Racz G, Noe C. Somatic blocks of the head and neck. In: Raj P, et al., editors. *Interventional pain management, image-guided procedures*. Philadelphia: Saunders; 2008.
18. Candido K, Batra M. Nerve blocks of the head and neck. In: Benzon H, et al., editors. *Raj's practical management of pain*. Philadelphia: Mosby; 2008.
19. Stubblefield MD. Radiation fibrosis syndrome: neuromuscular and musculoskeletal complications in cancer survivors. PM&R. 2011;3(11):1041–54.

20. Dolly JO, Aoki KR. The structure and mode of action of different botulinum toxins. Eur J Neurol. 2006;12(Suppl 4):1–9.
21. Stubblefield MD, Levine A, Custodio CM, Fitzpatrick T. The role of botulinum toxin type A in the radiation fibrosis syndrome: a preliminary report. Arch Phys Med Rehabil. 2008;89(3):417–21.
22. Sarin A, Safar B. Management of radiation proctitis. Gastroenterol Clin N Am. 2013;42(4):913–25.
23. Kurdali B, Sterban S, Siefferman J. Spinal cord stimulator lead placement via sacral hiatus in the treatment of post radiation proctitis. 16th annual North American neuromodulation society. From innovation to reality. 2012.
24. Krames E. Spinal cord stimulation: indications, mechanism of action, and efficacy. Curr Rev Pain. 1999;3(6):419–26.
25. Hunter C, Dave N, Diwan S, Deer T. Neuromodulation of pelvic visceral pain: review of the literature and case series of potential novel targets for treatment. Pain Pract. 2013;13(1):3–17.
26. Delanian S, Lefaix JL, Pradat PF. Radiation-induced neuropathy in cancer survivors. Radiother Oncol. 2012;105(3):273–82.
27. Delanian S, et al. Radiation-induced neuropathy in cancer survivors. Radiother Oncol. 2012;105:273–82.
28. Pfeilschifter J, Diel IJ. Osteoporosis due to cancer treatment: pathogenesis and management. J Clin Oncol. 2000;18(7):1570–93.
29. Lustberg MB, Reinbolt RE, Shapiro CL. Bone health in adult cancer survivorship. J Clin Oncol. 2012;30(30):3665–74. https://doi.org/10.1200/JCO.2012.42.2097. Epub 2012 Sep 24
30. Schiff D, Jensen ME. Kyphoplasty in cancer: an encouraging step. Lancet Oncol. 2011;12(3):202–3. https://doi.org/10.1016/S1470-2045(11)70032-8.
31. Burton AW, Mendel E. Vertebroplasty and kyphoplasty. Pain Physician. 2003;6:335–43. I
32. Hoh BL, Rabinov JD, Pryor JC, Hirsch JA. Balloon kyphoplasty for vertebral compression fracture using a unilateral balloon tamp via a uni-pedicular approach: technical note. Pain Physician. 2004;7:111–4.
33. Melvin Hu M, Eskey CJ, Tong SC, Nogueira RG, Pomerantz SR, Rabinov JD, Pryor JC, Hirsch JA. Kyphoplasty for vertebral compression fracture via a uni-pedicular approach. Pain Physician. 2005;8:363–7.
34. Cho CH, Mathis JM, Ortiz O. Sacral fractures and sacroplasty. Neuroimaging Clin N Am. 2010;20:179–86.
35. Shah RV. Sacral kyphoplasty for the treatment of painful sacral insufficiency fractures and metastases. Spine J. 2012;12(2):113–20.
36. Burton AW, Fanciullo GJ, Beasley RD, Fisch MJ. Chronic pain in the cancer survivor: a new frontier. Pain Med. 2007;8(2):189–98.
37. Stubblefield MD, Keole N. Upper body pain and functional disorders in patients with breast cancer. *PM&R*. 2013;6:170–83.
38. Rajput K. Painful neuromas. Clin J Pain. 2012;28(7):639–45.
39. Friedman T, Adler R. Sonographically guided cryoneurolysis: preliminary experience and clinical outcomes. Ultrasound Med. 2012;31(12):2025–34.
40. Rathmell JP. Atlas of image-guided intervention in regional anesthesia and pain medicine. Philadelphia: Lippincott Williams & Wilkins; 2011.
41. Hardy PA. Anatomical variation in the position of the proximal intercostal nerve. Br J Anaesth. 1988;61:338–9.
42. Byas-Smith MG, Gulati A. Ultrasound-guided intercostal nerve cryoablation. Anesth Analg. 2006;103(4):1033–5.
43. Karmakar MK. Ultrasound-guided thoracic paravertebral block. In: *Atlas of ultrasound-guided procedures in interventional pain management*. New York: Springer; 2011. p. 133–48.
44. Freynet A, Falcoz PE. Is transcutaneous electrical nerve stimulation effective in relieving postoperative pain after thoracotomy? *Interact Cardiovasc Thorac Surg*. 2010;*10*(2):283–8.
45. Tremont-Lukats IW, Teixeira GM, Backonja MM. Systemic administration of local anesthetic agents to relieve neuropathic pain. Cochrane Database of Systematic Reviews. 2005
46. Fishman SM. Bonica's management of pain. Philadelphia: Lippincott Williams & Wilkins; 2012.
47. Visser E, Schug SA. The role of ketamine in pain management. *Biomed Pharmacother*. 2006;*60*(7):341–8.
48. Graybill J, Conermann T, Kabazie AJ, Chandy S. Spinal cord stimulation for treatment of pain in a patient with post thoracotomy pain syndrome. Pain Physician. 2011;14:441–5.
49. Wininger KL, Bester ML, Deshpande KK. Spinal cord stimulation to treat postthoracotomy neuralgia: non–small-cell lung cancer: a case report. Pain Manag Nurs. 2012;13(1):52–9.
50. Borsje S, Bosmans JC, Vander Schans CP, Geertzen JHB, Dijkstra PU. Phantom pain: a sensitivity analysis. Disabil Rehabil. 2004;26(14–15):905–10.
51. Cohen SP, Gambel JM, Raja SN, Galvagno S. The contribution of sympathetic mechanisms to postamputation phantom and residual limb pain: a pilot study. J Pain. 2011;12(8):859–67.
52. Ilfeld BM, Moeller-Bertram T, Hanling SR, Tokarz K, Mariano ER, Loland VJ, Wallace MS. Treating intractable phantom limb pain with ambulatory continuous peripheral nerve blocks: a pilot study. Pain Med. 2013;14(6):935–42.
53. Kern U, Martin C, Scheicher S, Müller H. Botulinum toxin type A influences stump pain after limb amputations. J Pain Symptom Manag. 2003;26(6):1069–70.
54. Wu H, Sultana R, Taylor KB, Szabo A. A prospective randomized double-blinded pilot study to examine the effect of botulinum toxin type A injection versus lidocaine/depomedrol injection on residual and phantom limb pain: initial report. Clin J Pain. 2012;28(2):108.
55. Nielson KD, Adams JE, Hosobuchi Y. Phantom limb pain: treatment with dorsal column stimulation. J Neurosurg. 1975;42:301–7.
56. Viswanathan A, Phan PC, Burton AW. Use of spinal cord stimulation in the treatment of phantom limb pain: case series and review of the literature. Pain Pract. 2010;10(5):479–84.

Part V

Surgical Techniques and Neuromodulation

22 Intracranial Neuroablation

Roy Hwang, Ashwin Viswanathan, Ahmed M. Raslan, and Erich Richter

Introduction

Though ablative techniques are more commonly applied to spinal pain pathways, lesions can also be applied to intracranial targets for the treatment of cancer-related pain. In this chapter we will discuss the rationale, techniques, and outcomes for cingulotomy, hypophysectomy, trigeminal nucleotractotomy, and thalamotomy.

Cingulotomy

Rationale and Patient Selection

Cingulotomy has a long history as an ablative intervention in the treatment of psychiatric illnesses including obsessive-compulsive disorder, anxiety disorders, and depression. The anterior cingulate cortex (ACC) has been targeted in patients with intractable benign and cancer-related pain. The cingulate gyrus is located along the medial aspect of bilateral cerebral hemispheres and travels around the corpus callosum. The cingulate cortex can be divided into the anterior cingulate cortex (ACC) and the posterior cingulate cortex (PCC). The ACC is thought to play a dominant role in cognitive and emotional processing and in the descending modulation of pain [1]. It is well accepted that the ACC and its connection to the prefrontal cortex play an important role in the perception of pain [2]. Several retrospective studies have described cingulotomy in the treatment of intractable pain, with evidence suggesting pain improvement may result from interrupting the emotional response to pain.

Historically, patients undergoing cingulotomy for psychiatric illness have coincidentally experienced significant improvement in intractable pain. In patients with cancer-related pain, appropriate candidates for cingulotomy are patients with widespread pain with a significant emotional suffering component. The incidence of depression and anxiety approaches 50% in terminally ill cancer patients [3], emphasizing the importance of treating mental illness in this population. A cingulotomy generally improves the patient's affective component related to their pain and not their actual nociception. Therefore, patients suffering from an acute pain syndrome are not thought to be as likely to benefit from cingulotomy.

Operative Technique

Early series of cingulotomy employed ventriculography to delineate the ventricular anatomy and target the anterior cingulate for radiofrequency ablation. Recently, modern techniques use MRI-based stereotactic targeting [4]. Though some variability in targeting exists, a common strategy is to target 20 mm posterior to the tip of the frontal horn of the lateral ventricle, 10 mm from midline, and 1–2 mm above the roof of the lateral ventricle (Fig. 22.1). Two radiofrequency lesions are made at 80° C for 90 s each

R. Hwang
West Virginia University, Department of Neurosurgery, Morgantown, WV, USA
e-mail: rhwang@hsc.wvu.edu

A. Viswanathan
Baylor College of Medicine, Department of Neurosurgery, Houston, TX, USA
e-mail: AViswanathan@mdanderson.org

A. M. Raslan
Oregon Health & Science University, Department of Neurosurgery, Portland, OR, USA

Portland VA Medical Center, Neurological Surgery, Portland, OR, USA
e-mail: raslana@ohsu.edu

E. Richter (✉)
New Orleans Neurosurgical Associates, Marrero, LA, USA
e-mail: doctor@nolaneuro.com

A. Gulati et al. (eds.), *Essentials of Interventional Cancer Pain Management*, https://doi.org/10.1007/978-3-319-99684-4_22

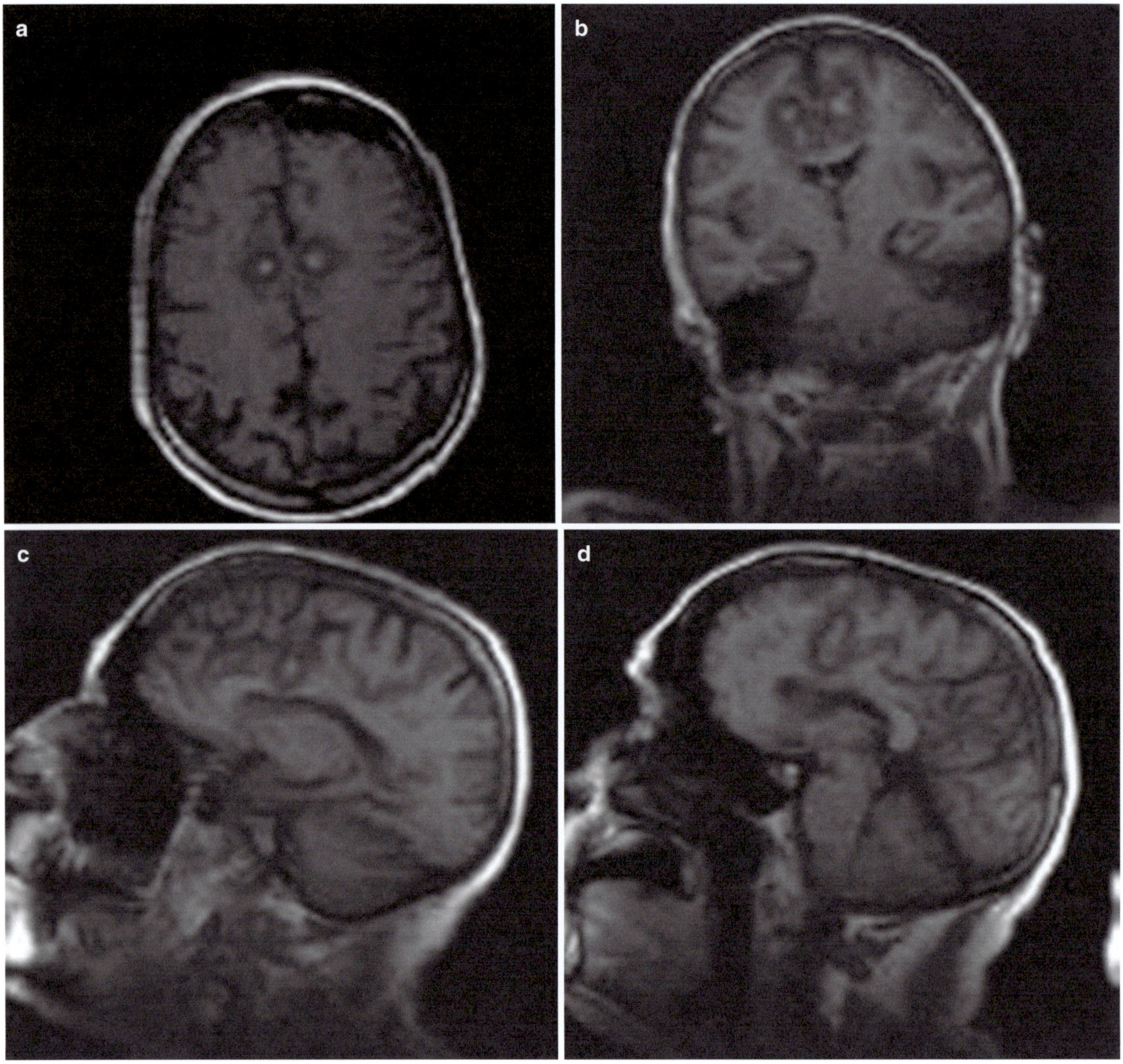

Fig. 22.1 (**a**) Axial, (**b**) coronal, and (**c**), (**d**) sagittal views of bilateral cingulotomy lesions

using a radiofrequency electrode with a 10 mm exposed tip. After creation of the first lesion, the radiofrequency probe is withdrawn by 10 mm to create the second lesion. The patient is treated bilaterally [4] (Fig. 22.1).

Outcomes

To date, 8 case series reporting 87 patients have been published focusing on cingulotomy in the treatment of cancer-related pain [5–11]. Though the studies are limited by quality and variability in reported pain outcomes, most series report that more than 50% of patients will experience a meaningful improvement in their pain condition (Table 22.1). Reported complications include rare transient hemiparesis, bleeding, ataxia, bowel bladder dysfunction, seizures, and memory problems. No deaths have been reported, but seizures and frontal lobe syndromes have been reported in literature and are approximately in the range of 1% [4, 7, 12].

Table 22.1 Cingulotomy for cancer pain

Authors and year	No. of pts	Procedure/target	Outcome	Follow-up
Foltz & White, 1962	6	Unilat or bilat air ventriculography-guided cingulotomy (1–2.5 cm pst to tip of frontal horn)	83% good or excellent outcome	4 days–9 months
Faillance et al., 1974	7	Bilat stereotactic cingulotomy (3.5–4 cm pst to tip of frontal horn)	45% improvement lasting from 3 days to 3 months	>2 years
Hurt & Ballantine, 1974	32	Stereotactic ant cingulate lesion (2–4 cm pst to tip of frontal horn); 1 lesion 2 cm above ventricle roof and 1 lesion 1 cm below the first	9% complete relief; 23% marked relief; 19% moderate relief; 44% slight or no relief	<3 months
Voris & Whisler, 1975	5	Bilat stereotactic cingulotomy (separate lesions 13 and 17 mm pst to tip of frontal horn, 12 mm from midline, 6 mm above ventricle)	All had pain relief until death	1–12 months
Pillay & Hassenbush, 1992	9	MRI-guided stereotactic cingulotomy (24 mm pst to tip of frontal horn, CCG chosen as target); 1 lesion made on each side (75 Celsius for 60 sec)	Pain relief: excellent 4; good 2; fair 1; poor 2	1 year
Wong et al., 1997	3	MRI-guided stereotactic cingulotomy (24 mm pst to tip of frontal horn, CCG chosen as target); 1 lesion made on each side	2 of 3 pts. had excellent outcome	N/a
Yen et al., 2005	15	Stereotactic bil ant cingulotomy (24 mm pst to tip of frontal horn); 1–2 lesions made on each side (80 Celsius for 80 sec)	53% significant pain relief; 27% meaningful pain relief; 20% no relief	1 week
			33% significant pain relief; 25% meaningful pain relief; 42% no relief	3 months
Yen et al., 2009	10	Stereotactic bil ant cingulotomy (24 mm pst to tip of frontal horn); 1–2 lesions made on each side (80 Celsius for 80 sec)	40% of pts had >75% relief; 20% of pts had 25–75% relief; and 40% of pts had <25% relief	Assessment at 1 week and 3 months post-op

Trigeminal Nucleotractotomy

Rationale and Patient Selection

Ablation of the descending trigeminal tract and nucleus caudalis can be utilized to treat multiple craniofacial pain syndromes that develop from head and neck tumors. Trigeminal afferent fibers carrying nociceptive information enter the pons and send descending fibers along the trigeminal tract into the caudal medulla and upper cervical cord. The descending trigeminal tract overlies and is lateral to the spinal trigeminal nucleus at the cervicomedullary junction. Primary sensory fibers from the 7th, 9th, and 10th cranial nerves also enter the descending tract of the trigeminal nerve and run behind and slightly medial in the tract. The trigeminal nucleus is divided into the oral (pons/medulla), interpolaris (medulla), and caudalis (cervicomedullary) nuclei from the pons to the upper cervical cord at approximately C2–4. Topographic organization of the nucleus caudalis runs centrally from the upper portion to peripherally at the caudal portions. Therefore, the target in tractotomy is in the posterolateral part of the spinal cord at the cervicomedullary junction. The descending trigeminal tract is in the lateral space and the rostral nucleus caudalis is medial. Lesioning this area will target the descending fiber tracts laterally and the nucleus caudalis medially [13]. Patients with both nociceptive and neuropathic facial pain syndromes, including deafferentation pains due to cancer and its treatment, can be candidates for trigeminal nucleotractotomy.

Operative Technique

Though open surgical techniques can be used, in the patient with cancer, CT-guided percutaneous trigeminal nucleotractotomy is usually the technique of choice [13]. The procedure is performed at the occiput-C1 level to target both the descending trigeminal tract and nucleus caudalis of the spinal trigeminal nucleus. Prior to the procedure, a lumbar puncture is performed to instill intrathecal contrast which will allow visualization of craniocervical junction. The procedure may be performed in either the prone or the lateral position in the diagnostic CT scan venue. A 20-gauge needle is inserted into the skin 6–8 mm lateral to the midline at the C1-occiput level. The target is located at the first third lateral to midline and the lateral surface of the upper spinal cord, at a depth of 3–3.5 mm from the surface of the spinal cord. Functional confirmation of the target is obtained by electrical stimulation confirming paresthesias of the painful region. Ipsilateral sensory stimulation of the arm indicates medial localization at the cuneus nucleus, and contralateral responses indicate spinothalamic tract stimulation anteriorly. Lesions can be achieved with a tip temperature of greater than 60 °C within 30 s. A maximum of two or three

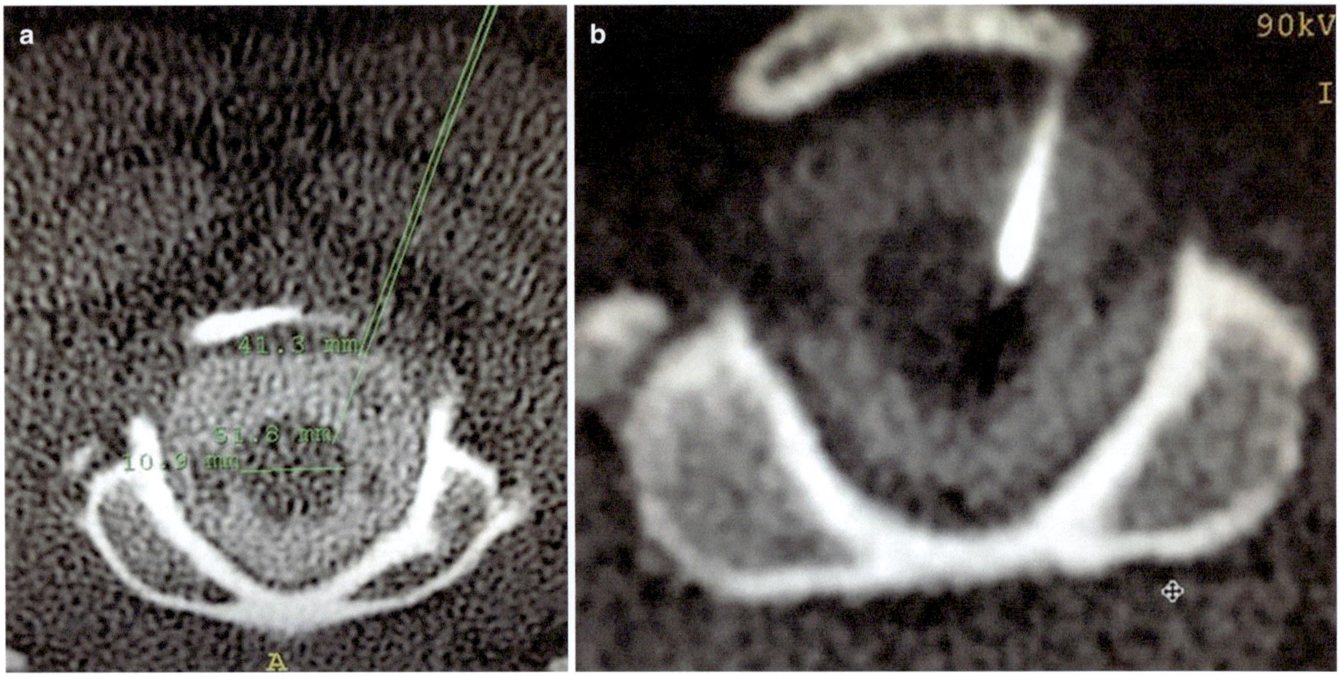

Fig. 22.2 Trigeminal tractotomy. (**a**) Measurement. (**b**) Needle placement

lesions should be performed, and the final lesion is made at 70 °C–80 °C for 60 s [14] (Fig. 22.2).

Outcomes

In 2008, Kanpolat reported on his series of 65 patients who had undergone trigeminal tractotomy for pain. Among all etiologies, 49 patients had no pain following the procedure. In the subset of 13 patients with craniofacial malignancies, 11 patients had no pain postoperatively, and 2 patients had partial nonsatisfactory pain relief. In Raslan's series of ten patients who had undergone trigeminal tractotomy-nucleotomy, 80% of patients had sustained benefit 6 months post-procedure [15, 16]. Complications include transient ataxia in 25–61% of patients and dysesthetic sensations in 25% of patients. Most studies reported recurrence with follow-up between 2 and 60 months [14, 15].

Thalamotomy

Rationale and Patient Selection

The intralaminar nuclei, the lateral portion of the medial dorsal nucleus, the centrum medianum, and parafascicular nuclear complexes are target nuclei for thalamic ablation for intractable pain. These target locations confer pain relief without sensory loss and risk of central pain and represent the medial thalamic system [17]. The medial thalamus has diffuse projections to prefrontal cortex and is important in the perceptive and affective component of pain [18]. Conceptually, therefore, relative activation of the lateral thalamic system or inhibition of the medial thalamic system can alleviate the suffering from central pain syndromes.

In 1952 Mark and Ervin verified the anatomical locations of stereotactic thalamic lesioning in 11 patients who succumbed to metastatic disease. They placed electrodes stereotactically and used radiofrequency ablation for permanent lesioning. Several clinical syndromes were detailed and correlated with postmortem sectioning. They defined three syndromes. The first consisted of sensory loss with mediocre or no relief of pain and resulted from ablation of VPL and VPM. The second syndrome produced little loss of sensation but good pain relief; this resulted from lesioning the parafascicular nucleus and the intralaminar nuclei. The third syndrome was characterized by changes in affect and neglect of external stimuli and resulted from lesioning the anterior nucleus and components of the medial dorsal nucleus. Based on this work, the current paradigm of thalamic ablation focuses on the parafascicular, centromedian, intralaminar, and medial dorsal nuclei.

Operative Technique

Jeanmonod et al. described their technique using a stereotactic frame compatible with magnetic resonance imaging

(MRI) to localize the target. The electrode is passed through a prefrontal approach under impedance monitoring. The target is 5 mm anterior to the posterior commissure, 4 mm above the AC-PC line, and 8–10 mm lateral to midline. Stimulation of the parvocellular regions of the medial thalamus yields contralateral painful burning as well as the patient's respective chronic pain sensation [19]. After achieving this physiologic confirmation in an awake patient, a radiofrequency lesion is placed at that target [20]. Alternatively, Young et al. described a technique using Gamma Knife radiation with radiosurgical doses of 140–180 Gy targeting the parafascicular, intralaminar, mediodorsal, and centromedian nuclei [21].

Outcomes

All published studies are case series, but most report significant improvement in symptoms in better than 50% of patients. Unfortunately, most report that recurrence is common several months later [22]. Reported complication rates for thalamotomy are approximately 10% and include primarily transient neurologic manifestations (somatosensory, motor deficits, ophthalmoplegia) and intraparenchymal hemorrhage [20]. Permanent sequelae appear to be rare.

Hypophysectomy

Rationale and Patient Selection

Surgical, chemical, and radiosurgical hypophysectomy is another option for intractable cancer pain and can relieve cancer pain if tumor regression is achieved and in patients with non-hormone-dependent tumors [23]. Initially proposed as a mechanism to control metastatic breast and prostate carcinoma by Charles Huggins in the 1950s, hypophysectomy was a logical extension of gonadectomy/adrenalectomy. In 1952 Perrault and colleagues in France and Scott in the United States were the first to report total hypophysectomies for metastatic disease [24]. Coincidentally several studies showed pain relief even without tumor regression ([25], [26]). In 1984 Ramierz et al. published a review with Levin including 10 publications accounting for 334 patients (43%) with breast cancer and the remainder with prostate cancer. Overall 70% of patients had significant pain relief immediately after the procedure [27]. The mechanism of pain relief is unknown; however, it appears that hypothalamic changes are responsible. Postmortem examinations of 59 patients who underwent hypophysectomy showed significant changes in the supraoptic and paraventricular nuclei, likely due to retrograde degeneration [28]. Similar pain relieving effects from adrenalectomy and oophorectomy have been noted. Pain relief from hypophysectomy does not seem to be related to endogenous opiate activity as naloxone does not reverse the effect [29]. It appears that patients with terminal breast or prostate cancer (and perhaps other widely metastatic cancers) with intractable pain may expect reasonable benefit in pain control from this procedure (Table 22.2).

Operative Technique

The procedure can be performed by surgical, chemical, or radiosurgical hypophysectomy. The open procedure is a well-tolerated transsphenoidal approach which usually requires general anesthesia. In a patient with end-stage metastatic carcinoma, chemical or minimally invasive hypophysectomy may be the preferred approach. Levin published a technique for chemical hypophysectomy. Patients are placed in a stereotactic holder, and an 18-gauge spinal needle is passed through the sphenoid sinus followed by a 20-gauge needle. Alcohol is instilled approximately 5–6 mL, 2 mL each at various depths. All patients received hormone replacement with thyroid and hydrocortisone and vasopressin as needed [30]. Hayashi et al. reported a Gamma Knife technique for hypophysectomy. The Leksell frame is applied to the head parallel with the optic nerves. Images for dose planning were obtained from both MR imaging and CT scanning. The target center was located at the border between the

Table 22.2 Hypophysectomy for cancer pain

Authors and year	No. of pts	Procedure	Outcome	Duration of pain relief
Miles J 1979	122	Chemical hypophysectomy	46% complete, 37% partial pain relief	Only 10% with greater than 3 months pain relief
Madrid 1979	329	Chemical hypophysectomy	67% complete, 27% partial pain relief	N/a
Levin 1980	29	Chemical hypophysectomy	93% excellent response	Most had lasting pain relief through remainder of life (longest survivor 9 months)
Levin 1984	82 (including 1980 data)	Chemical hypophysectomy	84% good response	Most had lasting pain relief (mean survival 5 months)
Hayashi 2002	9	Gamma Knife pituitary stalk ablation	100% good response; no complications	Lasted for all patients until they died (longest survivor 24 months)

pituitary gland and the stalk, at a maximum dose of 160 Gy at one isocenter using an 8 mm collimator. The 50% isodose covered both the lower part of the pituitary stalk and more than half of the pituitary gland. The optic pathway was kept below a maximum of 8 Gy [31].

Outcomes

In 1978 Miles performed chemical hypophysectomy in 122 cancer patients with 75% of patients receiving excellent to sufficient pain relief [32]. Madrid treated 329 patients with chemical hypophysectomy with 70–80% of patient receiving partial to complete relief of pain [33]. Levin et al. used stereotactic instillation of absolute alcohol into the sella turcica for pituitary destruction in 82 patients; 84% of patients reported good results [30]. Pain relief occurs immediately after chemical hypophysectomy and lasts for several weeks to years [23]. However, most patients develop endocrine disorders and half develop diabetes insipidus. In 2002 Hayashi reported the high-dose Gamma Knife technique. After several days, nine patients all had satisfactory pain relief. No patients developed panhypopituitarism, diabetes insipidus, or visual disturbances. 24-month follow-up showed no recurrence of pain [31].

References

1. Tracey I, Mantyh PW. The cerebral signature for pain perception and its modulation. Neuron. 2007;55:377–91.
2. Rolls ET, O'Doherty J, Kringelbach ML, Francis S, Bowtell R, McGlone F. Representations of pleasant and painful touch in the human orbitofrontal and cingulate cortices. Cereb Cortex. 2003;13:308–17.
3. Rosenstein D. Depression and end-of-life care for patients with cancer. Dialogues Clin Neurosci. 2011;13:101–8.
4. Viswanathan A, Harsh V, EAC P, Aziz TZ. Cingulotomy for medically refractory cancer pain. Neurosurg Focus. 2013;35:E1.
5. Faillace LA, Allen RP, JD MQ, Northrup B. Cognitive deficits from bilateral cingulotomy for intractable pain in man. Dis Nerv Syst. 1971;32:171–5.
6. Foltz EL, White LE Jr. Pain "relief" by frontal cingulumotomy. J Neurosurg. 1962;19:89–100.
7. Hurt RW, Thomas Ballantine H Jr. Stereotactic anterior cingulate lesions for persistent pain: a report on 68 cases. Clin Neurosurg. 1974;21:334–51.
8. Voris HC, Whisler WW. Results of stereotaxic surgery for intractable pain. Confin Neurol. 1975;37:86–96.
9. Yen CP, Kuan CY, Sheehan J, Kung SS, Wang CC, CK L, Kwan AL. Stereotactic bilateral anterior cingulotomy for intractable pain. J Clin Neurosci. 2005;12:886–90.
10. Yen CP, Kuan CY, Sheehan J, Kung SS, Wang CC, Liu CK, Kwan AL. Impact of bilateral anterior cingulotomy on neurocognitive function in patients with intractable pain. J Clin Neurosci. 2009;16:214–9.
11. Wong ET, Gunes S, Gaughan E, Patt RB, Ginsberg LE, Hassenbusch SJ, Payne R. Palliation of intractable cancer pain by MRI-guided cingulotomy. Clin J Pain. 1997;13:260–3.
12. Cosgrove GR, Rauch SL. Stereotactic cingulotomy. Neurosurg Clin N Am. 2003;14:225–35.
13. Kanpolant Y. Percutaneous Cordotomy and Trigeminal Tractotomy-Nucleotomy. In: Alterman RL, Youmans LA, editors. Neurological Surgery. Philadelphia: Elsiver; 2011. p. 1851–8.
14. Teixeira MJ, Fonoff ET. Technique of trigeminal nucleotractotomy. In: Lozano AM, Gildenberg PL, Tasker RR, editors. Textbook of stereotactic and functional neurosurgery. Berlin: Springer; 2009. p. 2097–123.
15. Thompson EM, Burchiel KJ, Raslan AM. Percutaneous trigeminal tractotomy-nucleotomy with use of intraoperative computed tomography and general anesthesia: report of 2 cases. Neurosurg Focus. 2013;35:E5.
16. Raslan A. Percutaneous computed tomography-guided radiofrequency ablation of upper spinal cord pain pathways for cancer-related pain. Neurosurgery. 2008;62:ONS226–33.
17. Vernon H, Mark MD, Frank R, Ervin MD, Thomas P, Hackett MD. clinical aspects of stereotactic thalamotomy in the human part I. The treatment of chronic severe pain. Arch Neurol. 1960;3(4):351–67. https://doi.org/10.1001/archneur.1960.00450040001001.
18. Jeanmonod D, Magnin M, Morel A. Thalamus and neurogenic pain: physiological, anatomical, and clinical data. Neuroreport. 1993;4:475–8.
19. Sano K. Intralaminal thalamotomy (thalamolaminotomy) and posterior-medial hypothalamotomy in the treatment of intractable pain. Prog Neurol Surg. 1977;8:50–103.
20. Jeanmonod D, Morel A. The central lateral thalamotomy for neuropathic pain. In: Lozano AMGPTR, editor. Textbook of stereotactic and functional neurosurgery. Berlin/Heidelberg: Springer; 2009. p. 2081–96.
21. Young RF, Vermeulen SS, Grimm P, Posewitz AE, Jacques DB, Rand RW, Copcutt BG. Gamma knife thalamotomy for the treatment of persistent pain. Stereotact Funct Neurosurg. 1995;64:172–81.
22. Richardson DE. Thalamotomy for control of chronic pain. Acta Neurochir. 1974;21:77–88.
23. Takeda F. Neurosurgical treatment of chronic pain. Postgrad Med J. 1984;60:905–13.
24. Perrault M, Le Beau J, Klotz B, Sicard J, Clavel B. L'hypohysectomie totale dans le traitment du cancer du sein: premier cas francais: avenir de la methode. Therapie. 1952;7:290–300.
25. Pearson OH, West CD, Hollander VP, Treves NE. Evaluation of endocrine therapy for advanced breast cancer. JAMA. 1954;154:234–9.
26. Kennedy BJ, French LA, Peyton WT. Hypophysectomy in advanced breast cancer. NEJM. 1956;255:1165–72.
27. Ramirez LF, Levin AB. Pain Relief after Hypophysectomy. Neurosurgery. 1984;4:499–504.
28. Daniel PM, Prichard MM. The human hypothalamus and pituitary stalk after Hypophysectomy or pituitary stalk section. Brain. 1972;95:813–24.
29. Hosobuchi Y, Adams JE, Linchitz R. Pain relief by electrical stimulation of the central Gray matter in humans and its reversal by naloxone. Science. 1977;197:183–6.
30. Levin AB, Ramirez LF, Katz J. The use of stereotaxic chemical Hypophysectomy in the treatment of thalamic pain syndrome. J Neurosurg. 1983;59(6):1002–6.
31. Hayashi M, Taira T, Ochiai T, Chernov M, Takasu Y, Izawa M, Kouyama N, Tomida M, Tokumaru O, Katayama Y, Kawakami Y, Hori T, Takakura K. Gamma knife surgery of the pituitary: new treatment for thalamic pain syndrome. J Neurosurg. 2005;102(Suppl):38–41.
32. Miles J. Neurological advances in the relief of pain. Br J Hosp Med. 1983;30:348. 350, 353.
33. Madrid JL. Chemical hypophysectomy. Adv Pain Res Ther. 1979;2:381–91.

Spinal Neuroablation for Cancer Pain

23

William S. Rosenberg, Parag G. Patil,
and Ahmed M. Raslan

Introduction

Surgically, two approaches are taken when targeting the brain or spinal cord to treat pain. The first, a nondestructive procedure, either uses electrical stimulation of neural targets, which is thought to modulate the process of pain perception, or uses pharmacological agents, which, when introduced into ventricular or intrathecal spaces, target pain-modulating receptors. Targets for electrical stimulation include the spinal cord, the thalamic nuclei, the periventricular gray matter, the periaqueductal gray matter, and the motor cortex. Generally, nondestructive surgical procedures are used for nonmalignant-type pain; however, intrathecal pharmacotherapy is also used for cancer pain treatment. The second, a destructive procedure known as neuroablation is used with the goal of interrupting signals that lead to pain perception at various levels.

Neuroablation performed on neuronal structures, such as nuclei or gyri, or on white matter tracts, aims to disrupt ascending sensory signals or destroy limbic pathways involved in the emotional processes associated with pain. Neurosurgical procedures to treat pain can be performed at the level of the spinal cord or the brain. The focus of this chapter is spinal cord neuroablation.

W. S. Rosenberg (✉)
Center for the Relief of Pain, Kansas City, MO, USA
e-mail: wsr@post.harvard.edu

P. G. Patil
University of Michigan Medical Center, Ann Arbor, MI, USA
e-mail: pgpatil@med.umich.edu

A. M. Raslan
Oregon Health & Science University, Department of Neurosurgery, Portland, OR, USA

Portland VA Medical Center, Neurological Surgery, Portland, OR, USA
e-mail: raslana@ohsu.edu

Spinal Cord Neuroablation

Spinal cord ablation is deeply rooted in the history of neurosurgery. The notion that sectioning pain pathways could achieve pain control was first introduced by Spiller in 1912 [1]. This was followed by the development of a whole array of surgical procedures aimed at the interruption of ascending pain signals throughout different parts of the central nervous system.

Only a few decades ago, spinal cord ablation was a routine surgical procedure in neurosurgical operating rooms. However, the introduction of opioids, with their varied methods of administration (e.g., intrathecal or transdermal delivery), leads to a drastic contraction in the art and science of ablative spinal cord surgery to treat pain. Decades of opioid use has demonstrated unanticipated disadvantages for cancer pain patients, and there is now a renewed and reinvigorated interest in the use of neuroablation to treat cancer pain.

Currently, spinal cord targets for neuroablative procedures to treat pain include: [1] the spinothalamic tract, [2] trigeminal spinal nucleus, [3] the midline ascending polysynaptic visceral pain pathway, and [4] the dorsal root entry zone (DREZ). A summary of these procedures is provided below.

Cordotomy

Cordotomy is the lesioning, sectioning, or interruption of the lateral spinothalamic tract (LST). This procedure was historically performed in the upper thoracic spine using an open posterior approach or less commonly high in the cervical spine [2]. The spinal cord anterolateral ascending pain transmission system carries information about pain and temperature from the contralateral side of the body. Fibers forming the LST decussate within the spinal cord (two to five segments higher than the level of entry), carrying signals to the thalamus and onward to the sensory cortex. The LST has a

A. Gulati et al. (eds.), *Essentials of Interventional Cancer Pain Management*, https://doi.org/10.1007/978-3-319-99684-4_23

somatotopic arrangement, with the sacral segments posterolateral and the cervical segments anteromedial [3]. Separated by intervening white matter, the pyramidal tract lies posterior to the LST. The ventral spinocerebellar tract overlies the LST, and inadvertent injury to this tract may cause ipsilateral ataxia of the arm. Human autonomic pathways for vasomotor and genitourinary control, in addition to the reticulospinal tract that controls ipsilateral automatic respiration, are also part of the anterolateral quadrant of the spinal cord. The ideal cordotomy candidate is a patient who requires treatment of somatic cancer pain of a nociceptive nature, localized below the neck, and confined to one half of the body [3].

From the beginning of the twentieth century through the early 1970s, cordotomy was performed as an open procedure, undertaken at various spinal levels, including the upper thoracic spine, in an effort to avoid complications such as ataxia and sleep apnea [4]. Mullan and Rosomoff introduced the percutaneous approach; this changed the risk-benefit equation and made it possible for the procedure to be performed on patients of poor general health, such as terminally ill cancer patients [5, 6]. Despite this technical improvement, advances in opioid pharmacology, as well as the introduction of reversible neuromodulatory techniques in the mid-1980s and early 1990s, the number of cordotomy procedures performed worldwide was significantly reduced. Kanpolat [7–9] introduced computed tomography (CT) guidance for cordotomy in the late 1980s. This technical advancement again improved safety and possibly efficacy. High-quality clinical outcome data still needs to be accrued.

Currently, cordotomy is performed using a lateral percutaneous approach to the spinal cord at the level of C2. However, a more caudal anterior transdiscal cervical approach can be used to avoid sleep apnea, the greatest risk coming after bilateral procedures at the same cervical level. In a recent clinical study, anterior CT-guided cordotomy, to avoid sleep apnea, was used to control cancer pain in six of eight patients with pulmonary-pleural malignancy [10].

A CT-guided cordotomy procedure involves a lumbar puncture and the injection of a water soluble dye into the patient's intrathecal space, 30 min prior to ablation. A CT scan guides the placement of a cordotomy radiofrequency electrode, which is isolated throughout the entire shaft excepting the tip (2 mm in length and 0.3–0.4 mm in diameter). After measurement of the skin-dura distance, an electrode is introduced just under the mastoid process, targeting the C2 foramen and the anterolateral quadrant of the spinal cord. Confirmation of placement within the spinothalamic tract, thereby avoiding a lesion within the corticospinal tract, is essential and is obtained through electrophysiological testing. Low frequency stimulation through the correctly placed electrode will produce only ipsilateral neck contractions through direct stimulation at the level of the electrode (as opposed to a motor response in the limbs, which would indicate corticospinal tract placement). Higher-frequency stimulation should produce a contralateral sensory response in the desired region of analgesia. Two lesions at a temperature range of 60–75 degrees centigrade for 60–90 sec are usually sufficient to produce the desired contralateral loss of pin prick sensation, which is the hallmark of successful spinothalamic ablation. CT-guided cordotomy has a higher success rate compared with fluoroscopy-guided cordotomy and fewer side effects. Cancer pain control is reported to be greater than 95%.

Cordotomy procedure complications include weakness, hypotension, dysesthesia, mirror image pain, ataxia, incontinence, and sleep apnea. Many of these complications are based on clinical data from open cordotomy, however, and the available data on complications with CT-guided cordotomy suggest they are minimal and transient [11].

The most recent technological advances include use of endoscopic guidance through a small port in the upper cervical spine [12] and the use of intraoperative imaging such as flat panel fluoroscopy (O-arm) to guide needle placement [13].

A recent evidence-based review argued that the case for cordotomy was unique among all cancer pain procedures; the procedure received a GRADE 1C (strong recommendation based on low-/very low-quality evidence) based on the international Grading of Recommendations Assessment, Development and Evaluation (GRADE) and had the most evidence of all other ablative procedures [14]. Another systematic review of cordotomy in mesothelioma-related pain recommended a national procedure registry, given the procedure's apparent effectiveness despite the lack of high-level evidence [15].

Trigeminal Tractotomy-Nucleotomy

Cranial sensory information is carried in the fifth, seventh, ninth, and tenth cranial nerves, which then converge on the trigeminal tract and branch into the spinal nucleus extending caudally to C2. This anatomic detail is exploited surgically in the many pain procedures that center around ablation of the trigeminal tract and/or nucleus [16]. The trigeminal tract has been considered a target for surgically treating facial pain since the 1930s, when Sjoqvist performed a transverse stab incision into the dorsal medullary cervical junction [17]. Crue and Hitchcock developed a stereotactic technique to lesion the trigeminal tract and the nucleus using radiofrequency, which was named trigeminal nucleotomy [18, 19]. As with CT-guided cordotomy, the stereotactic principle of approaching the trigeminal tract is what leads to the current version of trigeminal tractotomy-nucleotomy (TR-NC), which is also CT-guided (another contribution from Kanpolat and colleagues in the late 1980s) [20].

CT-guided TR-NC is performed using the same principles and techniques utilized with CT-guided cordotomy, except it is undertaken in a prone or occasionally in a lateral position. Verification of the target is performed both anatomically and electrophysiologically; however, sensory stimulation using radiofrequency electrodes of the trigeminal nucleus and tract is extremely painful, and, in certain patients, prone positioning is not possible while a patient is awake due to extreme hypersensitivity. These difficulties with awake TR-NC lead to the introduction of TR-NC under general anesthesia using intraoperative CT such as described by use of a CereTom CT scanner [21]. In this variation of TR-NC, anatomic and motor stimulation alone is used to confirm electrode placement, foregoing patient-reported sensory feedback. Indications for TR-NC include anesthesia dolorosa, postherpetic neuralgia, neuropathic facial pain, facial cancer pain, and glossopharyngeal and geniculate neuralgia [9, 20]. The procedure can be considered a miniature caudalis DREZ procedure. The nucleus caudalis DREZ operation involves the same concept as the TR-NC procedure but includes destruction of the whole substantia gelatinosa of the nucleus caudalis. Pain relief from TR-NC is reported as complete or satisfactory in 80% of cases [2]. Complications include ataxia due to injury of the spinocerebellar tract (rare and temporary occurrence) and contralateral hypoalgesia if the spinothalamic tract is included in lesioning [2, 9–11, 20].

Open caudalis DREZ ablation was introduced by Nashold [22] for control of deafferentation pain and neuropathic pain in the face. With this procedure, a radiofrequency or mechanical lesion of the nucleus caudalis portion of the spinal nucleus of the trigeminal nerve is created down to the level of C2 and caudally to the level of the obex. This procedure is rarely performed, and has been mostly replaced by percutaneous TR-NC.

Extralemniscal Myelotomy

Hitchcock was the first to describe the extralemniscal myelotomy (ELM) procedure where he aimed to stereotactically destroy the decussating fibers of the spinothalamic tract to control pain in the neck and both arms, a procedure then called a "commissural" myelotomy [23]. To achieve this, he created a lesion in the central medullary region at the cervicomedullary junction using a stereotactic apparatus designed to target this region of the skull.

It was noted that the ELM procedure controlled pain below the expected level of the lesion, and Schvarcz added the term "extralemniscal," anticipating that the target was an ascending non-specific polysynaptic pathway as described by Nauta [24]. This tract was confirmed later, and its presence has been described by several authors, who published reports of performing open midline punctate myelotomy at various spinal cord levels. This polysynaptic ascending pathway is thought to carry visceral nociceptive impulses and lies deep within the midline dorsal column [25–27]. Building on this notion, Kanpolat used CT-guidance to essentially replicate what Hitchcock and Schvarcz had performed and thus pioneered the percutaneous ELM procedure currently used today [28]. Extralemniscal myelotomy, both open and percutaneous, is a procedure for midline pain of visceral origin. Indications include patients with abdominal visceral, pelvic, sacral, or retroperitoneal pain.

Dorsal Root Entry Zone Surgery

Following the introduction of the gate theory of pain in the 1960s, [29] the dorsal horn received a lot of attention, which resulted in consideration as a target for both stimulation and ablation. In 1972, Sindou [30] first attempted DREZ destruction, although for spasticity not for pain. Nashold et al. soon followed and introduced radiofrequency to perform DREZ lesioning [31]. Other methods, such as laser and ultrasound probes, have also been used [31, 32]. When the large lemniscal afferents in peripheral nerves or dorsal roots are altered, as with plexus or root avulsions, there is a reduction in the inhibitory control of the dorsal horn [33]. The resulting disinhibition and excessive firing of dorsal horn neurons, which is thought to be the cause of deafferentation pain, makes DREZ lesioning a potential treatment for such pain [34]. The technical details of the procedure and its variants are beyond the scope of this chapter, but DREZ lesioning is performed as an open surgical procedure using general anesthesia, often using intraoperative neurophysiologic monitoring to prevent complications such as dorsal column injury. The DREZ operation is conceptually a transformation of an incomplete injury to the dorsal root/dorsal horn into a complete injury of the dorsal horn and essentially the five most superficial laminae of Rexed. This mechanism of action determines surgical candidacy. Ideal patients have brachial plexus avulsion, Pancoast tumor with brachial plexus invasion, pain due to spinal cord or cauda equina lesions, postherpetic neuralgia, peripheral nerve injury pain, and pain accompanying hyperspastic states [34].

Lack of functional use of the limb served by the spinal cord levels lesioned in the DREZ procedure is, in general, a prerequisite for the spinal DREZ procedure, since complete sensory denervation will render the limb useless, even if there is residual motor function. When patients are carefully selected and the lesions accurately performed, the success rate can be as high as 90% (with follow-up success rates reported for up to 4 years) [35]. DREZ procedure complications and side effects include cerebrospinal fluid fistula, meningitis, ataxia, increased neurological deficits, and dysesthesias [35].

Conclusion

Neuroablation of spinal cord pathways is one of the most effective methods for control of intractable pain. It is not considered a first-line treatment, but can be an effective strategy in the right context for severe, refractory pain. There is a renewed interest in neuroablation procedures, due to technological advances and the emergence of new indications for patients who fail neuromodulation therapy.

References

1. Spiller WG, Martin E. The treatment of persistent pain of organic origin in the lower part of the body by division of the anterolateral column of the spinal cord. JAMA. 1912;LVIII(20):1489–90.
2. Kanpolat Y. Percutaneous cordotomy, tractotomy, and midline myelotomy: minimally invasive stereotactic pain procedures. In: Fisher W, Burchiel K, editors. Seminars in neurosurgery: pain management for the neurosurgeon, vol. 2. New York: Thieme Medical Publishers Inc.; 2005. p. 203–19.
3. Walker A. The spinothalamic tract in man. Arch Neurol Psychiatr. 1940;43(2):284–98.
4. Hodge C, Christensen M. Anterolateral cordotomy. In: Burchiel K, editor. Surgical management of pain. Stuttgart/New York: Thieme Medical Publishers Inc; 2002. p. 732–44.
5. Mullan S, Harper PV, Hekmatpanah J, Torres H, Dobbin G. Percutaneous interruption of spinal-pain tracts by means of a Strontium90 needle. J Neurosurg. 1963;20:931–9.
6. Rosomoff HL, Brown CJ, Sheptak P. Percutaneous radiofrequency cervical cordotomy: technique. J Neurosurg. 1965;23(6):639–44.
7. Kanpolat Y, Akyar S, Caglar S. Diametral measurements of the upper spinal cord for stereotactic pain procedures: experimental and clinical study. Surg Neurol. 1995;43(5):478–82. discussion 482–473
8. Kanpolat Y, Akyar S, Caglar S, Unlu A, Bilgic S. CT-guided percutaneous selective cordotomy. Acta Neurochir. 1993;123(1–2):92–6.
9. Kanpolat Y, Savas A, Batay F, Sinav A. Computed tomography-guided trigeminal tractotomy-nucleotomy in the management of vagoglossopharyngeal and geniculate neuralgias. Neurosurgery. 1998;43(3):484–9. discussion 490
10. Raslan AM. Percutaneous computed tomography-guided transdiscal low cervical cordotomy for cancer pain as a method to avoid sleep apnea. Stereotact Funct Neurosurg. 2005;83(4):159–64.
11. Kanpolat Y, Savas A, Akyar S, Cosman E. Percutaneous computed tomography-guided spinal destructive procedures for pain control. Neurosurg Q. 2004;14:229–38.
12. Fonoff ET, de Oliveira YS, Lopez WO, Alho EJ, Lara NA, Teixeira MJ. Endoscopic-guided percutaneous radiofrequency cordotomy. J Neurosurg. 2010;113(3):524–7.
13. Collins KL, Patil PG. Flat-panel fluoroscopy O-arm-guided percutaneous radiofrequency cordotomy: a new technique for the treatment of unilateral cancer pain. Neurosurgery. 2013;72(1 Suppl Operative):27–34. discussion 34
14. Raslan AM, Cetas JS, McCartney S, Burchiel KJ. Destructive procedures for control of cancer pain: the case for cordotomy. J Neurosurg. 2011;114(1):155–70.
15. France BD, Lewis RA, Sharma ML, Poolman M. Cordotomy in mesothelioma-related pain: a systematic review. BMJ Support Palliat Care. 2014;4(1):19–29.
16. Taren JA, Kahn EA. Anatomic pathways related to pain in face and neck. J Neurosurg. 1962;19:116–21.
17. Sjogvist O. Studies on pain conduction in the trigeminal nerve: a contribution to the surgical treatment of facial pain. JAMA. 1940;115(5):408.
18. Crue BL, Carregal EJA, Felsoory A. Percutaneous stereotactic radiofrequency trigeminal Tractotomy with neurophysiological recordings. Stereotact Funct Neurosurg. 1972;34(6):389–97.
19. Hitchcock E. Stereotactic trigeminal tractotomy. Ann Clin Res. 1970;2(2):131–5.
20. Kanpolat Y, Deda H, Akyar S, Caglar S, Bilgic S. CT-guided trigeminal tractotomy. Acta Neurochir. 1989;100(3–4):112–4.
21. Thompson EM, Burchiel KJ, Raslan AM. Percutaneous trigeminal tractotomy-nucleotomy with use of intraoperative computed tomography and general anesthesia: report of 2 cases. Neurosurg Focus. 2013;35(3):E5.
22. Bernard EJ Jr, Nashold BS Jr, Caputi F, Moossy JJ. Nucleus caudalis DREZ lesions for facial pain. Br J Neurosurg. 1987;1(1):81–91.
23. Hitchcock E. Stereotactic cervical myelotomy. J Neurol Neurosurg Psychiatry. 1970;33(2):224–30.
24. Nauta HJ, Hewitt E, Westlund KN, Willis WD Jr. Surgical interruption of a midline dorsal column visceral pain pathway. Case report and review of the literature. J Neurosurg. 1997;86(3):538–42.
25. Al-Chaer ED, Lawand NB, Westlund KN, Willis WD. Pelvic visceral input into the nucleus gracilis is largely mediated by the postsynaptic dorsal column pathway. J Neurophysiol. 1996;76(4):2675–90.
26. Al-Chaer ED, Lawand NB, Westlund KN, Willis WD. Visceral nociceptive input into the ventral posterolateral nucleus of the thalamus: a new function for the dorsal column pathway. J Neurophysiol. 1996;76(4):2661–74.
27. Kanpolat Y, Atalag M, Deda H, Siva A. CT guided extralemniscal myelotomy. Acta Neurochir. 1988;91(3–4):151–2.
28. Schvarcz JR. Stereotactic extralemniscal myelotomy. J Neurol Neurosurg Psychiatry. 1976;39(1):53–7.
29. Melzack R, Wall PD. Pain mechanisms: a new theory. Science. 1965;150(3699):971–9.
30. Sindou M, Mertens P. Surgery in the dorsal root entry zone for pain. In: Fisher W, Burchiel K, editors. Seminars in neurosurgery: pain management for the neurosurgeon, vol. 2. New York: Thieme medical publishers Inc.; 2005. p. 221–32.
31. Dreval ON. Ultrasonic DREZ-operations for treatment of pain due to brachial plexus avulsion. Acta Neurochir. 1993;122(1–2):76–81.
32. Powers SK, Adams JE, Edwards MS, Boggan JE, Hosobuchi Y. Pain relief from dorsal root entry zone lesions made with argon and carbon dioxide microsurgical lasers. J Neurosurg. 1984;61(5):841–7.
33. Wall P. Presynaptic control of impulses at the first central synapse in the cutaneous pathway. In: Eccles J, Schade J, editors. Physiology of spinal neurons. Amsterdam: Elsevier; 1964. p. 92–118.
34. Guenot M, Bullier J, Sindou M. Clinical and electrophysiological expression of deafferentation pain alleviated by dorsal root entry zone lesions in rats. J Neurosurg. 2002;97(6):1402–9.
35. Emery E, Blondet E, Mertens P, Sindou M. Microsurgical DREZotomy for pain due to brachial plexus avulsion: long-term results in a series of 37 patients. Stereotact Funct Neurosurg. 1997;68(1–4 Pt 1):155–160.

Radiosurgery

24

Simon S. Lo, Tithi Biswas, Rodney J. Ellis, and Peter C. Gerszten

Introduction

In the past decade, there has been a significant advancement of radiotherapy technologies and techniques. These sophisticated radiotherapy technologies and techniques, including image-guidance capabilities, have facilitated the capability to deliver highly conformal radiation to a target volume with very high precision and accuracy. Gamma Knife-based stereotactic radiosurgery (SRS) was pioneered by Lars Leksell in Sweden about 50 years ago, and its success in the treatment of various intracranial conditions has aspired investigators from Sweden and Japan to explore the application of stereotactic radiation delivery in extracranial tumors, which has marked the birth of stereotactic body radiotherapy (SBRT), also named extracranial radiosurgery or stereotactic ablative radiotherapy (SABR) [1, 2]. In recent years, SBRT has been increasingly utilized to treat primary and metastatic tumors from various sites and has been established as one of the standard treatment options for stage I medically inoperable non-small cell lung cancer with excellent local control and relatively low toxicities [1–3]. Its use has been extended to other primary tumors such as renal cell carcinoma, prostate cancer, primary liver tumors, pancreatic cancer, and limited metastases in the liver, lung, adrenal, spine, and non-spinal bone [1, 4]. In this chapter, we will only cover the use of SBRT in the context of cancer pain control. Therefore, SBRT for liver and lung metastases, where most patients do not have pain symptoms and are treated with some curative intent, will not be included.

Brief Overview of the Technical Aspects of SBRT

The key components of the SBRT process include very robust immobilization, respiratory motion control, sophisticated treatment planning, pretreatment verification under image guidance, intrafractional motion control, and efficient, precise, and accurate treatment delivery [1, 2, 5]. With such a tedious process, a rigorous quality assurance program is essential. Several commercially available radiotherapy treatment devices carry SBRT capabilities. No matter what treatment device one is using to deliver SBRT, the training and the experience of the treatment team are likely the most important determining factors for successful treatment delivery [1].

Robust immobilization can be achieved using commercially available stereotactic body frames, body cradles, or vacuum cushions [2, 6]. A vacuum cushion with a dual vacuum system can provide extra accuracy in the setup, and this is essential in spinal SBRT. Some body frames have built-in abdominal compression capability (see below), rendering it a dual function device. There are three broad groups of respiratory motion control methods [1, 2] and they are:

1. Motion dampening – examples are abdominal compression and active breathing control (ABC).
2. Target gating.
3. Target tracking – example is robotic radiosurgery with the CyberKnife (Accuray, California, USA).

Targets requiring respiratory motion control include lung, liver, kidney, and adrenal tumors. When target gating or tracking techniques are used, surrogate markers such as fiducials are usually implanted to facilitate the process.

S. S. Lo (✉)
University of Washington School of Medicine, Department of Radiation Oncology, Seattle, WA, USA
e-mail: simonslo@uw.edu

T. Biswas · R. J. Ellis · P. C. Gerszten
University Hospitals Seidman Cancer Center, Case Comprehensive Cancer Center, Department of Radiation Oncology, Cleveland, OH, USA
e-mail: Biswas@UHhospitals.org; Rodney.Ellis@UHhospitals.org; gersztenpc@upmc.edu

A. Gulati et al. (eds.), *Essentials of Interventional Cancer Pain Management*, https://doi.org/10.1007/978-3-319-99684-4_24

Different treatment planning techniques have been employed, and the selection usually depends on multiple factors including the site and shape of tumor, the proximity of the tumor to organs at risk (OARs), availability of resources, and machine slot availability. Regardless of the technique used, the goal is to achieve a highly conformal isodose distribution while minimizing the radiation dose to the OARs [1, 2]. In the case of spinal SBRT, given the need to create a very steep dose gradient from the spinal target to the spinal cord and to contour the complex shape of spinal target, techniques such as intensity-modulated radiotherapy (IMRT) or volumetric modulated arc therapy (VMAT) are used if linear-accelerator-based SBRT or robotic radiosurgery with CyberKnife (Accuray, California, USA) is considered [5, 6].

To ensure that a patient is accurately set up prior to radiation treatment delivery, pretreatment verification via image guidance is necessary. Image guidance can be achieved using cone beam computerized tomography (CBCT), megavoltage CT, or stereoscopic X-rays, depending on the treatment device used [1]. Robust immobilization should minimize intrafractional movement, but it is prudent practice to perform a midway CBCT to ascertain that there are no shifts during treatment and appropriate adjustments are made if there are intrafractional shifts. This is important in spinal SBRT since the spinal cord is only 1–2 mm away from the spinal target and even a slight shift can significantly increase the spinal cord dose exposure, resulting in an increased risk of radiation myelopathy [5, 7]. Colleagues from the University of Toronto found that even with an immobilization device with a dual vacuum system, which attained the best setup accuracy, the possible shift could be up to 2 mm intrafractionally [8]. One important factor that can affect the setup accuracy is the amount of time needed for treatment delivery. It is more likely that a patient can lie still in the immobilization device throughout the whole treatment if the treatment time is relatively short. In the case of robotic radiosurgery (CyberKnife-based SBRT), which typically takes a longer time to deliver the radiation dose, the potential increase in intrafractional positional shift is partially mitigated by the near real-time tracking. Newer machines from major manufacturers now can deliver radiation with a very high dose rate, resulting in substantial shortening of the treatment time. This shorter treatment time theoretically translates into a decrease in intrafractional patient movement.

Non-spinal Bone Metastasis

For uncomplicated bone metastasis, the standard treatment is external beam radiation therapy, and there is level I evidence from multiple randomized trials and the American Society for Radiation Oncology (ASTRO) bone metastasis guideline to support the use of a single 8 Gy fraction for palliation of pain [9]. Given critical structures are usually remote from the treatment field, highly conformal techniques delivering high dose or ablative radiotherapy has not been routinely recommended. However, in patients with bone metastases from renal cell carcinoma, melanoma, and sarcomas, which are regarded as radioresistant tumors, conventional radiotherapy may not be as effective in pain and local control, and SBRT may be offered to improve pain and local control. However, the data on the use of SBRT in painful non-spinal bone metastasis is scarce.

In a series from the Methodist Hospital, 18 patients with 24 painful renal cell carcinoma bone metastases were treated with SBRT with a dose of 24–40 Gy in 3–5 fractions [4]. The investigators observed a radiation dose response for pain control. Overall, 78% of patients experienced pain relief after SBRT. Patients treated to a dose of 40 Gy in 5 fractions experienced a shorter time to achieve pain relief compared to those receiving lower radiation doses [4]. Patients who received a biologically effective dose (BED) of >85 Gy achieved a faster and more durable pain relief compared to those who received lower BED [4]. There were no grade 2 or higher toxicities. According to the current American College of Radiology (ACR) Appropriateness Criteria guidelines, SBRT is not routinely recommended for painful non-spinal bone metastases [10]. Rigorous testing of SBRT in a clinical trial setting is required before it can be regarded as the standard of care for patients with painful non-spinal bone metastases.

Table 24.1 summarizes selected studies of SBRT for painful non-spinal bone metastasis.

Spinal Metastases

There is abundant data from prospective trials and retrospective studies in the literature on the use of SBRT for spinal metastases in a variety of settings [7, 10–18]. Pain control is the primary endpoint reported in many of these studies. In one of the largest series from the University of Pittsburgh Medical Center, 393 patients with 500 spinal metastases were treated with single-fraction SBRT to 20 Gy (median dose). Long-term pain improvement was attained in 290 out of 336 evaluable cases based on assessment using a 10-point visual analog scale [15]. In a study from the University of California, San Francisco, 38 patients with 60 spinal metastases were treated with CyberKnife-based SBRT using 1–5 fractions to a median dose of 24 Gy in 3 fractions, and the investigators observed an improvement of pain in 31 of 46 painful sites [19]. The group from Memorial Sloan-Kettering Cancer Center treated 93 patients with 103 spinal metastasis lesions with single-fraction SBRT to a dose of 18–24 Gy, and at a median follow-up of 15 months, the actuarial local con-

Table 24.1 Selected studies of SBRT for bone, spinal, and adrenal metastases with pain control as one of the endpoints

Series/type/institution	No. of patients/ tumors/no. of tumors with prior EBRT	Site	Dose (Gy)	Follow-up	Pain control
Jhaveri [4]/ retrospective/Houston Methodist Hospital	18/24/0	Bone (both non-spinal and spinal) metastases from renal cell carcinoma	24–40 Gy in 3–5 fxs, 18–30 Gy in 3–5 fxs or 30–40 Gy in 3–4 fxs	38 weeks	BED < 85: 54% BED > 85: 88%
Gerszten [15]/ retrospective/University of Pittsburgh Medical Center	393/500/344	Spine	20 in 1 fx (range, 12.5–25)	21 months	86%
Gibbs [16]/ retrospective/Stanford University	74/102/50	Spine	14–25 in 1–5 fxs	9 months	84% of symptomatic patients
Sheehan [17]/ retrospective/University of Virginia	40/110/0	Spine	17.3 in 1 fx (range, 10–24)	12.7 months	85%
Wang [18]/phase I and II trial/MD Anderson Cancer Center	149/166/79	Spine	30 in 5 fxs of 27 in 3 fxs	15.9 months	No pain based on BPI: 26% increased to 54% at 6 months Opioid use: 28·9% decreased to 20·0% at 6 months
Amdur [11]/phase I and II trial/University of Florida	21/25/12	Spine	15 in 1 fx	N/A	43%
Garg [14]/phase I and II trial/MD Anderson Cancer Center	60/61/0	Spine	16–24 Gy in 1 fx	20 months (mean)	18 vs. 13 patients pain free at 3 and 6 months vs. baseline Reduced pain levels (based on BPI) at 3 and 6 months vs. baseline
Mahadevan [24]/ retrospective/Beth Israel Deaconess Hospital	60/81/81	Previously irradiated spine	24 in 3 fxs or 25–30 in 5 fxs (if tumor touched cord)	12 months	65%
Damast [13]/ retrospective/Memorial Sloan-Kettering Cancer Center	94/97/97	Previously irradiated spine	20–30 Gy in 5 fxs	12.1 months	Some pain relief: 85% Significant pain relief: 46% Mild pain relief: 31% No pain relief/ worsening of symptoms: 23%
Choi [12]/retrospective/ Stanford University	42/51/51	Previously irradiated spine	10–30 Gy in 1–5 fxs	7 months	65%
Balagamwala [33]/ retrospective/Cleveland Clinic Foundation	57/88 (67 lesions with pain)/18	Spine (from renal cell carcinoma)	15 Gy (range 8–16 Gy) in 1 fx	5.4 months (whole group of 57 patients with 88 lesions)	Complete pain relief: 15.4% at 2 weeks 66.7% by 9 months
Chawla [27]/ retrospective/University of Rochester	3/3/0	Adrenal	40 Gy (range 16–50 Gy) in 10 fxs (range 4–16 fxs) (whole group of 30 patients)	0.8–35 months (whole group of 30 patients)	100% complete and durable pain relief (4–5 out of 10 to 0 out of 10)
Guiou [28]/ retrospective/the Ohio State University	4/4/0	Adrenal (from lung cancer)	20–37.5 Gy in 5 fxs (whole group of 9 patients)	4.3 months (whole group of 9 patients)	100% (decreased narcotic usage)

EBRT external beam radiation therapy, *fx* fraction, *BPI* Brief Pain Inventory, *N/A* not applicable trol rate was 90% [20]. Even though pain control was not used as an endpoint, they observed that durable symptom palliation was achieved in all patients with no local failure. Prospective data on SBRT for spinal metastasis with pain control as one of the endpoints are scarce.

Investigators from MD Anderson Cancer Center conducted a phase I/II trial of SBRT for spinal metastasis and treated 149 patients with 166 uncomplicated spinal metastases with SBRT to either 30 Gy in 5 fractions or 27 Gy in 3 fractions [18]. Patients' symptoms were evaluated via the use of the Brief Pain Inventory (BPI) and the MD Anderson Symptom Inventory (MDASI) before SBRT and at several time points up to 6 months after SBRT. The frequency and duration of complete pain relief were the primary endpoints of this trial. The number of patients reporting no pain from bone metastases, based on BPI, increased from 26% to 54% 6 months after SBRT at a median follow-up of 15.9 months [18]. The BPI-based pain reduction from baseline to 4 weeks after SBRT was observed to be clinically meaningful. The use of opioid medications was reduced from 28.9% to 20% during the first 6 months post-SBRT. Significant pain reduction according to the MDASI during the first 6 months after SBRT was reported, and there were significant reductions in a composite score of the six MDASI symptom interferences with daily life items [18].

In another phase I/II trial of single-fraction SBRT for radiation-naïve spinal metastasis from MD Anderson Cancer Center, 61 patients with 63 non-cervical spinal or paraspinal metastases were enrolled and treated with SBRT to a dose of 16–24 Gy in one fraction. More patients were pain free at 3 and 6 months compared to baseline, and the pain levels were lower at 3 and 6 months compared those at baseline after SBRT [14]. The investigators also observed that the pain level was correlated with local control. Amdur et al. from the University of Florida conducted a phase II trial of single-fraction SBRT for spinal metastasis, enrolling 25 patients, and pain control was recorded as one of the endpoints [11]. A single dose of 15 Gy was used for the SBRT. Local tumor control and pain control rates were 95% and 43%, respectively [11]. Table 24.1 summarizes selected studies of SBRT for spinal metastases with pain control as one of the endpoints.

The treatment options for patients with painful but previously irradiated spinal metastasis are limited given the prior radiation exposure to the spinal cord and other OARs.

SBRT has provided a means for re-irradiation of a metastatic spinal lesion for pain control and is very attractive option for this group of patients [21]. Interestingly, the reported pain response rates did not appear to be significantly worse than those patients who received SBRT for radiation-naïve spinal metastases [19]. Data in the literature showed very low toxicity rates (though one should monitor for radiation-induced myelopathy despite re-irradiation with ablative radiation). Sahgal et al. analyzed five reported cases of radiation myelopathy with dosimetric correlations in patients who had SBRT and prior external beam radiotherapy [22]. The total spinal cord tolerance was estimated to be approximately 70 Gy based on the assumption that the dose per fraction was 2 Gy per fraction and the alpha-beta ratio was 2 Gy [22, 23]. Dosing guidelines for re-irradiation with SBRT have been suggested [22], and interested readers are encouraged to go to the original publication for further details.

Mahadevan et al. from Beth Israel Deaconess Hospital treated 60 patients with 81 previously irradiated spinal metastases with SBRT to 24–50 Gy in 3–5 fractions, yielding a pain response rate of 65% [24]. Investigators from Memorial Sloan-Kettering Cancer Center treated 94 patients with 97 previously irradiated spinal metastases with SBRT to 20–30 Gy in 5 fractions. At a median follow-up of 12.1 months, 85% of the patients experienced some pain relief, and 46% had significant pain relief [13]. Table 24.1 summarizes selected studies of SBRT for recurrent spinal bone metastasis with pain control as one of the endpoints.

Debate exists as to whether a single-dose or multisession SBRT is more desirable in terms of pain control for spinal metastasis. Although prospective data is nonexistent, there was a pooled data analysis from the University of Pittsburgh Medical Center and Georgetown University comparing single-fraction and multisession SBRT for spinal metastases [25]. In the study, 228 patients with 348 spinal metastases were treated with SBRT to a median dose of 16.3 Gy in 1 fraction or multisession SBRT to a dose 20.6–24.5 Gy in 3–5 fractions. The pain control was significantly improved in patients who were treated with single-fraction SBRT for all measured time points up to 1 year after treatment compared to those who received multisession SBRT (100% vs. 88%) [25]. However, the local tumor control was significantly better in patients receiving multisession SBRT up to 2 years after SBRT compared to patients receiving single-fraction SBRT treatment (96% vs. 70%). Moreover, the need for retreatment was significantly lower in patients who had multisession SBRT (1% vs. 13%) [25]. The rates of toxicity and neurological deficit improvement were similar between the two groups. These findings seem to suggest that single-fraction SBRT offers better short-term pain control but multisession SBRT provides more durable local tumor control. Patients with painful spinal metastases and with shorter life expectancy may benefit from single-fraction SBRT given its better short-term pain control and shorter treatment course.

In patients with symptomatic pathologic fracture of the vertebrae with moderate spinal canal compromise, Gerszten and Monaco described a unique approach involving percutaneous transpedicular coblation corpectomy immediately followed by balloon kyphoplasty through the same 8-gauge cannula under fluoroscopic guidance and subsequent single-dose SBRT to 19 Gy in 1 fraction within a mean time interval of 14 days [26]. This approach provided long-term pain improvement and radiographic tumor control in all the 11 patients treated at follow-up times ranging from 7 to 44 months. There was no radiation-induced toxicity or new neurologic deficits observed [26]. Based on these findings, this approach appears to be a reasonable alternative to a corpectomy although it is subject to rigorous clinical testing.

Adrenal Metastases

Most adrenal metastases are asymptomatic lesions and in most cases, found on diagnostic imaging scans during the staging work-up of the primary cancer. However, some patients may have visceral or somatic pain due to bulky adrenal lesions, and palliative radiation therapy may be offered for pain control. SBRT has been used to treat adrenal metastasis either as a local therapy for oligometastatic disease or for rapid pain control. In most studies, patients with pain at baseline experienced pain relief. In the study from the University of Rochester, 3 out of 30 patients treated with SBRT for adrenal metastasis had severe pain for the lesion (4–5 out of 10) and experienced complete and durable pain relief after treatment [27]. In the study from the Ohio State University, all the patients with baseline pain achieved pain control [28]. Table 24.1 summarizes selected studies of SBRT for adrenal metastasis with pain control.

Toxicities Associated with SBRT

Since the data on SBRT for pain control pertains mainly to spinal metastases, only toxicities associated with spinal SBRT will be discussed in this section. The major complications associated with spinal SBRT include radiation-induced myelopathy, nerve injury, subsequent vertebral compression fracture, and pain flare.

The overall incidence of all complications after SBRT is very low, even in the setting of re-irradiation. Sahgal et al. have published two seminal reports of radiation myelopathy in radiation-naïve and re-irradiation settings [22, 29]. In the report on radiation-naïve patients, nine cases of radiation myelopathy with dosimetric details were analyzed. It was determined the risk of radiation myelopathy should be ≤5% if the maximum dose to the thecal sac, a surrogate of spinal cord, was 12.4 Gy in one fraction, 17.0 Gy in 2 fractions, 20.3 Gy in 3 fractions, 23.0 Gy in 4 fractions, or 25.3 Gy in 5 fractions [29]. The spinal cord tolerance in the re-irradiation setting has already been discussed earlier in this chapter.

Spinal nerves and nerve plexuses are near the vertebrae, rendering these structures susceptible to injury by the ablative doses of radiation delivered via SBRT. The overall incidence of radiation-induced injury to these structures is also very low. In a phase I/II trial of SBRT for radiation-naïve spinal metastases from MD Anderson Cancer Center where doses of 16–24 Gy were given in 1 fraction, 10 out of 61 patients developed mild (grade 1 or 2) numbness and tingling, and 1 developed grade 3 radiculopathy at L5 after SBRT [14]. Investigators from Beth Israel Deaconess Hospital observed 4 cases of persistent or new radiculopathy out of 60 patients with recurrent epidural spinal metastases treated with SBRT. However, since all of those patients developed radiologic disease progression, it is uncertain whether the complications were caused by tumor progression, radiation-induced nerve injury, or both [24]. In another study from MD Anderson Cancer Center, 2 cases of grade 3 lumbar plexopathy were observed after re-irradiation with SBRT for recurrent spinal metastases in 59 patients [30].

Vertebral compression fracture is not an uncommon complication after SBRT, especially after a single dose of ≥20–24 Gy, according to the data in the literature [31]. Baseline vertebral compression fracture, lytic tumor, and spinal deformity also increase the risk of vertebral compression fracture. Most vertebral compression fracture cases occur within the first 4 months after SBRT [31].

Another relatively common complication associated with SBRT is pain flare. In a study from Sunnybrook Health Science Centre, pain flare occurred in two thirds of patients undergoing SBRT for spinal metastases, most commonly on day 1 after treatment [32]. They have identified risk factors including higher Karnofsky performance status and cervical/lumbar levels. Steroid therapy is effective in control of pain flare in most cases.

Conclusions

Based on the data available to date, SBRT or "extracranial radiosurgery" appears to be a very effective treatment for pain control, particularly for spinal metastases, and has a very favorable toxicity profile. Current data presented are from retrospective studies and single-arm prospective studies. The question remains whether conventional external beam radiotherapy is as effective as SBRT for palliation of cancer pain. Radiation Therapy Oncology Group (RTOG) is currently conducting the phase III portion of RTOG 0631 trial randomizing patients into receiving external beam radiation therapy to 8 Gy in 1 fraction and SBRT to 16–18 Gy in 1 fraction for painful spinal metastasis (www.rtog.org). Hopefully, the results of this seminal international trial will help better define the role of SBRT in the management of painful spinal metastases.

References

1. Lo SS, Fakiris AJ, Chang EL, Mayr NA, Wang JZ, Papiez L, et al. Stereotactic body radiation therapy: a novel treatment modality. Nat Rev Clin Oncol. 2010;7(1):44–54.

2. Timmerman RD, Kavanagh BD, Cho LC, Papiez L, Xing L. Stereotactic body radiation therapy in multiple organ sites. J Clin Oncol. 2007;25(8):947–52.
3. Timmerman R, Paulus R, Galvin J, Michalski J, Straube W, Bradley J, et al. Stereotactic body radiation therapy for inoperable early stage lung cancer. JAMA. 2010;303(11):1070–6.
4. Jhaveri PM, Teh BS, Paulino AC, Blanco AI, Lo SS, Butler EB, et al. A dose-response relationship for time to bone pain resolution after stereotactic body radiotherapy (SBRT) for renal cell carcinoma (RCC) bony metastases. Acta Oncol. 2012;51(5):584–8.
5. Lo SS, Sahgal A, Wang JZ, Mayr NA, Sloan A, Mendel E, et al. Stereotactic body radiation therapy for spinal metastases. Discov Med. 2010;9(47):289–96.
6. Lo SS, Chang EL, Yamada Y, Sloan AE, Suh JH, Mendel E. Stereotactic radiosurgery and radiation therapy for spinal tumors. Expert Rev Neurother. 2007;7(1):85–93.
7. Sahgal A, Larson DA, Chang EL. Stereotactic body radiosurgery for spinal metastases: a critical review. Int J Radiat Oncol Biol Phys. 2008;71(3):652–65.
8. Li W, Sahgal A, Foote M, Millar BA, Jaffray DA, Letourneau D. Impact of immobilization on intrafraction motion for spine stereotactic body radiotherapy using cone beam computed tomography. Int J Radiat Oncol Biol Phys. 2012;84(2):520–6.
9. Lutz S, Berk L, Chang E, Chow E, Hahn C, Hoskin P, et al. Palliative radiotherapy for bone metastases: an ASTRO evidence-based guideline. Int J Radiat Oncol Biol Phys. 2011;79(4):965–76.
10. Lutz ST, Lo SS, Chang EL, Galanopoulos N, Howell DD, Kim EY, et al. ACR Appropriateness Criteria(R) non-spine bone metastases. J Palliat Med. 2012;15(5):521–6.
11. Amdur RJ, Bennett J, Olivier K, Wallace A, Morris CG, Liu C, et al. A prospective, phase II study demonstrating the potential value and limitation of radiosurgery for spine metastases. Am J Clin Oncol. 2009;32:515.
12. Choi CY, Adler JR, Gibbs IC, Chang SD, Jackson PS, Minn AY, et al. Stereotactic radiosurgery for treatment of spinal metastases recurring in close proximity to previously irradiated spinal cord. Int J Radiat Oncol Biol Phys. 2010;78(2):499–506.
13. Damast S, Wright J, Bilsky M, Hsu M, Zhang Z, Lovelock M, et al. Impact of dose on local failure rates after image-guided reirradiation of recurrent paraspinal metastases. Int J Radiat Oncol Biol Phys. 2011;81(3):819–26.
14. Garg AK, Shiu AS, Yang J, Wang XS, Allen P, Brown BW, et al. Phase 1/2 trial of single-session stereotactic body radiotherapy for previously unirradiated spinal metastases. Cancer. 2012;118:5069–77.
15. Gerszten PC, Burton SA, Ozhasoglu C, Welch WC. Radiosurgery for spinal metastases: clinical experience in 500 cases from a single institution. Spine (Phila Pa 1976). 2007;32(2):193–9.
16. Gibbs IC, Kamnerdsupaphon P, Ryu MR, Dodd R, Kiernan M, Chang SD, et al. Image-guided robotic radiosurgery for spinal metastases. Radiother Oncol. 2007;82(2):185–90.
17. Sheehan JP, Shaffrey CI, Schlesinger D, Williams BJ, Arlet V, Larner J. Radiosurgery in the treatment of spinal metastases: tumor control, survival, and quality of life after helical tomotherapy. Neurosurgery. 2009;65(6):1052–61. discussion 61–2.
18. Wang XS, Rhines LD, Shiu AS, Yang JN, Selek U, Gning I, et al. Stereotactic body radiation therapy for management of spinal metastases in patients without spinal cord compression: a phase 1–2 trial. Lancet Oncol. 2012;13(4):395–402.
19. Sahgal A, Ames C, Chou D, Ma L, Huang K, Xu W, et al. Stereotactic body radiotherapy is effective salvage therapy for patients with prior radiation of spinal metastases. Int J Radiat Oncol Biol Phys. 2009;74(3):723–31.
20. Yamada Y, Bilsky MH, Lovelock DM, Venkatraman ES, Toner S, Johnson J, et al. High-dose, single-fraction image-guided intensity-modulated radiotherapy for metastatic spinal lesions. Int J Radiat Oncol Biol Phys. 2008;71(2):484–90.
21. Masucci GL, Yu E, Ma L, Chang EL, Letourneau D, Lo S, et al. Stereotactic body radiotherapy is an effective treatment in reirradiating spinal metastases: current status and practical considerations for safe practice. Expert Rev Anticancer Ther. 2011;11(12):1923–33.
22. Sahgal A, Ma L, Weinberg V, Gibbs IC, Chao S, Chang UK, et al. Reirradiation human spinal cord tolerance for stereotactic body radiotherapy. Int J Radiat Oncol Biol Phys. 2012;82(1):107–16.
23. Huang Z, Mayr NA, Yuh WT, Wang JZ, Lo SS. Reirradiation with stereotactic body radiotherapy: analysis of human spinal cord tolerance using the generalized linear-quadratic model. Future Oncol. 2013;9(6):879–87.
24. Mahadevan A, Floyd S, Wong E, Jeyapalan S, Groff M, Kasper E. Stereotactic body radiotherapy reirradiation for recurrent epidural spinal metastases. Int J Radiat Oncol Biol Phys. 2011;81(5):1500–5.
25. Heron DE, Rajagopalan MS, Stone B, Burton S, Gerszten PC, Dong X, et al. Single-session and multisession CyberKnife radiosurgery for spine metastases-University of Pittsburgh and Georgetown University experience. J Neurosurg Spine. 2012;17(1):11–8.
26. Gerszten PC, Monaco EA 3rd. Complete percutaneous treatment of vertebral body tumors causing spinal canal compromise using a transpedicular cavitation, cement augmentation, and radiosurgical technique. Neurosurg Focus. 2009;27(6):E9.
27. Chawla S, Chen Y, Katz AW, Muhs AG, Philip A, Okunieff P, et al. Stereotactic body radiotherapy for treatment of adrenal metastases. Int J Radiat Oncol Biol Phys. 2009;75(1):71–5.
28. Guiou M, Mayr NA, Kim EY, Williams T, Lo SS. Stereotactic body radiotherapy for adrenal metastases from lung cancer. J Radiat Oncol. 2012;1:155–63.
29. Sahgal A, Weinberg V, Ma L, Chang E, Chao S, Muacevic A, et al. Probabilities of radiation myelopathy specific to stereotactic body radiation therapy to guide safe practice. Int J Radiat Oncol Biol Phys. 2013;85(2):341–7.
30. Garg AK, Wang XS, Shiu AS, Allen P, Yang J, McAleer MF, et al. Prospective evaluation of spinal reirradiation by using stereotactic body radiation therapy: The University of Texas MD Anderson Cancer Center experience. Cancer. 2011;117(15):3509–16.
31. Sahgal A, Atenafu EG, Chao S, Al-Omair A, Boehling N, Balagamwala EH, et al. Vertebral compression fracture after spine stereotactic body radiotherapy: a multi-institutional analysis with a focus on radiation dose and the spinal instability neoplastic score. J Clin Oncol. 2013;31(27):3426–31.
32. Chiang A, Zeng L, Zhang L, Lochray F, Korol R, Loblaw A, et al. Pain flare is a common adverse event in steroid-naive patients after spine stereotactic body radiation therapy: a prospective clinical trial. Int J Radiat Oncol Biol Phys. 2013;86:638–42.
33. Balagamwala EH, Angelov L, Koyfman SA, Suh JH, Reddy CA, Djemil T, et al. Single-fraction stereotactic body radiotherapy for spinal metastases from renal cell carcinoma. J Neurosurg Spine. 2012;17(6):556–64.

25 Deep Brain Stimulation and Motor Cortical Stimulation for Malignant Pain

Joshua M. Rosenow and Jonathan Miller

Introduction

Neurostimulation for the treatment of chronic pain has a long history. Deep brain stimulation (DBS) has been used to treat medically refractory pain syndromes (both neuropathic and nociceptive) for over 40 years. The initial impetus for exploring the utility of this strategy arose from rodent experiments that demonstrated positive reinforcement of self-stimulation of the deep paramedian septal regions [1]. Additional rodent experiments suggested that stimulation of the periventricular (PVG) and periaqueductal (PAG) gray regions could produce pain relief [2]. Based on these observations, early clinical studies by Heath and Mickle [3] and Gol [4] confirmed that stimulation of the septal areas in humans could reduce chronic pain associated with malignancies. The modern era of DBS for neuropathic pain began with Hosobuchi and Adams' [5] report of success treating anesthesia dolorosa with stimulation of the ventrocaudal (Vc) thalamus. This was followed by the work of Richardson and Akil [6] that showed PAG stimulation was also effective in relieving refractory pain in patients with phantom-limb and thalamic pain syndromes. Subsequent investigators have evaluated other deep brain targets such as the internal capsule and the medial thalamic nuclei [7], including the centromedian-parafascicular (CM-Pf) complex [8] for the treatment of intractable pain.

Early research into neuropathic pain revealed the contributive role of the motor cortex and the possibility that manipulation of this area might be associated with improvement in these symptoms [9]. This knowledge gained clinical application with the advent of epidural stimulation of the primary motor cortex (MCS) for the treatment of central pain syndromes, first reported by Tsubokawa et al. in 1991 [10]. Unfortunately, the long-term results of both DBS and MCS have not been as durable as originally anticipated. Thus, the use of DBS or MCS for the treatment of chronic pain of various etiologies may be considered relatively effective because of limited availability of alternative treatment options [11]. An increasing body of literature supports this procedure as an option for the treatment of otherwise uncontrolled neuropathic pain [12, 13].

Deep Brain Stimulation

Traditionally, pain has been classified into two distinct categories: nociceptive and neuropathic. However, it is now recognized that a substantial proportion of patients who experience pain have elements of both, with mixed components; this is particularly true of cancer pain. In the past, multiple authors have advocated using PAG/PVG as the stimulation target for nociceptive pain and Vc thalamus for neuropathic pain, but it has become common to implant both PAG/PVG and Vc electrodes simultaneously and perform trial stimulation of both before determination of the final implant configuration [14].

DBS electrodes are implanted using stereotactic guidance with magnetic resonance imaging (MRI) or MRI guidance combined with CT. Local anesthesia with intravenous sedation is utilized in the operating room. A frontal incision and burr hole are made based on stereotactic planning. Often microelectrode recording is used for physiologic targeting of the electrodes, especially in the Vc nucleus where identification of neural activity correlated to sensory signals can be helpful to confirm localization. This region is organized so that areas serving the face are more medial while those serving the leg more lateral, with the upper extremity fibers

J. M. Rosenow (✉)
Northwestern Memorial Hospital, Department of Neurosurgery, Neurology and Physical Medicine and Rehabilitation, Chicago, IL, USA
e-mail: jrosenow@nm.org

J. Miller
University Hospitals Case Medical Center, Case Western Reserve University, Cleveland, OH, USA
e-mail: jonathan.miller@uhhospitals.org

A. Gulati et al. (eds.), *Essentials of Interventional Cancer Pain Management*, https://doi.org/10.1007/978-3-319-99684-4_25

between them. This knowledge may be helpful in identifying optimal lead placement. Direct stimulation may also be used to refine the Vc target. The PVG/PAG electrode does not always require microelectrode (stimulation) recording as it is a more straightforward anatomic location. After the target is identified, the permanent macroelectrodes are placed and intraoperative stimulation is performed to confirm adequate response to stimulation. During Vc stimulation, patients report paresthesias that ideally should cover of the painful area without side effects. The PAG/PVG target is usually involved with the affective component of pain so patients may report a generalized feeling of warmth or wellbeing when stimulation is activated.

Many centers conduct a trial of stimulation to determine if it is effective before implanting the programmable pulse generator (IPG). This trial usually lasts from several days to a week. There are no firm criteria for declaring a trial a success, but most centers will use a pain reduction level of 50% as measured by verbal or visual analog scale.

Published rates of long-term pain control after DBS vary from 19% to 79% [15]. The first multicenter trial of DBS for pain was conducted in 1976 using the now outdated Medtronic Model 3380 electrode (Medtronic, Minneapolis, MN) and enrolled 196 patients. This study was plagued by poor enrollment, a high attrition rate, a mixture of diagnoses with unclear patient-selection criteria, and wide variation in stimulation parameters used [16]. A second multicenter trial was completed in 2001 using the Medtronic Model 3387. This study enrolled only 50 patients and used standardized visual analog scores to rate pain intensity but was limited by very small case volume per center. These studies did not meet the primary outcome for efficacy, which was defined as greater than 50% pain relief 1 year after surgery. As a result, Medtronic did not apply for US Food and Drug Administration approval of DBS for the treatment of pain [17].

The concept that nociceptive pain responds to PAG/PVG stimulation and neuropathic pain responds to Vc thalamic stimulation is based on the understanding that the PVG region interacts with the endogenous opioid system, while the Vc thalamus is the relay for second-order nerve fibers that project from the dorsal column/medial lemniscal system, which is also targeted in spinal cord stimulation. In one study of Vc stimulation, 56% of patients with neuropathic pain obtained long-term benefit, compared with 0/51 patients who had nociceptive pain [15]. On the other hand, PVG stimulation was shown to be effective in only 23% of patients with neuropathic pain compared with 59% of patients with nociceptive pain [15]. In practice, many surgeons target both sites with separate electrodes at implantation given the frequency of combined pain syndromes [15]. Both the PVG/PAG and VC targets have been shown to be effective in treatment of cancer pain [18, 19]. A trial of stimulation prior to permanent implantation provides the opportunity to assess these differential effects.

In a recent large retrospective analysis of patients treated with DBS for pain, 62% of patients had a successful stimulation trial leading to IPG implantation, but long-term pain control rates were much lower, with only 38% of patients who had a successful trial still experiencing benefit from stimulation at last follow-up. However, the authors noted a relatively positive predictive value for patients with pain improvement from initial electrode implantation before stimulation, suggesting that response to the microlesion created by implantation may predict benefit from stimulation [17]. A meta-analysis showed that about 50% of patients achieve long-term pain control using DBS. For neuropathic pain, 42% of patients with neuropathic pain experience relief, compared with 61% of those with nociceptive pain [15].

The recent large series from Boccard et al. [20] reported on 85 patients who underwent a trial of either PVG, Vc, or combined PVG/Vc DBS for neuropathic pain. Seventy-four of the patients achieved enough pain reduction during a trial of stimulation to merit system implantation. Long-term outcomes were obtained for 59 of the patients. No patients in this series were specifically mentioned as having pain of malignant origin. Mean follow-up of implanted patients was 27.9 months. Mean VAS improvement at 10 months was 38.7%, although mean scores on the SF-36, EQ-5D, and McGill pain questionnaire (MPQ) all did not differ significantly from baseline at 12-month follow-up. However, those patients who did obtain significant relief maintained that relief at up to 4 years postoperatively.

Patients with spinal cord injury with central pain may benefit from DBS, but the efficacy is low, with only 16% of patients in one study reporting long-term relief [21]. DBS also may benefit patients with limb or plexus injuries, such as stump pain after amputation and phantom limb pain [22]. Pain after stroke also has been shown to be successfully treated with DBS [23].

Boccard et al. [24] have also recently published a series of 16 patients who underwent trial stimulation of the bilateral anterior cingulate cortex. This target is intended to influence only the affective component of the patients' pain syndrome, rather than reduce their VAS score, building on the experience of lesioning this region for treatment of intractable psychiatric disease. Almost all (15/16) patients passed a trial of stimulation and underwent system implantation. In the 11 patients with significant follow-up, VAS scores declined a mean of 24.5 mm. However, the functional scale results were mixed, with the entire SF-36 score not improving significantly but with some significant improvements on the physical functioning and bodily pain domains. EQ-5D scores did improve significantly. None of these patients were reported as having pain resulting from cancer.

Epidural Motor Cortex Stimulation

While the mechanism of pain modulation by epidural motor cortex stimulation (MCS) is not fully understood, it is believed that excitation of the motor cortex results in inhibition of nociceptive neurons in somatosensory areas of the postcentral gyrus, and this may interrupt pain sensation via corticocortical or corticothalamic connections. This inhibition extends to involve dorsal horn neurons [25].

PET and electrophysiological studies demonstrate regional activity differences during MCS [26]. MCS increases regional cerebral blood flow in the thalamus, brainstem, and anterior cingulate/orbitofrontal cortices. The most significant increases are seen in the ventrolateral thalamus, which is the relay nucleus for sensory information from the spinal cord and brain stem. Regional blood flow changes are greatest and correlate most closely to pain relief during the period after discontinuation of stimulation, and this helps explain the clinical extension of effect between intermittent stimulations [26]. MCS also increases endogenous opioid production in the anterior middle cingulate cortex and PAG region, as determined by PET imaging of opioid antagonist activity. This increased endogenous opioid production correlates with the level of pain relief [25]. Modulation of functional activity in the posterior insula may affect secondary sensation and affective aspects of the pain response [26]. Interestingly, during MCS, blood flow in the region of the somatosensory cortex remains unchanged, as do somatosensory evoked potentials. Importantly, the notion that corticospinal neurons from the motor cortex are involved in modulating descending pain transmission is supported by the finding that MCS is less effective for those patients with significant motor function loss in the painful region [27].

Numerous neuropathic pain conditions have been reported to be successfully treated with MCS. The technique was originally noted to be effective for central pain syndromes such as poststroke pain, spinal cord injury pain, and thalamic pain syndromes. Other pain disorders treated with MCS include trigeminal neuralgia, trigeminal neuropathic pain, and trigeminal deafferentation pain (anesthesia dolorosa). Cortical stimulation also has been used to treat peripheral pain syndromes such as complex regional pain syndrome type I, nerve root avulsion pain, stump and phantom limb pain, and postherpetic neuralgia [15].

Certain patient populations are less optimal candidates for MCS. For example, patients with large areas of motor cortical damage may have insufficient substrate for a substantial response. Moreover, those patients with significant cortical atrophy will have increased subarachnoid space, which may lead to a suboptimal response to stimulation due to excessive current spread through the CSF and less penetration to the cortex [27]. Not surprisingly, MCS best treats pain involving those areas of the body that have large areas of the motor cortex devoted to them, such as the face and arm/hand. The foot is a difficult area to target, mostly due to its motor cortical location in the interhemispheric fissure at some distance from the dura. These patients may be better candidates for DBS.

Several studies have attempted to identify preoperative criteria that accurately predict response to MCS. A positive response to barbiturates or ketamine has been shown to be a good predictor of response to cortical stimulation, but this is not an absolute requirement before a trial of stimulation. A positive response to transcranial magnetic stimulation has been associated with a successful outcome from epidural stimulation, but the predictive value of this relationship has not been firmly established. Minimal sensory loss and at least some preserved corticospinal function have been reported as prognostic factors for favorable results. However, these correlations have not been consistent across studies, and more rigorous evaluation is necessary [27].

The electrode implantation operation procedure may be performed either with general anesthesia or local anesthesia with sedation. The incision location approximates the central sulcus, as determined by traditional scalp reference lines or, more recently, image-guided stereotactic navigation. Burr holes or a small craniotomy, typically 4–6 cm in diameter, is used to expose the dura over the precentral gyrus and central sulcus. Frameless stereotactic navigation is used for anatomic localization of the central sulcus and precentral gyrus. Once the dura is exposed, intraoperative physiologic localization is performed by recording somatosensory evoked potentials elicited by peripheral stimulation, though this can be limited in conditions with significant sensory deafferentation. The reversal point of the phase from the negative postcentral N20 wave to the positive precentral P20 wave (evoked potential waves with a 20 ms latency) is used to localize the central sulcus. The somatotopic organization of the motor cortex (and the localization of the cortical region subserving motor function of the painful area) is determined using preoperative functional MRI and intraoperative transdural stimulation.

After placing the epidural electrodes in the estimated location over the motor cortex, the stimulation intensity is gradually increased while observing the affected body region for either visible contractions or the more sensitive electromyographic response. The implanted electrodes then are sutured to the dura. Some patients may eventually require electrode repositioning, although with modern stereotactic techniques, the number is low, generally less than 20% [28]. The electrode array may be positioned either perpendicular or parallel to the precentral gyrus and central sulcus. The lead placed is typically a paddle electrode such as that used for spinal cord stimulation. Many configurations have been used, including a single 4-contact paddle, two parallel 2-contact paddles, and the newer 16-contact paddles with electrodes in arrangements such as 2×8 and 5-6-5. No trials have compared the relative benefits of different arrangements.

Stimulation parameters and electrode configurations are determined by individual patient response during a 1-week externalized trial. Bipolar stimulation, with precentral cathode and postcentral anode placement, may preferentially excite cortical efferent neurons [29]. Wide internodal distances may increase the area of stimulation within the motor cortex. Pain reduction may be noted even at stimulation amplitudes less than 50% of the motor threshold [30]. Intermittent stimulation (or cycling mode on some generators) for a total of several hours throughout the day, often is used, and many patients report pain relief that may greatly outlast the actual stimulation time.

Studies supporting and refuting the effectiveness of the procedure have been published. In one study, 70% of patients with MCS reported that they would undergo the procedure again for similar results [31]. A recent meta-analysis of MCS trials found a good overall response rate, with 64% of patients with various types of central neuropathic pain reporting significant pain relief [13]. However, the first randomized trial of MCS [32], employing both open and crossover designs, suggested MCS efficacy from analysis of the open study data but failed to demonstrate significant results in the primary pain outcome scores in the crossover portion, possibly secondary to study design limitations including carry-over and ceiling effects from relief and a small study population. Even early adopters of the procedure are now finding long-term results to be disappointing and are turning away from the procedure [33].

A recent cost-effectiveness analysis found MCS to be more cost-effective in a 5-year model than transcranial stimulation for neuromodulation of chronic pain [34]. Over time, some patients experience a reduction in stimulation efficacy, possibly due to neuroplasticity or increased tissue impedance as scar builds up around the electrode paddles. Stimulation voltage may need to be increased, and reprogramming often is effective in re-establishing pain control [35].

There is very little in the published literature about MCS for the treatment of malignant pain. A single case report describes the apparently successful use of the technique to treat neuropathic facial pain following resection of a malignant glioma infiltrating the trigeminal nerve in a 3-year-old child [36].

Conclusions

Intracranial stimulation could potentially be effective for the treatment of malignant pain in selected patients. Deep brain stimulation can improve both nociceptive and neuropathic pain via the PAG/PVG and Vc thalamus targets, respectively; most patients have a mixture of both types of pain, so stimulation of both structures can be tested during an externalized trial. Motor cortex stimulation is effective for certain types of neuropathic pain, particularly pain due to deafferentation; though there is limited evidence for its effectiveness in malignant pain, pain associated with numbness (particularly in the face) may respond to this therapy. While relatively few cancer pain patients will be candidates for intracranial stimulation, it can be very effective in certain circumstances. As a result, it is important to be aware of these options when treating patients who have malignant pain.

References

1. Olds J, Milner P. Positive reinforcement produced by electrical stimulation of septal area and other regions of rat brain. J Comp Physiol Psychol. 1954;47(6):419–27. PubMed PMID: 13233369.
2. Reynolds DV. Surgery in the rat during electrical analgesia induced by focal brain stimulation. Science. 1969;164(878):444–5. PubMed PMID: 4887743.
3. Heath RG, Mickle WA. Evaluation of seven years' experience with depth electrode studies in human patients. In: Ramey ER, O'Doherty DS, editors. Electrical studies on the unanesthetized brain, vol. 1. New York: Paul B Hoeber; 1960. p. 214–28.
4. Gol A. Relief of pain by electrical stimulation of the septal area. J Neurol Sci. 1967;5(1):115–20. PubMed PMID: 6061755.
5. Hosobuchi Y. Subcortical electrical stimulation for control of intractable pain in humans. Report of 122 cases (1970–1984). J Neurosurg. 1986;64(4):543–53. PubMed PMID: 3485191.
6. Richardson DE, Akil H. Long term results of periventricular gray self-stimulation. Neurosurgery. 1977;1(2):199–202. PubMed PMID: 308192.
7. Adams JE, Hosobuchi Y, Fields HL. Stimulation of internal capsule for relief of chronic pain. J Neurosurg. 1974;41(6):740–4. PubMed PMID: 4609304.
8. Thoden U, Doerr M, Dieckmann G, Krainick JU. Medial thalamic permanent electrodes for pain control in man: an electrophysiological and clinical study. Electroencephalogr Clin Neurophysiol. 1979;47(5):582–91. PubMed PMID: 91485.
9. Lende RA, Kirsch WM, Druckman R. Relief of facial pain after combined removal of precentral and postcentral cortex. J Neurosurg. 1971;34(4):537–43. PubMed PMID: 5554359.
10. Tsubokawa T, Katayama Y, Yamamoto T, Hirayama T, Koyama S. Treatment of thalamic pain by chronic motor cortex stimulation. Pacing Clin Electrophysiol. 1991;14(1):131–4. PubMed PMID: 1705329.
11. Wallace JM. Update on pharmacotherapy guidelines for treatment of neuropathic pain. Curr Pain Headache Rep. 2007;11(3):208–14. PubMed PMID: 17504648.
12. Fontaine D, Hamani C, Lozano A. Efficacy and safety of motor cortex stimulation for chronic neuropathic pain: critical review of the literature. J Neurosurg. 2009;110(2):251–6. PubMed PMID: 18991496.
13. Lima MC, Fregni F. Motor cortex stimulation for chronic pain: systematic review and meta-analysis of the literature. Neurology. 2008;70(24):2329–37. PubMed PMID: 18541887.
14. Young R, Rinaldi P. Brain stimulation. In: Levy RM, North RB, editors. Neurosurgical management of pain, vol. 1. New York: Springer-Verlag; 1996. p. 65–83.

15. Levy R, Deer TR, Henderson J. Intracranial neurostimulation for pain control: a review. Pain Physician. 2010;13(2):157–65. PubMed PMID: 20309382.
16. Coffey RJ. Deep brain stimulation for chronic pain: results of two multicenter trials and a structured review. Pain Med. 2001;2(3):183–92. PubMed PMID: 15102250.
17. Hamani C, Schwalb JM, Rezai AR, Dostrovsky JO, Davis KD, Lozano AM. Deep brain stimulation for chronic neuropathic pain: long-term outcome and the incidence of insertional effect. Pain. 2006;125(1–2):188–96. PubMed PMID: 16797842.
18. Levy RM, Lamb S, Adams JE. Treatment of chronic pain by deep brain stimulation: long term follow-up and review of the literature. Neurosurgery. 1987;21(6):885–93. PubMed PMID: 3325851.
19. Mundinger F, Salomao JF. Deep brain stimulation in mesencephalic lemniscus medialis for chronic pain. Acta Neurochir Suppl (Wien). 1980;30:245–58. PubMed PMID: 7008520.
20. Boccard SG, Pereira EA, Moir L, Aziz TZ, Green AL. Long-term outcomes of deep brain stimulation for neuropathic pain. Neurosurgery. 2013;72(2):221–30. discussion 31. PubMed PMID: 23149975.
21. Previnaire JG, Nguyen JP, Perrouin-Verbe B, Fattal C. Chronic neuropathic pain in spinal cord injury: efficiency of deep brain and motor cortex stimulation therapies for neuropathic pain in spinal cord injury patients. Ann Phys Rehabil Med. 2009;52(2):188–93. PubMed PMID: 19909709.
22. Bittar RG, Otero S, Carter H, Aziz TZ. Deep brain stimulation for phantom limb pain. J Clin Neurosci. 2005;12(4):399–404. PubMed PMID: 15925769.
23. Owen SL, Green AL, Stein JF, Aziz TZ. Deep brain stimulation for the alleviation of post-stroke neuropathic pain. Pain. 2006;120(1–2):202–6. PubMed PMID: 16359796.
24. Boccard SG, Pereira EA, Moir L, Van Hartevelt TJ, Kringelbach ML, FitzGerald JJ, et al. Deep brain stimulation of the anterior cingulate cortex: targeting the affective component of chronic pain. Neuroreport. 2014;25(2):83–8. PubMed PMID: 24100411.
25. Garcia-Larrea L, Peyron R. Motor cortex stimulation for neuropathic pain: from phenomenology to mechanisms. NeuroImage. 2007;37(Suppl 1):S71–9. PubMed PMID: 17644413.
26. Peyron R, Faillenot I, Mertens P, Laurent B, Garcia-Larrea L. Motor cortex stimulation in neuropathic pain. Correlations between analgesic effect and hemodynamic changes in the brain. A PET study. NeuroImage. 2007;34(1):310–21. PubMed PMID: 17055297.
27. Pirotte B, Voordecker P, Brotchi J, Levivier M. Anatomical and physiological basis, clinical and surgical considerations, mechanisms underlying efficacy and future prospects of cortical stimulation for pain. Acta Neurochir Suppl. 2007;97(Pt 2):81–9. PubMed PMID: 17691293.
28. Canavero S, Bonicalzi V. Extradural cortical stimulation for central pain. Acta Neurochir Suppl. 2007;97(Pt 2):27–36. PubMed PMID: 17691286.
29. Lazorthes Y, Sol JC, Fowo S, Roux FE, Verdie JC. Motor cortex stimulation for neuropathic pain. Acta Neurochir Suppl. 2007;97(Pt 2):37–44. PubMed PMID: 17691287.
30. Holsheimer J, Lefaucheur JP, Buitenweg JR, Goujon C, Nineb A, Nguyen JP. The role of intra-operative motor evoked potentials in the optimization of chronic cortical stimulation for the treatment of neuropathic pain. Clin Neurophysiol. 2007;118(10):2287–96. PubMed PMID: 17765605.
31. Nuti C, Peyron R, Garcia-Larrea L, Brunon J, Laurent B, Sindou M, et al. Motor cortex stimulation for refractory neuropathic pain: four year outcome and predictors of efficacy. Pain. 2005;118(1–2):43–52. PubMed PMID: 16214292.
32. Lefaucheur JP, Drouot X, Cunin P, Bruckert R, Lepetit H, Creange A, et al. Motor cortex stimulation for the treatment of refractory peripheral neuropathic pain. Brain. 2009;132(Pt 6):1463–71. PubMed PMID: 19336459.
33. Sachs AJ, Babu H, Su YF, Miller KJ, Henderson JM. Lack of efficacy of motor cortex stimulation for the treatment of neuropathic pain in 14 patients. Neuromodulation. 2014;17(4):303–11. PubMed PMID: 24773411.
34. Zaghi S, Heine N, Fregni F. Brain stimulation for the treatment of pain: a review of costs, clinical effects, and mechanisms of treatment for three different central neuromodulatory approaches. J Pain Manag. 2009;2(3):339–52. PubMed PMID: 20585474. Pubmed Central PMCID: 2888303.
35. Henderson JM, Boongird A, Rosenow JM, LaPresto E, Rezai AR. Recovery of pain control by intensive reprogramming after loss of benefit from motor cortex stimulation for neuropathic pain. Stereotact Funct Neurosurg. 2004;82(5–6):207–13. PubMed PMID: 15583465. Epub 2004/12/08. eng.
36. Delavallee M, Rooijakkers H, Koerts G, Raftopoulos C. Motor cortex stimulation in a three-year-old child with trigeminal neuropathic pain caused by a malignant glioma in the cerebellopontine angle: case report. Neurosurgery. 2011;69(2):E494–6. PubMed PMID: 21792145.

26 Spinal Cord Stimulation and Oncologic Pain Management

Neel D. Mehta and Mohammad M. Piracha

History and the Gate Control Theory of Pain

In 1965, Melzack and Wall had established the gate control theory (GCT) of pain [1]. GCT revolutionized the concept of pain management and has propelled the constant evolution and implementation of new techniques to treat pain. Spinal cord stimulation (SCS) is one such application of this theory. Shealy and colleagues implanted the first spinal cord stimulator device on the dorsal column of the spinal cord for the treatment of chronic pain [2]. A mere 2 years later, in 1971, Shimogi and colleagues demonstrated the analgesic potential of direct epidural spinal cord stimulation [3].

The concept of the gate control theory involves the premise that transmission of signals from the external environment to the central nervous system (CNS) can be modulated [4–6].

When a painful stimulus is detected at the nociceptor peripherally, the small A-delta and C fibers override the inhibitory neurons, thereby allowing the pain signal to be transmitted, opening the "gate," to the CNS [6]. Activation of the large, non-noxious information-carrying nerve fibers can lead to the inhibitory neurons being reactivated allowing for the gate to "close." This large fiber activation then can result in decreasing, or elimination, of signals being transmitted from the noxious carrying nerve fibers. The application of GCT for pain control in the modern era focuses on closing the gate by manipulating the large nerve fibers. An example of the application of the GCT is the advent of transcutaneous electrical nerve stimulation (TENS) [7].

N. D. Mehta (✉) · M. M. Piracha
Joan and Sanford I. Weill Cornell Medical College of Cornell University, New York Presbyterian Hospital, Division of Pain Management, Department of Anesthesiology, New York, NY, USA
e-mail: nem9015@med.cornell.edu

SCS Application, Placement, Patient Selection, and Contraindications

SCS is indicated for a variety of disease processes, including complex regional pain syndrome (CRPS), postherpetic neuralgia, neuropathic pain, visceral pain, post-laminectomy syndrome, phantom limb pain, ischemic pain, and nerve root injury. However, new applications for SCS are a continued area of research. Among these areas are modulation of end-organ perfusion, consciousness, and cancer or tumors [8, 9].

In its simplest form, a SCS consists of an implantable pulse generator and electrodes. Electrodes, with the aid of fluoroscopy, are usually placed in the epidural space and designed to stimulate the dorsal columns of the posterior spinal cord. Newer systems have electrodes placed nearer individual dorsal roots, specifically dorsal root ganglia, for more precision in stimulation. Once a patient confirms appropriate stimulation, the level of intensity, usually defined as current applied to the electrodes, can be performed, with changes in amplitude, pulse width, frequency, and waveform characteristics available to modulate the signal for improved pain relief.

Selection criteria for patients amenable for SCS trial and implant include failure of conservative medical management of painful symptoms, failed back pain syndrome, and complex regional pain syndrome. In the oncologic population, while no specific criteria exist, we recommend considering stimulation techniques for treating pain arising from stable neurologic pain syndromes. For example, active cancer patients with progression of disease may be poor candidates since the pain syndrome may evolve, perhaps rendering stimulation insufficient to adapt to the changing pain characteristics. While psychological instability, history of drug addiction, presence of active sepsis or entry site infection, derangement of coagulation, and anatomical obliteration of the spinal canal or spina

A. Gulati et al. (eds.), *Essentials of Interventional Cancer Pain Management*, https://doi.org/10.1007/978-3-319-99684-4_26

bifida are common contraindications for placement, in the oncologic population, treatment considerations should be discussed with the oncologist prior to trial and implant of SCS devices [10]. Furthermore, we recommend an MRI of the total spine to evaluate the epidural space for spinal disease and lead placement. If a trial is recommended and performed, it is expected patient's adequate pain relief (usually >50% improvement in symptoms), improved functional status, and overall patient satisfaction with hopefully decreased use of systemic analgesics [10]. Finally, risks of coagulopathy, current anticoagulation, and infection should be addressed with the oncologist prior to consideration of SCS trial and/or implant.

The American Society of Interventional Pain Physicians (ASIPP) also has further guidelines for SCS placement [11].

Common Indications for SCS Implant in the Chronic Pain Population

1. Neuropathic pain, preferred over nociceptive pain [12].
2. CRPS – types 1 and 2 [10, 13].
3. Painful peripheral mononeuropathies [10, 13].
4. Anatomically limited pain, rather than diffuse pain syndromes [10, 13] (i.e., arachnoiditis, post-laminectomy pain, epidural fibrosis, degenerative disc disease).
5. Unilateral, usually easier to treat over bilateral pain syndromes [12].
6. Radicular, generally easier to treat than central pain [12, 10, 13] – cervical, lumbar.
7. Nonmalignant pain indications in the literature [14].
8. Angina pectoris refractory to conventional drug therapy and not amenable to surgical bypass [10, 13].
9. Painful ischemic peripheral vascular disease not amenable to conventional drug therapy or surgical bypass [10, 13].
10. Peripheral causalgia; postherpetic neuralgia, traumatic nerve injury, post-amputation syndromes, brachial plexopathy, and facial pain in the mandibular nerve distribution [14, 15].
11. Poor response to conservative treatment for at least 6 months [16].
12. Contraindications for remedial surgery [16] or failed back surgery.
13. Consider no major psychiatric disorders, including somatization disorder [16].
14. Consider no history of illicit drug use [16].
15. Consider no secondary gain or pending litigation for their condition [16].

SCS Placement

When SCS electrodes are placed, a trial usually ensues to determine optimal stimulation settings for pain control. The prevailing goal is to have stimulation which correlates with the somatotopy at the level of the spinal cord where the pain is distributed (of note, newer waveforms may redefine our understanding of this relationship). Therefore, a thorough understanding of the dermatomal distribution is required to allow for optimal pain relief. Table 26.1 illustrates the most common coverage areas desired with SCS. Some common pearls include placing leads nearer to the midline of the spinal cord to stimulate the dorsal columns. More lateral leads may cause dorsal root and motor stimulation, which may alter neuromodulation settings for successful pain control. While certain waveforms and settings may have improved pain relief in treating failed back syndrome and axial back pain, in the oncologic population, pain responses to variations in neuromodulation settings have not been well studied.

The Procedure for Trial and Implant

Most SCS kits (Fig. 26.1) for placement of percutaneous leads require syringes and local anesthetic for focal anesthesia on the skin, marking pen for planning, usually a 14G Tuohy epidural needle, loss of resistance syringe, occasionally contrast to confirm epidural space, the actual percutaneous (or paddle for surgical placement) leads, stylets, guide wire, tunneling tools, lead anchors, and a screening cable for paresthesia testing. In general, the implantable pulse generator (IPG or "battery") is separate from the lead kit so that the leads may be tested prior to IPG implantation.

Table 26.1 Dermatomal distribution for SCS

Lead placement targets	
Cervical	*Body distribution*
C2	Face, below the maxillary region
C2–C4	Neck and shoulder to hand
C4–C7	Forearm to hand
C7-T1	Anterior shoulder
Thoracic	
T1–T2	Chest wall
T5–6	Abdomen
T7–T9	Back and legs
T10–T12	Limb
L1	Pelvis
T12, L1	Foot
L5-S1	Foot, lower limb
S2–S4	Pelvic, rectum
Sacral hiatus	Coccyx

Usually, fluoroscopy is utilized to establish anatomic access to the epidural space. Bony landmarks, such as the pedicle and facet joints, are routinely used to plan access for lead placement using large gauge needles. Techniques in lead placement may differ between practitioners and device used. Nonetheless, anterior-posterior (AP), lateral, and oblique views are needed to correctly position needles (usually 14 gauge Tuohy needles) in shallow angles with relation to the epidural space (Fig. 26.2). Once percutaneous leads are positioned in the epidural space (via the needle), the patients, who are usually under light sedation, are routinely awoken and asked whether stimulation is an appropriate location. During a trial, the wires are externalized and attached to pulse generator, whereas a permanent placement internalizes a lead with an implantable and programmable battery.

If a patient is not arousable or general anesthesia is utilized, intraoperative neuromonitoring may be considered to determine sidedness of lead placement. In certain instances, paddle leads, electrodes placed in the epidural space via a laminectomy, are used instead of percutaneous leads. This may be helpful for the oncologic population if the epidural space is compromised because of spinal disease, precluding placement of percutaneous leads (Fig. 26.3).

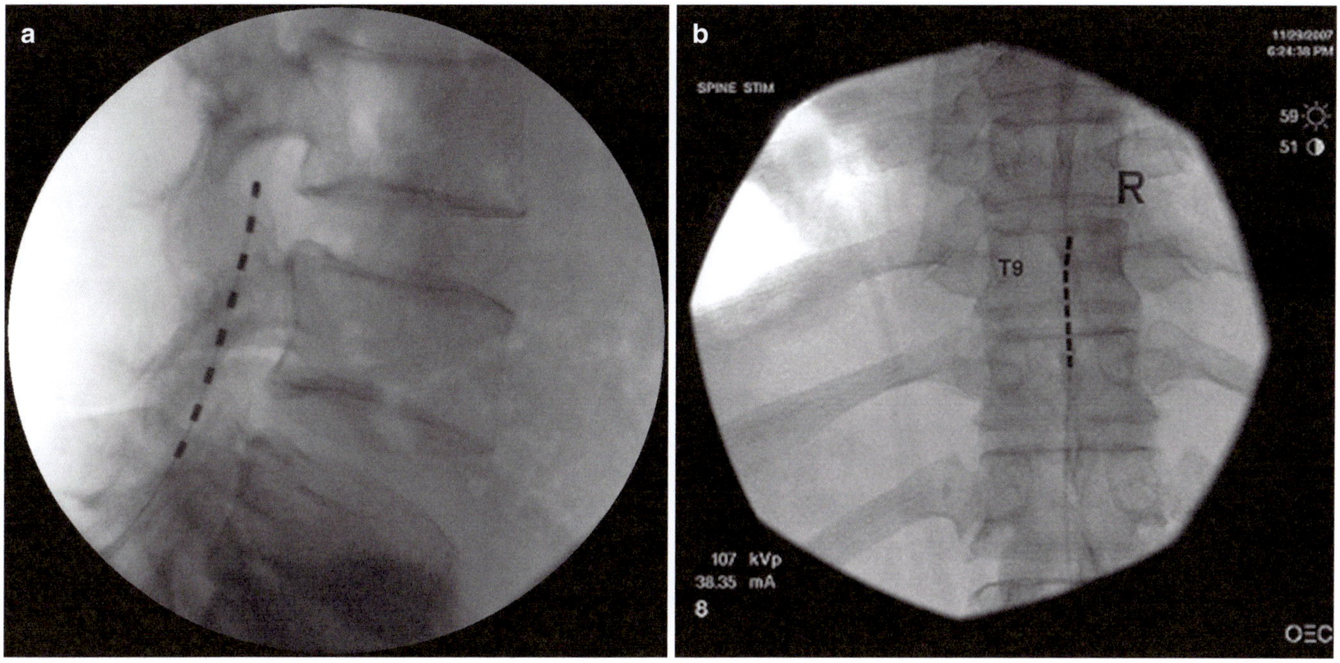

Fig. 26.1 (**a, b**) Table setup showing epidural kit and single-lead SCS pack

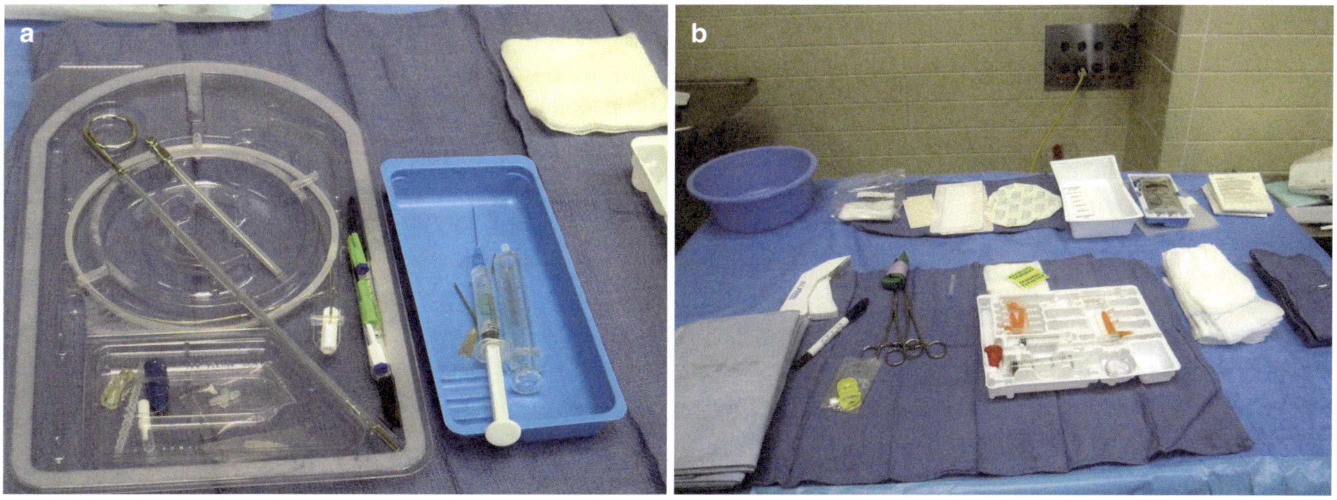

Fig. 26.2 (**a, b**) Lateral and anterior-posterior views of SCS placement. Percutaneous leads are shown

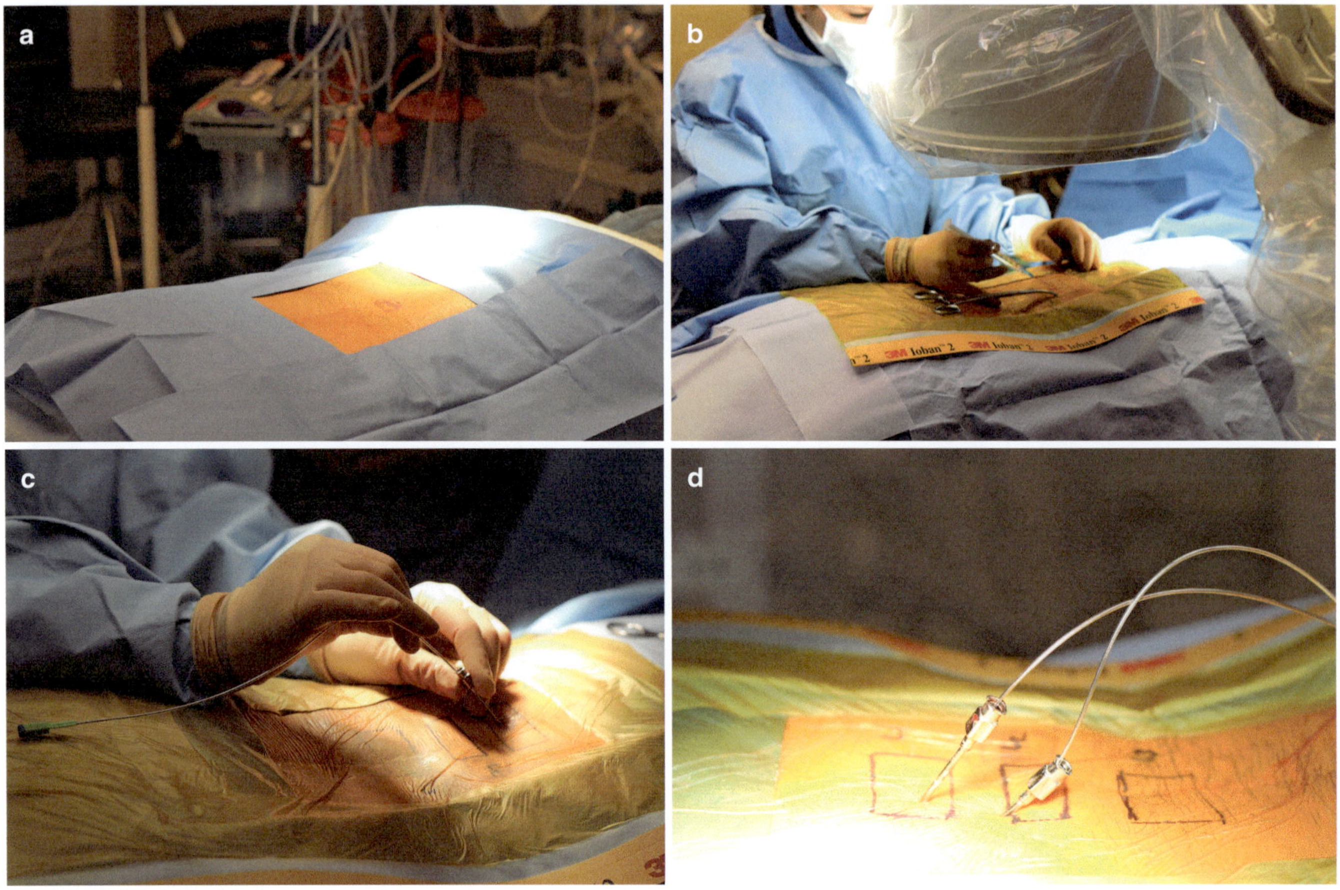

Fig. 26.3 (**a–d**) Step-by-step placement of SCS. (**a**) Patient is placed in a prone position which should minimize lumbar lordosis. (**b**) Shows the physician marking the interspinous intervals of interest for the SCS placement with the aid of a clamp to illustrate entry point. (**c**) Practitioner demonstrates local anesthetic injection and trajectory of needle entry. Then a loss of resistance, to air or saline, technique is utilized to elicit the epidural space and then confirmed with fluoroscopy. Electrode is then threaded through the needle and positioned in desired position. (**d**) Insert SCS lead into Tuohy needle and use steering device to advance lead under fluoroscopic guidance. Note two lead entry on ipsilateral side

Oncologic Pain

Estimates demonstrate that approximately one third of patients with cancer have some form of pain at the time of their diagnosis [7]. Studies have shown that of the patients suffering pain secondary to their cancer, up to 40% may suffer from neuropathic pain [7]. Furthermore, it is estimated that as much as 50% of patients that are diagnosed with cancer have pain as their presenting symptom [17]. Multiple modalities exist for the treatment of pain of an oncologic source. This includes, but is not limited to, opioids, antidepressants, nonsteroidal anti-inflammatory drugs (NSAIDs), and other classes of adjuvants. The World Health Organization (WHO) has established guidelines specifically for management of pain related to cancer [18].

In the past, spinal cord stimulation has been rarely considered as a treatment option for active cancer patients. In these patients, as disease evolves, so does the pain syndrome; making stimulation less ideal to modulate changing pain patterns. However, as cancer becomes chronic in nature, pain syndromes, especially neuropathic cancer-related pain, may become amenable to treatments with stimulation. Consideration for SCS in treatment-related pain syndromes may be more appropriate. This may include postsurgical (thoracotomy and mastectomy) as well as radiation-related neuropathic pain.

A thorough evaluation of oncologic patients is crucial in ensuring satisfactory pain relief. As a result, knowledge of the contraindications and concerns when placing SCS in these patients is paramount. Access to the epidural space as well as threading percutaneous leads in the epidural space may be evaluated with either CT myelogram or MRI of the spine. Discussion with the patient's treating oncologist should be considered to balance risks of procedure and side effects from oncologic treatment. In many cases, oncologic treatment may have effects on wound healing, bleeding, and risk of infection.

In any patient considering SCS implant, hardware complications may occur. The most common hardware concerns include lead migration, representing 13.2%, followed by lead breakage at 9.1%, infection at 3.4%, hardware malfunction at 2.9%, and unwanted stimulation at 2.4% [19]. Risks inherent to surgical procedure also apply, including surgical site infection, and/or pain, at the generator site. Epidural hematoma, epidural hemorrhage, CSF leak, and paralysis, albeit rare, are also possibilities. Both infection and bleeding complications may be more pronounced in the oncologic population given the propensity for infections and coagulopathies during various treatments. A discussion with the primary oncology team is important to balance risks and benefits for neuromodulation.

As discussed previously, one of the concerns unique to oncologic patients is the potential for recurrence of cancer, or metastatic spread. This implies that pain targets are at risk for change and may not be treatable with current SCS lead locations. For example, a patient suffering from breast cancer with metastatic disease may complain of severe chest wall pain, which could be targeted by SCS placed in the thoracic spine. However, should the patient develop metastatic spine lesions in the lumbar spine, and present with severe lower extremity pain, stimulation may not adequately reach the spinal cord locations to treat the pain symptoms. One must consider that cancer pain is rarely treated by solely one modality, and commonly used medications may help treat other distinct areas of pain.

Effects of Radiation on Implantable Pulse Generators

Unlike other patient subpopulations, radiotherapy becomes a very possible future in the lifetime of the oncologic patient. SCS implantable pulse generators might be susceptible to damage from ionizing radiation, such as radiotherapy, as well the electrical immittance generating the radiation. Walsh et al. published a case report involving a 46-year-old female with chronic back and leg pain, status post SCS implantation, who was found to have ductal carcinoma in situ (DCIS). A left mastectomy and axillary node dissection was performed with plan to perform radiotherapy. The patient had a Medtronic® SCS device and upon direct communication with the company, was recommended to avoid ionizing radiation. The patient was subsequently successfully irradiated by contouring the radiation field to reduce radiation exposure to the pulse generator [20]. Using cardiac pacemakers as a reference device, damage seems to be dependent on the total radiation dose delivered [21]. Guidelines based on total ionizing radiation dose to the pulse generator are correlated to the cardiac pacemaker guidelines in this field. Their case study determined a 5 Gy limit for the given pulse generator. Walsh's study illustrates that radiotherapy treatment in those patients with SCS can be safely performed, especially if the guidelines they proposed are implemented.

MRI Compatibility

Another concern for SCS placement in oncologic population is the potential of continued imaging to monitor cancer progression, particularly magnetic resonance imaging (MRI). Until recently, MRI-safe SCS was not available, which concerned many practitioners to avoid SCS in oncologic patients. MRI, aside from SCS failure or damage, also poses direct risk to patient's health, a consequence of thermal injury. Magnetic fields when directed at the leads in the SCS can lead to severe overheating of the wires with resultant potential burn injury and even neurological damage. Furthermore, the magnetic force produced by modern MRI scanners can move objects that are in any way ferromagnetic. As a result, the SCS may be moved within the patient or dislodged from its leads [22]. The currents produced by the MRI scanner may also alter the devices function or activity.

Recently, MRI conditional systems have been developed, reducing the risk of thermal tissue injury by allowing distribution of the MRI radio-frequency energy along the course of the entire lead. This dispersion of heat over a large area significantly reduces focal thermal tissue damage. The devices have been modified to prevent MRI energy from entering the device allowing for the energy to be redistributed outside the SCS, reducing internal damage to the device. Furthermore, the newer devices have a controllable MRI mode which switches the device off preventing it from being accidentally activated, or settings altered, by MRI interference. The device has also been redesigned to reduce the amount of ferromagnetic material, thereby reducing risk of dislodgment or movement of the device.

Case Studies

Unfortunately, current literature and research have a paucity of randomized controlled trials (RCTs) to truly test the efficacy of SCS in oncologic patients. However, the best examples of successful implementation of SCS in oncologic patients have been demonstrated by an array of case studies, case series, and reviews. Despite the lack of RCTs, these reports do provide a vast amount of information regarding the potential benefits for early consideration of SCS in this patient subpopulation.

Yakolev et al. had demonstrated the application of SCS in two cancer patients, as depicted in Table 26.2, a patient with anal cancer and one with an epidural cancer. The first of these patients was a 51-year-old male with a past history of anterior-posterior resection and intraoperative radiation ther-

Table 26.2 Case report data summarized

Author	Cancer type	Pain location	SCS location	Pre-VAS	Post-VAS
Yakolev [23]	Anal cancer	Left groin	T8–T9	2–4/10	1–2/10
Yakolev [25]	Epidural cancer	Lower right extremity and lower back	T9–T10	5–9/10	1/10
Dutta	Renal cell cancer	Bilateral lower extremity	T10–T11	8–9/10	1/10

apy for squamous cell carcinoma of the anus [23]. The course of the patient's pain was described as hot, burning, and sharp in the left groin. Pain was assessed using a visual analog scale (VAS) [24]. The patient indicated a VAS of 2–4, with exacerbations of pain (VAS of 8) due to activity. After the failure of conservative pharmacologic therapy, SCS was chosen as the next option for pain relief. The patient underwent a successful SCS trial with a quadripolar SCS device with two quadripolar epidural leads placed at T8–T9. His VAS score was reassessed posttrial and was decreased to 1–2 out of 10. The permanent implant had stimulation set to an amplitude of 3–6 volts with a pulse width of 210 ms and frequency of 100 hz. Reassessment of the patient 1 year postoperatively confirmed continued adequate pain relief with the patient utilizing the stimulator 100% of the time. The patient also had much improved functional status and able to successfully perform activities of daily living with significantly less pain on average.

The second patient examined by Yakolev was a 43-year-old female who presented with burning and shooting pain in her lower right extremity post resection and debulking of a metastatic epidural tumor. The patient had failed conservative pharmacologic therapy with opioids and adjuncts and rated the pain at 5 to 9 on the VAS. Additionally, multiple epidural steroid injections were also attempted with no relieve of pain. After determining no disease spread, it was decided that a SCS implantation be attempted. A SCS trial was then implemented at the T9–T10 with the patient reporting a VAS of 1 out of 10 post placement. As a result, a permanent SCS and a generator were then planned and placed. At a 1-year follow-up appointment, patient had sustained pain relief and increased daily function. Of further note, patient had also stopped using all supplemental opioids [25].

Dutta et al. published a case study in which a 70-year-old woman starting to experience neuropathic pain down both her legs secondary to renal cell cancer metastasis to the sacrum, depicted in Table 26.2. Opioids had failed to relieve her pain, and she was considered for placement trial of SCS. The patient was rating her pain 8–9 on the VAS. A SCS trial was planned and an octrode electrode was placed at the T10–T11 level. Patient's VAS score was reduced to 1–2. Her functionality also significantly improved and was now able to perform activities of daily living relatively pain free. A permanent SCS was placed and after 1 year follow-up patient reported 90% pain relief [26].

A larger review of SCS in cancer patients was performed by Lihua et al. The authors used the Cochrane Central Register of Controlled Trials, MEDLINE, EMBASE, and Chinese Biomedical Database (CBM) for their data collection dating from July 2012. Their search yielded 412 articles; however, no randomized controlled trials were found that met their inclusion criteria. Eighteen nonrandomized trials were eventually found and reviewed, and 13 of these trials were excluded.

Comprehensive review by Linhua (and subsequent review by Peng in 2015) resulted in four studies that met inclusion criteria. The first of these studies was a retrospective study by Meglio that analyzed 109 patients with chronic pain, among which 11 had cancer-related pain, summarized in Table 26.3. Meglio placed percutaneous electrodes with subsequent stimulation through a laminectomy to assess pain relief. Three of the 11 patients reported relief with trial stimulation, with these 3 reporting a mean level of reduction of pain of 75%.

Like Meglio, Shimoji retrospectively analyzed 454 patients with chronic pain and SCS implantation. Of the 454 patients in the study, 52 had pain related to cancer, and 45 of the 52 patients resulted in 50% reduction of pain-based VAS, summarized in Table 26.3. Based on a chi-squared analysis, Shimoji further analyzed the patient VAS data and concluded that of the patients that had a 50% reduction in pain, a significant proportion were cancer patients. Furthermore, pain medication in the study population was either significantly de-escalated or ceased, indicated adequate pain relief by SCS implantation.

The third study included by Linhua was by Yakovlev who performed two separate case series, as shown in Table 26.4. The first study included 14 patients with cancer-related pain. Subsequently, these patients received SCS implantation for pain control. Post-SCS implantation a significant decline in opioid use and VAS scores was noted. Furthermore, the VAS score continued to decline 12 months post implant. The second case series included 15 patients, and results were in congruence with the first case series, with a significant decline in VAS scores and opioid dose requirement.

The overall assessment of these cases reviewed by Linhua illustrated that 80% of patients with SCS implanted had 50% or greater reduction of pain. Major complications are similar as previously presented such as infection and pain at electrode or pulse generator sites. Conclusions based on their review revealed that evidence based on nonrandomized controlled trials were positive, with patients with oncologic diagnoses greatly benefiting from SCS implantation.

As evidenced by the cases presented, SCS provides oncologic patients with improved pain control, increased daily functionality, improved quality of life, and decreased need

Table 26.3 Summary of case series with VAS as endpoint

Author	Case series participants	Number of patients with benefit (at least 50% VAS reduction)	Proportion of patients benefiting
Meglio	11	3	3/11
Shimoji	52	45	45/52

Table 26.4 Yakolev studies with pre- and post-SCS implantation VAS scores and corresponding opioid use

Author	Case series participants	Pre-SCS VAS average	Post-SCS VAS average	Pre-SCS opioid use	Post-SCS opioid use
Yakolev [23]	14	7.43	2.07	14/14 (100%)	4/14 (29%)
Yakolev [25]	15	7.07	1.87	15/15 (100%)	7/15 (47%)

for pharmacologic adjuncts. Despite the lack of randomized controlled trials, the cases that are present in the literature demonstrate an overall benefit and low side effect profile. Indeed, future randomized controlled trials will bolster the evidence for SCS implantation and allow for continued adaptation by practitioners.

Cost-Effectiveness of Spinal Cord Stimulation

A variety of economic data and studies illustrate that by using SCS for pain treatment, the overall cost of pain management was reduced post implantation. For example, for chronic regional pain syndromes alone, SCS was found to be an effective therapy with lifetime cost saving of $60,800 [27]. At the same time, 20–40% of patients do report loss of analgesia within 24 months of implantation [28]; thus careful patient selection and technique are essential for initial success, and lifetime supervision are important for adjustment of pain treatments as needed. Currently, spinal cord stimulation is approved for CRPS types 1 and 2, arachnoiditis, failed back surgery syndrome, post-thoracotomy pain, peripheral neuropathy, postherpetic neuralgia, phantom limb pain, and ilioinguinal neuralgia [29].

Cost-effectiveness has also been evaluated by Kumar et al. [30]. Their study examined 104 patients with history of failed back surgery syndrome. Sixty patients were implanted with SCS and then monitored for a 5-year period. Annual cost was assessed and the SCS group had a total cost of $29,000 vs $38,000 in the non-SCS group. Higher cost of the non-SCS group was thought to be the result of medications, emergency center visits, imaging, and physician follow-up [31]. Again, these cost-benefit analysis studies are not involving cancer pain patients and are merely speculative in this population.

Conclusions

SCS has been proven effective for a variety of chronic pain conditions in many studies. However, SCS application in oncologic pain, as shown in multiple case reports, may be an excellent method to improve a patient's ailments. With constant advancement, the current generation of devices has overcome technical problems and high failure rates common in earlier devices. The evaluation of patients with oncologic pain should include the potential for SCS for management. In the case studies included in this section, along with others found in the literature, SCS appears to decrease opioid use post implant, increase daily functionality, and improve quality of life. Furthermore, cost analysis has repeatedly shown that SCS has a greater benefit economically when used appropriately. With routine trial stimulation, improved understanding of need for SCS in these patients, and knowledge of improved quality of life, SCS, if not contraindicated, can serve as an adjunct to oncologic pain management.

References

1. Melzack R, Wall PD. Pain mechanisms: a new theory. Science. 1965;150(3699):971–9.
2. Shealy CN, Mortimer JT, Resnick J. Electrical inhibition of pain by stimulation of the dorsal columns: preliminary reports. J Int Anesth Res Soc. 1967;46:489–91.
3. Shimoji K, Higashi H, Kano T, Asai S, Morioka T. Electrical management of intractable pain. Masui. 1971;20(5):444–7.
4. Melzack R, Katz J. The gate control theory: reaching for the brain. In: Craig KD, Hadjistavropoulos T, editors. Pain: psychological perspectives. Mahwah: Lawrence Erlbaum Associates, Publishers; 2004.
5. Basbaum, et al. Cellular and molecular mechanisms of pain. Cell. 2009;139:267. https://doi.org/10.1016/j.cell.2009.09.028.
6. Marchand S. Applied pain neurophysiology. In: Beaulieu P, Lussier D, Porreca F, Dickenson A, editors. Pharmacology of pain. Seattle: International Association for the Study of Pain Press; 2010.
7. Nachum Dafny, Ph.D. Pain modulation and mechanisms (Section 2, Chapter 8) Neuroscience online: an electronic textbook for the neurosciences |Department of Neurobiology and Anatomy – The University of Texas Medical School at Houston. N.p., n.d. Web. 5 Apr 2014. http://neuroscience.uth.tmc.edu/s2/chapter
8. Dilorenzo DJ, Bronzino JD. Neuroengineering. Boca Raton: CRC Press; 2008. Chapter 7.
9. Kunnumpurath S, Srinivasagopalan R, Vadivelu N. Spinal cord stimulation: principles of past, present and future practice: a review. J Clin Monit Comput. 2009;23:333–9.
10. Deer T. Spinal cord stimulation for the treatment of chronic pain. Pain Med News. 2010;2010:P1–8.
11. ASIPP–IPM Guidelines. Comprehensive evidence-based guidelines for interventional techniques in the management of chronic pain. Pain Physician. 2009;12(750):751.
12. North RB, Wetzel FT. Spinal cord stimulation for chronic pain of spinal origin: a valuable long-term solution. Spine. 2002;27(22):2584–91.
13. Deer T, Masone R. Selection of spinal cord stimulation candidates for the treatment of chronic pain. Pain Medicine. 2008;2009(s1):S82–92.

14. Kumar K, Nath R, Wyant GM. Treatment of chronic pain by epidural spinal cord stimulation: a 10-year experience. J Neurosurg. 1991;75(3):402–7.
15. Kumar K, Toth C, Nath RK, Laing P. Epidural spinal cord stimulation for treatment of chronic pain – some predictors of success. A 15-year experience. Surg Neurol. 1998;50(2):110–20.
16. Lee AW, Pilitsis JG. Spinal cord stimulation: indications and outcomes. Neurosurg Focus. 2006;21(6):E3.
17. Flagg A, Mcgreevy K, Williams K. Spinal cord stimulation in the treatment of cancer-related pain: "back to the origins". Curr Pain Headache Rep. 2012;16(4):343–9.
18. Schug SA, Zech D, Dörr U. Cancer pain management according to WHO analgesic guidelines. J Pain Symptom Manag. 1990;5(1):27–32.
19. Cameron T. Safety and efficacy of spinal cord stimulation for the treatment of chronic pain: a 20-year literature review. J Neurosurg. 2004;100(3 Suppl Spine):254–67.
20. Walsh L, Guha D, Purdie TG, et al. Spinal cord stimulators and radiotherapy: first case report and practice guidelines. Radiat Oncol. 2011;6:143.
21. Calfee RV. Therapeutic radiation and pacemakers. Pacing Clin Electrophysiol. 1982;5(2):160–1.
22. De Andres J, Valía JC, Cerda-Olmedo G, Quiroz C, Villanueva V, Martinez-Sanjuan V, de Leon-Casasola O. Magnetic resonance imaging in patients with spinal neurostimulation systems. Anesthesiology. 2007;106(4):779–86.
23. Yakovlev AE, Ellias Y. Spinal cord stimulation as a treatment option for intractable neuropathic cancer pain. Clin Med Res. 2008;6(3–4):103–6.
24. Bijur PE, Silver W, Gallagher EJ. Reliability of the visual analog scale for measurement of acute pain. Acad Emerg Med. 2001;8(12):1153–7.
25. Yakovlev AE, Resch BE, Karasev SA. Treatment of cancer-related chest wall pain using spinal cord stimulation. Am J Hosp Palliat Care. 2010;27(8):552–6.
26. Implantation of spinal cord stimulator in a patient with cancer pain. Dr Rajib Dutta Dr S P Ward Specialist Registrar in Anaesthesia and Chronic Pain, King's College Hospital NHS Foundation Trust, Denmark Hill, London, SE5 9RS Consultant in Pain Medicine, Princess Royal Hospital, Haywards Heath, West Sussex RH16 4EX.
27. Taylor RS, Van Buyten JP, Buchser E. Spinal cord stimulation for complex regional pain syndrome: a systematic review of the clinical and cost-effectiveness literature and assessment of prognostic factors. Eur J Pain. 2006;10(2):91–101.
28. Doleys DM. Psychological factors in spinal cord stimulation therapy: brief review and discussion. Neurosurg Focus. 2006;21(6):E1.
29. Lihua P, Su M, Zejun Z, Ke W, Bennett MI. Spinal cord stimulation for cancer-related pain in adults. Cochrane Database Syst Rev. 2013;2:CD009389.
30. Kumar K, Malik S, Demeria D. Treatment of chronic pain with spinal cord stimulation versus alternative therapies: cost-effectiveness analysis. Neurosurgery. 2002;51(1):106–15.
31. Bell GK, Kidd D, North RB. Cost-effectiveness analysis of spinal cord stimulation in treatment of failed back surgery syndrome. J Pain Symptom Manag. 1997;13(5):286–95.

Peripheral Nerve Stimulation for the Treatment of Cancer Pain

27

Jennifer A. Sweet and Nicholas M. Boulis

Background of Stimulation for Chronic Pain

Stimulation for the treatment of chronic pain has been utilized for over 60 years [1]. However, the types of stimulation and their respective targets vary largely depending on the etiology of the pain. Deep brain stimulation (DBS) has been reported in the anterior cingulate cortex, the periaqueductal gray area, and the ventral posterior thalamus to relieve nociceptive and neuropathic pain syndromes, including post-stroke pain and pain due to brain, spinal cord, or brachial plexus injury [1]. Motor cortex stimulation (MCS) is another modality of stimulation, frequently used for medically refractory facial pain syndromes, particularly deafferentation pain [2, 3]. Perhaps the most ubiquitous form of stimulation is spinal cord stimulation (SCS) for the management of chronic back pain and neuropathic pain of the extremities resulting from complex regional pain syndrome, post-laminectomy syndrome, peripheral vascular disease, and other pain states arising from a spinal or neural origin [4].

When pain is confined to a focal distribution, treatment with peripheral nerve stimulation (PNS) and subcutaneous peripheral nerve stimulation (SPNS) can be effective neuromodulation techniques. Neuropathic pain in a dermatomal or neurotomal distribution, such as the occipital neuralgia, can be significantly improved with peripheral nerve stimulation. Traditionally, occipital nerve stimulation (ONS) has been used for medically refractory occipital neuralgia; however, in recent years more widespread indications have been implemented, including migraines, cluster headaches, and other craniofacial pain syndromes [4]. Other commonly targeted nerves include the supraorbital nerve, infraorbital nerve, femoral nerve, and sciatic nerve. SPNS has also gained popularity for the management of intractable pain. Neuropathic or nociceptive pain that is focally distributed in regions of the body such as the abdomen or limb may be treated with SPNS which may relieve pain by stimulating regional dermatomal and visceral nerve endings [4]. SPNS is often used as an adjunctive treatment to PNS or SCS.

The primary benefits of PNS and SPNS are the specificity of treatment, the ability to modify stimulation therapy, and the reversibility of treatment. This contrasts with lesioning procedures, which can result in permanent numbness, dysesthesias, weakness, or other sequelae. In summary, PNS and SPNS can deliver targeted therapy to specific nerve distributions or other focal areas, potentially improving pain that is otherwise refractory to alternative treatments.

Stimulation for Cancer Pain

With respect to the management of cancer pain, the use of stimulation is far less common. Historically, lesioning of the anterior cingulate cortex rather than DBS was reported for intractable pain as seen in cancer patients with mixed results [1, 5–7]. However, the application of stimulation techniques over lesioning in cancer-related pain remains sparse. This is perhaps in part due to the limitations of obtaining magnetic resonance imaging (MRI) to monitor tumor progression or disease recurrence once the devices are implanted, thus frequently precluding the implantation of stimulators entirely. Even with the advent of MRI-compatible DBS and SCS, the image quality is diminished due to metal artifact, and the safety restrictions are numerous, making the utilization far less feasible. The use of peripheral nerve stimulation has an advantage over spinal cord stimulation in that it better allows for subsequent MRI scanning that may be indicated with malignancies under the right circumstances. The introduction of MRI-safe electrodes will enhance the capacity to use these devices in such circumstances.

J. A. Sweet (✉)
University Hospitals Case Medical Center, Cleveland, OH, USA
e-mail: Jennifer.sweet@uhhospitals.org

N. M. Boulis
Neurosurgery, Emory University Hospital, Atlanta, GA, USA
e-mail: NBOULIS@emory.edu

A. Gulati et al. (eds.), *Essentials of Interventional Cancer Pain Management*, https://doi.org/10.1007/978-3-319-99684-4_27

Another limitation of stimulation for pain due to malignancy is the extensive postoperative programming of stimulators, which is often required for optimal control of symptoms. In the setting of cancer patients, who may have shortened life expectancies, this labor-intensive process may not be warranted. Similarly, a poor prognosis may prevent insurance companies from assuming the high coverage costs of the implants in these patients. Finally, while stimulation techniques, including PNS and SPNS, have been applied in cases of non-neuropathic pain, they are most effective for pain of a neuropathic origin, thus further restricting their use in the cancer population.

Despite the restrictions described above, there are certain situations in the oncologic setting in which PNS and SPNS may be a valuable treatment option. This includes unresectable tumors entrapping or involving neural elements. For instance, head and neck tumors, resulting in chronic headaches or facial pain, abdominal or pelvic tumors producing visceral pain, and tumors of the extremities or intercostal nerves causing neuropathic pain may all benefit from PNS and/or SPNS treatment. In addition, patients with tumors previously treated by surgery or radiation may also be good candidates for PNS or SPNS, as such prior interventions may have resulted in nerve injury that is refractory to medical management.

PNS Techniques

The technique for implantation of PNS varies considerably depending on the nerve distribution to be targeted. Craniofacial pain can be treated with stimulation of the occipital, trigeminal, supraorbital, and infraorbital nerves or any combination of the above. If a trial is performed prior to permanent implantation, a percutaneous electrode is often used. Permanent implants can be done using percutaneous or paddle leads, depending on the location of stimulation and the surgeon's preference. An example of a trigeminal nerve stimulator electrode is shown in Fig. 27.1, in which a patient with medically refractory cranial nerve V1 distribution pain is treated with a percutaneous electrode placed through the foramen ovale to target the gasserian ganglion.

Percutaneous electrodes are typically placed with patients under mild sedation and local anesthetic. A curved Tuohy needle is carefully passed into the subcutaneous space using fluoroscopy for guidance of the needle relative to bony landmarks. For example, a supraorbital nerve stimulator is directed over the supraorbital ridge from lateral to medial [4], whereas an occipital nerve stimulator can be placed subcutaneously over the occipital ridge or in the subcutaneous plane overlying the posterior arch of C1 [8–10]. A percutaneous electrode, often with four or eight contacts, is then passed through the needle and tested with the patient awake to confirm adequate pain coverage [4]. Once the lead is determined to be in the correct location, it is tunneled away from the site of stimulation and either externalized for a trial or anchored to the fascia and connected to a generator that is placed in the subcutaneous space in the chest, buttocks, or abdomen.

Open techniques for insertion of paddle leads can also be used for ONS. If placement of the electrode is desired

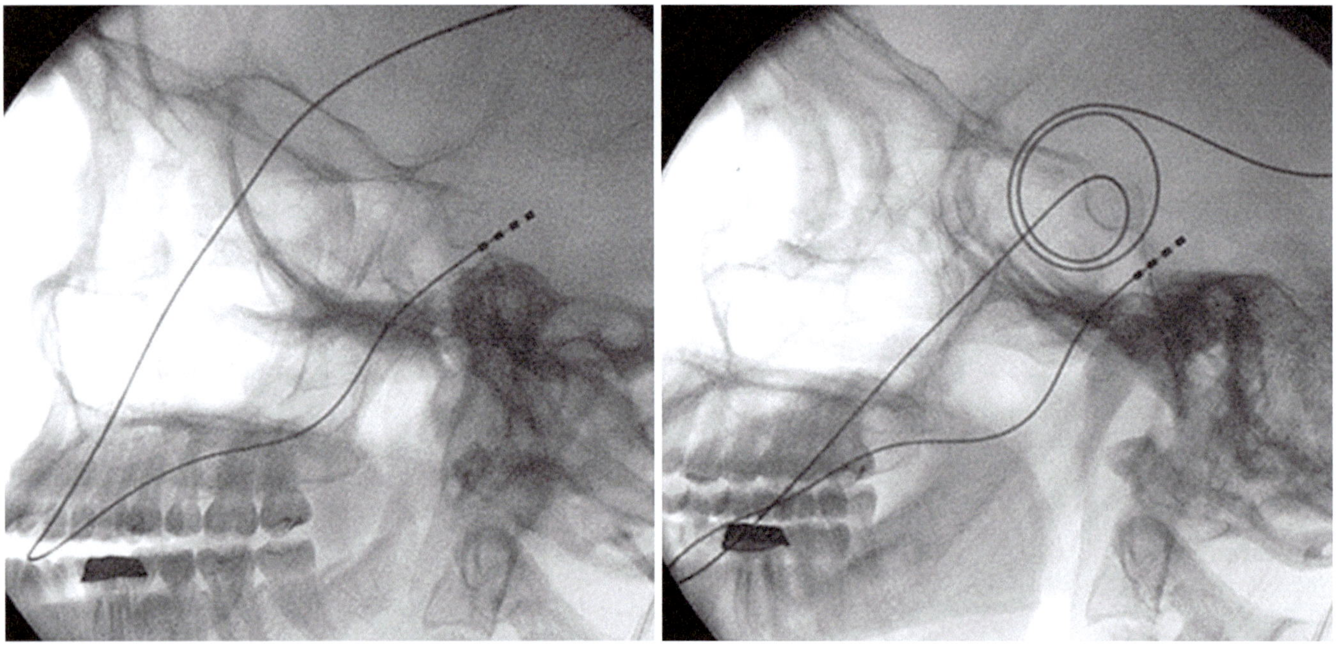

Fig. 27.1 Placement of a Medtronic 3387 DBS electrode (Minneapolis, MN) in the foramen ovale for V1 distribution medically refractory neuropathic pain. The image on the left is the percutaneous electrode used for intraoperative testing, and the image on the right is the tunneled percutaneous lead for the permanent implant

unilaterally over the occipital ridge to target the greater occipital nerve, with the patient under conscious sedation and local anesthetic, an incision can be made adjacent to the mastoid and below the superior nuchal line [11, 12]. A path can be tunneled in the subcutaneous space, and a paddle electrode can then be passed, again using fluoroscopy for guidance, from lateral to medial across the occiput. If bilateral paddle electrodes are inserted, a midline incision is made with tunneling of the leads from medial to lateral on either side over the occipital ridge or over the arch of C1, for targeting of the lesser occipital nerve [11, 12]. Figure 27.2a demonstrates bilateral percutaneous occipital nerve stimulators, and Fig. 27.2b shows a unilateral paddle occipital nerve stimulator. Just as with percutaneous electrodes, the patient is then awakened and tested to confirm coverage of pain, and the leads are then anchored to the fascia and tunneled away from the site of stimulation where they are connected to the implanted generator. Among the primary disadvantages to PNS include lead migration and fracture [4].

When placing PNS leads over peripheral nerves in the extremities, open techniques may be more effective, as this allows for a wide surgical exposure of the nerve in question to provide adequate visualization. Moreover, the use of paddle electrodes in such cases better facilitates anchoring of the lead to the adjacent fascia and soft tissue to help minimize the risk of lead migration. Figure 27.3 demonstrates a slightly larger surgical exposure required to access the proximal sciatic nerve, distal to the gluteal fold, for placement of a peripheral nerve stimulator on the sciatic nerve for treatment of medically refractory foot and leg pain. In Fig. 27.4, the importance of a wide dissection for safe electrode placement is also shown, as is securing the lead to the surrounding fascia in this patient with medically refractory palmar pain undergoing placement of a peripheral nerve stimulator electrode on the median nerve in the upper arm.

SPNS Techniques

Implantation of SPNS electrodes also depends on the location of pain, as well as on the extent of the area involved. In general, one or more leads are placed under local anesthesia overlying the area of maximal discomfort. If the patient had prior surgery for tumor resection, then the surgical scar can be used to guide placement of the electrode. A needle, such as a 14-gauge Tuohy needle, is introduced subcutaneously, and an electrode is then passed through the needle to the desired location, which can be confirmed with fluoroscopy if necessary. With the patient awake, correct lead placement can be further corroborated by testing the area of stimulation. Once lead position is verified, the distal portion of the electrode is tunneled beneath the skin, away from the region of stimulation. Typically, an external trial is performed for several days, and if patients experience greater than 50% pain relief, then permanent implantation occurs, with the generator placed subcutaneously in the chest, abdomen, or flank.

Pain localized to the inguinal region may only require one or two electrodes, inserted at the superolateral aspect of the inguinal region directed inferomedially in the subcutaneous

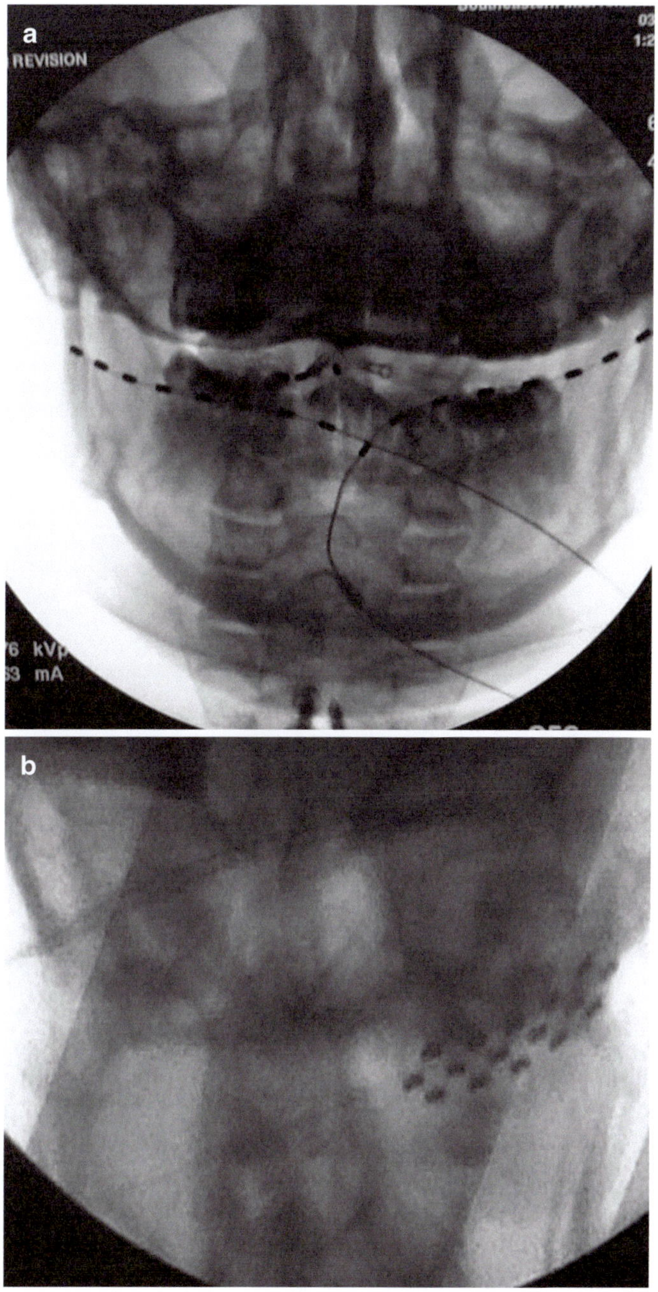

Fig. 27.2 (**a**) Placement of bilateral percutaneous occipital nerve stimulators at the C1 arch for intractable occipital neuralgia, (**b**) Placement of a unilateral paddle occipital nerve stimulator at the occipital ridge for a patient with intractable occipital neuralgia

tissue overlying the inguinal canal, as shown in Fig. 27.5. In contrast, a patient with hepatic cancers status postsurgical resection may have more extensive postsurgical pain, necessitating the placement of multiple electrodes oriented obliquely from the right intercostal margin to the right anterior iliac spine [13]. However, the lack of any randomized controlled studies or other well-designed trials evaluating the efficacy of SPNS should not be discounted [4].

PNS Specific Devices

More recently, devices that are specific to stimulation of peripheral nerves are being developed. A novel system has been described by Deer TR et al. using a smaller unipole lead which may be placed near a peripheral nerve. As opposed to a pulse generator that is implanted, an external pulse generator may be used. In this particular study, the responder rate

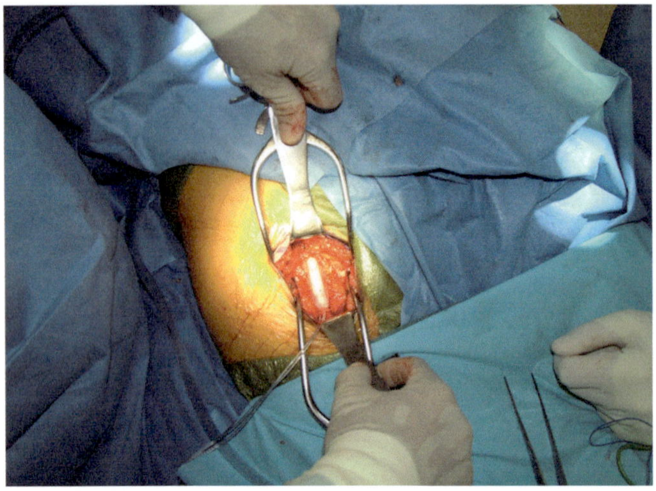

Fig. 27.3 Placement of a Medtronic 3987A On-Point Peripheral Nerve Stimulator (Minneapolis, MN) on the proximal sciatic nerve, distal to the gluteal fold, for treatment of medically refractory foot and leg pain

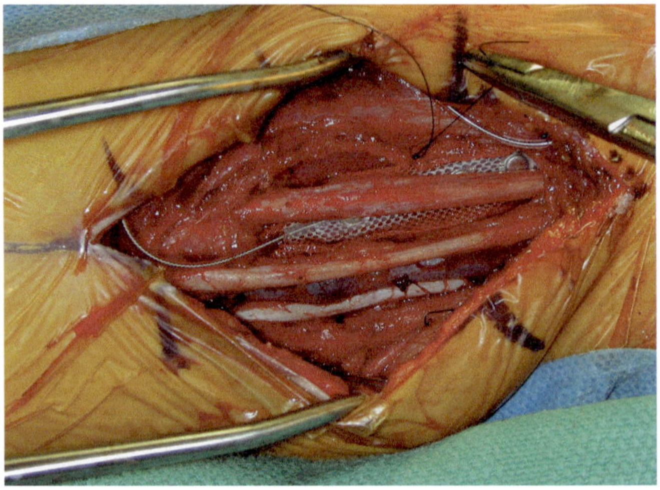

Fig. 27.4 Placement of a Medtronic 3987A On-Point Peripheral Nerve Stimulator (Minneapolis, MN) underneath the median nerve in the upper arm for treatment of medically refractory palmar pain. The lead is being secured with an anchoring stitch to the surrounding fascia

Fig. 27.5 Placement of two, staggered subcutaneous peripheral field stimulation for intractable inguinal pain

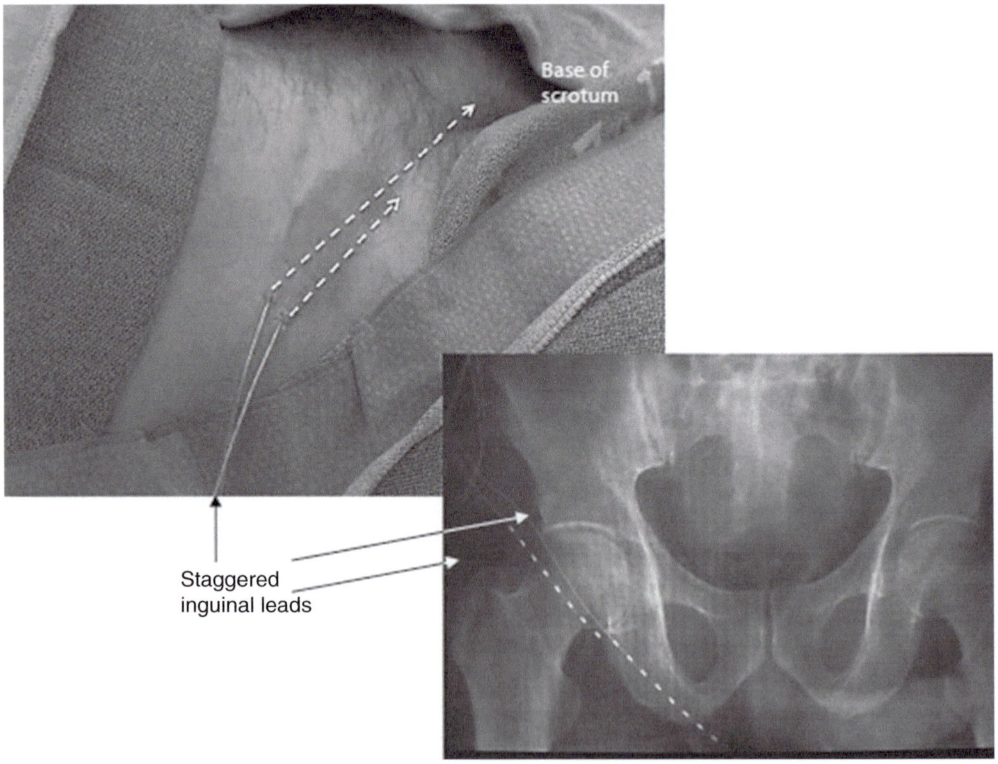

was 38% of patients receiving at least 30% pain relief for 3 months [14]. It is conceivable that image guidance, such as ultrasound technology, may help a pain practitioner localize a nerve and the optimal location for placement of future PNS devices, obviating an open technique [15].

Conclusions

Targeted stimulation therapy has become an increasingly accepted treatment modality for patients with chronic, medically intractable pain. The use of PNS and SPNS for focal distributions of both neuropathic and nociceptive pain syndromes is also gaining popularity. The application of such techniques in the treatment of cancer pain represents an important therapeutic modality in properly selected patients.

References

1. Boccard SGJ, Fitzgerald JJ, Pereira EAC, et al. Targeting the affective component of chronic pain: a case series of deep brain stimulation of the anterior cingulated cortex. Neurosurgery. 2014;74:628–37.
2. Esfahani DR, Pisanksy MT, Dafer RM, et al. Motor cortex stimulation: functional magnetic resonance imaging–localized treatment for three sources of intractable facial pain. J Neurosurg. 2011;114:189–95.
3. Lefaucheur JP, Drouot X, Cunin P, et al. Motor cortex stimulation for the treatment of refractory peripheral neuropathic pain. Brain. 2009;132:1463–71.
4. Stuart RM, Winfree CJ. Neurostimulation techniques for painful peripheral nerve disorders. Neurosurg Clin N Am. 2009;20(1):111–20.
5. Wong ET, Gunes S, Gaughan E, et al. Palliation of intractable cancer pain by MRI-guided cingulotomy. Clin J Pain. 1997;13(3):260–3.
6. Ballantine HT, Cosgrove GR, Giriunas IE. Surgical treatment of intractable psychiatric illness and chronic pain by stereotactic cingulotomy. In: Schmidek HH, Sweet WH, editors. Operative neurosurgical techniques: indications, methods, and results, vol. 2. Philadelphia: Saunders; 1995. p. 1423–30.
7. Hurt RW, Ballantine HT Jr. Stereotactic anterior cingulate lesions for persistent pain: a report on 68 cases. Clin Neurosurg. 1974;21:334–51.
8. Slavin KV, Nerseyan H, Wess C. Peripheral neurostimulation for the treatment of intractable occipital neuralgia. Neurosurgery. 2006;58:112–9.
9. Melvin EA, Jordan FR, Weiner RL, et al. Using peripheral stimulation to reduce the pain of C2-mediated occipital headaches: a preliminary report. Pain Physician. 2007;10:453–60.
10. Palmisani S, Al-Kaisy A, Arcioni R, et al. A six year retrospective review of occipital nerve stimulation practice: controversies and challenges of an emerging technique for treating refractory headache syndromes. J Headache Pain. 2013;14:67.
11. Oh MY, Ortega J, Bellotte JB, et al. Peripheral nerve stimulation for the treatment of occipital neuralgia. Neuromodulation. 2004;7(2):103–12.
12. Magown P, Garcia R, Beauprie I, et al. Occipital nerve stimulation for intractable occipital neuralgia: an open surgical technique. Clin Neurosurg. 2009;56:119–24.
13. Paicius RM, Bernstein CA, Lempert-Cohen C. Peripheral nerve field stimulation in chronic abdominal pain. Pain Physician. 2006;9:261–6.
14. Deer TR, Pope J, Benyamin R, et al. Prospective, multicenter, randomized, double-blinded, partial crossover study to assess the safety and efficacy of the novel neuromodulation system in the treatment of patients with chronic pain of peripheral nerve origin. Neuromodulation. 2016;19(1):91–100.
15. Huntoon MA1, Burgher AH. Ultrasound-guided permanent implantation of peripheral nerve stimulation (PNS) system for neuropathic pain of the extremities: original cases and outcomes. Pain Med. 2009;10(8):1369–77.

Transcutaneous Electrical Nerve Stimulation for Cancer Pain

28

Jeffrey Loh

Background

Initial attempts at electrical neuromodulation included the use of devices that stimulated sensations on the skin, transcutaneous electrical nerve stimulation (TENS). The use of electrical stimulation for the treatment of pain and as an anesthetic has been present since the mid-1800s; however acceptance of TENS for pain relief was only better accepted by the medical field in 1967 upon the publication of the gate theory of pain by Wall and Sweet [1, 2].

The original Wall and Sweet publication demonstrated that high-frequency (100 Hz) stimulation at an intensity that activates large afferent fibers reduced neuropathic pain in eight patients; however the actual mechanism of action by which TENS produced pain relief remained unclear for many years following this publication [1, 2]. While the exact mechanism remains unclear, multiple studies have addressed the efficacy of TENS on different pain conditions, with TENS improving various pain states from acute postsurgical pain to chronic conditions including back pain, neuropathic pain, and cancer pain.

Mechanism of Action

The original gate control theory involves the stimulation of large diameter afferent nerves which inhibit nociceptive fiber-evoked responses in the dorsal horn of the spinal cord. Recent studies support mechanisms with greater complexity, including anatomic pathways, involving neurotransmitters and their receptors in certain types of neurons [2].

J. Loh (✉)
Queen's Medical Center, Department of Anesthesiology & Pain Management, Honolulu, HI, USA
e-mail: jloh@queens.org

Original research supported high-frequency TENS stimulation resulting in conduction block or fatigue of A-beta and A-delta fibers. However, further analysis found that the afferent barrage from a pain stimulus remains intact during and after TENS. Thus, high-frequency TENS does not necessarily interrupt input from the peripheral site to the central nervous system. Anti-hyperalgesic effects of TENS was also found to outlast the stimulation time of TENS by greater than 8 hours, highlighting additional methods by which TENS may provide benefit [2].

One potential compound that may mediate pain inhibition produced by TENS is adenosine. The use of caffeine prior to the initiation of TENS seems to mitigate the response to TENS. As caffeine blocks adenosine receptors, adenosine has been targeted as a mediator for TENS-related pain control [2–4].

TENS may also improve pain symptoms with the release of endogenous opioids. Studies have shown that concentrations of beta-endorphins increase in the bloodstream and cerebrospinal fluid of healthy subjects after administration of either high- (greater than 80 Hz) or low-frequency (usually 2–20 Hz) TENS. Increased concentrations of opioid agonists, including methionine, enkephalin, and dynorphin A, have been found in lumbar cerebrospinal fluid following TENS application [5]. Given these findings, several potential endogenous opioids and their associated receptors are thought to mediate TENS associated pain relief.

In animal models, when opioid receptor antagonists were administered directly to the spinal cord, the anti-hyperalgesic effect of TENS was prevented. Blockade of mu opioid receptors with naloxone inhibited the anti-hyperalgesia of high-frequency TENS, while delta opioid receptor blockade with naltrindole inhibited the anti-hyperalgesia effects of low-frequency TENS. Blockade of opioids in the rostral ventral medulla (RVM) showed similar effects as spinal blockade in inhibiting the anti-hyperalgesia effects of TENS [6, 7].

A. Gulati et al. (eds.), *Essentials of Interventional Cancer Pain Management*, https://doi.org/10.1007/978-3-319-99684-4_28

Application and Use

A TENS unit typically consists of an electrical-signal generator, a battery, and a set of electrodes. The TENS unit is programmable such that the generator can deliver stimuli with variable current strengths, pulse rates, and pulse widths. To avoid the electrolytic and iontophoretic effects seen with a unidirectional current, a biphasic waveform is typically utilized. The settings on a TENS unit that are typically modifiable by the user are the amplitude, frequency (or pulse rate), and the pulse width. Most modern devices allow for changes in the delivery in the stimulation, from continuous, burst, and some form of intensity modulation.

When determining the amplitude (intensity) to use, patients increase the current to a level that provides a "buzzing" sensation without causing discomfort. Typical amplitudes used range from 0 to 100 mA on most TENS generators, with most patients sensing at 3–4 mA using pads between 1 and 3 inches apart.

The pulse width is the duration of time the stimulus is applied. The typical pulse width is microseconds in duration. While a higher pulse width (usually greater than 100 ms) conveys greater stimulation feel, a pulse width set too high will cause a muscle contraction, which is not a desired result with TENS. Conversely, too low of a pulse width will result in lack of perception of stimulus by the patient.

Pulse rate, also known as frequency, ranges from 1 to 250 Hz. The pulse rate is important, as this variable determines which nerve group is targeted, potentially affecting whether the gate theory or endorphin theory of TENS is utilized.

Due to the multiple different possible settings, patients are typically instructed to try different frequencies and intensities until they can find a setting that provides optimal pain control. In addition to the settings utilized, placement of the TENS electrode can affect the patient's pain relief.

> Note: We recommend high-frequency TENS (greater than 40 Hz) in the oncologic population. High-frequency TENS is associated with sensory nerve stimulation, leaving motor fibers minimally affected. Sensory stimulation usually does not lead to increased blood flow, as opposed to muscle contraction associated with low-frequency TENS.

Placement of the TENS electrodes is typically on the skin overlying the region of pain. However, other locations have been utilized, including cutaneous nerves/dermatomes, trigger points, and acupuncture sites. With each of the application sites, effective pain control has been seen.

The pulse duration is often short, up to 50 ms. With these settings, the onset of analgesia is typically rapid. Pain relief will last while the stimulus remains active and usually abates when the stimulation stops.

With acupuncture-like TENS, a low-frequency stimulus at 1–10 Hz, with a high intensity, is often applied. Due to the high stimulus intensity utilized, patients may find this application less comfortable, limiting its use. Thus, the use of acupuncture-like TENS is often considered after patients show a lack of response with conventional TENS. In contrast to the gate control theory postulated with conventional TENS, acupuncture-like TENS is thought to stimulate A-delta and C fibers, achieving pain control through descending pain suppression systems, which closes the gateway of pain transmission.

In addition to conventional and acupuncture-like TENS, pulsed (burst) TENS is another form of TENS that may be utilized by patients. In pulsed TENS, a low-intensity stimulus with high-frequency bursts is used. The recurrent bursts are usually discharged at 1–2 Hz, with the frequency of impulses within each burst set at 100 Hz. The efficacy of this modality remains unclear, as no advantage of pulsed TENS has been seen over conventional TENS.

Benefit

While multiple studies discuss the efficacy of TENS for treating cancer pain syndromes, few are randomized and controlled, comparing active TENS stimulation to placebo, with either no active stimulation or no treatment. Currently, two studies are reported in the literature. The benefit of TENS on cancer pain was conducted either on a select type of cancer or in a small patient population.

In one study assessing the efficacy of TENS for the treatment of breast cancer pain, Robb et al. found no significant difference in pain improvement between TENS and placebo. While pain improvement between the two groups was not significantly different, patients in the TENS group showed a greater continued use of TENS after study completion for continued pain control [8, 9].

In a randomized clinical trial by Gadsby et al., acupuncture-like TENS was studied to assess the efficacy in treating cancer pain or nausea and vomiting in 15 terminally ill patients. Like the breast cancer TENS study, acupuncture-like TENS did not show statistically significant differences in pain control or nausea and vomiting. However, due to the small sample size of this study, the study was lacking adequate power; thus the benefit of acupuncture-like TENS remains unclear [8, 10].

A study conducted by Bennett et al. in 2010 found conventional TENS providing statistically significant differences in pain control between active and placebo TENS for the treatment of cancer bone pain. The proportion of patients experiencing good or very good pain relief on movement with active TENS compared to placebo TENS showed statistical significance; however numerical rating scale (NRS) scores for pain relief and pain intensity on movement did not. Pain relief at rest showed no significant difference between active and placebo TENS [11].

While no randomized controlled trials of TENS have been studied assessing pain control for all types of cancer pain, a recent retrospective study by Loh et al. found benefit in the treatment of many types of cancer pain when TENS was utilized as a goal-directed therapy and when patients were initially trialed to determine whether they would be a suitable candidate. Patients showed a statistically significant change in reported pain levels in numerical rating scale (NRS) scores. Patients also reported subjective improvements in pain descriptions. While this study was not a randomized controlled trial, this study did show that appropriate training, goal-directed therapy, and initial trialing of TENS better increases the benefit for patients [12].

Risks/Limitations

TENS overall remains a safe treatment modality. The greatest limitation encountered by users is difficulty with application of TENS electrodes to inaccessible body regions. Patients with cancer-related back pain will typically report difficulty with application of the TENS pads in the region of their pain, limiting use. Thus, when starting use of TENS in a patient, ease of application or availability of a provider to help with application is important to address.

Other common complications encountered include skin burns or irritation when too strong of an electrical intensity is applied. Patients sensitive to adhesives may develop skin irritation or a rash from the electrical pads. Due to the electrical current utilized with TENS, patients that contain a pacemaker or who have a history of seizures are counseled against TENS use for fear of possibly disrupting pacemaker function or worsening of seizures.

One area of risk specific to the use of TENS in cancer patients is the theoretical risk of cancer recurrence in the site of TENS use. Tumor growth is dependent on angiogenesis and blood flow, which ultimately affects a tumor's oxygen and nutrient supply. Studies indicate that certain TENS settings can increase muscle activity and elevate blood flow. However, if TENS settings remain at a level below motor threshold, this risk of increased blood flow and cancer recurrence is unlikely [13–15].

Conclusions

TENS provides an alternative treatment modality beyond medications and interventional procedures for the treatment of cancer pain. While no definitive studies have proven active TENS to be more beneficial over placebo TENS in the treatment of cancer pain, initial studies using TENS as a goal-directed treatment appear promising. In patients that have known cancerous lesions at the site of their pain, TENS should be used cautiously, due to the theoretical risk of increased blood flow associated with TENS use, which may result in promotion of metastatic disease.

Transcranial Direct Current Stimulation and Repetitive Transcranial Magnetic Simulation for Cancer Pain

Background

The use of transcranial direct current stimulation (tCDS) for the treatment of depression was initially utilized in the 1960s. More recently, the use of tDCS for the treatment of chronic pain has been studied. tDCS has shown efficacy in treating fibromyalgia and spinal cord injury pain [16]. Unfortunately, the use of tDCS for the treatment of cancer pain remains unstudied currently. Cranial electrotherapy stimulation (CES), initially developed for the treatment of anxiety and depression, is similar to tDCS and has been studied for the treatment of chronic pain primarily in breast cancer patients [17].

While the tDCS and CES are technically two different techniques, both involve the application of low-intensity (typically <2 mA) electrical current to the cerebral cortex of the brain. tDCS uses large electrodes that are applied to the scalp over the targeted cerebral cortex to deliver a weak constant current. In contrast, CES utilizes a pulsed electrical current applied via clip electrodes attached to the patient's earlobes. Due to the paucity of studies detailing the efficacy of these treatments for cancer pain, the information detailed will focus more on the potential application of these treatments for cancer pain [17].

Similar to tDCS and CES, repetitive transcranial magnetic stimulation (rTMS) utilizes varying magnetic fields to induce electrical currents in focused parts of the brain. rTMS first gained prevalence in the 1980s when used to map the cerebral cortex and its connections. To induce electrical currents in the brain, a stimulating coil is applied to an individual's scalp. By applying rapidly changing magnetic fields, an electrical current is produced. Stimulation applied to the target region of the cortex induces alterations in brain activity in both local and remote brain regions. No current studies have examined the use of rTMS in the treatment of cancer pain; however rTMS has shown efficacy in the treatment of neuropathic pain conditions originating from a central etiology [17, 18].

Mechanism of Action

Central stimulation techniques, like tDCS, rTMS, and CES, modulate activity in the brain by directly altering the level of neuronal activity. Modulating brain activity reduces pain by altering neuronal activity involved in pain processing. With rTMS, low-frequency (<1 Hz) stimulation results in decreased cortical excitability, while high-frequency stimulation (>5 Hz) results in increased cortical excitability. A similar effect can be seen with tDCS treatments. Placement of the anode electrode over the cortical target results in increased excitability, while cathode stimulation results in decreased excitability. These induced alterations in excitability beyond the time of stimulation suggest electrochemical changes that result in long-term synaptic modulation [18, 19].

Cranial electrotherapy stimulation is also thought to modulate brain network activity, by direct activation on the hypothalamus, limbic system, and the reticular activating system. With tDCS, rTMS, and CES, stimulation of the motor cortex may reduce pain by modulating the thalamus and facilitating descending pain inhibitory mechanisms. Studies have shown that targeting the dorsolateral prefrontal cortex helps influence top-down pain perception. The ability for brain stimulation techniques to modulate an individual's pain perception highlights the complexity in determining the mechanisms by which these treatments function [18].

Benefit

Only one study has been published evaluating the efficacy of noninvasive brain stimulation for the treatment of cancer pain. Lyon et al. analyzed the effects of CES in the treatment of breast cancer pain and its associated cognitive symptoms. Though this study claimed to examine the effects of CES on the treatment of breast cancer pain, evaluation of patient pain levels using known quantitative scales was not performed. Instead, this study focused more on patient cognitive symptoms, including depression, anxiety, and fatigue, examining the efficacy of CES in improving these complaints [17].

The ability for CES to treat cognitive complaints in patients did not show a statistical difference between both active and placebo treatment groups, and both groups overall showed a worsening in depressive symptoms. However, the treatment group receiving active CES treatment had a smaller increase in depressive symptoms compared to placebo, and data appeared to indicate a trend toward statistical significance. Thus, the authors of this study felt that treatments like CES show potential benefit for the treatment of breast cancer pain and its associated symptoms; however, further studies on this subject are required [17].

While few studies have been performed evaluating the use of tDCS, rTMS, or CES in the treatment of cancer pain, this modality has shown proven benefit in the treatment of fibromyalgia, neuropathic pain, and depression. As cancer pain often entails many of these same pain states, the use of noninvasive brain stimulation for the treatment of cancer pain and its related states shows great potential.

Risks/Limitations

Common side effects experienced with tDCS treatments include mild headache, dizziness, nausea, and itching at the electrode site. Sink lesion and burns have also been reported, with care needed in examining and preparing the skin-electrode interface. No studies have reported seizures with the use of tDCS; however this adverse outcome is plausible given the use of electrical current applied to an individual's brain. Long-term safety associated with the use of tDCS remains unknown. Similar to tDCS, side effects associated with CES include mild skin irritation, dizziness, and headaches. Patients may also experience transient blurring of vision, giddiness, and tooth pain.

With rTMS, the main reported adverse effects are temporary auditory changes if no protection is used. This outcome stems from the clicking sound generated by the device. Mild transient headaches and neck pain are often associated with rTMS use. Seizures associated with the use of rTMS have been reported; however this side effect is rare and highly dependent on stimulation parameters and clinical characteristics of the patient receiving rTMS [18].

Conclusions

The application of noninvasive brain stimulation for the treatment of cancer pain remains untested. However, the use of these treatment modalities for many pain states commonly associated with cancer pain has proven successful. Further studies evaluating quantitative improvement in pain as well as patient quality of life are needed to validate the use of this treatment modality in cancer pain patients. In addition, studies determining the mechanism by which these treatments provide effect will help in improving the safety and efficacy of these treatments.

References

1. Wall PD, Sweet WH. Temporary abolition of pain in man. Science. 1967;155(3758):108–9.
2. Sluka KA, Walsh D. Transcutaneious electrical nerve stimulation: basic science mechanisms and clinical effectiveness. J Pain. 2003;4(3):109–21.
3. Salter MW, Henry JL. Evidence that adenosine mediates the depression of spinal dorsal horn neurons induced by peripheral vibration in the cat. Neuroscience. 1987;22(2):631–50.
4. Marchand S, Li J, Charest J. Effects of caffeine on analgesia from transcutaneous electrical nerve stimulation. N Engl J Med. 1995;333:325–6.
5. Han JS, Chen XH, Sun SL, Xu XJ, Yuan Y, Yan SC, Hao JX, Terenius L. Effect of low- and high-frequency TENS on Met-enkephalin-Arg Phe and dynorphin A immunoreactivity in human lumbar CSF. Pain. 1991;47(3):295–8.

6. Leonard G, Goffaux P, Marchand S. Deciphering the role of endogenous opioids in high-frequency TENS using low and high doses of naloxone. Pain. 2010;151(1):215–9. https://doi.org/10.1016/j.pain.2010.07.012. Epub 2010 Aug 21
7. Kalra A, Urban MO, Sluka KA. Blockage of opioid receptors in rostral ventral medulla prevents antihyperalgesia produced by transcutaneous electrical nerve stimulation (TENS). J Pharmacol Exp Ther. 2001;298(1):257–63.
8. Hurlow A, Bennett MI, Robb KA, Johnson MI, Simpson KH, Oxberry SG. Transcutaneous electric nerve stimulation (TENS) for cancer pain in adults. Cochrane Database Syst Rev. 2012;3:CD006276. https://doi.org/10.1002/14651858.CD006276.pub3.
9. Robb KA, Newham DJ, Williams JE. Transcutaneous electrical nerve stimulation vs. transcutaneous spinal electroanalgesia for chronic pain associated with breast cancer treatments. J Pain Symptom Manag. 2007;33(4):410–9.
10. Gadsby JG, Franks A, Jarvis P, Dewhurst F. Acupuncture like transcutaneous electrical nerve stimulation within palliative care: a pilot study. Complement Ther Med. 1997;5:13–8.
11. Bennett MI, Johnson MI, Brown S, Searle RD, Radford H, Brown JM. Feasibility study of transcutaneous electrical nerve stimulation (TENS) for cancer bone pain. J Pain. 2010;11(4):351–9.
12. Loh J, Gulati A. The use of transcutaneous electrical nerve stimulation (TENS) in a major cancer center for the treatment of severe cancer-related pain and associated disability. Pain Med. 2013; https://doi.org/10.1111/pme.12038. Epub ahead of print
13. Carmeliet P, Jain RK. Principles and mechanisms of vessel normalization for cancer and other angiogenic diseases. Nat Rev Drug Discov. 2011;10(6):417–27. https://doi.org/10.1038/nrd3455.
14. Cramp FL, McCullough GR, Lowe AS, Walsh DM. Transcutaneous electric nerve stimulation: the effect of intensity on local and distal cutaneous blood flow and skin temperature in healthy subjects. Arch Phys Med Rehabil. 2002;83(1):5–9.
15. Chen CC, Johnson MI, McDonough S, Cramp F. The effect of transcutaneous electrical nerve stimulation on local and distal cutaneous blood flow following a prolonged heat stimulus in healthy subjects. Clin Physiol Funct Imaging. 2007;27(3):154–61.
16. O'Connell NE, Wand BM, Marston L, Spencer S, Desouza LH. Non-invasive brain stimulation techniques for chronic pain. A report of a Cochrane systematic review and meta-analysis. Eur J Phys Rehabil Med. 2011;47(2):309–26. Epub 2011 Apr 14
17. Lyon DE, Schubert C, Taylor AG. Pilot study of cranial stimulation for symptom management in breast cancer. Oncol Nurs Forum. 2010;37(4):476–83. https://doi.org/10.1188/10.ONF.476-483.
18. Plow EB, Pascual-Leone A, Machado A. Brain stimulation in the treatment of chronic neuropathic and non-cancerous pain. J Pain. 2012;13(5):411–24. https://doi.org/10.1016/j.jpain.2012.02.001. Epub 2012 Apr 7
19. Rokyta R, Fricová J. Neurostimulation methods in the treatment of chronic pain. Physiol Res. 2012;61(Suppl 2):S23–31.

Part VI

Intrathecal Drug Delivery

29 Indications for Intrathecal Pump Therapy

Mercy A. Udoji and Helen M. Blake

Abbreviations

CSF	Cerebrospinal fluid
FDA	Food and Drug Administration
IT	Intrathecal
ITDD	Intrathecal drug delivery
ITP	Intrathecal pump
NMDA	N-methyl-D-aspartate
WHO	World Health Organization

Introduction

In the majority of cases, cancer pain is effectively managed with oral pain medications, utilizing the World Health Organization's (WHO) analgesic ladder as a guide. However, with time and disease progression, a significant number of patients require increasing doses of potent opioids, experience decreased levels of pain relief, and may not tolerate side effects of opioid medications [1]. Intrathecal drug delivery (ITDD) delivers potent analgesia while potentially decreasing systemic side effects. Intrathecal drug administration usually drastically reduces the systemic dose of opioids which are administered to the patient, thereby decreasing side effects.

History of Intrathecal Drug Therapy

The first documented injection of medication into the intrathecal space was performed by August Bier in 1898 for a series of lower extremity operations [2]. Despite a high degree of interest in this new technique within the scientific community, it took another century (1973) to discover the presence of opiate receptors on the spinal cord which may explain Bier's observations. Six years later, Wang reported the first successful use of an opiate (morphine) in the spinal cord to treat intractable cancer pain, documenting remarkable improvement in pain with absence of sedation, respiratory depression, and other deleterious side effects associated with systemic opioid therapy [3]. The first intrathecal drug delivery device was introduced to clinical use and used to treat severe pain secondary to cancer in 1981 [1, 3].

First-generation intrathecal pumps were approved by the Food and Drug Administration (FDA) exclusively for the treatment of patients with severe pain secondary to malignancy. Initially, only constant rate, non-programmable pumps were available. Over time, technological advancement has made it possible to have multidrug, intermittent infusion, programmable intrathecal pumps.

Multiple system types (Table 29.1) can be implemented depending upon the patient's life expectancy and clinical condition. The simplest device is a tunneled or non-tunneled percutaneous catheter attached to an external pump. These systems are easier to place but are only suitable for patients

Table 29.1 Types of intrathecal drug delivery systems

Percutaneous catheter used with external pump
Percutaneous catheter with subcutaneous access port and external pump
Implanted fixed-rate intrathecal pump (InfusAID, Codman 3000)
Implanted programmable intrathecal pump (Medtronic SynchroMed™)
Implanted programmable intrathecal pump (Flowonix Prometra™)

M. A. Udoji
Emory University/Atlanta Veterans' Administration, Department of Anesthesiology, Decatur, GA, USA
e-mail: mercy.udoji@va.gov

H. M. Blake (✉)
Pain and Rehabilitation Specialists of Saint Louis, LLC, St. Louis, MO, USA

A. Gulati et al. (eds.), *Essentials of Interventional Cancer Pain Management*, https://doi.org/10.1007/978-3-319-99684-4_29

with a limited life expectancy due to their association with high risk of infection. They require regular monitoring to assess infection risk and are suitable in an inpatient environment where nursing and ancillary staff is present. Due to connection to an external pump, this strategy may limit the patient's mobility and independence [3, 4].

A second type of delivery system tunnels an intrathecal catheter which is connected to an implanted subcutaneous port and subsequently an external pump. This system type is also only suitable for patients with a limited life expectancy. Due to the port connection to an external pump, similar restraints on the patient's mobility must be considered prior to implantation. Because this system is subcutaneous, close monitoring for infection at the access port is advised. Trained nursing staff must be available to prevent inadvertent delivery of medications inappropriate for intrathecal therapy through the access port.

The third class of intrathecal delivery systems includes implanted intrathecal pumps with either constant rate or programmable functions. These pump systems have the advantage of being fully implanted and percutaneously accessed for refill, commonly at intervals of 30–60 days. Implanted systems have decreased exposure to pathogens which allows for long-term management of a patient's pain. The patient's mobility is minimally affected with these devices [4].

Various intrathecal pumps are available on the market today including the SynchroMed infusion system (Medtronic), InfusAid pump (Strato/InfusAid), Prometra (Flowonix), and the Codman 3000 drug pump (Codman and Shurtleff) [3–5]. These pumps differ in reservoir volume, mechanism of delivery (internal vs external), and programmable characteristic. Intrathecal drug delivery systems consist of a pump (containing the reservoir and other programmable parts) which is implanted in the subcutaneous tissue, usually the anterior abdomen. A flexible spinal catheter is placed percutaneously and tunneled to connect to the reservoir and pump. The pump can be accessed with a noncoring Huber needle using a template to facilitate localization of the access port. It is controlled by an external programming device or a handheld device (personal therapy manager) given to the patient to allow for intermittent bolus dosing. Once in place, a variety of opioid and non-opioid adjuvant medications may be administered via the pump [3, 4, 6].

Intrathecal drug delivery allows the pharmacologic therapy to bypass the blood-brain barrier and directly affect receptors located in the dorsal horn of the spinal cord, modifying pre- and postsynaptic transmission [7]. Receptor targets include opioid (G-protein-coupled receptors), local anesthetics (sodium channel receptor blockers), alpha-2 agonists (alpha-2 receptors), ziconotide (calcium channel blocker), and N-methyl-D-aspartate (NMDA) receptor antagonists (G-protein coupled or ionotropic receptors) [8]. Morphine was and remains the gold standard agent for intrathecal drug delivery. Though medications from other classes described above are routinely used, only morphine, baclofen, and ziconotide are FDA approved for intrathecal use [6, 9]. Medications appropriate for intrathecal delivery and their unique applications are addressed more thoroughly in the chapter titled *Medication Choices.*

Indications for Intrathecal Therapy

Proper patient selection is the most important consideration for implantation. If the practitioner is considering intrathecal opioids, patient should not undergo trial and implantation if they have had little response to oral or intravenous opioid medications. Additionally, opiate-naïve patients are not considered optimal candidates for ITP placement due to risk of respiratory and other complications (relative and absolute contraindications are listed in Table 29.2). The physician must carefully consider multiple patient and disease factors prior to instituting intrathecal drug therapy. The indications for ITP placement are listed in Table 29.3.

Inadequate Analgesia

Persistent moderate to severe pain despite escalating doses of oral or parenteral opioids is the most common indication for intrathecal pump placement in the cancer pain population. The first major study to evaluate the effects of IT medications in this population was performed by Smith et al., a randomized controlled study comparing comprehensive

Table 29.2 Relative and absolute contraindications for IT pump therapy

Relative
Psychosocial factors (i.e., drug abuse, depression, dementia)
Unstable spine
Obstructive metastasis in the spine
Absolute
Bloodstream infection
Coagulopathy, uncorrectable
Skin infection at planned pocket, epidural, or tunneled sites
Intravenous drug abuse (intrathecal abuse potential)
Elevated cerebrospinal fluid pressure

Table 29.3 Indications for intrathecal pump (ITP) placement

Failure of conservative management
Favorable degree of pain relief with ITP trial
Inadequate analgesia with oral medications
Intolerable side effects from oral medications
Nondiffuse pain
No absolute contraindications (see Table 29.1)

medical management to IT drug delivery. Patients managed with intrathecal drug delivery had a trend for better treatment success and interestingly greater survival at the 6-month follow-up period (though this was not a primary outcome of the study). Not surprisingly, the incidence of therapy-related side effects was significantly reduced in the intrathecal drug delivery population [10, 11]. In 1997, Gestin et al. evaluated the effects of intrathecal analgesia (with available patient delivered boluses) on rate of infection and opioid side effects [12]. Their study showed intrathecal opioid infusions were not associated with higher incidence of side effects and provided satisfactory analgesia without an increase in infection or other complications [12]. Burton et al. followed a group of patients with refractory cancer pain after initiation of neuraxial analgesia (including epidural and intrathecal opioids). Published results demonstrated significant decrease in pain scores as well as decrease in symptoms such as drowsiness and mental clouding [13]. Other reports by Onofrio and Yaksh [14] as well as Rauck et al. [15] have validated the efficacy of intrathecal drug delivery in management of refractory cancer pain [14, 15].

Intolerable Side Effects

The presence of opioid-related side effects is the second most common indication for intrathecal drug delivery in the oncologic population. Side effects range from pruritus, nausea, vomiting, decreased appetite, and constipation to life-threatening respiratory depression and death [10]. In a prospective study by Rauck et al., cancer patients with intolerable side effects or inadequately controlled pain underwent implantation of intrathecal drug delivery systems and were evaluated over a period of 12 months [15]. Results demonstrated superior analgesia with intrathecal drug delivery [10, 15]. It is also worth noting that the studies by Burton, Gestin, and Smith (see "inadequate analgesia" above) have all demonstrated reductions in opioid-related side effects in patients treated with intrathecal opioids [12, 13, 15].

Other Considerations

Localized Pain Intrathecal analgesia is usually not appropriate for pain that is diffuse or in different quadrants of the body (i.e., left leg and right-hand pain). Diffuse pain may be better managed by oral or parenteral opioids since intrathecal medications have variable spread around the catheter tip based on various drug chemical properties (usually a few vertebral levels cephalad and rostral to the catheter tip) [16]. In addition, patients who experience pain at the shoulder level or higher are not considered optimal candidates for intrathecal drug delivery because of difficulties threading the catheter above the thoracic spine and higher risk of adverse effects from intrathecal medications [16].

Comorbid Conditions Medical conditions such as obstructive sleep apnea, diabetes, and morbid obesity may impact a practitioner's decision to transition from oral to intrathecal therapy. Patients with these conditions may have an increased risk of oral opioid-related side effects [1, 17] Consulting with the patient's primary oncologist to discuss risk factors is recommended prior to trial and implantation. As an example, the available evidence suggests that patients with lower Hgb A1C levels experience lower morbidity and infection rates in the diabetic population [1, 18]. Additionally, patients are often immunocompromised and require surveillance for infections (local or systemic) [1].

Life Expectancy In an increasingly cost-conscious healthcare environment, practitioners should consider cost of placement relative to a patient's projected life expectancy prior to offering intrathecal drug delivery. Commonly, a life expectancy of less than 3 months has been discussed as a time frame to consider for implantation of an internal system. For patients with a life expectancy less than 3 months, perhaps an external catheter may be implanted (e.g., an epidural placement). Recent consensus-based guidelines by Deer et al. support intrathecal drug delivery in any patient with cancer and concomitant inadequate analgesia or intolerable side effects, irrespective of expected survival [1, 3, 6].

Type of Pain Cancer pain syndromes may result from tissue infiltration of tumor, inflammation, obstruction chemotherapy, radiotherapy, etc. Historically, neuropathic pain has been thought to respond poorly to oral opioid medications. Opioids in the intrathecal space may have similar efficacy to treat neuropathic pain [1]. Becker et al.'s article retrospective examination of the efficacy of intrathecal opioids for the management of neuropathic and nociceptive pain in cancer patients supports this assertion. Initially, patients with both types of pain responded well to IT opioid therapy. However, over time, the neuropathic pain group showed very poor response to intrathecal opioids, whereas the nociceptive pain group continued to show good response to therapy [19]. The authors also noted that nociceptive pain in the "trunk" responded better than that in in the extremities [10, 19]. More recent reports have shown that neuropathic pain may respond to intrathecal ziconitide in some populations; however this claim has not been specifically evaluated in the cancer pain population. Intrathecal medications may relieve neuropathic pain associated with tumor invasion of nerve plexi and other structures [1]. Agents such as tricyclic antidepressants are being explored as adjuncts to morphine in the intrathecal space not only for their opioid-sparing effects but also for their increased efficacy in control of neuropathic pain [5].

Conclusion

Intrathecal drug delivery systems represent an evidence-based strategy to administer medications to improve pain control in the cancer patient. This therapeutic strategy offers significant advantages over traditional oral or parenteral opioid therapies including extension of life expectancy, decreased side effects otherwise associated with systemic medications, and improvement in patient mobility and function. Intrathecal drug delivery systems are likely underutilized in cancer patients. Appropriate patient selection is imperative in ensuring the efficacy of the therapy. Widely educating the medical community on the use and application of this therapy has the potential to identify more patients who may benefit from its implementation and improve patient outcome and satisfaction.

References

1. Deer TR, Smith HS, Burton AW, Pope JE, Doleys DM, Levy RM, et al. Comprehensive consensus based guidelines on intrathecal drug delivery systems in the treatment of pain caused by cancer pain. Pain Physician. 2011;14:E283–312.
2. Larson MD. History of anesthetic practice. In: Miller RD, editor. Miller's anesthesia. Philadelphia: Elsevier; 2005. p. 25–9.
3. Knight KH, Brand FM, Mchaourab AS, Veneziano G. Implantable intrathecal pumps for chronic pain: highlights and updates. Croat Med J. 2007;48:22–34.
4. Williams JE, Towlerton G, Louw G. Intrathecal pumps for giving opioids in chronic pain; a systematic review. Health Technol Assess. 2000;4(32):iii–iv, 1–65.
5. Wilson J, Stack C, Hester J. Recent advances in cancer pain management. F1000 Prime Rep. 2014;6:10.
6. Osenbach RK. Intrathecal drug delivery in the management of pain. In: Fishman S, Ballantyne J, Rathmell J, editors. Bonica's management of pain. Philadelphia: Lippincott, Williams, and Wilkins; 2010. p. 1437–57.
7. Cope DK, Zhao Z. Interventional management for cancer pain. Curr Pain Headache Rep. 2011;15:237–43.
8. Cohen SP, Dragovich A. Intrathecal analgesia. Anesthesiol Clin. 2007;25(4):863–82.
9. Penn RD, Paice JA. Chronic intrathecal morphine for intractable pain. J Neurosurg. 1987;67:182–6.
10. Hayek SM, Deer TR, Pope JE, Panchal SJ, Patel V. Intrathecal therapy for cancer and non-cancer pain. Pain Physician. 2011;14:219–48.
11. Smith TJ, Staats PS, Deer T, Stearns LJ, Rauck RL, Boortz-Marx RL, Buchser E, Catala E, Bryce DA, Coyne PJ, Pool GE. Implantable drug delivery systems study group. Randomized clinical trial of an implantable drug delivery system compared with comprehensive medical management for refractory cancer pain: impact on pain, drug-related toxicity and survival. J Clin Oncol. 2002;20(19):4040–9.
12. Gestin Y, Vainio A, Pegurier AM. Long term intrathecal infusion of morphine in the home care of patients with advanced cancer. Acta Anesthesiol Scand. 1997;41:12–7.
13. Burton AW, Rajagopal A, Shah HN, Mendoza T, Cleeland C, Hassenbusch SJ, et al. Epidural and intrathecal analgesia is effective in treating refractory cancer pain. Pain Med. 2004;5(3):239–47.
14. Onofrio BM, Yaksh TL. Long term pain relief produced by intrathecal morphine infusion in 53 patients. J Neurosurg. 1990;72:200–9.
15. Rauck RL, Cherry D, Boyer MF, Kosek P, Dunn J, Alo K. Long term intrathecal opioid therapy with a patient-activated implanted delivery system for the treatment of refractory cancer pain. J Pain. 2003;4:441–7.
16. Gulati A, Puttanniah V, Hung J, Malhotra V. Considerations for evaluating the use of intrathecal drug delivery in the oncologic patient. Curr Pain Headache Rep. 2014;18:391–6.
17. Upadhyay SP, Mallick PN. Intrathecal drug delivery system (IDDS) for cancer pain management: a review and updates. Am J Hosp Palliat Care. 2012;29:388–98.
18. Engle MP, Vinh BP, Harun N, Koyyalagunta D. Infectious complications related to intrathecal drug delivery system and spinal cord stimulator system implantations at a comprehensive cancer pain center. Pain Physician. 2013;16:251–7.
19. Becker R, Jakob D, Uhle E, Riegel T, Bertalanffy H. The significance of intrathecal opioid therapy for the treatment of neuropathic cancer pain conditions. Streotact Funct Neurosurg. 2000;75:16–26.

Intrathecal Drug Delivery System Trialing for Cancer Pain Management

30

Namrata Khimani and Sanjeet Narang

IDDS Trial

IDDS trials serve as the final step in the selection process prior to permanent implantation. Trials have become commonplace in the treatment of both malignant and nonmalignant pain as they are often mandated by insurance companies. Under current Medicare guidelines, a preliminary trial must be done with a temporary intrathecal/epidural catheter "to substantiate adequately acceptable pain relief and degree of side effects (including effects on the activities of daily living) and patient acceptance" [3]. However, as we will discuss later in the chapter, the necessity of trials in patients with cancer pain has become a topic of debate.

IDDS trials have traditionally been used for several reasons: (1) establish the efficacy of analgesic response, (2) create an initial dose estimation, (3) assess a reduction in opioid-related side effects, and (4) determine individual tolerability. Trialing can also contribute to the psychological assessment by giving insight into a patient's expectations and the consistency of a patient's analgesic response [4]. In fact, patients should be encouraged to define quantifiable goals prior to the trial. Doing so can help create realistic individualized expectations for a patient's own pain management as complete termination of pain is rarely achieved.

While trialing can provide useful information, limited data exists regarding the predictive value of a trial for successful post-implantation therapeutic response, and a direct correlation has yet to be established. A prospective study of 18 patients receiving a trial of intrathecal morphine or sufentanil reported that all patients received a 50% reduction in pain. But after a mean follow-up of 2.4 years after implantation, 39% no longer had any reduction in pain [5]. However, a study examining 53 patients with terminal metastatic cancer suggested a standard trialing technique may have a prognostic benefit [6]. To our knowledge, no study has examined the outcomes of patients who failed a trial and still went on to be implanted with an IDDS. Given the paucity of data, it may be wise for the implanting physician to simply use the trial as one criterion in a multitude of factors that must equally be considered when deciding which patients are appropriate candidate for permanent IDDS implantation.

Trialing Techniques

Several trialing techniques have been described: bolus versus continuous infusion, single versus multiple bolus injections, and epidural versus intrathecal routes. There is no consensus on an optimal trialing technique. In fact, recent guidelines and consensus panels highlight the fact that no study has shown a single trialing method to be superior to another in predicting long-term outcome [4, 7–9].

Furthermore, there is no standardized outcome measure that is used to declare a trial as successful. The usual criteria used in both clinical practice and research protocols are a 50% or greater reduction in pain score as measured by an accepted rating scale (i.e., visual analog scale). Many clinicians also attempt to quantify improvements in functionality and a decrease in opioid side effects. However, for many cancer patients, particularly those at end of life, assessing improvement in function may not be as essential.

The 2012 (and subsequent 2017) Polyanalgesic Consensus Conference (PACC), an expert panel composed of clinicians with extensive experience in the use of intrathecal analgesics for pain management, outlined a potential trialing algorithm

N. Khimani (✉)
Department of Anesthesiology, Perioperative and Pain Medicine, The Pain Management Center at Brigham and Women's Hospital, Chestnut Hill, MA, USA

S. Narang
Department of Anesthesiology, Perioperative and Pain Medicine, The Pain Management Center at Brigham and Women's Hospital, Harvard Medical School, Chestnut Hill, MA, USA
e-mail: snarang@partners.org

A. Gulati et al. (eds.), *Essentials of Interventional Cancer Pain Management*, https://doi.org/10.1007/978-3-319-99684-4_30

for nonmalignant pain [4]. While recommendations such as these are vital for the establishment of best practices, several questions, regarding the appropriate length of the trial or tapering of systemic opioids during the trial, still remain. Therefore, there is great variation in technique, and the decision to use one method over another is largely based on physician preference, infrastructure of the practice environment, patient condition, and insurance coverage. It is ultimately up to the implanting physician to consider the benefits and limitations of each method and decide which technique is best suited for the individual patient.

Each trialing technique has its potential advantages and disadvantages. A retrospective multicenter survey from 1987 examined various trialing methods in cancer and non-cancer patients and found that the most commonly employed method was a continuous epidural infusion (35%), followed by intrathecal bolus injection (34%), epidural bolus injection (25%), and finally continuous intrathecal infusion (6%) [10]. No recent studies have surveyed the current trialing practices of physicians. All trial methods, though arguably to varying degrees, are also potentially subject to placebo effect.

Intuitively, one would think it best to choose a trialing method that most closely resembles intrathecal drug delivery through the implanted system. Using this logic, a continuous intrathecal catheter trial would be the method of choice. However, as evident by the multicenter survey [10], continuous intrathecal catheters are usually not the modality of choice for trialing. Based on our experience, intrathecal catheter trials are often not used as the infrastructure and monitoring required for safe intrathecal drug delivery through an external catheter are simply not available in many hospital and/or clinic settings. Furthermore, there is no data to justify the use of intrathecal catheters, which have the potential for more severe consequences if not used correctly, over other methods.

Intrathecal trialing can also be done with single or intermittent boluses. Single and intermittent bolus trials can establish efficacy of analgesic response. Intermittent boluses are sometime used as they potentially allow for better control of placebo response as compared to a single bolus injection. However, continuous infusion trials are more often employed as they are thought to establish more information while avoiding the fluctuating drug levels seen with intermittent boluses. A recent prospective, randomized outcomes study of 40 patients showed that intrathecal intermittent boluses and continuous infusions showed no clinically significant difference in predicting trial success or long-term outcomes [11].

Epidural administration, whether it be through boluses or infusions, does not mimic an implanted IDDS. It requires up to a tenfold higher dose of opioid due to different drug kinetics in the epidural space and excludes any contribution of the CSF fluid dynamics [4]. However, epidural trials avoid the need for a dural puncture and potential post-dural puncture headache. Moreover, by selecting an epidural infusion, the catheter tip can be placed as close as possible to the dermatomal level involved in pain and may more accurately mimic the actual analgesia achieved by the IDDS as compared to boluses via any route.

At our institution, trials are considered advantageous with the majority of patients undergoing a continuous epidural infusion trial. Often, by the time we are consulted, patients are on high-dose opioid therapy with inadequate pain control suffering from sedative and cognitive side effects in a complicated psychosocial setting. We employ a continuous epidural trial usually done over a 2–4 day period during which time the patient is admitted to our inpatient service. The epidural catheter may be placed at bedside or in the operating room with fluoroscopic guidance depending on the anatomic target, the patient's spinal anatomy and ability to maintain the appropriate position, and physician comfort level. Our practice is to define the upper and lower horizontal extent of the maximal pain affected area and attempt to place the epidural within the middle dermatomal level. Once the epidural catheter is in place, systemic opioid therapy is reduced, often by 50%. The dose of intrathecal opioids is increased every 12–24 h until analgesia is established, systemic side effects are minimized, and the patient's trust and willingness in this form of therapy is gained.

Implantation Without a Trial

The unique nature of cancer pain is evident in the fact that approximately 90% of patients suffering from nonmalignant chronic pain and spasticity receive a psychological assessment as part of the preimplantation selection process, while only 10% of cancer patient are similarly assessed [12]. IDDS trials may play an important role for patients requiring long-term therapy, but the utility of trials in cancer patients has been questioned as cancer pain and its treatments can differ from chronic non-cancer pain in a multitude of ways. Cancer pain patients often have a much poorer prognosis, multiple sites and/or types of pain, and different goals for improvements in function.

Many patients who are considered for IDDS implantation have limited life expectancies and are often receiving palliative care in the setting of high-dose opioid therapy. For these patients, undergoing an IDDS trial may be of limited value as there is a need to evaluate treatment options quickly and efficiently. The utility of trialing has also become debatable as issues surrounding rapid disease progression and opioid-induced hyperalgesia are critical and often difficult to adequately assess in a brief trialing period. A trial could potentially even lead to underestimation of the failure rate with long-term infusion [4]. Determining which patients are appropriate candidates for an IDDS trial is ultimately up to the implanting physician as specific criteria do not exist.

Unfortunately, the reality of the matter is that many cancer patients who fail comprehensive medical management often are not referred to an interventional specialist until late in the disease process when they are experiencing significant side effects, poor pain control, and limited life expectancy. The purpose of the IDDS trial in this population is usually to determine an effective intrathecal starting dose as well as the patient's willingness to proceed. If an IDDS trial was to be forgone in certain cancer patients, the dilemma arises as to how to determine the starting dose of therapy.

The consensus statement by PACC suggested that trialing may not be needed if the patient has tolerated the same drug by another route [4]. However, there is sparse data regarding what constitutes an appropriate method for conversion from systemic to intrathecal opioids. While it is likely that patients who had a 50% or greater improvement in pain with systemic opioids will benefit from IDDS therapy, studies have not shown a direct correlation between a patient's response to oral opioids and subsequent analgesic response to intrathecal opioids [13].

Du Pen et al. sought to describe a conversion tool, specifically for epidural dosing, by assigning relative weights to various pain characteristics and examined its efficacy in a limited sample of four cases [14]. More recently, Malhotra and colleagues used statistical analysis to examine independent factors that could be used to calculate the initial intrathecal dose without an epidural trial. Using pre- and post-IDDS data from 46 cancer patients receiving systemic opioids who had undergone an epidural trial, the authors created an equation that predicts an appropriate initial dose predicted solely on preimplantation daily systemic opioid requirements that also allow for intermittent bolus dosing. Given the broad 95% prediction interval (−122.7–147.6%), the authors recognize the value of utilizing a trial when feasible [15]. It must be kept in mind that many other factors may influence opioid conversion from oral and intravenous preimplantation doses to post-implantation intrathecal doses, including disease progression, medication tolerance, and increased postsurgical pain. Therefore, patients who are not trialed will likely require close clinical follow-up with ongoing adjustments.

In 2011 an expert panel published the Comprehensive Consensus Based Guidelines on Intrathecal Drug Delivery Systems in the Treatment of Pain Caused by Cancer. Although the practice of trialing was supported, the panel did recommend the reconsideration of mandatory trials in certain patients, particularly for those at end of life [8]. Recognizing the lack of a proven correlation between trial response and post-implantation outcomes is important when deciding the need for trialing in cancer patients in whom life expectancy is limited and urgency is warranted.

Drugs Used in Trials

Choosing the initial medications for IDDS is not standardized and can be confusing. The medications used in the trial for intrathecal pumps are often chosen to reflect the eventual intrathecal medication mixture. However, this practice varies with institution and practitioner and can be influenced by the evolution of cancer pain therapy within a geographical location. As morphine and ziconotide are the only agents approved by the US Food and Drug Administration for intrathecal analgesia, individual institution/pharmacy rules and practices are important to consider when using off-label medications. The PACC outlined an evidence-based algorithm regarding the utilization of different medications in an IDDS to help guide the safe and effective use of intrathecal analgesics [4]. At our institution, cancer patients are often referred late in their disease process compelling us to use a triple mix of opioid, local anesthetic, and clonidine from the outset, rather than the stepwise approach recommended by PACC for chronic refractory pain. We find that the administration of intrathecal opioid alone for cancer pain management often does not provide sufficient pain relief without compromising an improved side effect profile, thus requiring the addition of local anesthetics and clonidine. Though custom mixtures are available in our institution, the initial choice is determined by the availability of premade infusions in the hospital pharmacy. Hydromorphone is commonly the initial drug of choice, unless contraindicated. For postoperative pain control, our pharmacy offers 10 mcg/ml and 20 mcg/ml concentrations off the shelf. This is usually combined with varying concentrations of bupivacaine (0.0625–0.2%) and clonidine. When pain is in the chest or pelvic area, more dilute concentrations of local anesthetic are initially employed, whereas abdominal pain often requires higher amount of daily local anesthetic, such as bupivacaine 4–6 mg/day.

Conclusion

Intrathecal drug delivery systems (IDDS) play an important role in cancer pain management with early placement leading to improved pain control, decreased side effects, and even increased life expectancy. IDDS trials often serve as the final step in patient selection and have traditionally been used to establish the efficacy of analgesic response, create an initial dose estimation, assess a reduction in opioid-related side effects, and determine individual tolerability. Several trialing techniques have been described: bolus versus continuous infusion, single versus multiple bolus injections, and epidural versus intrathecal routes. However, no method has been shown to be superior in predicting post-implantation outcomes. Furthermore, the necessity of a trial in cancer patients, in whom life expectancy is limited and urgency is warranted, has come into question. Ultimately, determining which patients are appropriate candidates for an IDDS trial is up to the implanting physician as specific criteria do not exist.

References

1. Smith TJ, Coyne PJ, Staats PS, et al. An implantable drug delivery system (IDDS) for refractory cancer pain provides sustained pain control, less drug-related toxicity, and possibly better survival compared with comprehensive medical management (CMM). Ann Oncol. 2005;16:825–33.
2. Smith TJ, Staats PS, Deer T, et al. Randomized clinical trial of an implantable drug delivery system compared with comprehensive medical management for refractory cancer pain: impact on pain, drug-related toxicity, and survival. J Clin Oncol. 2002;20:4040–9.
3. Medicare Coverage Issues Manual. Coverage issues—durable medical equipment. www.cms.hhs.gov/manuals/downloads/Pub06_PART_60.pdf. Accessed 19 Oct 2015.
4. Deer TR, Prager J, Levy R, et al. Polyanalgesic Consensus Conference-2012: recommendations on trialing for intrathecal (intraspinal) drug delivery: report of an interdisciplinary expert panel. Neuromodulation. 2012;15(5):420–35.
5. Yoshida GM, Nelson RW, Capen DA, Nagelberg S, Thomas JC, Rimoldi RL, Haye W. Evaluation of continuous intraspinal narcotic analgesia for chronic pain from benign causes. Am J Orthop. 1996;25:693–4.
6. Onofrio BM, Yaksh TL, et al. Long-term pain relief produced by intrathecal morphine infusion in 53 patients. J Neurosurg. 1990;72:200–9.
7. Bolash R, Mekhail N. Intrathecal pain pumps indications, patient selection, techniques, and outcomes. Neurosurg Clin N Am. 2014;25:735–42.
8. Deer TR, Smith HS, Burton AW, et al. Comprehensive consensus based guidelines on intrathecal drug delivery systems in the treatment of pain caused by cancer pain. Pain Physician. 2011;14:E283–312.
9. Grider JS, Harned ME, Etscheidt MA, et al. Patient selection and outcomes using a low-dose intrathecal opioid trialing method for chronic nonmalignant pain. Pain Physician. 2011;14(4):343–51.
10. Penn RD, Paice JA. Chronic intrathecal morphine for intractable pain. J Neurosurg. 1987;67:182–6.
11. Hamza M, Doleys DM, Saleh IA, et al. A prospective, randomized, single-blinded, head-to-head long-term outcome study, comparing intrathecal (IT) boluses with continuous infusion trialing techniques prior to implantation of drug delivery systems (DDS) for the treatment of severe intractable chronic nonmalignant pain. Neuromodulation. 2015;18(7):636–48.
12. Ahmed SU, Martin NM, Chang Y, et al. Patient selection and trial methods for intraspinal drug delivery for chronic pain: a national survey. Neuromodulation. 2005;8:112–20.
13. Krames ES, Olson K. Clinical realities and economic considerations: patient selection in intrathecal therapy. J Pain Symptom Manag. 1997;14:S3–S13.
14. Du Pen SL, Williams AR. The dilemma of conversion from systemic to epidural morphine: a proposed conversion tool for treatment of cancer pain. Pain. 1994;56:113–8.
15. Malhotra VT, Root J, Kesselbrenner J, et al. Intrathecal pain pump infusions for intractable cancer pain: an algorithm for dosing without a neuraxial trial. Anesth Analg. 2013;116:1364–70.

Intrathecal Pump Implantation Technique

31

Shane E. Brogan and Christina Bokat

The delivery of intrathecal therapy for the management of cancer related pain has become an accepted modality that is associated with high success and a low complication rate [1]. Obtaining favorable outcomes while minimizing complications depends largely upon skillful catheter and implantation technique, in addition to meticulous management of the infused medications.

This chapter will focus on the implantation process, with an emphasis on presurgical preparation, the surgical procedure itself, and the immediate postoperative period. The following technical descriptions are the opinions of the authors and are intended to serve merely a guideline for the reader to develop his or her own preferences.

Presurgical Considerations

While it is possible to do a pump implant under sedation and copious local anesthesia, general anesthesia is preferred. Ensure that the patient is in an optimal state of health before proceeding to implantation. Avoid implanting a pump when there is an active infection present, and delay the case until the infection has been satisfactorily treated. Patients should be screened for staphlococcus aureus using a nasal swab culture and a positive result (whether it mehicillin resistant or not) should be treated with nasal muciporin and chlorhexidine skin decontamination [2, 3]. In diabetics, glycemic control should be optimized [4].

Imaging

In patients with known spinal metastatic disease, a recent lumbar MRI should be reviewed so that an appropriate, safe, lumbar space is identified. The intrathecal needle placement should avoid areas of significant spinal stenosis and enter at a level with sufficient CSF volume for easy catheter advancement.

Anticoagulation and Hemostasis

Because an intrathecal catheter placement involves placement of a needle into the neuraxis, there is an inherent risk of epidural hematoma formation. To mitigate this potentially catastrophic risk, every effort should be made to optimize the patient's hemostasis perioperatively. In the cancer patient, this may be particularly difficult given that many individuals will be on anticoagulants for various reasons or be thrombocytopenic secondary to their cancer treatments.

There are no specific guidelines for intrathecal catheter placement and anticoagulation, but many practitioners use the American Society of Regional Anesthesia (ASRA) recommendations [5]. Coumadin (warfarin) should be held sufficiently long to allow the INR to reach 1.4 or lower. In the setting of intravenous heparin infusions, the heparin should be discontinued for at least 4 h and a normal prothrombin time (PTT) demonstrated. For low molecular weight heparins, full-dose (therapeutic) regimens should be held for 24 h. For prophylactic regimens, the LMWH should be held for 12 h.

Guidelines regarding platelet count and neuraxial procedures are lacking. In the cancer setting, thrombocytopenia is often related to recent chemotherapy, so it is best to discuss the timing of pump implantation with the patient's oncologist so that a platelet count "nadir" is avoided. It is also important not only to simply consider the platelet count alone but also to consider the trajectory of recent platelet counts and the platelet response to previous chemotherapy cycles. Our group avoids placing an intrathecal catheter when the platelet count is less than 80,000 platelets per microliter of blood [6].

Rarely, if thrombocytopenia is persistent, a preoperative platelet transfusion may be necessary.

S. E. Brogan (✉) · C. Bokat
University of Utah, Department of Anesthesiology, Salt Lake City, UT, USA
e-mail: shane.brogan@hsc.utah.edu; christina.bokat@hsc.utah.edu

A. Gulati et al. (eds.), *Essentials of Interventional Cancer Pain Management*, https://doi.org/10.1007/978-3-319-99684-4_31

The Operating Room

An operating room with laminar air flow and restricted access is mandatory.

Drug

Prior to implantation, consider what intrathecal regimen is indicated, and the appropriate drug should be ordered in advance and be available in the operating room.

Marking

In the preoperative area, examine the patient's abdomen and decide upon an appropriate pump location. If a colostomy is present, the pump should be implanted on the contralateral side of the abdomen. Find a pump position that is acceptable to the patient, avoiding the costal margin, the iliac crest, and the beltline if possible. Mark the proposed incision with an ink skin marker.

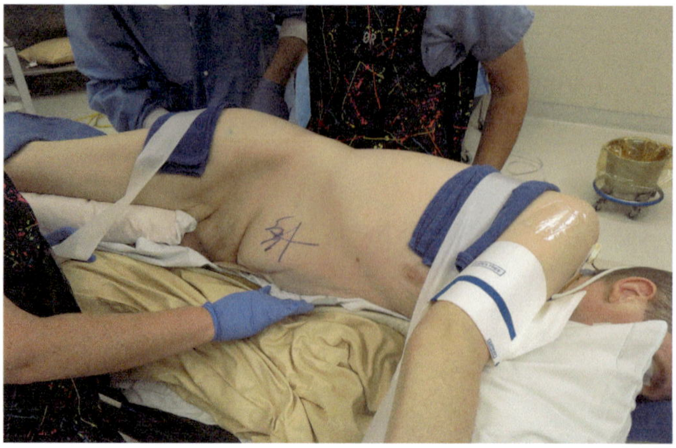

Fig. 31.1 Positioning, anterior view. Note the ample access to the abdominal surgical site and the position of the non-dependent arm

The Procedure

Positioning

The patient is positioned in the lateral decubitus position allowing ample access to the lumbar spine and the abdominal wall (Figs. 31.1 and 31.2). A "bean bag" can help with the security of positioning. An axillary roll should be placed and all pressure points padded. The non-dependent arm can be placed on pillows. Remember that a C-arm fluoroscope will be used, so ensure that the unit can easily image the lumbar and thoracic spine.

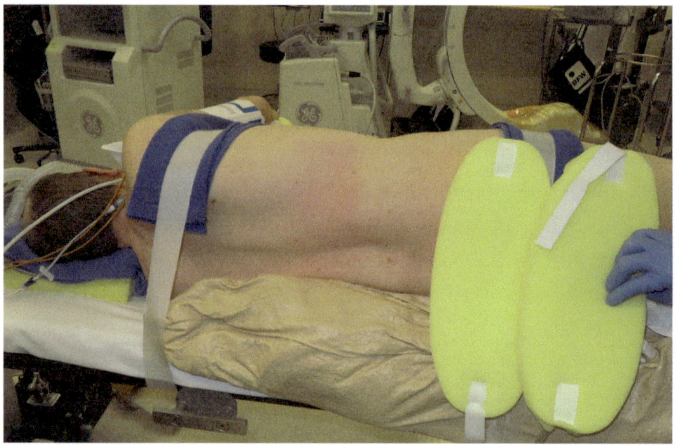

Fig. 31.2 Positioning, posterior view

Skin Preparation

The authors use alcohol as the first preparation, allowing it to completely dry. Next a chlorhexidine/alcohol solution is used (ChloraPrep®), again allowing complete drying. Always prepare a larger area than you think necessary.

Draping

Standard draping techniques are used to ensure adequate access to both surgical sites (Figs. 31.3 and 31.4). An antimicrobial adhesive material such as Ioban® can be used to minimize contact with the skin. During draping do not touch the prepped skin, if contact occurs, consider changing sterile gloves. The C-arm should also be fully draped. See Fig. 31.5 for a suggested final positioning of the surgeon and the C-arm.

Lumbar Incision and Dissection

Using anteroposterior fluoroscopy, identify the L3/4 or L4/5 interspace. Just lateral (on non-dependent side) and caudal to the desired interspace, approximating a line drawn between the pedicles, place a surgical instrument parallel to the spine, verify with fluoroscopy, and draw a line (see Fig. 31.6). Anesthetize the area with local anesthetic. With a scalpel, make a 2 cm incision (in obese patients, may need to be 3–4 cm), and obtain hemostasis with electrocautery. Place a Weitlaner, or other similar types of retractor, into the incision and retract the edges. While pulling the Weitlaner firmly toward the operator, perform electrocautery down to the dorsal fascia, taking care not to migrate too medially or laterally. The very robust

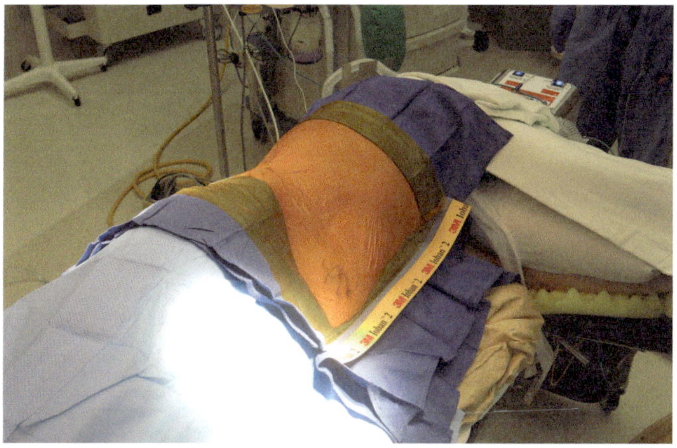

Fig. 31.3 Draping process

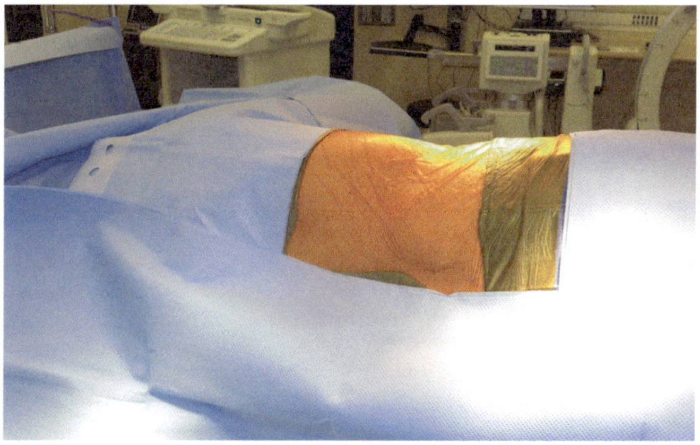

Fig. 31.4 Completed draping process, posterior view

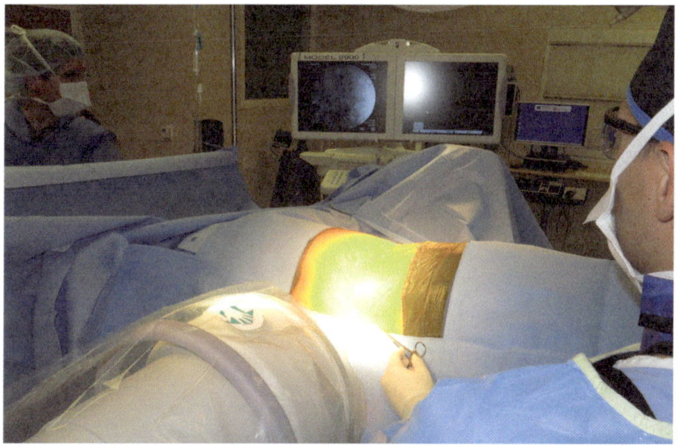

Fig. 31.5 Fluoroscopy and surgeon positioning

dorsal fascia is easily identified by its whitish color and will have muscle palpable just deep to it. Using finger dissection, expose enough fascia to allow easy anchoring of the catheter. Ensure good hemostasis.

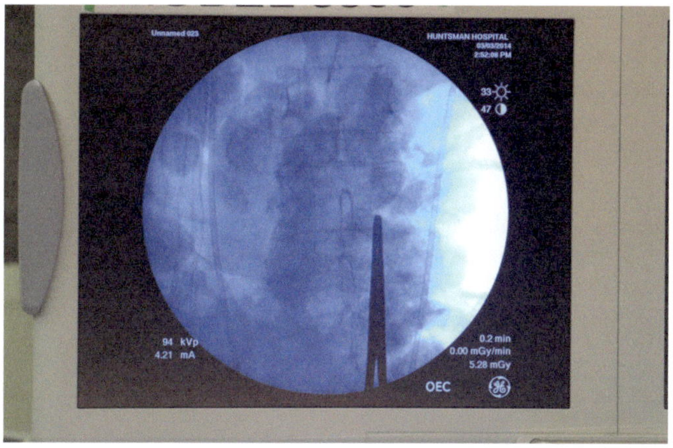

Fig. 31.6 Fluoroscopy imaging of the lumbar spine, with the instrument indicating the proposed incision site, with a suitable interspace (L3/4) just cephalad

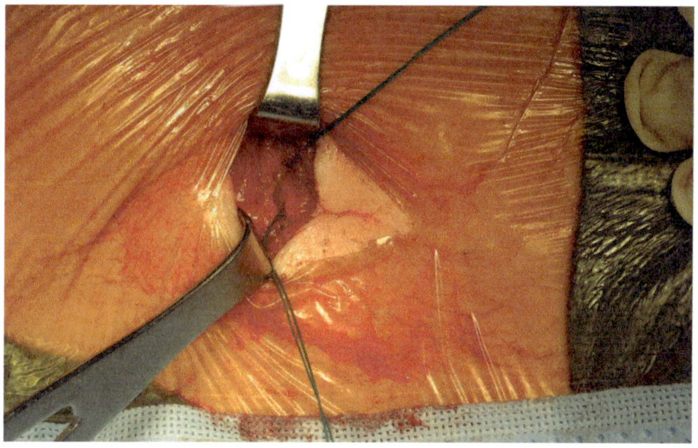

Fig. 31.7 The lumbar incision showing exposed dorsal fascia with two anchoring sutures in place. The left side of the photograph is cephalad

Anchor Placement

The authors prefer to place the anchor sutures before the needle placement because it is easier not to work around the needle (see Fig. 31.7). It should be remembered the any unnecessary movement of the needle, once intrathecal, may inadvertently enlarge the dural puncture and possible increase the likelihood of CSF leak around the catheter. Lateral to the midline, two braided and nonabsorbable sutures, such a 0-Ethibond®, are placed through the fascia about 1.5 cm apart and tied down.

Intrathecal Access

The 14-gauge intrathecal needle is then introduced between, to the anchoring sutures in a medial and cephalad direction (see Fig. 31.8). The use of fluoroscopy is preferred so that a single pass can be made into the intrathecal space, thereby minimizing the risk of multiple dural punctures and trauma to neural structures (see Fig. 31.9). Some practitioners use a loss of resistance technique to first identify the epidural space, but this is not necessary.

Advance the needle slowly, checking for CSF return intermittently. With experience, the resistance of the ligamentum flavum will be noted, and then a "pop" as the dura is pierced. Once the needle is in a subarachnoid position, clear CSF should return briskly. Re-stylet the needle to avoid excessive CSF loss.

Catheter Placement

Remove the stylet and introduce the catheter (see Fig. 31.10). Advance under intermittent or continuous fluoroscopy, watching for appropriate cephalad movement without any kinking (see Fig. 31.11). The ultimate catheter tip location is a matter of anecdotal physician preference, but most providers aim to place the catheter tip in a position appropriate to treat the dermatomal distribution of the patient's pain location. For example, abdominal pain may respond best to a catheter tip in the T1-4 range, so that if local anesthetics are used, the splanchnic nerve roots are targeted, with minimal risk of local anesthetic effect on the lumbar nerve roots and the development of lower extremity weakness. See Table 31.1 for further suggestions.

Once the catheter tip is an appropriate position, carefully remove the needle, taking care to maintain the catheter in the same position. Next, the catheter stylet is removed. After a couple of minutes, CSF should be seen slowly dripping from the proximal orifice of the catheter.

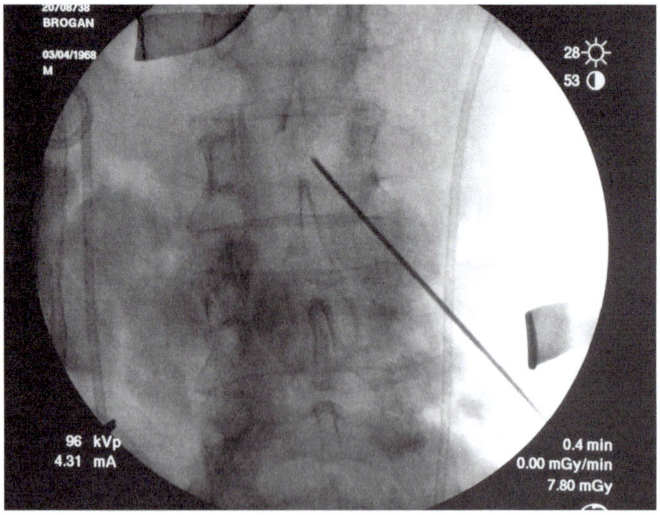

Fig. 31.9 Flouroscopic view of the needle being advanced toward the L2/3 interlaminar space

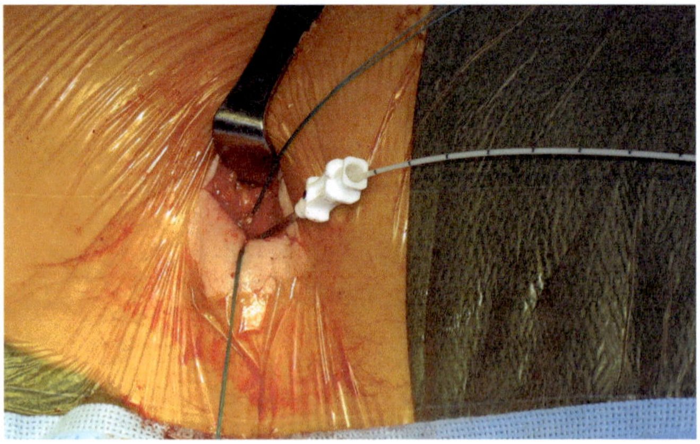

Fig. 31.10 The catheter has been placed through the needle and into the intrathecal space

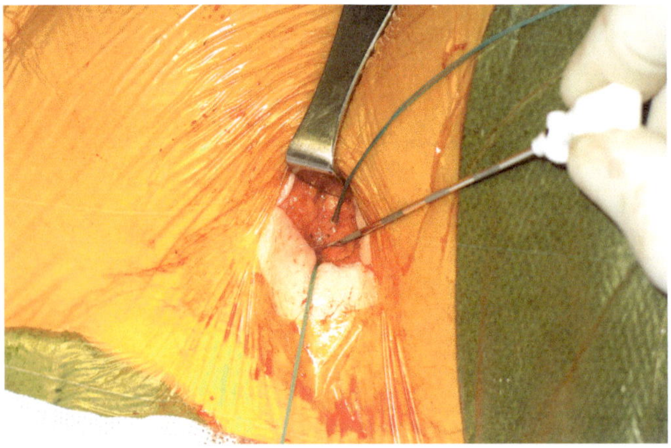

Fig. 31.8 The needle is being introduced between the two anchoring sutures and angled cephalad

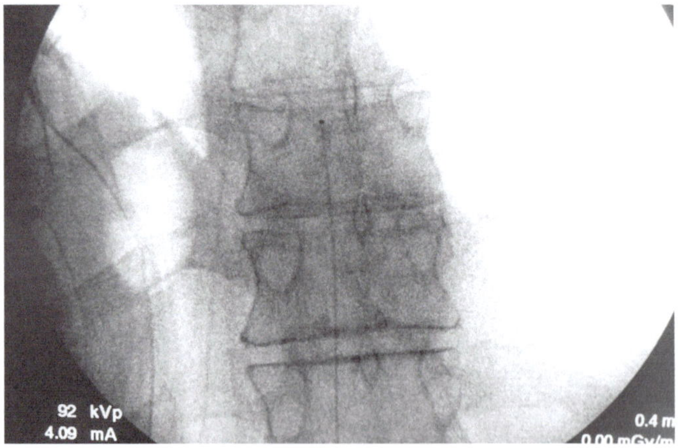

Fig. 31.11 Note the presence of the catheter in the spinal canal with the tip more prominent due to its obvious radiopaque "bead" at T9/10

Table 31.1 Suggested intrathecal catheter tip locations for the management of selected regional pain location

Worst pain location	Catheter tip location
Head and neck	C1-C2
Upper extremity	C3-C6
Abdominal and thoracic	C7-T6
Lower extremity and pelvic	T6 and below

Note that there is no clinical data on this, and this information is based more on anecdotal experience

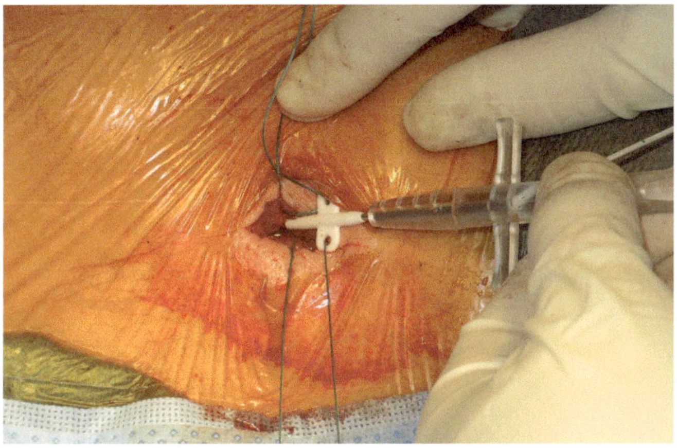

Fig. 31.12 The anchoring device has been placed on the catheter and is being advanced toward the dorsal fascia. Note that the anchoring sutures have been loaded through the eyelets at this point

Catheter Anchoring

Use the manufacturer's supplied anchoring device and fix to the fascia using the anchoring sutures placed previously. See Figs. 31.12, 31.13, and 31.14 for additional information. Ensure that there is the least possible distance between the catheter anchoring site and the catheter point of entry through the fascia – this minimizes the risk of spontaneous catheter migration out of the intrathecal space.

Myelogram

The myelogram is optional but confirms satisfactory intrathecal placement of the catheter and rules out an inadvertent epidural, subdural, or intravascular location. A 3 ml syringe may be attached to the catheter by carefully introducing a 25-gauge needle into the catheter lumen. Inject 1–3 ml of myelographically safe contrast solution under live AP fluoroscopy. A myelogram should be observed with the contrast layering in the dependent (down) lateral margin of the intrathecal space in a "scalloping" pattern (see Figs. 31.15 and 31.16). Observe for any intravascular uptake or a contrast pattern that looks more typical for epidural or subdural

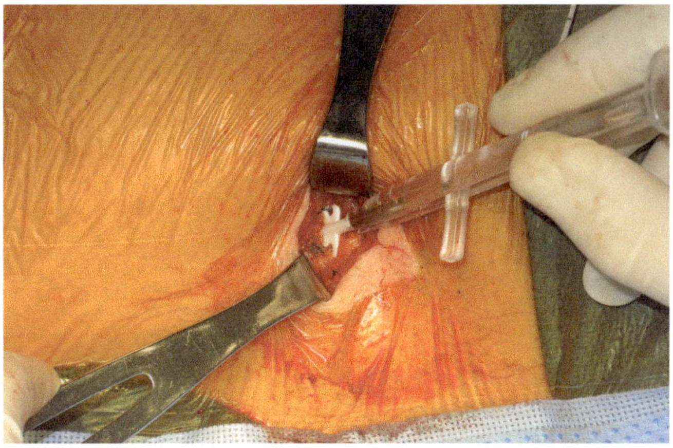

Fig. 31.13 The tip of the anchoring device has been advanced into the dorsal fascia and the anchoring suture tied and cut

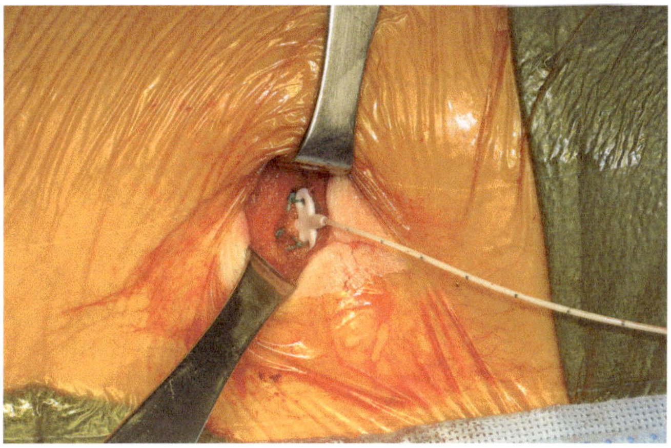

Fig. 31.14 The anchoring device has been deployed and removed, completing the anchoring process

spread. It will be noted that the contrast dissipates over several minutes.

Pump Pocket Creation

A 7–8 cm incision is made over the location decided upon in the preoperative area, and good hemostasis is achieved using electrocautery. Using retractors, simultaneously retract and pull the skin edges outward. In a thin patient, dissect directly down to the rectus fascia (see Fig. 31.17), which can be easily identified by its twitching response to electrocautery. In an obese patient, the rectus fascia will be too deep to allow for easy pump refills, so a more superficial plane 1–3 cm deep into the skin should be identified. Using blunt dissection, extend the plane of the pocket caudally approximately 8–10 cm. Also dissect in a cephalad direction for a couple of centimeters – this allows for eas-

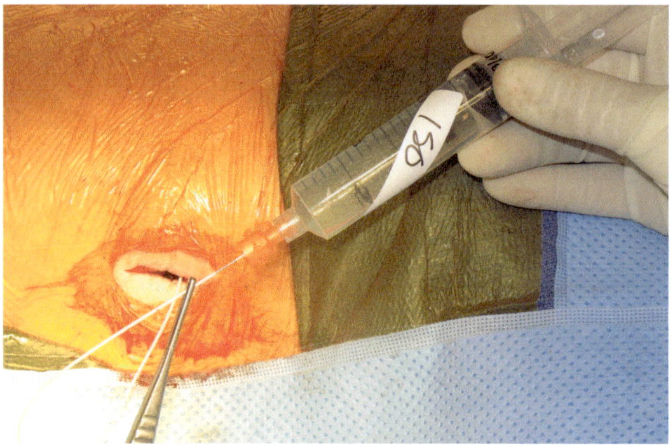

Fig. 31.15 A syringe of radiopaque contrast is attached to the intrathecal catheter

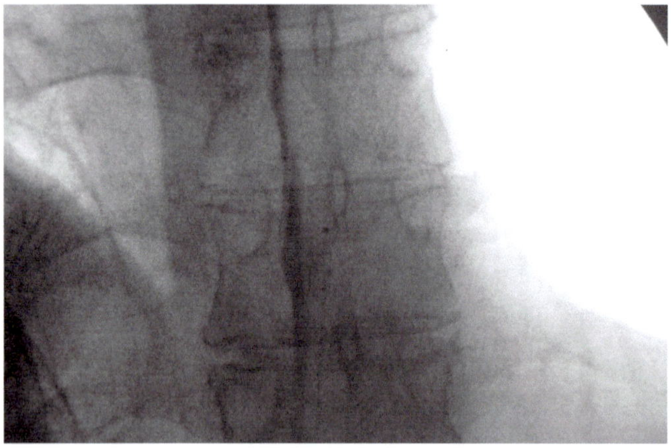

Fig. 31.16 Demonstrated is a typical myelogram on the dependent side

ier anchoring and skin closure. A useful guide is that four fingers should be easily introduced into the pocket. Ensure good hemostasis.

Anchor Placement

Next, nonabsorbable sutures should be placed in the fascia for anchoring of the pump (Fig. 31.18). Some practitioners skip this step, but this is not recommended, as good anchoring prevents rotational movement of the pump and kinking of the catheter and ensures that the pump does not flip upside-down. Three to four anchoring sutures are generally used, often in the approximate 4, 8, and 10 o'clock positions. Tie each suture to the fascia and clip to the drapes to avoid tangling.

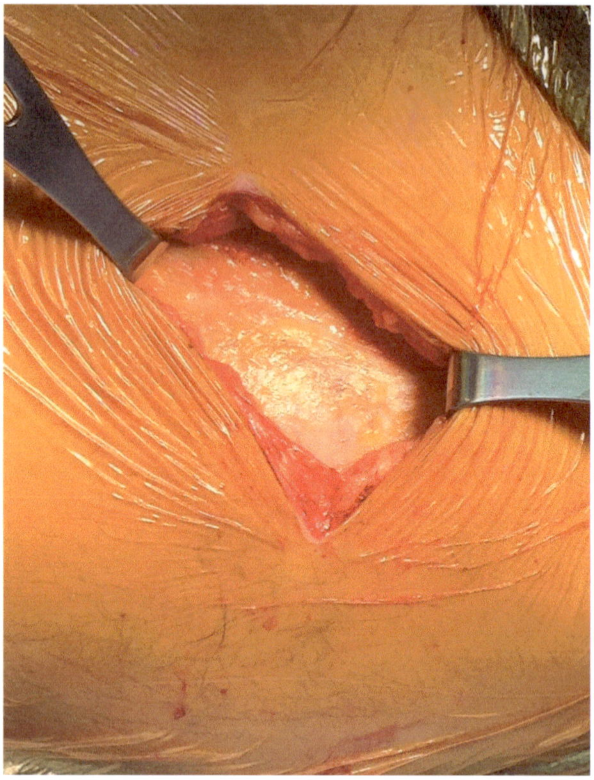

Fig. 31.17 The abdominal incision after dissection down to the rectus fascia

Tunneling

First, ensure that the supplied tunneling tool is long enough to connect the lumbar and abdominal incisions. It is best to tunnel from the lumbar incision, starting as caudal as possible (to avoid acute angles with the catheter) and in the same fascial plane as the anchoring (Figs. 31.18 and 31.19). Placing a gentle curve in the tunneling tool will facilitate easier advancement around the flank. Firm pressure should be applied, and the tool should advance without excessive force if in an appropriate plane. It is very important to keep track of the tool's tip and ensure that it does not dive too deep. Keep cephalad to the iliac crest so that a future hip operation does not jeopardize the catheter. When approaching the pump pocket, try to enter the pocket as deep as possible. Remove the handle and stylet and advance the catheter through the tunneling tool until visible in the pocket and carefully withdraw the tool from the abdominal side. Pull the catheter through until a loose "J" is observed in the lumbar incision. Trim the proximal catheter so that 6–10 cm is visible in the pocket – the discarded catheter segment must be measured so that the final catheter volume is accurately known. Ensure ongoing flow of CSF through the catheter.

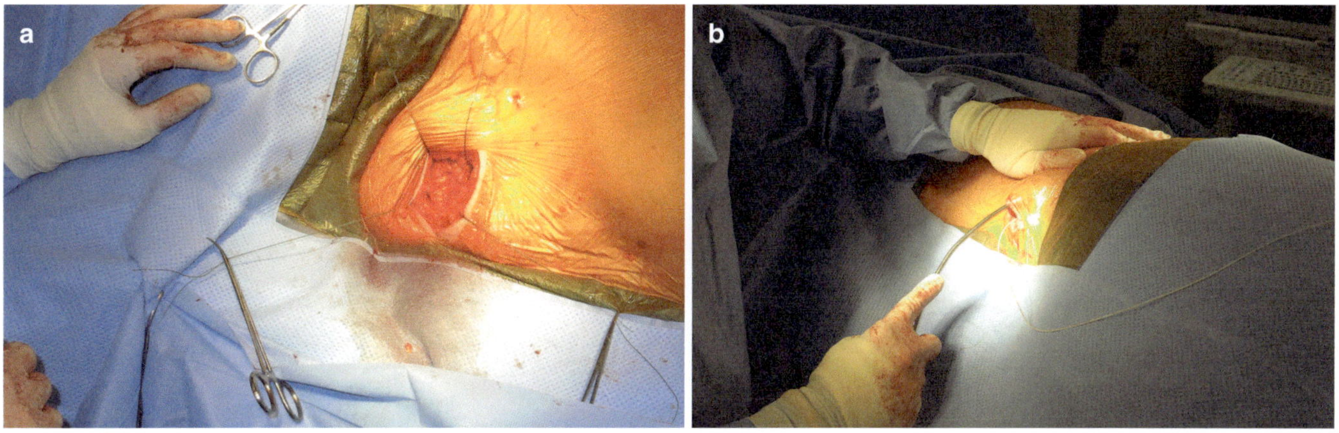

Fig. 31.18 (**a**) The pump pocket with placement of three anchoring sutures. (**b**) Tunneling from the lumbar incision to the pump pocket

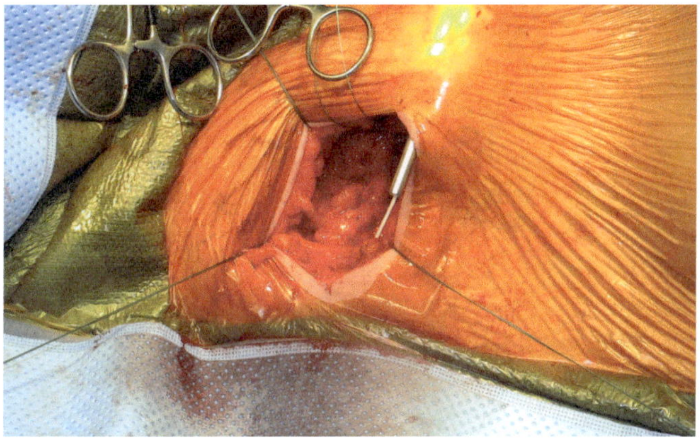

Fig. 31.19 The tunneling tool in the pump pocket, with the intrathecal catheter visible

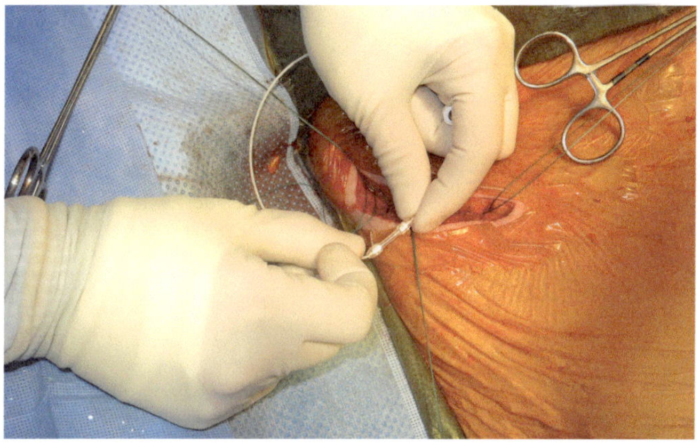

Fig. 31.20 Attaching the intrathecal segment to the pump segment

Pump Insertion

During the steps the pump should be loaded with the appropriate drug to the manufacturer's specifications. Copiously irrigate the pump pocket with saline or antibiotic solution. Before handling the pump, consider changing to a new pair of sterile gloves. Connect the pump to the catheter using the manufacturer's connector device (Figs. 31.20 and 31.21). Place the previously placed anchoring sutures through the appropriate pump eyelets, and insert the pump into the pocket (Figs. 31.22 and 31.23). The pump fit should be snug yet allow for easy closure of the fascia and skin with minimal tension. The excess catheter should be loosely coiled behind the pump so that future pump refills do not place the catheter at risk for puncture. Tie the anchoring sutures sufficiently to keep the pump in position.

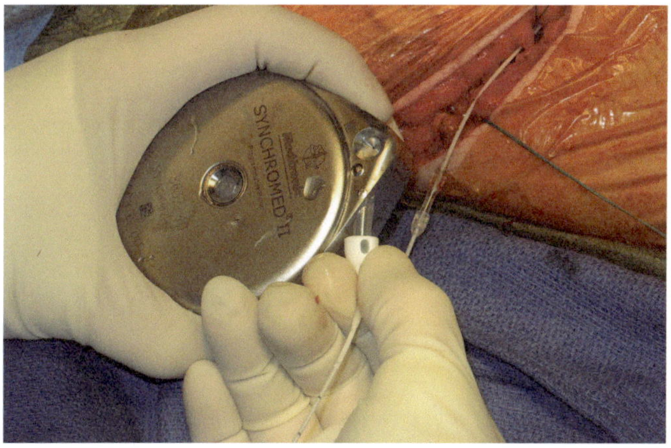

Fig. 31.21 Connecting the catheter to the pump

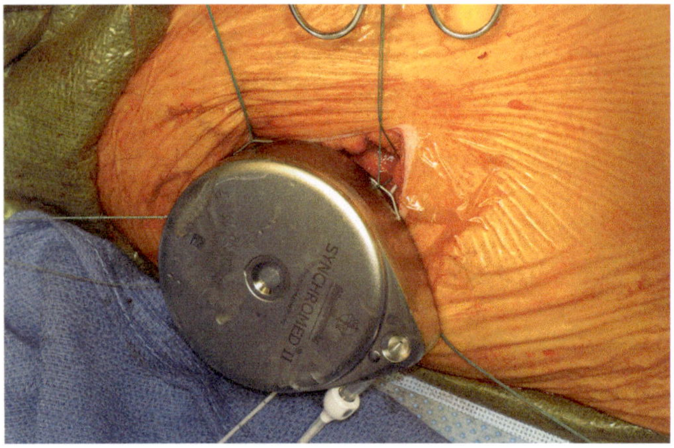

Fig. 31.22 The anchoring sutures have been placed through the pump eyelets in preparation for anchoring to the fascia

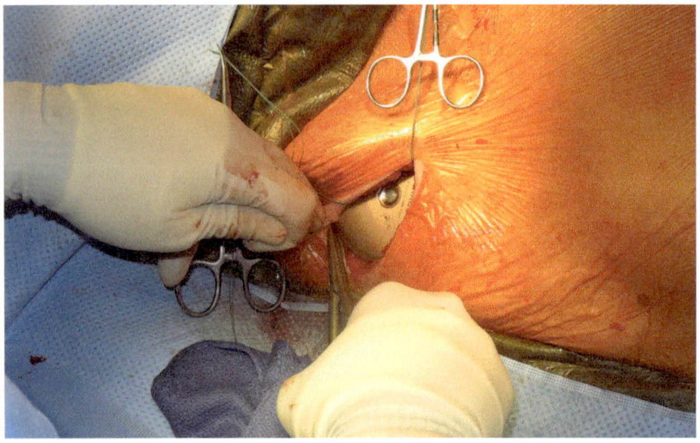

Fig. 31.23 The pump is placed in the pocket and the anchor sutures are tied and cut

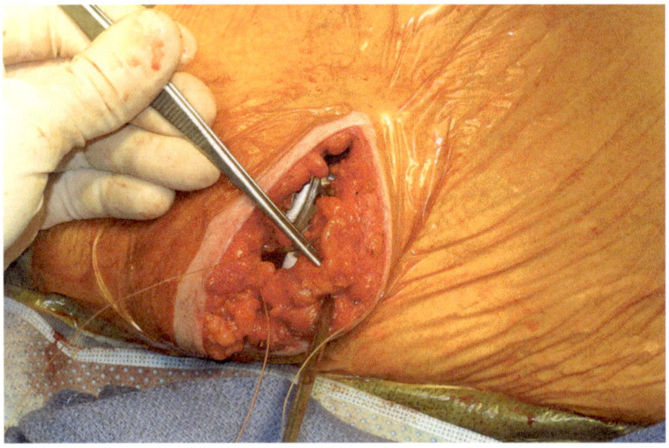

Fig. 31.24 Closing the deep layer

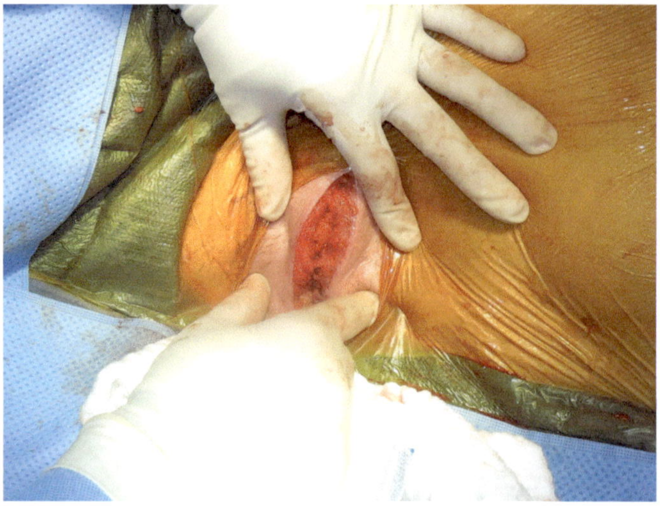

Fig. 31.25 The deep layer is closed. Note that traction of the incision does not reveal any of the pump elements

Skin Closure

Closure is performed in three layers to ensure optimal microbial resistance, wound integrity, and cosmetic appearance.

The deep fascial layers are closed with an absorbable, braided suture like 0 Vicryl® (Fig. 31.24). The goal with closure of the deep layers is that, when complete, the pump or catheter elements are neither visible nor palpable (Fig. 31.25).

The lumbar incision deep layer should include a bite of the prevertebral fascia (taking care not to damage or kink the catheter) so that a potential space for seroma development is minimized. Two-to-three interrupted sutures typically are sufficient for the lumbar deep layers.

For the abdominal deep layer, good approximation can be obtained using either interrupted sutures or a running suture.

Closure of the skin is more an issue of surgeon preference. Staples, simple nonabsorbable sutures, and an absorbable technique are all acceptable closure techniques. The authors prefer the latter because of a better cosmetic appearance and the fact that suture or staple removal is not required. Our skin closure technique is an interrupted deep dermal suture with 3-0 Vicryl® or equivalent, then a running subcuticular suture with 4-0 Monocryl® or equivalent. Finally, liquid cyanoacrylate tissue adhesive (Dermabond®) is used to provide additional closure integrity and microbial resistance (Fig. 31.26). With this technique a dressing is not required, but we often apply a clear adhesive dressing to keep the area clean.

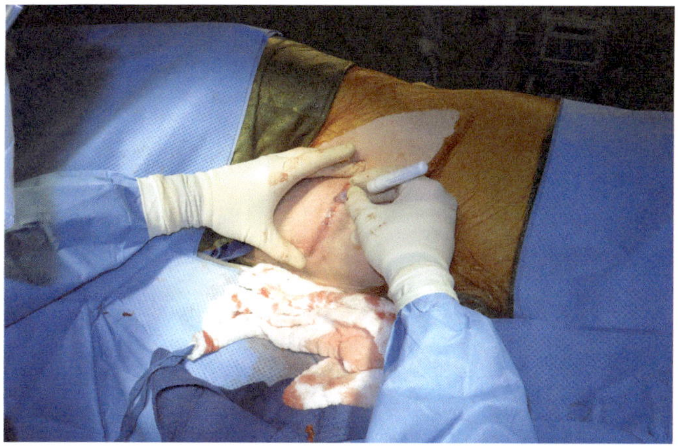

Fig. 31.26 The closure is complete and a tissue adhesive is being applied

Postoperative Period

An abdominal binder is placed snuggly around the abdomen to minimize the risk of seroma in the pump pocket, and patients are advised to wear it for 2 weeks.

The pump is programmed in the postoperative area taking care to calculate the implanted catheter length accurately and initiate appropriate basal and patient-activated intrathecal dosing.

We routinely admit our patients overnight for the following reasons: (1) safety concerns after initiation of intrathecal opioids, (2) frequent medical comorbidities including obstructive sleep apnea, and (3) allow for rapid and safe transition from conventional opioids to intrathecal opioids only.

Follow-Up

Patients are discharged with careful instructions regarding being vigilant for signs of infection or other complications. It is advisable to see patients in follow-up within a week or less to ensure intrathecal drug efficacy and screen for concerning side effects or complications. Given that the highest incidence of pump infection is in the 2–4-week postoperative period, it is also advisable to see patients during this time.

References

1. Smith TJ, Staats PS, et al. Randomized clinical trial of an implantable drug delivery system compared with comprehensive medical management for refractory cancer pain: impact on pain, drug-related toxicity, and survival. J Clin Oncol. 2002;20(19):4040–9.
2. Bode LG, Klyuymtans JA, Wertheim HF et al. Preventing surgical-site infections in nasal carriers of Staphylococcus aureus. N Engl J Med. 2010;362(1):9–17.
3. Epstein NE. Preoperative, intraoperative, and postoperative measures to further reduce spinal infections. Surg Neurol Int. 2011;2:17.
4. Deer TR, Levy R, et al. Polyanalgesic consensus conference – 2012: recommendations to reduce morbidity and mortality in intrathecal drug delivery in the treatment of chronic pain. Neuromodulation. 2012;15(5):467–82.
5. Horlocker TT, Wedel DJ, et al. Executive summary: regional anesthesia in the patient receiving antithrombotic or thrombolytic therapy: American society of regional anesthesia and pain medicine evidence-based guidelines (third edition). Reg Anesth Pain Med. 2010;35(1):102–5.
6. van Veen JJ, Nokes TJ, et al. The risk of spinal haematoma following neuraxial anaesthesia or lumbar puncture in thrombocytopenic individuals. Br J Haematol. 2010;148(1):15–25.

32 Medications in Intrathecal Pumps

Grant H. Chen

There are currently three medications approved by the Food and Drug Administration (FDA) for intrathecal (IT) drug use [1]. Of the three medications, morphine and ziconotide are approved for the treatment of pain, while baclofen is approved for severe spasticity. However, there are many other medications such as bupivacaine and clonidine that can be used intrathecally for the treatment of cancer pain. When considering and adjusting IT medication in cancer pain, one should keep in mind that the dosing may fall outside the standard recommended practice.

Opioids

In 1979, Wang et al. demonstrated significant pain relief using IT morphine in humans [2]. Opioids commonly used for IT therapy include morphine, hydromorphone, fentanyl, and sufentanil. Other opioids such as meperidine, methadone, and tramadol have demonstrated neurotoxicity and are not recommended for IT use [3].

Morphine

Morphine is a mu-opioid receptor agonist with its primary pain modulation in the dorsal horn of the spinal cord. It has been administered as IT therapy for decades [4] and is most commonly used as first-line IT therapy for cancer. Morphine is effective for nociceptive or mixed pain, both neuropathic and nociceptive pain.

Multiple retrospective and prospective studies support the efficacy of long-term intrathecal monotherapy morphine in the reduction of visual analog scale scores in non-cancer pain [5, 6]. A randomized control trial by Smith et al. for IT morphine in patients with cancer pain concluded that patient who received medication intrathecally demonstrated improved clinical success in pain control, reduced pain, relieved drug toxicities, and improved survival [7]. However, in this trial, patients were switched to other IT medications if morphine was unsuccessful in controlling pain. In addition, the patients did not strictly adhere to the treatment that they were randomized into. In a prospective study, Rauck et al. showed a significant, long-term decrease in pain scores in patients with refractory cancer pain using a patient-controlled analgesia intrathecal delivery system with IT morphine [8].

There are also multiple studies evaluating the efficacy of IT morphine as a combination therapy with other medications such as bupivacaine, ziconotide, and clonidine. Several studies demonstrated the effectiveness of IT morphine with bupivacaine in long-term pain control for patients with refractory pain secondary to cancer [9–12].

Starting dose of morphine varies when considering cancer patient. Often, oncologic patients are on high doses of opioids and thus, opioid tolerant. In addition, direct conversion of oral or parental opioid varies depending on different resources and literature. While a conservative starting dose conversation of 300:1 oral to intrathecal morphine ratio has been recommended, a more aggressive 100:1 ratio may be more appropriate for cancer patients with overnight monitoring after the placement of the pump. Starting dose for IT morphine may range anywhere from 0.1 to 50 mg/day depending on the patient's opioid tolerance. In a retrospective review of cancer patients receiving chronic IT morphine, increases in opioid dosing was noted over time [13] which may be secondary to tolerance but may also be due to other factors such as physician practice preferences or worsening development of cancer. For patients with concerns of current or future opioid tolerance, a pump with larger reservoir is recommended to hold more volume. Higher concentration of IT morphine should be used as well in anticipation of rapid increases in infusion rate post pump placement.

G. H. Chen (✉)
Memorial Sloan Kettering Cancer Center, Department of Anesthesiology and Critical Care Medicine, New York, NY, USA
e-mail: cheng@mskcc.org

A. Gulati et al. (eds.), *Essentials of Interventional Cancer Pain Management*, https://doi.org/10.1007/978-3-319-99684-4_32

Most side effects of IT morphine are dose dependent. The most common side effect is pruritus and is likely localized to the face, neck, or upper chest [14]. Other side effects of IT morphine include sedation, nausea, sexual dysfunction, immunosuppression, respiratory depression, peripheral edema, constipation, and urinary retention [15]. Prolong use of IT morphine can also lead to granuloma formation, hyperalgesia, and tolerance to the medication. Higher concentration and lower flow rates of IT morphine have been postulated as a risk factor for granuloma but not definitively proven.

In addition, adverse events such as withdrawal symptoms can occur because of pump dysfunction. Rare cases of naloxone-reversible nystagmus have been reported with IT morphine. Risks of IT morphine should be discussed with all patients considering long-term therapy.

Hydromorphone

Like morphine, hydromorphone acts on the opioid receptors. A conservative starting dose of IT hydromorphone in patients taking oral hydromorphone is 300:1, oral to intrathecal. However, like morphine, a possible more aggressive starting dose of 100:1 may be necessary in cancer patients [16]. Hydromorphone can also be used as opioid rotation in patients who are tolerant to morphine.

Fentanyl

Fentanyl is another opioid medication that is more lipophilic compared to morphine and hydromorphone. Due to the lipophilic nature of fentanyl and its short duration in the cerebrospinal fluid, the medication should be delivered as close to the affected dermatome as possible. There are reports that lower extremity edema secondary to IT morphine or hydromorphone can be resolved by switching to IT fentanyl infusion [17]. Starting dose can range from 25 to 500mcg/day with no known maximum daily dose.

Sufentanil

Like fentanyl, sufentanil is lipophilic and thus cephalad migration is less common. However, the medication should also be delivered as close to the affected dermatome as possible. Starting dose can range anywhere between 10 and 100 mcg/day. Again, a maximum daily dose has not been described and likely limited by side effects and infusion concentrations and flow rates of the infusion device.

Ziconotide

Ziconotide is a non-opioid analgesic approved by the FDA only for intrathecal use. The drug is a synthetic derivative of the toxin from the venomous predatory cone snail, *Conus magus* [18]. The peptides bind to presynaptic N-type voltage-sensitive calcium channels and block nociceptive signals in the Rexed lamina I and II of the spinal cord's dorsal horn [19]. A multicenter, randomized, placebo-controlled trial involving patients with chronic pain from either cancer or AIDS showed that the IT ziconotide received a significant reduction in mean VAS scores compared to the placebo group. Another study of 20 patients with bone metastasis showed that the combination of IT ziconotide and morphine was rapidly effective in the treatment of pain [20]. The former study also showed that ziconotide produced vestibular adverse events including confusion (more common in the elderly), somnolence, fever, and urinary retention than placebo [21]. In addition, patients on IT ziconotide can experience increase in creatinine kinase so serum levels should be monitored periodically.

Acute psychotic events have been documented in patients on ziconotide including hallucination, paranoia, delirium, and psychosis [22]. Also, ziconotide has been associated with an increased risk of suicidality even in patient without symptoms of depression [23]. Given the multitude of psychiatric and cognitive problems that may arise with IT ziconotide, the medication may not be ideal as the first-line therapy for cancer patients. On the other hand, unlike IT opioid infusion, animal studies have suggested that chronic infusion of ziconotide produces minimal tolerance due to their mechanism of action [24].

Recommended starting dose according to the fourth Polyanalgesic Consensus Conference (PACC) report in 2012 for ziconotide is 0.5–2.4 mcg/day with a maximum of 19.2 mcg/day. Given the medication's narrow therapeutic window, a slow titration is necessary to limit dose-limiting side effects. There are no reports of respiratory depression in patients receiving IT ziconotide. In addition, a benefit of ziconotide is that the medication can be stopped abruptly without any adverse withdrawal effects [25].

Local Anesthetics

Bupivacaine

Bupivacaine is an amide local anesthetic that is often used as a combination therapy with opioid for cancer pain. Dose escalation of opioid may lead to significant side effects so adding bupivacaine at the appropriate level may be beneficial. Starting dose for bupivacaine varies depending on the patient as well as location of the pain. Recommended starting dose for patient is 3–6 mg/day [26]. However, physicians should be cognizant of multiple factors that can increase or decrease the dose. As with opioids, standard guidelines should not be strictly applied to oncology patients. For end-stage and severe cancer pain, consider a higher starting dose of 8–10 mg/day. On the other hand, patient with lumbar or sacral catheter tips who are susceptible to falls or those with neurologic dysfunction should be started on a lower dose [27]. Lower thoracic and lumbar catheters may be started at a lower dose, while sacral catheters should be started at 1–2 mg/day with close monitoring of bladder and lower extremity weakness. Cervical catheters also should also be started at a decreased dose (4 mg/day) secondary to possible upper extremity weakness. Of note, patient with severe terminal pain may need a higher starting dose regardless of the location of the catheter simply to provide numbness without consideration of weakness. At our institution, inpatients with a catheter at the conus may start as high as 8 mg/day of bupivacaine. This may cause weakness or paralysis of the lower extremities, but it will also provide some comfort for end-of-life care.

The maximum dose of the medication can vary depending on the level of the catheter tip, but at around 20 mg/day of bupivacaine, side effects are often experienced. Side effects include reversible upper and lower extremity weakness and sensory deficits, urinary retention, hypotension, respiratory depression, seizures, and cardiotoxicity [28].

Ropivacaine

Ropivacaine is another amide local anesthetic developed with less cardiotoxicity than bupivacaine [29]. With a similar onset, potency, and block time as bupivacaine, the reduced toxicity of ropivacaine is very favorable. However there have not been many published studies regarding longer-term IT ropivacaine for use in chronic pain or cancer pain.

Clonidine

Clonidine is an α_2-adrenergic agonist that has been shown to be effective in the treatment of cancer pain especially in the treatment of neuropathic pain [30]. The Polyanalgesic Consensus Conference 2012 considers intrathecal clonidine as a second-line medication for the treatment or nociceptive and neuropathic pain. Clonidine has been postulated to stimulate cholinergic interneurons in the spinal cord by increasing cerebrospinal fluid acetylcholine levels as well as increase acetylcholine in the dorsal horn [31]. There are also increasing evidence that clonidine may mitigate pain using immunomodulation by blocking neuroimmune activation associated with neuropathic pain [32]. In addition, IT clonidine does not interact with opioid [33] receptors making it a good medication to use synergistically with opioids.

IT clonidine should be started at a rate of 25–50 mcg/day and titrated up barring any side effects. Hypotension was the most commonly observed side effect affecting approximately 25% of patients [34]. Other side effects include malaise, impotence, headache, dry mouth, sedation, and confusion. Notably, the abrupt cessation of clonidine can lead to rebound systemic hypertension which may be an emergency. In a survey of pain physician using IT pumps, the mean highest dose of clonidine was 474 mcg/day [35]. Clonidine can be increased to a maximum of 700 mcg/day.

Dexmedetomidine

Like clonidine, dexmedetomidine acts as an α_2-adrenergic agonist. There are no large systematic studies for IT dexmedetomidine. There are reports that IT dexmedetomidine augments the effects of IT morphine in cancer patients [36]. However, the drug has been found to be neurotoxic in animal models [37].

Baclofen

Baclofen is an agonist at the γ-aminobutyric acid B receptor site. The medication is FDA approved for intrathecal use and inhibits sensory information to the motor neurons of the spinal cord for the treatment of severe spasticity of spinal [38] or cerebral [39] origin as well as neuropathic pain. Baclofen is 5th in line for neuropathic pain according to the PACC and not recommended for nociceptive pain. In a 10-year study of over 300 patients on IT baclofen for spasticity of spinal or cerebral origin, most patients were found to have improvements in spasticity without any observable tolerance to the medication [40]. On the other hand, tolerance was noted in 22% of patient on long-term IT therapy in a study for 37 patients [41]. A major risk factor for IT baclofen is that abrupt discontinuation can be life-threatening [42]. It can cause a variety of symptoms including spasticity, hyperthermia, hemodynamic instability, seizures, rhabdomyolysis, disseminated intravascular coagulation, and multisystem organ failure. Treatment is primarily baclofen and benzodiazepine, while other adjunctive medications such as antiepileptics, beta blockers, cyproheptadine, and clonidine can also be used. The patient should also be admitted as an inpatient to monitor for hemodynamic changes. Baclofen has been implicated in the development and mild progression of scoliosis [43]. Typical starting dose for baclofen in the treatment of spasticity is 10–100 mcg/day.

Ketamine

Ketamine is a noncompetitive N-methyl-D-aspartate (NMDA) receptor antagonist that, when infused intrathecally, has been shown to cause demyelination and lesions to the spinal cord in canines [44] as well as forebrain apoptosis in rats [45]. Postmortem finding in a case report of an oncology patient with IT ketamine showed extensive subpial vacuolation and near circular loss of myelin staining [46]. It is not recommended for chronic IT administration but may be considered for terminal cancer pain. In a double-blinded, crossover trial of 20 patients comparing IT morphine with 1 mg of ketamine versus morphine only, the group with ketamine performed better over a brief period of time [47]. Recommended starting dose for IT ketamine is 25–1000 mcg/day [48]. (Tables 32.1 and 32.2).

Table 32.1 Dosing for intrathecal medications

Drug	Recommended starting dose	Recommended maximum dose for cancer pain[a]
Morphine	0.1–50 mg/day	50 mg/day
Hydromorphone	0.1–50 mg/day	50 mg/day
Fentanyl	25–500 mcg/day	No known maximum
Sufentanil	10–100 mcg/day	No known maximum
Ziconotide	0.5–2.4 mcg/day	19.2 mcg/day
Bupivacaine[b]	3–6 mg/day	20 mg/day
Clonidine	25–50 mcg/day	700 mcg/day
Baclofen[c]	10–100 mcg/day	

[a]At the Memorial Sloan Kettering Cancer Center
[b]Dependent on catheter location
[c]Curr Pain Headache Rep (2014) 18:391

Table 32.2 Maximum concentration for intrathecal medication

Drug	Maximum concentration for non-cancer pain[a]	Maximum concentration for cancer pain[b]
Morphine	20 mg/ml	90 mg/ml
Hydromorphone	15 mg/ml	90 mg/ml
Fentanyl	10 mg/ml	10 mg/ml
Sufentanil	5 mg/ml	5 mg/ml
Ziconotide	100 mcg/ml	100 mcg/ml
Bupivacaine[a]	30 mg/ml	40 mg/ml
Clonidine	1000 mcg/ml	2000 mcg/ml
Baclofen		4 mg/ml

[a]Recommendations from Polyanalgesic Consensus Conference 2012
[b]At Memorial Sloan Kettering Cancer Center and compounded by MasterPharm™

Titration and Bolus of Intrathecal Medications

Opioid

Multiple adjustments of IT medication are usually necessary post intrathecal pump placement. Aggressive daily adjustments will require inpatient monitoring for signs of weakness, respiratory depression, and drug toxicity. At our institution with single-agent, opioid-only medication, the daily dose can be increased every 24 h by up to 25% as necessary. Bolus dosing can begin at approximately 5–10% of the daily dose with a minimum lockout time of every 4 h. Following evaluation, the lockout time can then be decreased as needed based on the severity of the patient's pain and how frequently the patient uses the bolus dosing.

Bupivacaine

In patients with IT bupivacaine, the increases should be prudent. Side effects such as weakness and numbness should be evaluated with each increase in dosing especially with catheter tips near the cervical or sacral spine.

As for maintenance of the patient's breakthrough pain, a bolus of up to 10% of the daily bupivacaine dose is recommended with a lockout period of 3 h. This is usually started on post-op day 2 as needed. Again, the dosing and lockout period should be tailored to the patient's specific situation while being cognizant of the bupivacaine's side effects. For example, in a patient with a very limited lifespan, the IT bupivacaine rate can be increased more rapidly for comfort care and pain control.

Ziconotide

Ziconotide can be titrated up by a maximum of 2.4 mcg/day up to three times per week until the maximum dose of 19.2 mcg/day is reached. The use of bolus dosing in IT ziconotide has been demonstrated to be useful in pain control [49] despite controversy regarding ziconotide's label stating its contraindication for bolus dosing [50]. However, the use of bolus dosing has not been well evaluated with ziconotide. Given ziconotide's narrow therapeutic window, care must be taken to ensure that the patients do not get more than the maximum allowable daily dose of the medication. According to PACC, the recommended dosing is 1–5 mcg initially.

References

1. Bottros MM, Christo PJ. Current perspectives on intrathecal drug delivery. J Pain Res. 2014;7:615–26.
2. Wang JK, Nauss LA, Thomas JE. Pain relief by intrathecally applied morphine in man. Anesthesiology. 1979;50(2):149–51.
3. Deer TR, Prager J, Levy R, et al. Polyanalgesic consensus conference 2012: recommendations for the management of pain by intrathecal (intraspinal) drug delivery: report of an interdisciplinary expert panel. Neuromodulation. 2012;15(5):436–64.
4. Hassenbusch SJ, Pillay PK, Magdinec M, et al. Constant infusion of morphine for intractable cancer pain using an implanted pump. J Neurosurg. 1990;73(3):405–9.
5. Atli A, Theodore BR, Turk DC, et al. Intrathecal opioid therapy for chronic nonmalignant pain: a retrospective cohort study with 3-year follow-up. Pain Med. 2010;11(7):1010–6.
6. Reig E, Abejon D. Continuous morphine infusion: a retrospective study of efficacy, safety, and demographic variables. Neuromodulation. 2009;12(2):122–9.
7. Smith TJ, Staats PS, Deer T, et al. Randomized clinical trial of an implantable drug delivery system compared with comprehensive medical management for refractory cancer pain: impact on pain, drug-related toxicity, and survival. J Clin Oncol. 2002;20(19):4040–9.
8. Rauck RL, Cherry D, Boyer MF, et al. Long-term intrathecal opioid therapy with a patient-activated, implanted delivery system for the treatment of refractory cancer pain. J Pain. 2003;4(8):441–7.
9. Sjöberg M, Appelgren L, Einarsson S, et al. Long-term intrathecal morphine and bupivacaine in "refractory" cancer pain. I. Results from the first series of 52 patients. Acta Anaesthesiol Scand. 1991;35(1):30–43.
10. Sjöberg M, Nitescu P, Appelgren L, et al. Long-term intrathecal morphine and bupivacaine in patients with refractory cancer pain. Results from a morphine: bupivacaine dose regimen of 0.5:4.75 mg/ml. Anesthesiology. 1994;80(2):284–97.
11. Mitchell A, McGhie J, Owen M, et al. Audit of intrathecal drug delivery for patients with difficult-to-control cancer pain shows a sustained reduction in pain severity scores over a 6-month period. Palliat Med. 2015;29(6):554–63.
12. Mercadante S, Intravala G, Villari P, et al. Intrathecal treatment in cancer patients unresponsive to multiple trials of systemic opioids. Clin J Pain. 2007;23(9):793–8.
13. Yaksh TL, Onofrio BM. Retrospective consideration of the doses of morphine given intrathecally by chronic infusion in 163 patients by 19 physicians. Pain. 1987;31(2):211–23.
14. Chaney MA. Side effects of intrathecal and epidural opioids. Can J Anaesth. 1995;42:891–903.
15. Ruan X. Drug-related side effects of long-term intrathecal morphine therapy. Pain Physician. 2007;10(2):357–66.
16. Malhotra VT, Root J, Kesselbrenner J, et al. Intrathecal pain pump infusions for intractable cancer pain: an algorithm for dosing without a neuraxial trial. Anesth Analg. 2013;116(6):1364–70.
17. Veizi E, Tornero-Bold M, Hayek SM. Resolution of intrathecal hydromorphone or morphine-induced peripheral edema by opioid rotation to fentanyl: a case series. Pain Pract. 2016;16(6):E94–8.
18. Olivera B, Gray WR, Zikus R, et al. Peptide neurotoxins from fish-hunting cone snails. Science. 1985;230(4732):1338–43.
19. Bowersox SS, Gadbois T, Singh T, et al. Selective N-type neuronal voltage-sensitive calcium channel blocker, SNX-111, produces spinal antinociception in rat models of acute, persistent and neuropathic pain. J Pharmacol Exp Ther. 1996;279:1243–9.
20. Alicino I, Giglio M, Manca F, et al. Intrathecal combination of ziconotide and morphine for refractory cancer pain: a rapidly acting and effective choice. Pain. 2012;153(1):245–9.
21. Staats PS, Yearwood T, Charapata SG, et al. Intrathecal ziconotide in the treatment of refractory pain in patients with cancer or AIDS: a randomized controlled trial. JAMA. 2004;291(1):63–70.
22. Prilat. Ziconotide intrathecal infusion. [prescribing information]. San Diego: Jazz Pharmaceuticals, Inc.; 2016.
23. Maier C, Cockel HH, Gruhn K, et al. Increased risk of suicide under intrathecal ziconotide treatment? – a warning. Pain. 2011;152(1):235–7.
24. Malmberg AB, Yaksh TL. Effect of continuous intrathecal infusion of omega-conopeptides, N-type calcium-channel blockers, on behavior and antinociception in the formalin and hot-plate tests in rats. Pain. 1995;60(1):83–90.
25. Prialt (ziconotide) Solution, Intrathecal Infusion [package insert]. Palo Alto: Jazz Pharmaceuticals, Inc.; 2013.
26. Fishman S, Ballantyne J, Rathmell JP, Bonica JJ. Bonica's management of pain. 4th ed. Baltimore: Lippincott, Williams & Wilkins; 2010.
27. Gulati A, Puttanniah V, Hung J, et al. Considerations for evaluating the use of intrathecal drug delivery in the oncologic patient. Curr Pain Headache Rep. 2014;18(2):391.
28. Sloan PA. Neuraxial pain relief for intractable cancer pain. Curr Pain Headache Rep. 2007;11(4):238–9.
29. Graf BM, Abraham I, Eberbach N, et al. Differences in cardiotoxicity of bupivacaine and ropivacaine are the result of physicochemical and stereoselective properties. Anesthesiology. 2002;96(6):1427–34.
30. Eisenach JC, DuPen S, Dubois M, et al. Epidural clonidine analgesia for intractable cancer pain. Pain. 1995;61:391–9.
31. Klimscha W, Tong C, Eisenach JC. Intrathecal α_2-adrenergic agonists stimulate acetylcholine and norepinephrine release from the spinal cord dorsal horn in sheep. An in vivo microdialysis study. Anesthesiology. 1997;87(1):110–6.
32. Feng X, Zhang F, Dong R, et al. Intrathecal administration of clonidine attenuates spinal neuroimmune activation in a rat model of neuropathic pain with existing hyperalgesia. Eur J Pharmacol. 2009;614(1–3):38–43.
33. Yaksh TL. Pharmacology of spinal adrenergic systems which modulate spinal nociceptive processing. Pharmacol Biochem Behav. 1985;22:845–58.
34. Hassenbusch SJ, Gunes S, Wachsman S, et al. Intrathecal clonidine in the treatment of intractable pain: a phase I/II study. Pain Med. 2002;3(2):85–91.
35. Hassenbusch SJ, Portenoy RK. Current practices in intraspinal therapy – a survey of clinical trends and decision making. J Pain Symptom Manag. 2000;20(2):S4–11.
36. Ugur F, Gulcu N, Boyaci A. Intrathecal infusion therapy with dexmedetomidine-supplemented morphine in cancer pain. Acta Anaesthesiol Scand. 2007;51(3):388.
37. Konakci S, Adanir T, Yilmax G, et al. The efficacy and neurotoxicity of dexmedetomidine administered via the epidural route. Eur J Anaesthesiol. 2008;25(5):403–9.
38. Coffey RJ, Cahil D, Steers W, et al. Intrathecal baclofen for intractable spasticity of spinal origin: results of a long-term multicenter study. J Neurosurg. 1993;78:226–32.
39. Albright AL, Gilmartin R, Swift D, et al. Long-term intrathecal baclofen therapy for severe spasticity of cerebral origin. J Neurosurg. 2003;98:291–5.
40. Koulousakis A, Kuchta J. Intrathecal antispastic drug application with implantable pumps: results of a 10 year follow-up study. Acta Neurochir Suppl. 2007;97.(Pt 1:181–4.
41. Heetla HW, Staal MJ, Kliphuis C, et al. The incidence and management of tolerance in intrathecal baclofen therapy. Spinal Cord. 2009;47(10):751–6.

42. Coffey RJ, Edgar TS, Francisco GE, et al. Abrupt withdrawal from intrathecal baclofen: recognition and management of a potentially life-threatening syndrome. Arch Phys Med Rehabil. 2002;83:735–41.
43. Ginsburg GM, Lauder AJ. Progression of scoliosis in patients with spastic quadriplegia after the insertion of an intrathecal baclofen pump. Spine (Phila Pa 1976). 2007;32(24):2745–50.
44. Yaksh TL, Tozier N, Horais KA, et al. Toxicology profile of N-methyl-D-aspartate antagonists delivered by intrathecal infusion in the canine model. Anesthesiology. 2008;108(5):938–49.
45. Wang C, Sadovova N, Fu X, et al. The role of the N-methyl-d-aspartate receptor in ketamine-induced apoptosis in rat forebrain culture. Neuroscience. 2005;132:967–77.
46. Vranken JH, Troost D, Wegener JT, et al. Neuropathological findings after continuous intrathecal administration of S(+)-ketamine for the management of neuropathic cancer pain. Pain. 2005;117(1–2):231–5.
47. Yang CY, Wong CS, Chang JY, et al. Intrathecal ketamine reduces morphine requirements in patients with terminal cancer pain. Can J Anaesth. 1996;43(4):379–83.
48. Osenbach RK. Intrathecal drug delivery in the management of pain. In: Fishman S, Ballantyne J, Rathmell J, editors. Bonica's management of pain. Philadelphia: Lippencott, Williams, & Wilkins; 2010. p. 1437–57.
49. Pope JE, Deer TR. Intrathecal pharmacology update: novel dosing strategy for intrathecal monotherapy ziconotide on efficacy and sustainability. Neuromodulation. 2015;18(5):414–20.
50. Medtronic Inc. http://professional.medtronic.com/pt/neuro/idd/prod/myptm-personal-therapy-manager/features-specifications/index.htm#.V9CNejf2ZaQ. September 7, 2016.

33 Compounding Drugs for Intrathecal Use

Shalini Shah

Introduction

Physicians should understand the safety and efficacy of compounding and administering novel analgesic combinations into the intrathecal space. A clear understanding of the toxicities and risk is necessary. Compounding involves preparing products that are not readily available for commercial use. Solutions prepared from powders of single-entity salts (such as morphine sulfate) are compounded in sterile environments and generally prepared for same day administration, not for shelf life unless testing has been done to assure stability for longer periods. Many of these drugs and combinations of drugs are not specifically approved for intrathecal administration.

Currently, there are no Food and Drug Administration (FDA)-suggested recommendations for mixed or blended compounds of two or more agents. A paucity of literature exists describing compound admixtures and methodological regulations. Therefore, it is necessary for physicians to understand the principles of customizing blends of medications for intrathecal drug infusion systems. In addition, the compounding pharmacist that is consulted must have a thorough knowledge of the pharmacokinetics of each of the agents, while the facilities used to prepare these compounds must comply with the highest standards of practice.

Understanding Targeted Receptors

Compounding therapy should be targeted to activation and/or inhibition of specific receptors, specifically polyanalgesia for receptors involved in pain transmission (Table 33.1). For example, mu receptor activation specifically activates inhibitory signals, while NMDA or sodium channel antagonists will modify the pain signal differently. The polyanalgesic approach provides aggressive pain control while minimizing drug-related side effects of a high concentration of a single agent and may reduce pain and improve quality of life [1].

Table 33.1 Receptors for pain transmission and FDA approval

Commonly used intrathecal agent by class	Medication	FDA approved for intrathecal injection
Opioid	Morphine	Approved
	Hydromorphone	Not Approved
	Fentanyl	Not Approved
	Sufentanil	Not Approved
	Meperidine	Not Approved
	Methadone	Not Approved
Local anesthetics	Lidocaine	Not Approved
	Bupivacaine	Not Approved
	Ropivacaine	Not Approved
	Tetracaine	Not Approved
GABA-receptor agonist	Baclofen	Approved
	Midazolam	Not Approved
Calcium channel antagonist	Ziconotide	Approved
Adrenergic agonists	Clonidine	Not Approved

Combination Therapy

The practice of blending or "cocktailing" includes an understanding of achieving a response by different receptor site activations while minimizing risks of adverse effects such as respiratory depression, sedation, and granuloma formation. Common admixtures of two opioids or opioids and local anesthetic agents are created to minimize the maximal dose of a single agent to avoid toxicity, possible allergy to the drug, adverse drug events, and inflammatory reactions. Popular combinations include morphine + fentanyl, morphine + hydromorphone, morphine + clonidine, and morphine + bupivacaine + fentanyl + clonidine. The addition of a local anesthetic, for example, has been shown to be very effective in treating phantom limb pain

S. Shah (✉)
University of California, Irvine, Department of Anesthesiology and Perioperative Care, Irvine, CA, USA

A. Gulati et al. (eds.), *Essentials of Interventional Cancer Pain Management*, https://doi.org/10.1007/978-3-319-99684-4_33

where denervation of central pain fibers can contribute to peripheral nerve pain. Baclofen may be added for tremors [2]. Midazolam has been shown to be effective against persistent nausea and vomiting from opioid infusions [3]. Pitfalls to single-entity delivery systems do exist, as in the example of morphine where inflammatory masses may arise causing a mass effect on the spinal cord. In such a situation, it may be advisable to infuse an admixture of clonidine + morphine which has extensively been shown to reduce the inflammatory response while achieving the same level of analgesia [4, 5]. This chapter outlines current standard of polyanalgesic admixtures for first-line, second-line, and third-line therapies.

Preparation of Agents and Sterile Technique

A "compounded sterile preparation" (CSP) is defined in United States Pharmacopeia (USP) Chapter 797 as a dosage unit that (1) is prepared according to manufacturer's labeled instructions, (2) contains non-sterile ingredients or employs non-sterile components and devices that must be sterilized before administration, or (3) is biologic, diagnostic, drug, nutrient, or pharmaceutical agent that possesses either of the two previous characteristics and which includes, but is not limited to, baths and soaks for live organs and tissues, implants, inhalations, injections, powder for injection, irrigations, metered sprays, and ophthalmic and otic preparations [6]. Powders derived from high-grade USP-approved chemicals are combined according to the chemical formula for mixture, are weighted and dissolved in sterile water, and are filtered for injection. The USP-National Formulary (USP-NF) has required all sterile compounding comply with mandatory requirements to prepare sterile injectables. USP-NF defines designs of environment: clean room with and without glove boxes or hoods and outlines procedures for gowning, gloving, and masking during sterilization. End-product testing for sterility, pyrogenicity, and endotoxin and potency testing are also regulated.

Microbial Contamination Risk Level

To compound level 3/highest-risk drugs, such as sterile intrathecal agents, preparation begins with compliance of Chapter 797 regulations and risk level determination. Appropriate risk level (low, level 1; moderate, level 2; high, level 3) assigned according to corresponding probability of contamination with microbial (organisms, spores, endotoxins) or chemical or physical (foreign chemicals or physical matter).

Previously, infused intrathecal medications were considered level 2/moderate risk as were all medications delivered over several days without containing a broad-spectrum bacteriostatic substance. Current literature, however, agrees that all intrathecal medications are level 3 (high) risk as they lack bacteriostatic preservatives and include products exposed to an inadequately controlled environment even if the final preparation is sterilized before use. Preparations of a sterile solution, such as intrathecal agents, from a non-sterile powder are always at a level 3 risk.

Key High-Risk Level Requirements [7]

- CSPs compounded from sterile commercial drugs using commercial sterile devices.
- Compounding occurs in International Organization for Standardization (ISO) Class 5 (formerly known as Class 100) environment at all times.
- Compounding procedures involve only a few closed system basic, simple aseptic transfers, and manipulations.
- Routine disinfection and air quality testing to maintain ISO Class 5 occur.
- There is adequate personnel garb for sterile preparation.
- A review for correct identity and amounts of components occurs before and after compounding.
- There is a final visual inspection of each sterile preparation.
- Semiannual media-fill test procedure for each person who compounds is performed to validate proper aseptic technique.

An example of low-risk agents are hydration fluids, produced for extemporaneous intravenous piggyback use; moderate risk includes prepackaged syringes or TPN formulations, while high risk involves measuring raw chemicals, weighing, dissolving, and finalizing with filtered technique in a standardized clean room.

A clean room is a controlled environment that has a low level of environmental pollutants such as dust, airborne microbes, aerosolized particles, and chemical vapors. More accurately, a clean room has a controlled level of contamination that is specified by the number of particles per cubic meter at a specified particle size and is categorized accordingly into classes (Table 33.2). All agents prepared for intrathecal use must be prepared in at least a Class 100 clean room. The ambient air outside in a typical urban environment contains 35,000,000 particles per cubic meter, 0.5 micron and larger in diameter, corresponding to a Class 1,000,000 clean room.

Class 100 of Chapter 797 is mandated protocol for a production environment of intrathecal agents. Class 100 environment, also known as International Standardization Organization (ISO) Class 5 (i.e., maximally 100 particles 0.5 micron and larger in diameter are allowed per cubic foot), compliance may include a sterile hood within a sterile room or only a sterile isolator within a clean room.

Table 33.2 International Organization for Standardization for clean rooms

ISO	≥0.1 μm	≥0.2 μm	≥0.3 μm	≥0.5 μm	≥5 μm	Class
ISO 3	35	7	3	1		**1**
ISO 4	350	75	30	10		**10**
ISO 5		750	300	100		**100**
ISO 6				1000	7	**1000**
ISO 7				10,000	70	**10,000**
ISO 8				100,000	700	**100,000**

Table adapted from US Department of Commerce FED-STD-209E standard which was officially canceled in 2001 but still widely used. Clean rooms are classified according to the number and size of particles permitted per volume of air. "Class 100" or "Class 1000" denotes the number of particles of size 0.5 micrometer or larger permitted per cubic foot of air. Intrathecal preparations require Class 100 or ISO 5 standards at minimum

Filtration

Once medications are prepared and filtered in lab, they are filtered again by the physician prior to delivery to CSF. As intrathecal medications have no barrier, physicians are relying on the assumption that pharmacy is preparing the agent sterilely and pyrogen-free, therefore a double filtration process is the final step. Sterile filtration requires a 0.22-micron-size filter or smaller. A filter with 0.22 pore size can prevent most forms of bacteria and some very large viruses from passing through the filter since bacteria tend to range from about 0.1 micron to 600 microns. Many viruses are less than 0.1 micrometers, so a 0.22-micron filter is not nearly as effective for viruses. High-flow 0.22-micron pore size filter was specifically designed for sterilization and bacteria retentive applications.

Responsibility of Compounding Labs

USP Chapter 797 sets standards, guidance, and examples for compounding sterile preparations. However, it does not provide specific and comprehensive information describing how to meet those standards. Therefore, pharmacists who compound sterile preparations should exercise their professional judgment to obtain the education and training necessary to prove their competence in managing sterile compounding facilities and in sterile compounding processes and quality assurance. Each compounding lab writes its own policies and procedures necessary to meet Chapter 797 standards for intrathecal medications based on its individual lab facilities [6].

The FDA has long expressed concern about the quality of compounded medications [8]. Recent deaths caused by microbial contamination of injectable steroids have prompted several state boards of pharmacy to strengthen compounding regulations. Although the American Society of Health-System Pharmacists (ASHP) published the profession's first sterile compounding standards in 1992, sterile compounding practices have potential for low compliance with voluntary standards. Enforceable standards, once seriously implemented, will improve compliance and greatly enhance patient safety [7].

Stability and Solubility

It is well known that stability of intrathecal agents at physiological temperature is important to the ultimate success of the analgesic therapy. Some agents are not stable at certain concentrations, certain temperatures, or when mixed in combination with other agents. While most pharmacologic agents are intended for use within 1–2 weeks of manufacture date, intrathecal agents are not intended for shelf life and must be administered either on the date of preparation or the beyond use date that has been established for the drug because of stability testing. Furthermore, since an agent will remain within the pump chamber, it is important to test the agent for stability at 25 °C and 37 °C for 90–120 days. Refill intervals should not exceed the period of stability. Morphine, hydromorphone, clonidine, and baclofen are stable at room and body temperature for 3 months [4, 9–11]. Bupivacaine is stable for 60 days and may lead to consideration of more frequent refills if used in combination with opioids [12]. Again, concentration, particularly high concentrations of single agents, has the potential for decreased stability over agents with lower concentrations.

Polyanalgesic therapy admixtures are injected sooner, so stability is tested for 60–75 pump day run.

There are currently three medications approved by the FDA for intrathecal infusions for chronic pain: morphine, baclofen, and ziconotide. While an agent may be approved for intraspinal injection, the concentration given for chronic intrathecal delivery systems is too high than is commercially prepared and packaged. This is known as "off-label use." All infusion admixtures of single- and mixed-entity agents are off label. There are no instructions or approved monograph by the FDA. Physicians who administer the medications typically give patients instructions on maintenance of pump and how to prepare for adverse effects. Physicians have the obligation to explain the off-label use of compounded medications and document such discussions.

There may be issues of stability when certain agents are compounded for clinical use. The definition of stability is an agent that is stable when 90% or more of the active form of the drug remains at the time point specified [13]. Stability is also a function of solubility at 25 ° C room temperature up to physiological temperature at 37 °C. All agents indicated for intrathecal use are prepared and maintained at this temperature (see Table 33.3). The challenge in compounding agents

Table 33.3 Solubility and pKa coefficients for commonly used intrathecal agents

Drug	Octanol: Buffer (oil: water) solubility coefficient	pKa	Solubility at physiological pH
Morphine	1.42	7.9	Water
Hydromorphone	0.32	8.2	Water
Fentanyl	860	8.4	Lipid
Bupivacaine	346	8.1	Lipid
Clonidine	114	8.05	Lipid
Ziconotide	1.4	Unpublished	Water

for intrathecal drug delivery systems is customizing admixtures as appropriate for each patient on an individual basis, so solubility and stability testing should be determined for the exact admixture before infusion.

Each individual laboratory has determined its own proprietary data of stability testing for 6-month infusions of single agent and multiple agent mixtures. The clinician may readily attain these data from the compounding lab supplying the intrathecal medications for review before starting therapy. This is important to prevent precipitations of solution which may cause corrosive damage and ultimately lead to pump failure. For example, bupivacaine at 4% is the highest concentration one can solubilize the drug. If this concentration is exposed to temperatures below room temp, it will crystallize out of solution [14]. This is in contrast with morphine which may remain in solution up to 55 mg/ml. Therefore, stability is a function of temperature, concentration, and solubility coefficients. Ziconotide at less than 1 microgram/mL concentration is not very stable, but appears to have molecular stability at concentrations higher than 1 microgram/mL. Morphine and hydromorphone accelerate the rate of ziconotide degradation, so combinations of ziconotide with lower concentrations of the compounded opioid agents are expected to be more stable [11].

All medications intended for intrathecal infusion systems are prepared preservative-free. Preservatives are neurotoxic and should not be used for any agent intended for neuraxial use. Common preservatives include benzyl alcohol, mercuries, and ethylenediaminetetraacetic acid (EDTA).

Pump Stability and Failure

Pump failure is also a concern with high concentrations of opioids. The average life expectancy of most intrathecal pump systems is 5–7 years. Pump failure secondary to high concentrations within the pump chamber can corrode the mechanism of the delivering system leading to failure of the pump earlier, 3–5 years. In cancer pain, the clinician is far less concerned with the life of the pump than in patients with chronic nonmalignant pain. Unfortunately, since the average life expectancy of cancer patients implanted with intrathecal pumps is 18–24 months, the clinician may choose to be more aggressive with higher concentrations as the issue is quality of life rather than pump mechanism failure in these selected patients.

For patients with chronic nonmalignant pain, one major concern is how often patients can make time for follow-up appointments for pump refills. Ideally, higher concentrations of medications are favored to lengthen the time period between pump refills, however not always advisable due to potential risks of inflammatory masses as well as stability of the drug. Since the pump chamber contains higher concentrations of opioids, the volume delivered daily is at lower, and the patient may achieve the similar analgesia with a greater time between refills.

Risks of Intrathecal Therapy

There are a variety of risks of intrathecal therapy. Briefly, complication can occur with the pump and catheter, or with the drugs, implantation of the device, or pump refill.

Insertion of the Device

At the time of the insertion of the device, one needs to take great care to avoid infection and avoid damage of the spinal cord with insertion of the catheter. The pump needs to be stabilized at the correct level in the abdomen to avoid pump flipping or being placed to deeply or superficially. In this situation, the pump may flip, rotate, and dislodge the catheter, and it may not be able to be refilled (if placed to deeply) or if placed too superficially can erode through the skin wall.

A greater concern is malfunction of the pump. While a stalled pump is unlikely to release medications into the intrathecal space, it is possible for malfunction to occur resulting in infusion of all of the remaining solution from the reservoir. This obviously would lead to life-threatening respiratory failure and overdose of intrathecal medications.

The catheters can also kink or break, leading to no extravasation of drugs or drugs being slowly released in to the subcutaneous tissue. An infusion into the subcutaneous tissue may still lead to drug overdose and side effect and will need to be monitored.

Medication Problems

Problems with medications include adverse drug reactions, allergic reactions, respiratory and neurologic depression, and suppression of testosterone and possibly lead to the development of osteoporosis. Neurotoxicity of the spinal cord could occur with off-label use of drugs. In addition, if the compounding pharmacy does not use appropriate technique, it is possible to refill the pump with incorrect or unstable drugs. Suppression of natural killer (NK) cell activity has also been reported in animal models leading to a concern of increasing the chance of metastatic spread [15]. Currently the most feared complication is the development of inflammation around the catheter tip site.

Inflammatory Mass Formation

Granulomas are inflammatory masses that can form inside the spinal canal with infusions of intrathecal agents. In extreme cases, they can cause cord compression and paralysis. Granulomas are most commonly seen with intrathecal opiates but have been also seen with non-opioids including baclofen [16].

Intrathecal morphine was the first drug to be associated with granulomatous masses from continuous intrathecal therapy. They can occur from weeks to years after initiating therapy and have been seen at low doses as well as higher doses of intrathecal therapy. They seem to be associated with high concentration and low flow rate pump settings.

Safety of chronic intrathecal morphine infusion has been extensively studied for potential neurotoxic effects and demonstrated to be dose dependent determined by the amount of morphine infused [17]. Intrathecal morphine doses of 12–18 mg/day produced inflammatory masses extending from the catheter tip down the length of the catheter within the intrathecal space in sheep model within 28 days of infusion [17]. A dose of 3 mg/day produced no neurotoxicity, and spinal histopathologic changes were equivalent to those observed in saline-treated animals [17]. Nevertheless, concentration-dependent neurotoxicity is well established, with dose-dependent allodynia usually presenting as the initial sign soon after initiation of high-dose morphine (morphine dose >9 mg/day), ultimately leading to motor weakness secondary to mass evolution and compression [10]. Morphine at doses 12 mg/day or greater for greater than 28 days of infusion produces inflammatory masses in all animal models studied consisting of multifocal immunoreactive cells (macrophages, neutrophils, cytokines), most often observed between the dura and arachnoid layers, and aseptic in nature [10, 17]. Human cases have been reported in patients receiving intrathecal opioids alone or in combination with other intrathecal agents or in patients receiving investigational agents not intended for long-term intrathecal use [4, 18].

Future Directions

Intrathecal therapy can be a very effective therapy for patients with chronic pain. However, a thorough understanding of the various agents utilized, and expected doses are necessary when managing implantable pumps. While there are risks associated with intrathecal therapy, they can relieve pain, lower side effects, and improve the quality of life in patients with intractable pain.

References

1. Stearns L, Boortz-Marx R, Du Pen S, et al. Intrathecal drug delivery for the management of cancer pain: a multidisciplinary consensus of best clinical practices. J Support Oncol. 2005;3:399–408.
2. Weiss N, North RB, Ohara S, et al. Attenuation of cerebellar tremor with implantation of an intrathecal baclofen pump: the role of gamma-aminobutyric acidergic pathways. Case report. J Neurosurg. 2003;99:768–71.
3. Ho KM, Ismail H. Use of intrathecal midazolam to improve perioperative analgesia: a meta-analysis. Anaesth Intensive Care. 2008;36:365–73.
4. Yaksh TL, Hassenbusch S, Burchiel K, et al. Inflammatory masses associated with intrathecal drug infusion: a review of preclinical evidence and human data. Pain Med. 2002;3:300–12.
5. Siddall PJ, Gray M, Rutkowski S, et al. Intrathecal morphine and clonidine in the management of spinal cord injury pain: a case report. Pain. 1994;59:147–8.
6. Convention USP. 2009; Chapter 797, United States Pharmacopeia/National Formulary 1st ed. US Pharmacopeia; 4139.
7. Kastango E. The ASHP discussion guide for compounding sterile preparations: summary and implementation of USP Chapter 797 2004. ASHP Publishing.
8. Outterson K. Regulating compounding pharmacies after NECC. N Engl J Med. 2012;367:1986–72.
9. Yaksh TL, Horais KA, Tozier NA, et al. Chronically infused intrathecal morphine in dogs. Anesthesiology. 2003;99:174–87.
10. Deer T, Krames ES, Hassenbusch SJ, et al. Polyanalgesic Consensus Conference 2007: recommendations for the management of pain by intrathecal (Intraspinal) drug delivery: report of an interdisciplinary expert panel. Neuromodulation. 2007;10:300–28.
11. Hildebrand KR, Elsberry DE, Anderson VC. Stability and compatibility of hydromorphone hydrochloride in an implantable infusion system. J Pain Symptom Manag. 2001;22:1042–7.
12. Deer TR, Serafini M, Buchser E, et al. Intrathecal bupivacaine for chronic pain: a review of current knowledge. Neuromodulation. 2002;5:196–207.
13. Trissel L, editor. Trissel's stability of compounded formulations. 4nd ed. Washington, DC: APHA Publications; 2009.
14. O'Neil M, Smith A, Heckelman P, et al., editors. Merck index. 13th ed. New York: Wiley; 2001.
15. Yeager MP, Colacchio TA, Yu CT, et al. Morphine inhibits spontaneous and cytokine-enhanced natural killer cell cytotoxicity in volunteers. Anesthesiology. 1995;83(3):500–8.
16. Deer TR, Raso LJ, Coffey RJ, et al. Intrathecal baclofen and catheter tip inflammatory mass lesions (granulomas): a reevaluation of case reports and imaging findings in light of experimental, clinicopathological, and radiological evidence. Pain Med. 2008;9:391–5.
17. Gradert TL, Baze WB, Satterfield WC, et al. Safety of chronic intrathecal morphine infusion in a sheep model. Anesthesiology. 2003;99:188–98.
18. Coffey RJ, Burchiel K. Inflammatory mass lesions associated with intrathecal drug infusion catheters: report and observations on 41 patients. Neurosurgery. 2002;50:78–86. discussion 86-77.

Part VII

Interventional Oncology

Image Guidance and Planning

34

Ramon Go and Jeffrey Prinsell Jr.

Introduction

Image Guidance

The concept of interrupting nociceptive impulses of an abdominal nerve plexus originated in 1914 when Max Kappis of Germany performed a transcutaneous splanchnic nerve block using bony landmarks [1]. The technique of being able to isolate an abdominal or retroperitoneal nerve plexus percutaneously using a needle provided a less invasive approach to "blocking" nociceptive impulses. Popper et al. further described the use of splanchnic nerve block as a diagnostic tool to differentiate between somatic and visceral abdominal pains [2]. Thereafter, ethanol-induced neurolysis of celiac plexus was demonstrated by Jones and colleagues for long-term pain relief. As the number of studies showing the efficacy and benefits of percutaneous nerve plexus block and neurolysis increased, so did the number of complications associated with this landmark-based technique [3, 4]. The risks associated with previous landmark-based techniques eventually led to the use of imaging guidance.

Fluoroscopic guidance was first introduced in the 1950s, followed by computed tomography (CT) guidance, and eventually ultrasound (US) guidance in the 1990s [5]. While each modality possesses individual benefits and limitations which will be discussed below, it is more important to understand patient-specific characteristics, such as tolerating positioning, managing anticoagulation, and understanding anatomic causes for a patient's pain symptoms. Diagnostic images such as CT scans may allow physicians to preplan a therapeutic plan for the interventions. Various plexus blocks and neurolyses, such as celiac, splanchnic, superior hypogastric, and lumbar sympathetic, have become an essential therapeutic option in the management of cancer-related abdominal and pelvic pain.

Anatomy

In addition to improving the evaluation of cancer progression, the technological advancement of various imaging modalities has expanded our understanding of internal anatomical structures and potentially improves the effectiveness of interventional procedures in providing pain relief. In order to effectively utilize the technological advancement of radiological studies, the application of advanced imaging to provide analgesia is needed to shift the approach of utilizing "external landmarks" as described by Max Kappis in 1914 to using "internal landmarks" which can be successfully visualized by using any number of imaging techniques such as traditional CT, MRI, and US.

In order to make this transition successfully, the evaluation, anatomical appreciation, and strategy for approach are all important. These imaging techniques, which are used to evaluate disease progression, can also be used to aid and map our interventional approach. The targets (i.e., celiac plexus and superior hypogastric) have all been well described anatomically, including their variations between individuals [6]. More specifically, Zhang et al. reported that 94% of the celiac ganglia are located at the level of T12 or L1 [7]. Although the target for a nerve block or neurolysis can be reliably predictable, the surrounding anatomy (i.e., vital organs, tumor, and vascular supply) and individual patient factors (i.e., positioning, pain, ascites, and postsurgical changes) prove to be the biggest obstacles.

Vascular

The most important feeding artery of the thoracolumbar spinal cord is the great anterior radiculomedullary artery, also

R. Go (✉) · J. Prinsell Jr.
Pain Management, Memorial Sloan Kettering Cancer Center, New York, NY, USA

A. Gulati et al. (eds.), *Essentials of Interventional Cancer Pain Management*, https://doi.org/10.1007/978-3-319-99684-4_34

known as the artery of Adamkiewicz. It originates from a left intercostal or lumbar artery 68–73% of the time and at the level of the 9th to 12th intercostal artery in only 62–75% of the time and averages about 1 mm in diameter [8]. The most extensive research evaluating the detection and anatomical assessment of the artery of Adamkiewicz has occurred in the radiology literature evaluating for thoracoabdominal aortic aneurysm repair. In the preoperative evaluation of patients with aortic aneurysms, routine cost-effective conventional CT or magnetic resonance imaging (MRI) angiography is used to evaluate the vascular anatomy of each individual. In 2002, Kieffer et al. reported a detection rate of 86% in 480 cases when evaluating how well they could identify the artery of Adamkiewicz [9]. The variability of the location of the artery of Adamkiewicz and its collaterals remain a real and significant concern when performing any number of percutaneous blocks, but technology is improving to better identify these variations and hopefully provide clinically safer outcomes.

Radiologic Modalities

Fluoroscopy is an imaging modality commonly used for interventional procedures not only for the treatment of cancer pain but also other pain syndromes. Compared to MRI and CT, fluoroscopy is simple to use and operate. It provides the freedom to operate and obtain multiple images at various angles to achieve optimal needle positioning. Disadvantages include poor anatomic resolution (with an emphasis on bony anatomy) and the inability to distinguish a nerve or nerve plexus from its surrounding structures (including blood vessels, vital organs, tumors, etc.). Consequently, fluoroscopic guidance alone is user dependent and often associated with higher rates of complications [10].

US has been described as a simple and cost-effective modality allowing for real-time visualization of retroperitoneal structures. In addition, the user is able to potentially visualize spread of any local anesthetic or neurolytic agent without the need for contrast [11]. However, US technique is user dependent, requires a high degree of operator skill, and favors patient body habitus to view retroperitoneal structures [11]. Furthermore, US resolution is limited to the footprint of the probe (usually in centimeters), and ultrasound cannot penetrate boney anatomy; thus, only superficial bony anatomy may be visualized.

Haaga and colleagues first described the role of interventional CT imaging in 1977 and then later the value of CT in guiding neurolytic celiac plexus block in 1984 [12, 13]. Since then, CT-guided percutaneous neurolysis, particularly the celiac plexus, has surpassed the other imaging modalities for visualizing surrounding anatomical structures leading to an improved safety profile [11]. In addition to better visualization of retroperitoneal structures compared to US and fluoroscopy, CT guidance can demonstrate the extent of tumor spread and potential other etiologies for pain such as bowel obstruction, bone destruction, and muscle invasion [11]. One of the more important distinguishing characteristics of CT guidance is to account for any variability in anatomy from patient to patient. Regardless of the imaging modality used for any interventional procedure, determining the etiology of the pain, the ability to accurately visualize the desired location of the needle tip, and the anatomical variation obstructing your approach will factor into the success and potentially minimize adverse events. CT guidance also allows for confirmation with contrast dye injection and visualization of local anesthetic or neurolytic agent spread. Radiation exposure is a significant risk factor, especially in a cancer patient. It is often a realistic expectation to have to repeat the interventional procedure in the future if the pain returns, and this has also contributed to the limited use of CT guidance.

Along with CT and fluoroscopy guidance for celiac plexus blockade, MRI guidance has recently been introduced. Hol et al. reported successful results in 57–93% of patients who underwent MRI-guided celiac plexus block with similar safety profile [14]. More data will be needed to determine its role in the future, especially in combination with other modalities, such as high-intensity focused ultrasound.

Mapping Strategies

The anatomic considerations of any nerve block or neurolysis should be taken into account when planning a percutaneous intervention. According to De Cicco et al., one of the most common reasons for failure of neurolysis is inadequate spread of the neurolytic agent [15]. This potential failure is believed to be a result of regional anatomic disruptions, which result from tumor infiltration, postoperative changes, or postradiation therapy changes [15]. These factors in addition to anatomic variations can potentially alter therapeutic success. Many physicians review previous CT and MRI scans before any therapeutic intervention, and we suggest taking this practice a step further.

Interventional pain management physicians may become adept in fluoroscopy-guided interventions, and access to a CT scanner may be difficult. These factors potentially limit the utility of CT-guided procedures. However, the previous CT or MRI imaging studies may be used to guide the site of entry and needle path when procedures are performed under fluoroscopy. Typical neurolytic procedures (i.e., celiac plexus, superior hypogastric, or lumbar sympathetic) should be individualized for each patient and each procedural episode, with the needle entry site and needle tip end point reevaluated for every procedure due to the multiple anatomical changes that may occur over the course of a cancer patient's treatment. Using a previous CT/MRI scan to evaluate "internal landmarks" in addition to the "external landmarks" with a focus on the needle tip's journey instead of just the destination can potentially provide more successful treatments and fewer complications to each individual patient.

An Example: Lumbar Sympathetic Block

Generally, the lumbar sympathetic chain consists of three to five paired ganglia that lie over the anterolateral surface of the second through fourth lumbar vertebrae [16]. Using previous CT imaging for surveillance of anatomy and surrounding structures helps to determine the percutaneous entry point. This can be determined by direct visualization of the imaging to determine how lateral from midline to begin as well as the cranial or caudal internal trajectory. Moreover, we recommend precisely measuring the lateral distance from midline spinous process and determining cranial and caudal trajectory based on scrolling through the CT/MR images, determining how many millimeters (based on slice thickness) separates the needle entry and needle end point. It is important to understand that the eventual needle tip end point under fluoroscopic guidance will be the same regardless of imaging modality, and our main objective is using internal landmarks based on CT imaging, especially in a cancer patient who may have altered anatomy from tumor infiltration, radiation, or previous surgery.

To begin, we recommend first viewing available CT or MRI studies as normally performed but with the focus not only on the end point of the needle but the entire trajectory of your needle. This means gaining an appreciation not only for lateral to medial but also cranial and caudal needle position. The goal is to not only provide a greater appreciation for the surrounding anatomy but also to evaluate your three-dimensional approach, which will ultimately be performed visualizing a two-dimensional fluoroscopic screen.

Methods

Lumbar Sympathetic Block

The lumbar sympathetic plexus is composed of a flattened network of intercommunicating nerve fibers that descend over the aortic bifurcation [16]. Traditionally, the goal of the block is for local anesthetic or neurolytic agent to spread anteriorly at L2 through L4. We recommend a five-step process in performing this procedure (see Figs. 34.1, 34.2, 34.3, 34.4 and 34.5).

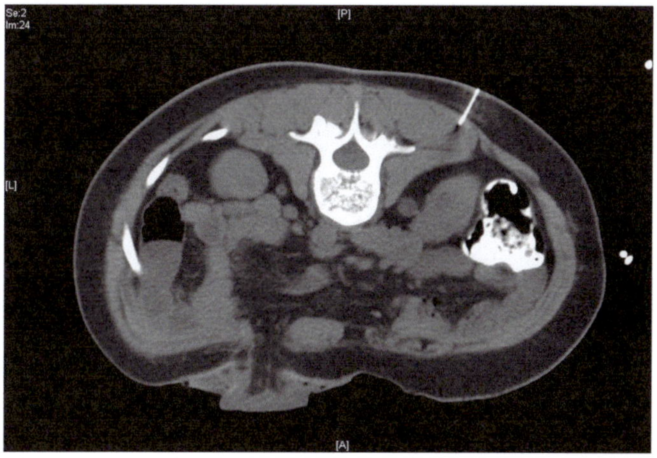

Fig. 34.1 An ideal percutaneous entry point is made by creating intersecting two lines. The first line from the target site to the skin and the second line are made by identifying midline as indicated by the spinous process

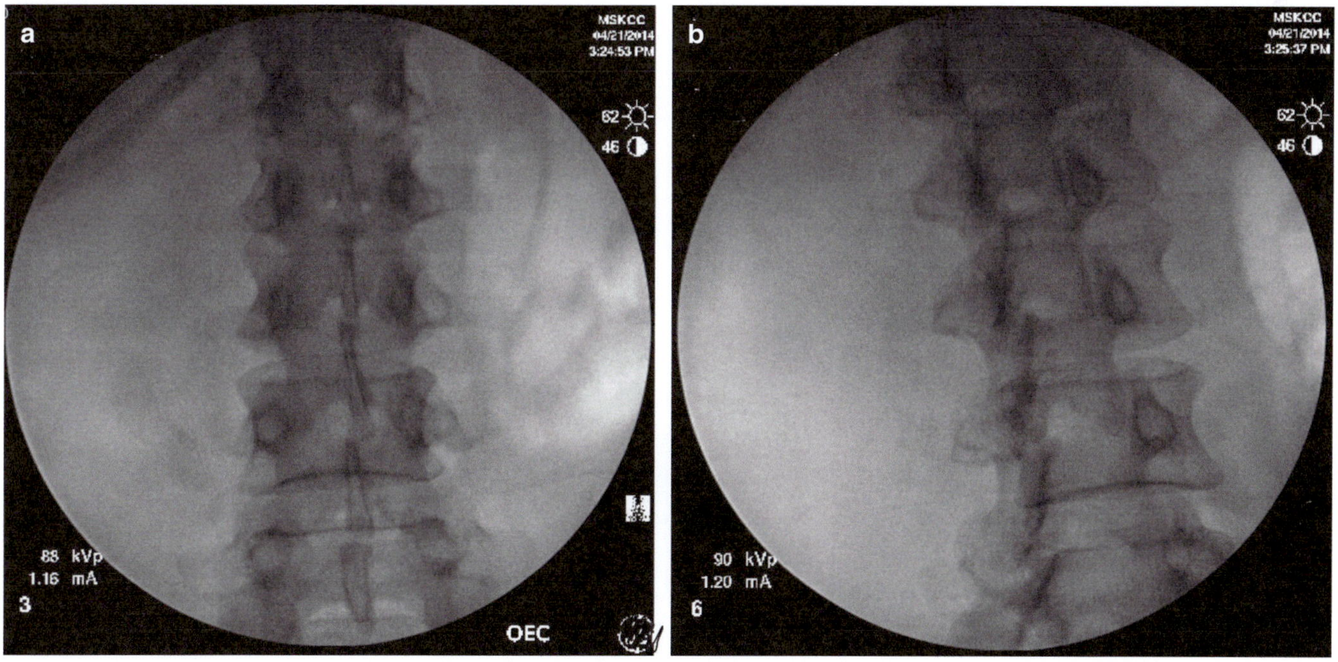

Fig. 34.2 (**a**) The vertebral body end plates are lined up. Confirmation of the vertebral levels is performed by counting from T12 down to L2 or sacrum to L2. (**b**) Oblique rotation of the fluoroscope beam is performed to reproduce a similar angle from the CT imaging

Step 1: Review Radiological Studies
Reviewing available radiological studies of the patient is crucial in understanding potential sources of pain, anatomic variations, and procedure mapping. The L2 to L4 vertebrae should be evaluated, and the safest needle trajectory identified at the L2 level. The pedicles should be present on the image to prevent potential nerve root injury. Next, measure the ideal percutaneous entry point to the needle end point (anterolateral L2 vertebral body) taking careful note of the potential needle trajectory and avoiding critical structures. Last, measure the distance from the spinous process (midline) to the theoretical percutaneous entry point, providing the distance from the patient's midline to the needle entry site. The angle created by these two lines should be near 45 degrees (Fig. 34.1). By reviewing previous radiological studies and pre-procedural mapping, exposure to radiation and procedural related complications may be minimized.

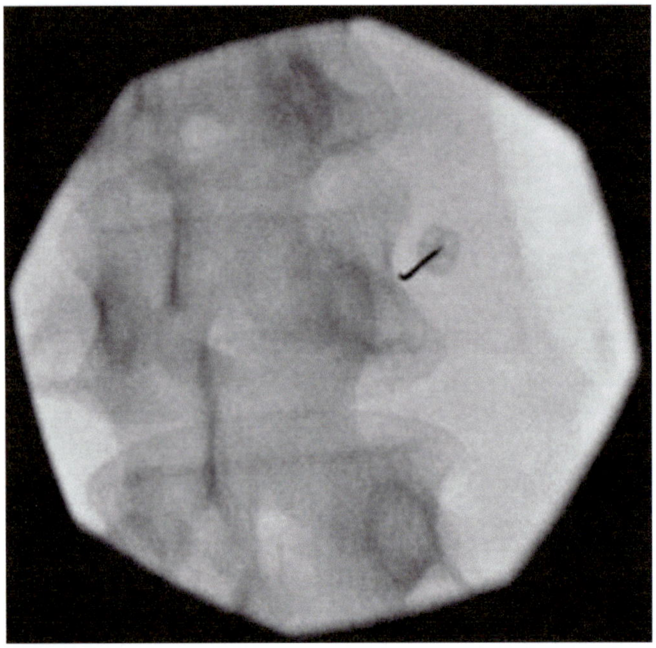

Fig. 34.3 A coaxial technique is used to approach the target site in the oblique view

Step 2: Evaluate Anatomy Under Fluoroscopy
The patient is placed in a prone positioning with a pillow placed under the patient's abdomen. External landmarks are used to identify the L2 vertebral body. With the patient laying prone and prepped, the external landmarks should be used to identify the lumbar vertebral levels under fluoroscopy to minimize radiation exposure. The L2 vertebral body end plates are lined up. Confirmation of the vertebral levels is performed by counting from T12 down to L2 or sacrum to L2 (see Fig. 34.2a). The distance lateral from midline to entry point from previous step is marked. Oblique rotation of the fluoroscope beam is performed to reproduce a similar angle from the CT imaging (see Fig. 34.2b).

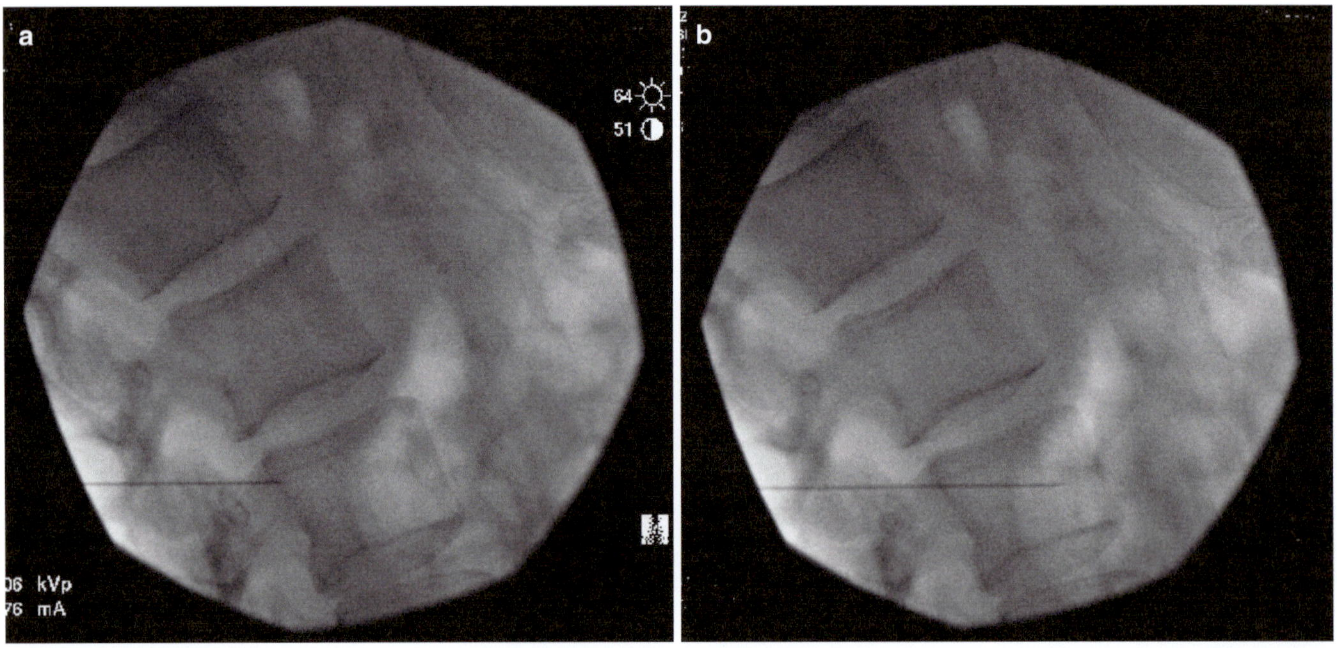

Fig. 34.4 (**a**) A radiograph in the lateral view shows the needle tip posterior to the vertebral body. (**b**) The needle is further advanced to the anterior one third of the vertebral body. (**c**) A CT image of the lumbar sympathetic nerve block is shown with the needle along the anterolateral aspect of L2 vertebrae

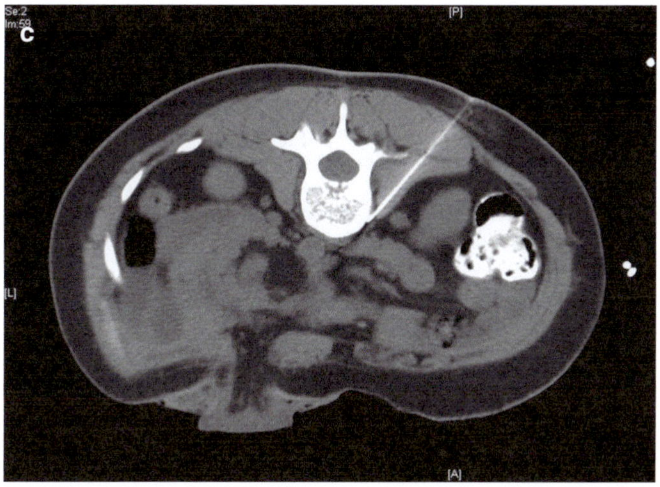

Fig. 34.4 (continued)

Step 3: Needle Insertion

A 1-inch 30-gauge needle is used to create a skin wheal over the marked entry site. Next, a 5-inch 22-gauge needle is inserted coaxially cephalad to the transverse process. Collimation may be performed to decrease radiation exposure and to improve image resolution (see Fig. 34.3).

Step 4: Engaging Target Site

Once the needle is coaxial and directed toward the respective target, the fluoroscope is then rotated to a true lateral position. The distance from needle tip to target site should be noted, and the needle should be advanced with caution to avoid periosteum which may be painful. If periosteum is reached, the needle may be turned lateral with the bevel facing laterally and advanced. If turning the bevel lateral does not allow for the needle advancement, then the needle is

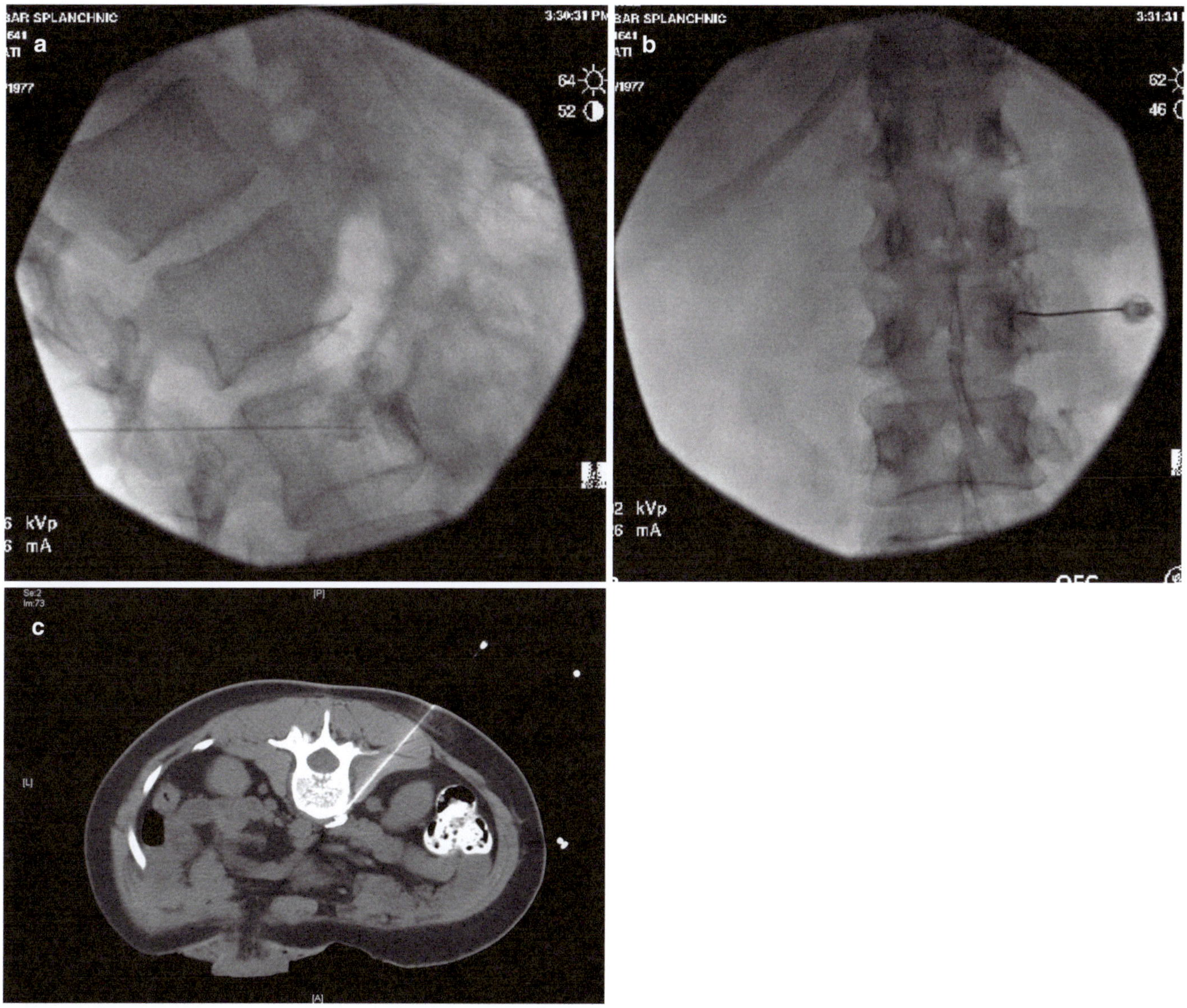

Fig. 34.5 (**a**) The radiograph in the lateral view shows the needle tip positioned at the anterior L2 vertebral body and contrast injected. (**b**) The spread of the contrast is then visualized in the anterior view. (**c**) A view of the needle in the correct position and the surrounding structures is visualized in a CT image

withdrawn near skin and advanced in a slightly lateral plane. A CT image of the needle at the target location is shown in panel C. Critical anatomical structures such as the right kidney, bowel, and vascular structures such as the inferior vena cava and the aorta are avoided in the CT image (see Fig. 34.4).

Step 5: Confirmation and Injection of Agents
Once the needle is in the correct position at the anterior one third of the L2 vertebral body (see panel A), contrast should be injected to demonstrate adequate linear spread without intravascular uptake or injection into the psoas muscle and further confirmed with the anteroposterior view (see panel B). About 10 mL of local anesthetic or neurolytic agent is then injected. A CT image of the needle with contrast injection at the target site is shown in panel C. Scanning the CT image in a cranial and to caudal manner will display contrast spread. This entire process may be repeated on the left lumbar plexus if indicated (see Fig. 34.5).

Discussion

An appreciation for anatomical variation, especially in cancer patients, is an important factor in determining successful interventional analgesia. Clinicians should view previous images to determine the "internal landmarks" in addition to the external approach to provide a more accurate diagnostic block or neurolysis. There are multiple anatomical variations among individuals, and this may become more complex in patients with malignancy. By using these precise and specific steps, important vascular (IVC and spinal artery) and anatomical structures may be avoided, and radiation exposure lessened. Therefore, combining standardized techniques and utilizing previous CT or MRI imaging can optimize block techniques.

References

1. Fujita Y, Sari A. Max Kappis and the celiac plexus block. Anesthesiology. 1997;86(2):508.
2. Popper HL. Acute pancreatitis; an evaluation of the classification, symptomatology, diagnosis and therapy. Am J Dig Dis. 1948;15(1):1–4.
3. Bridenbaugh LD, Moore DC, Campbell DD. Management of upper abdominal cancer pain: treatment with celiac plexus block with alcohol. JAMA. 1964;190:877–80.
4. Jacobs JB, Jackson SH, Doppman JL. A radiographic approach to celiac ganglion block. Radiology. 1969;92(6):1373–3.
5. Wiersema MJ, Wiersema LM. Endosonography-guided celiac plexus neurolysis. Gastrointest Endosc. 1996;44(6):656–62.
6. Loukas M, Klaassen Z, Merbs W, Tubbs RS, Gielecki J, Zurada A. A review of the thoracic splanchnic nerves and celiac ganglia. Clin Anat. 2010;23(5):512–22.
7. Zhang XM, Zhao QH, Zeng NL, et al. The celiac ganglia: anatomic study using MRI in cadavers. AJR Am J Roentgenol. 2006;186(6):1520–3.
8. Yoshioka K, Niinuma H, Ehara S, Nakajima T. MR angiography and CT angiography of the artery of Adamkiewicz: state of the art. Radiographics. 2006;26(1):S63–73.
9. Kieffer E, Fukui S, Chiras J, Koskas F, Bahnini A, Cormier E. Spinal cord arteriography: a safe adjunct before descending thoracic or thoracoabdominal aortic aneurysmectomy. J Vasc Surg. 2002;35(2):262–8.
10. Wang PJ, Shang MY, Qian Z, Shao CW, Zhao XH. CT-guided percutaneous neurolytic celiac plexus block technique. Abdom Imaging. 2006;31(6):710–8.
11. Kambadakone A, Thabet A, Gervais D, Mueller P, Arellano R. CT-guided celiac plexus neurolysis: a review of anatomy, indications, technique, and tips for successful treatment. Radiographics. 2011;31:1599–621.
12. Haaga JR, Reich NE, Havrilla TR, Alfidi RJ. Interventional CT scanning. Radiol Clin N Am. 1977;15(3):449–56.
13. Haaga JR, Kori SH, Eastwood DW, Borkowski GP. Improved technique for CT-guided celiac ganglia block. AJR Am J Roentgenol. 1984;142(6):1201–4.
14. Hol PK, Kvarstein G, Viken O, Smedby O, Tonnessen TI. MRI-guided celiac plexus block. J Magn Reson Imaging. 2000;12(4):562–4.
15. De Cicco M, Matovic M, Balestreri L, Fracasso A, Morassut S, Testa V. Single-needle celiac plexus block: is needle tip position critical in patients with no regional anatomic distortions? Anesthesiology. 1997;87(6):1301–8.
16. Rathmell J. Atlas of image-guided intervention in regional anesthesia and pain medicine. Philadelphia: Lippincott Williams & Wilkins; 2006. p. 135–45.

Ablative Techniques for Painful Metastasis (Radiofrequency ablation, Microwave ablation, Cryoablation, Chemical ablation, and HIFU)

35

Hooman Yarmohammadi

Introduction

Cancer pain remains a major issue despite the WHO recommendations, and it has been estimated that approximately 30% of cancer patients have poor pain control, particularly in their last year of life [1, 2]. External beam radiation is currently the most accepted first line of treatment for painful metastatic bone lesions. However, radiation is successful in relieving pain in 60% of patients and is often temporary [3]. Radiation therapy is also associated with the risk of injuring the adjacent tissue [3]. Ablative techniques using image guidance have emerged as safe and efficacious palliative treatment for painful lesions in cancer patients [4–10]. These techniques have evolved during the recent years [5, 6]. Additionally, most recent reports indicate that these techniques are cost-effective and may also be able to improve the overall survival rate [11].

The most common palliative interventional radiology (IR) techniques that are implemented for treatment of intractable pain secondary to cancer include radiofrequency ablation (RFA), microwave ablation (MWA), cryoablation, chemical ablation (CA), and high-intensity focused ultrasound (HIFU). These techniques have been used for the treatment of painful osseous metastatic disease, head and neck lesions, ablation of painful soft tissue lesions, neurolysis, and ablation for decreasing mass effect. In this chapter, these techniques will be described, and their applications will be elucidated through multiple cases using pertinent evidence from the literature.

H. Yarmohammadi (✉)
Department of Radiology, Memorial Sloan Kettering Cancer Center, New York, NY, USA
e-mail: yarmohah@mskcc.org

General Considerations Prior to Percutaneous Image-Guided Ablation

The first step in applying image-guided ablation techniques to cancer patients is patient and lesion selection. Complete and thorough physical examination should be performed to determine the location of pain and its severity. The patient's cross-sectional images should be thoroughly reviewed to determine the safest approach for ablation. Tumors that are less than 1 cm away from the spinal cord, major motor nerves, and arteries supplying the bladder, bowel, or central nervous system are considered relative contraindications to ablation [12]. Osteolytic and mixed osteolytic/osteoblastic osseous metastatic lesions are the most suitable for ablation therapy. Ablation is less effective in pure osteoblastic lesions. Due to the high density of the pure osteoblastic lesions, access to them is difficult and there is poor RFA energy deposition [13].

Most authors recommend pretreatment pain assessment utilizing the Brief Pain Inventory Short Form or Memorial Pain Assessment Card (MPAC) [7]. This scale is used for quantitative posttreatment evaluation. Prior to the ablation treatment, the treatment expectations should be discussed in detail with the patient, patient's family, and other caregivers.

Most ablations can be performed with conscious/moderate sedation, local anesthetics, and as an outpatient procedure. At our institution, general anesthesia is used in patients with elevated baseline pain that are on large doses of opioids.

Computed tomography (CT) scan is the most common modality used for image guidance. Ultrasound can be used as image guidance in more superficial lesions. MRI-guided ablation has been used less frequently due to the need for special MRI compatible probes.

The ultimate objective of ablation is to destroy the sensory afferent nerves in the region of involvement which could be a lytic bone cortex, involved periosteum or a soft tissue mass.

A. Gulati et al. (eds.), *Essentials of Interventional Cancer Pain Management*, https://doi.org/10.1007/978-3-319-99684-4_35

Radiofrequency Ablation (RFA)

Background

Radiofrequency refers to the frequencies ranging from 350 to 500 kHz in the electromagnetic spectrum. This high frequency is delivered in alternating currents through a shielded electrode, and the electromagnetic energy induces thermal injury to the tissue surrounding the electrode, producing temperatures in excess of 50–100 °C. The heat results in coagulation necrosis and protein denaturation. The amount of cell death is dependent on the distance of the tissue from the electrode (most important factor), the intensity of current generated, and the duration of radiofrequency current application [14–16].

Advantages and Limitations

The Main Advantages of RFA over Other Thermal Ablation Techniques:

1. Immediate cell death
2. Well-controlled focal area of coagulation necrosis around the needle tip or electrodes
3. Ability to accurately monitor the ablation temperature
4. Can be performed with local anesthesia and moderate (conscious) sedation
5. Probe placement is achieved using percutaneous image guidance [16].

The Limitations of RFA

1. *Heat sink* effect. RFA efficacy decreases when the treating lesion is adjacent to a high-flow vessel due to the thermal modulation from the blood flow [17–19].
2. *Charred tissue* effect. If the power is increased too high too fast, the tissue around the probe becomes desiccated producing significant gas. This tissue will act as an insulating sleeve around the probe limiting transmission of the temperature and limiting the effect of RFA.
3. RFA is contraindicated in tumors that come in contact with metallic objects.
4. The ablation margin cannot be visualized with CT scan.

Description of the Technique

Heating the tissue at 50°–55 °C for 4–6 min results in irreversible cellular damage [20]. The ablation zone should cover the entire tumor and extend 5–10 mm into the normal surrounding tissue resulting in an ablation margin of 5–10 mm thickness [16, 20]. For a more effective ablation zone, a methodical increase in energy is recommended than a quick rise in temperature. Rapid rise to temperatures greater than 105 °C will result in carbonization, boiling, and vaporization of the tissue around the probe resulting in decreased energy transmission and consequently limiting larger ablation zone. Ultimately, the goal is to heat the tissue to 50°–100 °C for 4–6 min without causing vaporization or charring of the tissue [21]. Following 5 min of coiling, the probes may be repositioned and subsequent ablation can be performed if deemed necessary. Depending on the size of the tumor, a single probe/antenna (ranging from 14 to 17 gauges) or multiple probes may be used. Figure 35.1 demonstrates a patient with painful metastatic bone lesion from lung cancer that RFA was performed and his pain was relieved.

Application of Technique to Cancer Patients and Literature Review

RFA was initially used for treatment of benign skeletal lesions like osteoid osteoma but has rapidly emerged into the treatment of choice for palliation of painful metastatic skeletal lesions that are not responsive to pain medications and external beam radiation therapy [22]. RFA may relieve cancer pain in patients with soft tissue metastasis from a variety of malignancies including rectal cancer, fallopian tube carcinoma, and bladder carcinoma [8, 23–25]. The effectiveness and safety of RFA in managing painful osseous metastasis has been documented in two multicenter prospective studies. A multicenter trial involved 9 sites in the United States and Europe with 43 patients [26]. The second study was performed by the American College of Radiology Imaging Network in 9 sites in the United States on 55 patients [10]. In this study, Dupuy et al. demonstrated that RFA effectively relieved pain from osseous metastatic disease up to 3 months following ablation with less than 5% complication rate [10]. In a more recent study performed by Guenette et al., RFA

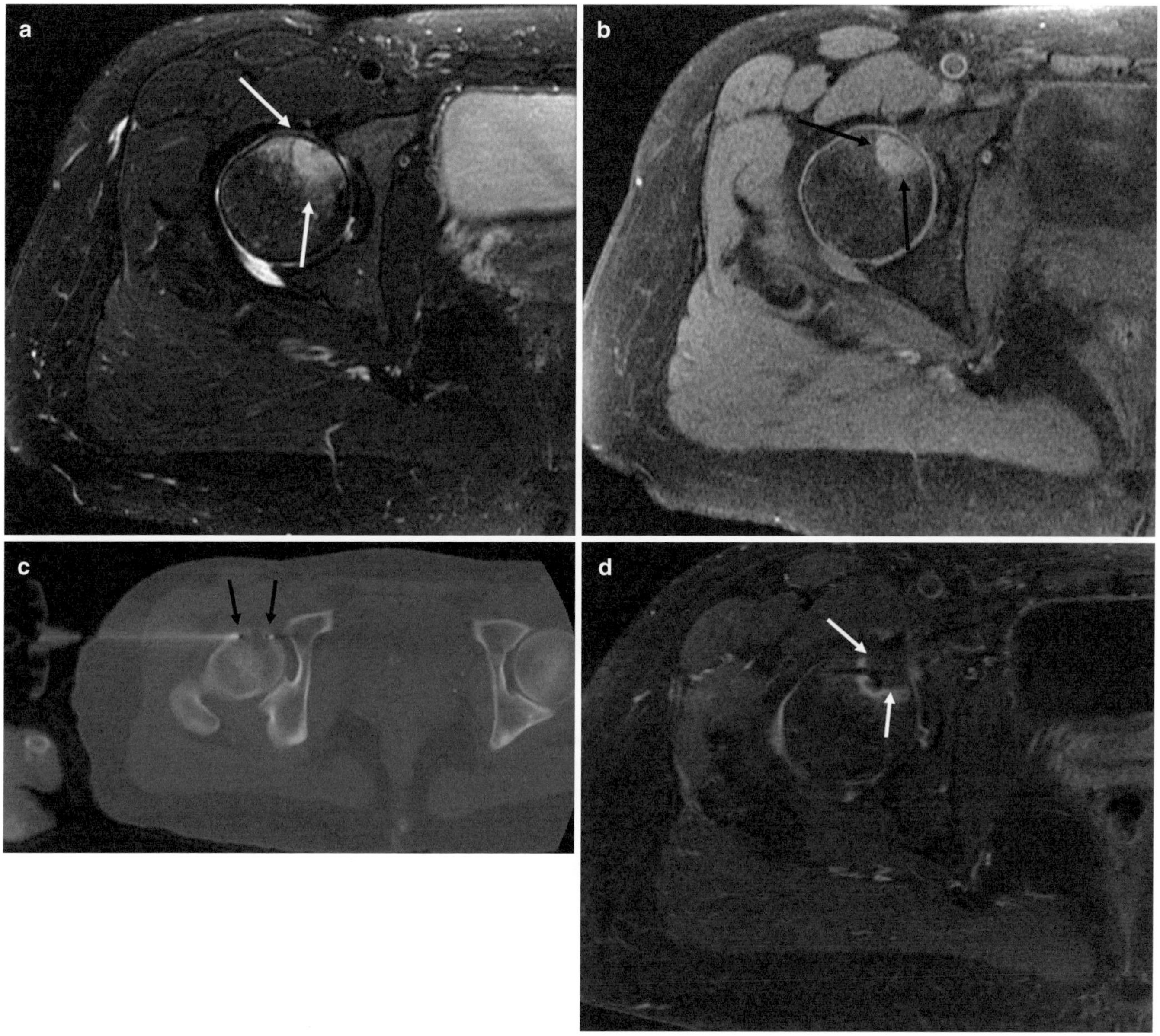

Fig. 35.1 (**a**) T2 axial fat saturation MR image of the right femur demonstrating a hyperintense lesion in the anteromedial aspect of the femoral head (white arrows). (**b**) Same lesion demonstrating enhancement on T1-post-contrast images (black arrows). (**c**) RFA probe inside the lesion (black arrow). (**d**) Three-month follow-up MRI of the right hip demonstrates post-ablation changes with no enhancement (white arrows)

was performed in 49 subjects with painful osseous metastasis. The aim of this study was to identify any correlation between the pre- and post-ablation imaging features and pain relief [27]. Guenette et al. concluded that existing pathologic fracture and smaller tumor size were predictive parameters of success.

Table 35.1 demonstrates the list of the most recent studies on the efficacy of RFA in relieving cancer pain.

Table 35.1 Review of literature of different ablation techniques

Author	Year	Study design	Modality	# of pt.	Efficiency in pain relief	Complication rate
Callstrom et al. [28]	2002	Prospective	RFA	12	Both worst pain score in a 24-hr period and mean pain significantly decreased at 4 weeks posttreatment	None
Goetz et al. [26]	2004	Prospective Multicenter	RFA	43	Average pain decreased from 6.6 of 10 at baseline to 3.7 at week 4, 2.9 at week 12, and 1.3 at week 24	7%
Thanos et al. [29]	2008	Retrospective	RFA	30	Significant decrease in the mean past-24-h Brief Pain Inventory (BPI) score for worst pain, for average pain, and for pain interference during daily life (4.7, 4.8, and 5.3 units, respectively) 4 and 8 weeks after treatment Marked decrease (3 out of 30 patients 4 and 8 weeks after treatment) in the use of analgesics	None
Carrafiello et al. [30]	2009	Prospective	RFA	10	3-month follow-up showed a statistically significant reduction of pain	None
Dupuy et al. [10]	2010	Prospective Multicenter	RFA	55	The average improvement in pain relief was 26.3 at 1 month on a 100-point scale (0, no relief; 100, complete relief) and 16.4 at 3 months	Grade 3 < 5%
Thacker et al. [8]	2011	Retrospective	RFA	22	Decrease in pain score at 24-h post-procedure from 6.0 ± 1.41 to 5.0 ± 2.04	4.5%
Guenette et al. [27]	2013	Prospective multicenter	RFA	49	RFA was more effective in patients with existing pathologic fracture and patients with smaller tumor size	Not reported
Clarencon et al. [31]	2013	Prospective	RFA	24	Pain was significantly reduced at 6 months FU (mean VAS reduction = 4.1; $P < 0.00001$)	12.5%
Pusceddu et al. [32]	2012	Retrospective	MWA	21	On average, the mean BPI score during the 3-month follow-up period was reduced by 92% (41–100%)	None
Kastler et al. [33]	2013	Retrospective	MWA	25	Immediate pain reduction in 93% of patients with a mean duration of 5.5 months	4%
Callstrom et al. [34]	2006		Cryo			
Masala et al. [35]	2011	Prospective	Cryo	20	Quantitative analysis provided by PET correlated with the response to cryoablation as assessed by CT data and clinical VAS evaluation	Not mentioned
Thacker et al. [8]	2011	Retrospective	Cryo	36	Decrease in pain score at 24 h post-procedure from 6.5 to 3.5	None
Callstrom et al. [36]	2013	Prospective multicenter	Cryo	61	Mean score worst pain in 24-h period decreased from 7.1/10 to 5.1/10, 4.0/10, 3.6/10, and 1.4/10 in 1, 4, 8, and 24 weeks after the procedure, respectively	2%
Prologo et al. [37]	2014	Retrospective	Cryo	50	Statistically significant decreases in the median VAS score and narcotic usage at both 24 h and 3 months	11%
Gangi et al. [38]	1994	Retrospective	CA	25	Within 24–48 h 74% of the cases demonstrated reduction in analgesic needs	
Catane et al. [39]	2007	Prospective	HIFU	13	MRI-guided HIFU provided safe and effective noninvasive alternative for palliation of pain	0%
Liberman et al. [40]	2009	Prospective Multicenter	HIFU	31	Significant pain improvement in 72% of the patients	0%
Napoli et al. [41]	2013	Prospective	HIFU	18	Statistically significant decrease in pain between baseline and follow-up findings	0%

Microwave Ablation (MWA)

Background

Microwave applies electromagnetic waves and produces alternating electric fields. This causes rotational movements in the water molecules within the tissue surrounding the microwave probes resulting in frictional heat [42]. This heat ultimately causes coagulation necrosis in the ablated tissue, similar to RFA. Bone tissue has low conductivity and high impedance. Therefore, theoretically, since microwave is relatively insensitive to impedance, it may be advantageous in bone tissue [43].

Advantages and Limitations

Main Advantages of Microwave

1. Since microwave uses frictional heat and is not dependent on convection of electrical current, the microwave generators do not require ground pads.
2. Microwave produces larger tumor ablation volumes compared to RFA due to higher intratumoral temperatures [44, 45].
3. MWA is faster than RFA [44].
4. Ability to use multiple applicators [46].

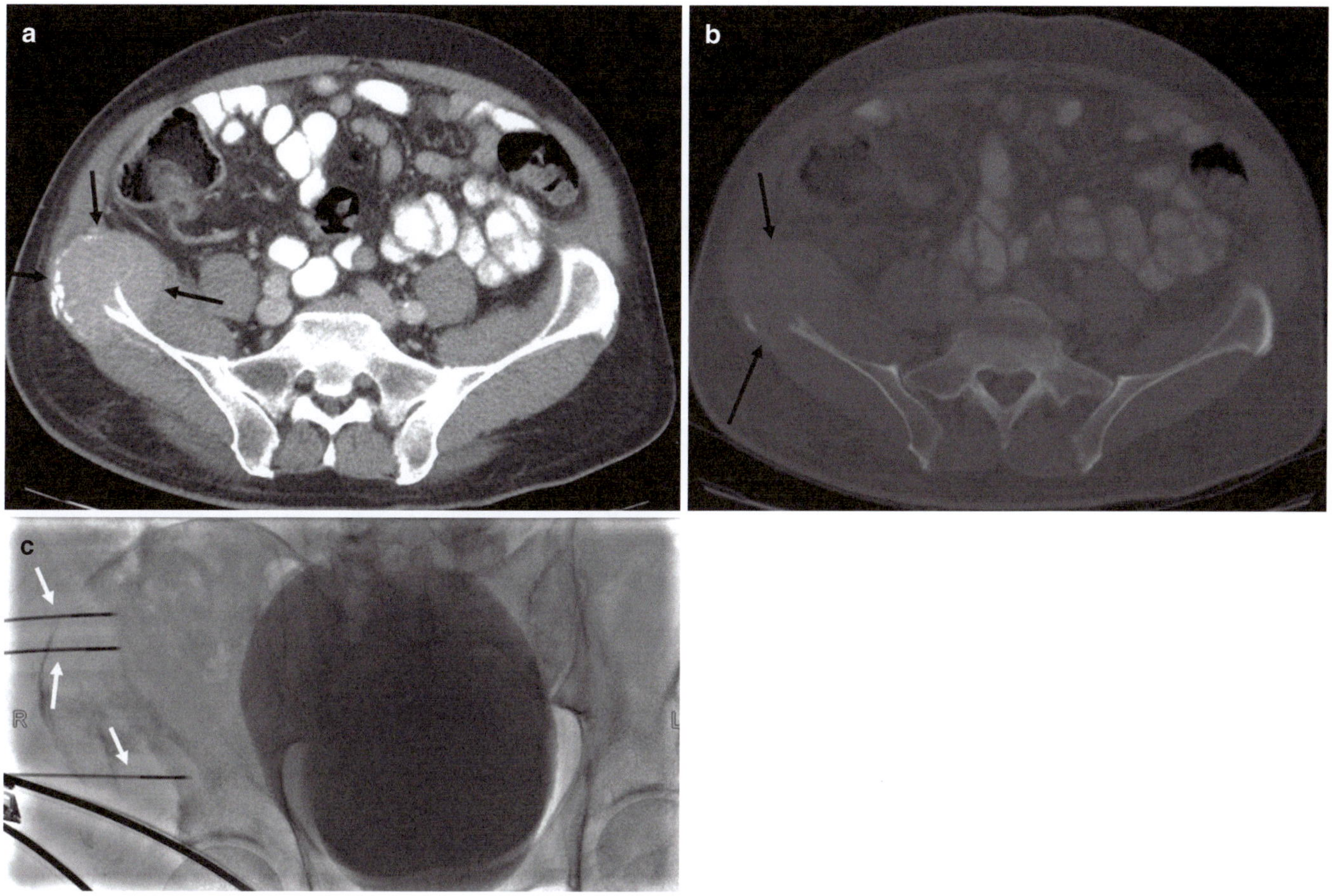

Fig. 35.2 CT scan of a patient with hepatocellular carcinoma and painful metastasis to the right iliac bone. (**a**) Mixed lytic/sclerotic lesion in the right iliac bone in soft tissue window (black arrows). (**b**) The metastatic lesion in bone window (black arrows). (**c**) Fluoroscopic lesion with multiple microwave probes in the lesion (17 G probe, NeuWave Medical, Madison, WI; white arrows)

5. Due to electromagnetic nature of microwaves, there is no *heat sink* effect or *charred tissue* effect. Therefore, optimal heating of cystic masses and tumor close to large vessels (>3 mm in diameter) can be achieved [43, 46, 47].
6. Less procedural pain probably because there is not flow of current within the patients' body.

Main Limitations of MWA

1. The ablation margin cannot be visualized with CT scan.

Description of the Technique

Microwave uses frequencies of at least 915 MHz–2.45 GHz [48]. A single 14.5-gauge antenna is usually used when the tumor is less than 3.5 cm in maximal diameter, and more than two antennas are used when the tumor is larger than 3.5 cm. In order to pierce the cortex, a 13-G bone biopsy needle can be used and can serve as a coaxial introducer for the antenna. The introducer is then retracted prior to delivery of energy. Percutaneous approach can be achieved using ultrasound or CT guidance. If the lesion is too close to the skin (<3 cm), skin precaution should be performed to avoid skin burn.

Figure 35.2 demonstrates a patient with painful metastatic bone lesion from lung cancer that MWA was performed, and her pain completely improved.

Application of Technique to Cancer Patients and Literature Review

MWA is independent on tissue conduction, produces high tissue temperatures, and is less sensitive to "heat sink" effect. Therefore, theoretically MWA should be effective in bone lesions. Early reports have demonstrated that MWA can efficiently decrease pain in cancer patients [32, 33]. In a retrospective study performed by Pusceddu et al., 21 patients with metastatic bone lesions were treated with MWA. Patients reported a significant reduction in their pain with improved quality of life as early as 1 week after the procedure, as measured by BPI score [32]. In another retrospective study, performed on 15 patients, Kastler et al. concluded that MWA is a safe and effective method of treating painful refractory bone and soft tissue tumors [33]. MWA is a powerful tool, and precaution should be used when the lesion is located near vital structures or close to the skin. Kastler et al. recommended multiple, short, relatively low-powered heating cycles, especially in cases of small lesions. Table 35.1 demonstrates the list of the most recent studies on the efficacy of MWA in relieving cancer pain.

Cryoablation

Background

Cryoablation causes cytotoxic effect through formation of intracellular ice crystals. These ice crystals cause protein denaturation, cell membrane rupture, and shearing of the intracellular structures. A liquid gas, commonly argon or nitrous oxide, runs through the cryoablation probes. This gas rapidly cools the tip of the cryoablation probe and forms an ice ball around the probe. Ice formation is followed by a thawing phase, commonly by using helium. The freezing and thawing phases cause water to rush into the tumor cells resulting in swelling and bursting of the cells [49]. The temperature necessary to cause cellular necrosis depends on the cell type and tissue type. Tissue destruction is complete at −20 °C to −40 °C. This temperature is achieved approximately 3–5 mm deep to the visible edge of the ice ball, which corresponds to 0 °C [50, 51]. The mechanism by which cryoablation reduces pain has not been studied. However, it most likely reduces pain by reducing tumor burden and osteolysis. The size of the ablation zone is dependent on the size of the cryoprobe, the length of the uninsulated tip, and the freezing time.

Advantages and Limitations

Main Advantages of Cryoablation

1. The main advantage of cryoablation over other ablation techniques is that cryoablation forms a distinct ice ball that can be seen with CT scan, MRI, or ultrasound and can be used to precisely monitor tumor coverage [52, 53]. The ice ball boarder also confirms proper exclusion of critical structures adjacent to the ablation margin [54]. Any structure/tissue beyond the low-attenuation ice ball is safe from the thermal injury.
2. Decreased intra-procedural and post-procedural pain [8]. Compared to RFA, patients treated with cryoablation do not experience increased pain during the procedure or immediately after the ablation [8].
3. Multiple probes can be used because each probe acts independent to others.

Main Limitations of Cryoablation

1. More time-consuming than RFA and MWA, typically takes 25–30 min. This is because unlike radiofrequency and microwave ablation, cryoablation provides no zone of direct or active cooling, and so the surface area of the cryoablation probe limits cooling efficiency.
2. Risk of cryoshock: This systemic complication that includes hypotension, multi-organ failure, respiratory compromise, and disseminated intravascular coagulopathy happens when the ablation zone is reperfused after the ice ball is melted. The rapid release of the cellular debris into the systemic circulation causes cryoshock. This is rarely seen with heat-based ablation techniques [50].
3. May be more expensive than RFA. More probes are needed during cryoablation, therefore increasing the cost.
4. Since cryoablation does not use heat, there is no cautery effect which may result in bleeding complications.
5. Organ fracture may happen due to the fact that frozen tissue is more brittle.

Description of the Technique

Cryoablation of the bone or soft tissue is performed under moderate conscious sedation or general anesthesia. The probes are larger than those used for RFA ranging from 11 to 17 gauges. Multiple probes can be used to provide synergistic effect and increase the size of the ice ball. Like other ablation methods, CT scan is the most common modality used for guidance in placement of the cryoprobes. The probe(s) should be placed approximately 1 cm from the margins in order to provide complete coverage of the tumor. When using multiple probes, the probes should be placed 2 cm from each other. The probes should be placed in parallel along the long axis of the tumor. If the mass is larger than 8 cm in diameter, it should be treated in two sessions on sequential days. If the area of ablation is in close proximity to the bowel, bladder, or skin, hydrodissection can be performed to displace them [55]. Non-contrast CT scan should be performed every 2–5 min throughout the freezing phase of the ablation to monitor the size, location, and extent of the ice ball coverage. The ablation zone is identified as a well-marginated low-attenuation area seen on non-contrast CT scan and best visualized on body window and level settings of (W400, L40). As mentioned earlier the visible edge of the ice ball corresponds to 0 °C, and therefore cell death occurs approximately 3 mm deep to this edge. After the freezing process, the probes should be actively thawed for 10–15 min. The probes should only be removed once the temperature reaches approximately +25 °C.

There are numerous reported variations on freeze–thaw–freeze cycles that depend on tumor type and size; however the most common method for cryoablation involves a 10-min freeze, 5-min thaw, and then a second 10-min freeze (10-5-10 min). Figure 35.3 demonstrates a patient with breast cancer with painful osseous lesion in her hip. Cryoablation was performed and was able to relieve her pain.

Application of Technique to Cancer Patients and Literature Review

Cryoablation has been reported to be an effective and safe method in the treating painful osseous metastases [8, 34, 36]. In a retrospective study, Thacker et al. reviewed 58 patients with painful osseous metastasis [8]. These patients were divided into 2 groups of 36 (cryoablation) and 22 (RFA). Patients who had undergone cryoablation had significantly less short-term analgesic requirement and shorter hospital stay compared to the group that received RFA [8]. In a multicenter clinical trial, 61 patients with 1 or 2 painful osseous metastasis were evaluated [36]. This study reported highly significant reduction in pain scores (75% of the patients achieved 90% or higher pain relief) and

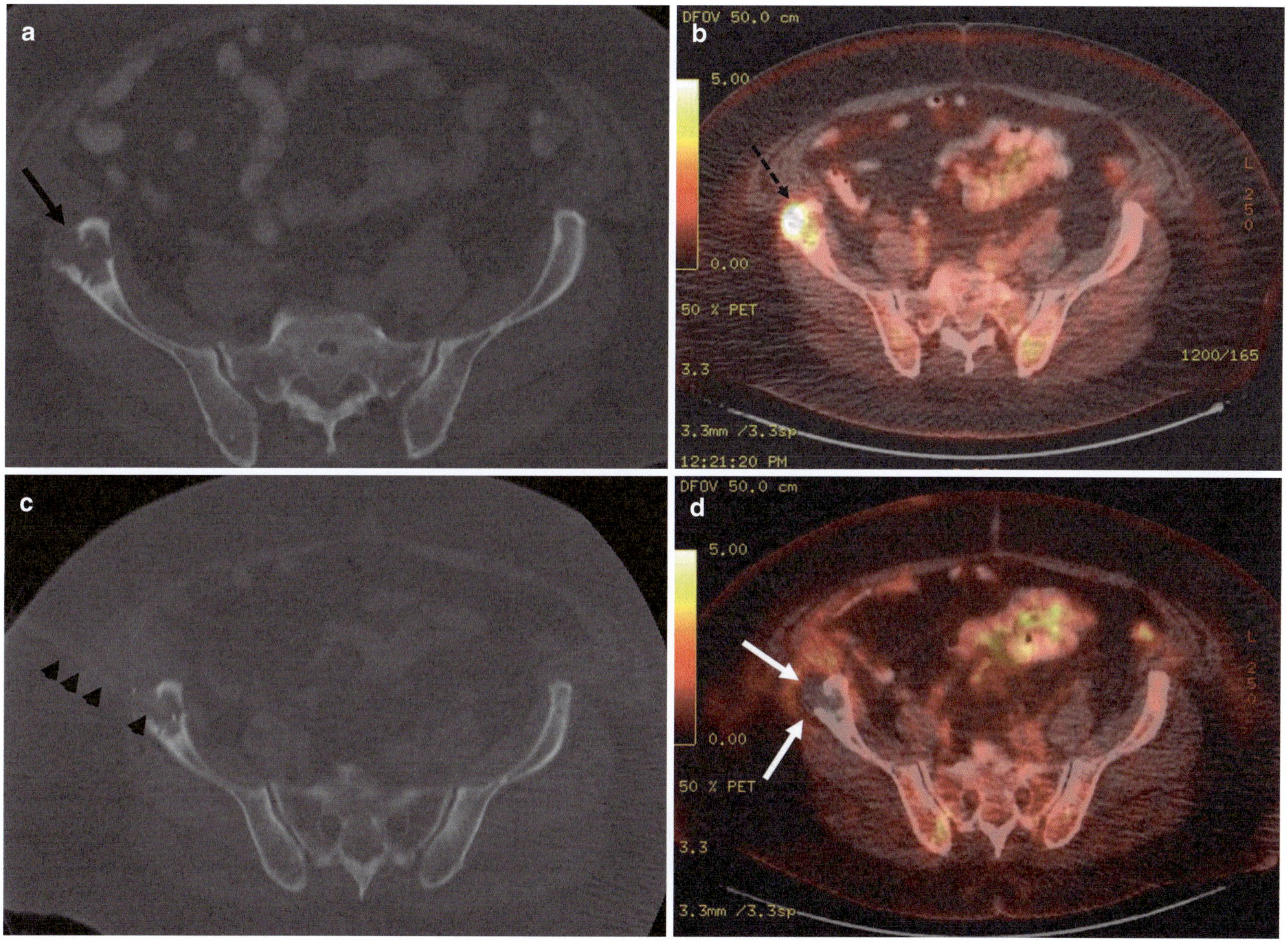

Fig. 35.3 (**a**) CT scan demonstrates a lytic lesion with cortical destruction in the right iliac bone (black arrow). (**b**) Same lesion is shown on a PET/CT scan which demonstrates FDG uptake in the lesion and the adjacent soft tissue component (dashed black arrow). (**c**) Cryoablation probe (Ice Force 2.1 CX probe, Galil Medical Inc., Arden Hills, MN; black arrow heads) inside the lesion. (**d**) PET/CT scan performed 3 months post-ablation demonstrating the lesion that is no longer FDG avid (white arrows)

improvement in the quality of life at 1, 4, 8, and 24 weeks after treatment with cryoablation [36]. The pain relief was durable in 86% of the patients. In a similar study, Masala et al. demonstrated significant pain relief after cryoablation for painful osseous metastases in 20 patients [35]. In another recent study on cryoablation in 50 patients with osseous metastasis, pain was significantly decreased at 24 h and 3-month follow-up [37]. Finally, Rosenthal and Callstrom published a comprehensive review of case studies and small series on efficiency and safety of cryoablation for painful osseous metastases [56]. Cryoablation has also been effective in relieving pain from celiac plexus involvement by pancreas cancer and intractable pudendal nerve involvement [57, 58].

Chemical Ablation (CA)

Background

Chemical ablation (CA) is achieved by percutaneous injection of chemical agents that induce cell death. Cell death happens due to vascular and cellular effects. There are two main chemical agents that are used in clinical practice including ethanol and acetic acid. Acetic acid diffuses better than ethanol and produces a bigger area of necrosis compared to ethanol, and therefore it may be preferred to treat large tumors [59]. Ethanol and acetic acid cause denaturation of the cell protein and dehydration of the cytoplasm. Additionally, they result in endothelial cell necrosis and platelet aggregation which leads to vascular thrombosis and ischemia.

Advantages and Limitations

Main Advantages of CA

1. Cheapest method of ablation.
2. Rapid relief of pain: pain relief occurs in 24–48 h.

Main Limitations of CA

1. CA is a painful procedure, particularly in the bone.
2. Diffusion of the chemical agent is not predictable and uncontrollable; therefore it may result in injury to the adjacent nervous structures and intravascular injection.
3. Degree of necrosis is highly variable.
4. Potential complication is massive tumor necrosis specifically after injection of more than 30 ml of alcohol.

Description of the Technique

Procedure is performed under CT guidance. Ethanol 95% is mixed with contrast and injected. A 22-gauge spinal needle is used to inject the ethanol into the lesion. The non-necrotic part of the tumor is targeted. Therefore, a contrast-enhanced CT is usually performed prior to the procedure to identify areas of necrosis in the lesion. Initially, lidocaine diluted with 25% contrast medium is injected into the lesion. This reduces the pain provoked by alcohol injection. CT scan is performed to evaluate the distribution of the contrast media. The distribution of the contrast within the tumor is used to predict the dispersal of the injected alcohol. If contrast diffuses beyond the tumor margins and approaches a critical structure like nerves, injection of ethanol or acetic acid cannot be performed. Depending on the size of the tumor and the type of chemical agent used, 5–25 ml is instilled into the tumor [38].

Application of Technique to Cancer Patients and Literature Review

Although CA is the cheapest and the easiest ablation method, the use of other ablation techniques has reduced the utilization of this technique. This ablation technique is utilized mainly when other ablation techniques are not feasible. Gangi et al. reported 74% reduction in pain in 25 patients with 27 bone metastases after 24–48 h of 95% ethanol injection [38].

High-Intensity Focused Ultrasound (HIFU)

Background

High-intensity focused ultrasound (HIFU) is a noninvasive ablative technique using ultrasound waves within an area of human tissue, generating local heat, leading to cellular death. HIFU was first used in human in the 1950s in treatment of patients with Parkinson's disease [60]. Real-time US or MRI is used for guidance. MRI can provide additional information that can be used for precise treatment mapping. Focused ultrasound waves are generated and focused for 15–25 s. These focused waves result in tissue heating in an elliptical-shaped spot measuring up to 7 cm. Bone absorbs ultrasound waves approximately 50 times more than soft tissues, and thermal conductivity of the bone is minimal. Therefore, when HIFU is used to treat osseous metastatic disease, the focus point is placed behind the targeted bone to allow a larger field of heating. Bone procedures are typically 2 h long. The procedure is painful and should be performed under deep sedation or locoregional anesthesia.

Advantages and Limitations

Main Advantages of HIFU

1. The main advantage of this modality is that the treatment is performed under real-time MRI guidance. The tumor can be precisely localized using real-time MRI, and thermal dose can be accurately deposited.
2. Noninvasive thermal ablation modality.

Main Limitations of HIFU

1. Time-consuming. Bone procedures typically take 2 h.

Description of The Technique

Patients are placed on the MRI table and positioned in a way that the target lesion is aligned with ultrasound transducer. The transducer is located in the MRI table within an oil bath. The transducer is coupled to the patient's skin using a gel pad to eliminate air across the path of the ultrasound beam. Since MRI is used for guidance, the treatment planning is performed in three dimensions, coronal, sagittal, and axial planes.

Application of Technique to Cancer Patients and Literature Review

MRI-guided focused ultrasound ablation was effective in treating soft tissue tumors such as uterine fibroids [61]. Additionally, this modality has been used as a noninvasive treatment for benign and malignant breast tumors [62]. HIFU with or without MRI guidance has been reported among different studies to significantly reduce pain from osseous metastasis disease [39–41, 63]. Catane et al. used MRI-guided HIFU in 13 patients with symptomatic bone metastases and were successful in improving pain score and reducing analgesic dose in these patients [39]. In a multi-center study, Liberman et al. used MRI-guided HIFU in 31 patients and reported significant improvement in pain in 72% of their patients [40]. In a recent study performed by Napoli et al., 18 consecutive patients with painful bone metastases were treated with MRI-guided focused ultrasound [41]. Pain was significantly decreased when compared to baseline, and no treatment-related adverse event was reported.

Conclusion

Palliative treatment of painful metastatic disease can be efficiently and safely achieved by percutaneous ablation techniques. The therapeutic armamentarium includes radiofrequency ablation, microwave ablation, cryoablation, chemical ablation, and HIFU. Multiple studies have demonstrated the efficiency and safety of these techniques. Thorough knowledge of indications, limitations, and protective techniques of each ablation technique is mandatory for a successful treatment.

References

1. Valeberg BT, Miaskowski C, Hanestad BR, Bjordal K, Moum T, Rustoen T. Prevalence rates for and predictors of self-reported adherence of oncology outpatients with analgesic medications. Clin J Pain. 2008;24(7):627–36.
2. Fitzgibbon D. Interventional procedures for cancer pain management: selecting the right procedure at the right time. J Support Oncol. 2010;8(2):60–1.
3. Wu JS, Wong R, Johnston M, Bezjak A, Whelan T. Meta-analysis of dose-fractionation radiotherapy trials for the palliation of painful bone metastases. Int J Radiat Oncol Biol Phys. 2003;55(3):594–605.
4. Patel IJ, Pirasteh A, Passalacqua MA, Robbin MR, Hsu DP, Buethe J, et al. Palliative procedures for the interventional oncologist. AJR Am J Roentgenol. 2013;201(4):726–35.
5. Bhaskar AK. Interventional management of cancer pain. Curr Opin Support Palliat Care. 2012;6(1):1–9.
6. McCullough HK, Bain RM, Clark HP, Requarth JA. The radiologist as a palliative care subspecialist: providing symptom relief when cure is not possible. AJR Am J Roentgenol. 2011;196(2):462–7.
7. Foster RC, Stavas JM. Bone and soft tissue ablation. Semin Interv Radiol. 2014;31(2):167–79.
8. Thacker PG, Callstrom MR, Curry TB, Mandrekar JN, Atwell TD, Goetz MP, et al. Palliation of painful metastatic disease involving bone with imaging-guided treatment: comparison of patients' immediate response to radiofrequency ablation and cryoablation. AJR Am J Roentgenol. 2011;197(2):510–5.
9. Requarth J. Image-guided palliative care procedures. Surg Clin North Am. 2011;91(2):367–402. i35
10. Dupuy DE, Liu D, Hartfeil D, Hanna L, Blume JD, Ahrar K, et al. Percutaneous radiofrequency ablation of painful osseous metastases: a multicenter American College of Radiology Imaging Network trial. Cancer. 2010;116(4):989–97.
11. Bang HJ, Littrup PJ, Currier BP, Goodrich DJ, Aoun HD, Klein LC, et al. Percutaneous cryoablation of metastatic lesions from non-small-cell lung carcinoma: initial survival, local control, and cost observations. J Vasc Interv Radiol. 2012;23(6):761–9.
12. Nazario J, Hernandez J, Tam AL. Thermal ablation of painful bone metastases. Tech Vasc Interv Radiol. 2011;14(3):150–9.
13. Dupuy DE, Hong R, Oliver B, Goldberg SN. Radiofrequency ablation of spinal tumors: temperature distribution in the spinal canal. AJR Am J Roentgenol. 2000;175(5):1263–6.

14. Nahum Goldberg S, Dupuy DE. Image-guided radiofrequency tumor ablation: challenges and opportunities--part I. J Vasc Interv Radiol. 2001;12(9):1021–32.
15. Simon CJ, Dupuy DE. Percutaneous minimally invasive therapies in the treatment of bone tumors: thermal ablation. Semin Musculoskelet Radiol. 2006;10(2):137–44.
16. Dupuy DE, Goldberg SN. Image-guided radiofrequency tumor ablation: challenges and opportunities--part II. J Vasc Interv Radiol. 2001;12(10):1135–48.
17. Patterson EJ, Scudamore CH, Owen DA, Nagy AG, Buczkowski AK. Radiofrequency ablation of porcine liver in vivo: effects of blood flow and treatment time on lesion size. Ann Surg. 1998;227(4):559–65.
18. Goldberg SN, Hahn PF, Tanabe KK, Mueller PR, Schima W, Athanasoulis CA, et al. Percutaneous radiofrequency tissue ablation: does perfusion-mediated tissue cooling limit coagulation necrosis? J Vasc Interv Radiol. 1998;9(1 Pt 1):101–11.
19. Lu DS, Raman SS, Vodopich DJ, Wang M, Sayre J, Lassman C. Effect of vessel size on creation of hepatic radiofrequency lesions in pigs: assessment of the "heat sink" effect. AJR Am J Roentgenol. 2002;178(1):47–51.
20. Rhim H, Goldberg SN, Dodd GD 3rd, Solbiati L, Lim HK, Tonolini M, et al. Essential techniques for successful radio-frequency thermal ablation of malignant hepatic tumors. Radiographics. 2001;21 Spec No:S17–35; discussion S6–9.
21. Goldberg SN, Solbiati L, Halpern EF, Gazelle GS. Variables affecting proper system grounding for radiofrequency ablation in an animal model. J Vasc Interv Radiol. 2000;11(8):1069–75.
22. Woertler K, Vestring T, Boettner F, Winkelmann W, Heindel W, Lindner N. Osteoid osteoma: CT-guided percutaneous radiofrequency ablation and follow-up in 47 patients. J Vasc Interv Radiol. 2001;12(6):717–22.
23. Thanos L, Mylona S, Kalioras V, Pomoni M, Batakis N. Palliation of painful perineal metastasis treated with radiofrequency thermal ablation. Cardiovasc Intervent Radiol. 2005;28(3):381–3.
24. Sanou R, Bazin C, Krakowski I, Boccaccini H, Mathias J, Beot S, et al. Radiofrequency ablation for palliation of soft tissue tumor pain. J Radiol. 2010;91(3 Pt 1):281–6.
25. Rosenthal DI, Alexander A, Rosenberg AE, Springfield D. Ablation of osteoid osteomas with a percutaneously placed electrode: a new procedure. Radiology. 1992;183(1):29–35.
26. Goetz MP, Callstrom MR, Charboneau JW, Farrell MA, Maus TP, Welch TJ, et al. Percutaneous image-guided radiofrequency ablation of painful metastases involving bone: a multicenter study. J Clin Oncol Off J Am Soc Clin Oncol. 2004;22(2):300–6.
27. Guenette JP, Lopez MJ, Kim E, Dupuy DE. Solitary painful osseous metastases: correlation of imaging features with pain palliation after radiofrequency ablation—a multicenter American college of Radiology Imaging Network study. Radiology. 2013;268(3):907–15.
28. Callstrom MR, Charboneau JW, Goetz MP, Rubin J, Wong GY, Sloan JA, et al. Painful metastases involving bone: feasibility of percutaneous CT- and US-guided radio-frequency ablation. Radiology. 2002;224(1):87–97.
29. Thanos L, Mylona S, Galani P, Tzavoulis D, Kalioras V, Tanteles S, et al. Radiofrequency ablation of osseous metastases for the palliation of pain. Skelet Radiol. 2008;37(3):189–94.
30. Carrafiello G, Lagana D, Pellegrino C, Fontana F, Mangini M, Nicotera P, et al. Percutaneous imaging-guided ablation therapies in the treatment of symptomatic bone metastases: preliminary experience. Radiol Med. 2009;114(4):608–25.
31. Clarencon F, Jean B, Pham HP, Cormier E, Bensimon G, Rose M, et al. Value of percutaneous radiofrequency ablation with or without percutaneous vertebroplasty for pain relief and functional recovery in painful bone metastases. Skelet Radiol. 2013;42(1):25–36.
32. Pusceddu C, Sotgia B, Fele RM, Melis L. Treatment of bone metastases with microwave thermal ablation. J Vasc Interv Radiol. 2013;24(2):229–35.
33. Kastler A, Alnassan H, Pereira PL, Alemann G, Barbe DA, Aubry S, et al. Analgesic effects of microwave ablation of bone and soft tissue tumors under local anesthesia. Pain Med (Malden Mass). 2013;14(12):1873–81.
34. Callstrom MR, Atwell TD, Charboneau JW, Farrell MA, Goetz MP, Rubin J, et al. Painful metastases involving bone: percutaneous image-guided cryoablation—prospective trial interim analysis. Radiology. 2006;241(2):572–80.
35. Masala S, Schillaci O, Bartolucci AD, Calabria F, Mammucari M, Simonetti G. Metabolic and clinical assessment of efficacy of cryoablation therapy on skeletal masses by 18F-FDG positron emission tomography/computed tomography (PET/CT) and visual analogue scale (VAS): initial experience. Skelet Radiol. 2011;40(2):159–65.
36. Callstrom MR, Dupuy DE, Solomon SB, Beres RA, Littrup PJ, Davis KW, et al. Percutaneous image-guided cryoablation of painful metastases involving bone: multicenter trial. Cancer. 2013;119(5):1033–41.
37. Prologo JD, Passalacqua M, Patel I, Bohnert N, Corn DJ. Image-guided cryoablation for the treatment of painful musculoskeletal metastatic disease: a single-center experience. Skelet Radiol. 2014;43(11):1551–9.
38. Gangi A, Kastler B, Klinkert A, Dietemann JL. Injection of alcohol into bone metastases under CT guidance. J Comput Assist Tomogr. 1994;18(6):932–5.
39. Catane R, Beck A, Inbar Y, Rabin T, Shabshin N, Hengst S, et al. MR-guided focused ultrasound surgery (MRgFUS) for the palliation of pain in patients with bone metastases--preliminary clinical experience. Ann Oncol. 2007;18(1):163–7.
40. Liberman B, Gianfelice D, Inbar Y, Beck A, Rabin T, Shabshin N, et al. Pain palliation in patients with bone metastases using MR-guided focused ultrasound surgery: a multicenter study. Ann Surg Oncol. 2009;16(1):140–6.
41. Napoli A, Anzidei M, Marincola BC, Brachetti G, Noce V, Boni F, et al. MR imaging-guided focused ultrasound for treatment of bone metastasis. Radiographics. 2013;33(6):1555–68.
42. Simon CJ, Dupuy DE, Mayo-Smith WW. Microwave ablation: principles and applications. Radiographics. 2005;25(Suppl 1):S69–83.
43. Skinner MG, Iizuka MN, Kolios MC, Sherar MD. A theoretical comparison of energy sources—microwave, ultrasound and laser—for interstitial thermal therapy. Phys Med Biol. 1998;43(12):3535–47.
44. Yu J, Liang P, Yu X, Liu F, Chen L, Wang Y. A comparison of microwave ablation and bipolar radiofrequency ablation both with an internally cooled probe: results in ex vivo and in vivo porcine livers. Eur J Radiol. 2011;79(1):124–30.
45. Izzo F. Other thermal ablation techniques: microwave and interstitial laser ablation of liver tumors. Ann Surg Oncol. 2003;10(5):491–7.
46. Wright AS, Lee FT Jr, Mahvi DM. Hepatic microwave ablation with multiple antennae results in synergistically larger zones of coagulation necrosis. Ann Surg Oncol. 2003;10(3):275–83.
47. Wright AS, Sampson LA, Warner TF, Mahvi DM, Lee FT Jr. Radiofrequency versus microwave ablation in a hepatic porcine model. Radiology. 2005;236(1):132–9.
48. Brace CL. Microwave tissue ablation: biophysics, technology, and applications. Crit Rev Biomed Eng. 2010;38(1):65–78.
49. Hoffmann NE, Bischof JC. The cryobiology of cryosurgical injury. Urology. 2002;60(2 Suppl 1):40–9.
50. Rubinsky B. Cryosurgery. Annu Rev Biomed Eng. 2000;2:157–87.
51. Rubinsky B, Lee CY, Bastacky J, Onik G. The process of freezing and the mechanism of damage during hepatic cryosurgery. Cryobiology. 1990;27(1):85–97.
52. Silverman SG, Tuncali K, Adams DF, Nawfel RD, Zou KH, Judy PF. CT fluoroscopy-guided abdominal interventions: techniques, results, and radiation exposure. Radiology. 1999;212(3):673–81.

53. Tacke J, Speetzen R, Heschel I, Hunter DW, Rau G, Gunther RW. Imaging of interstitial cryotherapy--an in vitro comparison of ultrasound, computed tomography, and magnetic resonance imaging. Cryobiology. 1999;38(3):250–9.
54. Weber SM, Lee FT Jr, Warner TF, Chosy SG, Mahvi DM. Hepatic cryoablation: US monitoring of extent of necrosis in normal pig liver. Radiology. 1998;207(1):73–7.
55. Farrell MA, Charboneau JW, Callstrom MR, Reading CC, Engen DE, Blute ML. Paranephric water instillation: a technique to prevent bowel injury during percutaneous renal radiofrequency ablation. AJR Am J Roentgenol. 2003;181(5):1315–7.
56. Rosenthal D, Callstrom MR. Critical review and state of the art in interventional oncology: benign and metastatic disease involving bone. Radiology. 2012;262(3):765–80.
57. Yarmohammadi H, Nakamoto DA, Azar N, Hayek SM, Haaga JR. Percutaneous computed tomography guided cryoablation of the celiac plexus as an alternative treatment for intractable pain caused by pancreatic cancer. J Cancer Res Ther. 2011;7(4):481–3.
58. Fanucci E, Manenti G, Ursone A, Fusco N, Mylonakou I, D'Urso S, et al. Role of interventional radiology in pudendal neuralgia: a description of techniques and review of the literature. Radiol Med. 2009;114(3):425–36.
59. Xiao YY, Tian JL, Li JK, Yang L, Zhang JS. CT-guided percutaneous chemical ablation of adrenal neoplasms. AJR Am J Roentgenol. 2008;190(1):105–10.
60. Fry WJ, Barnard JW, Fry FJ, Brennan JF. Ultrasonically produced localized selective lesions in the central nervous system. Am J Phys Med. 1955;34(3):413–23.
61. Stewart EA, Rabinovici J, Tempany CM, Inbar Y, Regan L, Gostout B, et al. Clinical outcomes of focused ultrasound surgery for the treatment of uterine fibroids. Fertil Steril. 2006;85(1):22–9.
62. Gianfelice D, Khiat A, Boulanger Y, Amara M, Belblidia A. Feasibility of magnetic resonance imaging-guided focused ultrasound surgery as an adjunct to tamoxifen therapy in high-risk surgical patients with breast carcinoma. J Vasc Interv Radiol. 2003;14(10):1275–82.
63. Chen W, Zhu H, Zhang L, Li K, Su H, Jin C, et al. Primary bone malignancy: effective treatment with high-intensity focused ultrasound ablation. Radiology. 2010;255(3):967–78.

36 Introduction to Radiation Therapy

Shayna E. Rich and Kavita V. Dharmarajan

Radiation therapy is a complex treatment modality that is frequently used for palliative treatment for advanced cancers, including up to 50% of patients in a typical radiation oncology practice. Radiation therapy can be used with palliative intent to reduce pain, neurological dysfunction, bleeding, fungating wounds, nausea, vomiting, or obstructive symptoms [1]. It is considered most frequently for bony metastatic disease, but it can be used to treat a wide variety of sites including the brain, head and neck, liver, pelvis, thorax, and skin. Palliative radiation therapy is often given using shorter courses with larger doses at each treatment, instead of lengthier treatment courses delivered with curative intent. The length and total dose of treatment may be adjusted based on the patient's cancer prognosis, treatment goals and preferences, and other indicators of life expectancy. In this chapter, we provide an overview of the concepts in physics and biology that underlie the use of radiation therapy. We then describe the process of planning and delivering radiation therapy. Finally, we describe the indications, doses, and toxicities associated with common sites for palliative radiation therapy.

Introduction to Radiation Therapy

Radiation Physics

Radiation dose is defined in units of gray (Gy), which is determined by the amount of energy deposited by a radiation beam. One Gy is defined as one joule of dose absorbed per kilogram of irradiated material. Dose is not uniformly deposited throughout a material, but the effect will depend on the type of radiation and its energy. The most common type of radiation machine in use today is a linear accelerator or *linac* that can produce either an electron beam with energies of 4–20 MeV (mega electron volts) or a corresponding photon beam with a distribution of energies but a similar maximum energy (Fig. 36.1). Lower energy treatments can be given with contact therapy, superficial therapy, or orthovoltage therapy units (Fig. 36.2). These machines are not commonly used for radiation therapy in the modern day given their limited dose range; however they may be useful for treating more superficial lesions such as skin cancers.

Megavoltage photon x-ray beams have dose buildup at the material surface to reach a maximal value, followed by a gradual falloff within the tissue (Fig. 36.3). Electron beams have a higher dose deposited near the surface, followed by a gradual increase in dose to a maximum within a few centimeters. The falloff for electron beams is sharp, meaning that virtually no dose is deposited beyond a certain depth within the material. Particle radiation beams such as proton beams deposit dose over a relatively narrow range of depths. This type of radiation beam is useful for avoiding irradiation of sensitive organs located both superficial and deep to the tumor (Fig. 36.4).

Radiation Biology

Radiation therapy is designed to kill cancerous cells by causing damage to the cell's DNA, either directly or indirectly, in the form of DNA strand breaks. Radiation can damage all cell types as it passes through tissues within the body, but the response of individual tissue types differs. This quality is known as *radiosensitivity*, and it depends on how quickly the cells within the respective tissues are dividing. Radiosensitivity also depends on the type of radiation beam used, the dose, fractionation, and the conditions under which radiation is given. Cancer cells differ in their inherent radiosensitivity based on their histology. For instance, leukemia and lymphoma are considered to be highly radiosensitive

S. E. Rich
Haven Hospice, Gainesville, FL, USA

K. V. Dharmarajan (✉)
Icahn School of Medicine at Mount Sinai, New York, NY, USA
e-mail: kavita.dharmarajan@mountsinai.org

A. Gulati et al. (eds.), *Essentials of Interventional Cancer Pain Management*, https://doi.org/10.1007/978-3-319-99684-4_36

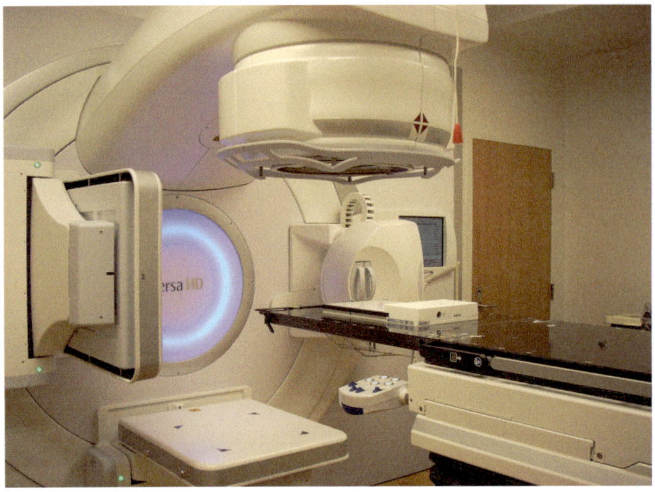

Fig. 36.1 Typical linear accelerator

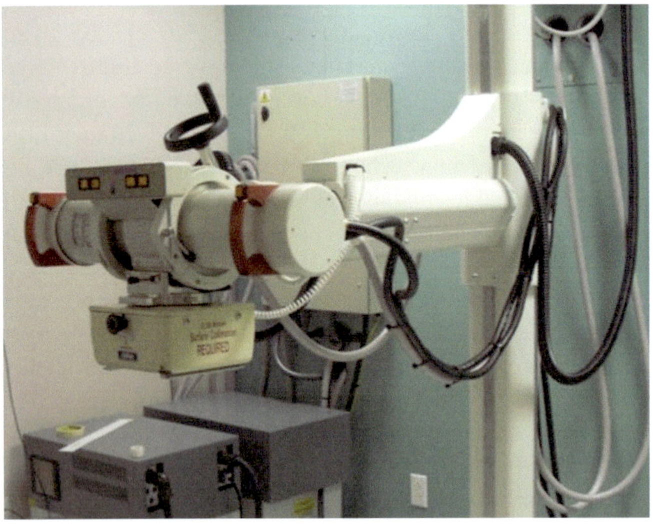

Fig. 36.2 Typical orthovoltage therapy unit

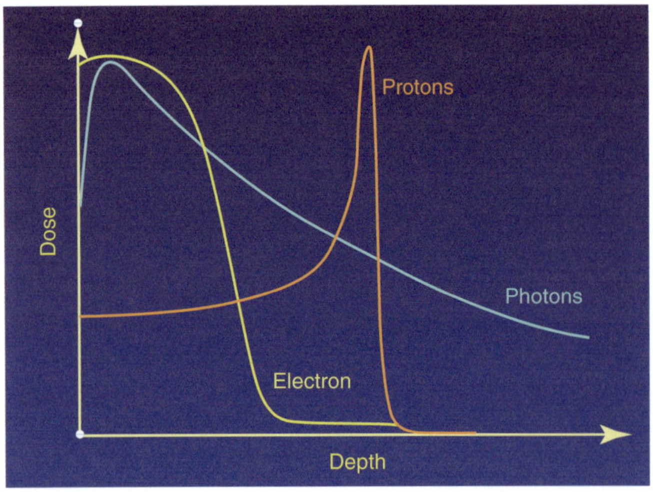

Fig. 36.3 Typical percentage depth-dose curves comparing photons, electrons, and protons

tumor types, but renal cell carcinoma and melanoma are considered highly radioresistant. Nonetheless, all cells will die if a sufficiently high dose of radiation is given.

Tissues can be categorized as early-reacting or late-reacting. At low doses, early-reacting tissues (including tumors) are more sensitive than late-reacting tissues, and thus cells within early-reacting tissues die or are damaged. At high doses, late-reacting tissues are unable to repair sufficiently to compensate for radiation-induced damage. Thus late-reacting tissues are increasingly radiosensitive compared to early-reacting tissues as higher doses are used. Examples of early- and late-reacting tissues are seen in Table 36.1.

Dose fractionation is the concept of delivering a total therapeutic dose of radiation divided over several treatments. Dose fractionation is important because of differences in radiosensitivity of tissues. It is impossible to provide radiation therapy to a tumor without irradiating neighboring normal tissues, but the effects on these tissues can be spared in part by dose fractionation. Early-reacting tissues (including tumorous tissues) are sensitive to small changes in the dose per fraction, whereas late-reacting tissues will only be substantially damaged with a large increase in the total dose. Thus, the use of conventional fractionation (1.8–3 Gy/fraction in once-daily fractions) or even hyperfractionation (defined as doses <1.8 Gy/fraction) ensures that the maximal total dose can be given, with only minimal increase to the toxicity to late-reacting tissues. Hypofractionation (defined as doses >3Gy/fraction) is generally used to complete a treatment in fewer fractions by delivering larger radiation doses in each fraction. This is particularly relevant in the palliative setting when patients may have a limited life expectancy or cannot tolerate a long treatment course for logistical or other clinical reasons. Of note, fractionation is often of minimal benefit if the neighboring normal tissue is also early-reacting (e.g., gastrointestinal tract). In this case, the total dose will be limited regardless of the fractionation.

Biologically equivalent dose (BED) is a radiobiologic principle used to compare the theoretical biological impact of different fractionation schemes on a tissue type. BED calculations consider number of fractions, dose per fraction, and the repair capacity of a particular tissue. It is assumed two radiation treatment courses with identical BED values will result in similar probability of tumor control or normal tissue effect.

The Process of Radiation Treatment

Radiation therapy generally requires a preparatory CT scan, called a simulation, and treatment planning procedures prior to a patient beginning treatment. Radiation treatment plans are customized based on each patient's anatomy and target

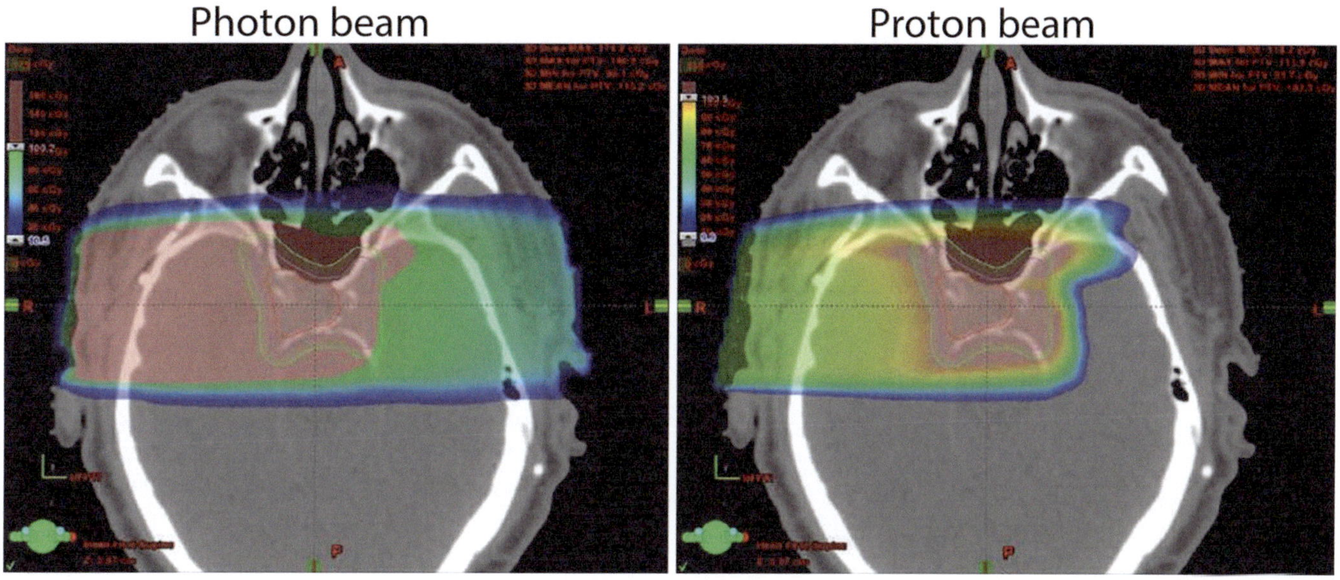

Fig. 36.4 Comparing plans using a photon vs proton beam targeting a cavernous sinus tumor

Table 36.1 Examples of early-reacting and late-reacting tissues

Early-reacting tissues	Late-reacting tissues
Gastrointestinal mucosa	Kidney
Skin (epidermis)	Skin (dermis)
Bone marrow	Lung
Spermatogenic cells	Spinal cord
Melanocytes	Liver
Tumors	Bone/cartilage
	Bladder

areas for treatment. During simulation, the patient will be placed in a position that is as comfortable and easily reproducible as possible for their daily treatment. Positioning also takes into consideration possible beam arrangements that might be used to limit normal organ toxicity as much as possible. Immobilization devices such as thermoplastic masks or body molds are made to ensure anatomic positioning that varies minimally from day to day (Fig. 36.5). A variety of localizing techniques may be used to ensure proper targeting of the tissues to be treated by enhancing visualization of the tissues, including placement of fiducial markers within or near the tumor, use of barium contrast in body cavities, radiopaque stickers or wires on skin, or use of intravenous contrast. Techniques may also be used to account for motion, such as 4D scanning which tracks respiratory motion, abdominal compression, coached breathing techniques, or breath-holding.

Following CT simulation, additional imaging such as MRI or PET may be fused to the planning CT scan to improve tumor and normal tissue visualization during treatment preparation. For example, MRI scans may be fused to ensure improved localization of the spinal cord or brain tumors. PET scans may be used to determine the appropriate sites of disease. Scans prior to chemotherapy or surgery may also be used to identify areas at risk of residual disease. The radiation oncologist then uses this information to contour the target treatment areas and organs at risk for toxicity. The physician will account for the disease that is grossly visible on imaging (defined as the gross tumor volume or GTV, Fig. 36.6), as well as regions thought to harbor microscopic disease (defined as the clinical target volume or CTV). An additional margin is then added to account for the daily setup variation and uncertainty (defined as the planning target volume or PTV).

Contours and the underlying CT data are used to optimize an individualized plan for the patient, including defining the location, timing, and dose rate of each beam. This plan is then checked for quality assurance, and physics calculations are performed. The process of treatment planning and quality assurance often takes up to 7–10 days. For emergent treatments, such as in patients with malignant spinal cord compression or superior vena cava compression, simple beam arrangements can be set up based on a clinician's identification of anatomic (usually bony) landmarks using fluoroscopic or CT imaging (Fig. 36.7). Dosimetric calculations and quality assurance for these simple beam arrangements can be performed within a few minutes, and treatment can be provided immediately. For patients requiring complex treatment plans, it is generally not possible to simulate and treat in the same day due to the quality assurance, dosimetry, and therapy checks necessary to assure treatment accuracy and safety.

Treatments are usually delivered on a once-daily basis, 5 days per week. Studies of radiation therapy delivered 7 days per week have demonstrated intolerable acute toxicity

[2, 3]. Some patients may be treated twice daily, 5 days per week, if they are receiving hyperfractionated treatment or need to complete treatment quickly. To allow for cellular repair within normal tissues, twice-daily treatments are performed at least 6 hours apart. This time gap allows normal tissues to recover sufficiently between treatments. At each treatment, patients are placed into the appropriate position using the devices made at CT simulation. The proper positioning is confirmed using radiographs or cone-beam CT at the time of treatment (Fig. 36.8). A patient is typically on the treatment machine for 15–30 min for each treatment.

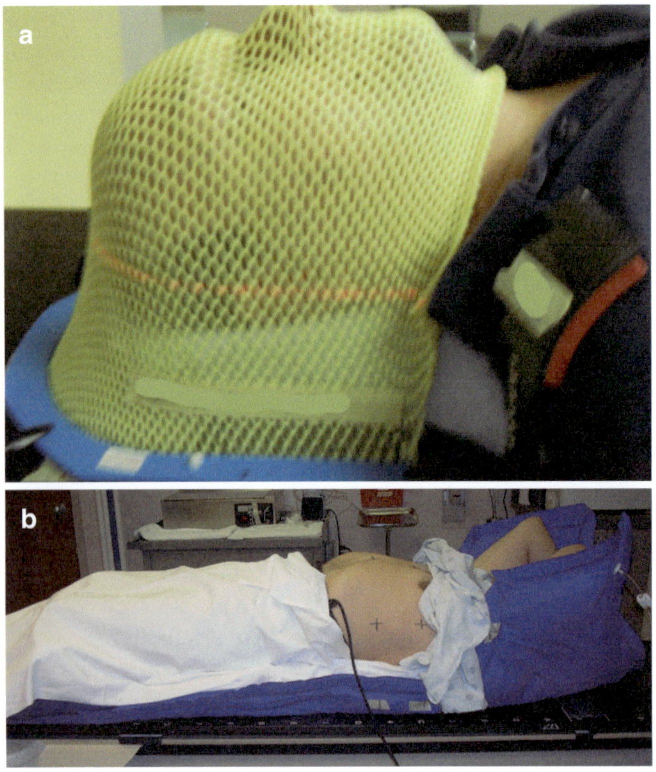

Fig. 36.5 Immobilization devices. (**a**) Thermoplastic mask and (**b**) body mold

Overview of Radiation Treatment Planning and Dosimetry

A dosimetrist performs radiation treatment planning to ensure the dose prescribed by the radiation oncologist is properly given. A computerized plan for the radiation is prepared using the Hounsfield units from the planning CT scan. A set of isodose lines is drawn on the CT imaging, and this is used to evaluate the quality of the plan (Fig. 36.9). The dosimetrist and radiation oncologist ensure that (1) sufficient dose is given to the target tissue, (2) dose hot spots and cold spots are limited, and (3) dose to critical organs at risk is below a set of predefined constraints. In some cases, it is not possible to meet these goals simultaneously. For these patients, the radiation oncologist must make an individual judgment.

Dose-limiting organs include the nearby tissues that are most radiosensitive or those with the risk of catastrophic toxicity, such as blindness, paralysis, or death. Dose constraints for critical organs at risk are determined based on theoretical models, randomized trials, and historical standards with known levels of toxicity. Constraints may be defined in terms of the maximal dose to an organ or the volume of an organ receiving a particular dose. In many cases, both types of constraints are used to ensure the dose delivered to an organ at risk is appropriately limited and toxicity is minimized.

Conformality in Radiation Therapy

A variety of techniques have been developed to maximize *conformality* of the treatment, i.e., maximize radiation dose to the target tissues and limit dose to normal tissues. Historically, all radiation treatments were defined by conventional planning, in which a set of beams are arranged at angles to each other to maximize coverage of the targets (Fig. 36.10). The set of beams chosen is usually standardized for a specific tumor site. The most basic arrangement of beams is AP/PA, which has one beam directed anterior to posterior and a second beam directed from posterior to

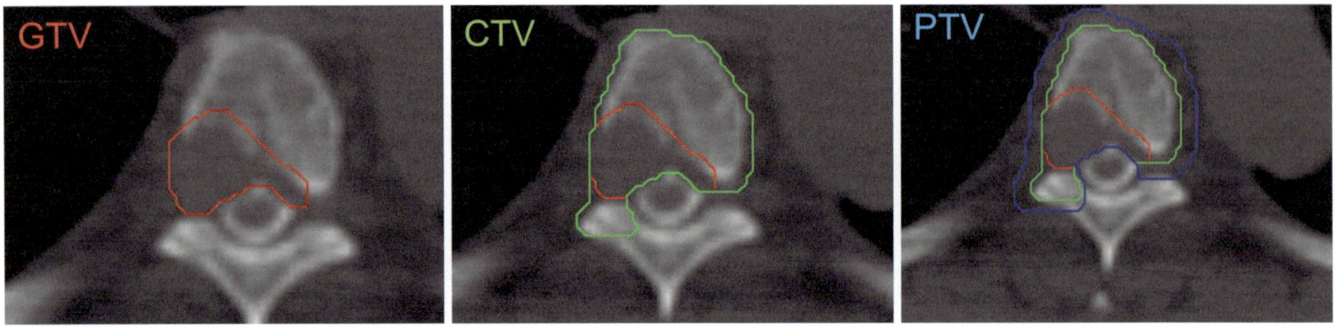

Fig. 36.6 Typical contours for the gross tumor volume (GTV), clinical target volume (CTV), and planning target volume (PTV) for a spinal tumor

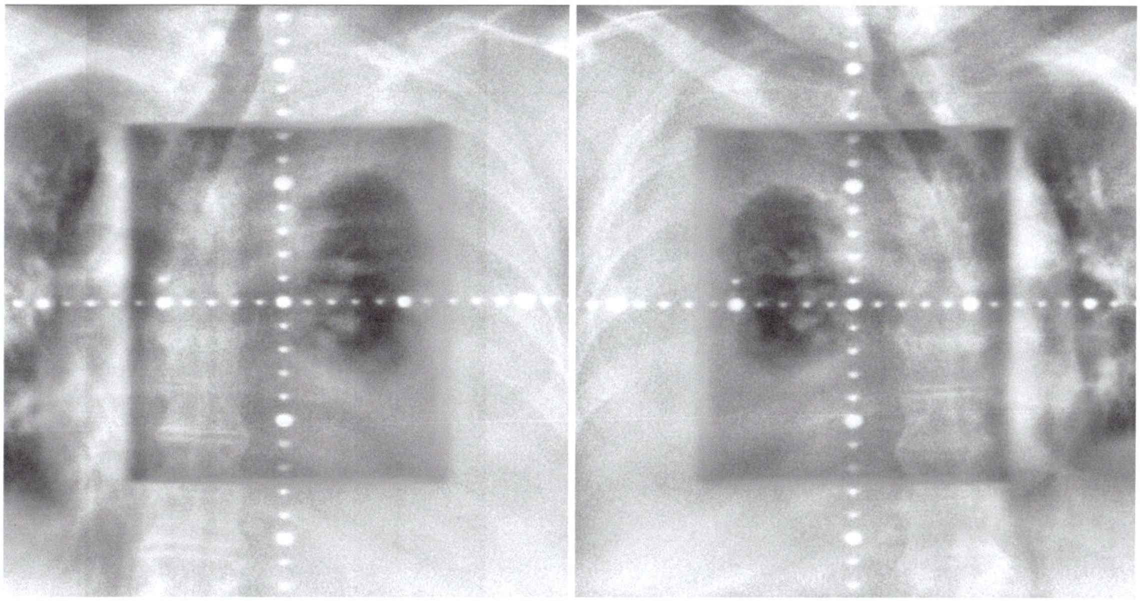

Fig. 36.7 Simple AP/PA treatment plan setup by portal imaging (darkened area on each image represents treated region)

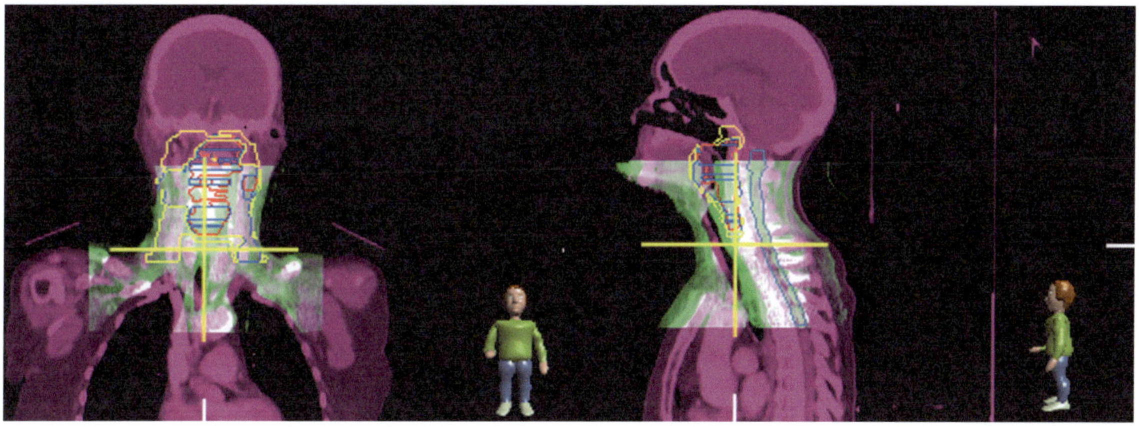

Fig. 36.8 Images used to confirm proper positioning during a treatment

anterior (Fig. 36.11). To improve conformality of the treatment to the target tissues, plans can be defined using three-dimensional conformal radiation, which uses multiple beams of varying energies that are shaped to match the target region (Fig. 36.12).

Inverse planning uses a computer algorithm based on the data from the CT simulation and tumor and organ contouring to optimize a plan based upon prespecified dosing criteria to maximize conformality around the target and minimize extraneous radiation dose to critical tissues adjacent to the target. The computer algorithm models the dose deposited by the beam, considering any scattering of dose. Intensity-modulated radiation therapy (IMRT) determines the angles, outlines, and intensities for a set of beams that best meet these goals. Unlike beams in conventional planning, the beams used in IMRT typically have very complex outlines and intensities, far beyond the practical computa-

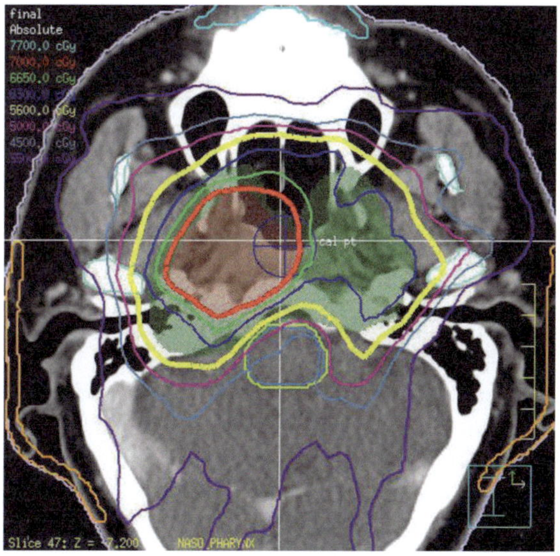

Fig. 36.9 Typical isodose plan for a head and neck cancer

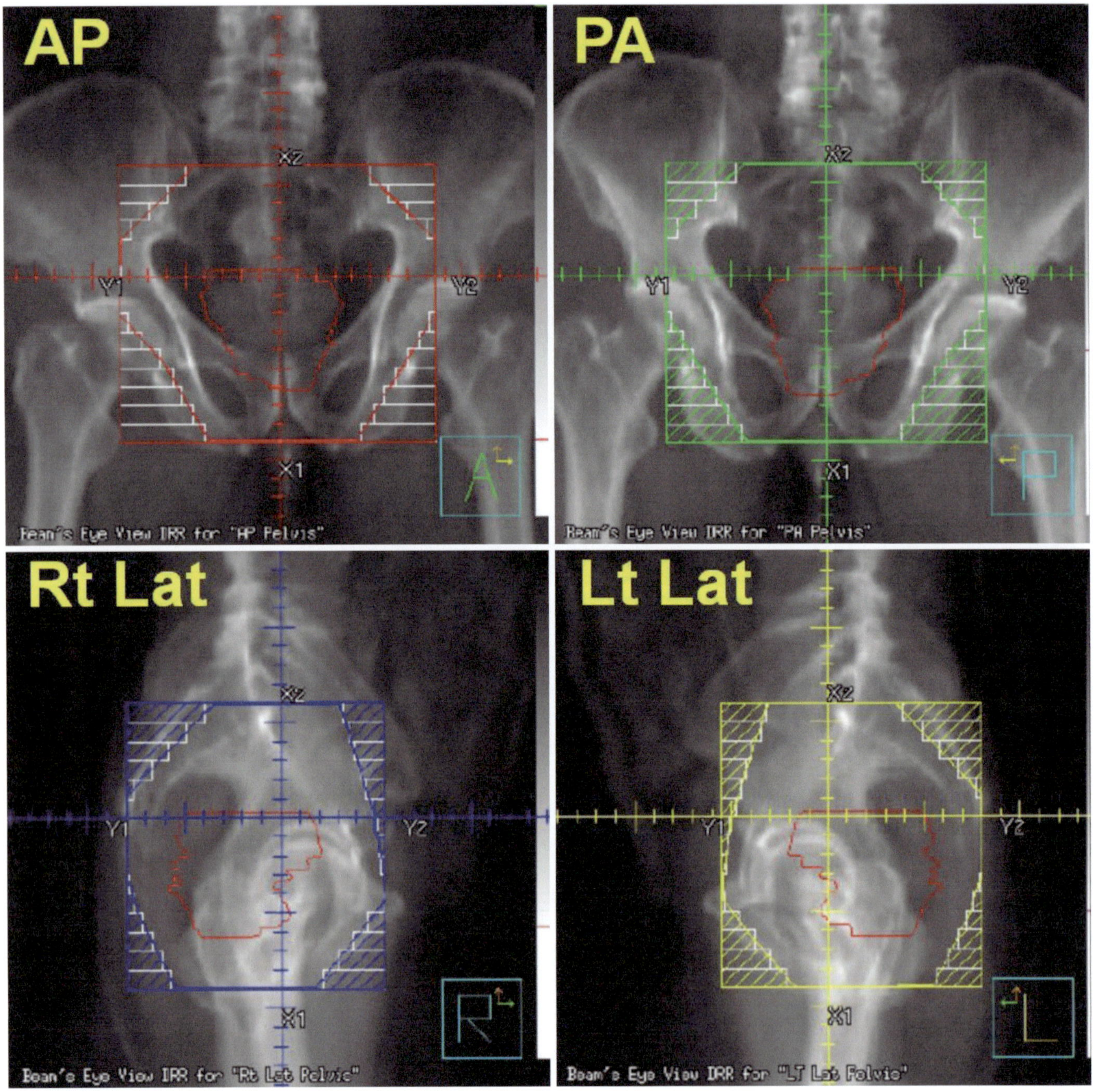

Fig. 36.10 Conventional plan for treatment of a rectal tumor (PTV delineated by red outline)

tion by a human (Fig. 36.13). Stereotactic radiosurgery (SRS), delivered in a single very high-dose treatment, and stereotactic body radiation therapy (SBRT), usually delivered over three to five fractions, employ very precise imaging, motion control, and the division of dose into a multitude of small beamlets to ensure that the radiation dose to normal tissue outside the target is kept to a minimum (Fig. 36.14).

Brachytherapy

Brachytherapy is a type of radiation delivered using sealed radioactive sources. It allows for a very high dose of radiation to regions of tumor and a very sharp falloff of dose over a short distance beyond the regions of tumor thereby keeping neighboring normal tissues safe. A radiation oncologist directly places a radioactive source on, in, or very near the target tissue, usually

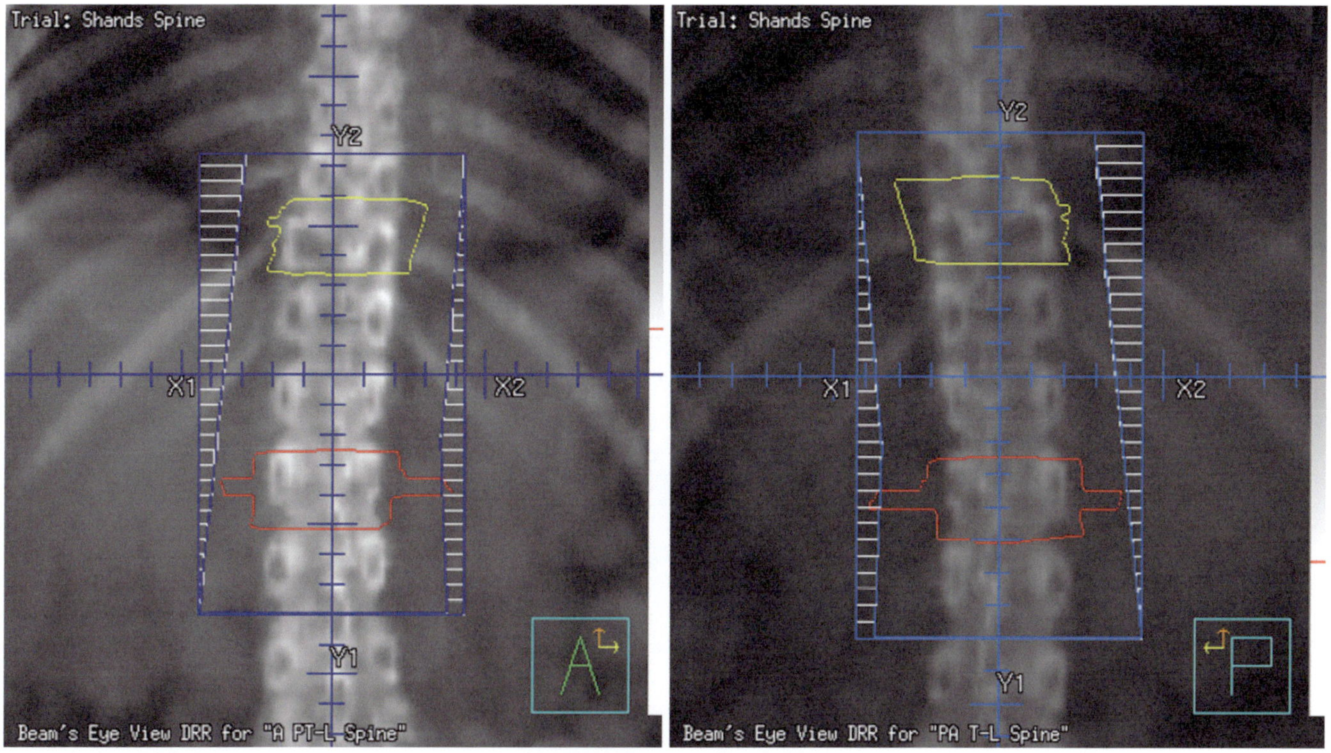

Fig. 36.11 AP/PA plan for treatment of spinal metastasis (PTV delineated by red outline)

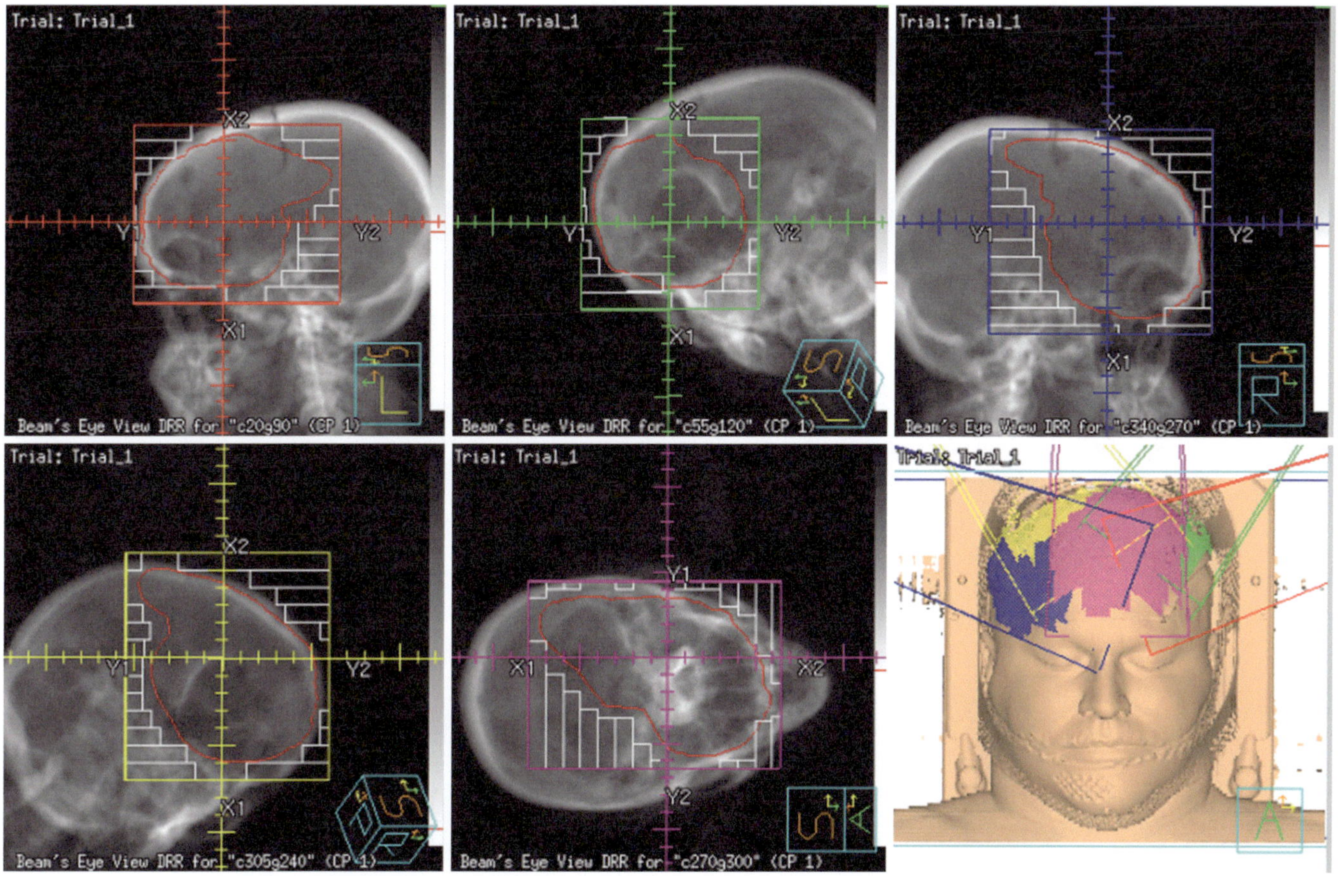

Fig. 36.12 Three-dimensional conformal plan for brain tumor (PTV delineated by red volume)

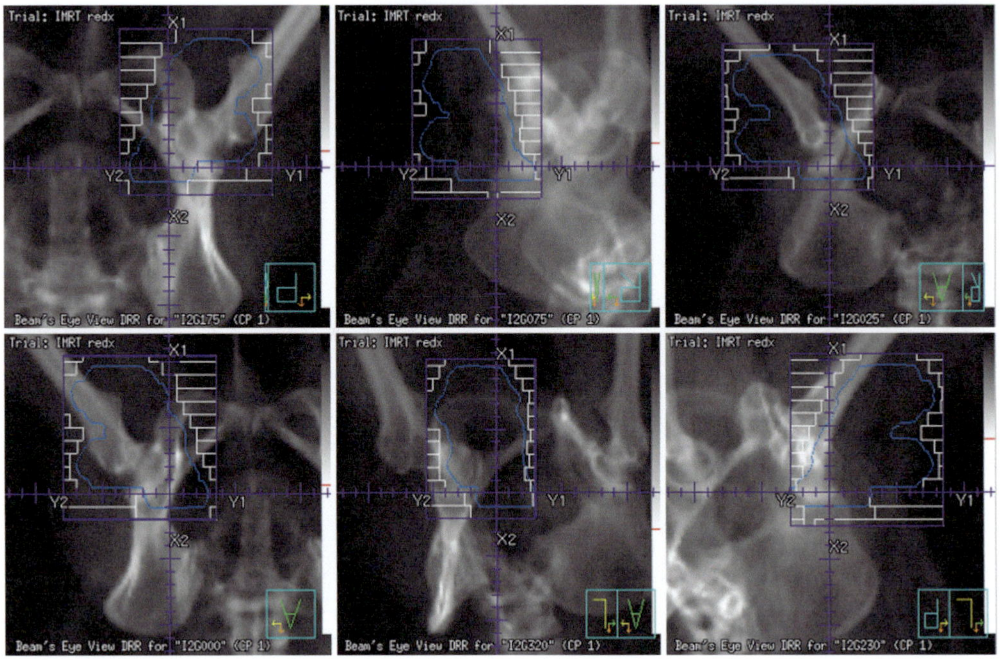

Fig. 36.13 Typical intensity-modulated radiation therapy plan

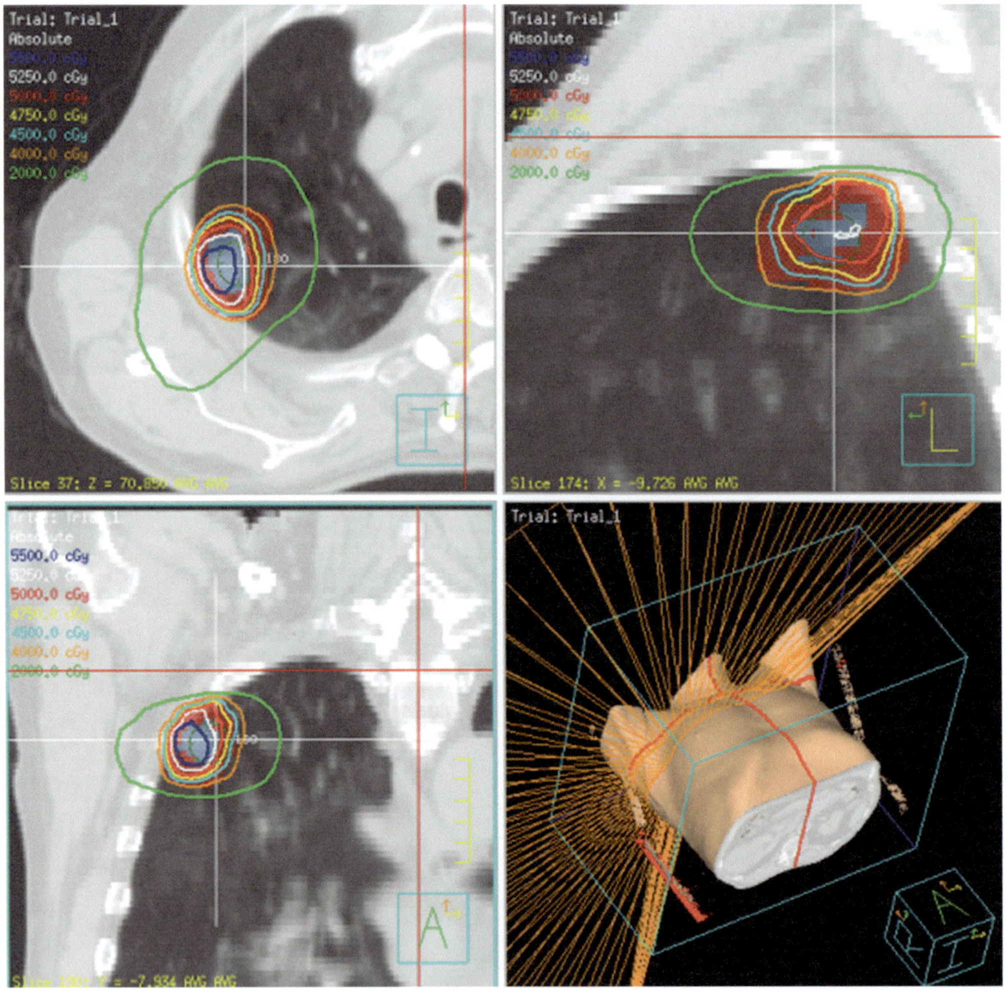

Fig. 36.14 Typical stereotactic body radiation therapy isodose plan in axial, sagittal, and coronal projections and treatment plan. (Note: individual beams are too complex to illustrate)

involving a surgery or invasive procedure. Brachytherapy can be used with molds or plaques to allow treatment of skin or mucosal lesions (Fig. 36.15), with needles to directly insert sources called "seeds" into deeper tissues such as a nasal vestibule (Fig. 36.16) or prostate gland (Fig. 36.17), or with catheters or cylinders to insert sources into body cavities such as the vagina (Fig. 36.18). The radiation sources can be kept permanently in place or can be placed temporarily and removed after the desired dose of radiation has been achieved. If patients are undergoing surgery, intraoperative radiation therapy can be delivered into the cavity that the surgeon creates during resection (Fig. 36.19).

Brachytherapy is categorized based on the source's dose rate into low-dose rate (LDR, with a dose rate of 0.4–2 Gy/h), medium-dose rate (rarely used), or high-dose rate (HDR, with a dose rate > 12 Gy/h). LDR treatment involves the insertion of a radioactive source that decays over days to weeks. Iodine-125, palladium-103, and cesium-137 are examples of sources used in LDR brachytherapy. Iridium-192 is a commonly used source in HDR brachytherapy that is inserted through catheters for a few minutes and then removed. Patients with cervical, breast, or skin cancer can be treated effectively with brachytherapy in the palliative setting. It can be used instead of external beam radiation therapy to quickly palliate bleeding, fungating wounds, or pain.

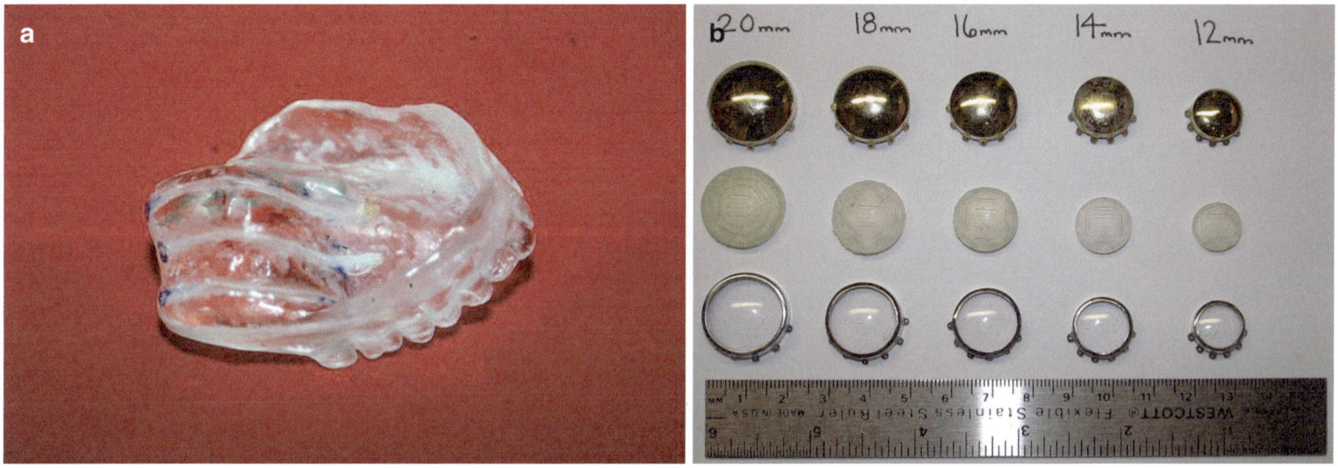

Fig. 36.15 Brachytherapy treatment appliances. (**a**) Soft palate mold for intraoral treatment, (**b**) eye plaques for intraocular treatment

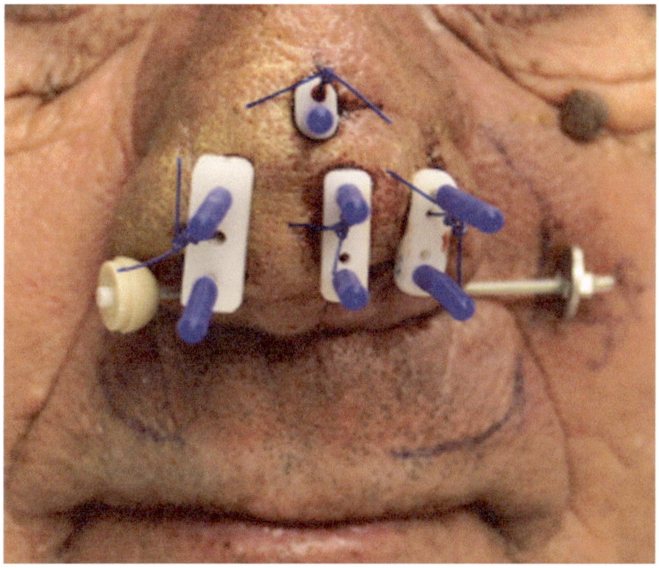

Fig. 36.16 Brachytherapy treatment of a nasal vestibule cancer using needles and catheters

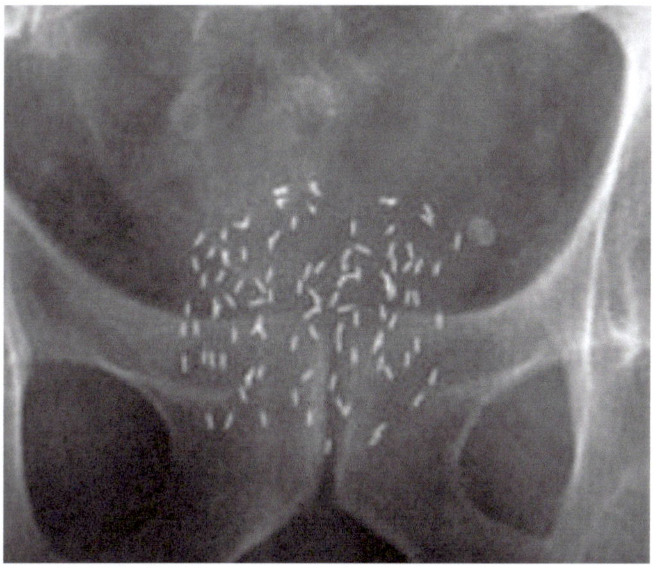

Fig. 36.17 Fluoroscopic image of prostate gland with implanted brachytherapy seeds

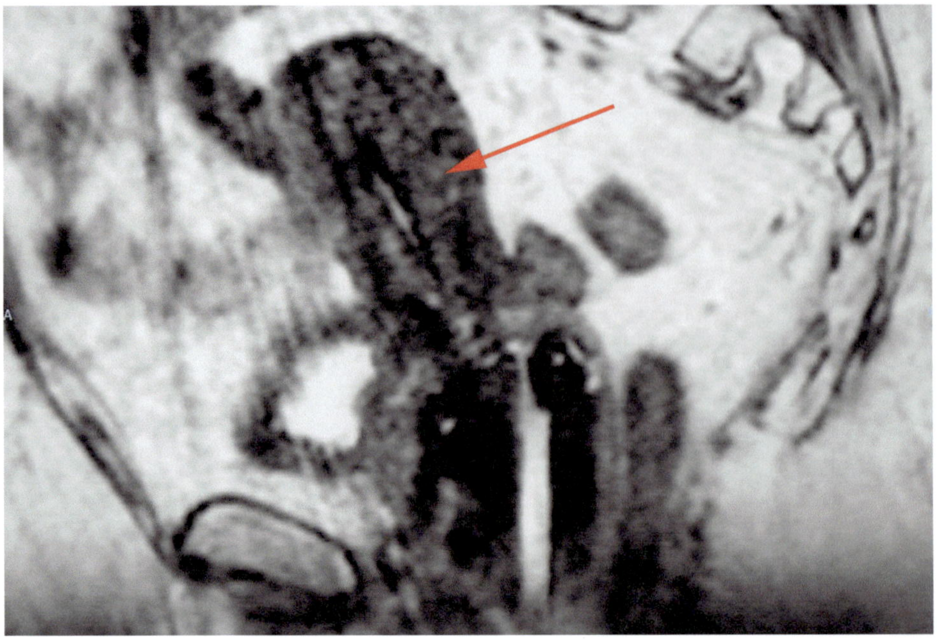

Fig. 36.18 Sagittal MRI of pelvis with tandem and ring in place for brachytherapy treatment of endometrial cancer (red arrow points to tandem inside uterus)

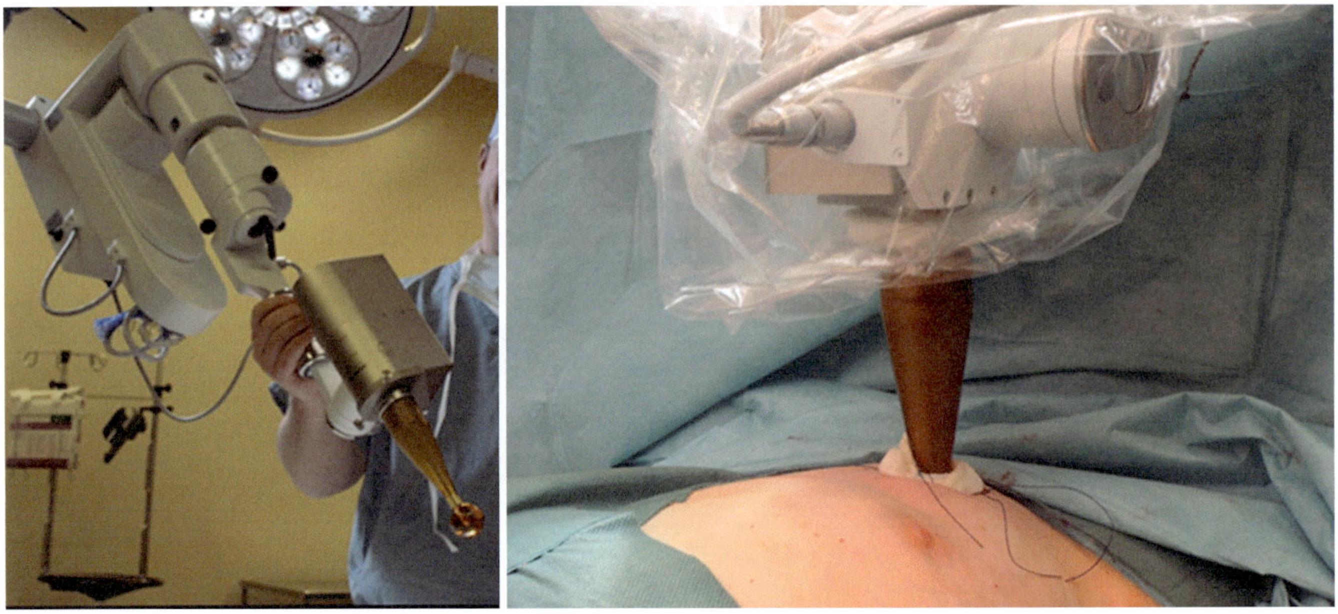

Fig. 36.19 Intraoperative brachytherapy for breast cancer. (**a**) Intrabeam applicator and (**b**) applicator in place for treatment. (Reprinted with permission from University of Florida Health. Credit: Stephen Grobmyer, MD., UF College of Medicine professor of surgery, and Judith Lightsey, MD, UF College of Medicine radiation oncology assistant professor, University of Florida Health, 2001)

References

1. Lutz ST, Jones J, Chow E. Role of radiation therapy in palliative care of the patient with cancer. J Clin Oncol. 2014;32(26):2913–9.
2. Horiot JC, Bontemps P, van den Bogaert W, Le Fur R, van den Weijngaert D, Bolla M, Bernier J, Lusinchi A, Stuschke M, Torrecilla JL, Begg AC, Pierart M, Collette L. Accelerated fractionation (AF) compared to conventional fractionation (CF) improves loco-regional control in the radiotherapy of advanced head and neck cancers: results of the EORTC 22851 randomized trial. Radiother Oncol. 1997;44:111–21.
3. Bernier J, Denekamp J, Rojas A, Minatel E, Horiot JC, Hamers H, Antognoni P, Dahl O, Richaud P, van Glabbeke M, Pierart M. ARCON: accelerated radiotherapy with carbogen and nicotinamide in head and neck squamous cell carcinomas. Radiother Oncol. 2000;55(2):111–9.

37 Palliative Radiation Therapy

Shayna E. Rich and Kavita V. Dharmarajan

Overview of Palliative Radiation Therapy

Radiation therapy is delivered with palliative intent in up to 40–50% of radiation oncology patients. Palliative radiation usually involves shorter treatment courses delivered for symptom management. Palliative radiation therapy may be chosen based on the patient's cancer prognosis, treatment goals, and other indicators of life expectancy including performance status, comorbidities, and prior and concurrent treatments [1]. The risks of early toxicity in palliative treatments are considered carefully to ensure that treatment has an appropriate risk-benefit ratio. Patient preferences also play a critical role in determining the appropriate treatment course.

Radiation therapy can be used with palliative intent to reduce pain, neurological dysfunction, bleeding, fungating wounds, nausea, vomiting, or obstructive symptoms. Pain can improve as disease is reduced or controlled or as tumor-related inflammation is quelled. Neurological dysfunction can be controlled or ameliorated by reducing tumor compression upon nerves, brain, or spinal cord from an intraaxial tumor or external compression. Bleeding and fungating wounds from the tumor or invasion of blood vessels can be controlled by radiation, because treatment causes vasoconstriction, tumor shrinkage, scarring, and fibrosis of vasculature. Nausea or vomiting can be controlled if they are caused by tumor mass in the liver, bowels, or brain. Obstructive symptoms can be relieved by the reduction of tumor burden, regardless of whether the obstruction is in an airway (e.g., due to head and neck cancer), in the esophagus or bowels, in the bile duct (e.g., due to pancreatic cancer), in the ureters or bladder (e.g., due to renal cell carcinoma), or in the superior vena cava (e.g., due to lung cancer or lymphoma).

S. E. Rich
Haven Hospice, Gainesville, FL, USA

K. V. Dharmarajan (✉)
Icahn School of Medicine at Mount Sinai, New York, NY, USA
e-mail: kavita.dharmarajan@mountsinai.org

Palliation for Vertebral and Other Bone Metastases

Painful bone metastases are the most common reason for palliative radiation therapy. For example, palliative radiation therapy to a vertebral bone tumor can relieve symptoms of spinal cord compression, including focal weakness, numbness, or bowel and bladder dysfunction. Multiple series have found response rates of 70–80%, with similar results for treatment of bone metastases in the peripheral skeleton or spinal sites [2–6]. Radiation therapy can be provided in the form of external beam radiation therapy or using unsealed sources in the form of radiopharmaceuticals designed to target diffuse bony disease (e.g., Samarium-153, Strontium-89, or the newer Radium-223 specifically for prostate cancer patients).

Effective dose-fractionation schemes for external beam radiation therapy include 8 Gy in a single fraction, 20 Gy at 4 Gy/fraction, and 30 Gy at 3 Gy/fraction. Large randomized studies comparing these fractionations have not found a significant difference in short-term outcomes, other than an increased rate of re-irradiation among patients receiving 8 Gy in a single fraction (Table 37.1). However, data regarding treatment patterns among radiation oncologists in the United States have shown that only a small percentage of patients treated with palliative radiation for bone metastases are treated with 8 Gy in a single fraction and most undergo treatment courses lasting 2 or more weeks [7]. Table 37.1 summarizes data from several bone metastases trials.

Acute complications of palliative radiation therapy for bone metastases include a temporary increase in pain a few days after radiation treatment (i.e., pain flare) and fatigue. Pain flare may be prevented by the use of anti-inflammatory medications, commonly in the form of an oral steroid, and it can be treated with an increased dose of standard pain medications [8]. Pain relief is expected to occur gradually starting at 1 week after treatment and maximizing at 4–6 weeks after treatment [5, 9–11]. A further course of treatment may be required to control pain.

A. Gulati et al. (eds.), *Essentials of Interventional Cancer Pain Management*, https://doi.org/10.1007/978-3-319-99684-4_37

Table 37.1 Results of recent randomized clinical trials of the treatment of bone metastases

Investigator	Patients (n)	Fractionation	Overall pain relief (%)	Re-irradiation rate (%)
Anter 2015 [6]	100	8 Gy in 1 fx 20 Gy in 5 fx	75 75	Not reported
Gutierrez Bayard 2014 [2]	90	8 Gy in 1 fx 30 Gy in 10 fx	79 88	13 9
Howell 2013 [3]	235	8 Gy in 1 fx 30 Gy in 10 fx	70 62	15 5
Majumder 2012 [4]	64	8 Gy in 1 fx 30 Gy in 10 fx	77 85	Not reported
Chow 2012 [10]	5617	Single Multiple	60 61	20 8
Meeuse 2010 [11]	1157	8 Gy in 1 fx 24 Gy in 6 fx	53 56	7 2

fx fraction

Radiation therapy can be used in conjunction with other treatments including surgical decompression, stabilization, laminectomy, or kyphoplasty [12]. These treatments are indicated particularly in the setting of fracture, impending fracture, or unstable bone structure, because reduction of tumor burden may further destabilize the bone. Radiation therapy following these surgical interventions is usually treated with a fractionation scheme of 30 Gy at 3 Gy/fraction for more durable tumor control. Radio-frequency ablation can also be used before or after palliative radiation therapy to enhance tumor control. Finally, radiation therapy can also be given in conjunction with bisphosphonates to reduce the risk of fracture, spinal cord compression, or the need for surgical stabilization.

Palliation for Brain Metastases and Leptomeningeal Disease

The primary goal of radiation therapy for brain metastases and leptomeningeal disease is the control of neurological symptoms, such as seizures, and focal symptoms, like weakness and problems with speech. Patients treated with whole brain radiation therapy (WBRT, Fig. 37.1) have improved symptoms in approximately 60–90% of patients, and complete response in up to 25% [13]. Radiation therapy is usually used in conjunction with medical supportive care including steroids and antiepileptic medications. Radiation therapy for control of brain metastases may lead to improved overall survival [14].

Radiation therapy options for treatment of brain metastases include stereotactic radiosurgery (SRS) to individual lesions, fractionated partial brain irradiation, and WBRT. SRS is generally recommended for patients with five or fewer lesions, inoperable lesions, older individuals, or those with a longer life expectancy, given that the risk of late neurocognitive deficits is greater after WBRT [15]. Patients may be scored using the recursive partitioning analysis (RPA, Table 37.2) or graded prognostic assessment (GPA, Table 37.3) to determine their probable life expectancy, before determining their appropriateness for SRS [16]. Patients with symptomatic leptomeningeal disease are generally treated with WBRT [17].

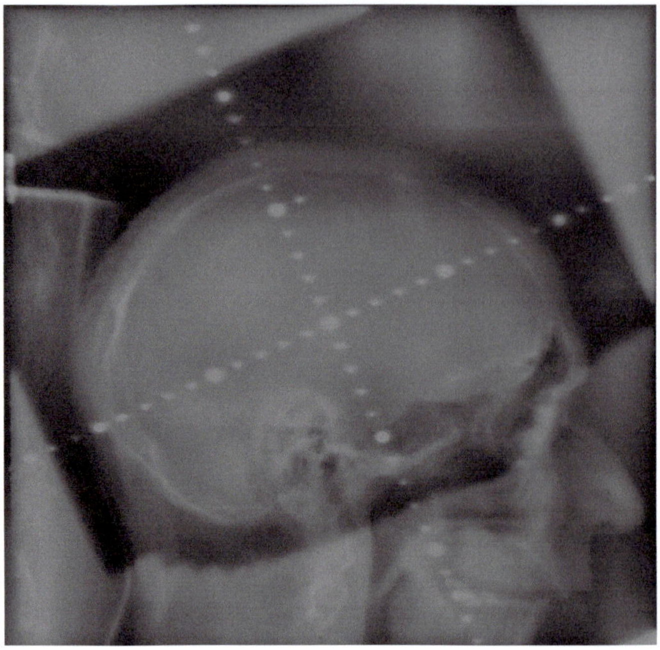

Fig. 37.1 Typical portal image of whole brain radiation therapy

For patients receiving SRS, the optimal dose depends on the size and location of the lesions. The dose range is typically between 15 and 24 Gy given in a single fraction [18]. Fractionated radiation with palliative intent is typically given to 30 Gy at 3 Gy/fraction, although 20 Gy at 4 Gy/fraction is sometimes used for patients with a very short life expectancy [14]. Other fractionation schemes include 35.5 Gy at 2.5 Gy/fraction and 40 Gy at 2 Gy/fraction. The first two studies performed by the Radiation Therapy Oncology Group (RTOG) examined the effectiveness of a variety of different fractionation schemes for the palliative of patients with brain metastases [19–21]. These studies, designated RTOG 6901 and 7361, demonstrated no significant differences in survival, progression, or symptom control between fractionation schemes including 30 Gy at 3 Gy/fraction, 20 Gy at 4 Gy/fraction, and longer fractionation regimens [19, 21]. These studies showed that whole brain ultra-rapid hypofractionation such as 10 Gy in a single fraction or 12 Gy at 6 Gy/fraction had increased toxicity and worse time to progression [20].

Acute-onset toxicity from WBRT includes fatigue, headache, nausea, vomiting, alopecia, and ototoxicity. These toxicities are typically controlled with an increased dose of steroids, or with antiemetics for nausea/vomiting. More con-

Table 37.2 Recursive partitioning analysis (RPA) for patients with brain metastases

Class	Patient characteristics
I	Age < 65 years, Karnofsky Performance Score ≥ 70, controlled primary tumor, and no extracranial metastases
II	All patients not in class I or III
III	Karnofsky Performance Score < 70

Table 37.3 Graded prognostic assessment (GPA) for lung cancer patients with brain metastases

Patient characteristic	0	0.5	1.0	
Age	>60	50–59	<50	
Karnofsky Performance Score	<70	70–80	90–100	
Number of central nervous system metastases	>3	2–3	1	
Extracranial metastases	Present	–	Absent	
Total points	0–1	1.5–2	2.5–3	3.5–4
Median survival in months	3.0	5.5	9.4	14.8

cerning is the potential for late-onset toxicity. There is a known risk for decline in short-term memory, brain atrophy, and even radionecrosis [22]. Radionecrosis is possible with SRS but uncommon with WBRT. Approximately 5–10% of patients will develop symptomatic brain necrosis after SRS [22], which can be treated with steroid therapy and surgical resection.

Radiation therapy can be used as an adjuvant treatment following surgery to improve control of brain tumors, particularly in the cases of subtotal resection or with the risk of catastrophic recurrence. Studies have shown improved outcomes for patients with surgical resection of metastases followed by WBRT compared to those with WBRT alone [23] or those with surgery alone [24]. It can also be used in conjunction with some chemotherapy drugs. Patients who have received WBRT who have progressive intracranial metastases may undergo additional radiation to the brain with either repeat WBRT or SRS [14, 15].

Palliation for Head and Neck Cancers

Patients presenting with advanced cancers of the head and neck typically have symptoms of pain, bleeding (including hemoptysis), facial disfigurement, fungating masses, odynophagia, and dysphagia to solids and liquids. They may also present with an increased risk of airway obstruction. Most head and neck primary neoplasms are squamous cell carcinomas. Given the significant radiosensitivity of squamous cell carcinoma of the head and neck, these cancers may respond rapidly to short courses of palliative radiation therapy. One study showed that 38% of patients with advanced head and neck primaries had sustained improved symptoms at 1 year after as little as two doses of radiation therapy [25]. Palliative radiation is similar when used to treat cancers in this anatomic region of all histologies, including squamous cell carcinomas, gastrointestinal, and salivary gland cancers. Because radiation therapy may cause acute transient edema, patients at risk of airway compromise should undergo tracheostomy or another procedure to protect the airway prior to undergoing radiation therapy.

Conventional courses for palliative treatment of advanced head and neck cancers include 30 Gy at 3 Gy/fraction over 10 days, the "quad shot" technique of 14 Gy at 3.5 Gy/fraction given twice daily on 2 consecutive days, or a hypofractionation regimen to 20 Gy at 10 Gy/fraction given 1 week apart. The "quad shot" is designed to be delivered once every 4 weeks for up to three cycles, based on toxicity and progression [26]. This treatment can be delivered safely as primary therapy with or without chemotherapy or as re-irradiation.

Because mucosal tissues are early-reacting, the potential complications of head and neck radiation therapy are similar in both palliative and curative settings and include mucositis, dysphagia, and xerostomia. Conformal radiation therapy techniques such as intensity modulated radiation therapy (IMRT) are typically used in the curative or re-irradiation settings to minimize the toxicity and morbidity associated with head and neck radiation.

Palliative Radiation for Primary or Metastatic Hepatic Cancers

Patients with primary or metastatic liver cancers can be treated with palliative radiation therapy for relief of symptoms related to parenchymal disease, vascular obstruction, or biliary obstruction. These symptoms can include abdominal pain, jaundice, ascites, and pruritus. Treatment options include surgical resection, transcatheter arterial chemoembolization (TACE), ablation, or radiation therapy. Historically, radiation therapy was not frequently used, due to the low median liver tolerance. There is increasing interest in using radiation therapy with advanced techniques including conformal radiation therapy (e.g., IMRT) and stereotactic body radiation therapy (SBRT).

Patients with a limited life expectancy and a large hepatic disease burden can be treated with whole liver radiation therapy (Fig. 37.2). Approximately one-quarter of these patients will have a clinically meaningful improvement in quality of life after 1 month [26]. Commonly prescribed fractionation schedules for these patients include 21 Gy at 3 Gy/fraction, 10 Gy in two fractions, or 8 Gy in one fraction for patients with a very poor prognosis. Patients with good performance status and limited disease should be treated with a highly conformal treatment plan that spares as much healthy liver tissue as possible. These patients are also often treated with concurrent systemic or hepatic artery chemotherapy.

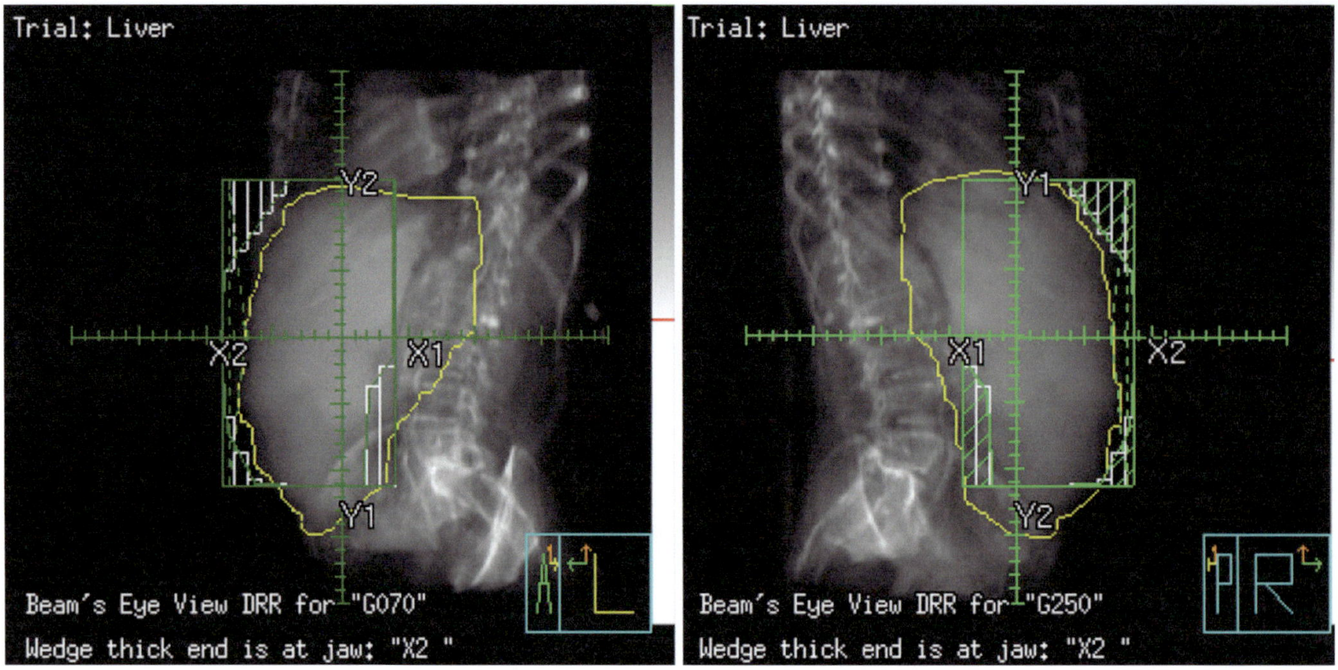

Fig. 37.2 Typical plan for whole liver radiation therapy

Patients receiving whole liver radiation therapy may develop significant nausea and vomiting on the day of treatment, and they should be pretreated with steroids and antiemetics [27]. Many patients will also develop a transient mild fatigue. The main concerning toxicity of radiation therapy to the liver is the risk of late liver injury particularly radiation-induced liver disease (RILD). However, an RTOG dose-escalation study showed that late toxicity due to liver injury up to 10% of patients only when they were treated with 33 Gy [28]. It is believed that the low rate of palliative radiation treatment for liver metastases (as compared to metastatic disease in the bone, brain, or lung) is due to an incorrect belief that liver radiation inevitably leads to RILD, whereas RILD may be rare in patients treated with palliative hypofractionation [29].

Palliation for Pelvic Tumors

Palliative pelvic radiation is indicated for control of pain, malignant obstruction of the bowels or ureters, or tumor-related bleeding. Patients may require pelvic radiation for gynecologic cancers, colorectal cancer, genitourinary cancers, or even lymphoma. As with other sites, palliative pelvic radiation can result in rapid improvement of symptoms. Radiation therapy can also be used to reduce the burden of disease prior to surgery and reduce risk of local recurrence [30].

A variety of radiation fractionation schemes may be appropriate depending on the primary tumor site, disease burden, and overall prognosis. For example, patients with locally advanced prostate cancer or lymphoma may have a long life expectancy, even if cure is no longer possible. These patients may be treated with longer-duration treatment courses like those used for curative intent using conventional fractionation. In patients with limited life expectancy, fractionation schemes for pelvic metastases tend to be significantly shorter and include 30 Gy at 3 Gy/fraction, 20 Gy at 4 Gy/fraction, 10 Gy/fraction in a single monthly fraction or a quad shot fractionation to 14.8 Gy at 3.7 Gy/fraction given twice daily for 2 days. (Note that total dose for the quad shot differs slightly from the quad shot given for head and neck palliation.) The single monthly and quad shot fractionation regimens have been used primarily to palliate bleeding [31, 32].

Radiation to the pelvis will generally involve dose to the large and small intestines, which are particularly radiosensitive. Thus, the major potential toxicities of pelvic radiation include diarrhea, nausea, and vomiting acutely, or bowel obstruction and fistula chronically. Interventions including surgical resection, stenting, or laser ablation should be performed preferentially over radiation therapy to avoid the potential bowel complications [33]. Patients may also develop irritation of the bladder including minor hematuria.

If disease in the abdomen and pelvis is limited, conformal radiation therapy can be used to limit bowel toxicity, with IMRT being the preferred modality [34]. In most cases, however, the burden of disease in the pelvis is sufficient to require a large dose to the bowels. Conventional radiation planning including use of a four-field box (AP/PA and right and left laterals) is typically used for palliative radiation therapy to the pelvis.

Palliation for Superior Vena Cava (SVC) Syndrome

SVC syndrome is defined by symptoms including swelling of the face and upper extremities (Fig. 37.3), cough or dyspnea, and dilated chest veins. Causes include cancers such as small cell lung carcinoma or lymphoma and benign lesions such as thrombosis, goiter, aortic aneurysm, or congestive heart failure. Palliative radiation therapy is effective in treating SVC syndrome caused by cancer, which is only about 60% of all cases of SVC syndrome [35]. If the patient does not have a known diagnosis of cancer prior to presentation, radiation therapy may obscure the histologic diagnosis and should be deferred until diagnostic biopsy is obtained whenever possible.

First choice for treatment of SVC syndrome should be stent placement, as this will provide immediate relief of symptoms. It will also keep the vascularity patent during radiation therapy, even though radiation may cause transient swelling and exacerbate the SVC compression. For cancer patients with impending SVC compression, or those who cannot undergo stent placement, radiation therapy can provide effective palliation of symptoms. Premedication with steroids (after the histologic diagnosis is determined) can minimize radiation-induced edema. Even in a study of a hypofractionated regimen for SVC syndrome in elderly patients older than 70 years, overall response rate was 87% [36]. Symptomatic response time for radiation therapy is typically 7–15 days, but it can be seen as quickly as 3 days after radiation [37]. Patients presenting with SVC syndrome causing central airway compromise, severe laryngeal edema, or coma due to cerebral edema may require emergent treatment other than radiation therapy, particularly because radiation therapy will not restore normal vascular flow.

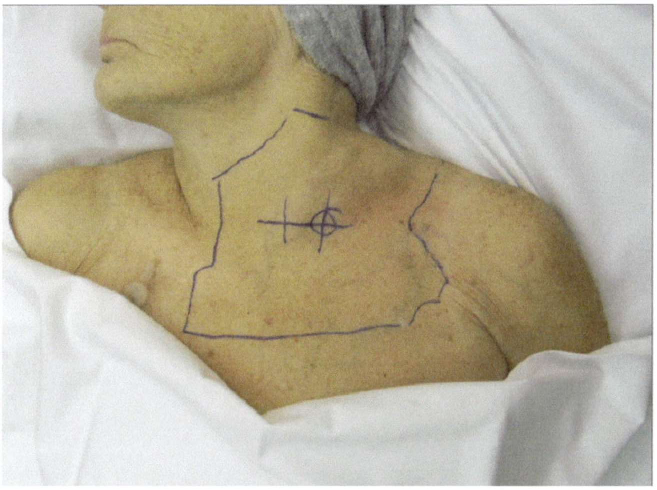

Fig. 37.3 Upper body swelling due to superior vena cava syndrome (AP field for radiation treatment marked on skin)

Patients with SVC syndrome will also have widely varied prognosis based on their underlying tumors, including a significant chance of cure for some diagnoses. Appropriate dose will also vary based on prognosis. Regimens for SVC syndrome have varied widely, including 40 Gy at 2 Gy/fraction, 30 Gy at 3 Gy/fraction, 20 Gy at 4 Gy/fraction, and 16 Gy at 8 Gy/fraction given 1 week apart [38].

The most bothersome acute complications of palliative radiation therapy to the SVC and thorax are dysphagia and esophagitis, which may result in reduced oral intake causing dehydration and weight loss. Some patients will require feeding tube placement, although this is usually temporary. Patients with lymphoma are also at risk for tumor lysis syndrome, and they should be well-hydrated and carefully monitored to avoid the risk of severe kidney damage. With a hypofractionated regimen, patients may have chest pain, rigors, and fever that can be treated with a steroid or nonsteroidal anti-inflammatory drug [36]. Long-term complications may be related to the dose to the lungs (causing a risk of radiation pneumonitis or pulmonary fibrosis), heart (causing a risk of pericarditis), or esophagus (causing stenosis).

Patients with SVC syndrome usually receive multiple concurrent modalities of treatment, depending on the specific cancer diagnosis. For example, patients with lymphoma will typically be treated with high-dose steroids and thoracic radiation therapy in the emergent setting, followed by more definitive treatment including chemotherapy and additional radiation as indicated. Patients with small cell lung cancer will usually receive concurrent chemotherapy and radiation therapy.

Palliation of Skin Cancers

Advanced skin cancers can cause fungating wounds, bleeding, increased risk of wound infections, and pain. For treatment purposes, skin cancers are divided into melanoma, Merkel cell carcinoma, cutaneous lymphomas (including mycosis fungoides), squamous cell carcinomas, and basal cell carcinomas. Melanoma treatment is primarily by surgical resection including lymph node dissection, but radiation therapy is effective for microscopic residual, unresectable, recurrent, or metastatic disease [39, 40]. Immunotherapy can also effectively control disease in patients whose tumors harbor target mutations. Merkel cell carcinoma treatment is similarly surgical resection with regional lymph node dissection, followed by radiation therapy to the primary site and at-risk nodes [41]. Chemotherapy may be added based on the extent of disease and the medical oncologist's preference. Cutaneous lymphomas should be treated preferentially with topical agents, chemotherapy, and ultraviolet A phototherapy (PUVA) [42]. Radiation can be used for treatment to tumors and plaques that are localized and painful. Some institutions use total skin electron therapy to treat diffuse, symptomatic mycosis fungoides and cutaneous B-cell lymphoma (Fig. 37.4) [43].

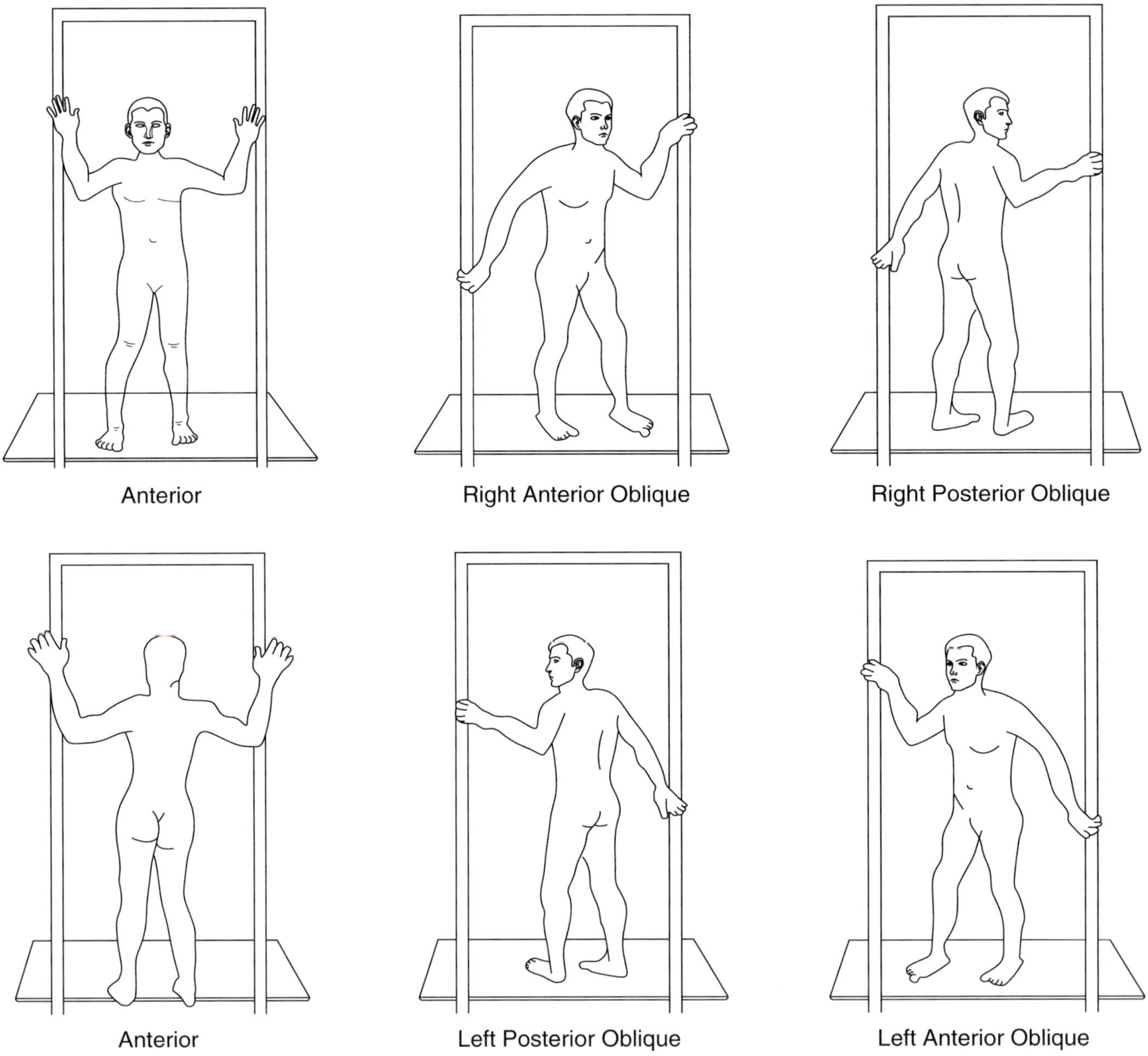

Fig. 37.4 Body positions used to ensure full coverage for total skin electron therapy

The most common skin cancers are squamous cell carcinoma and basal cell carcinoma. Although there are important differences in the details of treatment for these diseases, treatment algorithms are generally similar: surgery is the primary treatment if possible and cosmesis will be good, radiation therapy is reserved for poor surgical candidates or adjuvant treatment of extensive disease, and chemotherapy is usually not given because it is not clearly effective [44]. Topical agents should not be used concurrently with radiation therapy given the risk of increased acute adverse effects.

Skin cancers can be treated with superficial radiation including orthovoltage or electrons or with photon radiation as needed for sufficient depth of treatment coverage. Radiation should be avoided for skin cancers with limited vascularity that are directly over bone and may have poor healing after radiation (e.g., over tibia). The type of radiation will differ based on the organs deep to the target lesion, as well. For example, skin cancers of the scalp should not be treated with orthovoltage due to a large exit dose that could cause brain necrosis. Special care must be taken to shield the eye, ear, or nasal cavity (Fig. 37.5).

Melanomas are often treated with a fractionation scheme of 30 Gy at 6 Gy/fraction given at two fractions/week. Merkel cell carcinoma doses are typically 60–70 Gy at 2 Gy/fraction for definitive cases, but the melanoma fractionation can be used if transportation is problematic. Cutaneous lymphomas are treated to 8 Gy at 4 Gy/fraction for patches and plaques, 12 Gy at 4 Gy/fraction for tumors, and 15 Gy at 3 Gy/fraction for larger fields. Historically, numerous fractionation schemes have proven effective for squamous cell and basal cell skin cancers [45]. Fractionations can be categorized based on whether cosmetic outcome is a concern; in the palliative setting in which life expectancy is short, dose options include 40 Gy at 10 Gy/fraction, 30 Gy at 5 Gy/fraction, and 20 Gy in a single fraction. Patients with skin cancers in the head and neck region may also be treated with the quad shot dose or 20 Gy at 10 Gy/fraction weekly, as this has proven effective.

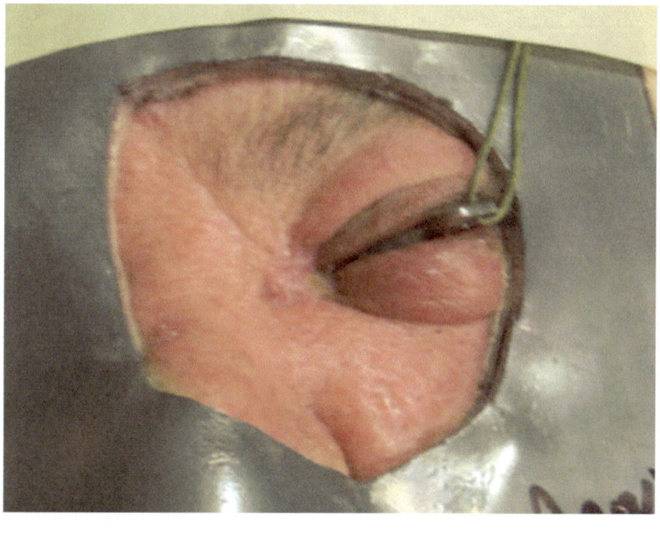

Fig. 37.5 Orthovoltage treatment of medial canthus skin cancer, with lead skin shield and lead eye shield in place

Skin is categorized as an early-reacting tissue, so acute adverse effects of radiation therapy are similar for palliative treatment and more definitive treatments. In particular, skin erythema and desquamation are common, and patients may develop a non-healing wound following radiation therapy. For many palliative patients, however, a fungating wound is present prior to undergoing radiation, and the adverse effects of radiation therapy are minimal compared to the problems associated with the cancer. Late complications may include poor cosmesis, fibrosis, and permanent changes in skin pigmentation. Other acute and late adverse effects will differ based on the location of the skin lesion.

Challenges of Re-irradiation

Cells have differential ability to repair radiation damage. However, cellular damage is never fully repaired; a tissue that has been irradiated in the past will have a lower tolerance for additional radiation regardless of the interval between the two doses of radiation. Of course, tissue repair improves the longer the interval between treatments, and some tissues have better capability of repair after radiation compared to other tissues. For dose-limiting organs such as the spinal cord, kidneys, and small intestine, it is important to consider the cumulative dose over all treatment courses.

Palliative radiation treatment is often given at a dose-fractionation far below the constraints of the dose-limiting organs. In this case, re-irradiation can be provided without much concern for toxicity. For example, numerous studies have examined the treatment of patients who have been irradiated to bony metastases and subsequently required re-irradiation to the same lesions [46, 47]. If both radiation courses are given at low doses, there is minimal risk of toxicity even after the second treatment, and the treatment may be effective. A systematic review showed an overall pain response in 58% of patients receiving re-irradiation for painful bone metastases, regardless of the prior response to radiation therapy [46]. This study and a prospective retreatment trial have shown good responses and limited toxicity even with a repeat single fraction dose of 8 Gy [46, 47].

Re-irradiation of the spinal cord is of concern given the catastrophic potential harm of radiation myelopathy. Studies of re-irradiation typically account for differences in the fractionation schedules by determining biologically equivalent dose (BED) for each course and cumulative BED. Although there is still some uncertainty regarding the specific contraindications of re-irradiation to the spinal cord, studies have shown that patients

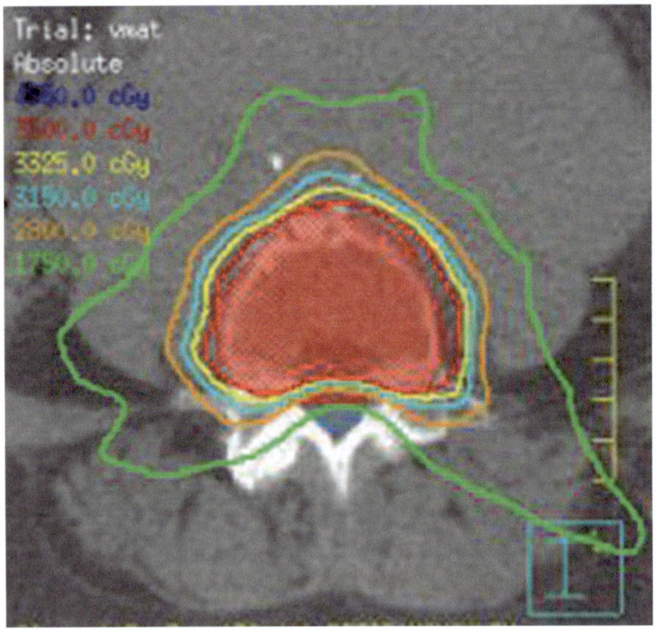

Fig. 37.6 Axillary slice of isodose plan for SBRT for vertebral body lesions

can be reliably categorized for their risk of radiation myelopathy [48]. Thus, patients can be identified for re-irradiation who are unlikely to experience significant toxicity.

With the development of highly conformal techniques, it has become possible to dramatically localize radiation. Thus, the risks of re-irradiation may be limited if the target region is sufficiently small. Although not necessary in all cases, SRS and SBRT may often be useful to limit toxicity in re-irradiation (Fig. 37.6). Similarly, brachytherapy can limit radiation dose outside of the target tissue, given the rapid drop-off of dose. Thus, brachytherapy may be particularly useful in the re-irradiation setting.

References

1. Lutz ST, Jones J, Chow E. Role of radiation therapy in palliative care of the patient with cancer. J Clin Oncol. 2014;32(26):2913–9.
2. Gutierrez Bayard L, Salas Buzon Mdel C, Angulo Pain E, de Ingunza Baron L. Radiation therapy for the management of painful bone metastases: results from a randomized trial. Rep Pract Oncol Radiother. 2014;19(6):405–11.
3. Howell DD, James JL, Hartsell WF, Suntharalingam M, Machtay M, Suh JH, Demas WF, Sandler HM, Kachnic LA, Berk LB. Single-fraction radiotherapy versus multifraction radiotherapy for palliative of painful vertebral bone metastases-equivalent efficacy, less toxicity, more convenient: a subset analysis of Radiation Therapy Oncology Group trial 97–14. Cancer. 2013;119(4):888–96.
4. Majumder D, Chatterjee D, Bandyopadhyay A, Mallick SK, Sarkar SK, Majumdar A. Single fraction versus multiple fraction radiotherapy for palliation of painful vertebral metastases: a prospective study. Indian J Palliat Care. 2012;18(3):202–6.
5. Rich SE, Chow R, Raman S, Zeng KL, Lutz S, Lam H, Silva MF, Chow E. Update of the systematic review of palliative radiation therapy fractionation for bone metastases. Radiother Oncol. 2018;126(3):547–57.
6. Abeer Hussien A. Single Fraction versus multiple fraction radiotherapy for treatment of painful bone metastases: a Prospective Study; Mansoura experience. Forum Clin Oncol. 2015;6(2):8–13.
7. Fairchild A, Barnes E, Ghosh S, Ben-Josef E, Roos D, Hartsell W, Holt T, Wu J, Janjan N, Chow E. International patterns of practice in palliative radiotherapy for painful bone metastases: evidence-based practice? Int J Radiat Oncol Biol Phys. 2009;75(5):1501–10.
8. Hird A, Zhang L, Holt T, Fairchild A, DeAngelis C, Loblaw A, Wong R, Barnes E, Tsao M, Danjoux C, Chow E. Dexamethasone for the prophylaxis of radiation-induced pain flare after palliative radiation therapy for symptomatic bone metastases: a phase II study. Clin Oncol (R Coll Radiol). 2009;21(4):329–35.
9. Chow E, Harris K, Fan G, Tsao M, Sze WM. Palliative radiotherapy for bone metastases: a systematic review. J Clin Oncol. 2007;25(11):1423–36.
10. Chow E, Zeng L, Salvo N, Dennis K, Tsao M, Lutz S. Update on the systematic review of palliative radiotherapy trials for bone metastases. Clin Oncol (R Coll Radiol). 2012;24(2):112–24.
11. Meeuse JJ, van der Linden YM, van Tienhoven G, Gans RO, Leer JW, Reyners AK. Dutch bone metastasis study group. Efficacy of radiotherapy for painful bone metastases during the last 12 weeks of life: results from the Dutch bone metastasis study. Cancer. 2010;116(11):2716–25.
12. Lutz S, Berk L, Chang E, Chow E, Hahn C, Hoskin P, Howell D, Konski A, Kachnic L, Lo S, Sahgal A, Silverman L, von Gunten C, Mendel E, Vassil A, Bruner DW, Hartsell W. American Society for Radiation Oncology. Palliative radiotherapy for bone metastasis: an ASTRO evidence-based guideline. Int J Radiat Oncol Biol Phys. 2011;79(4):965–76.
13. Khuntia D, Brown P, Li J, Mehta MP. Whole-brain radiotherapy in the management of brain metastasis. J Clin Oncol. 2006;24(8):1295–304.
14. Tsao MN, Rades D, Wirth A, Lo SS, Danielson BL, Gaspar LE, Sperduto PW, Vogelbaum MA, Radawski JD, Wang JZ, Gillin MT, Mohideen N, Hahn CA, Chang EL. Radiotherapeutic and surgical management for newly diagnosed brain metastasis(es): an American Society for Radiation Oncology evidence-based guideline. Pract Radiat Oncol. 2012;2(3):210–25.
15. Eichler AF, Loeffler JS. Multidisciplinary management of brain metastases. Oncologist. 2007;12(7):884–98.
16. Sperduto PW, Berkey B, Gaspar LE, Mehta M, Curran W. A new prognostic index and comparison to three other indices for patients with brain metastases: an analysis of 1,960 patients in the RTOG database. Int J Radiat Oncol Biol Phys. 2008;70(2):510–4.
17. Kak M, Nanda R, Ramsdale EE, Lukas RV. Treatment of leptomeningeal carcinomatosis: current challenges and future opportunities. J Clin Neurosci. 2015;22(4):632–7.
18. Shaw E, Scott C, Souhami L, Dinapoli R, Kline R, Loeffler J, Farnan N. Single dose radiosurgical treatment of recurrent previously irradiated primary brain tumors and brain metastases: final report of RTOG protocol 90–05. Int J Radiat Oncol Biol Phys. 2000;47(2):291–8.
19. Borgelt B, Gelber R, Kramer S, Brady LW, Chang CH, Davis LW, Perez CA, Hendrickson FR. The palliation of brain metastases: final results of the first two studies by the Radiation Therapy Oncology Group. Int J Radiat Oncol Biol Phys. 1980;6(1):1–9.
20. Borgelt B, Gelber R, Larson M, Hendrickson F, Griffin T, Roth R. Ultra-rapid high dose irradiation schedules for the palliation of brain metastases: final results of the first two studies by the Radiation Therapy Oncology Group. Int J Radiat Oncol Biol Phys. 1981;7(12):1633–8.

21. Gelber RD, Larson M, Borgelt BB, Kramer S. Equivalence of radiation schedules for the palliative treatment of brain metastases in patients with favorable prognosis. Cancer. 1981;48(8):1749–53.
22. Sneed PK, Mendez J, Vemer-van den Hoek JG, Seymour ZA, Ma L, Molinaro AM, Fogh SE, Nakamura JL, McDermott MW. Adverse radiation effect after stereotactic radiosurgery for brain metastasis: incidence, time course, and risk factors. J Neurosurg. 2015;123(2):373–86.
23. Patchell RA, Tibbs PA, Walsh JW, Dempsey RJ, Maruyama Y, Kryscio RJ, Markesbery WR, Macdonald JS, Young B. A randomized trial of surgery in the treatment of single metastases to the brain. N Engl J Med. 1990;322(8):494–500.
24. Patchell RA, Tibbs PA, Regine WF, Dempsey RJ, Mohiuddin M, Kryscio RJ, Markesbery WR, Foon KA, Young B. Postoperative radiotherapy in the treatment of single metastases to the brain: a randomized trial. JAMA. 1998;280(17):1485–9.
25. Erkal HS, Mendenhall WM, Amdur RJ, Villaret DB, Stringer SP. Squamous cell carcinomas metastatic to cervical lymph nodes from an unknown head and neck mucosal site treated with radiation therapy with palliative intent. Radiother Oncol. 2001;59:319–21.
26. Corry J, Peters LJ, Costa ID, Milner AD, Fawns H, Rischin D, Porceddu S. The "QUAD SHOT"—a phase II study of palliative radiotherapy for incurable head and neck cancer. Radiother Oncol. 2005;77(2):137–42.
27. Soliman H, Ringash J, Jiang H, Singh K, Kim J, Dinniwell R, Brade A, Wong R, Brierley J, Cummings B, Zimmermann C, Dawson LA. Phase II trial of palliative radiotherapy for hepatocellular carcinoma and liver metastases. J Clin Oncol. 2013;31(31):3980–6.
28. Russell AH, Clyde C, Wasserman TH, Turner SS, Rotman M. Accelerated hyperfractionated hepatic irradiation in the management of patients with liver metastases: results of the RTOG dose escalating protocol. Int J Radiat Oncol Biol Phys. 1993;27(1):117–23.
29. Hoyer M, Swaminath A, Bydder S, Lock M, Mendez Romero A, Kavanagh GKA, Okunieff P, Dawson LA. Radiotherapy for liver metastases: a review of evidence. Int J Radiat Oncol Biol Phys. 2012;82(3):1047–57.
30. Herman J, Messersmith W, Suh WW, Blackstock W, Cosman BC, Mohiuddin M, Poggi MM, Regine WF, Saltz L, Small W Jr, Zook J, Konski AA. ACR appropriateness criteria: rectal cancer-metastatic disease at presentation. Curr Probl Cancer. 2010;34(3):201–10.
31. Halle JS, Rosenman JG, Varia MA, Fowler WC, Walton LA, Currie JL. 1000 cGy single dose palliation for advanced carcinoma of the cervix or endometrium. Int J Radiat Oncol Biol Phys. 1986;12(11):1947–50.
32. Spanos WJ Jr, Perez CA, Marcus S, Poulter CA, Doggett RL, Steinfeld AD, Grigsby PW. Effect of a rest interval on tumor and normal tissue response—a report of phase III study of accelerated split course palliative radiation for advanced pelvic malignancies (RTOG-8502). Int J Radiat Oncol Biol Phys. 1993;25(3):399–403.
33. Smith SC, Koh WJ. Palliative radiation therapy for gynaecological malignancies. Best Pract Res Clin Obstet Gynaecol. 2001;15(2):265–78.
34. Hymel R, Jones GC, Simone CB 2nd. Whole pelvic intensity-modulated radiotherapy for gynecological malignancies: a review of the literature. Crit Rev Oncol Hematol. 2015;94(3):371–9.
35. McCurdy MT, Shanholtz CB. Oncologic emergencies. Crit Care Med. 2012;40(7):2212–22.
36. Lonardi F, Gioga G, Agus G, Coeli M, Campostrini F. Double-flash, large-fraction radiation therapy as palliative treatment of malignant superior vena cava syndrome in the elderly. Support Care Cancer. 2000;10(2):156–60.
37. Wan JF, Bezjak A. Superior vena cava syndrome. Emerg Med Clin North Am. 2009;27(2):243–55.
38. Luppattelli M, Maranzano E, Bellavita R, Chionne F, Darwish S, Piro F, Latini P. Short-course palliative radiotherapy in non-small-cell lung cancer: results of a prospective study. Am J Clin Oncol. 2000;23(1):89–93.
39. Harwood AR, Dancuart F, Fitzpatrick PJ, Brown T. Radiotherapy for nonlentiginous melanoma of the head and neck. Cancer. 1981;48(12):2599–605.
40. Burmeister BH, Henderson MA, Ainslie J, Fisher R, Di Iulio J, Smithers BM, Hong A, Shannon K, Scolyer RA, Carruthers S, Coventry BJ, Babington S, Duprat J, Hoekstra HJ, Thompson JF. Adjuvant radiotherapy versus observation alone for patients at risk of lymph-node field relapse after therapeutic lymphadenectomy for melanoma: a randomized trial. Lancet Oncol. 2012;13(6):589–97.
41. Mojica P, Smith D, Ellenhorn JD. Adjuvant radiation therapy is associated with improved survival in Merkel cell carcinoma of the skin. J Clin Oncol. 2007;25(9):1043–7.
42. Kaye FJ, Bunn PA Jr, Steinberg SM, Stocker JL, Ihde DC, Fischmann AB, Glatstein EJ, Schechter GP, Phelps RM, Foss FM, Parlette HL, Anderson MJ, Sausville EA. A randomized trial comparing combination electron-beam radiation and chemotherapy with topical therapy in the initial treatment of mycosis fungoides. N Engl J Med. 1989;321(26):1784–90.
43. Smith BD, Glusac EJ, McNiff JM, Smith GL, Heald PW, Cooper DL, Wilson LD. Primary cutaneous B-cell lymphoma treated with radiotherapy: a comparison of the European Organization for Research and Treatment of Cancer and the WHO classification systems. J Clin Oncol. 2004;22(4):634–9.
44. Stratigos A, Garbe C, Lebbe C, Malvehy J, Del Marmol V, Pehamberger H, Peris K, Becker JC, Zalaudek I, Saiag P, Middleton MR, Bastholt L, Testori A, Grob JJ, European Dermatology Forum, European Association of Dermato-Oncology, European Organization for the Research and Treatment of Cancer. Diagnosis and treatment of invasive squamous cell carcinoma of the skin: European consensus-based interdisciplinary guideline. Eur J Cancer. 2015;51:1989–2007.
45. Mendenhall WM. Radiotherapy for cutaneous squamous and basal cell carcinomas. In: Cognetta AB, Mendenhall WM, editors. Radiation therapy for skin cancer. New York: Springer; 2013. p. 160.
46. Huisman M, van den Bosch MA, Wijlemans JW, van Vulpen M, van der Linden YM, Verkooijen HM. Effectiveness of reirradiation for painful bone metastases: a systematic review and meta-analysis. Int J Radiat Oncol Biol Phys. 2012;84(1):8–14.
47. Chow E, van der Linden YM, Roos D, Hartsell WF, Hoskin P, Wu JS, Brundage MD, Nabid A, Tissing-Tan CJ, Oei B, Babington S, Demas WF, Wilson CF, Meyer RM, Chen BE, Wong RK. Single versus multiple fractions of repeat radiation for painful bone metastases: a randomized, controlled, non-inferiority trial. Lancet Oncol. 2014;15(2):164–71.
48. Nieder C, Grosu AL, Andratschke NH, Molis M. Update of human spinal cord reirradiation tolerance based on additional data from 38 patients. Int J Radiat Oncol Biol Phys. 2006;66(5):1446–9.

External Beam Radiotherapy in the Treatment of Painful Bone Metastases

38

Candice Johnstone, Amol J. Ghia, and Anussara Prayongrat

Introduction

Tumors from primary sites such as the breast, prostate, and lung as well as hematologic malignancies such as multiple myeloma spread to the bone [1]. External beam radiation therapy (EBRT) plays a role in the multidisciplinary management of symptomatic and asymptomatic lesions. This multidisciplinary team generally consists of surgeons, radiologists, interventional radiologists, radiation oncologists, medical oncologists, and pathologists, though others may also be involved. Memorial Sloan Kettering Cancer Center (MSKCC) has developed a decision framework for metastatic spine disease, neurologic, oncologic, mechanical instability, and systemic disease (NOMS), to provide a score to determine the appropriate treatment for an individual patient [2].

Bone metastasis typically cause symptoms earlier in the patient's course than visceral metastasis. Symptoms range from localized pain and pathologic fracture to compression of nerves, nerve roots, or the spinal cord [3, 4]. Bones suffer the direct effects of tumor invasion as well as altered remodeling mediated by osteoblasts and osteoclasts. The perception of pain may therefore include descriptions by the patient such as "sharp," "burning," "shock-like," "cramping," "achy," or "unrelenting." Systemic effects of osseous metastases include nausea, vomiting, fatigue, anorexia, and psychological changes caused by hypercalcemia. Bone metastases that are asymptomatic may also require treatment if there is impending spinal cord compromise or significant involvement of weight-bearing bones. This may be especially true in the management of lesions of the acetabulum, where surgical options are limited.

C. Johnstone (✉)
Department of Radiation Oncology, Medical College of Wisconsin, Milwaukee, WI, USA
e-mail: cjohnstone@mcw.edu

A. J. Ghia
University of Texas MD Anderson Cancer Center, Department of Radiation Oncology, Houston, TX, USA
e-mail: ajghia@mdanderson.org

A. Prayongrat
King Chulalongkorn Memorial Hospital and Chulalongkorn University, Department of Radiation Oncology, Bangkok, Thailand

Radiotherapy for Pain

Between 50% and 75% of radiographically evident bone metastases will cause discomfort during a patient's disease course. Treatment of painful bone metastases is the most common indication for palliative radiation therapy. External beam radiotherapy (EBRT) provides effective and time-efficient pain relief with a low risk of complications. Overall response rates range from 60% to 80% for EBRT with complete response rates of 25–30% [5, 6]. Even painful metastases caused by tumors thought to be less radioresponsive, such as sarcomas, respond quite well to treatment.

Pain relief typically does not begin until several days after the start of EBRT and may take several weeks for the full palliative effect to become evident. The mean time to the onset of pain relief is 3 weeks [7]. Thus, a patient must have a reasonable pain medication regimen in place until the palliative effect of radiotherapy is manifested. Due to the logistics of radiation therapy planning and treatment delivery, patients must also be reasonably comfortable lying flat for 15–20 min. The World Health Organization has described a stepwise approach to pain management to help patients achieve sufficient pain relief during this interval [8]. These regimens often include nonsteroidal anti-inflammatory agents, narcotic analgesics, or adjuvant pain medicines such as corticosteroids, nerve-stabilizing medicines, or antidepressants.

Pain control or pain response typically lasts several months, which in many cases is the patients' entire remaining life. In a subgroup analysis of long-term survivors of patients treated for painful osseous metastasis, the mean duration of response was approximately 5 months [9]. Unfortunately, approximately 55% of patients have progression of pain at the treated site at a mean interval of

A. Gulati et al. (eds.), *Essentials of Interventional Cancer Pain Management*, https://doi.org/10.1007/978-3-319-99684-4_38

16–17 weeks. If pain recurs, re-treatment can generally be performed safely with good palliative effect [10]. (See Re-treatment below.)

Radiation response occurs because of photon interactions with DNA and other molecules, such as water, that create double-stranded DNA breaks. Normal cells have intact DNA repair mechanisms and more easily repair the damage caused by radiation. Cancer cells are defined by aberrant growth, and the resultant DNA damage typically results in cell death. Pain relief following EBRT may occur faster than tumor cell death, suggesting a more complex process that may include the production of factors, e.g., cytokines, that lead to stimulation of nociceptors on adjacent nerves.

Impending or Pathologic Fracture, Spinal Instability, and the Need for Surgical Evaluation

Patients with bone metastases should be evaluated for radiographic findings that suggest a risk for pathologic fracture. The morbidity and mortality of a completed fracture are much higher than for a properly managed impending fracture. Unfortunately, definitively determining the true risk of pathologic fracture from clinical and radiographic information can be difficult for even the most experienced physicians [11, 12]. Pathologic fractures most commonly occur in weight-bearing bones under torsional forces, though bones weakened by a large tumor burden may fracture by simple adjustments of position. Surgical stabilization of weakened bones can prevent pathologic fracture with postoperative EBRT doses of 20–30 Gy given to promote healing and minimize persistent pain [13, 14]. Radiation delivered to a bone at risk for a pathologic fracture decreases the tumor burden and promotes remineralization. Bisphosphonates can reduce the risk of pathologic fracture, are complementary to, and can be used in combination with EBRT.

One reason commonly cited against the use of higher dose per fraction EBRT regimens is the potential for pathologic fracture. A meta-analysis of multiple randomized trials of fractionation comprising more than 5000 patients did not demonstrate a difference in the long-term risk of pathologic fracture between single and multi-fraction EBRT regimens [6].

There are criteria for determining the risk of pathologic fracture (Harrington's [15] and Mirels' [16]) and spinal instability [17] in the setting of osseous metastasis. Harrington lists four criteria that increase the risk of pathologic fracture: destruction of the metaphysis (>50–75%) or diaphysis (>50% or 2.5 cm), destruction of the subtrochanteric femoral region, and persistent pain following radiation therapy [15]. Mirels' criteria assign a score to each of four factors: site, type and size of the lesion, and the type of pain. Prophylactic fixation should be considered for a score > 8 [16]. The Spinal Instability Neoplastic Score (SINS) assigns a score for the location of the lesion, type of pain and spinal alignment, extent of vertebral body collapse, and presence of involvement of the posterolateral spinal elements. The composite score places patients tinto groups of spinal stability. Patients with a score of 7 or greater should be evaluated for prophylactic stabilization [17]. Bilsky et al. proposed a magnetic resonance imaging (MRI)-based grading system for metastatic spinal cord compression (MSCC) [18]. (See Table 38.1.) Patients with grade 0 (bone only) and grade 1 (epidural impingement without spinal cord compression) in the absence of mechanical instability are appropriate candidates for EBRT. Those with grade 2 (partial MSCC) and grade 3 (complete MSCC) should be evaluated for surgical decompression followed by radiation, unless the tumor is considered highly radiosensitive. The management of grade 1c (deformation of the thecal sac without cord compression) is controversial (See Table 38.2). Ryu et al., proposed a grading system based on MRI and neurological criteria to determine the use of surgery versus SBRT [19]. Surgical intervention may be most appropriate when there is rapid or progressive neurological deficit (neurological grade d and e) to achieve immediate decompression of the spinal cord and restore the neurological function, while EBRT or SBRT are appropriate when neurological function is intact. Tables 38.1 and 38.2 summarize both grading systems. Short-course EBRT may be appropriate for those patients with MSCC with short life expectancy [20, 21].

Table 38.1 Grading system of metastatic epidural spinal cord compression (MSCC) by Bilsky et al. [18]

Radiographic grade	Description	Recommendations
0	Spinal bone involved only	Radiotherapy (RT)
1a	Epidural impingement, without deformation of the thecal sac	
1b	Deformation of the thecal sac without spinal cord abutment	
1c	Deformation of the thecal sac with spinal cord abutment but without cord compression	RT or surgery
2	Spinal cord compression with cerebrospinal fluid(CSF) visible around the cord	Surgery followed by postoperative RT
3	Spinal cord compression without CSF visible around the cord	

Table 38.2 Grading system of metastatic epidural spinal cord compression (MSCC) by Ryu et al. [19]

Radiographic grade	Description	Recommendations
0	Spinal bone involved only	Radiotherapy (RT)
I	Thecal sac impingement	
II	Thecal sac compressed, or ≤ 50% of spinal canal compressed at cauda level	
III	Spinal cord impinged	RT or surgery
IV	Spinal cord displaced, CSF visible between cord and tumor, or >50% of spinal canal compressed at cauda level	Surgery followed by postoperative RT
V	Spinal cord compressed, CSF not visible between cord and tumor	
Neurological grade	**Description**	**Recommendations**
a	No abnormality	Stereotactic body radiation therapy (SBRT)
b	Focal minor symptom (pain, radiculopathy, sensory change)	
c	Functional paresis with ≥4/5 muscle power Nerve root sign (involved functional muscle) Spinal cord sign (ambulatory, functional upper extremity)	
d	Nonfunctional paresis with ≤3/5 muscle power Nerve root sign (involved functional muscle) Spinal cord sign (nonambulatory, nonfunctional upper extremity)	Surgery followed by postoperative RT
e	Paralysis and/or incontinence	

Dose Fractionation

More than 100 radiation fractionation schemes are used to treat metastatic bone pain worldwide [22]. Multiple prospective, randomized trials analyzed the equivalency of specific regimens in the treatment of uncomplicated bone metastasis during the past three decades. The majority of these studies compare single-fraction (SF) regimens such as 8 Gy in a single fraction to other multi-fraction (MF) regimens. Short-term pain relief, mean time to response, and mean duration of response are equivalent with courses of 30 Gy in 10 fractions, 24 Gy in 6 fractions, 20 Gy in 5 fractions, and a single 8 Gy fraction for uncomplicated bone metastasis. There is very little support in the literature for choosing a MF regimen over a SF regimen in the treatment of uncomplicated bone metastasis. When SF radiation therapy is employed, there is a threshold effect. SF doses of 6 or 8 Gy are required for therapeutic effect [23]. Eight Gy has become the standard SF dose. Results from the three largest randomized trials of fractionation are illustrated in Table 38.3 [7, 24–26].

SF treatment is more convenient for patients and their caregivers and is associated with fewer short-term side effects [24]. Though many physicians believe that this approach should be reserved for patients with a short life expectancy, an unplanned subgroup analysis of patients surviving >52 weeks in the Dutch Bone Metastasis trial suggests that MF treatment with higher total doses offers no additional benefit over a SF [9, 27]. This lack of added therapeutic benefit is compounded by the fact that physicians routinely overestimate patient survival [9, 28]. Another theoretical advantage of the higher dose per fraction in SF treatment is the increase in double-stranded DNA breaks seen with increased dose per fraction and the potential to overcome the relative radioresistance of certain tumor histologies, e.g., renal cell carcinoma, though there is limited data in this setting as the majority of patients enrolled in these trials have breast, lung, or prostate primary tumors.

A higher total dose of 20–30 Gy can be considered when bone metastases are associated with a large extraosseous component, osteolytic lesions with impending pathologic fracture in medically inoperable patients, and lesions with spinal canal or cauda equina compression or neuropathic pain [29]. The goal of the longer course in these circumstances extends beyond pain control to maximizing tumor control, functional status, and remineralization, issues that are more relevant in patients who will survive at least several months. A single trial of patients with neuropathic pain from bone metastases did not show superiority for either 20 Gy in 5 fractions or a single 8 Gy fraction, though the proper fractionation for this clinical circumstance remains somewhat controversial [30]. At least one randomized trial did not demonstrate a difference in functional outcome between SF and MF treatment of MSCC [31].

A SF course is more commonly associated with re-treatment to the same painful site than fractionated courses, with rates of 20% versus 8%, respectively. This may be due in part to reluctance on the part of radiation oncologists to give additional fractionated radiation after a fractionated course, as randomized trials indicate that long-term survivors are equally likely (55%) to experience recurrent pain regardless of initial fractionation regimen [9]. A randomized trial of re-treatment with either 20 Gy in 5 fractions or a

Table 38.3 EBRT fractionation schemes and response rates of the three largest randomized trials of fractionation in the treatment of painful bone metastasis

Trial (Ref)	Number of patients	Randomization dose/ fraction number	Response rate SF (%)	Response rate MF (%)	Retreatment rate SF/MF	Complete response SF	Complete response MF
Bone pain trial working party [25]	761	8 Gy/1 vs. 20 Gy/5	274/351 (78%)	257/330 (78%)	23%/10%	57%	58%
Dutch Bone Metastasis Study [7, 26]	1171	8 Gy/1 vs. 24 Gy/6	395/556 (71%)	396/543 (73%)	24%/6%	37%	33%
RTOG 97–14 (24)	898	8 Gy/1 vs. 30 Gy/10	187/455 (41%)	188/443 (42%)	18%/9%	15%	18%

SF single fraction, *MF* multi-fraction

single 8 Gy fractions in patients who had varying initial fractionation schemes treatments showed equivalence of the SF regimen to the MF regimen. Since single-fraction RT is equally efficacious, less expensive, and more convenient, it is recommended as the favored re-treatment regimen.

Process of Radiation Therapy Planning and Delivery

Radiation oncologists commonly consult on patients with bone metastases following a definitive diagnosis and evaluation by other oncology physicians. Therefore, the radiation oncologist must gather and interpret relevant clinical data and radiographic studies while optimizing communication with those other healthcare providers. Once EBRT has been determined to be appropriate by the radiation oncologist and has been accepted in an informed fashion by the patient, the patient is scheduled for a simulation or radiation planning session. One purpose of the simulation is to establish a comfortable and reproducible patient position that allows treatment of the affected area without giving unnecessary radiation dose to other body parts, e.g., the arms. At simulation, the patient's body shape and anatomy are captured in the treatment position either by fluoroscopy or a quick CT scan to allow for dose calculation and reproducible setup for subsequent treatment(s). While simulation may be completed by clinically assessing bony landmarks or using fluoroscopy to visualize bony anatomy, the most common mechanism for simulation involves a 20–30-min-long CT-based simulation of the patient in the same position that treatment will be delivered.

The dosimetry, or dose planning, is completed next and involves computerized measurement of the best means by which to deliver dose to the intended target while minimizing treatment to adjacent normal tissues. For patients who do not live near a radiation facility or who suffer pain with transfer to and from CT scanners and treatment tables, it is most efficient to complete the consultation, simulation, and initiation of single-fraction therapy during the same day. The physicist and physician review the radiation plan to ensure accurate delivery of radiation. Prior to treatment, portal images are obtained to verify that the setup of the patient is correct and that the correct area is in the treatment field. The delivery of radiotherapy commonly takes only 10–15 min per dose, and it is painless other than discomfort that may be associated with transfer to or lying on the treatment table. Figures 38.1, 38.2 and 38.3 demonstrate the radiation treatment plans for patients requiring EBRT treatment to the whole pelvis (x.1), L4 (x.2) and shoulder (x.2).

Side Effects of EBRT

Radiation therapy for bone metastases may cause acute side effects that are most often predictable, mild, manageable with conservative measures, and dependent upon the area of the body irradiated. Fatigue is the main systemic side effect associated with treatment; it is usually less significant than that which is caused by the disease or other treatment modalities. Local side effects can include skin irritation, gastrointestinal complaints like nausea or diarrhea, or dysphagia. Factors such as the daily dose and total dose delivered can influence the risk for acute, subacute, and long-term toxicity. Previous trials have suggested a slightly higher risk of acute side effects following multiple fractions of radiotherapy when compared to a single, larger fraction for bone metastases [27, 32]. Tumor cell kill can cause a transient increase in bone pain around the time of the first few fractions of radiotherapy in 20–40% of patients [33]. When it occurs, this pain flare may be minimized using nonsteroidal anti-inflammatory drugs or oral dexamethasone.

The late effects of radiotherapy, which may occur several months to years after treatment, are relatively rare but can be more serious than acute side effects. These symptoms may involve targeted and nearby tissue and may include pain from neuritis and myositis. While the acute effects of treatment depend mostly upon the total dose of

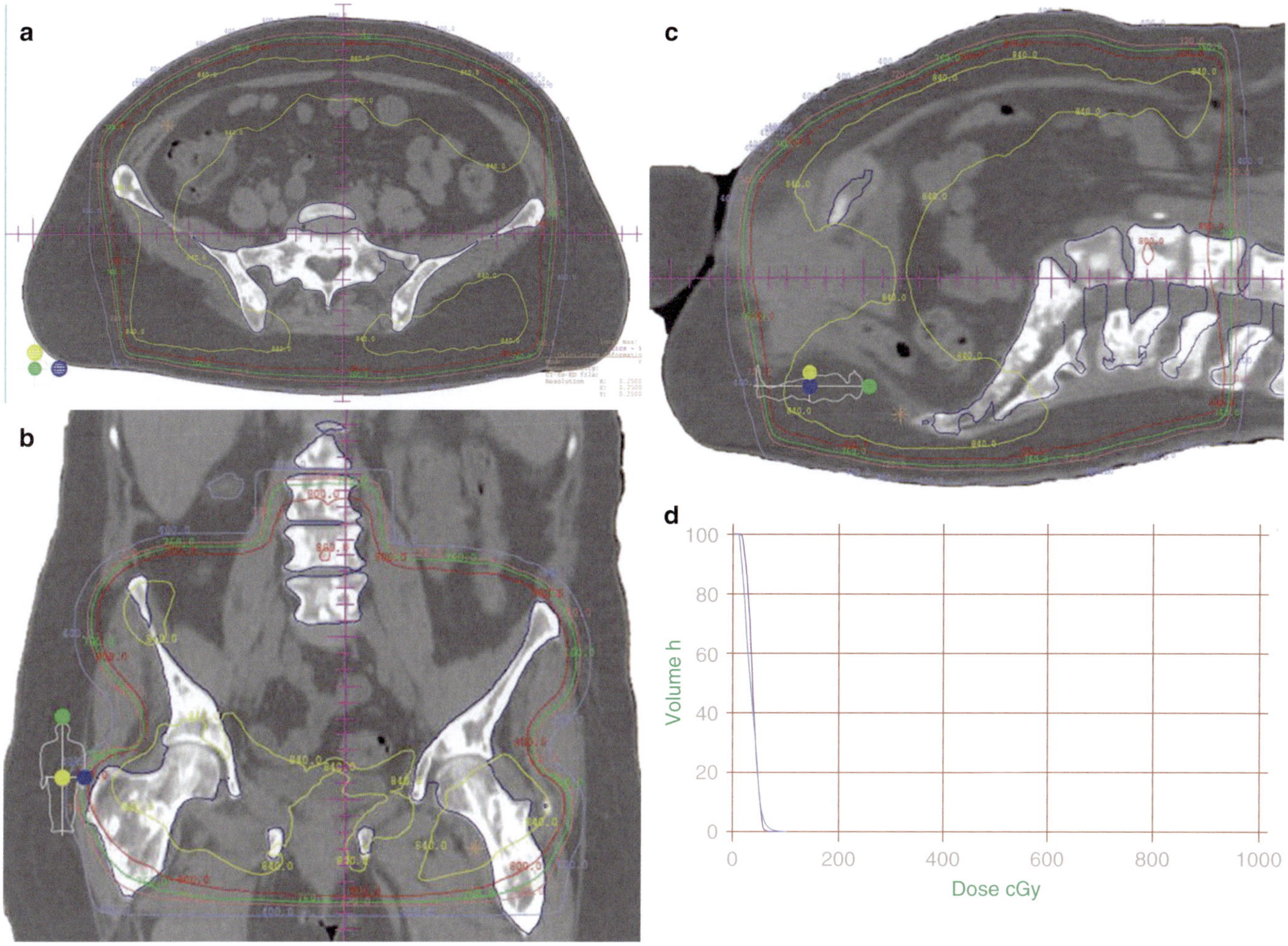

Fig. 38.1 Depicts the axial (**a**), coronal (**b**), and sagittal (**c**) planes with RT isodose curves in a patient with small cell lung cancer treated to the whole pelvis for extensive painful osseous metastasis. Also shown is a dose-volume histogram (**d**)

delivered radiotherapy, the late side effects of radiation depend upon both the total dose delivered and the size of dose delivered per treatment. In other words, larger daily doses of radiation correlate with a higher risk of long-term side effects. Patients with bone metastases have historically not lived a sufficiently lengthy time to commonly suffer late side effects. Improvements in systemic treatment have allowed some patients with bone metastases to live longer and potentially put them at risk for long-term toxicity that can be associated with short course, high dose per fraction therapy. To date, this hasn't been clinically significant given the relatively short survival in metastatic cancer and modest total dose delivered when larger fraction sizes are used. In the Dutch Bone Metastasis Study, a separate stratification and randomization was performed for patients who were thought to have a better prognosis; after 1 year, only 53% of those patients were alive [9]. Factors that are associated with improved survival include histology (breast or prostate), absence of visceral metastasis, Karnofsky Performance Status, and the Functional Assessment of Cancer Therapy (FACT) [28].

Re-treatment with EBRT

Patients who have been previously treated with EBRT receive re-treatment to that same painful site with some frequency. If the first course of palliative radiation was a multi-fraction course, the re-treatment rates are about 8%. For those whose first course was a single fraction of 8 Gy, the re-treatment rate is 20% [5]. Approximately 55% of patients experience recurrent pain at the treated site, regardless of the initial regimen. At least one trial demonstrated less benefit from re-treatment after multi-fraction regimens [7]. The true incidence of recurrent pain is uncertain, given that re-treatment in most trials was given at the discretion of the

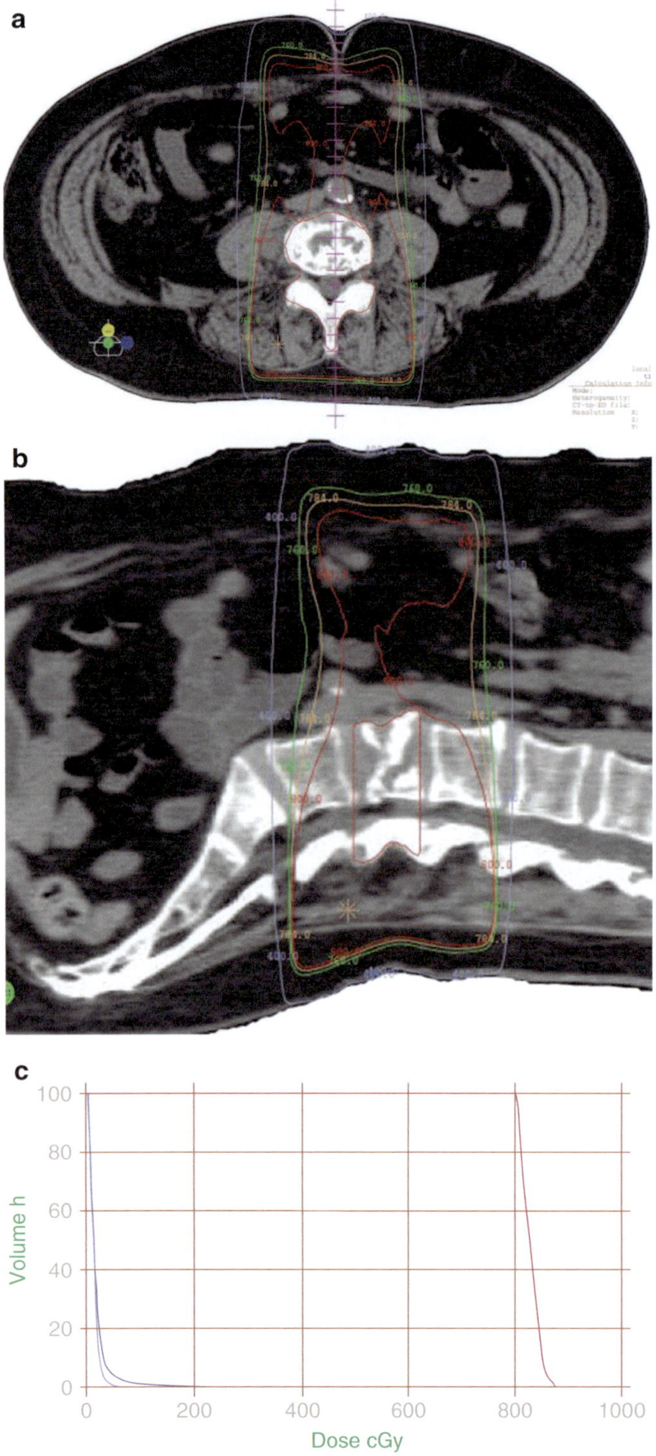

Fig. 38.2 Depicts the axial (**a**) and sagittal (**b**) planes with RT isodose curves in a patient with breast cancer treated to the L4 which includes one vertebral body above and one below for painful L4 osseous metastasis. Also shown is a dose-volume histogram (**c**)

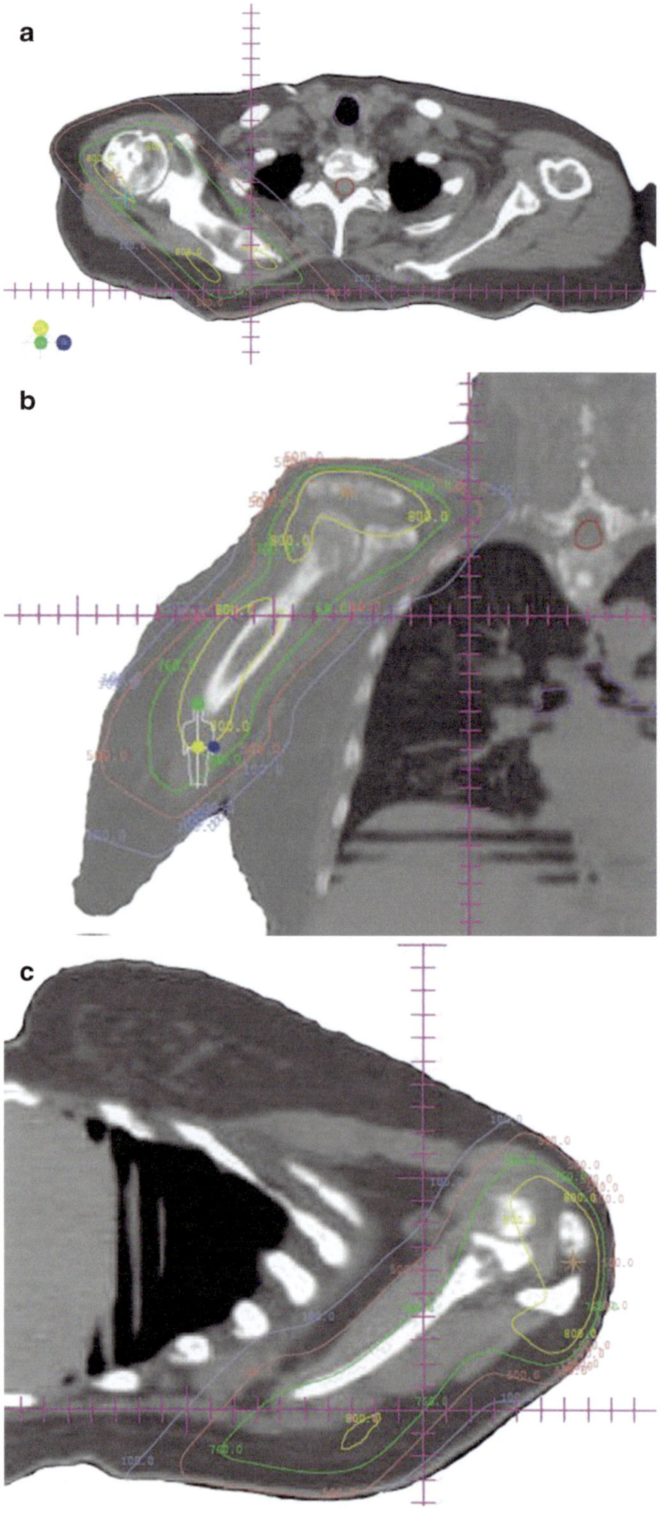

Fig. 38.3 Depicts the axial (**a**), coronal (**b**), and sagittal (**c**) planes with RT isodose curves in a patient with lung cancer treated to the scapula

treating physician. In general, both patients and physicians are more likely to accept re-treatment after an initial single fraction versus a more prolonged radiotherapy course [7]. Recent consensus conference groups have therefore begun to better define the criteria by which re-treatment should be considered. Given that pain sometimes recedes slowly following radiotherapy over a period of days to weeks, the minimum interval before re-treatment should be considered is 4 weeks [34]. There is little prospective data available to predict the risk for combined side effects from initial treatment and re-treatment of painful bone metastases, though retrospective studies suggest that re-treatment can be given with relatively safety and a 50–70% chance for pain relief [35]. A prospective randomized international study demonstrated that SF (8 Gy) was non-inferior to the MF (20 Gy in 5 fractions) regimen and less toxic. Therefore 8 Gy SF was recommended as the preferred re-treatment regimen [10].

Highly Conformal Therapy

Several emerging technologies are capable of producing EBRT that is considered highly conformal [36]. The goal of these techniques is to deliver high doses to the target while minimizing damage to adjacent structures. These approaches include intensity-modulated radiation therapy (IMRT), which uses an inverse planning process with dose constraints for organs at risk (OAR) in the treated volume. Stereotactic body radiation therapy (SBRT) involves the delivery of large, highly conformal doses with fastidious attention paid to dose planning, patient setup, and localization. This technique may be especially useful in the re-treatment of an area where the spinal cord has reached tolerance due to their initial definitive course of radiation therapy. Image-guided radiation therapy (IGRT) can help to optimize patient positioning [37]. Proton beam therapy takes advantage of spatial qualities of radiation dose delivery to maximize dosing to the intended target [38].

SBRT has been used for painful bone metastases involving the spine, both as a primary treatment and as a method for delivering re-treatment to spine bones that have previously received standard external beam radiotherapy [39]. SBRT fractionation regimens include 30 Gy in 5 fractions, 27 Gy in 3 fractions, 40 Gy in 5 fractions, or 16–24 Gy in a single fraction [40–42]. The results of these early trials are promising with prospective, randomized data likely to further define the best use of this technology [43]; SBRT may be used for the primary treatment or re-treatment of spine metastases. However, the relative lack of information about the long-term effects of very large single doses through innovative delivery systems may create a higher risk of long-term side effects than would be true for more established treatment approaches, so care must accompany this approach [44]. Routine use should not be employed until sufficient evidence from clinical trials justifies the substantive increase in cost when compared to standard EBRT.

Stereotactic Body Radiation Therapy for Spinal Metastases

Stereotactic body radiation therapy (SBRT) is an emerging advanced technology that combines sophisticated computerized treatment planning; advanced imaging such as magnetic resonance imaging (MRI), immobilization devices, treatment delivery with beam intensity, or beam gantry modulation; and image-guided radiation therapy (IGRT) to alleviate pain, improve local control, prevent or improve neurological dysfunction, and improve quality of life while minimizing possible toxicity. SBRT is typically defined as fewer than 5 fractions, though longer courses of up to 7–8 fractions may accomplish the same goals.

The advantages of SBRT broadly belong to one of three categories: physical, biological, and clinical aspects.

1. **Physical aspects**: High conformality achieved by complicated beam arrangements or intensity modulation and precise and accurate targeting localization due to image guidance resulting in tumor dose escalation with adjacent normal tissue sparing achieved due to steep dose falloff outside the target volume.
2. **Biological aspects**: SBRT allows treatment with higher doses per fraction resulting in a higher biological equivalent dose (BED). The BED, calculated using linear-quadratic (LQ) model, is as high as 41.6–81.6 Gy_{10} for SBRT regimens of 16–24 Gy in SF to 24–27 Gy in 3 fractions compared with 14.4–39 Gy_{10} for 8 Gy in SF to 30 Gy in 10 fractions with conventional radiotherapy. The precise mechanism of cell death is controversial and is likely multifactorial [45–47]. Indirect cell death by high-dose fractionation is not accounted for the LQ model resulting in underestimation of tumor control [47, 48].
3. **Clinical aspects**: Conventional external beam radiotherapy (EBRT) has been historically utilized for palliation of pain and other symptoms. SBRT with IGRT allows delivery of a potentially ablative radiation dose and the potential for durable pain relief particularly for radioresistant tumors. However, there is limited data concerning the long-term normal tissue toxicity [49]. Pain control and freedom from progression in spinal metastatic patients are reported in 84–97% of patients treated with SBRT [39, 49–58]. In the postoperative setting, SBRT may decrease rates of the instrument failure, though these rates are generally quite low [59]. SBRT is especially useful in patients for whom re-irradiation to areas that have previ-

ously been treated to doses at spinal cord tolerance by the attempt at curative therapy. Like conventional EBRT, SBRT is a noninvasive outpatient procedure that can be delivered in a single fraction.

Decision-making for spine SBRT is similar to the process for conventional EBRT and other therapies. One consideration that may be more important in the selection of patients for SBRT is the extent of systemic disease, specifically the lack of significant systemic disease and the chance for prolonged >1 year survival. SBRT, which delivers an ablative dose of radiation, may be more appropriate in the setting of oligometastatic disease when tumor ablation is the goal rather than pure palliation.

Prognostic Prediction Spinal Metastasis

Various scoring systems are applied in attempt to select the proper treatment modality for each individual patient with spinal metastasis. Most of these prognostic tools were developed in the context of surgical intervention [60–64]. There is high concordance among 83 specialists from 44 hospitals using the Tomita score and modified Bauer scores in the treatment of spine metastases [65]. A revised version demonstrated that the score of 0–8, 9–11, and 12–15 predicted a life expectancy of less than 6 months, 6 months or more, and 12 months or more, respectively. Therefore, a patients' life expectancy can guide the clinical management [66, 67]. There are many other tools that help determine the prognosis of patients with advanced cancer in other settings. Two of the most generalizable to general palliative radiotherapy are the NRF and the TEACHH models [68, 69]. Two prognostic models specifically assess survival after spine SBRT: recursive partitioning analysis (RPA) index for patients undergoing spine SBRT and prognostic index for spine metastasis (PRISM) [68, 69]. See Table 38.4.

RPA was developed by Chao et al. [67] who analyzed 174 patients receiving SBRT for spinal metastasis to assess survival after treatment. The authors classified patients into three classes: Class 1 defined as patients with a time from primary diagnosis (TPD) of >30 months and a Karnofsky Performance Status (KPS) of > 70, Class 2 defined as those with a TPD of > 30 months and a KPS of ≤ 70 or a TPD of < 30 months and age < 70 years, and Class 3 defined as a TPD of ≤ 30 months and age ≥ 70 years. Median overall survival (OS) was 21.1 months, 8.7 months, and 2.4 months for Classes 1, 2, and 3, respectively [70]. Recently, Tang et al. developed a new survival stratification system using seven pretreatment parameters as presented in Table 38.4. This model was proposed to identify patient subgroups with poor (Group 4) and excellent (Group 1) prognosis after spine SBRT with the median OS of 9.1 months and > 70 months, respectively [71].

Table 38.4 Survival score and patient subgroups in prognostic index for spine metastasis (PRISM) model [71]

Score parameter	Score
Female	+2
Every 10 points over KPS 60	+1 per 10 KPS
Previous surgery at SBRT site	+2
Previous radiation at SBRT site	-2
Every organ system involved with metastasis (outside of bone)	−1 per system
SBRT site represents solitary metastasis	+3
Time of diagnosis to metastasis >5 years	+3
Survival groups	**Score range**
Group 1 (excellent prognosis)	>7
Group 2	4–7
Group 3	1–3
Group 4 (poor prognosis)	<1

Abbreviations: *KPS* Karnofsky performance status, *SBRT* stereotactic body radiation therapy

SBRT for spinal metastasis is not cost-effective compared with EBRT at a 100,000 per quality-adjusted life years (QALYs) gained willingness-to-pay (WTP) threshold. If used in patients whose median survival is ≥11 months, SBRT costs ≤$100,000 per QALY gained, emphasizing that SBRT should be selectively used in patients with longer survival [72].

Clinical Applications of Spine SBRT

Tumor and/or pain control in patients treated with SBRT for spinal metastases ranging from 77% to 100% with median time to pain relief of 2–4 weeks after treatment. The median duration of tumor and pain control was 6–13.6 months. This compares favorably with conventional EBRT as described earlier in the chapter. Duration of control is longer in these series, but these series are single-institution reports of well-selected patients compared with patients treated on large randomized clinical trials.

There are three clinical scenarios where spine SBRT is used.

1. Primary Treatment in Unirradiated Patients
   Spine SBRT provides favorable tumor control and pain relief in selected patients. This technology is being evaluated in a current Radiation Therapy Oncology Group (RTOG) trial [73] where patients with painful bone metastasis are randomized to 8 Gy SF with EBRT vs. 16 Gy SF with SBRT. SBRT in previously unirradiated patients may be best reserved for those in whom ablative doses may prove beneficial, such as those with oligometastatic disease and projected prolonged survival.
   The role of SBRT in malignant spinal cord compression MSCC is controversial and still limited to the context of

a clinical trial. Ryu et al. reported the outcome of 62 patients with 85 spinal MSCC lesions treated with SBRT 12–20 Gy (median dose of 16 Gy) SF [19]. All patients had ≥4/5 muscle power (neurological grade c or better). The mean epidural volume was reduced by 65% at 2 months with complete disappearance of 35%, and the thecal sac patency improved after SBRT. A promising result of 81% improvement in neurological function indicated that radiosurgical decompression may be an alternative noninvasive treatment option for MSCC, though further study is needed.

Radioresistant tumors might be benefit from SBRT. Two series reported 89–96% pain control in RCC and melanoma patients treated with SBRT 17.5–25 Gy SF [74–76]. In primary and metastatic spinal sarcoma treated with 16–45 Gy in 1–3 fractions, pain control rate was 89% and 68% at 6 and 12 months, respectively [77].

2. Salvage Treatment in Reirradiated Patients

Patients who have previously received RT to the spine can develop new, recurrent, or progressive disease at any time. The incidence of in-field recurrence varies from 2.5% to 11%, and time to failure ranges from 2 to 40 months after first radiotherapy [78–80]. Depending on the total dose, dose per fraction, and part of the spine irradiated, SBRT may be the best re-treatment strategy, though an additional 8 Gy in 1 fraction or 20 Gy in 5 fractions can safely be delivered to most areas of the body with EBRT after initial palliative radiation therapy [10]. There were some areas of the spine when combined with some initial MF schemes that required dose modifications or who were not eligible for enrollment.

Patients who have previously completed radiation therapy with curative intent, especially those with head and neck or thoracic cancers, may develop painful tumors in the spine in the previously irradiated area. The goals of treatment are pain relief and prevention of further complications due to local tumor progression without inducing radiation myelopathy. Treatment options include surgical decompression with or without EBRT or SBRT.

Spine SBRT results in tumor control or palliation of symptoms in 77–100% of reirradiated patients [75, 81–89]. In one of the largest series, 500 lesions in 393 patients were treated with SBRT, 69% of whom had received prior RT. Ninety percent of patients achieved pain and neurological improvement as well as local tumor control [86]. Higher radiotherapy doses, larger doses per fraction, and previous exposure to radiation are associated with an increased risk of developing radiation-induced myelopathy, a late effect that develops months or years after radiotherapy [78, 79, 90].

3. Postoperative SBRT for Spinal Metastases

Postoperative SBRT results in tumor control of 81–94.4% [91–93]. SBRT is performed 1–2 weeks after radical resection, decompressive surgery, or stabilization procedures. The target volume includes residual tumor and surgical bed. Two disadvantages of postoperative SBRT are poor image quality for tumor and normal tissue delineation and dosimetric uncertainty due to artifact from spinal instrumentation. This approach remains investigational.

Spine Stereotactic Body Radiation Therapy Techniques

Stereotactic radiotherapy represents an emerging treatment modality with advanced target determination, patient immobilization, complex radiation planning, and verification to deliver relatively high doses of radiation while minimizing surrounding critical normal tissue dose. The radiosurgery target volume is contoured based on potential anatomical extension according to routes of spread within the spinal segment [80, 85, 94].

Toxicity of SBRT

Acute Toxicity

Acute toxicities are relatively uncommon but include dysphagia, esophagitis, laryngitis, nausea and vomiting, fatigue, skin hyperpigmentation, pain flare, and postoperative wound complications [84, 85, 95, 96]. Development of a pain flare from SBRT varies from 23% to 68.3% [97, 98]. Prophylactic treatment with dexamethasone in patients treated with spine SBRT remains controversial in the absence of prospective randomized data.

Late Toxicity

Overall late toxicity from spine SBRT is not common but not completely defined due to the newness of this approach. However, late toxicities such as radiation myelopathy (RM) are devastating. RM occurs 3–25 months after RT, although the incidence of RM after SBRT is rare (<1%) when conservative constraints for the spinal cord are utilized [80, 84, 85, 88, 91, 96, 99–101].

Vertebral compression fracture (VCF) is more common ranging from asymptomatic fractures to severe mechanical pain due to spine instability. The pathophysiology of VCF development can be described by tumor-induced demineralization through abnormal bone turnover, architectural changes, radiation-induced collagen damage, and necrosis of bone and tumor tissue. These mechanisms affect the bone quality in terms of bone strength, ductility, and toughness leading to increased risk of fracture [102]. The incidence of radiographic VCF after SBRT is significantly higher at 11–39% when compared with 5% after EBRT. It generally occurs at 1.6–3.3 months after SBRT [103–106]. Predictive factors for VCF include tumor location at or below T10, lytic lesions especially those involving >40% of the vertebral body, kyphotic deformity, radiation dose ≥20 Gy per fraction, age > 55 years, preexisting fracture, and baseline pain [103–106]. There is no consensus on criteria for high-risk patients who may benefit from prophylactic spine stabilization. Surgical management or percutaneous cement augmentation procedures, such as vertebroplasty and kyphoplasty, is required in one third of patients.

Guidelines and Quality Measures

Though the optimal treatment of bone metastases with radiotherapy has been evaluated in multiple prospective randomized trials, there has been a great deal of variability in the dose fractionation regimens employed by radiation oncologists. One survey revealed that 101 different dose fractionation schemes were employed worldwide for this single clinical circumstance [22]. These disparities have led to the formation of treatment guidelines by the American Society for Radiation Oncology (ASTRO) and the American College of Radiology (ACR) [107–109]. These guidelines confirm that the available data reveal four fractionation schemes that are equivalent in the successful management of painful bone metastases: 30 Gy in 10 fractions, 24 Gy in 6 fractions, 20 Gy in 5 fractions, and a single 8 Gy fraction. The guidelines acknowledge a trade-off between increased convenience and a higher re-treatment rate with single-fraction therapy. Additionally, the publications differentiate between treatment approaches that have proven to be effective through clinical trials and those approaches that require further investigation before being used in a routine, non-protocol setting. The use of one of the four approved fractionation schemes is considered a measure of quality as determined by the National Quality Forum (NQF) [110]. The NQF is a nonprofit organization that is tasked to assess healthcare priorities in the United States while providing a means to measure and report on the performance of healthcare providers and healthcare facilities. Furthermore, the choice to offer appropriate length fractionation schemes for patients with painful bone metastases is under review in an initiative called "Choosing Wisely" [111], a program started to help physicians become better financial stewards of healthcare use.

Summary

Bone metastases continue to be a significant clinical problem, with pain being the most common symptom requiring intervention. External beam radiation therapy continues to serve as the main form of treatment for painful bone metastases, with good coordination required between the radiation oncologist and other specialists including medical oncologists, surgeons, palliative medicine specialists, and physiatrists. Short-course treatments effectively provide symptom relief, with many patients best treated by a single fraction. The acute and long-term side effect rates from EBRT are minimal and usually self-limited. Highly conformal therapy for bone metastases shows great promise, especially in patients with recurrent pain in the spine after previous conventionally fractionated curative therapy. Bone metastases treatment guidelines and quality measures provide data-derived direction to the management of patients with this clinical condition.

References

1. Galasko CS. Then anatomy and pathways of bone metastasis. In: Weiss L, Gilbert A, editors. Bone metastasis. Boston: GK Hall; 1981. p. 49–63.
2. Laufer I, Rubin DG, Lis E, Cox BW, Stubblefield MD, Yamada Y, et al. The NOMS framework: approach to the treatment of spinal metastatic tumors. Oncologist. 2013;18(6):744–51. PubMed PMID: 23709750. Pubmed Central PMCID: 4063402. eng.
3. Coleman RE. Skeletal complications of malignancy. Cancer. 1997;80(8 Suppl):1588–94. PubMed PMID: 9362426. Epub 1997/11/15. eng.
4. Kamby C, Vejborg I, Daugaard S, Guldhammer B, Dirksen H, Rossing N, et al. Clinical and radiologic characteristics of bone metastases in breast cancer. Cancer. 1987;60(10):2524–31. PubMed PMID: 3664434. Epub 1987/11/15. eng.
5. Chow E, Harris K, Fan G, Tsao M, Sze WM. Palliative radiotherapy trials for bone metastases: a systematic review. J Clin Oncol. 2007;25(11):1423–36.
6. Chow E, Zeng L, Salvo N, Dennis K, Tsao M, Lutz S. Update on the systematic review of palliative radiotherapy trials for bone metastases. Clin Oncol (R Coll Radiol). 2012;24(2):112–24. PubMed PMID: 22130630. Epub 2011/12/02. eng
7. van der Linden YM, Lok JJ, Steenland E, Martijn H, van Houwelingen H, Marijnen CAM, et al. Single fraction radiotherapy is efficacious: a further analysis of the Dutch bone metastasis study controlling for the influence of retreatment. Int J Radiat Oncol Biol Phys. 2004;59(2):528–37. PubMed PMID: 15145173
8. WHO. World Health Organization Pain Ladder 2010 [cited 2013 9 Feb 3013]. Available from: http://www.who.int/cancer/palliative/painladder/en/.
9. van der Linden YM, Steenland E, van Houwelingen HC, Post WJ, Oei B, Marijnen CAM, et al. Patients with a favourable prognosis are equally palliated with single and multiple fraction radiotherapy: results on survival in the Dutch bone metastasis study. Radiother Oncol. 2006;78(3):245–53.
10. Chow E, van der Linden YM, Roos D, Hartsell WF, Hoskin P, Wu JS, et al. Single versus multiple fractions of repeat radiation for painful bone metastases: a randomised, controlled, non-

inferiority trial. Lancet Oncol. 2014;15(2):164–71. PubMed PMID: 24369114.
11. Nielsen OS, Munro AJ, Tannock IF. Bone metastases: pathophysiology and management policy. J Clin Oncol. 1991;9(3):509–24.
12. Springfield D. Pathologic fractures. Rockwood and Green's fractures in adults. 5th ed. Philadelphia: Lippincott Williams Wilkins; 2001.
13. Koswig S, Budach V. [Remineralization and pain relief in bone metastases after after different radiotherapy fractions (10 times 3 Gy vs. 1 time 8 Gy). A prospective study]. Strahlentherapie und Onkologie : Organ der Deutschen. Rontgengesellschaft [et al]. 1999 Oct;175(10):500–8. PubMed PMID: 10554645. Epub 1999/11/11. Remineralisation und Schmerzlinderung von Knochenmetastasen nach unterschiedlich fraktionierter Strahlentherapie (10 mal 3 Gy vs. 1 mal 8 Gy). Eine prospektive Studie. ger.
14. Townsend PW, Smalley SR, Cozad SC, Rosenthal HG, Hassanein RE. Role of postoperative radiation therapy after stabilization of fractures caused by metastatic disease. Int J Radiat Oncol Biol Phys. 1995;31(1):43–9. PubMed PMID: 7995767. Epub 1995/01/01. eng
15. Harrington KD. Impending pathologic fractures from metastatic malignancy: evaluation and management. Instr Course Lect. 1986;35:357–81. PubMed PMID: 3819423.
16. Mirels H. Metastatic disease in long bones. A proposed scoring system for diagnosing impending pathologic fractures. Clin Orthop Relat Res. 1989;249:256–64. PubMed PMID: 2684463.
17. Fourney DR, Frangou EM, Ryken TC, Dipaola CP, Shaffrey CI, Berven SH, et al. Spinal instability neoplastic score: an analysis of reliability and validity from the spine oncology study group. J Clin Oncol. 2011;29(22):3072–7. PubMed PMID: 21709187.
18. Bilsky MH, Laufer I, Fourney DR, Groff M, Schmidt MH, Varga PP, et al. Reliability analysis of the epidural spinal cord compression scale. J Neurosurg Spine. 2010;13(3):324–8. PubMed PMID: 20809724. eng.
19. Ryu S, Rock J, Jain R, Lu M, Anderson J, Jin JY, et al. Radiosurgical decompression of metastatic epidural compression. Cancer. 2010;116(9):2250–7. PubMed PMID: 20209611. eng.
20. Maranzano E, Bellavita R, Rossi R, De Angelis V, Frattegiani A, Bagnoli R, et al. Short-course versus split-course radiotherapy in metastatic spinal cord compression: results of a phase III, randomized, multicenter trial. J Clin Oncol. 2005;23(15):3358–65. PubMed PMID: 15738534.
21. Maranzano E, Latini P, Perrucci E, Beneventi S, Lupattelli M, Corgna E. Short-course radiotherapy (8 Gy x 2) in metastatic spinal cord compression: an effective and feasible treatment. Int J Radiat Oncol Biol Phys. 1997;38(5):1037–44. PubMed PMID: 9276370.
22. Fairchild A, Barnes E, Ghosh S, Ben-Josef E, Roos D, Hartsell W, et al. International patterns of practice in palliative radiotherapy for painful bone metastases: evidence-based practice? Int J Radiat Oncol Biol Phys. 2009;75(5):1501–10. PubMed PMID: 19464820. Epub 2009/05/26. eng.
23. Jeremic B, Shibamoto Y, Acimovic L, Milicic B, Milisavljevic S, Nikolic N, et al. A randomized trial of three single-dose radiation therapy regimens in the treatment of metastatic bone pain. Int J Radiat Oncol Biol Phys. 1998;42(1):161–7. PubMed PMID: 9747834.
24. Hartsell WF, Scott CB, Bruner DW, Scarantino CW, Ivker RA, Roach M, et al. Randomized trial of short- versus long-course radiotherapy for palliation of painful bone metastases. J Natl Cancer Inst. 2005;97(11):798–804.
25. Party BPTW. 8 Gy single fraction radiotherapy for the treatment of metastatic skeletal pain: randomised comparison with a multifraction schedule over 12 months of patient follow-up. Bone Pain Trial Working Party. Radiother Oncol. 1999;52(2):111–21. PubMed PMID: 10577696.
26. Steenland E, Leer JW, van Houwelingen H, Post WJ, van den Hout WB, Kievit J, et al. The effect of a single fraction compared to multiple fractions on painful bone metastases: a global analysis of the Dutch bone metastasis study. Radiother Oncol. 1999;52(2):101–9. PubMed PMID: 10577695.
27. Foro Arnalot P, Fontanals AV, Galceran JC, Lynd F, Latiesas XS, de Dios NR, et al. Randomized clinical trial with two palliative radiotherapy regimens in painful bone metastases: 30 Gy in 10 fractions compared with 8 Gy in single fraction. Radiother Oncol. 2008;89(2):150–5. PubMed PMID: 18556080. Epub 2008/06/17. eng
28. Hartsell WF, Desilvio M, Bruner DW, Scarantino C, Ivker R, Roach M 3rd, et al. Can physicians accurately predict survival time in patients with metastatic cancer? Analysis of RTOG 97-14. J Palliat Med. 2008;11(5):723–8. PubMed PMID: 18588404. Epub 2008/07/01. eng.
29. Van der Linden YM, Dijkstra PD, Kroon HM, Lok JJ, Noordijk EM, Leer JW, et al. Comparative analysis of risk factors for pathological fracture with femoral metastases. J Bone Joint Surg. 2004;86(4):566–73. PubMed PMID: 15174555. Epub 2004/06/04. eng
30. Roos DE, Turner SL, O'Brien PC, Smith JG, Spry NA, Burmeister BH, et al. Randomized trial of 8 Gy in 1 versus 20 Gy in 5 fractions of radiotherapy for neuropathic pain due to bone metastases (Trans-Tasman Radiation Oncology Group, TROG 96.05). Radiother Oncol. 2005;75(1):54–63. PubMed PMID: 15878101. Epub 2005/05/10. eng.
31. Maranzano E, Trippa F, Casale M, Costantini S, Lupattelli M, Bellavita R, et al. 8Gy single-dose radiotherapy is effective in metastatic spinal cord compression: results of a phase III randomized multicentre Italian trial. Radiother Oncol. 2009;93(2):174–9. PubMed PMID: 19520448.
32. Hartsell W, Scott C, Bruner DW, et al. Phase III randomized trial of 8 Gy in 1 fraction vs. 30 Gy in 10 fractions for palliation of painful bone metastases: preliminary results of RTOG 97–14. Int J Radiat Oncol Biol Phys. 2003;57(Supplement):124.
33. Loblaw DA, Wu JS, Kirkbride P, Panzarella T, Smith K, Aslanidis J, et al. Pain flare in patients with bone metastases after palliative radiotherapy—a nested randomized control trial. Support Care Cancer. 2007;15(4):451–5. PubMed PMID: 17093912. Epub 2006/11/10. eng
34. Chow E, Hoskin P, Mitera G, Zeng L, Lutz S, Roos D, et al. Update of the international consensus on palliative radiotherapy endpoints for future clinical trials in bone metastases. Int J Radiat Oncol Biol Phys. 2012;82(5):1730–7. PubMed PMID: 21489705. Epub 2011/04/15. eng.
35. Huisman M, van den Bosch MA, Wijlemans JW, van Vulpen M, van der Linden YM, Verkooijen HM. Effectiveness of reirradiation for painful bone metastases: a systematic review and meta-analysis. Int J Radiat Oncol Biol Phys. 2012;84(1):8–14. PubMed PMID: 22300568.
36. Lo SS, Fakiris AJ, Chang EL, Mayr NA, Wang JZ, Papiez L, et al. Stereotactic body radiation therapy: a novel treatment modality. Nat Rev Clin Oncol. 2010;7(1):44–54. PubMed PMID: 19997074. Epub 2009/12/10. eng.
37. Jaffray D, Kupelian P, Djemil T, Macklis RM. Review of image-guided radiation therapy. Expert Rev Anticancer Ther. 2007;7(1):89–103. PubMed PMID: 17187523. Epub 2006/12/26. eng
38. Allen AM, Pawlicki T, Dong L, Fourkal E, Buyyounouski M, Cengel K, et al. An evidence based review of proton beam therapy: the report of ASTRO's emerging technology committee. Radiother Oncol. 2012;103(1):8–11. PubMed PMID: 22405807. Epub 2012/03/13. eng.

39. Sahgal A, Larson DA, Chang EL. Stereotactic body radiosurgery for spinal metastases: a critical review. Int J Radiat Oncol Biol Phys. 2008;71(3):652–65. PubMed PMID: 18514775. Epub 2008/06/03. eng
40. Wang XS, Rhines LD, Shiu AS, Yang JN, Selek U, Gning I, et al. Stereotactic body radiation therapy for management of spinal metastases in patients without spinal cord compression: a phase 1–2 trial. Lancet Oncol. 2012;13(4):395–402. PubMed PMID: 22285199. Epub 2012/01/31. eng
41. Garg AK, Shiu AS, Yang J, Wang XS, Allen P, Brown BW, et al. Phase 1/2 trial of single-session stereotactic body radiotherapy for previously unirradiated spinal metastases. Cancer. 2012;118(20):5069–77. PubMed PMID: 22511344. Epub 2012/04/19. eng.
42. Jhaveri PM, Teh BS, Paulino AC, Blanco AI, Lo SS, Butler EB, et al. A dose-response relationship for time to bone pain resolution after stereotactic body radiotherapy (SBRT) for renal cell carcinoma (RCC) bony metastases. Acta Oncol. 2012;51(5):584–8. PubMed PMID: 22248089. Epub 2012/01/18. eng.
43. RTOG. RTOG 0618: A Phase II trial of Stereotactic Body Radiation Therapy (SBRT) in the treatment of patients with operable Stage I/II non-small cell lung cancer 2006. Available from: http://www.google.com/url?sa=t&rct=j&q=&esrc=s&frm=1&source=web&cd=2&ved=0CDYQFjAB&url=http%3A%2F%2Fwww.rtog.org%2FClinicalTrials%2FProtocolTable%2FStudyDetails.aspx%3Faction%3DopenFile%26FileID%3D4650&ei=9b4TUaD7B6yE2QXYooCgCA&usg=AFQjCNH3XRG72GBwcAqbx2WYC37kQV-SoQ&sig2=M25iWW62dHbnx_PJnOTUtQ.
44. Lo SS, Sahgal A, Chang EL, Mayr NA, Teh BS, Huang Z, et al. Serious complications associated with stereotactic ablative radiotherapy and strategies to mitigate the risk. Clin Oncol (R Coll Radiol). 2013;25(6):378–87.
45. Brown JMCD, Brenner DJ. The tumor radiobiology of SRS and SBRT: are more than the 5 Rs involved? Int J Radiat Oncol Biol Phys. 2014;88(2):254–62.
46. Song CW, Kim MS, Cho LC, Dusenbery K, Sperduto PW. Radiobiological basis of SBRT and SRS. Int J Clin Oncol. 2014;19(4):570–8. PubMed PMID: 24993673. eng.
47. Song CW, Cho LC, Yuan J, Dusenbery KE, Griffin RJ, Levitt SH. Radiobiology of stereotactic body radiation therapy/stereotactic radiosurgery and the linear-quadratic model. Int J Radiat Oncol Biol Phys. 2013;87(1):18–9. PubMed PMID: 23608235. eng.
48. Kirkpatrick JP, KMJ M, Marks LB. The linear-quadratic model is inappropriate to model high dose per fraction effects in radiosurgery. Semin Radiat Oncol. 2008;18(4):240–3. 20080826 DCOM-20081009. eng.
49. Yu HH, Hoffe SE. Beyond the conventional role of external-beam radiation therapy for skeletal metastases: new technologies and stereotactic directions. Cancer Control. 2012;19(2):129–36. PubMed PMID: 22487975. Epub 2012/04/11. eng.
50. Lutz S, Lo SS, Chow E, Sahgal A, Hoskin P. Radiotherapy for metastatic bone disease: current standards and future prospectus. Expert Rev Anticancer Ther. 2010;10(5):683–95. PubMed PMID: 20470001.
51. Guckenberger M, Sweeney RA, Flickinger JC, Gerszten PC, Kersh R, Sheehan J, et al. Clinical practice of image-guided spine radiosurgery—results from an international research consortium. Radiat Oncol. 2011 20120227 DCOM- 20120615;6(1748-717X (Electronic)):172. PubMed PMID: 22172095. Pubmed Central PMCID: 3286433. eng.
52. Sahgal A, Bilsky M, Chang EL, Ma L, Yamada Y, Rhines LD, et al. Stereotactic body radiotherapy for spinal metastases: current status, with a focus on its application in the postoperative patient. J Neurosurg Spine. 2011;14(2):151–66. PubMed PMID: 21184635. Epub 2010/12/28. eng.
53. Sahgal A, Roberge D, Schellenberg D, Purdie TG, Swaminath A, Pantarotto J, et al. The Canadian Association of Radiation Oncology scope of practice guidelines for lung, liver and spine stereotactic body radiotherapy. Clin Oncol (R Coll Radiol). 2012;24(9):629–39. PubMed PMID: 22633542. eng.
54. Sohn S, Chung CK. The role of stereotactic radiosurgery in metastasis to the spine. J Korean Neurosurg Soc. 2012;51(1):1–7. PubMed PMID: 22396835. Pubmed Central PMCID: 3291699. eng.
55. Chawla S, Schell MC, Milano MT. Stereotactic body radiation for the spine: a review. Am J Clin Oncol. 2013;36(6):630–6. PubMed PMID: 22134513. Epub 2011/12/03. eng
56. Ejima Y, Matsuo Y, Sasaki R. The current status and future of radiotherapy for spinal bone metastases. J Orthop Sci. 2015.;(1436–2023 (Electronic)). PubMed PMID: 25860575. eng.
57. Ryu S, Yoon H, Stessin A, Gutman F, Rosiello A, Davis R. Contemporary treatment with radiosurgery for spine metastasis and spinal cord compression in 2015. Radiat Oncol J. 2015;33(1):1–11. PubMed PMID: 25874172. Pubmed Central PMCID: 4394063. eng.
58. Park HJ, Kim HJ, Won JH, Lee SC, Chang AR. Stereotactic body radiotherapy (SBRT) for spinal metastases: who will benefit the most from SBRT? Technol Cancer Res Treat. 2015;14(2):159–67. PubMed PMID: 24502552. Epub 2014/02/08. eng.
59. Gerszten PC, Mendel E, Yamada Y. Radiotherapy and radiosurgery for metastatic spine disease: what are the options, indications, and outcomes? Spine. 2009;15(22 Suppl):S78–92. 20091015 DCOM-20100126. eng.
60. Bauer HWR. Survival after surgery for spinal and extremity metastases. Acta Orthop Scand. 1995;66(2):143–6.
61. Wibmer C, Leithner A, Hofmann G, Clar H, Kapitan M, Berghold A, et al. Survival analysis of 254 patients after manifestation of spinal metastases: evaluation of seven preoperative scoring systems. Spine. 2011;36(23):1977–86. PubMed PMID: 21304424. eng.
62. Leithner A, Radl R, Gruber G, Hochegger M, Leithner K, Welkerling H, et al. Predictive value of seven preoperative prognostic scoring systems for spinal metastases. Eur Spine J. 2008;17(11):1488–95. PubMed PMID: 18787846. Pubmed Central PMCID: 2583181. eng.
63. Tomita K, Kawahara N, Kobayashi T, Yoshida A, Murakami H, Akamaru T. Surgical strategy for spinal metastases. Spine. 2001;26(3):298–306. PubMed PMID: 11224867. eng.
64. Tokuhashi Y, Matsuzaki H, Toriyama S, Kawano H, Ohsaka S. Scoring system for the preoperative evaluation of metastatic spine tumor prognosis. Spine. 1990;15(11):1110–3. PubMed PMID: WOS:A1990EJ57700005. English.
65. Arana E Kovacs FM, Royuela A, Asenjo B, Pérez-Ramírez Ú, Zamora J; Spanish Back Pain Research Network Task Force for the improvement of inter-disciplinary management of spinal metastasis. Agreement in the assessment of metastatic spine disease using scoring systems. Radiother Oncol. 115(1):135-140 2015 20150516:pii: S0167-8140(15)00155-3. doi: https://doi.org/10.1016/j.radonc.2015.03.016. [Epub ahead of print]. Eng.
66. Tokuhashi Y, Matsuzaki H, Oda H, Oshima M, Ryu J. A revised scoring system for preoperative evaluation of metastatic spine tumor prognosis. Spine. 2005;30(19):2186–91. PubMed PMID: 16205345. eng.
67. Wang M, Bunger CE, Li HS, Wu CS, Hoy K, Niedermann B, et al. Predictive value of Tokuhashi scoring systems in spinal metastases, focusing on various primary tumor groups evaluation of 448 patients in the Aarhus spinal metastases database. Spine. 2012;37(7):573–82. PubMed PMID: WOS:000302266400014. English.
68. Krishnan MS, Epstein-Peterson Z, Chen YH, Tseng YD, Wright AA, Temel JS, et al. Predicting life expectancy in patients with

metastatic cancer receiving palliative radiotherapy: the TEACHH model. Cancer. 2014;120(1):134–41. PubMed PMID: 24122413.
69. Chow E, Abdolell M, Panzarella T, Harris K, Bezjak A, Warde P, et al. Validation of a predictive model for survival in metastatic cancer patients attending an outpatient palliative radiotherapy clinic. Int J Radiat Oncol Biol Phys. 2009;73(1):280–7. PubMed PMID: 18676092.
70. Chao ST, Koyfman SA, Woody N, Angelov L, Soeder SL, Reddy CA, Rybicki LA, Djemil T, Suh JH. Recursive partitioning analysis index is predictive for overall survival in patients undergoing spine stereotactic body radiation therapy for spinal metastases. Int J Radiat Oncol Biol Phys. 2012;82(5):1738–43. 20120320 DCOM- 20120511. eng.
71. Tang C, Hess K, Bishop AJ, Pan HY, Christensen EN, Yang JN, et al. Creation of a prognostic index for spine metastasis to stratify survival in patients treated with spinal stereotactic radiosurgery: secondary analysis of mature prospective trials. Int J Radiat Oncol Biol Phys. 2015;93(1):118–25. PubMed PMID: 26130231. eng.
72. Kim H, Rajagopalan MS, Beriwal S, Huq MS, Smith KJ. Cost-effectiveness analysis of single fraction of stereotactic body radiation therapy compared with single fraction of external beam radiation therapy for palliation of vertebral bone metastases. Int J Radiat Oncol Biol Phys. 2015;91(3):556–63. PubMed PMID: 25680599. eng.
73. RTOG. RTOG 0631: a phase II/III study of image-guided radiosurgery/SBRT for localized spine metastasis—RTOG CCOP study 2006 [Jan 31 2016]. Available from: https://www.rtog.org/ClinicalTrials/ProtocolTable/StudyDetails.aspx?study=0631.
74. Gerszten PC, Burton SA, Ozhasoglu C, Vogel WJ, Welch WC, Baar J, et al. Stereotactic radiosurgery for spinal metastases from renal cell carcinoma. J Neurosurg Spine. 2005;3(4):288–95. PubMed PMID: 16266070. eng.
75. Gerszten PC, Burton SA, Quinn AE, Agarwala SS, Kirkwood JM. Radiosurgery for the treatment of spinal melanoma metastases. Stereotact Funct Neurosurg. 2005;83(5–6):213–21. 20060407 DCOM- 20060829. PubMed PMID: 16534253. eng.
76. Sohn SCC, Sohn MJ, Chang UK, Kim SH, Kim J, Park E. Stereotactic radiosurgery compared with external radiation therapy as a primary treatment in spine metastasis from renal cell carcinoma: a multicenter, matched-pair study. J Neuro-Oncol. 2014;119(1):121–8. 20140812 DCOM- 20151019. eng.
77. Chang UK, Cho WI, Lee DH, Kim MS, Cho CK, Lee SY, et al. Stereotactic radiosurgery for primary and metastatic sarcomas involving the spine. J Neuro-Oncol. 2012;107(3):551–7. PubMed PMID: 22246201. eng.
78. Maranzano E, Trippa F, Pacchiarini D, Chirico L, Basagni ML, Rossi R, et al. Re-irradiation of brain metastases and metastatic spinal cord compression: clinical practice suggestions. Tumori. 2005;91(4):325–30. PubMed PMID: 16277098. eng.
79. Nieder C, Grosu AL, Andratschke NH, Molls M. Update of human spinal cord reirradiation tolerance based on additional data from 38 patients. Int J Radiat Oncol Biol Phys. 2006;66(5):1446–9. PubMed PMID: 17084560.
80. Ryu S, Rock J, Rosenblum M, Kim JH. Patterns of failure after single-dose radiosurgery for spinal metastasis. J Neurosurg. 2004;101(Suppl 3) (0022–3085 (Print)):402–5. PubMed PMID: 15537196. eng.
81. Hamilton AJ, Lulu BA, Fosmire H, Stea B, Cassady JR. Preliminary clinical experience with linear accelerator-based spinal stereotactic radiosurgery. Neurosurgery. 1995;36(2):311–9. PubMed PMID: 7731511. eng.
82. Milker-Zabel S, Zabel A, Thilmann C, Schlegel W, Wannenmacher M, Debus J. Clinical results of retreatment of vertebral bone metastases by stereotactic conformal radiotherapy and intensity-modulated radiotherapy. Int J Radiat Oncol Biol Phys. 2003;55(1):162–7. PubMed PMID: 12504049. eng.
83. Mahan SL, Ramsey CR, Scaperoth DD, Chase DJ, Byrne TE. Evaluation of image-guided helical tomotherapy for the retreatment of spinal metastasis. Int J Radiat Oncol Biol Phys. 2005;63(5):1576–83. PubMed PMID: 16125871. eng.
84. Yamada Y, Lovelock DM, Yenice KM, Bilsky MH, Hunt MA, Zatcky J, et al. Multifractionated image-guided and stereotactic intensity-modulated radiotherapy of paraspinal tumors: a preliminary report. Int J Radiat Oncol Biol Phys. 2005;62(1):53–61. PubMed PMID: 15850902. eng.
85. Chang EL, Shiu AS, Mendel E, Mathews LA, Mahajan A, Allen PK, et al. Phase I/II study of stereotactic body radiotherapy for spinal metastasis and its pattern of failure. J Neurosurg Spine. 2007;7(2):151–60. PubMed PMID: 17688054. eng.
86. Gerszten PC, Burton SA, Ozhasoglu C, Welch WC. Radiosurgery for spinal metastases: clinical experience in 500 cases from a single institution. Spine. 2007;32(2):193–9. PubMed PMID: 17224814. eng.
87. Gibbs IC, Kamnerdsupaphon P, Ryu MR, Dodd R, Kiernan M, Chang SD, et al. Image-guided robotic radiosurgery for spinal metastases. Radiother Oncol. 2007;82(2):185–90. PubMed PMID: 17257702. eng.
88. Sahgal A, Chou D, Ames C, Ma L, Chuang C, Lambom K, et al. Proximity of spinous/paraspinous radiosurgery metastatic targets to the spinal cord versus risk of local failure. Int J Radiat Oncol. 2007;69(3):S243. PubMed PMID: WOS:000249950200431. English.
89. Wang XS, Rhines LD, Shiu AS, Yang JN, Selek U, Gning I, Liu P, Allen PK, Azeem SS, Brown PD, Sharp HJ, Weksberg DC, Cleeland CS, Chang EL. Stereotactic body radiation therapy for management of spinal metastases in patients without spinal cord compression: a phase 1–2 trial. Lancet Oncol. 2012;13(4):395–402. 20120403 DCOM- 20120622. eng.
90. Supe SS, Ganesh KM, Naveen T, Jacob S, Sankar BN. Spinal cord response to altered fractionation and re-irradiation: radiobiological considerations and role of bioeffect models. J Cancer Res Ther. 2006;2(3):105–18. PubMed PMID: 17998688. eng.
91. Gerszten PC, Germanwala A, Burton SA, Welch WC, Ozhasoglu C, Vogel WJ. Combination kyphoplasty and spinal radiosurgery: a new treatment paradigm for pathological fractures. J Neurosurg Spine. 2005;3(4):296–301. 20051103 DCOM- 20051115. eng.
92. Moulding HD, Elder JB, Lis E, Lovelock DM, Zhang Z, Yamada Y, et al. Local disease control after decompressive surgery and adjuvant high-dose single-fraction radiosurgery for spine metastases. J Neurosurg Spine. 2010;13(1):87–93. PubMed PMID: 20594023. eng.
93. Rock JP, Ryu S, Shukairy MS, Yin FF, Sharif A, Schreiber F, et al. Postoperative radiosurgery for malignant spinal tumors. Neurosurgery. 2006;58(5):891–8. discussion -8. PubMed PMID: 16639323. eng.
94. Ryu S, Pugh SL, Gerszten PC, Yin FF, Timmerman RD, Hitchcock YJ, et al. RTOG 0631 phase 2/3 study of image guided stereotactic radiosurgery for localized (1-3) spine metastases: phase 2 results. Pract Radiat Oncol. 2014;4(2):76–81. PubMed PMID: 24890347. Pubmed Central PMCID: 3711083.
95. Degen JW, Gagnon GJ, Voyadzis JM, McRae DA, Lunsden M, Dieterich S, et al. CyberKnife stereotactic radiosurgical treatment of spinal tumors for pain control and quality of life. J Neurosurg Spine. 2005;2(5):540–9. PubMed PMID: 15945428. eng.
96. Sahgal A, Chou D, Ames C, Ma L, Lamborn K, Huang K, et al. Image-guided robotic stereotactic body radiotherapy for benign spinal tumors: the University of California San Francisco preliminary experience. Technol Cancer Res Treat. 2007;6(6):595–604. PubMed PMID: 17994789. eng.
97. Pan HY, Allen PK, Wang XS, Chang EL, Rhines LD, Tatsui CE, et al. Incidence and predictive factors of pain flare after spine stereotactic body radiation therapy: secondary analysis of phase 1/2

trials. Int J Radiat Oncol Biol Phys. 2014;90(4):870–6. PubMed PMID: 25227497. Epub 2014/09/18. eng

98. Chiang A, Zeng L, Zhang L, Lochray F, Korol R, Loblaw A, et al. Pain flare is a common adverse event in steroid-naive patients after spine stereotactic body radiation therapy: a prospective clinical trial. Int J Radiat Oncol Biol Phys. 2013;86(4):638–42. PubMed PMID: 23664326. Epub 2013/05/15. eng.
99. Ryu S, Fang Yin F, Rock J, Zhu J, Chu A, Kagan E, et al. Image-guided and intensity-modulated radiosurgery for patients with spinal metastasis. Cancer. 2003;97(8):2013–8. PubMed PMID: 12673732. eng.
100. Rades D, Stalpers LJ, Veninga T, Hoskin PJ. Spinal reirradiation after short-course RT for metastatic spinal cord compression. Int J Radiat Oncol Biol Phys. 2005;63(3):872–5. PubMed PMID: 15939549. eng.
101. Hall WA, Stapleford LJ, Hadjipanayis CG, Curran WJ, Crocker I, Shu HK. Stereotactic body radiosurgery for spinal metastatic disease: an evidence-based review. Int J Surg Oncol. 2011 20120207 DCOM- 20120823;2011(2090–1410 (Electronic)):979214. PubMed PMID: 22312536. Pubmed Central PMCID: 3263656. eng.
102. Sahgal A, Whyne CM, Ma L, Larson DA, Fehlings MG. Vertebral compression fracture after stereotactic body radiotherapy for spinal metastases. Lancet Oncol. 2013;14(8):e310–20. PubMed PMID: 23816297. eng.
103. Rose PS, Laufer I, Boland PJ, Hanover A, Bilsky MH, Yamada J, et al. Risk of fracture after single fraction image-guided intensity-modulated radiation therapy to spinal metastases. J Clin Oncol. 2009;27(30):5075–9. PubMed PMID: 19738130. Pubmed Central PMCID: 3664037. eng.
104. Cunha MV, Al-Omair A, Atenafu EG, Masucci GL, Letourneau D, Korol R, et al. Vertebral compression fracture (VCF) after spine stereotactic body radiation therapy (SBRT): analysis of predictive factors. Int J Radiat Oncol Biol Phys. 2012;84(3):e343–9. PubMed PMID: 22658511. eng.
105. Boehling NS, Grosshans DR, Allen PK, McAleer MF, Burton AW, Azeem S, et al. Vertebral compression fracture risk after stereotactic body radiotherapy for spinal metastases. J Neurosurg Spine. 2012;16(4):379–86. PubMed PMID: 22225488. eng.
106. Thibault I, Al-Omair A, Masucci GL, Masson-Cote L, Lochray F, Korol R, et al. Spine stereotactic body radiotherapy for renal cell cancer spinal metastases: analysis of outcomes and risk of vertebral compression fracture. J Neurosurg Spine. 2014;21(5):711–8. PubMed PMID: 25170656. eng.
107. Lo SS, Lutz ST, Chang EL, Galanopoulos N, Howell DD, Kim EY, et al. ACR Appropriateness Criteria((R)) spinal bone metastases. J Palliat Med. 2013;16(1):9–19. PubMed PMID: 23167547. Epub 2012/11/22. eng.
108. Lutz S, Berk L, Chang E, Chow E, Hahn C, Hoskin P, et al. Palliative radiotherapy for bone metastases: an ASTRO evidence-based guideline. Int J Radiat Oncol Biol Phys. 2011;79(4):965–76. PubMed PMID: 21277118. Epub 2011/02/01. eng
109. Lutz ST, Lo SS, Chang EL, Galanopoulos N, Howell DD, Kim EY, et al. ACR appropriateness criteria(R) non-spine bone metastases. J Palliat Med. 2012;15(5):521–6. PubMed PMID: 22536988. Epub 2012/04/28. eng
110. NQF. #1822 External beam radiotherapy for bone metastasis. American Society for radiation oncology; Fairfax VA USA. 2012; pp. 1–23.
111. "Choosing Wisely" ABIM foundation; Philadelphia PA USA. 2014.

Non-opioid Intravenous Infusions for Management of Cancer-Associated Pain

39

Yury Khelemsky and Mourad M. Shehabar

Introduction

Cancer-associated pain, which results from the disease process or as sequelae of treatment, is often challenging to control and may not respond to standard analgesic regimens. Opioids are the cornerstone therapy for cancer pain in most patients; however, these medications may not always provide adequate pain control [1]. Administration of opioids may produce tolerance and hyperalgesia [2]. Furthermore, opioid therapy can lead to other untoward side effects such as sedation, myoclonus, respiratory depression, constipation, immunosuppression, and suppression of hypothalamo-pituitary axis [1]. In order to mitigate these effects, clinicians have implemented various techniques including opioid rotation, addition of adjuvant medications, as well as interventional procedures [3–5]. In this chapter we will discuss the utility of intravenous infusions of ketamine, lidocaine, bisphosphonates, and various radioisotopes as adjuncts in the management of malignancy-related pain.

Ketamine

Ketamine, a phencyclidine derivative, is a dissociative anesthetic that can be utilized in the operating room for both sedation and general anesthesia cases [6, 7]. Ketamine infusions are an excellent adjuvant in cases of chronic intractable cancer pain when there may be a narrowing therapeutic window between pain relief and side effects of opioids [8]. Administration of ketamine has been shown to reduce opioid requirements, as well as enhance the efficacy of the opioids administered [9]. Decreasing doses of opioids along with infusing ketamine may decrease cognitive impairment, which is highly prevalent in patients with advanced malignancy [8].

Y. Khelemsky (✉) · M. M. Shehabar
Icahn School of Medicine at Mount Sinai, Department of Anesthesiology, New York, NY, USA

Ketamine is a noncompetitive N-methyl-D-aspartate (NMDA) receptor antagonist, can bind to μ receptors enhancing opioid-induced conformations (not antagonized by naloxone), as well as an agonist at nicotinic and muscarinic receptors [8, 10–12]. Its action is thought to eliminate central sensitization via NMDA antagonism along with inhibiting primary and secondary hyperalgesia in response to repetitive nociceptive stimulation [13]. Ketamine's alpha half-life lasts just a few minutes, while the beta half-life is 2–3 h [10]. It is metabolized to norketamine (one third–one fifth as potent as ketamine) via the CYP3A4 cytochrome p450 enzyme in the liver, and thus its metabolism may be altered by substances inhibiting or inducing CYP3A4 [14, 15].

Ketamine may be used in both short- and long-term infusions. During short-term infusions, ketamine is administered for a duration of a few hours. During the longer infusions, ketamine is usually administered with other analgesics and eventually tapered off or in some cases continued until the end of a patient's life. When using ketamine alone, a wide range of infusion dosages are found in the literature with successful usage of infusions at 0.05 mg/kg/h–4.1 mg/kg/h from 1 to 350 days, with most studies not recommending more than 0.5 mg/kg/h as a starting dose [16]. In one pediatric case report of a patient with intractable pain from AML, ketamine 0.1 mg/kg was given as an intravenous bolus followed by an infusion at 0.1 mg/kg/hour. Titration of this infusion went up to as high as 1.7 mg/kg/hour as an outpatient providing this patient with adequate analgesia and meaningful time with his family [7]. In another case report, a patient with metastatic osteosarcoma was given 0.24 mg/kg/h ketamine bolus followed by an infusion of 0.05 mg/kg/h, which eventually was titrated to 0.14 mg/kg/h [7]. With clear instructions and oversight from the clinician, patients' families may adjust and titrate the ketamine dosages at home. In one retrospective study, 14 patients were infused with ketamine, midazolam, and fentanyl. When combined with fentanyl (5 μg/mL), midazolam (0.1 mg/mL), and ketamine (2 mg/mL), infusions

A. Gulati et al. (eds.), *Essentials of Interventional Cancer Pain Management*, https://doi.org/10.1007/978-3-319-99684-4_39

were set at 2 mL/h to 13 mL/h with some patients having the ability to bolus 3–4 mL/every 10 min via a PCA [8]. When encountering patients with refractory cancer-related pain in the intensive care unit, successful use has been shown with increasing doses of ketamine from 0.09 mg/kg/h to 0.65 mg/kg/h while simultaneously decreasing morphine over a 27-day period [10].

Overall, a slow bolus of ketamine at a loading dose of 0.1 mg/kg/h to 0.5 mg/kg/h has been demonstrated to be an effective starting point with titration according to symptoms followed by a low dose of 0.05 mg/kg/h to 0.1 mg/kg/h. Given that the beta elimination half-life of ketamine is 2–3 h, titration can take place two to three times daily [10]. Titrations up to 1.5 mg/kg/h usually correspond to a sufficient response. Maximum dosages range from 450 to 700 mg/day. Additionally, many pediatric patients have a standing dose of lorazepam 0.025 mg/kg every 12 h. In the adult population, lorazepam 1 mg prior to the start of the ketamine infusion followed by 1 mg every 6–8 h thereafter has been employed [1]. Premedication with a small dose of an anticholinergic (e.g., glycopyrrolate) may reduce salivation secondary to the ketamine.

With an onset occurring in less than 30 s after initiating ketamine infusions, it is important to continuously monitor heart rate, blood pressure, respiratory rate, and oxygen saturation levels [1]. Ketamine infusions have successfully been administered as an outpatient for greater than 30 days with side effects monitored by visiting healthcare professionals in conjunction with a pain clinician. This allows the patient to remain at home and maintain dignity at the end of life [7, 10].

Ketamine infusions for chronic cancer pain are usually subanesthetic, which correlates to tolerable side effect profile [10]. As it is associated with an increased sympathetic outflow, ketamine may cause hypertension and tachycardia. Ketamine possesses well-known side effects, including sedation, somnolence, sensory illusions/hallucinations, blurred vision/nystagmus, abdominal pain, nausea/vomiting, increased salivation, anorexia, and rarely hemorrhagic cystitis [10, 17]. With higher doses (above 2 mg/kg intravenous), panic attacks, impaired motor function, amnesia, and hypertension can occur [15]. Hallucinations tend to occur with more acute administration of ketamine (less than 4 days), but benzodiazepines can help mitigate these symptoms [18, 19]. It has been demonstrated that the administration of less than 150 μg/kg/hour and gradual titration of ketamine can both help prevent psychotomimetic effects in patients with advanced cancer [7, 20]. Although mild transaminitis can occur after 4 days of infusion, hepatic failure has been rarely noted in patients with underlying liver disease receiving ketamine [15, 21].

Ketamine when combined with midazolam and fentanyl infusions in patients with metastatic cancer has also been shown to exhibit qualitative improvement with pain control, functionality in environment, and cognitive agitation [8]. In the pediatric population, ketamine has been successfully utilized demonstrating better pain control with decreased opioid use in 73% of patients. Ketamine has been also thought to assist in major depressive symptoms, which can be concurrent with the underlying diagnosis of cancer [22, 23]. The response to ketamine has been shown to endure past the cessation of the infusion, with apparent effects lasting up to 8 weeks [24].

Lidocaine

Lidocaine was first introduced in 1948 and has been widely used since [25]. Intravenous lidocaine can be utilized for a number of different pain syndromes including nonmalignant (i.e., CRPS I and CRPS II, peripheral nervous system injury, neuralgia, thalamic pain, etc.), as well as malignant pain [25, 26]. With its quick onset, lidocaine infusions can alleviate severe rapidly progressing pain in patients with opioid-resistant malignancy-induced neuropathy [28]. These patients tend to be hospital bound due to their refractory pain [27, 28]. It is an especially effective therapeutic intervention for malignancy at end of life when the ability of the patient to interact with friends and family may be fundamental [25]. Prior to the conversion from high-dose opioids to intravenous lidocaine, patients may also be taking numerous medications to counteract opioid-induced side effects such as constipation and nausea, which can now be amended [25].

Both central and peripheral sensitization can play a role in malignant neuropathic pain with peripheral sensitization occurring by abnormal activation of sodium channels on damaged nerves [29]. At low concentrations, lidocaine can block these sodium channels while allowing normal neurotransmission [29]. Studies have shown that patients with pain emanating from dysfunctional dorsal roots, dorsal root ganglia, or peripheral nerves are more likely to respond to intravenous lidocaine than injuries from the central nervous system [25]. Lidocaine, with its anti-inflammatory and analgesic properties, has a pharmacological plasma half-life of 60–90 min [30, 31]. It has been shown to block nerve conduction, as it depresses both myelinated A-D and unmyelinated C fibers significantly along with decreasing heat-I capsaicin-induced secondary hyperalgesia via its central effect [32–34]. Additionally, lidocaine blocks the accumulation of inflammatory mediators including cytokines and neutrophils at the injury site [30, 35].

Although lidocaine infusion can be given perioperatively with success, long-term infusions for cancer pain are of growing interest. Lidocaine is usually infused over a short duration of time (hours), which can have lasting potential relief (weeks) or can be infused long term over days at a steady state for viable outpatient treatment [36]. The average starting infusion rate administered to adults by clinicians range from 1.5 to 5 mg/kg/h over 30 min–1 h, which can be converted to 25–83 μg/kg/min [37]. At this dose, the plasma level of lidocaine is about 1–3 μg/mL, which is the lower level of the antiarrhythmic range [25]. Few side effects were to be shown at this clinical scale [25]. Many clinicians use 1–3 mg/kg for an infusion over 20–30 min. Pain intensity tends to decrease significantly quite promptly, which will merit an initiation of an infusion 1–3 mg/kg/hour that can be titrated to effect over hours to days.

The dosing of lidocaine infusion in the pediatric population has not been well-established with one study reporting successful titrating dose of 35–63 μg/kg/min [25]. In another case report, lidocaine infusion (when combined with ketamine) at slightly lower rate of 9.3–14 μg/kg/min for 45 days was successfully utilized in a 5-year-old with intractable pain secondary to malignant T-cell lymphoma [28]. Of note, methadone at 0.3 mg/kg/h with bolus doses of 0.6 mg/kg every 15 min has been shown to be helpful in preventing opioid withdrawal while converting to a lidocaine infusion from a high-dose opioid regimen [25].

Although there is potential for systemic local anesthetic toxicity (LAST) with infusion of lidocaine, it does not appear to be a significant issue when employing average infusion dosages [38, 39]. Some case reports have shown patients experiencing perioral numbness (an early sign of LAST) and tinnitus, which were self-resolving after termination of the infusion [31]. Sedation or drowsiness was noted in one study to be the most common side effect [31]. Side effects tend to be dose-dependent with higher infusions (greater than 3 mg/kg/min) and lidocaine toxicity at plasma concentration of greater than 5 μg/mL, which usually correlates with complaints of light-headedness, perioral numbness, or dizziness. Plasma levels of greater than 8 μg/mL may result in auditory or visual hallucinations, hypotension, and muscle twitching. With a lidocaine plasma level of 12 μg/mL, convulsions may occur; in 16 μg/mL, coma may develop; and finally above 20 μg/mL, respiratory or cardiovascular collapse can take place [40]. Tricyclic antidepressants should be stopped for at least 48 h prior to the infusion to minimize the risk of arrhythmias. Patients who have a history of cardiac dysfunction may warrant a proper cardiac evaluation prior to initiating a local anesthetic infusion. Rapid boluses rather than steady-state infusions can also lead to mild to moderate side effects [25]. Vigilance and close patient observation is important factors whenever infusing lidocaine.

Baseline laboratory work, which may include electrolytes, liver function tests, as well as an ECG, should be done prior to initiating the lidocaine infusion. Neurologic and cardiovascular monitoring with a three-lead ECG, pulse oximeter, noninvasive blood pressure, and respiratory rate every 10 min should be employed during inpatient lidocaine infusions [25, 31]. Intravenous alcohol (ETOH 5% IV solution 2 mL/hr) can be made available to counteract any neurological symptoms as an inpatient by its sedative effect via inhibiting the neuronal excitability and heart rate, while clonazepam 0.25 mg twice daily can alleviate those symptoms as an outpatient [25]. Close interaction with healthcare personnel is recommended when outpatient lidocaine is implemented [25]. Although there is no need to obtain lidocaine levels during an infusion, if there is concern for toxicity, it may be warranted with levels drawn 8–12 h after the initiation of infusion or a dosing change. Since lidocaine is metabolized in the liver, toxicity can be seen in patients with comprised hepatic function [25]. Doses should be reduced by 50% in patients with liver disease or heart failure.

A phase II randomized, double-blind, placebo-controlled, crossover study of intravenous lidocaine in opioid-refractory cancer pain illustrated statistically significant pain relief with decrease in analgesic requirements with a 2 mg/kg bolus followed by 2 mg/kg infusion for 1 h [31]. Pain relief with lidocaine infusion had an earlier onset and longer duration compared to placebo. An average duration of pain relief was 9.34 days well beyond the period of infusion of just 80 min, thus demonstrating potential relief beyond the plasma half-life and time of administration [31].

In another randomized control study, the lidocaine group had statistically significant less pain during movement, restoring bowel function status post-abdominal surgery and reducing hospital length of stay when comparing to the placebo group [38]. When dealing with patients exhibiting refractory neuropathic cancer pain, lidocaine is an excellent adjuvant to assist in reducing the unwanted side effects of increasing opioid requirements along with postoperative analgesic consumption [28, 37]. Studies have demonstrated patients' overall mental status and appetite improving with intravenous lidocaine infusion when comparing to opioid alone [25]. Overall, lidocaine is an excellent adjuvant for treating cancer-related neuropathic pain.

Bisphosphonates

Bisphosphonates, or bone-modifying agents, are selective inhibitors of osteoclastic bone resorption and have been successfully used in Paget's disease, primary hyperparathyroidism, myelomatosis, tumor-induced hypercalcemia, and skeletal metastasis from both osteolytic lesions as well as solid tumors [41]. Metastatic bone disease and resulting pain are common in patients with breast, prostate, and lung cancer, thus creating an important quality-of-life issue [42, 43]. This type of pain can be intermittent and progressive emanating from structural damage, nerve entrapment, or periosteal damage [43].

Each generation of bisphosphonates has increased potency and efficacy over the previous one. Zoledronic acid has a broader indication and is a newer and highly potent nitrogen-containing bisphosphonate. It has been successfully utilized for bone pain and is 100–850 more times as potent as pamidronate, thus being a preferable choice for clinicians [43, 44]. Although pamidronate, a second-generation bisphosphonate, is eliminated exclusively by renal excretion, patients with renal comorbidities do not require a decreased dose as the infusions are separated by weeks [45]. In two rat models, zoledronic has been shown to be less nephrotoxic than pamidronate, but pamidronate should still be infused slower to minimize potential nephrotoxicity [46, 47]. Creatinine should be monitored prior to either zoledronic or pamidronate infusions as both medications should be held upon evidence of renal insufficiency (i.e., creatinine >3.0 mg/dL or 265 μmol/L) [48, 49]. After rapid intravenous administration, 40–50% of ibandronate, a third-generation bisphosphonate similar to zoledronic acid, will bind rapidly to the bone with the remaining being eliminated unchanged via urine and feces [50].

Zoledronic acid 4 mg can be administered every 3–4 weeks over 15 min intravenously, whereas pamidronate infusion 90 mg is over 2–4 h every 3–4 weeks for at least two to three treatments, thus allowing more convenience for an outpatient with zoledronic acid [43, 47]. Ibandronate 6 mg has been successfully infused monthly and can be given as a bolus over a few minutes with no need to monitor for creatinine as it does not possess the same renal toxicity of the other bisphosphonates therefore making it even more suitable for outpatients [51–53]. There is no need for tapering bisphosphonates as they can be stopped at any time.

Often during the time period patients are receiving bisphosphonates, supplemental calcium 500 mg and vitamin D 1000–2000 IU will be given daily [43]. Serum creatinine, hematocrit/hemoglobin, calcium, magnesium, phosphate, and electrolytes should also be monitored when receiving bisphosphonate infusions on a regular basis [54]. Urinary bone resorption markers (NTX, PYD, DPYD) tend to decrease upon administration of bisphosphonates and can be used a prognostic factor [47, 54].

Although occurring less than 2% of the time, acute systemic inflammatory reaction, ocular inflammation, renal failure, osteonecrosis of the jaw, and hypocalcemia have all been reported as adverse reactions after the administration of bisphosphonates [55]. Although reported as an uncommon occurrence, risk factors for osteonecrosis of the jaw include dental extraction, local infection or trauma, and systemic chemotherapy [56]. As mentioned previously, renal toxicity occurs more frequently via rapid infusions of pamidronate. More common side effects include skeletal pain, nausea, headaches, fatigue, upper respiratory infections, constipation, and occasional fever [47].

When treating osteoblastic skeletal metastasis in prostate carcinoma, bisphosphonate infusion decreased bone pain within 3 days as well as reduced hypercalcemia by up to 67% [41, 57]. Zoledronic acid has been shown to significantly decrease pain on movement and at rest from baseline, reduced skeletal-related events by 20%, as well as increase quality of life and survival when compared to pamidronate [58–61]. Ibandronate and other bisphosphonates exhibit antitumor activity by reducing tumor spread and invasion while preventing bone metastasis [53]. Increasing bone mass and density, preserved bone strength, and maintained bone quality are all features of bisphosphonates [62]. Multiple myeloma patients who received 90 mg of pamidronate over a 4 h infusion every 4 weeks for nine cycles had significantly decreased skeletal pain, prolonged time until first skeletal fracture, and reduction in skeletal fractures when compared to placebo [63, 64]. High doses of ibandronate 4 mg for four consecutive days have been shown to be effective in opioid-resistant bone pain [65]. Overall, with bisphosphonate infusions, patients had a better quality of life, pain score and performance status, decreased incidence of fractures by approximately 25–50%, and decreased need for skeletal radiotherapy by 50% [57, 63, 66]. Additionally, bisphosphonates have been successfully utilized for up to 24 months in breast, lung, and other solid tumor patients [67, 68]. Furthermore, bisphosphonates has potential on decreasing the financial burden of tumor bone disease and can successfully be implemented as a home infusion with the appropriate supportive care [57, 61, 69].

Strontium

Strontium-89, a radioisotope, is an alternative to hemibody irradiation without the negative side effects such as nausea, mucositis, desquamation, and pneumonitis [70]. It has been shown to be effective for pain emanating from bony metastasis [70].

Strontium-89 is an electron-emitting radioisotope with a half-life of about 50 days [71]. Similar to the composition of calcium, strontium-89 is treated similarly by being incorporated into growing bone by osteoblasts [70]. Given that it has "bone-seeking" capabilities, strontium-89 will emit beta radiation locally (6–7 millimeters in local tissue and 3–4 millimeters in bone), thus being even more effective than calcium [72–74]. Patients with disseminated and painful skeletal metastasis are ideal candidates for this therapy [70]. Although plasma clearance can be variable (1–11 liters/day), total body retention after 90 days is about 20% [73].

The usual infusion dose of strontium-89 is 40–60 microCi (mCi) per kilogram of body weight or 1.5–2.2 MBq/kg as a single infusion over 1–2 min [70]. With pain occasionally increasing within the first 36 h, patients are encouraged to continue taking their analgesic medications [70]. This "flare" tends to have a positive prognostic indication that the patient will respond to the radioisotope [75]. It is recommended to continue strontium-89 infusions, if effective, but not to redose within 90 days.

Although there may be an insignificant decrease in platelets and leukocytes, acute side effects such as flushing are rare and can usually be avoided with slower injection time [70]. Caution is advised in patients with the presence of critical metastasis with spinal cord compression as strontium-89 may cause edema at these sites. The radioisotope may cause contamination in patients with urinary incontinence as it is excreted via urine. As the radiation is absorbed locally, there is no radiation risk for family members who are in close quarters with the patients; thus they can be educated about the lack of side effects which usually occur with radiation therapy [70].

Strontium-89 has been shown to relieve pain in over 70% of patients with prostate bone metastasis [76]. When comparing strontium-89 and samarium-153 combined with intravenous bisphosphonates versus bisphosphonates alone in patients with metastatic breast cancer, patients in the former group tend to have more effective therapy with greater pain relief by means of 30% decrease in pain medications [77]. Pain relief usually begins within 1–3 weeks after the intravenous infusion with maximum pain relief after 6 weeks with mean duration of 12 months [70]. The time frame should be thought about prior to initiating therapy as an actively dying patient may be better suited for traditional treatment modalities [70].

Newer radioisotopes such as 186Re-HEDP have been shown to be effective in alleviating bone pain secondary to metastasis [78]. In one study, 40–90-mCi of 186Re-HEDP was infused over 10 min with complete blood counts, analgesic intake, and visual analog scale recorded weekly. Over 78% of patients reported pain relief with a common adverse reaction of thrombocytopenia and leukopenia occurring [78]. Samarium-153, another radiopharmaceutical, has a shorter half-life of 1.9 days and lower incidence of severe myelosuppression when compared to strontium-89 [79].

Radium-223

Skeletal metastasis has been widely treated with external radiotherapy but may be limited secondary to its lack of selectivity. Normal cells are often being targeted along with cancerous cells leading to potential bone marrow suppression. A targeted radionuclide therapy would be beneficial in preferential destruction [80].

Radium-223 (*223Ra*), an isotope of radium, is a radiopharmaceutical known to treat metastatic cancer in bone [80]. It has been approved by the FDA for castration-resistant prostate cancer with symptomatic bone metastasis (up to 90% of patients) and no known visceral metastatic disease [81, 82]. Unlike other malignancies, death from prostate cancer is usually due to bone disease and its complications [83]. *223Ra* has also been recently shown to be effective in hormone-resistant breast cancer with metastasis to the bone (up to 80% of patients) [84].

223Ra has a similar structure to calcium allowing it to target and bind to areas of high bone turnover (i.e., sites of bone metastases or osteoblast activity) [81]. *223Ra* emits short-range (<100 micrometers), high-energy α-particles to produce a local cytotoxic effect by breaking double-stranded DNA in the target area [80, 81]. The α-particles carefully minimize damage to surrounding healthy tissue and bone marrow (allowing decreased myelosuppression) [85].

Following intravenous injection, *223Ra* is rapidly cleared from the blood; within 15 min, 80% radioactivity is removed; by 4 h, 2–4% remains in the blood; by 24 h, <1% of injected radioactivity remains in blood [86]. At 4 h after injection, 60% of the radioactivity remains in the bone and is retained there [86].

223Ra has an 11.4-day half-life and is not metabolized within the body, thus reducing interactions with other drugs [81]. 96% of the decay is emitted as α-particles with the excretion primarily in feces [80].

223Ra is distributed as a single-use solution of 6 mL, which contains radium-223 chloride (1000 kBq/mL = 27microcurie/mL) and sodium chloride for intravenous injection. The recommended regimen is six treatments of 50 kBq/kg (1.3 uCi per kg), repeated at 4-week intervals [81]. The intravenous injection should be administered over 1 min. In a phase I study, dosing of 46–250 kBq/kg has been utilized with well-tolerated, favorable effects, and no dose-limiting toxicity was noted [87].

Hematologic evaluations should be performed at baseline and prior to every injection. Before the first administration, the recommended absolute neutrophil count should be ≥1.5 × 109/L, platelet count ≥100 × 109/L, and hemoglobin ≥10 g/dL. Before subsequent administrations, the absolute neutrophil count should be ≥1 × 109/L and platelet count ≥50 × 109/L. Although reversible myelosuppression can occur with a nadir of 2–4 weeks, if counts do not recover to previous stated values after 6–8 weeks, treatment should be discontinued [88].

Patients are instructed to be well-hydrated and follow good hygiene skills, which includes flushing the toilet numerous times after usage within 1 week of injection, promptly washing soiled clothing separately, and using birth control and condoms for up to 6 months status post last injection [88]. *223Ra* cannot be given during chemotherapy and is contraindicated in patients with visceral *metastasis.*

223Ra has a low gamma-irradiation, which is favorable with handling and ensuring radiation protection [80]. When comparing *223Ra* vs. placebo, it exhibited less or no serious adverse reactions. [82] As *223Ra* has been shown to minimize any drop in hematologic parameters, it can be safely combined with other radiosensitizing therapies [84]. In a larger trial with 600 patients, the most frequent reported side effects (occurring in about 10% of patients) were mild and included nausea, vomiting, diarrhea, and peripheral edema [87].

In a phase II trial, *223Ra* demonstrated to reduce pain associated with bone metastasis and improve disease-related biomarkers such as bone alkaline phosphatase and prostate-specific antigen (PSA) [89]. A phase III, randomized, double-blind, multinational, placebo-controlled study of 921 men with castration-resistant prostate cancer with more than 2 bone metastases but no visceral metastasis was conducted. With receiving *223Ra* or placebo every 4 weeks for 6 injections, there was over a 30% reduction of death in the *223Ra* group, demonstrating *223Ra* to be statistically significant in overall survival (14.9 vs. 11.3 months) and effectively terminating this study early [82]. In the same study, *223Ra* also significantly prolonged the time to first skeletal event (15.6 vs. 9.8 months), the time to increase for alkaline phosphatase (7.4 vs. 3.8 months), and time to increase for PSA (3.6 vs. 3.4 months) when compared to placebo [81]. More importantly, 16 and 24 weeks after the initiation of *223Ra*, patients were shown to have significantly less pain than the placebo group [82].

A phase IIa trial involving 23 advanced breast cancer patients with metastasis to the bone has recently been conducted with *223Ra* injections being supplied every 4 weeks for 4 cycles [90]. This study showed a consistent decrease in urinary N-telopeptide of type 1 (uNTX-1) and serum bone alkaline phosphatase during the 16-week treatment period. Most adverse reactions were mild (grade 1 or 2) and self-limiting. A Brief Pain Inventory (BPI) was filled out at the end of the treatment and again at the 6-, 9-, and 12-month follow-up visits and showed a steady reduction in pain scores [90].

In one study utilizing wide ranges of dosages, *223Ra* demonstrated pain relief 52–60% of patients at 1–8 weeks, with no definite dose-response relationship [87]. In a similar study, there was mean pain relief duration of 44 days following injection of 50–100 kBq/kg [87]. When comparing changes in Functional Assessment Scale scores, *223Ra* improved quality of life especially with pain, which in turn led to improved social, familial, physical, and emotional well-being of patients [91].

223Ra has been shown to be a safe and effective treatment for bone metastasis in castration-resistant prostate cancer and began to show efficacy in breast cancer metastasis to the bone. *223Ra* is helpful in pain control and more significantly in decreasing skeletal-related events and increasing survival [87].

Denosumab

Denosumab is a newer human monoclonal antibody RANKL inhibitor which helps prevent the development of osteoclasts which are involved in bone destruction [92]. The dosing is 120 mg subcutaneously every 4 weeks with a mean elimination half-life of 28 days. It has also gained wide use for treatment of bone metastases, and a recent systematic review has shown a favorable significant impact on delaying the time to first skeletal-related event when compared to bisphosphonates [92].

Conclusion

Non-opioid intravenous infusions for management of cancer-associated pain can provide significant analgesia while decreasing opioid requirements. Minimization of opioid dosing leads to a decrease in opioid-related side effects such as constipation, sedation, nausea, pruritus, and respiratory depression, among others. This can significantly improve a patient's quality of life. As newer radioisotope infusions are developed by relying on preferential targeting of malignant cells while decreasing destruction of the surrounding healthy tissue, there is significant potential for further advancement in non-opioid infusions in the near future.

References

1. Finkel JC, Pestieau SR, Quezado ZM. Ketamine as an adjuvant for treatment of cancer pain in children and adolescents. J Pain. 2007;8:515–21.
2. Angst MS, Clark JD. Opioid-induced hyperalgesia: a qualitative systematic review. Anesthesiology. 2006;104:570–87.
3. Drake R, Longworth J, Collins JJ. Opioid rotation in children with cancer. J Palliat Med. 2004;7:419–22.
4. Shinde S, Gordon P, Sharma P, Gross J, Davis MP. Use of non-opioid analgesics as adjuvants to opioid analgesia for cancer pain management in an inpatient palliative unit: does this improve pain control and reduce opioid requirements? Support Care Cancer. 2014;23(3):695–703.
5. Eidelman A, White T, Swarm RA. Interventional therapies for cancer pain management: important adjuvants to systemic analgesics. J Natl Compr Canc Netw. 2007;5:753–60.
6. Reich DL, Silvay G. Ketamine: an update on the first twenty-five years of clinical experience. Can J Anaesth. 1989;36:186–97.
7. Conway M, White N, Jean CS, Zempsky WT, Steven K. Use of continuous intravenous ketamine for end-stage cancer pain in children. J Pediatr Oncol Nurs. 2009;26:100–6.
8. Berger JM, Ryan A, Vadivelu N, Merriam P, Rever L, Harrison P. Ketamine-fentanyl-midazolam infusion for the control of symptoms in terminal life care. Am J Hosp Palliat Care. 2000;17:127–34.
9. Clark JL, Kalan GE. Effective treatment of severe cancer pain of the head using low-dose ketamine in an opioid-tolerant patient. J Pain Symptom Manag. 1995;10:310–4.
10. Chung WJ, Pharo GH. Successful use of ketamine infusion in the treatment of intractable cancer pain in an outpatient. J Pain Symptom Manag. 2007;33:2–5.

11. Romero TR, Galdino GS, Silva GC, et al. Ketamine activates the L-arginine/Nitric oxide/cyclic guanosine monophosphate pathway to induce peripheral antinociception in rats. Anesth Analg. 2011;113:1254–9.
12. Gupta A, Devi LA, Gomes I. Potentiation of μ-opioid receptor-mediated signaling by ketamine. J Neurochem. 2011;119:294–302.
13. Arendt-Nielsen L, Mansikka H, Staahl C, et al. A translational study of the effects of ketamine and pregabalin on temporal summation of experimental pain. Reg Anesth Pain Med. 2011;36:585–91.
14. Hagelberg NM, Peltoniemi MA, Saari TI, et al. Clarithromycin, a potent inhibitor of CYP3A, greatly increases exposure to oral S-ketamine. Eur J Pain. 2010;14:625–9.
15. Bell RF. Ketamine for chronic non-cancer pain. Pain. 2009;141:210–4.
16. Bredlau AL, Thakur R, Korones DN, Dworkin RH. Ketamine for pain in adults and children with cancer: a systematic review and synthesis of the literature. Pain Med. 2013;14:1505–17.
17. Hardy J, Quinn S, Fazekas B, et al. Randomized, double-blind, placebo-controlled study to assess the efficacy and toxicity of subcutaneous ketamine in the management of cancer pain. J Clin Oncol. 2012;30:3611–7.
18. Bell RF, Eccleston C, Kalso E. Ketamine as adjuvant to opioids for cancer pain. A qualitative systematic review. J Pain Symptom Manag. 2003;26:867–75.
19. Gilliland HE, Prasad BK, Mirakhur RK, Fee JP. An investigation of the potential morphine sparing effect of midazolam. Anaesthesia. 1996;51:808–11.
20. Okamoto Y, Tsuneto S, Tanimukai H, et al. Can gradual dose titration of ketamine for management of neuropathic pain prevent psychotomimetic effects in patients with advanced cancer? Am J Hosp Palliat Care. 2013;30:450–4.
21. Noppers I, Niesters M, Aarts L, Smith T, Sarton E, Dahan A. Ketamine for the treatment of chronic non-cancer pain. Expert Opin Pharmacother. 2010;11:2417–29.
22. Cortiñas-Saenz M, Alonso-Menoyo MB, Errando-Oyonarte CL, Alférez-García I, Carricondo-Martínez MA. Effect of subanaesthetic doses of ketamine in the postoperative period in a patient with uncontrolled depression. Rev Esp Anestesiol Reanim. 2013;60:110–3.
23. Larkin GL, Beautrais AL. A preliminary naturalistic study of low-dose ketamine for depression and suicide ideation in the emergency department. Int J Neuropsychopharmacol. 2011;14:1127–31.
24. Jackson K, Ashby M, Martin P, Pisasale M, Brumley D, Hayes B. "Burst" ketamine for refractory cancer pain: an open-label audit of 39 patients. J Pain Symptom Manag. 2001;22:834–42.
25. Massey GV, Pedigo S, Dunn NL, Grossman NJ, Russell EC. Continuous lidocaine infusion for the relief of refractory malignant pain in a terminally ill pediatric cancer patient. J Pediatr Hematol Oncol. 2002;24:566–8.
26. Nagaro T, Shimizu C, Inoue H, et al. The efficacy of intravenous lidocaine on various types of neuropathic pain. Masui. 1995;44:862–7.
27. Ferrante FM, Paggioli J, Cherukuri S, Arthur GR. The analgesic response to intravenous lidocaine in the treatment of neuropathic pain. Anesth Analg. 1996;82:91–7.
28. Kajiume T, Sera Y, Nakanuno R, et al. Continuous intravenous infusion of ketamine and lidocaine as adjuvant analgesics in a 5-year-old patient with neuropathic cancer pain. J Palliat Med. 2012;15:719–22.
29. Baron R. Mechanisms of disease: neuropathic pain—a clinical perspective. Nat Clin Pract Neurol. 2006;2:95–106.
30. Hollmann MW, Durieux ME. Local anesthetics and the inflammatory response: a new therapeutic indication? Anesthesiology. 2000;93:858–75.
31. Sharma S, Rajagopal MR, Palat G, Singh C, Haji AG, Jain D. A phase II pilot study to evaluate use of intravenous lidocaine for opioid-refractory pain in cancer patients. J Pain Symptom Manag. 2009;37:85–93.
32. Groudine SB, Fisher HA, Kaufman RP, et al. Intravenous lidocaine speeds the return of bowel function, decreases postoperative pain, and shortens hospital stay in patients undergoing radical retropubic prostatectomy. Anesth Analg. 1998;86:235–9.
33. Rimbäck G, Cassuto J, Tollesson PO. Treatment of postoperative paralytic ileus by intravenous lidocaine infusion. Anesth Analg. 1990;70:414–9.
34. Dirks J, Fabricius P, Petersen KL, Rowbotham MC, Dahl JB. The effect of systemic lidocaine on pain and secondary hyperalgesia associated with the heat/capsaicin sensitization model in healthy volunteers. Anesth Analg. 2000;91:967–72.
35. Kuo CP, Jao SW, Chen KM, et al. Comparison of the effects of thoracic epidural analgesia and i.v. infusion with lidocaine on cytokine response, postoperative pain and bowel function in patients undergoing colonic surgery. Br J Anaesth. 2006;97:640–6.
36. McCleane G. Intravenous lidocaine: an outdated or underutilized treatment for pain? J Palliat Med. 2007;10:798–805.
37. Koppert W, Weigand M, Neumann F, et al. Perioperative intravenous lidocaine has preventive effects on postoperative pain and morphine consumption after major abdominal surgery. Anesth Analg. 2004;98:1050–5. table of contents.
38. Tikuisis R, Miliauskas P, Samalavicius NE, Zurauskas A, Samalavicius R, Zabulis V. Intravenous lidocaine for post-operative pain relief after hand-assisted laparoscopic colon surgery: a randomized, placebo-controlled clinical trial. Tech Coloproctol. 2014;18:373–80.
39. Kang JG, Kim MH, Kim EH, Lee SH. Intraoperative intravenous lidocaine reduces hospital length of stay following open gastrectomy for stomach cancer in men. J Clin Anesth. 2012;24:465–70.
40. Ferrini R, Paice JA. How to initiate and monitor infusional lidocaine for severe and/or neuropathic pain. J Support Oncol. 2004;2:90–4.
41. Adami S. Bisphosphonates in prostate carcinoma. Cancer. 1997;80:1674–9.
42. Rubens RD. Bone metastases—the clinical problem. Eur J Cancer. 1998;34:210–3.
43. Addeo R, Nocera V, Faiola V, et al. Management of pain in elderly patients receiving infusion of zoledronic acid for bone metastasis: a single-institution report. Support Care Cancer. 2008;16:209–14.
44. Green JR, Müller K, Jaeggi KA. Preclinical pharmacology of CGP 42′446, a new, potent, heterocyclic bisphosphonate compound. J Bone Miner Res. 1994;9:745–51.
45. Berenson JR, Rosen L, Vescio R, et al. Pharmacokinetics of pamidronate disodium in patients with cancer with normal or impaired renal function. J Clin Pharmacol. 1997;37:285–90.
46. Green JR, Seltenmeyer Y, Jaeggi KA, Widler L. Renal tolerability profile of novel, potent bisphosphonates in two short-term rat models. Pharmacol Toxicol. 1997;80:225–30.
47. Berenson JR, Vescio RA, Rosen LS, et al. A phase I dose-ranging trial of monthly infusions of zoledronic acid for the treatment of osteolytic bone metastases. Clin Cancer Res. 2001;7:478–85.
48. Body JJ. Breast cancer: bisphosphonate therapy for metastatic bone disease. Clin Cancer Res. 2006;12:6258s–63s.
49. Van Poznak CH, Temin S, Yee GC, et al. American Society of Clinical Oncology executive summary of the clinical practice guideline update on the role of bone-modifying agents in metastatic breast cancer. J Clin Oncol. 2011;29:1221–7.
50. Pecherstorfer M. Managing neoplastic bone disease with ibandronic acid: a preclinical and clinical data update. Expert Opin Pharmacother. 2008;9:3111–9.
51. Body JJ, Mancini I. Bisphosphonates for cancer patients: why, how, and when? Support Care Cancer. 2002;10:399–407.
52. Cameron D. Patient management issues in metastatic bone disease. Semin Oncol. 2004;31:79–82.

53. Guay DR. Ibandronate, an experimental intravenous bisphosphonate for osteoporosis, bone metastases, and hypercalcemia of malignancy. Pharmacotherapy. 2006;26:655–73.
54. Hillner BE, Ingle JN, Chlebowski RT, et al. American Society of Clinical Oncology 2003 update on the role of bisphosphonates and bone health issues in women with breast cancer. J Clin Oncol. 2003;21:4042–57.
55. Tanvetyanon T, Stiff PJ. Management of the adverse effects associated with intravenous bisphosphonates. Ann Oncol. 2006;17:897–907.
56. Migliorati CA, Schubert MM, Peterson DE, Seneda LM. Bisphosphonate-associated osteonecrosis of mandibular and maxillary bone: an emerging oral complication of supportive cancer therapy. Cancer. 2005;104:83–93.
57. Body JJ. Effectiveness and cost of bisphosphonate therapy in tumor bone disease. Cancer. 2003;97:859–65.
58. Cartenì G, Bordonaro R, Giotta F, et al. Efficacy and safety of zoledronic acid in patients with breast cancer metastatic to bone: a multicenter clinical trial. Oncologist. 2006;11:841–8.
59. Drudge-Coates L. Improving management of patients with advanced cancer. Patient Prefer Adher. 2010;4:415–24.
60. Ripamonti C, Fagnoni E, Campa T, et al. Decreases in pain at rest and movement-related pain during zoledronic acid treatment in patients with bone metastases due to breast or prostate cancer: a pilot study. Support Care Cancer. 2007;15:1177–84.
61. Wardley A, Davidson N, Barrett-Lee P, et al. Zoledronic acid significantly improves pain scores and quality of life in breast cancer patients with bone metastases: a randomised, crossover study of community vs hospital bisphosphonate administration. Br J Cancer. 2005;92:1869–76.
62. Bauss F, Russell RG. Ibandronate in osteoporosis: preclinical data and rationale for intermittent dosing. Osteoporos Int. 2004;15:423–33.
63. Berenson JR, Lichtenstein A, Porter L, et al. Efficacy of pamidronate in reducing skeletal events in patients with advanced multiple myeloma. Myeloma Aredia Study Group. N Engl J Med. 1996;334:488–93.
64. Coleman RE. Efficacy of zoledronic acid and pamidronate in breast cancer patients: a comparative analysis of randomized phase III trials. Am J Clin Oncol. 2002;25:S25–31.
65. Mancini I, Dumon JC, Body JJ. Efficacy and safety of ibandronate in the treatment of opioid-resistant bone pain associated with metastatic bone disease: a pilot study. J Clin Oncol. 2004;22:3587–92.
66. Body JJ, Bartl R, Burckhardt P, et al. Current use of bisphosphonates in oncology. International Bone and Cancer Study Group. J Clin Oncol. 1998;16:3890–9.
67. Lipton A, Theriault RL, Hortobagyi GN, et al. Pamidronate prevents skeletal complications and is effective palliative treatment in women with breast carcinoma and osteolytic bone metastases: long term follow-up of two randomized, placebo-controlled trials. Cancer. 2000;88:1082–90.
68. Rosen LS, Gordon D, Tchekmedyian NS, et al. Long-term efficacy and safety of zoledronic acid in the treatment of skeletal metastases in patients with nonsmall cell lung carcinoma and other solid tumors: a randomized, Phase III, double-blind, placebo-controlled trial. Cancer. 2004;100:2613–21.
69. Italiano A, Ciais C, Chamorey E, et al. Home infusions of biphosphonate in cancer patients: a prospective study. J Chemother. 2006;18:217–20.
70. Baumrucker S. Palliation of painful bone metastases: Strontium-89. Am J Hosp Palliat Care. 1998;15:113–5.
71. Mertens WC, Stitt L, Porter AT. Strontium 89 therapy and relief of pain in patients with prostatic carcinoma metastatic to bone: a dose response relationship? Am J Clin Oncol. 1993;16:238–42.
72. Mertens WC, Porter AT, Reid RH, Powe JE. Strontium-89 and low-dose infusion cisplatin for patients with hormone refractory prostate carcinoma metastatic to bone: a preliminary report. J Nucl Med. 1992;33:1437–43.
73. Zenda S, Nakagami Y, Toshima M, et al. Strontium-89 (Sr-89) chloride in the treatment of various cancer patients with multiple bone metastases. Int J Clin Oncol. 2013;19(4):739–43.
74. Taylor AJ. Strontium-89 for the palliation of bone pain due to metastatic disease. J Nucl Med. 1994;35:2054.
75. Hansen DV, Holmes ER, Catton G, Thorne DA, Chadwick DH, Schmutz DA. Strontium-89 therapy for painful osseous metastatic prostate and breast cancer. Am Fam Physician. 1993;47:1795–800.
76. Second-line treatment of metastatic prostate cancer. Prednisone and radiotherapy for symptom relief. Prescrire Int. 2013;22:74–8.
77. Baczyk M, Baczyk E, Sowiński J. Preliminary results of combined application of radioisotopes and biphosphonates in the management of pain associated with osteoblastic-osteolytic bone metastases of breast cancer. Ortop Traumatol Rehabil. 2003;5:234–7.
78. Pirayesh E, Amoui M, Mirzaee HR, et al. Phase 2 study of a high dose of 186Re-HEDP for bone pain palliation in patients with widespread skeletal metastases. J Nucl Med Technol. 2013;41:192–6.
79. Serafini AN. Samarium Sm-153 lexidronam for the palliation of bone pain associated with metastases. Cancer. 2000;88:2934–9.
80. Henriksen G, Fisher DR, Roeske JC, Bruland Ø, Larsen RH. Targeting of osseous sites with alpha-emitting 223Ra: comparison with the beta-emitter 89Sr in mice. J Nucl Med. 2003;44:252–9.
81. Radium – 223 (Xofigo) for prostate cancer. Med Lett Drugs Ther. 2013;55:79–80.
82. Parker C, Nilsson S, Heinrich D, et al. Alpha emitter radium-223 and survival in metastatic prostate cancer. N Engl J Med. 2013;369:213–23.
83. Lange PH, Vessella RL. Mechanisms, hypotheses and questions regarding prostate cancer micrometastases to bone. Cancer Metastasis Rev. 1998;17:331–6.
84. Takalkar A, Adams S, Subbiah V. Radium-223 dichloride bone-targeted alpha particle therapy for hormone-refractory breast cancer metastatic to bone. Exp Hematol Oncol. 2014;3:23.
85. Kerr C. (223)Ra targets skeletal metastases and spares normal tissue. Lancet Oncol. 2002;3:453.
86. Shirley M, McCormack PL. Radium-223 dichloride: a review of its use in patients with castration-resistant prostate cancer with symptomatic bone metastases. Drugs. 2014;74:579–86.
87. Pandit-Taskar N, Larson SM, Carrasquillo JA. Bone-seeking radiopharmaceuticals for treatment of osseous metastases, Part 1: α therapy with 223Ra-dichloride. J Nucl Med. 2014;55:268–74.
88. Den RB, Doyle LA, Knudsen KE. Practical guide to the use of radium 223 dichloride. Can J Urol. 2014;21:70–6.
89. Parker CC, Pascoe S, Chodacki A, et al. A randomized, double-blind, dose-finding, multicenter, phase 2 study of radium chloride (Ra 223) in patients with bone metastases and castration-resistant prostate cancer. Eur Urol. 2013;63:189–97.
90. Coleman R, Aksnes AK, Naume B, et al. A phase IIa, nonrandomized study of radium-223 dichloride in advanced breast cancer patients with bone-dominant disease. Breast Cancer Res Treat. 2014;145:411–8.
91. Zustovich F, Fabiani F. Therapeutic opportunities for castration-resistant prostate cancer patients with bone metastases. Crit Rev Oncol Hematol. 2014;91:197–209.
92. Menshawy A, et al. Denosumab versus bisphosphonates in patients with advanced cancers-related bone metastasis: systematic review and meta-analysis of randomized controlled trials. Support Care Cancer. 2018;26(4):1029–38. Epub Feb 1 2018.

Part VIII

Interventional Physiatry

Cancer Rehabilitation

40

Ameet Nagpal, Jacob Fehl, Brittany Bickelhaupt, Maxim S. Eckmann, Brian Boies, and Jon Benfield

Impairments Caused by Treatments

Contemporary innovations in the medical field have led to new cancer treatment methods, which have been able to increase survivability and cure rates. A leading trend in cancer management is the widespread use of combined modality treatment. This approach encourages a treatment plan, which may include chemotherapy, radiation, and surgery during the clinical course of the disease. Although multimodal treatment may improve the therapeutic window, patients are exposed to potentially diverse side effects.

Complications of Surgery

Despite surgical conservative efforts, healthy tissue will be damaged along with the neoplastic tissue. Aggressive surgery is often necessary for complete eradication and local disease control. The tissues with the greatest rehabilitation implications are bone, nerve, muscle, lung, heart, and lymphatics. Secondary surgical impairments result from patients' overcompensation of impairments leading to poor posture, gait, balance, muscle imbalances, and other maladaptive behaviors. With apposite identification and therapy, these secondary impairments are preventable [1].

A. Nagpal (✉) · M. S. Eckmann · B. Boies
University of Texas Health Science Center at San Antonio (UTHSCSA), UT Medicine Pain Consultants, Department of Anesthesiology, San Antonio, TX, USA

University of Texas Health Science Center at San Antonio (UTHSCSA), Department of Anesthesiology, San Antonio, TX, USA
e-mail: nagpala@uthscsa.edu; eckmann@uthscsa.edu; boies@uthscsa.edu

J. Fehl
Kansas City VA Medical Center, Kansas City, MO, USA

B. Bickelhaupt
University of Texas Health Science Center at San Antonio (UTHSCSA), Department of Physical Medicine and Rehabilitation, San Antonio, TX, USA
e-mail: Bickelhaupt@uthscsa.edu

J. Benfield
South Texas Spinal Clinic, San Antonio, TX, USA

Donor Graft Surgeries

Within the treatment course, postsurgical plans can include reconstructive surgery for function and cosmesis. Donor graft sites include the muscle, skin, bone, nerve, tendon, ligament, and fat. Notwithstanding, overall the procedures are beneficial to the patient to improve function or cosmesis at the graft site, but the donor site will inevitably undergo dysfunction. For example, with the advent of affordable genetic testing and increasing surveillance protocols, there is a high incidence of mastectomies due to risk or presence of breast cancer. The most commonly used flap for reconstruction is the transverse rectus abdominus muscle. Despite high cosmetic satisfaction, the donor site has a 4% risk of abdominal wall bulge, abdominal hernia, and dehiscence. These complications further predispose the patient to loss of truncal stability, loss of proprioception, exaggerated lumbar lordosis, and back pain [2].

Spinal Accessory Nerve Palsy

There has been a shift in antineoplastic culture to focus on individualistic functional outcomes instead of standardized aggressive treatment. In the past, head and neck cancers were treated primarily with large surgical debulking including removal of the sternocleidomastoid muscle and spinal accessory nerve. Popular practice now advocates for preservation of structures, which has led to significantly decreased incidence of shoulder pain and functional impairments [1]. If the spinal accessory nerve is injured during surgery, there is an inevitable weakness in the trapezius. The degree of dysfunction depends on the patient's anatomy as the trapezius can also receive innervation from the cervical plexus [3].

Reinnervation of the trapezius due to spinal accessory nerve regrowth can occur throughout the first year after

A. Gulati et al. (eds.), *Essentials of Interventional Cancer Pain Management*, https://doi.org/10.1007/978-3-319-99684-4_40

surgery due to neuroplasticity. The potential of neuroplasticity is optimal immediately after injury and amplified with rehabilitation. Rehabilitation should focus on prevention of frozen shoulder through active range of motion, strengthening of substitute scapular elevators and retractors, electrical stimulation of the remaining trapezius muscle, and teaching compensatory methods [4, 5].

Dysphonia

Patients with head and neck cancer should be monitored for progressive dysphonia. Their dysphonia is typically due to radiation but can likewise be due to tumor invasion of the recurrent laryngeal nerve. Radiation-induced complications such as trismus, pharyngeal edema, and fibrosis can lead to reduced oral expulsion and secretions and impaired phonation.

The dysphonia can be spontaneous if due to treatment methods or permanent and progressive if the patient's team opted for organ preservation. Inability to communicate can make the patient lose independence and overwhelmingly hamper quality of life. A speech pathologist should be consulted for progressive dysphonia to discuss communication options after considering prognosis and underlying pathology. Options for voiceless communication include writing, mouthing words, esophageal speech, tracheoesophageal speech, sign language, and an electrolarynx [6].

Amputations

Amputation was once the primary treatment for extremity and soft tissue sarcomas with prevalence as high as 50% three decades ago [7, 8]. Current radiation and chemotherapy regimens and conservative surgical techniques have reduced amputation rates to less than 15% [9–11]. Limb salvage osteotomy can utilize the distal lower extremity and ankle joint to improve residual limb function [12]. However, when a tumor invades proximal musculature, nerves, or bones, extremity amputation is unavoidable [13, 14]. Whether the surgery is palliative or an attempt to gain source control, there are associated complications.

The most common complications following amputation include cellulitis, abscess, pain, phantom limb pain (PLP), and flap necrosis [10]. Intractable pain and PLP have severe limitations and affect the patient's quality of life. PLP is defined as retained sensory perception of an amputated body part. These sensations include burning, stabbing, pressure, and aching [15, 16]. PLP occurs in up to 77% of amputation patients [10]. The pathophysiology is incompletely understood but is hypothesized to involve the neuroma acting as an ectopic generator of pain and driver of secondary central plasticity and sensitization, leading to increased sympathetic activity. This is known as the peripheral afferent theory [15].

PLP has been extensively studied in the general population, but little is known about pharmacological interventions for amputations due to malignancy. Morphine, gabapentin, and ketamine provide effective, temporary relief. Significant benefits in sleep, mood, quality of life, function, and pain have not been consistently demonstrated among studies [15–17]. For severe and recalcitrant cases of PLP associated with amputation due to malignancy, interventions such as aggressive mirror therapy, neurolytic injection, spinal cord stimulation, or continuous intrathecal drug delivery can be weighed against potential complications in patients with a favorable psychological profile.

Complications of Chemotherapy

Chemotherapy has a wide range of utilization with its applications including induction for advanced disease, adjunct treatment, or primary treatment [1, 18]. The widespread use of chemotherapy agents has led to high prevalence of their debilitating toxicities. All antineoplastic agents have distinct mechanisms of action and are synergistically or sequentially combined for multi-agent therapy to allow a comprehensive antineoplastic strategy. The most commonly seen side effects are neuropathy, cognitive dysfunction, pulmonary toxicity, pancytopenia, diarrhea, nausea, vomiting, and cardiomyopathy [18].

Neuropathy

Chemotherapy-induced neuropathy is a ubiquitous dysfunction among patients. The agents identified with the highest neuropathic potential are the vinca alkaloids, the platins, and the taxanes [19]. Peripheral neuropathy is dose dependent and is a limiting factor in guiding treatment [18, 20]. Patients, who have underlying peripheral neuropathy due to comorbid diseases such as diabetes mellitus, are at increased risk for neuropathic chemotherapy toxicity [21]. Toxicity is augmented by any existing neural ischemia, compression, or electrolyte disturbances. Neuropathy can vary from acute to chronic onset or a transient to progressive disease course [18].

The platin compounds, such as cisplatin and carboplatin, are typically used in lung, breast, ovarian, and colon cancers. Their predominating toxicity is sensory neuropathy and typically presents after treatment is completed. Proprioceptive impairments are secondary to direct platinum binding to the large sensory fibers' mitochondria [18, 19].

The vinca alkaloids inhibit microtubule and mitotic spindle apparatus assembly and axonal transport [18, 22]. Consequently, nerves with longer axons are more susceptible to damage. These agents are used for leukemia, lymphoma, and sarcoma treatment [18]. Their toxicity will accumulate as early as 3 months after starting treatment. Vinca alkaloid toxicity will present with distal extremity paresthesias and eventual lower extremity muscle stretch reflex loss [20]. Mononeuropathies, persistent muscle cramps, wrist extensor weakness, metatarsal dorsiflexor weakness, and cranial nerve lesions are not uncommon [18, 23, 24]. There is a potential of autonomic damage leading to paralytic ileus, bowel and bladder dysfunction, sexual dysfunction, and orthostatic hypotension [19, 25]. There is currently no successful pharmacological treatment or prophylaxis for vinca alkaloid-induced neuropathy.

Paclitaxel and docetaxel are used largely for breast, ovarian, or lung cancers [18]. Taxanes act to hyperstabilize the microtubule subunit linking, therefore inhibiting the ability of the cell to reorganize the cytoskeleton [18]. Taxanes produce paresthesias, loss of muscle stretch reflexes, decreased vibratory sensation, and gait disturbances [26]. There is no treatment for taxane-induced neuropathy, but lengthening time between cycles and lowering the dose may be effective.

Cognitive Disorders

Chemotherapy can have toxic effects on the central nervous system (CNS) including memory loss, impaired attention, processing speed, concentration, and executive function [27, 28]. These symptoms can continue to progress after therapy completion, and the patient may not return to their prior social and occupational level of functioning [29]. All classes of chemotherapeutic agents have the potential for CNS toxicity. The incidence of chemotherapy-induced cognitive impairments is climbing as malignancies are identified in earlier stages [30].

The pathophysiology in these neurocognitive disorders is not completely understood but may involve the hippocampus [28]. The hippocampus is largely responsible for new memory formation, learning, and spatial processing. Adult hippocampal neurogenesis, the process of generating new neurons, is responsible for maintenance of brain plasticity and memory [31, 32]. Chemotherapeutic agents disrupt neurogenesis in the hippocampus, which results in impaired cognitive functions [33].

Agents specifically implicated in disrupted hippocampal neurogenesis include DNA cross-linking agents (cisplatin, cyclophosphamide), antimetabolites (methotrexate, 5-fluorouracil), hormone antagonists (tamoxifen), anthracyclines (doxorubicine), and the taxanes (paclitaxel, docetaxel) [34–37]. Through magnetic resonance imaging (MRI) studies, these drugs are known to reduce hippocampal volume and functional recruitment compared to controls, corresponding to the cognitive impairments seen in patients [28, 38].

The physician should be prepared to monitor the patient for these neurocognitive impairments. Preemptive initiation of neuropsychological testing and speech pathology therapy can minimize the lasting neurocognitive effects and their implications on occupational and social participation.

Cardiomyopathy

Chemotherapy regimens can cause long-standing cardiovascular complications such as ventricular systolic dysfunction, pericarditis, hypertension, arrhythmias, and thromboembolism [39]. Anthracyclines, such as doxorubicin, have been known for decades to induce cardiomyopathy. The toxicity is dose dependent with a prevalence ranging from 2% in low dose regimens to 48% in high dose regimens [40]. Oxidative free radical-mediated damage is responsible for the cardiotoxicity. Cardiac dysfunction can present as acute pericarditis or lead to irreversible chronic progressive cardiomyopathy [41]. Dosing can be reduced or offered in bolus administrations, although no dose is considered safe against doxorubicin-induced cardiotoxicity.

Trastuzumab has gained increasing popularity with higher incidence rates of breast cancer. It is a monoclonal antibody to human epidermal growth factor 2 (HER-2/neu). The incidence of cardiomyopathy is 3% when given alone and 27% when given in combination with anthracyclines [42]. Patients present in New York Heart Association (NYHA) class III or IV heart failure. The antibody interferes with myocyte repair and anti-apoptosis pathways [43]. Fortunately, trastuzumab-induced cardiotoxicity is reversible once the treatment is completed.

Alkylating agents, such as cyclophosphamide, cross-link DNA strands and add alkyl groups to prevent replication in rapidly dividing cells. Cyclophosphamide causes a dose-dependent cardiomyopathy through left ventricular systolic dysfunction. The mechanism of damage is unknown but involves hemorrhagic myocardial necrosis with interstitial edema and fibrin deposition. Ventricular dysfunction happens more acutely compared to other agents and presents within days to weeks of initiating therapy [44].

Treatment of chemotherapy-induced cardiomyopathy has limited data. However, patients with left ventricular systolic dysfunction should be treated according to the same heart failure guidelines used in the general population [45]. There is a growing need for physicians to recognize symptomatic and asymptomatic heart failure in these patients and to initiate treatment early [46]. Patients can be referred to specific cardiopulmonary rehabilitation specialists who will focus on maintaining cardiac and physical conditioning.

Pulmonary Toxicity

Chemotherapy-induced pulmonary toxicity can be subdivided into early- and late-onset complications. Early complications are relatively straightforward and include inflammatory interstitial pneumonitis, pulmonary edema, bronchospasm, and pleural effusions. Most of this section will discuss the more prevalent and distressing late-onset complications.

Bleomycin is widely used for germ cell tumors, lymphomas, and squamous cell tumors. It is well known for its high risk of pulmonary fibrosis. Presentation includes nonproductive cough, dyspnea on exertion or rest, tachypnea, cyanosis, and bibasilar rales [47]. Bleomycin-induced lung injury occurs due to oxidative injury, dysfunctional repair, and unregulated proteolytic enzymes [48]. It specifically damages type I pneumocytes, which then stimulates fibroblasts with resultant collagen deposition. Pulmonary fibrosis has an incidence rate of 10% in patients receiving bleomycin with development 1–6 months after treatment [47, 49]. Toxicity is dose dependent and exacerbated by renal disease due to its renal excretion.

Cyclophosphamide induces early-onset pneumonitis and late-onset fibrosis. The late-onset fibrosis is indolent and progressive for years after treatment is completed [50]. Cyclophosphamide causes an upregulation of transforming growth factor-beta and subsequent increased collagen synthesis. Fibrosis soon becomes irreversible [47].

The taxanes and vinca alkaloids usually do not cause permanent pulmonary toxicity. The taxanes may cause acute-onset pulmonary type 1 hypersensitivity reactions, which can be mitigated with antihistamine or dexamethasone premedication [51]. The monoclonal antibodies (bevacizumab, rituximab, cetuximab) are associated with bronchospasm, hypoxia, and pulmonary infiltrates [47].

Complications of Radiation

Radiation is a mainstay of treatment and used for intent to cure, palliation, and improving quality of life [52, 53]. Approximately half of the 14 million cancer survivors in America receive radiation during their disease course [54, 55]. Radiation-induced toxicity is a considerable cause of long-term disability in cancer patients. Its consequences can be present for years after treatment and are often permanent.

Radiation utilizes photons, protons, neutrons, or electrons to penetrate tissue and cause tissue damage. Any rapidly dividing cell in the radiation field is susceptible to cell death, including the dermis, mucous membranes, and viscera [56, 57]. Radiation can produce acute injury, which is present during therapy, or late injury, which is slowly progressive and continues to mature years after radiation.

Late radiation injury takes the form of fibrosis and sclerosis of tissues, including neurons, muscles, tendons, and ligaments. Without continual range of motion, contractures will certainly develop in these structures. Ranging should be a central part of lifelong treatment to prevent the ongoing contracture formation. There has not been wide success in the pharmacological treatment of radiation fibrosis. However, the combination of pentoxifylline and tocopherol can attenuate radiation fibrosis but cannot reverse its damage [58].

Cognitive Disorders

Encephalopathy

Encephalopathy due to radiation is a delayed effect and is secondary to necrotic brain parenchyma [59]. Symptoms do not develop until 2 years after radiation therapy and are often misinterpreted as recurrence of the primary malignancy. The patient should undergo a positron emission tomography (PET) scan to differentiate radiation-induced necrosis versus primary malignancy recurrence. The distinguishing factor is the presence of hypermetabolic activity in malignancy compared to necrosis, which is easily identified in a PET scan [1]. Necrosis-induced encephalopathy carries a poor prognosis with little hope for return to prior level of functioning. The only current treatment available for necrosis-induced encephalopathy is resection with postsurgical therapy interventions to maximize outcomes [1].

Cerebral Atrophy

When patients undergo whole-brain radiation, they are vulnerable to radiation-induced cerebral atrophy. Executive functions, attention, mentation, judgment, and insight will be affected. The differential diagnosis on initial presentation includes vascular and Lewy body dementias [60]. The permanent effects of cerebral atrophy will drastically alter the patient's occupational participation and will subsequently benefit from vocational rehabilitation. Like radiation-induced encephalopathy, there is little potential for regain of prior functioning.

Radiation Fibrosis Syndrome

Radiation fibrosis syndrome (RFS) is a broad, collective term to describe the clinical manifestations of progressive fibrotic tissue sclerosis that transpires as a result of radiation [57]. All tissue types including the heart, lung, skin, muscle, nerve, ligament, tendon, and bone are susceptible to RFS [61–63]. RFS usually does not manifest until months to years after radiation therapy and follows an irreversible, slowly progressive trajectory [64, 65]. There are several risk factors for RFS, including age, health, degenerative spine disease, cancer staging, chemotherapy regimens, and the location and size of the radiation field [66].

The pathogenesis of RFS is not entirely understood but is theorized to involve the induction of apoptosis via free radical-mediated DNA damage [55]. Radiation stimulates changes in cell function and activates the coagulation system, inflammation, epithelial regeneration, and tissue remodeling via cytokines, chemokines, and growth factors [55, 57]. This results in a procoagulant, proinflammatory, mitogenic, and profibrogenic effect on smooth muscle cells and fibroblasts. Inflammatory mediators then provoke a positive feedback loop to sustain the chronic radiation injury and sclerosis [57, 67].

Neuromuscular

The progressive fibrosis of the brain, spinal cord, nerve roots, nerve plexi, peripheral nervous system (PNS), and muscle amasses into neuromuscular complications [62]. PNS dysfunction is due to compressive fibrosis of surrounding tissues and fibrosis-induced ischemia in the vasa nervorum [1, 68]. The most prominent symptoms are pain, sensory loss, weakness, numbness, and autonomic dysfunction with hypotension, bowel and bladder changes, and sexual dysfunction.

Neuropathic Pain

Neuropathic pain is common in RFS and is due to several interacting pathways. One theory involves the generation of ectopic activity in a radiation-exposed neural structure and damage to descending modulatory pathways. Since these ectopic pain signals are not grossly anatomical in etiology, the pain experienced is out of proportion to the stimulus [69, 70]. The ectopic signal can be due to radiation-induced compression or ischemia with resultant demyelination and axonal loss. Preexisting diabetes or spinal degeneration leaves these structures even more susceptible to neuropathic pain in RFS. If the neuropathic pain presents as sensory loss without pain, the patient will become more prone to other injuries, affect gait, and impair activities of daily living.

Funicular Pain

Funicular pain results from spinal cord radiation, which is a relatively common treatment regimen. Its pathophysiology involves ectopic activity in the ascending spinothalamic tracts with resultant excruciating and ambiguous pain. It does not follow a dermatomal or fixed nerve referral pattern, complicating diagnosis of the syndrome. For example, damage to the funiculi of the cervical spinal cord can cause pain in any part of the body caudal to the lesion. The pain can follow a radiculopathic, plexopathic, polyneuropathic, or mononeuropathic distribution causing the lesion to be difficult to localize [57, 71].

Neuropathies

Radiation will invariably affect nerves resulting in an array of presentations and disorders. Radiation-induced myopathy requires radiation damage to the nerve roots and will present as weakness in a myotomal pattern. If myelopathy develops, it may present 12–50 months after radiation therapy and progress toward paraparesis or quadriparesis [1]. Radiation-induced plexopathy can result in devastating pain and disability. Of the possible plexus involvements, the brachial plexus is most vulnerable to radiation damage due to its apical location [72]. The radiation-induced plexopathies are dose related and can be differentiated from malignant plexopathies by minimal pain, upper trunk involvement, and myokymia on electromyography [1]. Mononeuropathies due to radiation can involve large neural structures such as the sciatic or axillary nerves but can present among a composite of deficits due to damage to smaller neural structures. If treated with large radiation fields, patients may develop dysfunction in multiple neural and muscular structures. They can exhibit interconnected pathophysiologies of myelopathy, radiculopathy, plexopathy, mononeuropathy, and myopathy in a syndrome called myelo-radiculo-plexo-neuro-myopathy [72–74].

Spasms

Radiation damage to muscles permits them to be prone to spasms secondary to weakness, fatigability, and ectopic activity of the motor nerve [74]. The spasm may not be distinct and could exist as vague stiffness. If the spasms are not alleviated, then the patient is in jeopardy of permanent contracture [75]. The ectopic activity in the motor nerve allows for elevated activity at the motor endplate zone, excessive acetylcholine production, and sustained sarcomere shortening. The sustained contraction requires energy and oxygen, resulting in local acidity and constricted blood flow causing tissue hypoxia. Tissue hypoxia attracts inflammatory mediators and cytokines with sensitization of nociceptive nerve fibers and cyclical contraction, hypoxia, acidification, and pain. This RFS cycle can be mistaken for fibromyalgia or a rheumatological disease [76].

Tendons, Ligaments, and Bones

RFS in tendons and ligaments is due to gradual fibrosis with loss of elasticity, shortening, and contracture, which results in decreased range of motion and limited function. Areas most commonly affected are the shoulder, elbow, wrist, hip, knee, ankle, fingers, and neck [57]. Under radiation, bone becomes brittle and prone to injury and osteoradionecrosis. When children undergo radiation of the long bones, their growth plates become affected resulting in interrupted bone maturation. Patients may become vulnerable to endocrine-related growth abnormalities if the cranium is irradiated. Osteopenia and osteoporosis are delayed effects of radiation and require unremitting physician vigilance for fracture prevention [77–79].

Radiation Fibrosis Syndrome: Common Clinical Dysfunctions

RFS can present as a vague neuromuscular complaint or as a pathognomonic, radiation-specific clinical syndrome. These include neck extensor weakness, shoulder pain, cervical dystonia, or trismus.

Neck Extensor Weakness

Commonly known as "dropped head syndrome," neck extensor weakness presents with atrophy and weakness of the cervicothoracic paraspinal and shoulder girdle muscles [57, 80]. The heterogeneous pathophysiology is composed of neuropathic, myopathic, and mixed etiologies as demonstrated by electromyography findings [81]. The atrophy is due to damage of the anterior horn cell, nerve roots, cervical plexus, or peripheral nerves [57].

The discomfort of neck extensor weakness is caused by an amalgamation of muscle fatigue, spasms, and muscle imbalances due to atrophy and hypertrophy of denervated and innervated muscles, respectively. These factors predispose the patient to poor posture with the head and shoulders flexed forward relative to the spine in a kyphotic fashion. The cervicothoracic and rotator cuff muscles become prone to dysfunction due to poor kinetics and kinematics.

Neck extensor weakness is treated with postural retraining and reconditioning of cervicothoracic and rotator cuff muscles. Although nerve damage is usually irreparable, functional gains are probable with consistent, suitable therapy. Unfortunately, the progression of weakness due to denervation is inexorable, and compliance to a lifelong home exercise program is mandatory to maintain function and reduce pain. If the poor posture is incompletely responsive to conservative measures, a cervical orthotic can be applied for additional relief. The collar allows for rest of the weakened cervicothoracic musculature. As a second-line treatment, pregabalin or gabapentin can be offered [82]. Injected pain relievers and steroids should be used sparingly given the patient's predisposition to worsening weakness with these injections.

Shoulder Pain

If the shoulder girdle muscles, innervating nerves, or bony structures are exposed to radiation, significant dysfunction and pain can develop. For example, if C5 or C6 nerve roots are damaged, the rotator cuff muscles will become weak and refer pain in a dermatomal pattern to the lateral shoulder and arm. This mechanism places the shoulder at risk of anterior subluxation, tendon impingement, tendonitis, and adhesive capsulitis [83].

The diagnosis of shoulder pathologies does not differ from the general population and can be made on physical exam and history. The foundation of treatment in radiation-induced shoulder pain is physical therapy, which should address posture, shoulder and pectoral girdle tightness, neck extensor weakness, and rotator cuff weakness. NSAIDs, gabapentin, and pregabalin can be offered as adjunctive therapies. Surgery is a last resort since the underlying problem of these patients is neuromuscular and not structural [57].

Cervical Dystonia

In radiation-induced cervical dystonia, the sternocleidomastoid, scalene, and trapezius muscles are involved. This exposed region is susceptible to ectopic activity development in the spinal accessory nerve and cervical nerve roots. This allows for involuntary spasms and contracture of the neck musculature. These muscles will become painful and demonstrate neuropathic and myelopathic findings on electromyography. As the RFS progresses, the patient will have improper head positioning and consequent difficulty in swallowing, phonation, driving, and occupational tasks. If the anterior cervical soft tissues are irradiated, there is a possibility of RFS and subsequent kyphotic head positioning.

Patients may utilize physical therapy to prevent further loss of range of neck motion. Exercises should focus on maintenance of neck range of motion. The home exercise program should be continued for at least 2 years after therapy completion and possibly indefinitely. Patients can be instructed on self-massage techniques to augment their physical therapy with tissue release. Neuropathic and opioid agents can offer relief in a minority of patients. Botulinum toxin injections into the painful muscles, when combined with physical therapy, have demonstrated optimal improvement on range of motion [75].

Trismus

Trismus is reported to be prevalent in as many as 38% of head and neck cancers [84]. Trismus causes difficulties in chewing, swallowing, oral hygiene, and pulmonary function. The dysfunction can be due to many factors such as primary tumor invasion of adjacent tissues and neural structures, surgery, or radiation [85]. Ectopic activity in the trigeminal nerve causes altered mechanics from involuntary spasms within masseter and pterygoid muscles. These spasms lead to contracture of the tendons and ligaments and eventual RFS-induced trismus.

As in most neuromuscular disorders, physical therapy is the initial treatment approach for radiation-induced trismus. However, its long-term efficacy is limited [84]. Other more aggressive options, such as forced mouth opening under anesthesia and surgical coronoidectomy, have been studied. Surgical coronoidectomy has been effective and relatively safe. Forced mouth opening under anesthesia has short-lived effects and presents a high risk of alveolus fracture. Botulinum toxin injections into the masseter muscle have been shown to reduce pain, but not trismus [75]. If a patient is able to maintain compliance, there are a host of jaw-opening devices. Orthotics include stacked tongue depressors, corkscrew devices, TheraBite Jaw Motion Rehabilitation System, and the Dynasplint Trismus System. The TheraBite Jaw Motion Rehabilitation System has demonstrated efficacy in patients up to 5 years after the completion of radiation [86].

Vocational Rehabilitation and Disability

Vocational rehabilitation and disability is a process that enables an individual with functional, psychological, developmental, cognitive, and emotional impairments or health disabilities to overcome barriers to accessing, maintaining, or returning to employment or other useful occupation. In the case of cancer rehabilitation, vocational rehabilitation is unique to each patient and dependent on the type of cancer, timeline of the cancer progression, severity of the disease, and other unique deficits. These deficits can be attributable to the specific type of cancer itself and deficits that have resulted from surgeries, chemotherapy, or other treatments. Overall, the approach and implementation of vocational rehabilitation practices with cancer patients are the same as those with other diseases [87, 88].

General Strategies

The goal of vocational rehabilitation is to aid in integration back into daily life or to obtain as much independent function that their condition will permit. Often cancer patients have significant disabilities that will limit them to prolonged bed rest. Therapy may be aimed at maximizing a patient's limited physical activity to avoid complications associated with bed rest or immobility associated with prolonged hospitalization and medical treatment. Within the general population, bed rest has a dramatic impact on strength, decreasing by 1.0–1.5% per day and as much as 20–30% during only a week to 9 days of bed rest. Five weeks of total inactivity results in losing 50% of the patient's muscular strength. Muscle mass loss due to inactivity is estimated to be lost at 5–10% per week. Patients are encouraged to perform strengthening exercises using an elastic band or mild resistive exercises against gravity while in bed. One contraction a day at 50% of maximal strength is enough to prevent strength loss [89]. Due to inactivity and constant bed rest, pressure ulcers are of great concern. Those who are restricted to bed rest can be taught to self-monitor mobility. Frequent repositioning with cushions or pillow aids and tilt tables are used to decrease skin breakdown and risk of joint contractures.

Lymphedema

Lymphedema, also known as lymphatic obstruction, is a condition of localized fluid retention and tissue swelling caused by a compromised lymphatic system, which normally returns interstitial fluid to the thoracic duct and then the bloodstream. This results in an accumulation of protein which occurs in the interstitium, changing the colloidal pressure, and detracts fluid into the interstitial space [90]. Large protein molecules remain interstitial and continually change the colloidal pressure.

Damage or destruction to lymph nodes and vessels via surgical resection and radiation will result in this chronic fluid collection within the interstitial space. For example, lymphedema is a frequent complication of breast cancer management and is manifested by upper extremity swelling associated with a sense of arm fullness [89]. Lymphedema grading is as follows:

Grade 1 (mild) Pitting edema that can be reversed by elevation
Grade 2 (moderate) Non-pitting and unresponsive to elevation
Grade 3 (severe) Lymphostatic elephantiasis and cartilage-like
Grade 4 (gigantic) Elephantiasis

In Grade 4 lymphedema, the lymphatic channels are nearly completely obstructed, and without intervention, the limb will continue to progressively enlarge. Intervention measures focus on prevention by avoiding limb constriction in order to not interfere with lymph outflow, infection prevention, preventing excess scarring, and avoidance of vasodilation from extreme heat exposure [89].

Lymphedema Treatment Overview

Current treatment for chronic lymphedema is complete decongestive therapy (CDT). CDT has been shown to be effective in reducing lymphedema. CDT is accomplished in two phases. The first phase is manual lymphatic drainage followed by compression bandages, which are left in place for 21–24 hours/day. This process is repeated until maximal volume reduction has been achieved. The second phase is long-term maintenance including compressive garments and routine exercise and monitoring [91]. A specialist in wound care management often monitors this process. Throughout CDT skin care is strictly monitored to preclude infection and breakdown. Long-term management requires routine follow-up as lymphedema can develop slowly over time.

Compression garments achieve the following:

Improve lymphatic flow and reduce accumulated protein
Improve venous return
Shape and reduce the size of the limb
Maintain skin integrity
Protect the limb from potential trauma [91]

Pathological Fractures

Bone and musculoskeletal pain are common complaints in cancer patients. If a patient reports new changes in their pain, then metastasis, osteopenia, and possible pathologic fracture must be high considerations for the differential diagnosis. A patient may have multiple comorbidities that can also contribute to the risk of pathologic fractures such as prolonged bed rest. As previously discussed, bed rest and decreased physical activity dramatically reduce muscle strength and mass, and without resistance and impact training, bone density can decrease. This decrease in bone density places the patient at further risk of fracture, especially if the patient has concern for metastatic disease. If metastatic involvement is suspected, non-weight-bearing restrictions to the extremity in question should be observed, and a full workup completed [89]. Surgical treatment of pathologic fractures is directed at pain relief, preservation or restoration of function, skeletal stabilization, and local tumor control [92]. Indications for surgery include life expectancy of more than 1 month with a fracture of a weight-bearing bone and life expectancy of more than 3 months for a fracture of a non-weight-bearing bone [1].

Comprehensive Inpatient Rehabilitation

The decision for inpatient versus outpatient therapy is multifactorial. Often if a patient is already admitted to the hospital, daily therapies can be consulted for inpatient care; however, these services are limited. If the patient is stable enough to be discharged from an acute setting, however still requires physician supervision and can tolerate at least 3 hours of dedicated therapy daily, admission to an inpatient rehabilitation facility should be considered. If a patient already has an appropriate degree of functional independence but would still benefit from focused therapy, then outpatient visits may be appropriate.

A patient may be considered for inpatient rehabilitation if they can achieve significant functional gains in activities of daily living or benefit from teaching of compensatory techniques. Several studies have reported equal Functional Independence Measures (FIM) efficacies when patients with malignant squamous cell carcinoma (SCC) are compared with patients with similar but traumatic- and ischemic-induced impairments. Comparison of patients admitted for inpatient rehabilitation with wide-ranging cancer-related impairments noted no significant differences in FIM scores or length of stay relative to non-cancer patients. This suggests that inpatient admissions should be considered for patients with cancer whose debilities arise from impairments other than intracranial or epidural metastases [1, 93]. A patient must be able to participate in at least 3 hours of dedicated therapy within at least two therapy disciplines daily for at least 5 days of the week as follows:

Physical therapy evaluates and treats impaired functional mobility, strength, and endurance. Physical therapies occurs at least 5 days per week, for the duration of the inpatient rehab stay. Treatment is directed at improving and optimizing functional independence with gross motor control, bed mobility, transfers, balance and safety awareness, strengthening, endurance, progressive locomotion, and patient/family education. The patient is also evaluated for appropriate durable medical equipment.

Occupational therapy evaluates and treats for impaired activities of daily living management, upper extremity strength and dexterity, and ability to perform self-care tasks. Occupational therapies occurs at least 5 days per week, for the duration of the inpatient rehab stay. Treatment is directed at improving and optimizing functional independence with progressive strengthening and retraining with adaptive techniques for fine motor control, transfers, dressing, grooming, hygiene, toileting, bathing, safety awareness, other self-care tasks, and patient/family education. The patient is also evaluated for appropriate durable medical equipment.

Speech language pathology evaluates and treats for impaired cognition including memory, concentration, attention, problem-solving, reasoning, judgment, language, and communication skills. Speech therapies occurs at least 5 days per week, for the duration of the inpatient rehab stay. Treatment is directed at improving and optimizing functional independence with cognition, speech, language, communication, swallowing function, and patient/family education.

Prior to completion of inpatient rehabilitation, the patient is evaluated for continued outpatient physical therapy, occupational therapy, and speech language pathology. Other therapies that may be useful inpatient or outpatient include kinesiotherapy, recreational therapy, music therapy, psychiatry, psychology, and other integrative therapies depending on the patient's unique needs.

Cancer Rehabilitation Therapy approach to cancer rehabilitation can be divided into preventative, supportive, and palliative therapy [89].

Preventative Therapy Cancer rehabilitation should involve pre-planning therapies prior to chemotherapy, radiation or surgery. An essential part of preventative therapy is patient education, including setting appropriate expectations and goals of functional recovery. Preventative therapy, or prehabilitation, has been defined as a process on the cancer continuum of care that occurs between the time of cancer diagnosis and the beginning of acute treatment. It includes physical and psychological assessments that establish a baseline functional level, identify impairments, and provide interventions that promote physical and psychological health to reduce the incidence and severity of future impairments [94]. Establishment of a prehabilitation plan at the time of diagnosis or prior to invasive interventions may benefit the patient with physical recovery as well as psychological endurance. Pre and post treatment rehabilitation efforts can improve the physical and psychological health outcomes of a patient and may reduce work-related disability and the risk of early retirement in survivors [94]. Recent studies have shown that prior to major cancer surgery, exercise improved cardiorespiratory function with a tendency for responders to suffer fewer major postoperative complications [95]. Additionally, psychological prehabilitation can benefit a patient's quality of life, somatic symptoms, and psychological outcomes [96].

Supportive Therapy Supportive therapy is utilized throughout the course of a patient's cancer treatment. This includes evaluation for necessary adaptive equipment as the disease progresses, consults for psychological support, pain management and interventions, and consideration for inpatient rehabilitation for intensive recovery. Speech language pathology can play a vital role in many cancers that affect the brain, as well as treatments that can cause a decrease in cognitive function. A high index of suspicion for swallowing disorders should be maintained. Swallowing difficulty can be associated with cognitive impairment, central nervous system involvement, and radiation treatment and in patients with generalized deconditioning secondary to bed rest. When aspiration is suspected, a dysphagia evaluation is performed. A follow-up video fluoroscopic swallow study (VFSS) may be required. If silent aspiration is suspected, VFSS is necessary. Extremities with possible tumor involvement should be positioned for non-weight-bearing and range of motion withheld until a workup is completed [89].

Palliative Rehabilitation In palliative rehabilitation therapy, the goals are to improve or maintain comfort and function during the terminal stage of the disease. Pain interventions are especially appropriate due to the increased likelihood of pain due to cancer progression. Patients and family may work closely with psychology and psychiatry to manage chronic issues such as pain, long-term disability, and other chronic life changes. In patients with CNS, breast, lung, head, and neck tumors, physical medicine problems may occur in over 70%. Often, there is a gap in rehabilitative patient care, which is changed dramatically by introducing a physiatrist to the oncologic management team [89].

References

1. Braddom RL. Physical medicine & rehabilitation. Philadelphia: Elsevier; 2016.
2. Montiero M. Physical therapy implications following the TRAM procedure. Phys Ther. 1997;77:765–70.
3. Brown H. Anatomy of the spinal accessory nerve plexus: relevance to head and neck cancer and atherosclerosis. Exp Biol Med. 2002;227:570–8.
4. McNeely MI, Parlaiment MB, Seikaly H, et al. Effect of exercise on upper extremity pain and dysfunction in head and neck cancer survivors: a randomized controlled trial. Cancer. 2008;113:214–22.
5. Rogers LQ, Anton PM, Fogleman A, et al. Systematic review of the role of bisphosphonates on skeletal morbidity in metastatic cancer. BMJ. 2003;327:469.
6. Happ MB. Interpretation of nonvocal behavior and the meaning of voicelessness in critical care. Soc Sci Med. 2000;50:1247–55.
7. Abbas JS, et al. The surgical treatment and outcome of soft-tissue sarcoma. Arch Surg. 1981;116:765–9.
8. Shiu MH, et al. Surgical treatment of 297 soft tissue sarcomas of the lower extremity. Ann Surg. 1975;182:597–602.
9. Karakousis CP, Proimakis C, Walsh DL. Primary soft tissue sarcoma of the extremities in adults. Br J Surg. 1995;82:1208–12.
10. Parsons CM, et al. The role of radical amputations for extremity tumors: a single institution experience and review of the literature. J Surg Oncol. 2012;105:149–55.
11. Whelan JS, et al. Survival from high-grade localized extremity osteosarcoma: combined results and prognostic facts from three European Osteosarcoma Intergroup randomized controlled trials. Ann Oncol. 2011;23:1607–16.
12. Finn HA, Simon MA. Limb-salvage surgery in the treatment of osteosarcoma in skeletally immature individuals. Orthop Surg Rehab Med. 1991;262:108–18.
13. Carter SR, et al. Hindquarter amputation for tumors of the musculoskeletal system. J Bone Joint Surg Br. 1990;72:490–3.
14. Schwarz RE, et al. Long-term survival after radical operations for cancer treatment-induced sarcomas: how two survivors invite reflection on oncologic treatment concepts. Am J Clin Oncol. 2002;25:244–7.
15. McCormick Z, Chang-Chien G, Marshall B, Huang M, Harden RN. Phantom limb pain: a systematic neuroanatomical-based review of pharmacological treatment. Pain Med. 2014;15:292–305.
16. Alviar MJM, Hale T, Dungca M. Pharmacologic interventions for treating phantom limb pain: Review. Cochrane Syst Rev. 2011;12:CD006380.
17. Nikolajsen L, et al. Randomized trial of epidural bupivacaine and morphine in prevention of stump and phantom pain in lower-extremity limb amputation. Lancet. 1997;350:1353–7.
18. Soffietti R, Trevisan E, Ruda R. Neurologic complications of chemotherapy and other newer and experimental approaches. Handb Clin Neurol. 2014;121:1199–218.
19. Sioka C, Kryritsis AP. Central and peripheral nervous system toxicity of common chemotherapeutic agents. Cancer Chemother Pharmacol. 2009;63:761–7.
20. Carla C, Verstappen J, Heimans K, et al. Neurotoxin complications of chemotherapy in patients with cancer. Drugs. 2003;63:1549–63.
21. Chauvenet AR, et al. Vincristine-induced neuropathy as the initial presentation of Charcot-Marie-Tooth disease in acute lymphoblastic leukemia: a pediatric oncology group study. J Pediatr Hematol Oncol. 2003;25:316–20.
22. Paulson JC, McClure WO. Inhibition of axoplasmic transport by colchicine, podophyllotoxin, and vinblastine: an effect on microtubules. Ann N Y Acad Sci. 1975;253:517–27.
23. Sanderson PA, Kuwabara T, Cogan DG. Optic neuropathy presumably caused by vincristine therapy. Am J Ophthalmol. 1976;81:146–50.
24. Kalcioglu MT, et al. Bilateral hearing loss during vincristine therapy: a case report. J Chemother. 2003;15:290–2.
25. Moudgil SS, Riggs JE. Fulminant peripheral neuropathy with severe quadriparesis associated with vincristine therapy. Ann Pharmacother. 2000;34:1136–8.
26. Postma TJ, Vermorken JB, Liefting AJ, et al. Paclitaxel-induced neuropathy. Ann Oncol. 1995;6:489–94.
27. Wefel JS, Schagen SB. Chemotherapy-related cognitive dysfunction. Curr Neurol Neurosci Rep. 2012;12:267–75.
28. Dietrich J, Prust M, Kaiser J. Chemotherapy, cognitive impairment and hippocampal toxicity: Review. Neuroscience. 2015;309:224–32.
29. Collins B, MacKenzie J, Tasca GA, Scherling C, Smith A. Cognitive effects of chemotherapy in breast cancer patients: a dose-response study. Psychooncology. 2013;22:1517–27.
30. Dietrich J, Monje M, Wefel J, Meyers C. Clinical patterns and biological correlates of cognitive dysfunction associated with cancer therapy. Oncologist. 2008;13:1285–95.

31. Deng W, Almone JB, Gage FH. New neurons and new memories: how does adult hippocampal neurogenesis affect learning and memory? Nat Rev Neurosci. 2010;11:339–50.
32. Spalding KL, et al. Dynamics of hippocampal neurogenesis in adult humans. Cell. 2013;153:1219–27.
33. Seigers R, et al. Inhibition of hippocampal cell proliferation by methotrexate in rats is not potentiated by the presence of a tumor. Brain Res Bull. 2010;81:472–276.
34. Christie LA, Acharya MM, Parihar VK, Nguyen A, Martirosian V, Limoli CL. Impaired cognitive function and hippocampal neurogenesis following cancer chemotherapy. Clin Cancer Res. 2012;18:1954–65.
35. Nokia MS, Anderson ML, Shors TJ. Chemotherapy disrupts learning, neurogenesis and theta activity in the adult brain. Eur J Neurosci. 2012;36:3521–30.
36. Walker EA, Foley JJ, Clark-Vetri R, Raffa RB. Effects of repeated administration of chemotherapeutic agents tamoxifen, methotrexate, and 5-fluorouracil on the acquisition and retention of a learned response in mice. Psychopharmacology. 2011;217:539–48.
37. Yang M. Neurotoxicity of methotrexate to hippocampal cells in vivo and in vitro. Biochem Pharmacol. 2011;82:72–80.
38. De Ruiter MB, et al. Cerebral hyporesponsiveness and cognitive impairment 10 years after chemotherapy for breast cancer. Hum Brain Mapp. 2011;32:1206–19.
39. Higgins AY, O'Halloran TD, Chang JD. Chemotherapy-induced cardiomyopathy. Heart Fail Rev. 2015;20:721–30.
40. Swain SM, Whaley FS, Ewer MS. Congestive heart failure in patients treated with doxorubicin: a retrospective analysis of three trials. Cancer. 2003;11:2869–79.
41. Todaro MC, et al. Cardioncology: state of the heart. Int J Cardiol. 2013;168:680–7.
42. Seidman A. Cardiac dysfunction in the trastuzumab clinical trials experience. J Clin Oncol. 2002;20:1215–21.
43. Khouri MG, et al. Cancer therapy-induced cardiac toxicity in early breast cancer: addressing the unresolved issues. Circulation. 2012;126:2749–63.
44. Morandi P, et al. Serum cardiac troponin I levels and ECG/Echo monitoring in breast cancer patients undergoing high-dose (7g/m(2)) cyclophosphamide. Bone Marrow Transplant. 2002;28:277–82.
45. Hunt SA, American College of Cardiology F, American Heart A. 2009 focused update incorporated into the ACC/AHA 2005 guidelines for the diagnosis and management of heart failure in adults: a report of the American College of Cardiology Foundation/American Heart Association task force on practice guidelines developed in collaboration with the international society for heart and lung transplantation. J Am Coll Cardiol. 2009;53:e1–e90.
46. Yoon GF, et al. Left ventricular dysfunction in patients receiving cardiotoxic cancer therapies: are clinicians responding optimally? J Am Coll Cardiol. 2010;56:1644–50.
47. Meador M, Floyd J, Perry MC. Pulmonary toxicity of chemotherapy. Semin Oncol. 2006;33:98–105.
48. Fennell DA, Rudd RM. Pulmonary toxicity and cancer treatment. Hosp Med. 2004;65:462–4.
49. Sleijfer S. Bleomycin-induced pneumonitis. Chest. 2001;120:617–24.
50. Kreisman H, Wolkove N. Pulmonary toxicity of antineoplastic therapy. Semin Oncol. 1992;19:508–20.
51. Rowinsky EK, Donehower RC. Paclitaxel (Taxol). N Engl J Med. 1995;332:1004–14.
52. O'Meara WP, Thiringer JK, Johnstone PA. Follow-up of head and neck cancer patients post-radiotherapy. Radiother Oncol. 2003;66:323–6.
53. Tannock IF. Combined modality treatment with radiotherapy and chemotherapy. Radiother Oncol. 1989;16:83–101.
54. Mariotto AB, Yabroff KR, Shao Y, Feuer EJ, Brown MI. Projections of the cost of cancer care in the United States: 2010–2020. J Natl Cancer Inst. 2011;103:117–28.
55. Hauer-Jensen M, Fink LM, Wang J. Radiation injury and the protein C pathway. Crit Care Med. 2004;32:S325–30.
56. Stubblefield MD. Radiation fibrosis syndrome: neuromuscular and musculoskeletal complications in cancer survivors. PMR. 2011;3:1041–54.
57. Leduc O, Klein P, Demaret P, et al. Dynamic pressure variation under bandages with different stiffness. In: Vascular medicine: proceedings. Amsterdam: Elsevier Science; 1993. p. 465–8.
58. Liu AK, Macy ME, Foreman NK. Bevacizumab as therapy for radiation necrosis in four children with pontine gliomas. Int J Radiat Oncol Biol Phys. 2009;75:1148–54.
59. Marks JE, Wong J. The risk of cerebral radionecrosis in relation to dose, time, and fractionation: a follow-up study. Prog Exp Tumor Res. 1985;29:210–8.
60. Moretti M, Torre P, Antonello RM, et al. Neuropsychological evaluation of late-onset post-radiotherapy encephalopathy: a comparison with vascular dementia. J Neurol Sci. 2005;229–230:195–200.
61. Jr C, Shapiro CL, Ng A, et al. American society of clinical oncology clinical evidence review on the ongoing care of adult cancer survivors: cardiac and pulmonary late effects. J Clin Oncol. 2007;25:3991–4008.
62. Dropcho EJ. Neurotoxicity of radiation therapy. Neurol Clin. 2010;28:217–324.
63. Libschitz HI, DuBrow RA, Loyer EM, Charnsangavej C. Radiation change in normal organs: an overview of body imaging. Eur Radiol. 1996;6:786–95.
64. Johansson S, Svensson H, Denekamp J. Timescale of evolution of late radiation injury after postoperative radiotherapy of breast cancer patients. Int J Radiat Oncol Biol Phys. 2000;48:754–0.
65. Johansson S, Svensson H, Denekamp J. Dose response and latency for radiation-induced fibrosis, edema, and neuropathy in breast cancer patients. Int J Radiat Oncol Biol Phys. 2000;52:1207–19.
66. Zackrisson B, Mercke C, Strander H, Wennerberg J, Cavalin-Stahl E. A systematic overview of radiation therapy effects in head and neck cancer. Acta Oncol. 2003;42:443–61.
67. Fajardo LF. The pathology of ionizing radiation as defined by morphologic patterns. Acta Oncol. 2005;44:13–22.
68. Gillette EL, LaRue SM, Gillette SM. Normal tissue tolerance and management of radiation injury. Semin Vet Med Surg. 1995;10:209–13.
69. Baron R, Binder A, Wasner G. Neuropathic pain: diagnosis, pathophysiological mechanisms, and treatment. Lancet Neurol. 2010;9:807–19.
70. Heinricher MM, Tavares I, Leith JL, Lumb BM. Descending control of nociception: specificity, recruitment and plasticity. Brain Res Rev. 2009;60:214–25.
71. Chan CK, Lee HY, Choi WC, Cho JY, Lee SH. Cervical cord compression presenting with sciatica-like leg pain. Eur Spine J. 2011;20:S217–21.
72. Jaeckle KA. Neurologic manifestations of neoplastic and radiation-induced plexopathies. Semin Neurol. 2010;30:254–62.
73. Hsia AW, Katz JS, Hancock SL, Peterson K. Post-irradiation polyradiculopathy mimics leptomeningeal tumor on MRI. Neurology. 2003;60:1694–6.
74. Miller TM, Layzer RB. Muscle cramps. Muscle Nerve. 2005;32:431–42.
75. Stubblefield MD, Levine A, Custodio CM, Fitzpatrick T. The role of botulinum toxin type A in the radiation fibrosis syndrome: a preliminary report. Arch Phys Med Rehabil. 2008;89:417–21.
76. Shah JP, Danoff JV, Desai MJ, et al. Biochemicals associated with pain and inflammation are elevated in sites near to and remote from active myofascial trigger points. Arch Phys Med Rehabil. 2008;89:16–23.

77. Engleman MA, Woloschak G, Small W Jr. Radiation-induced skeletal injury. Cancer Treat Res. 2006;128:155–69.
78. Spoudes HA. Growth and endocrine function after chemotherapy and radiotherapy in childhood. Eur J Cancer. 2002;38:1748–59.
79. Stava CJ, Jimenez C, Hu MI, Vassilopoulou-Sellin R. Skeletal sequelae of cancer and cancer treatment. J Cancer Surviv. 2009;3:75–88.
80. Appels C, Geokoop R. Dropped-head syndrome due to high-dose irradiation. J Rheumatol. 2009;34:666–9.
81. Rowin J, Cheng G, Lewis SL, Meriggioli MN. Late appearance of dropped-head syndrome after radiotherapy for Hodgkin's disease. Muscle Nerve. 2006;34:666–9.
82. Stubblefield MD, Burstein HJ, Burton AW, et al. NCCN task force report: management of neuropathy in cancer. J Natl Compr Cancer Netw. 2009;7:S1–S26.
83. Herrera JE, Stubblefield MD. Rotator cuff tendonitis in lymphedema: a retrospective case series. Arch Phys Med Rehabil. 2004;85:1939–42.
84. Dijkstra PU, Kalk WW, Roodenburg JL. Trismus in head and neck oncology: a systematic review. Oral Oncol. 2004;40:879–89.
85. Ichimura K, Tanaka T. Trismus in patients with malignant tumours in the head and neck. J Laryngol Otol. 1993;107:1017–20.
86. Buchbinder D, Currivan RB, Kaplan AJ, Urken ML. Mobilization regimens for the prevention of jaw hypomobility in irradiated patients: an analysis and comparison of two techniques. Med Oral Patol Oral Cir Bucal. 2007;43:389–94.
87. Huang ME, Cifu DX, Keyser-Marcus L. Functional outcomes after brain tumor and acute stroke: a comparative analysis. Arch Phys Med Rehabil. 1998;79(11):1386–90.
88. O'Dell MW, Barr K, Spanier D, Warnick RE. Functional outcomes of inpatient rehabilitation in persons with brain tumors. Arch Phys Med Rehabil. 1998;79:1530–4.
89. Cuccurullo SJ. Physical medicine and rehabilitation board review. 3rd ed. New York: Demos Medical; 2014.
90. Casley-Smith JR. The pathophysiology of lymphedema and the action of benzopyrones in reducing it. Lymphology. 1988;21:190–4.
91. Casley-Smith JR. Modern treatment for lymphedema. 5th ed. Malvern: The Lymphoedema Association of Australia Inc; 1997.
92. Wood TJ, Racano A, Yeung H, et al. Surgical management of bone metastases: quality of evidence and systematic review. Ann Surg Oncol. 2014;21:4081–9.
93. McKinley WO, Huang ME, Tewksbury MA. Neoplastic vs. traumatic spinal cord injury: an inpatient rehabilitation comparison. Am J Phys Phys Med Rehabil. 2000;79:138–44.
94. Silver JK. Cancer rehabilitation and prehabilitation may reduce disability and early retirement. Cancer. 2014;120:2072–6.
95. Huang GH, Ismail H, Murnane A, Kim P, Riedel B. Structures exercise program prior to major cancer surgery improves cardiopulmonary fitness: a retrospective cohort study. Support Care Cancer. 2016;24(5):2277–85. Epub 2015 Nov 21
96. Tsimopoulou I, Pasquali S, Howard R, Dasai A, Gourevitch D, Tolosa I, Vohra R. Psychological prehabilitation before cancer surgery: a systematic review. Ann Surg Oncol. 2015;22(13):4117–23.

Neuromuscular Medicine: Cancer Pain

41

Eric Leung

Introduction

Neuromuscular dysfunction in cancer is well recognized and is a major cause of pain and disability in this population [1–5]. Pain can be due to a compressive injury secondary to underlying tumor (local expansion, hematogenous spread, or lymphatic spread), paraneoplastic effects, complications of treatment strategies, or indirect effects of chronic illness and underlying medical conditions. Despite recent advancements in oncologic care and treatment, the development of pain secondary to neuromuscular injury continues to negatively influence patients' quality of life [3–5]. Potential efforts to prevent or decrease pain have limited evidence or efficacy [2]. Current recommended treatment strategies include a multidisciplinary approach with a combination of pharmacological and psychosocial treatment, behavioral education, physical therapy, and interventional pain procedures [1, 2].

Clinical and Pathophysiology Neuromuscular Pain

The neuromuscular system encompasses the entire peripheral nervous system, including the sensory and motor fibers of the peripheral nerve, neuromuscular junction, and the muscle itself. Injury of any segment of this system can lead to potential dysfunction and pain. Tumor growth or its infiltration can compress or invade underlying peripheral nerves, nerve plexuses, or other nervous structures. Immune responses toward the tumor can secondarily affect neuromuscular structures. Complications in treatment strategies can cause neuromuscular injury. Chemotherapy and radiation therapy are well known for their potential toxic effects [6, 7]. Chronic illness and underlying medical conditions, such as diabetic neuropathy, may worsen in the setting of growing tumor burden. Other secondary nutritional, vitamin or electrolyte depletion may precipitate the onset or worsening of underlying peripheral neuropathy.

Patients often characterize their neuromuscular pain as spontaneous pain, which can be sharp, shooting, electrical, lancinating, and burning in nature. This may be accompanied by weakness or discoordination [6]. Identification and characterization of the pain pattern and localization are crucial for diagnosis; however, symptoms may vary in presentation and therefore can be inconsistent with classic presentations of pain syndromes. Electrodiagnostic tools, such as nerve conduction studies (NCS) and needle electromyography (EMG), assist in the confirmation and localization of injury to the neuromuscular system [8]. Nerve conduction studies and needle electromyography provide objective information to assess the function of the peripheral nervous system. In cancer survivors, injury to the neuromuscular system can occur in all levels, including the anterior horn cells, primary sensory neurons (dorsal root ganglion), nerve roots, nervous plexus (brachial and lumbosacral), peripheral nerves, neuromuscular junction, and the muscle. Electrodiagnostic testing, in conjunction with a detailed clinical evaluation, is useful in the localization of a lesion and determining the chronicity and severity of existing neuromuscular disorders [8, 9].

Electrodiagnosis: Nerve Conduction Studies and Needle Electromyography

Electrodiagnostic testing is generally divided into nerve conduction studies (NCS) and needle electromyography (EMG). NCS are routinely performed prior to needle examination; depending on the abnormalities found, muscle sampling can be planned. NCS are performed by stimulating the peripheral nerves through an electrical impulse, which generates an action potential via depolarization. The action potential is

E. Leung (✉)
Department of Physical Medicine and Rehabilitation,
Northwell Health, Manhasset, NY, USA
e-mail: eleung2@northwell.edu

A. Gulati et al. (eds.), *Essentials of Interventional Cancer Pain Management*, https://doi.org/10.1007/978-3-319-99684-4_41

detected by a recording electrode that transmits the impulse to an amplifier within the EMG machine to be analyzed.

Nerve conduction studies are subdivided into motor and sensory responses. Many peripheral nerves can be studied; however, there are some limitations. Large myelinated fibers can only be recorded in traditional NCS. Small myelinated fibers (Aδ) and unmyelinated fibers (C) that generally transmit pain cannot be recorded with these studies [9].

For motor NCS, a recording electrode is placed over the muscle innervated by the targeted peripheral nerve. The nerve is then stimulated proximally and distally with supramaximal stimulation. This generates an action potential (CMAP) that is amplified and displayed within the screen of the computer. Specialized software will document several measurements including amplitude, latencies, and conduction velocity. The amplitude (measured in millivolts) and area of the CMAP are related to the number and size of muscle fibers in the muscle group. The onset latency (measured in milliseconds) represents the nerve conduction time from the stimulus site to the neuromuscular junction (NMJ), the time delay across the NMJ, and the depolarization time across the muscle. The conduction velocity is a measure of speed of the fastest conducting motor axons and is calculated by comparing the difference in latency between the proximal and distal stimulation of the nerve being studied.

In contrast to motor NCS, in which the CMAP reflects conduction along the nerve, NMJ, and muscle, sensory nerve action potential (SNAP) only assess conduction along the nerve fiber. The SNAP represents the summated action potential of individual sensory nerve fibers, and the amplitude, generally much smaller than CMAP amplitude, is measured in microvolts. The smaller amplitudes, although technically more difficult to obtain, are more sensitive to peripheral nervous system disorders [9]. Other recorded parameters include onset and peak latency (measured in milliseconds) and conduction velocity. It is important to note that SNAP remain normal in lesions proximal to the dorsal root ganglia including lesions of the nerve roots, spinal cord, and brain. Patients may report sensory symptoms or sensory loss but may have normal SNAP [8].

Both motor and sensory NCS help assess the function of distal segments of the peripheral nervous system. Abnormalities in these studies can identify and localize focal sites of injury and characterize any pathophysiology of the distal peripheral nervous system. To evaluate more proximal segments, additional nerve conduction studies are performed. These studies are referred to as late responses, which consist of the F response and H response. F responses are small CMAPs recorded over distal muscles following motor nerve stimulation. When the nerve is stimulated, an action potential is generated which travels both orthodromically (along the path of normal nerve transmission) and antidromically (opposite the path of normal nerve transmission). The action potential traveling orthodromically will result in a standard CMAP. The antidromic action potential will travel toward the anterior horn cell, whereupon it will cause the adjacent anterior horn cells to depolarize. Subsequently, those action potentials will then travel orthodromically until they reach the recorded muscle, generating a CMAP of much smaller amplitude, about 1–5% of the amplitude. Each F response varies in latency and amplitude. Minimal F response latency is recorded and compared side to side. The H response (or H-reflex) involves a low submaximal stimulation to selectively activate Ia muscle fibers. The sensory action potential subsequently travels orthodromically to the spinal cord and synapses and creates a motor arc action potential that travels orthodromically to the muscle. Minimal H response latency is recorded and compared side to side. Both the F and H response helps assess proximal structures of the peripheral nerve. Careful consideration must be done when interpreting abnormalities of late responses. Although abnormal prolonged responses or asymmetry from side to side are seen in proximal lesions such as radiculopathy or plexopathy, these abnormalities are not specific to any given lesion, since they can also be abnormal in neuromuscular junction disorders and polyneuropathies [9].

There are a variety of additional nerve conduction studies, which can be performed in patients with other suspected neuromuscular disorders. Repetitive nerve conduction studies are a specialized technique that evaluates suspected neuromuscular junction disorders such as myasthenia gravis or Lambert-Eaton myasthenic syndrome. The blink reflex evaluates cranial nerves V (trigeminal) and VII (facial) along their proximal segments and connections in the pons and medulla. It is useful for detecting abnormalities along the cranial nerves as well as central lesions in the brainstem [9].

Following nerve conduction studies, intramuscular needle EMG is employed for further evaluation of the motor unit. EMG is the recording of electrical activity of muscle fibers within the motor unit action potentials (MUAP). A motor unit is defined as a single motor neuron, from the anterior horn cell body, the axon and its branches, the neuromuscular junction, and all of the muscle fibers it innervates [8]. EMG can distinguish motor neuron, peripheral nerve, NMJ, and muscle disease. Clinical evaluation and data gathered from NCS help guide which muscles are studied.

The needle EMG examination begins with the assessment of insertional activity. As the needle is advanced through the muscle, muscle fibers depolarize in a brief burst of activity, which is normal. Increased insertional activity lasting longer than 300 ms can been seen in both neuropathic and myopathic conditions. Insertional activity may be decreased if the muscle has been replaced by fat or fibrous connective tissue, as seen in certain myopathies.

From here, the needle EMG examination is typically divided into two sections. They are the analysis of spontaneous activity and recruitment of muscle fibers during muscle contractions. Spontaneous activity is the presence of any activity during muscle relaxation and originates from a variety of source generators with each source generator associated with a specific morphology. Table 41.1 lists abnormal spontaneous potential discharges and their characteristics.

After assessing for insertional and spontaneous activity, the examination proceeds to assess the morphology, stability, and firing characteristic of the MUAP. Muscle fibers are volitionally activated and recorded (this process is called recruitment). MUAP morphology parameters include stability, duration, amplitude, and number of phases and turns. As the muscle contracts, either motor units can increase their firing rate or additional motor units are recruited. Typically, the ratio of firing frequency to the number of different MUAP firing is approximately 5:1 (i.e., as the first MUAP firing frequency reaches 10 Hz, a second MUAP should begin to fire). Changes in the MUAP morphology or recruitment can indicate existence of a neuromuscular disorder (see Table 41.2).

It is important to note that electrodiagnostic testing has its limitations, and combinations of neuromuscular disorders may complicate the interpretation. Taken together, abnormalities seen with NCS and needle EMG in patients with cancer pain can help identify and characterize any potential peripheral nervous system disorder in the cancer patient.

Interpretation of Electrodiagnostic Studies in Cancer: Radiculopathies

Radiculopathy is defined as an injury to the spinal nerve root associated with either structural (compression) or nonstructural abnormalities. Like the general population, patients with cancer can develop radiculopathy secondary to compression (i.e., herniated nucleus pulposus, degeneration of uncovertebral joints or zygapophyseal joints, hypermobility of segments within the spine, stenosis of the spine). Other causes of radiculopathy in patients with cancer include tumors of the spine, tumors of adjacent soft tissue, and infection (secondary to a vulnerable immune system). Compression of the nerve root, particularly from vertebral metastasis, is the most common etiology of associated nerve root compression as a result of cancer, occurring in 5–10% of patients with malignancy [10]. The types of malignancy most commonly associated with this are breast, prostate, and lung cancer [11]. Primary spine tumors such as multiple myeloma typically spare the posterior ele-

Table 41.1 The below table is a summary of abnormal spontaneous activity, its morphology, source generator, and clinical correlates

Potential	Source generator	Characteristic	Causes
Fibrillations	Spontaneous discharge of muscle fiber	*Stability:* stable *Firing rate:* 0.5–10 Hz *Firing pattern:* regular	Active denervation associated with neuropathic disorders (i.e., radiculopathies); can also be seen in some muscle disorders (i.e., dystrophy)
Positive sharp waves	Spontaneous discharge of muscle fiber	*Stability:* stable *Firing rate:* 0.5–10 Hz *Firing pattern:* regular	Accompany fibrillations
Myotonic discharge	Spontaneous discharge of muscle fiber	*Stability:* wax/wanes *Firing rate:* 20–150 Hz *Firing pattern:* wax/wanes	Seen in myotonic dystrophy, paramyotonia congenita, and myopathies
Complex repetitive discharge	Time-linked multiple muscle fiber discharge	*Stability:* stable *Firing rate:* 5–100 Hz *Firing pattern:* regular	Chronic neuropathy and myopathic disorders
Fasciculation	Involuntary discharge of individual motor unit	*Stability:* stable *Firing rate:* 0.1–10 Hz *Firing pattern:* irregular	Anterior horn cell pathology, lower motor neuron disease (i.e., ALS) Can be seen in radiculopathy, polyneuropathy, and entrapment neuropathy
Doublets, triplets, multiplets	Motor unit action potential that fires in groups	*Stability:* stable *Firing rate:* 1–50 Hz *Firing pattern:* burst	Hypocalcemia, tetany Can also be present with fasciculations
Myokymic discharge	Grouped fasciculations	*Stability:* stable *Firing rate:* 1–5 Hz interburst 5–60 Hz intraburst *Firing Pattern:* burst	Radiation-induced nerve damage Can also be present infrequently in radiculopathy and entrapment neuropathy Facial myokymia can be seen in brain stem lesions (i.e., multiple sclerosis) and after radiation
Neuromyotinic discharge	Spontaneous activity generated at the motor unit	*Stability:* decrement *Firing rate:* 150–250 Hz *Firing pattern:* waning	Common in neuromyotonic syndromes but can also be seen in myasthenia gravis and various malignancies and inflammatory demyelinating polyneuropathies

Table 41.2 The below table summarizes the variability in the morphology and firing pattern of abnormal MUAP. Neuromuscular junction disorders are not listed.

Morphology			Firing pattern		
Duration	*Amplitude*	*Phases*	*Activation*	*Recruitment*	
NL	NL	NL	NL	NL	Neuropathic – demyelinating (slowing of CV)
NL	NL	NL	NL	Dec	Neuropathic – demyelinating (conduction block)
NL	NL	NL	NL	Dec	Acute neuropathy
Incr	Incr	Incr	NL	Dec	Chronic neuropathy
Dec	Dec	Incr	NL	NL/Early	Acute myopathic
Incr/Dec	Incr/Dec	Incr	NL	Dec	Chronic myopathic
Incr/Dec	Incr/Dec	Incr	NL	Significant Dec	End-stage myopathic
NL	NL	NL	Significant Dec	NL	CNS disorder

NL normal

ments in the spine; however, extradural extension with subsequent nerve root compression can occur [9]. Primary intradural spinal cord tumors (2–4% of all CNS neoplasms) can potentially extend along the nerve roots and cause radicular pain.

Non-compressive sources of radiculopathy include adverse effects from radiation or chemotherapy, paraneoplastic syndromes, and acute polyradiculoneuritis [10]. Clinical symptoms of radiculopathy include pain and sensory loss in a dermatomal distribution as well as weakness in the muscles innervated by the affected nerve. MRI is the most sensitive and specific test to evaluate spinal lesions caused by cancer; however, non-compressive lesions may not be seen by MRI. Electrodiagnostic studies typically demonstrate normal sensory responses, abnormal or delayed late responses (F waves and H-reflex), and needle EMG abnormalities depending on severity and timing of the lesion found.

In the acute to subacute period, there may be evidence of increased insertional activity and spontaneous activity, with acute neuropathic changes (see Tables 41.1 and 41.2). In the chronic period, spontaneous activity may be absent with chronic neuropathic changes on MUAP. The electrodiagnostic definition of radiculopathy is given when proximal and distal muscles innervated by the same myotome, but by different peripheral nerves, demonstrate needle abnormalities [9]. Evaluation of the paraspinal muscle during EMG sampling may also assist in the diagnosis of radiculopathy.

Ganglionopathy

Dorsal root ganglion dysfunction can occur as part of a subgroup of peripheral nervous system disorders in patients with cancer and is associated with a paraneoplastic neurological syndrome [11]. This syndrome is referred to as subacute sensory neuronopathy. Clinically, patients will present with a loss of vibratory sensation and proprioception, followed by paresthesia and pain. Other characteristics include ataxia, asymmetric distribution of sensory loss. Neurological deficits initially affect one extremity and can be misdiagnosed as radiculopathy or polyneuropathy. This syndrome is thought to be due to an antitumor immune reaction localized at the dorsal root ganglion and is associated with anti-Hu antibodies [12]. Tumors often associated with this syndrome include breast, prostate, and colon cancer, lymphoma, and small cell lung cancer (most common). Electrodiagnostic testing demonstrates reduced or absent sensory potentials (at least 3 SNAP with 30% normal amplitude) with normal or borderline motor nerve conduction velocities (less than 2 abnormal CMAP) [12].

Plexopathy

Nervous plexuses (cervical, brachial, and lumbosacral) may be significantly affected in patients with cancer. A plexus injury most commonly occurs from direct tumor infiltration and compression or via effects of radiation therapy. Direct tumor infiltration can be secondary to primary neoplastic plexopathies (i.e., schwannomas, neurofibromas) or external tumors that invade the plexus. Overall, the brachial plexus is most commonly affected, with the lumbosacral plexus being second [13, 14]. Clinical features of plexopathy reflect the location of injury and the nervous branches affected. In patients with metastatic plexopathies, severe pain is often the most significant clinical feature. Other impairments include weakness and decreased sensation. In the cervical plexus, pain radiating to the neck, shoulder, or throat is the primary symptom. Sensory dysfunction and weakness can occur, with weakness affecting the trapezius, sternocleidomastoid, and deep cervical muscles. In the brachial and lumbar plexus, the distribution pain and neurological deficits vary depending on the part of the plexus being most significantly affected. MRI imaging is the modality of choice to evaluate extent of the lesion. Electrodiagnostic testing can help further define and localize the lesion, as well as differentiate between tumor recurrence and radiation fibrosis. The studies typically have a variety of abnormal

Table 41.3 NCS and EMG findings of brachial plexopathy

Brachial plexopathy		
	NCS findings	EMG findings
Panplexus	Decreased/absent SNAP of all sensory nerves in the entire arm	Entire arm affected with sparing of muscles innervated directly from the nerve roots (rhomboids and serratus anterior, paraspinal muscles)
Upper trunk	Decreased/absent SNAP in axillary and lateral antebrachial cutaneous nerves, radial and median sensory branches to thumb and index finger Median and ulnar NCS and F responses are normal	Abnormal in C5–C6 innervated muscles (deltoid, biceps, brachioradialis, supraspinatus, and infraspinatus). Partial upper trunk innervations (protator, triceps may be affected). There is sparing of the muscles innervated by proximal C5 roots such as rhomboids and paraspinals
Middle trunk	Decreased/absent SNAP in the middle finger (sensory branch of median nerve) and posterior forearm (posterior cutaneous nerve of the forearm of radial nerve)	Abnormal in C7 innervated muscles (triceps, flexor carpi radialis, and pronator teres). There is sparing of paraspinals muscles innervated by C7
Lower trunk	Decreased/absent SNAP of the medial aspect of the arm, corresponding to the ulnar, dorsal ulnar, and medial antebrachial cutaneous nerves Median and ulnar motor NCS and F responses may be abnormal	Weakness in C8–T1 innervated muscles (abductor pollicis brevis, flexor digitorum profundus, extensor indicis proprius). There is sparing of the paraspinals innervated by C8 and T1
Lateral cord	Decreased/absent SNAP of the lateral antebrachial cutaneous nerve and median sensory to the thumb or middle finger	Abnormal in biceps and proximal forearm muscles Distal forearm and hand muscles such as flexor pollicis longus and abductor pollicis brevis are normal. Other C5 and C6 innervated muscles such as deltoid, triceps, and paraspinals are spared
Posterior cord	Decreased/absent SNAP of the radial sensory nerve. Radial motor NCS at the EIP may be abnormal	Abnormal in all radially innervated muscles, extensor indicis proprius, brachioradialis, and triceps. May also see abnormalities in deltoid, teres minor, and latissimus dorsi. There is sparing of the paraspinal muscles
Medial cord	Same as the lower trunk	Same as lower trunk *except* radially innervated C8 muscles are normal (extensor indicis proprius). There is sparing of the paraspinal muscles

Table 41.4 NCS and EMG findings of lumbosacral plexopathy

Lumbosacral		
	NCS findings	EMG findings
Upper plexus	Decreased/absent saphenous, lateral femoral cutaneous nerve sensory NCS Decreased/absent femoral motor NCS	Abnormal in muscles innervated by the femoral and obturator nerve (iliacus, vastus lateralis, vastus medialis oblique, adductor longus, brevis, and magus) Tibialis anterior and gluteus medius may be affected as they receive partial innervation from the upper plexus Normal paraspinal muscle sampling
Lower plexus	Decreased/absent superficial peroneal and sural sensory NCS Decreased/absent peroneal, tibial motor NCS and F, H response	Abnormal in muscles innervated by the sciatic, peroneal, tibial, and superior and inferior gluteal nerves (tibialis anterior, peroneus longus, medial gastrocnemius, tibialis posterior, biceps femoris, gluteus maximus, tensor fasciae latae, gluteus medius) Normal paraspinal muscle sampling

findings depending on location and extent of involvement (see Tables 41.3 and 41.4).

In addition to tumor infiltration and compression, nervous plexuses can be affected by radiation treatment. This condition was first described in 1964 and is commonly called radiation plexopathy [10]. Radiation-induced plexopathy can occur from 3 months to 26 years post radiation therapy (XRT) and is thought to be secondary to demyelination, impaired circulation, and fibrosis of the nerve fibers. Clinically, radiation plexopathy presents with paresthesia and pain typically developing later on the course. Risk factors include higher XRT doses and fraction size, utilization of three-field technique, concomitant chemotherapy, and susceptibility of the underlying tissue [13, 15]. In patients with history of malignancy and XRT, it can be difficult to distinguish between radiation plexopathy versus tumor recurrence. Features suggestive of radiation plexopathy in the electrodiagnostic evaluation include demyelinating conduction block, fasciculation, and, most classically, myokymic discharges [16]. MRI imaging can demonstrate homogenous enhancement or signal abnormality of muscles and other structures without nodularity [15]. The presence of these findings, however, does not rule out tumor recurrence as these conditions can occur concomitantly.

Mononeuropathy

Mononeuropathy is defined as a focal injury to a peripheral nerve and generally occurs in isolation. If several nerves are affected concomitantly, this systemic process is referred to as mononeuropathy multiplex. The diagnosis is established based on the clinical features and electrodiagnostic studies. Outside that of the general population, common causes of mononeuropathy in patients with cancer include compression or infiltration of a nerve from tumor, radiation therapy, and external compression of superficial nerves (especially in patients with history of weight loss and loss of subcutaneous tissue/fat) [10, 17]. Depending on the location of the compression, electrodiagnostic studies typically demonstrate abnormal NCS and EMG in the distribution of the affected nerve distal to the compressive lesion. Abnormal NCS will typically demonstrate axonal loss (decreased amplitudes) and/or demyelination (focal slowing, conduction block, or both) features across the site of lesion, such as in an entrapment neuropathy (i.e., CTS) [9]. Affected muscles will demonstrate neuropathic EMG findings (see Table 41.2). Myokymia may be present in radiation-induced neuropathy [16]. It is important to differentiate between mononeuropathy, plexopathy, and polyneuropathy as clinical and electrodiagnostic findings can be similar.

Peripheral Neuropathy

Peripheral neuropathy refers to a systemic symmetric nerve injury affecting the longest and most distal nerve endings [9]. These nerve endings can be motor, autonomic, sensory, or all three. Clinical features of peripheral neuropathy can include pain, sensory loss, dysesthesia, numbness, and imbalance. Other findings may include distal weakness and atrophy which represent motor nerve involvement. In patients with cancer, common etiologies of peripheral neuropathy include chemotherapy-induced peripheral neuropathy, neuropathy associated with monoclonal gammopathies/lymphoproliferative disease, and amyloid neuropathy [10]. Other causes of peripheral neuropathy include worsening systemic disease processes such as diabetes mellitus and electrolyte or vitamin deficiencies.

Abnormalities found in nerve conduction studies may be seen in both motor and sensory fibers, affecting some or all of the components of the NCS such as delayed distal latencies, decreased amplitudes, slow conduction velocities, and prolonged late responses. When CMAP amplitudes are decreased, needle abnormalities may be seen in the muscles affected by these fibers most commonly seen in the distal musculature of the limbs.

Chemotherapy-Induced Peripheral Neuropathy

Chemotherapy-induced peripheral neuropathy (CIPN) is a common cause of peripheral neuropathy and is an adverse effect of cytotoxic agents. Of the chemotherapy agents, the most common groups known to cause CIPN are the vinca alkaloids (i.e., vincristine), platinum compounds (i.e., cisplatin), Taxol (i.e., paclitaxel), and proteasome inhibitor bortezomib [18, 19]. CIPN occurs in about 30–40% of patients; however, the incidence has been reported to be as high as 70% [20]. Symptoms usually are consistent with sensory changes (pain and paresthesia) but may vary depending on the type of chemotherapy. Symptoms typically resolve following the cessation of treatment; however, CIPN may persist for months (coasting) and, in some cases, can be permanent [18, 20]. Depending on the severity and functional impairments, oncologists may decide to decrease or stop chemotherapy treatment [21]. Patients at increased risk for developing CIPN are those receiving high cumulative dose of chemotherapy, on long duration of therapy, on concomitant neurotoxic agents, older age, pre-existing nerve damage, renal and hepatic insufficiency, and patients with genetic vulnerability to these agents. Electrodiagnostic findings are consistent with symmetric peripheral sensorimotor polyneuropathy. A related syndrome named paclitaxel subacute pain syndrome [18] is a constitution of arthralgias and myalgias associated with initiation of placitaxol and typically resolves after 7 days of treatment. Although the exact cause of this syndrome is unknown, it is thought to be neuropathic in nature.

The research in the prevention of CIPN has been largely inconsistent [20]. Antidepressants such as duloxetine and venlafaxine has shown some efficacy in decreasing the incidence of CIPN [20, 22]. Other trials of anticonvulsants, calcium, magnesium, vitamin E, glutathione, acetyl-l-carnitine, and amitriptyline have demonstrated mixed results [20]. Treatment of CIPN in literature is also limited with inconsistent results. Overall, antidepressants (such as duloxetine and venlafaxine) and pregabalin demonstrate modest improvement in pain in patients with CIPN [20]. Other studies evaluating alternative neuropathic medications including gabapentin, tricyclic antidepressants demonstrate minimal or conflicting results. Topical creams such as menthol and baclofen/amitriptyline/ketamine mixture demonstrate improvement as compared to placebo in small studies [23]. Other treatment modalities that have been explored include acupuncture, transcutaneous electrical stimulation, and spinal cord stimulation for refractory neuropathic pain secondary to CIPN [24, 25]. Although the evidence is of low grade, initial studies seem promising. Larger, high-quality studies should be performed to evaluate the efficacy of these treatment modalities.

Neuromuscular Junction and Myopathy

Neuromuscular junction syndromes and myopathies typically present with progressive fatigue, proximal weakness, and sparing of sensory abnormalities; however, symptoms can also progress into myalgia and pain. The most common neuromuscular junction disorders in cancer patients are myasthenia gravis (seen more commonly in thymoma) and Lambert-Eaton myasthenic syndrome (seen more commonly in SCLC) [10]. These neuromuscular junction disorders are caused by autoantibodies directed against the NMJ. NCS may demonstrate fluctuant CMAP on repetitive stimulation with normal SNAP. Needle EMG may reveal motor unit instability and subtle myopathic change in proximal muscles.

Myopathy in cancer may occur directly secondary to tumor invasion, paraneoplastic effects (necrotizing myopathy, dermatomyositis, polymyositis, amyloid), or therapy-induced (such as steroid myopathy and chemotherapy-induced myopathy) [10]. NCS abnormalities may include low CMAP amplitudes if severe and normal SNAPs. Needle examination will reveal abnormal spontaneous activity in the presence of inflammatory myopathies with early recruitment, decreased duration, and amplitudes upon muscle activation.

Treatment

Neuromuscular pain disorders can be challenging to treat and require a multidisciplinary approach. A multimodal program with oral medications, physical therapy, modalities, psychosocial treatment, behavioral education, interventional pain procedures, and potential surgery is recommended. For those with metastatic disease, radiation therapy may also be a palliative option [2]. Treatment recommendations vary depending on the neuromuscular pain disorder. Pharmacologic agents include opioids, adjuvant analgesics, nonsteroidal anti-inflammatory drugs, and muscle relaxants. Overall, there is limited data for these agents in treatment of cancer-related neuromuscular pain [2, 26]. A systematic review found mixed evidence in the role of anticonvulsants, tricyclic antidepressants, and opioids for neuropathic pain in cancer [2]. Selective norepinephrine reuptake inhibitors (SNRI), such as duloxetine, have been recently studied and found to have some potential for treatment of painful chemotherapy-induced neuropathy. NSAIDs and muscle relaxants may help with pain control in patients with cancer. Topical analgesics, such as menthol cream and compounded creams (ketamine/amitriptyline/baclofen), demonstrate promise in treatment of neuromuscular pain [23].

Psychosocial support and behavioral interventions for neuropathic pain disorders include cognitive-based therapy, breathing exercises, relaxation, imagery or hypnosis, psychosocial support, and education [27–29]. There has been data supporting its positive benefit in cancer pain and in cancer survivors, although the significance of its effect is not clear [29]. Despite the limited data, it is recommended that these services should be offered.

Physical therapy and general exercise may be effective in treatment of myofascial pain and neuropathic pain [30–33]. Treatments employed by a physical therapist include therapeutic massage, activity modification, range of motion and strengthening exercises, energy conservation, and work simplification. Mobility of the affected area increases the strength of involved muscles as well as accessory muscles, which can improve coordination and sensory integration [30, 31]. Hypersensitivity can be treated with desensitization techniques, contrast baths, and contrast textures. Other modalities like decongestive therapy, transcutaneous electrical stimulation, magnetic therapy, and cold therapy may help with pain desensitization [34]. General exercise and physical activity has been shown to reduce neuropathic pain and sensory dysfunction in peripheral neuropathy [32].

Interventional pain procedures, like chemodenervation, peripheral nerve blocks and ablations, sympathetic nerve blocks, epidural injections, and neuromodulation, can aid in the treatment of neuromuscular pain. Chemodenervation with botulinum toxin has been shown to decrease neuropathic pain and muscle spasms in postsurgical and postradiation pain in cancer patients [35–37]. Peripheral nerve blocks, typically performed with image guidance, can aid in diagnosis of an affected nerve, and if successful in temporary pain relief, chemoneurolysis or thermoneurolysis can be performed for extended relief [38, 39]. Peripheral nerves typically targeted include intercostal nerves, spinal medial branches, and cutaneous sensory nerves. Sympathetic blocks and epidural steroid injections may transiently provide analgesia and decrease systemic medication use [38, 40]. Neuromodulation therapy includes spinal cord stimulation, peripheral nerve stimulation, deep brain stimulation, and motor cortex stimulation and is typically reserved for refractory neuropathic pain conditions [23, 24, 41]. Overall, there is limited data on the efficacy of these procedures in cancer-related pain, and current evidence is limited to mostly case reports and case series. Nevertheless, interventional options for neuromuscular pain are an expanding field and provide an alternative option if their pain is refractory to conventional methods.

Conclusion

Neuromuscular dysfunction in cancer is a major cause of pain and disability. Electrodiagnostics, in conjunction with a detailed clinical evaluation, can help localize and determine the chronicity and severity of neuromuscular disorders.

There is limited evidence on efficacy of all domains of treatment including pharmacological and psychosocial treatment, behavioral education, physical therapy, and interventional pain procedures. Thus, treatment may be challenging, and an interdisciplinary and multimodal program is recommended. Further studies should be performed to identify and expand on treatment for neuromuscular pain in patients with cancer.

References

1. Swarm RA, Abernethy AP, Anghelescu DL, et al. Adult cancer pain. J Natl Compr Cancer Netw. 2013;11(8):992–1022.
2. Denlinger CS, Ligibel JA, Are M, et al. Survivorship: pain version 1.2014. J Natl Compr Cancer Netw. 2014;12(4):488–500.
3. Pachman DR, Barton DL, Swetz KM, Loprinzi CL. Troublesome symptoms in cancer survivors: fatigue, insomnia, neuropathy, and pain. J Clin Oncol. 2012;30(30):3687–96.
4. Van den Beuken-van Everdingen MH, De rijke JM, Kessels AG, Schouten HC, Van kleef M, Patijn J. Prevalence of pain in patients with cancer: a systematic review of the past 40 years. Ann Oncol. 2007;18(9):1437–49.
5. Pachman DR, Barton DL, Watson JC, Loprinzi CL. Chemotherapy-induced peripheral neuropathy: prevention and treatment. Clin Pharmacol Ther. 2011;90(3):377–87.
6. Mehta N, Mehta A, Gulati A. Neuropathic pain in cancer. In: Stubblefield MD, O'Dell MW, editors. Cancer rehabilitation: principles and practice. New York: Demos Medical; 2009.
7. Jung BF, Herrmann D, Griggs J, Oaklander AL, Dworkin RH. Neuropathic pain associated with non-surgical treatment of breast cancer. Pain. 2005;118(1–2):10–4.
8. Custodio CM. Electrodiagnosis in cancer. In: Stubblefield MD, O'Dell MW, editors. Cancer rehabilitation: principles and practice. New York: Demos Medical; 2009.
9. Preston DC, Shapiro BE. Electromyography and neuromuscular disorders: clinical-electrophysiologic correlations. Philadelphia: Butterworth-Helnemann; 2005.
10. Stübgen JP. Neuromuscular disorders in systemic malignancy and its treatment. Muscle Nerve. 1995;18(6):636.
11. Sayko O, Dillingham T. Radiculopathy in cancer. In: Stubblefield MD, O'Dell MW, editors. Cancer rehabilitation: principles and practice. New York: Demos Medical; 2009.
12. Kuntzer T, Antoine JC, Steck AJ. Clinical features and pathophysiological basis of sensory neuronopathies (ganglionopathies). Muscle Nerve. 2004;30(3):255–68.
13. Ferrante MA. Plexopathy in cancer. In: Stubblefield MD, O'Dell MW, editors. Cancer rehabilitation: principles and practice. New York: Demos Medical; 2009.
14. Ladha SS, Spinner RJ, Suarez GA, Amrami KK, Dyck PJ. Neoplastic lumbosacral radiculoplexopathy in prostate cancer by direct perineural spread: an unusual entity. Muscle Nerve. 2006;34(5):659–65.
15. Delanian S, Lefaix JL, Pradat PF. Radiation-induced neuropathy in cancer survivors. Radiother Oncol. 2012;105(3):273–82.
16. Shin HY, Park HJ, Choi YC, Kim SM. Clinical and electromyographic features of radiation-induced lower cranial neuropathy. Clin Neurophysiol. 2013;124(3):598–602.
17. Stubblefield MD, Kim A, Riedel ER, Ibanez K. Carpal tunnel syndrome in breast cancer survivors with upper extremity lymphedema. Muscle Nerve. 2015;51(6):864–9.
18. Quasthoff S, Hartung HP. Chemotherapy-induced peripheral neuropathy. J Neurol. 2002;249(1):9–17.
19. Lehky TJ, Leonard GD, Wilson RH, Grem JL, Floeter MK. Oxaliplatin-induced neurotoxicity: acute hyperexcitability and chronic neuropathy. Muscle Nerve. 2004;29(3):387–92.
20. Hershman DL, Lacchetti C, Dworkin RH, et al. Prevention and management of chemotherapy-induced peripheral neuropathy in survivors of adult cancers: American Society of Clinical Oncology clinical practice guideline. J Clin Oncol. 2014;32(18):1941–67.
21. Postma TJ, Heimans JJ. Grading of chemotherapy-induced peripheral neuropathy. Ann Oncol. 2000;11:509–13.
22. Smith EM, Pang H, Cirrincione C, et al. Effect of duloxetine on pain, function, and quality of life among patients with chemotherapy-induced painful peripheral neuropathy: a randomized clinical trial. JAMA. 2013;309(13):1359–67.
23. Barton DL, et al. A double blind placebo controlled trial of a topical treatment for chemotherapy-induced peripheral neuropathy: NCCTG trial N06CA. Support Care Cancer. 2011;19:833–41.
24. Cata JP, Cordella JV, Burton AW, Hassenbusch SJ, Weng HR, Dougherty PM. Spinal cord stimulation relieves chemotherapy-induced pain: a clinical case report. J Pain Symptom Manag. 2004;27(1):72–8.
25. Abd-elsayed A, Schiavoni N, Sachdeva H. Efficacy of spinal cord stimulators in treating peripheral neuropathy: a case series. J Clin Anesth. 2016;28:74–7.
26. Koyyalagunta D, Bruera E, Solanki DR, et al. A systematic review of randomized trials on the effectiveness of opioids for cancer pain. Pain Physician. 2012;15(3 Suppl):ES39–58.
27. Cassileth BR, Keefe FJ. Integrative and behavioral approaches to the treatment of cancer-related neuropathic pain. Oncologist. 2010;15(Suppl 2):19–23.
28. Montgomery GH, Weltz CR, Seltz M, Bovbjerg DH. Brief presurgery hypnosis reduces distress and pain in excisional breast biopsy patients. Int J Clin Exp Hypn. 2002;50(1):17–32.
29. Sheinfeld gorin S, Krebs P, Badr H, et al. Meta-analysis of psychosocial interventions to reduce pain in patients with cancer. J Clin Oncol. 2012;30(5):539–47.
30. Santiago-Palma J, Payne R. Palliative care and rehabilitation. Cancer. 2001;92:1049–52.
31. Paice JA. Mechanisms and management of neuropathic pain in cancer. J Support Oncol. 2003;1(2):107–20.
32. Kumar SP, Adhikari P, Jeganathan PS, D'Souza SC. Physiotherapy management of painful diabetic peripheral neuropathy: a current concepts review of treatment methods for clinical decision-making in practice and research. Int J Curr Res Rev. 2010;2:29–39.
33. Dobson JL, Mcmillan J, Li L. Benefits of exercise intervention in reducing neuropathic pain. Front Cell Neurosci. 2014;8:102.
34. Raphael J, Hester J, Ahmedzai S, et al. Cancer pain: part 2: physical, interventional and complimentary therapies; management in the community; acute, treatment-related and complex cancer pain: a perspective from the British pain society endorsed by the UK

Association of Palliative Medicine and the Royal College of general practitioners. Pain Med. 2010;11(6):872–96.
35. Rostami R, Mittal SO, Radmand R, Jabbari B. Incobotulinum toxin-a improves post-surgical and post-radiation pain in cancer patients. Toxins (Basel). 2016;8(1):E22.
36. Dessy LA, Maruccia M, Mazzocchi M, Scuderi N. Treatment of post mastectomy pain syndrome after mastopexy with botulinum toxin. J Plast Reconstr Aesthet Surg. 2014;67(6):873–4.
37. Fabregat G, Asensio-samper JM, Palmisani S, Villanueva-pérez VL, De andrés J. Subcutaneous botulinum toxin for chronic post-thoracotomy pain. Pain Pract. 2013;13(3):231–4.
38. Andima L, Gulati A, Cubert K. Interventional pain management in the patient with cancer. In: Stubblefield MD, O'Dell MW, editors. Cancer rehabilitation: principles and practice. New York: Demos Medical; 2009.
39. Wisotzky EM, Saini V, Kao C. Ultrasound-guided intercostobrachial nerve block for intercostobrachial neuralgia in breast cancer patients: a case series. PM R. 2016;8(3):273–7.
40. Mishra S, Rana SP, Upadhyay SP, Bhatnagar S. Use of epidural steroid as an adjuvant in neuropathic cancer pain management: a case report. Am J Hosp Palliat Care. 2010;27(7):482–5.
41. Stadler JA, Ellens DJ, Rosenow JM. Deep brain stimulation and motor cortical stimulation for neuropathic pain. Curr Pain Headache Rep. 2011;15(1):8–13.

Cancer-Related Pelvic Pain

42

Sarah Hwang and Megan Clark

Introduction

Chronic pelvic pain (CPP) is defined as pain in the region of the pelvis for greater than 6 months. It may involve visceral or somatic system and encompass structures supplied by the nervous system from the tenth thoracic spinal level and below [1, 2]. More specifically, this pain can be located between the umbilicus and the thighs. Chronic pelvic pain carries a broad differential diagnosis, including gynecologic, urologic, gastrointestinal, neurologic, and musculoskeletal systems. Estimated prevalence for causes of CPP was reported to be 50–80% dysmotility disorders (including irritable bowel syndrome), 30–70% musculoskeletal disorders, 5–10% urological diagnoses, <5% advanced endometriosis and/or dense bowel adhesions, 30–50% multiple medical diagnoses, and <5% with no identifiable medical diagnosis [3].

One of the musculoskeletal causes of CPP is levator muscle spasm or high tone pelvic floor dysfunction. Literature suggests that the pelvic floor muscles contribute to CPP as both the primary pain generator and as a compensatory contributor [4, 5]. This theory also applies to cancer-related pelvic pain. Pelvic floor dysfunction (PFD) may occur because of inherent musculoskeletal causes in the pelvic floor muscles, ligaments, and tendons or as a functional adaptation to other disorders within the pelvis-hip-spine complex.

Gynecologic cancers were estimated to comprise over 94,000 new cases of cancer in the United States in 2015. Uterine cancer is the most common of the gynecologic cancers, followed by ovarian, cervical, and vulvar cancers. In males, cancers related to the reproductive organs were estimated to total over 230,000 cases in 2015, the great majority being prostate cancer, which is the second most diagnosed cancer in males. Less frequent are testicular and penile cancers [6].

Cancer-related pelvic pain is a symptom that can be seen at any point through the spectrum of a patient's pre-diagnosis, diagnosis, and treatment of certain cancers. In the cancer patient, pelvic pain can be related to the involvement of viscera and neural or pelvic musculature and develop as the only presenting feature for the patient prior to diagnosis, a symptom secondary to the involvement of the tumor itself, or side effect of treatments. Although most commonly seen in gynecologic cancers, pelvic pain has been described in multiple settings, including prostate and colorectal cancers. It is important to remember the potential comorbid psychological diagnoses, which are commonly present in cancer patients. In the general population, up to 60% of patients with referral for CPP were found to have psychological diagnoses (depression 25–50%, somatoform disorders 10–20%, anxiety disorders 10–20%, and multiple psychological diagnoses 20–30%) [3]. Depression, anxiety, and self-image disorders following a diagnosis of cancer are common and can impact a patient's subjective pain.

Anatomy

The pelvis is composed of a bony ring, which serves as a site for multiple cartilaginous, ligamentous, and tendon attachments [7]. The female pelvis is smaller, shallower, and wider than the male pelvis. While this is crucial for pregnancy and childbirth, it can also lead to an increase in injuries that can occur in the female pelvis. The sacroiliac joints are located posterior to the pelvis, while the pubic symphysis is located anteriorly; ligaments stabilize these joints. Extending from the sacrum is the coccyx, which acts as an important ligamentous and tendinous anchor.

The pelvic floor is composed of muscles, ligaments, and fascia that act as a sling to support the bladder, reproductive organs, and rectum. The pelvic floor muscles (PFM) are

S. Hwang (✉)
Shirley Ryan AbilityLab, Chicago, IL, USA
e-mail: shwang@sralab.org

M. Clark
University of Kansas, Department of Physical Medicine and Rehabilitation, Kansas City, KS, USA
e-mail: mclark11@kumc.edu

A. Gulati et al. (eds.), *Essentials of Interventional Cancer Pain Management*, https://doi.org/10.1007/978-3-319-99684-4_42

divided into three layers: the superficial perineal layer, the deep urogenital diaphragm layer, and the pelvic diaphragm. The superficial PFM are the bulbospongiosus, ischiocavernosus, and superficial transverse perineal muscles. The deep urogenital diaphragm contains the compressor urethra, the uterovaginal sphincter, and the deep transverse perineal muscles. The deep PFM that line the inner walls of the pelvis are the levator ani and coccygeus, which along with the endopelvic fascia comprise the pelvic diaphragm. The levator ani is muscle group composed of three muscles – the puborectalis, pubococcygeus, and iliococcygeus. The levator ani muscle originates lateral to the pubic symphysis on the posterior surface of the superior ramus and inserts onto the inner surface of the spine of the ischium. The muscle fibers of the levator ani attach to the coccyx and anus, the rectum and the sphincter muscles, and the sides of the vagina. The coccygeus muscle is triangular in shape and is located posterior to the levator ani. This muscle reinforces the posterior pelvic floor, arising from the ischial spine and inserting on the lower sacral-coccygeal bones and is contiguous with the sacrospinous ligament. The perineal body or central perineal tendon is located between the vagina and anus. This is a site where the pelvic muscles and sphincters converge to provide support to the pelvic floor. Lining the lateral walls of the pelvis, the piriformis muscle arises from the anterior sacrum, with the sacrotuberous ligament, and attaches on the superior border of the greater trochanter. The obturator internus arises from the pelvic surfaces of the ilium, ischium, and obturator membrane. It attaches just distally to the piriformis on the greater trochanter. Levator ani is separated from obturator internus by the arcus tendineus.

The PFM receive innervation through somatic, visceral, and central pathways. The skin of the lower trunk, perineum, and proximal thigh is innervated by the iliohypogastric, ilioinguinal, and genitofemoral nerves via the lumbar plexus. Arising from the ventral branches of S2–4 of the sacral plexus, the pudendal nerve passes between the piriformis and coccygeal muscles as it traverses through the greater sciatic foramen, over the spine of the ischium and back into the pelvis through the lesser sciatic foramen. It courses along the lateral wall of the ischiorectal fossa (Alcock's canal). The three main terminal branches of the pudendal nerve include the inferior rectal nerve, the perineal nerve, and the dorsal nerve of the penis/clitoris. The pudendal nerve innervates the penis/clitoris, the bulbospongiosus and ischiocavernosus muscles, the anterior portions of the levator ani muscles, the perineum, the anus, the external anal sphincter, and the urethral sphincter. This nerve contributes to many important functions, including external genital sensation, continence, orgasm, and ejaculation. Muscles of the levator ani are thought to have direct innervation from sacral nerve roots S3–5 [8].

History and Physical Exam

The history and physical exam are important tools in evaluating a person with CPP. A thorough history of the person's cancer diagnosis and treatments is important, including use of surgical intervention, chemotherapy, and radiation. Onset of pain in relation to these treatments can also help in diagnosis. The patient should be questioned about their pain – onset, mechanism of onset, location, quality, intensity, frequency, aggravating and relieving factors, quality, and radiation of pain. It is also very important to understand any previous treatments they have undergone to manage their pain. This may include medications, physical therapy, interventional procedures, or surgeries. Table 42.1 illustrates important questions regarding various organ systems that may be involved in the patient's pain complaints. A bladder diary may be beneficial in evaluating the patient's urinary habits and fluid intake. Another extremely important aspect of the history includes questioning the patient about any history of abuse, including physical, emotional, verbal, or sexual abuse.

The physical exam should be guided by the patient's complaints but should typically include a neurologic and musculoskeletal exam focusing on the lumbar spine, hips, pelvic girdle, lower extremities, and pelvic floor muscles. Palpation of the pubic symphysis as well as the muscular insertion sites should be included, as should an examination of the sacroiliac joints, including provocative testing. Gluteus medius and piriformis muscles should be palpated, evaluating for tenderness as well as spasm of the muscle. Disorders of the hip can mimic pelvic floor spasm or be a causative factor to the development of pelvic floor spasm. Evaluating for intra-articular hip disorder is important. Evaluation should include gait, range of motion, and provocative testing (may include log roll, FABER, hip impingement testing).

An abdominal exam should be included in any patient presenting with pelvic pain. Examiner should palpate for scar tissue, hernias, and masses. The iliopsoas tendon and iliacus should also be palpated.

A pelvic floor exam may include both vaginal and rectal exam to assess pelvic floor muscle function. Visceral structures are typically not examined during a pelvic floor exam. Verbal consent from the patient is required. The exam begins with inspection of the external genitalia to assess for any rashes, swelling, cysts, scars, or lesions. During external inspection, the examiner should also assess PFM function by having the patient perform a voluntary pelvic floor muscle contraction (known as a Kegel contraction) with voluntary relaxation after the contraction, perform an involuntary contraction (by coughing), and finally perform involuntary relaxation (using the Valsalva maneuver). The examiner should visualize the lift of the perineal body during contraction of the pelvic floor and the decent of the perineal body

Table 42.1 Important aspects of the history for patients with chronic pelvic pain

Bladder
How many times per day do you typically urinate or how often do you urinate (frequency)?
When you have to urinate, do you feel like you have to get to the toilet immediately (urgency)?
What do you drink throughout the day (specifically, how much and what beverages)? What do you drink after dinner?
Do you feel like you are emptying your bladder completely?
Do you have difficulty starting the flow of urine?
Do you have pain with urination?
Do you ever experience urinary incontinence or leaking?
With coughing and sneezing? With standing from a chair? With exercise?
Do you ever have difficulty making it to the toilet in time?
Do you have incontinence during intercourse?
Are you ever incontinent at night while sleeping?
How often are you incontinent?
Do you wear a pad? If yes, how often do you change the pad?
How many times do you get up at night to urinate?
Do you have frequent urinary tract infections?
Bowel
Are you constipated?
How often do you have a bowel movement (BM)?
Have you ever been diagnosed with irritable bowel syndrome (IBS)?
Do you have to strain to empty?
Do you ever have to push from your vagina in order to have a BM?
Do you feel like you have to continue to wipe more than normal in order to get yourself clean?
Are your stools hard or soft?
Do you have pain during or after a BM?
Gynecologic
Are your periods regular?
Do you wear tampons? Is it painful to wear tampons?
Are gynecologic exams painful for you?
Have you ever been diagnosed with endometriosis?
Do you have problems with chronic yeast infections?
Are you sexually active?
Do you have pain with intercourse?
When it is painful (initial penetration, deeper penetration)?
Do you have pain after intercourse? If so, how long does this last?
Is it painful when you orgasm?
Obstetric
How many times have you been pregnant?
How many children have you had?
What was the largest birth weight?
Did you have pain during pregnancy?
How long were you in labor? How long did you push?
Did you have tearing or an episiotomy?
Did the delivery require use of vacuum or forceps?
Any complications during labor and delivery?
Psychiatric
Do you have a history of depression or anxiety?
Have you ever been hospitalized for psychiatric illness?
Have you ever had thoughts of killing yourself?
Have you ever been the victim of abuse (physical, sexual, emotional, verbal)?

during relaxation or Valsalva. During this inspection, the examiner should also assess for pelvic organ prolapse. An external sensory exam of the S2–5 sacral dermatomes is performed, and the anal wink reflex is tested to assess the sacral reflex arc. The Q-tip test is performed to assess for vulvodynia by lightly touching a cotton swab inside the vestibule. The test is positive if it elicits allodynia. Finally, the superficial pelvic floor muscles (bulbospongiosus, ischiocavernosus, and superficial transverse perineal muscles) are palpated to assess for tenderness.

The internal pelvic floor exam is best performed on a flat table without the use of stirrups or speculum. The vaginal exam is performed with the patient supine with the knees bent and ankles hip-width apart. Once lubricated, a gloved finger is inserted into the vaginal introitus to palpate the pelvic floor muscles internally. A clock face diagram can be used to correctly describe the anatomic positions of the PFM, with the pubic bone being the 12 o'clock position and the anus and coccyx being the 6 o'clock position. The rectal exam is typically performed in the left lateral decubitus position. The levator ani can be palpated on vaginal from the 1 to 5 o'clock position on the patient's left and the 7 to 11 o'clock position on the patient's right side. Levator ani can also be palpated during the rectal exam. The obturator internus is located at the 3 o'clock and 9 o'clock positions and is separated from the levator ani by the arcus tendineus, which, on palpation, feels like a guitar string. Location of the obturator internus can be confirmed by having the patient externally rotate their hip to activate the muscle (which will cause it to bulge under the examiner's finger). Coccygeus, piriformis, and puborectalis muscles can be palpated on vaginal exam in certain patients but typically require rectal exam for further assessment. The tone of the anal sphincter is also assessed on rectal exam. Finally, the coccyx can be examined during the rectal exam, including assessment for tenderness, mobility, and any deviation.

The PFM are assessed for tenderness, spasm, trigger points, tone, taut bands, and scar tissue. Next, the examiner should perform an exam of the function of the PFM internally. Contraction of the PFM results in a squeezing and lifting of the muscles around the examiner's finger. Muscle strength testing should be performed in four quadrants. Endurance should be assessed up to 10 s, and the examiner should be mindful of relaxation after the contraction as well. Another assessment of muscle strength is to have the patient perform "quick flicks" where the patient attempts to contract-release-contract-release. After the strength exam is finished, the patient should be asked to bear down or attempt to push out the examiner's finger. This will allow the examiner to assess for PFM relaxation as well as the presence of pelvic organ prolapse.

Cancer-Related Pelvic Pain

Endometrial Cancer

Endometrial cancer is the most common gynecologic malignancy in Western countries with an estimated 54,870 new cases in the United States in 2015 [9]. Surgery is the primary treatment for most patients, with the standard surgical approach including hysterectomy and bilateral salpingo-oophorectomy (BSO), with surgical staging with selective pelvic and para-aortic lymphadenectomy [10]. The current standard of care involves minimally invasive surgery with improved blood loss, postoperative pain, complications, and length of hospital stay compared to laparotomy [11]. There have been several studies evaluating sexual dysfunction, particularly dyspareunia, in women with a history of endometrial cancer. Aerts et al. [12] found that women who underwent surgery without adjuvant therapy for endometrial cancer had significantly more entry dyspareunia at 1 and 2 years compared to women who had undergone hysterectomy for benign conditions. Adjuvant therapy with radiotherapy and/or chemotherapy is recommended in patients with higher risk of recurrence and higher stage disease. Radiation therapy is often completed with vaginal brachytherapy (VBT) or external beam radiotherapy (EBRT), but both have been noted to have significant side effects including vaginal stenosis and shortening, fibrosis, and dyspareunia [13, 14].

Cervical Cancer

Cancer of the cervix is the third most common cancer among women worldwide, with a higher incidence in developing countries as compared to developed countries [15]. In the United States, cervical cancer accounts for approximately 13% of all gynecologic cancers [6]. With the introduction of screening programs, the disease is often detected earlier thus leading to majority of patients being diagnosed at a relatively young age [16]. Most survivors therefore live for many years with the sequelae of the disease and its treatment [17].

Surgical treatment can include cervical conization, simple hysterectomy, or radical hysterectomy with pelvic lymphadenectomy depending on the stage of the cancer and tumor characteristics. Radical hysterectomy is associated with greater residual side effects including sexual function and bowel and bladder function [18]. The pelvic floor dysfunction that occurs after radical hysterectomy may be related to autonomic nerve damage during surgery [19]. Morbidities following surgery can be reduced with less radical, nerve-sparing surgery [10].

Radiation therapy with vaginal brachytherapy (VBT) or external beam radiation therapy (EBRT) can also be utilized as a primary and/or adjuvant treatment with or without chemotherapy. Research has shown that the addition of chemotherapy to radiotherapy results in not only an absolute improvement in overall survival but also a significant reduction in local recurrence for all stages of the disease [20–22]. Unfortunately, while beneficial to the overall survival, radiation therapy, whether used as primary or adjuvant treatment, has been associated with greater sexual dysfunction and vaginal toxicity compared to surgery alone [18]. Chemoradiation can result in ovarian failure and early menopause, leading to a decrease in vaginal lubrication, a decrease in tissue elasticity, and weakness of the pelvic floor muscles [23]. De Noronha et al. reported that women who underwent radical hysterectomy were less likely to report dyspareunia as compared to women who underwent radiotherapy or chemoradiation [24]. It is also not surprising that women in the radiotherapy and chemoradiation groups had significantly shorter vaginal length as compared to women in the radical hysterectomy group which may lead to the increased reports of dyspareunia in these groups.

Ovarian Cancer

Although it only accounts for 3% of cancers in women, ovarian cancer is responsible for more deaths than any other gynecologic cancer [6]. Because of the typically advanced stage at presentation, treatment consists of a sequence of surgery and chemotherapy. Surgical options include hysterectomy, bilateral salpingo-oophorectomy (BSO), omentectomy, lymphadenectomy, and tumor debulking. With any significant gynecological surgery, the risk of intraperitoneal adhesions is greater. Bukovic et al. reported that women who underwent chemotherapy alone or chemotherapy along with surgical treatment had more pronounced sexual dissatisfaction, with the most common complaint being dyspareunia [25]. Secondary effects of intraperitoneal adhesions can include chronic pelvic pain, dyspareunia, subfertility, and bowel obstruction. Although multiple agents have been trialed to prevent formation of adhesions after gynecological pelvic surgery, based on current reviews, there is not adequate data on subsequent pelvic pain, fertility outcomes, quality of life, or safety [26].

Vulvar Cancer

Vulvar cancer comprises approximately 5% of gynecologic malignancies [6]. Although previously seen primarily in older women, vulvar cancer has been increasing among younger women secondary to human papillomavirus infections [27]. Primary surgery, radiotherapy, or a combination of the two can be used depending on the size, location, and concern for metastases to lymph nodes [28]. Lymphadenectomy may also be needed as a part of surgical management, but complete groin dissection is associated with infection and wound breakdown in 20–40% of patients and secondary lymphedema in approximately 30% of patients [29]. After surgery, women may experience physical changes including vaginal narrowing, numbness along the scar, removal of the clitoris, and alterations in the tissue quality [30]. As noted above for the other types of gynecologic cancers, radiation therapy to the pelvic organs can result in vaginal toxicity and decreased sexual function.

Prostate Cancer

Prostate cancer is the second most common cancer in men, with an estimated 220,800 new cases in the United States in 2015 [6]. Treatment options vary based on stage and grade of the cancer as well as patient characteristics. In older men (over age 75 years) or those with less aggressive tumors, active surveillance is a reasonable option [31, 32]. More than half of men ages 64 or younger are initially treated with radical prostatectomy. The most common treatment in men ages 65–74 years is radiation therapy. Some men undergo a combination of surgery and radiation. Treatment may also involve hormonal therapy (androgen deprivation). More advanced disease may be treated with hormone therapy, chemotherapy, bone-directed therapy (zoledronic acid or denosumab), radiation therapy, or some combination of these. Over 90% of the time, diagnosis of prostate cancer is made while the disease is in the local or regional stages. In this group, 5-year survival rates approach 100% [15]. While the survival rate has improved greatly over the years, nearly half of all men treated with radiation for prostate cancer have sexual dysfunction [33, 34]. Urinary incontinence and erectile dysfunction have been well-described as side effects [35]. Although addressed less in the literature, pelvic pain after treatment of prostate cancer is seen clinically.

Other Sequelae of Cancer Treatment

Premature ovarian failure can be triggered by high doses of alkylating chemotherapy, moderate doses of radiation to the ovaries, or bilateral oophorectomy. When menopause symptoms are triggered by cancer treatment, the symptoms can occur abruptly, with higher intensity and more prolonged symptoms. Estrogen deprivation results in a decreased elasticity of genital tissue and loss of lubrication, which in turn leads to vaginal dryness and discomfort. Vaginal atrophy can interfere with sexual pleasure but also may make surveillance pelvic exams more painful and difficult for the women to tolerate [36].

Treatment

When determining treatment plans for pelvic pain, the ability to determine the etiology will help to guide management. However, for many cases the etiology will remain unknown or multifactorial. General treatment for chronic pelvic pain, as recommended by a Cochrane review, includes hormonal treatments, counseling after negative ultrasound, multidisciplinary approach to pain management, physical therapy, psychotherapy, diet, and environmental factors [37]. While this can provide a foundation for treatment options, the cancer patient can face additional treatment obstacles and comorbidities, which require individualized treatment plans.

Vaginal Dryness, Stenosis, and Atrophy

Following pelvic radiation, providers will often recommend the use of vaginal dilators to prevent vaginal stenosis. In some cases, dilators are used in the acute phase, either during or immediately after radiation. While there are few studies on this topic, results from studies of the effectiveness of dilators do not appear to support this practice [38]. Occasional penetration may prevent the walls of the vagina from adhering to each other; however regular dilation may increase the inflammatory response resulting in worsening of scarring and fibrosis. Dilators are likely more beneficial for long-term treatment of vaginal stenosis related to radiation therapy when used after the inflammatory phase immediately following radiation [38]. Regular sexual activity can also help maintain vaginal health. One study, by Carter et al., recommends using a vaginal dilator or having intercourse two to three times per week [36].

Topical vaginal moisturizers can be used several times a week to improve tissue quality, comfort, and overall vaginal health [36]. The goal of their use is to hydrate the vaginal mucosa by improving the balance of intracellular fluids in the vaginal epithelium and restore the vaginal pH [36]. Replens is a polycarbophil-based moisturizer that binds to the vaginal epithelium and allows for increased vaginal epithelium maturation. In a study by Bygdeman et al., Replens was compared to vaginal estrogen with equivalent improvement in dyspareunia and vaginal irritation [39]. While vaginal dryness was improved in both cases from baseline, vaginal estrogen was superior to Replens. Hyaluronic acid can also be used for water retention and lubricating properties [40]. In studies comparing vaginal estrogen and hyaluronic acid, there was improved vaginal atrophy and dryness with decreased vaginal symptoms and decreased pH with both.

Water- or silicone-based lubricants may also be used during sexual activity to reduce pain, dryness, irritation, and mucosal tears. These can be found over the counter and are recommended over petroleum-based lubricants, which are associated with increased risk of vaginal infection, damage to latex condoms, and vaginal odor. Similarly, lubricants with perfumes or flavors may also act as irritants [36]. These recommended lubricants can be used prior to sexual activity and can be reapplied several times as needed [36].

Currently, Osphena (ospemifene), a selective estrogen-receptor modulator, is the only FDA-approved, non-estrogen, oral pill for moderate to severe dyspareunia due to vulvovaginal atrophy in postmenopausal women. It has not been investigated in the cancer population at this time. Estrogen therapy, both vaginal and systemic, has been shown to be effective in the general population with dyspareunia and atrophy secondary to menopause [41]. However, reports from the Women's Health Initiative [42] stated the increased risks of coronary heart disease, stroke, and breast cancer outweigh the benefits from use of estrogen therapy. In patients with hormone-receptor-positive cancer, hormone replacement therapy is controversial. Although a few retrospective studies have previously not associated oral estrogen with increased risk of recurrence in early-stage endometrial cancer [43], further studies have been closed following the Women's Health Initiative results [44].

Topical lidocaine can be used in the treatment of severe penetrative dyspareunia. A small randomized controlled, double-blind trial was performed in breast cancer survivors. In these patients, the study concluded that lidocaine applied to the vulvar vestibular tissue prior to vaginal penetration reduced sexual distress and improved comfort with penetration [45]. No similar study has been completed in gynecologic cancer patients. Using lidocaine gel prior to physical therapy may reduce some of the discomfort associated with treatment.

Physical Therapy

Pelvic floor physical therapy including dilator training, pelvic floor muscle strengthening and relaxation exercises, intravaginal myofasical techniques, and biofeedback can help to correct muscle imbalance, improve blood flow, and increase flexibility of paravaginal tissue [46]. In a small prospective study of patient with vestibulodynia, patients who completed pelvic floor therapy had significant improvement in overall sexual function and reduction in pain with intercourse [46].

Pelvic floor physical therapy is used for myofascial pain and dysfunction with goals to restore muscle imbalance, improve function, and reduce pain. Often, therapy combines neuromuscular reeducation and soft tissue mobilization. Exercises to restore normal muscle movement patterns, strength, and range of motion can be utilized to help reeducate the patient [7]. Biofeedback can provide objective feedback about muscle activation with activity and at rest.

Trigger point manual release, acupressure, muscle energy, and strain-counterstrain can be used for myofascial trigger points. Trigger points can be in the pelvic floor muscles or the abdominal wall musculature.

Psychotherapy

It is important to address any comorbid depression and/or anxiety. Patients should be screened for depression, anxiety, and history of abuse. Appropriate patients should be referred to psychiatry, psychology, or cognitive behavioral therapy.

Pharmacology

In advanced stages of cancer, approximately 75% of patients report having pain [47]. Pharmacological therapy is the mainstay of cancer pain management. The World Health Organization (WHO) has a systematic analgesic ladder for management of cancer pain, and it has been noted to be 85–95% effective when used appropriately [48]. It should however be noted that chronic use of opioids has been reported to reduce the quality of life for cancer patients [49].

Generally, pharmacologic treatment in chronic pelvic pain is used to treat acute pain and secondary etiology such as depression, anxiety, and insomnia. Nonsteroidal anti-inflammatories may be used for acute onset of pelvic pain and musculoskeletal injuries. Neuropathic pain medications can be effective (gabapentin, pregabalin, serotonin-norepinephrine reuptake inhibitors, tricyclic antidepressants), especially when there is a neurogenic component to the patient's pelvic pain. These medications are also helpful in the treatment of central sensitization. Oral muscle relaxants may help reduce overall muscle tone that is perceived to be painful but is not specific for the pelvic floor.

Certain muscle relaxants, such as diazepam and baclofen, can be made into a suppository or compounded cream and used intravaginally. Vaginal diazepam is generally well tolerated, with the major side effect being drowsiness. In a retrospective review by Carrico and Peters, 67% of women reported no adverse effects from the vaginal diazepam, while 33% of women reported some drowsiness [50]. Lidocaine, as mentioned above, can be used topically. This medication is especially useful when used prior to intercourse. Lidocaine gel can also be used internally prior to physical therapy for patients that have trouble tolerating internal myofascial release of the pelvic floor muscles.

Interventional Management

Nerve Blocks

When therapeutic and medical management fails, alternative interventional pain management procedures may be required. Neurolytic blocks of ganglion can be effectively used in some cases. The ganglion impar, or ganglion of Walther, is found on the ventral surface of the coccyx where it forms the caudal origin of the bilateral sympathetic chain. It has sympathetic innervation to the perineal and anal regions, and block of this can disrupt afferent sympathetic and nociceptive signals from that area. In one small case study, nine patients with CPP who failed to respond to optimized pharmacologic management underwent block of the ganglion of Walther under fluoroscopic guidance with local anesthetic, steroid and pentoxifylline. In this study, four of the nine women had malignancy-related pelvic pain with a duration of their symptoms ranging from 1 to 7 years. The reported pain relief lasted from 4 weeks to 3 years and reported in four women to have "complete and permanent cessation of pain" [51].

Superior hypogastric plexus blocks (SHPB) with fluoroscopy or computed tomography (CT) guidance have also been used in malignant and non-oncological chronic pelvic pain [52]. The superior hypogastric plexus is a retroperitoneal structure extending below the aortic bifurcation in association with the common and internal iliac vessels. It innervates much of the pelvic viscera including the bladder, urethra, uterus, vagina, vulva, perineum, prostate, penis, testes, rectum, and descending colon. Classically a posterior approach to the SHPB had been used, but in 2005, Michalek and Dutka described two cases on an anterior approach for non-cancer pelvic pain [53]. Since that time, further studies have shown CT-guided anterior approach can be completed in a shorter duration with better patient satisfaction [54]. Anterior ultrasound-guided superior hypogastric plexus neurolysis (SHPN) has also been reported to be an effective option in pelvic cancer pain for patients with gynecological cancer. In a study by Mishra, 50 patients with advanced stage (stages III and IV) of gynecological malignancy were divided into two groups and given either oral morphine or underwent anterior ultrasonography (USG)-guided SHPN. Both groups continued to use as needed morphine for break through pain. The patients who had USG-guided SHPN showed greater improvement in baseline pain and decreased daily morphine consumption [55].

Pelvic Floor Trigger Point Injections

Trigger point injections have been described in myofascial pain, including CPP [56]. These injections can be beneficial when a patient presents with pelvic pain and is found to have a trigger point in the pelvic floor muscles. Trigger point injections are generally not used as a first-line treatment or monotherapy but are generally more beneficial when used alongside physical therapy, medication management, and behavioral therapy [56].

Pelvic Floor Botulinum Toxin Injections

For patients with refractory pelvic floor muscle spasm, botulinum toxin has been utilized to decrease spasm, therefore reducing pelvic pain. Botulinum toxin type A blocks the cholinergic transmission at the neuromuscular junction. Abbott et al. [57] performed a double-blinded randomized, placebo-controlled trial in patients with CPP and demonstrated a significant decrease in dyspareunia and non-menstrual pain in the botulinum toxin group. In addition, they reported a significant reduction in pelvic floor pressure in the botulinum toxin group when compared to the preinjection values. It is important to note that there were no statistically significant differences demonstrated between the groups in any of the previously mentioned parameters.

Neuromodulation

Neuromodulation has been also used as a treatment for CPP. Neuromodulation is a nondestructive technique that delivers electrical stimulation to the spinal cord or peripheral nerves for the treatment of pain. Patients with CPP may benefit from spinal cord stimulation, sacral stimulation, or peripheral nerve stimulation. Tibial nerve stimulation, which is an in-office weekly procedure, has shown some promise in the treatment of pelvic pain, fecal incontinence, and overactive bladder.

Conclusion

Chronic pelvic pain is a disorder that can be difficult to evaluate and treat. It is commonly seen in cancer patients and survivors and often requires a multidisciplinary approach. It is important to obtain a thorough history and physical to narrow down the cause or causes of the patient's pain. Once treatment is initiated, close follow-up is recommended to follow patient's progress.

References

1. Apte G, et al. Chronic female pelvic pain—part 1: clinical pathoanatomy and examination of the pelvic region. Pain Pract. 2012;12(2):88–110.
2. Stein SL. Chronic pelvic pain. Gastroenterol Clin N Am. 2013;42(4):785–800.
3. Reiter R. Evidence-based management of chronic pelvic pain. Clin Obstet Gynecol. 1998;41(2):422–35.
4. Tu FF, As-Sanie S, Steege JF. Musculoskeletal causes of chronic pelvic pain: a systematic review of diagnosis: part I. Obstet Gynecol Surv. 2005;60(6):379–85.
5. Mathias SD, et al. Chronic pelvic pain: prevalence, health-related quality of life, and economic correlates. Obstet Gynecol. 1996;87(3):321–7.
6. Howlader N, et al. SEER cancer statistics review, 1975–2012. Bethesda: National Cancer Institute; 2015.
7. Prather H, et al. Review of anatomy, evaluation, and treatment of musculoskeletal pelvic floor pain in women. PM R. 2009;1(4):346–58.
8. Barber MD, et al. Innervation of the female levator ani muscles. Am J Obstet Gynecol. 2002;187(1):64–71.
9. Siegel RL, Miller KD, Jemal A. Cancer statistics, 2015. CA Cancer J Clin. 2015;65(1):5–29.
10. Huffman LB, et al. Maintaining sexual health throughout gynecologic cancer survivorship: a comprehensive review and clinical guide. Gynecol Oncol. 2016;140(2):359–68.
11. Boggess JF, et al. A comparative study of 3 surgical methods for hysterectomy with staging for endometrial cancer: robotic assistance, laparoscopy, laparotomy. Am J Obstet Gynecol. 2008;199(4):360 e1–9.
12. L Aerts PE, J Verhaeghe W, Poppe I, Vergote FA. Sexual functioning in women after surgical treatment for endometrial cancer: a prospective controlled study. J Sex Med. 2015;12(1):198–209.
13. Katz A, et al. Early development of vaginal shortening during radiation therapy for endometrial or cervical cancer. Int J Gynecol Cancer. 2001;11(3):234–5.
14. Brand AH, Bull CA, Cakir B. Vaginal stenosis in patients treated with radiotherapy for carcinoma of the cervix. Int J Gynecol Cancer. 2006;16(1):288–93.
15. Jemal A, et al. Global cancer statistics. CA Cancer J Clin. 2011;61(2):69–90.
16. Jackson KS, Naik R. Pelvic floor dysfunction and radical hysterectomy. Int J Gynecol Cancer. 2006;16:354–63.
17. Park SY, et al. Quality of life and sexual problems in disease-free survivors of cervical cancer compared with the general population. Cancer. 2007;110(12):2716–25.
18. Greimel ER, et al. Quality of life and sexual functioning after cervical cancer treatment: a long-term follow-up study. Psychooncology. 2009;18(5):476–82.
19. Pieterse QD, et al. An observational longitudinal study to evaluate miction, defecation, and sexual function after radical hysterectomy with pelvic lymphadenectomy for early-stage cervical cancer. Int J Gynecol Cancer. 2006;16(3):1119–29.
20. Collaboration, C.f.C.C.M.-A. Reducing uncertainties about the effects of chemoradiotherapy for cervical cancer: a systematic review and meta-analysis of individual patient data from 18 randomized trials. J Clin Oncol. 2008;26(35):5802–12.
21. Green JA, et al. Concomitant chemotherapy and radiation therapy for cancer of the uterine cervix (review). Cochrane Database Syst Rev. 2005;3:CD002225.
22. Kirwan JM, et al. A systematic review of acute and late toxicity of concomitant chemoradiation for cervical cancer. Radiother Oncol. 2003;68:217–26.
23. Bruner DW, et al. Measurement of vaginal length: reliability of the vaginal sound—a gynecologic oncology group study. Int J Gynecol Cancer. 2006;16(5):1749–55.
24. Noronha AF, et al. Treatments for invasive carcinoma of the cervix: what are their impacts on the pelvic floor functions? Int Braz J Urol. 2013;39(1):46–54.
25. Buković D, et al. Sexual functioning and body image of patients treated for ovarian Cancer. Sex Disabil. 2008;26(2):63–73.
26. Hindocha A, Beere L, Dias S, Watson A, Ahmad G. Adhesion prevention agents for gynaecological surgery: an overview of Cochrane reviews. Cochrane Database Syst Rev. 2015. CD 011254.
27. Hampl M, et al. New aspects of vulvar cancer: changes in localization and age of onset. Gynecol Oncol. 2008;109(3):340–5.
28. Stehman FB, Look KY. Carcinoma of the vulva. Obstet Gynecol. 2006;107(3):719–33.
29. Gaarenstroom KN, et al. Postoperative complications after vulvectomy and inguinofemoral lymphadenectomy using separate groin incisions. Int J Gynecol Cancer. 2003;13(4):522–7.
30. Barlow EL, et al. Sexuality and body image following treatment for early-stage vulvar cancer: a qualitative study. J Adv Nurs. 2014;70(8):1856–66.
31. Albertsen PC, Hanley JA, Fine J. 20-year outcomes following conservative management of clinically localized prostate cancer. JAMA. 2005;293(17):2095–101.

32. Lu-Yao GL, et al. Outcomes of localized prostate cancer following conservative management. JAMA. 2009;302(11):1202–9.
33. Thor M, et al. Radiation dose to the penile structures and patient-reported sexual dysfunction in long-term prostate cancer survivors. J Sex Med. 2015;12(12):2388–97.
34. Budaus L, et al. Functional outcomes and complications following radiation therapy for prostate cancer: a critical analysis of the literature. Eur Urol. 2012;61:112–27.
35. Potosky AL, et al. Five-year outcomes after prostatectomy or radiotherapy for prostate cancer: the prostate cancer outcomes study. J Natl Cancer Inst. 2004;96(18):1358–67.
36. Carter J, Goldfrank D, Schover LR. Simple strategies for vaginal health promotion in cancer survivors. J Sex Med. 2011;8(2):549–59.
37. Stones RW, Mountfield J. Interventions for treating chronic pelvic pain in women. Cochrane Database Syst Rev. 2000. CD000387.
38. Johnson N, Miles TP, Cornes P. Dilating the vagina to prevent damage from radiotherapy: systematic review of the literature. BJOG. 2010;117(5):522–31.
39. Bygdeman M, Swahn ML. Replens versus Dienoestrol cream in the symptomatic treatment of vaginal atrophy in postmenopausal women. Maturitas. 1996;23(3):259–63.
40. Chen J, et al. Evaluation of the efficacy and safety of hyaluronic acid vaginal gel to ease vaginal dryness: a multicenter, randomized, controlled, open-label, parallel-group, clinical trial. J Sex Med. 2013;10(6):1575–84.
41. Suckling JA, et al. Local estrogen for vaginal atrophy in postmenopausal women. Cochrane Database Syst Rev. 2006. CD001500.
42. Writing Group for the Women's Health Initiative Investigators. Risks and benefits of estrogen plus progestin in healthy postmenopausal women principal results from the women's health initiative randomized controlled trial. JAMA. 2002;288(3):321–33.
43. Lee RB, Burke TW, Park RC. Estrogen replacement therapy following treatment for stage I endometrial carcinoma. Gynecol Oncol. 1990;36:189–91.
44. Barakat RR, et al. Randomized double-blind trial of estrogen replacement therapy versus placebo in stage I or II endometrial cancer: a gynecologic oncology group study. J Clin Oncol. 2006;24(4):587–92.
45. Goetsch MF, Lim JYC, B A. A practical solution for dyspareunia in breast cancer survivors: a randomized controlled trial. J Clin Oncol. 2015;33(30):3394–400.
46. Goldfinger C, et al. A prospective study of pelvic floor physical therapy: pain and psychosexual outcomes in provoked vestibulodynia. J Sex Med. 2009;6(7):1955–68.
47. Portenoy RK. Cancer pain. Epidemiology and syndromes. Cancer. 1989;63(11 Suppl):2298–307.
48. Schug SA, Zech D, Dorr U. Cancer pain management according to WHO analgesic guidelines. J Pain Symptom Manage. 1990;5(1):27–32.
49. Caraceni A, Portenoy RK. Pain management in patients with pancreatic carcinoma. Cancer. 1996;78(3 Suppl):639–53.
50. Carrico DJ, Peters KM. Vaginal diazepam use with urogenital pain/pelvic floor dysfunction: serum diazepam levels and efficacy data. Urol Nurs. 2011;31(5):279–84. 299
51. Malec-Milewska M, et al. Neurolytic block of ganglion of Walther for the management of chronic pelvic pain. Wideochir Inne Tech Maloinwazyjne. 2014;9(3):458–62.
52. de Leon-Casasola OA. Critical evaluation of chemical neurolysis of the sympathetic axis for cancer pain. Cancer Control. 2000;7(2):142–8.
53. Michalek P, Dutka J. Computed tomography-guided anterior approach to the superior hypogastric plexus for noncancer pelvic pain: a report of two cases. Clin J Pain. 2005;21(6):553–6.
54. Ghoneim AA, Mansour SM. Comparative study between computed tomography guided superior hypogastric plexus block and the classic posterior approach: a prospective randomized study. Saudi J Anaesth. 2014;8(3):378–83.
55. Mishra S, Bhatnagar S, Rana SP, Khurana D, Thulkar S. Efficacy of the anterior ultrasound-guided superior hypogastric plexus neurolysis in pelvic cancer pain in advanced gynecological cancer patients. Pain Med. 2013;14:837–42.
56. Moldwin RM, Fariello JY. Myofascial trigger points of the pelvic floor: associations with urological pain syndromes and treatment strategies including injection therapy. Curr Urol Rep. 2013;14(5):409–17.
57. Abbott JA, et al. Botulinum toxin type a for chronic pain and pelvic floor spasm in women: a randomized controlled trial. Obstet Gynecol. 2006;108(4):915–23.

Exercise Therapy and Fatigue Management

43

Jack B. Fu and Arash Asher

Abbreviations

CRF	Cancer-related fatigue
ECAM	Energy conservation and activity management
FACT-F	Functional Assessment of Cancer Therapy: Fatigue

Introduction

Fatigue is among the most common symptoms reported by cancer patients with an incidence between 25 and 99 [1]. A survey of 534 cancer patients and 91 physician experts revealed that fatigue was the most important symptom or concern for patients across all cancer types [2]. Cancer-related fatigue (CRF) may persist for years after cancer treatment in patients with no evidence of disease [1]. Most episodes of fatigue in the general population are self-limiting and are considered non-pathologic. Healthy fatigue is relieved by rest and sleep. Patients typically feel recharged and energized after sleep. Pathologic fatigue, e.g., CRF, causes severe impairments to an individual's functional activity and quality of life [3].

The National Comprehensive Cancer Network describes cancer-related fatigue as a distressing, persistent, and subjective sense of tiredness or exhaustion related to cancer or cancer treatment that is not proportional to recent activity and interferes with usual function [4]. It is markedly different in quality and severity from ordinary fatigue and is unrelieved by rest or sleep [5]. The term fatigue can encompass many subtypes that have different causes. Fatigue can be categorized into peripheral and central fatigue. Peripheral fatigue is due to a lack of response from the neuromuscular system after central stimulation (e.g., fatigability in the muscle itself). Central fatigue is characterized by a failure to transmit motor impulses or perform voluntary activities [6]. Cancer-related fatigue has been suggested to be both peripheral and central in nature [7].

CRF can have profound physical, psychosocial, and economic impacts. Cancer patients average 4.2 days of missed work per month, and caregivers average 4.5 days of missed work per month because of cancer-related fatigue [8].

Identification and Evaluation of Cancer-Related Fatigue

The National Comprehensive Cancer Network guidelines recommend that every cancer patient should be screened for fatigue [4]. Unfortunately, CRF is often underreported and overlooked by healthcare professionals [9–12]. The use of screening assessments can help clinicians assess the presence of fatigue, which is often included in many multi-symptom screening tools including the Edmonton Symptom and Assessment Scale and the MD Anderson Symptom Inventory. On a 1–10 scale, fatigue severity of more than 4 should be evaluated by further history and physical. Over 20 detailed fatigue measurement tools have been used to better delineate patient fatigue symptoms including the Brief Fatigue Inventory [13], Functional Assessment of Cancer Therapy: Fatigue or FACT-F [14], Revised Piper Fatigue Scale [15], and Multidimensional Fatigue Inventory [16].

In addition to fatigue measurement tools, a thorough history and physical are essential in the evaluation of CRF patients. Clinicians should discern the patient's cancer history including treatments and time since treatment. Current

J. B. Fu (✉)
Department of Palliative, Rehabilitation and Integrative Medicine, University of Texas MD Anderson Cancer Center, Houston, TX, USA
e-mail: jfu@mdanderson.org

A. Asher
Samuel Oschin Comprehensive Cancer Institute at Cedars-Sinai Medical Center, Los Angeles, CA, USA
e-mail: arash.asher@cshs.org

A. Gulati et al. (eds.), *Essentials of Interventional Cancer Pain Management*, https://doi.org/10.1007/978-3-319-99684-4_43

and past medications should be reviewed. Questions regarding confounding factors including sleep quality, stress, mood, etc. could be helpful. A physical examination should include a cardiac, pulmonary, neurologic, cognitive, and functional evaluation. A fatigue laboratory panel is among the initial screening tools for cancer-related fatigue. These fatigue panels may differ between institutions, but their purpose is to identify potentially treatable causes of fatigue. Elements of the fatigue laboratory panel used in the Supportive Care Center at MD Anderson Cancer Center include a cell blood count, electrolytes, folate, vitamin B12, thyroid-stimulating hormone, testosterone level (in males), erythrocyte sedimentation rate, and urinalysis.

Causes and Pathophysiology of Cancer-Related Fatigue

The causes of cancer-related fatigue are numerous. Most oncology patients are using medications that can be potentially sedating and contributing to fatigue. Medications for nausea, seizures, pain, anxiety, and depression are often culprits. Furthermore, these patients concurrently suffer from pancytopenia during treatment. Anemia and thrombocytopenia may contribute to fatigue [17]. Infections including urinary tract infections may cause fatigue, and genetic susceptibility to fatigue may play a role. Malnutrition, direct brain damage from cancer treatment, depression, and sleep disturbances may also lead to fatigue in cancer patients [18–21]. Hormonal changes including hypothyroidism, hypogonadism, and adrenal insufficiency during cancer treatment have also been implicated [22, 23]. Additionally, the effects of deconditioning and skeletal muscle weakness and atrophy are likely contributors [24]. Other implicated causes of cancer-related fatigue include electrolyte disturbances, cardiopulmonary dysfunction, renal dysfunction, and hepatic dysfunction [25].

Cancer fatigue is often found in association with other symptoms, which suggests a relationship due to common causative mechanisms. Research has found that systemic hyperinflammation may cause many symptoms including pain, insomnia, depression, anxiety, stress, poor appetite, cognitive dysfunction, loss of muscle mass, and fatigue. It is also important to note the interplay of these symptoms. While inflammation causes fatigue, the other associated symptoms (e.g., insomnia and depression) which could be caused by the same source are also contributing simultaneously. The cancer hyper-inflammatory state results in a polysymptom picture in patients [26–30].

The inflammatory process is regulated by immunomodulating proteins called cytokines. These proteins are released by immune and tumor cells during cancer treatment including chemotherapy and radiation therapy. It has also been found that these inflammatory cytokines are able to cross the blood-brain barrier through a variety of mechanisms which explains why patients who are receiving radiation in a peripheral extremity still experience fatigue [31].

Treatment of Cancer-Related Fatigue

Because of the interplay of cancer symptoms, treating conditions that could contribute to fatigue may improve fatigue. Insomnia, depression, and cachexia are commonly associated with fatigue and can intensify the feeling of fatigue. A nutrition evaluation and perhaps appetite stimulation for malnourished patients could be considered. Some research suggests that treating depression in cancer patients also results in improved fatigue [32–34]. Pain and fatigue often present together. Relaxation techniques, sleep hygiene, stimulus control (e.g., avoiding alcohol caffeine or alcohol shortly before bedtime), reduction of cognitive-emotional arousal (e.g., 1 h of pre-sleep relaxation routinely), and addressing sleep apnea may improve sleep quality and fatigue [35]. The use of sleep aids, antidepressants, appetite stimulants, and nutritional supplements has been studied with mixed results [7]. Neuro-stimulants, in particular methylphenidate, have also been studied in multiple placebo-controlled trials. The scientific evidence supporting the use of neuro-stimulants for CRF is still very preliminary with low absolute numbers. Further study is required [36].

A number of strategies have been used to try to reduce inflammation in hopes of treating cancer fatigue. Anti-inflammatory agents studies such as nonsteroid anti-inflammatory drugs have had conflicting results [37, 38].

The use of erythropoietic stimulants has been studied in multiple trials, and the evidence suggests that these agents do reduce fatigue in cancer patients with hemoglobin less than 10 grams/deciliter. The evidence is more limited in milder anemia [39–42].

Mechanism of Exercise as a Treatment for Fatigue

Exercise has multiple benefits in the general and cancer population. Heart and lung function, muscle strength, body composition, bone health, feelings of well-being, and perception of symptoms can all be positively affected through exercise. It may also play a role in cancer prevention and control [43]. Evidence supports physical activity in improving survival and reducing disease recurrence among cancer survivors [44]. The evidence is suggestive that exercise and rehabilitation programs result in sustained improvement in fatigue (in addition to other cancer symptoms) [45]. Exercise has been shown in multiple randomized control trials to be an effective treatment for CRF [46–48]. Exercise and physical activity in cancer patients has been shown to improve aerobic capacity, minimize muscle loss, improve body composition, and improve conditioning, in addition to psychologic benefits [49, 50].

One possible mechanism that has been gaining increased attention is the anti-inflammatory effects of exercise. Hyperinflammation likely causes many cancer symptoms. Exercise reduces inflammation through several factors:

1. Reduction in visceral fat mass: [51] TNF-α is a pro-inflammatory cytokine secreted by adipocytes, specifically visceral adipocytes. Conversely, there is some evidence that subcutaneous fat (i.e., not visceral) may secrete anti-inflammatory cytokines [52]. Studies have shown that visceral adipocyte-secreted pro-inflammatory cytokines are positively related to a sedentary lifestyle, adiposity, and low aerobic fitness [53]. Exercise can reduce visceral fat and waist circumference, thereby reducing pro-inflammatory cytokine release and resulting fatigue [54].
2. Contracting muscle produces IL-6, an anti-inflammatory cytokine: While visceral fat secretes pro-inflammatory cytokines, muscle produces anti-inflammatory cytokines, sometimes called myokines [55]. Studies have demonstrated up to a 12-fold increase in IL-6 (in this instance with an anti-inflammatory role) compared to rest in a study of patients on an exercise program [56].
3. Increasing levels of cortisol and adrenaline: Through stimulation of the hypothalamic-pituitary-adrenal axis, exercise has been shown to increase levels of cortisol and adrenaline through moderate- to high-intensity exercise [57, 58]. Both hormones have anti-inflammatory effects.
4. Inhibition of macrophage infiltration into adipose tissue: A sedentary lifestyle and accumulation of visceral adipose tissue leads to increased migration of macrophages into adipose tissue. These macrophages produce pro-inflammatory cytokines. This process has been implicated in the development of non-insulin-dependent diabetes mellitus and the metabolic syndrome [59, 60].
5. Downregulation of toll-like receptors on monocytes and macrophages: Toll-like receptors recognize pathogens and trigger the immune response. By reducing the expression of these receptors, the overall inflammatory state is reduced [61]. Reduction of C-reactive protein and IL-6 (both pro-inflammatory cytokines) has been demonstrated after therapeutic exercise programs for cancer patients [43, 62, 63].

Treating Fatigue with Exercise

Cancer patients with active disease can become deconditioned due to treatment, malnutrition, medical complications, and prolonged hospitalizations. Fatigue may be overwhelming and discourage patients from performing physical activity. Many cancer inpatients have been bed bound for extended periods of time. Encouraging patients to become active will help them with other medical considerations (including adequate pulmonary aeration, orthostasis, etc.) but also reduce their fatigue. Overcoming, the inertia of inactivity can be difficult for these patients. Initially, having severely debilitated patients sit in a chair and gradually increase the duration of sitting is helpful. Recumbent bikes which allow patients to exercise while sitting have been used in many cancer exercise programs. Figure 43.1 illustrates how inactivity and exercise can affect fatigue.

Organized group exercise programs can help encourage patient participation. Regularly administered physical and occupational therapy (at times under the supervision of a physiatrist) can also be of benefit.

For cancer survivors without evidence of disease, exercise guidelines have been developed by the American Heart Association, the American Cancer Society, the American College of Sports Medicine, and the United States Department of Health & Human Services. All the guidelines are fairly similar. With respect to aerobic exercise, the American College of Sports Medicine consensus statement recommends that cancer patients and survivors adhere to exercise guidelines for the general population. That recommendation consists of 150 min per week of moderate-intensity aerobic activity or 75 min of vigorous-intensity exercise or an equivalent combination. For strength training, 2–3 weekly sessions that include exercises for major muscle groups are recommended. For flexibility, stretching of major muscle

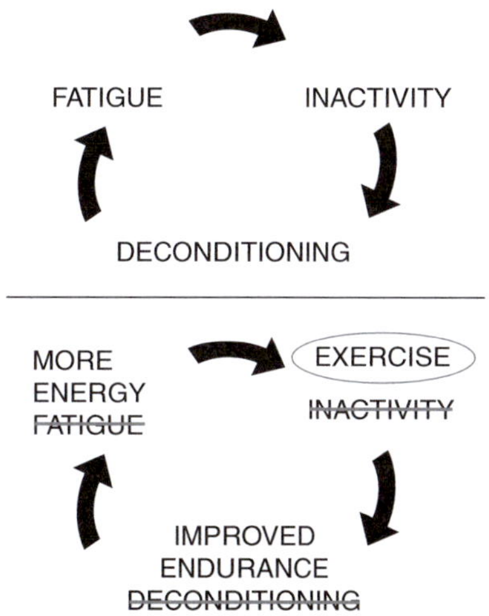

Fig. 43.1 An illustration of the effects of exercise on deconditioning and fatigue. The top diagram illustrates the cycle experienced by many cancer patients which consists of fatigue that discourages activity and worsens deconditioning. In the lower diagram, breaking this cycle with exercise can improve endurance, leading to more energy and greater tolerance of exercise [64]

groups and tendons occurs on days that other exercises are performed [43]. These guidelines are still fairly non-specific. Individualized treatment programs that are patient tailored by rehabilitation professionals are optimal.

Unfortunately, less than half of cancer survivors maintain their pre-diagnosis activity levels. It is often overlooked by healthcare professionals. Only 21.5% of cancer survivors can recall a discussion of exercise with their healthcare professional. This is compared to 24% of adults without cancer. However, 84% of survivors indicate that they would prefer to receive exercise counseling during their cancer experience [65]. Physical activity is a modifiable lifestyle with which the patient has significant control. Adequate education and support are needed to help the patient exercise adequately and safely.

Patient safety is an important consideration in any exercise plan. Cancer patients can suffer from numerous musculoskeletal and medical issues which affect exercise recommendations. However, excessive exercising may be detrimental. Gradual incremental increases in activity, including duration, frequency, and intensity, can improve both fatigue and mobility. Brown et al. found that exercise programs that were too intense led to worsening cancer fatigue [66].

The level of appropriate immune suppression can be challenging. While the negative effects of excessive hyperinflammation are quite clear, excessive immunosuppression in an already leukopenic patient could make the patient even more susceptible to infection. Runners who ran more than 866 miles/year have been found to have an increased rate of viral infection. These findings led to the proposal of a "J-shaped" curve to define the relationship of exercise and susceptibility to infection [67]. Patients should undergo an evaluation prior to starting an exercise program (Table 43.1).

Cancer patients undergoing rehabilitation and exercise program should be periodically monitored by healthcare professionals to insure optimal exercise programs and to address safety concerns. Communication between providers is vital. Letting therapists know what precautions are needed is critical. Structured prescriptions will help remind providers to mention necessary aspects of the exercise program including safety precautions [69].

Published exercise programs vary from group programs to supervised individual to self-directed individual programs. Structured rehabilitation programs result in sustained improvements in cancer survivors who have completed treatment without evidence of disease. A number of studies support the effectiveness of such programs [70].

Organized exercise programsoffer a variety of interventions including intense exercise, sports, psychoeducation, and physical modalities. The published evidence suggests that the psychological support and education associated with structured exercise programs can improve fatigue in cancer patients. Education consists of self-identifying fatigue and recommends optimizing sleep, exercise, and coping strategies [71]. An example of this type of educational framework is energy conservation and activity management (ECAM). ECAM encourages patients to perform the daily routine in an energy-efficient manner by performing them more efficiently, eliminating some activities, insuring adequate rest between activities, and preventing prolonged inactivity [72, 73]. These strategies should be incorporated into a rehabilitation plan of care for CRF.

Complementary treatments such as yoga [74, 75], acupuncture [76], relaxation techniques [77], and biofield therapies [78] may reduce cancer-related fatigue. Further research of these treatments is needed. {Can we have an exercise program example?}

A plethora of exercise programs have been studied. Resistive exercises, aerobic exercises (including walking, swimming, and cycling), and a combination of aerobic and combined exercises have been studied. Also the frequency, intensity, and duration can vary significantly from study to study. Intensities studied have ranged from 50% to 90% of the estimated maximum heart rate. Exercise frequencies have ranged from twice a day to twice a week. Exercise program durations have ranged from 2 weeks to a year. Many of the studies are pilot studies regarding feasibility and patient adherence. Because of the wide divergence of exercise programs studied, there is a lack of evidence-based knowledge about the type, intensity, and duration of exercise that is optimal in fatigue reduction.

Table 43.1 A list of common findings on history and physical during a patient evaluation

Findings on a patient evaluation	Considerations for an exercise program
Cardiopulmonary disease, pancytopenia	Limitation on intensity
Neuromuscular disorders	Fall precautions
Orthopedic concerns (i.e., impending fracture	Weight bearing and range of motion limitations Use of orthotics (include hip abduction braces, knee immobilizers, neck braces, and back braces
Neutropenia	Infection precautions (mask and gloves) Avoid public gymnasiums and pools
Lymphedema	Moderate resistance exercise is appropriate

Listed are common considerations before initiating an exercise program [68]

Conclusion and Future Directions

Prerehabilitation or preventative cancer rehabilitation (as described by Dietz) has becoming an area of increased interest [79]. Several studies suggest some improvement in medical outcomes, but the effects on cancer symptoms for fatigue and symptom reduction are still unclear. Further studies in this potentially exciting area of cancer rehabilitation are needed. Third party coverage for "cancer rehabilitation" in the United States needs to improve. More research is needed to show the cost-effectiveness of cancer rehabilitation programs [43].

The evidence to support exercise in reducing cancer-related fatigue is promising. It is one of the most effective treatments for treating cancer-related fatigue. Unfortunately, physical activity is often overlooked by clinicians. More research is necessary. In particular, elucidating the optimal duration, intensities, and types of exercise is badly needed. A better understanding of the inflammatory and hormonal contributions to cancer fatigue will help guide future exercise research.

References

1. Servaes P, Verhagen C, Bleijenberg G. Fatigue in cancer patients during and after treatment: prevalence, correlates and interventions. Eur J Cancer. 2002;38:27–43.
2. Butt Z, Rosenbloom SK, Abernethy AP, Beaumont JL, Paul D, Hampton D, Jacobsen PB, Syrjala KL, Von Roenn JH, Cella D. Fatigue is the most important symptom for advanced cancer patients who have had chemotherapy. J Natl Compr Cancer Netw. 2008;6(5):448–55.
3. Chanudrhuri A, Behan PO. Fatigue and basal ganglia. J Neurol Sci. 2000;179:34–42.
4. Cancer-related fatigue (version 1.2010). National Comprehensive Cancer Network; 2010. http://www.nccn.org/professionals/physician_gls/PDF/fatigue.pdf. Accessed 2 Jan 2010.
5. Cella D, Lai JS, Chang CH, Peterman A, Slavin M. Fatigue in cancer patients compared with fatigue in the general Untied States population. Cancer. 2002;94:528–38.
6. Chaudhuri A, Behan PO. Fatigue in neurological disorders. Lancet. 2004;363:978–88.
7. Mitchell SA. Cancer-related fatigue: state of the science. PM R. 2010;2(5):364–83.
8. Curt GA. The impact of fatigue on patients with cancer. Overview of fatigue 1 and 2. Oncologist. 2000;5:9–12.
9. Vogelzang NJ, Breitbart W, Cella D, Curt GA, Groopman JE, Horning SJ, Itri LM, Johnson DH, Scherr SL, Portenoy RK. Patient, caregiver, and oncologist perceptions of cancer-related fatigue: results of a tripart assessment survey. The fatigue coalition. Semin Hematol. 1997;34(3 Suppl 2):4–12.
10. Knowles G, Borthwick D, McNamara S, Miller M, Leggot L. Survey of nurses' assessment of cancer-related fatigue. Eur J Cancer Care (Engl). 2000;9(2):105–13.
11. Shun SC, Lai YH, Hsiao FH. Patient-related barriers to fatigue communication in cancer patients receiving active treatment. Oncologist. 2009;14(9):936–43.
12. Collins S, de Vogel-Voogt E, Visser A, van der Heide A. Presence, communication and treatment of fatigue and pain complaints in incurable cancer patients. Patient Educ Couns. 2008;72(1):102–8.
13. Mendoza TR, Wang XS, Cleeland CS, et al. The rapid assessment of fatigue severity in cancer patients: use of the brief fatigue inventory. Cancer. 1999;85:1186–96.
14. Yellen SB, Cella DF, Webster K, Blendowski C, Kaplan E. Measuring fatigue and other anemia-related symptoms with the Functional Assessment of Cancer therapy (FACT) measurement system. J Pain Symptom Manag. 1997;13(2):63–74.
15. Piper BF, Dibble SL, Dodd MJ, Weiss MC, Slaughter RE, Paul SM. The revised Piper fatigue scale: psychometric evaluation in women with breast cancer. Oncol Nurs Forum. 1998;25:677–84.
16. Smets EM, Garssen B, Bonke B, De Haes JC. The Multidimensional Fatigue Inventory (MFI) psychometric qualitifes of an instrument to assess fatigue. J Psychosom Res. 1995;39:315–25.
17. Paddison JS, Temel JS, Fricchione GL, Pirl WF. Using the differential from complete blood counts as a biomarker of fatigue in advanced non-small cell lung cancer: an exploratory analysis. Palliat Support Care. 2009;7:213–7.
18. Capuano G, Gentile PC, Bianciardi F, Tosti M, Palladino A, Di Palma M. Prevalence and influence of malnutrition on quality of life and performance status in patients with locally advanced head and neck cancer before treatment. Support Care Cancer. 2009;18:433–7.
19. Ray M, Rogers LQ, Trammell RA, Toth LA. Fatigue and sleep during cancer and chemotherapy: translation rodent models. Comp Med. 2008;58:234–45.
20. Sateia MJ, Lang BJ. Sleep and cancer: recent developments. Curr Oncol Rep. 2008;10:309–18. Francoeur RB. The relationship of cancer symptom clusters to depressive affect in the initial phase of palliative radiation. J Pain Symptom Manag. 2005;29:130–55.
21. Ancoli-Israel S, Liu L, Marler MR, et al. Fatigue, sleep, and circadian rhythms prior to chemotherapy for breast cancer. Support Care Cancer. 2006;14:201–9.
22. Strasser F, Palmer JL, Schover LR, et al. The impact of hypogonadism and autonomic dysfunction on fatigue, emotional functional and sexual desire in male patients with advanced cancer: a pilot study. Cancer. 2006;107:2949–57.
23. Bower JE, Ganz PA, Dickerson SS, Peterson L, Aziz N, Fahey JL. Diurnal cortisol rhythm and fatigue in breast cancer survivors. Psychoneuroendocrinology. 2005;30:92–100.
24. al-Majid S, McCarthy DO. Cancer-related fatigue and skeletal muscle wasting: the role of exercise. Biol Res Nurs. 2001;2:186–97.
25. Yavuzsen T, Davis MP, Ranganathan VK, et al. Cancer-related fatigue: central or peripheral? J Pain Symptom Manag. 2009;38:587–96.
26. Bower JE. Cancer-related fatigue: links with inflammation in cancer patients and survivors. Brain Behav Immun. 2007;21:863–71.
27. Collado-Hidalgo A, Bower JE, Ganz PA, Cole SW, Irwin MR. Inflammatory biomarkers for persistent fatigue in breast cancer survivors. Clin Cancer Res. 2006;12:2759–66.
28. Schubert C, Hong S, Natarajan L, Mills PJ, Dimsdale JE. The association between fatigue and inflammatory marker levels in cancer patients: a quantitative review. Brain Behav Immun. 2007;21:413–27.
29. Wood LJ, Nail LM, Gilster A, Winters KA, Elsea CR. Cancer chemotherapy-related symptoms: evidence to suggest a role for proinflammatory cytokines. Oncol Nurs Forum. 2006;33:535–42.
30. Jager A, Sleifer S, van der Rijt CC. The pathogenesis of cancer related fatigue: could increased activity of pro-inflammatory cytokines be the common denominator? Eur J Cancer. 2008;44:175–81.
31. Seruga B, Zhang H, Bernstein LJ, Tannock IF. Cytokines and their relationship to the symptoms and outcome of cancer. Nat Rev Cancer. 2008;8(11):887–99.
32. Strong V, Waters R, Hibberd C, et al. Management of depression for people with cancer (SMaRT oncology 1): a randomized trial. Lancet. 2008;372:40–8.
33. Savard J, Simard S, Giguere I, et al. Randomized clinical trial on cognitive therapy for depression in women with metastatic breast

cancer: psychological and immunological effects. Palliat Support Care. 2006;4:219–37.
34. Levesque M, Savard J, Simard S, Guathier JG, Ivers H. Efficacy of cognitive therapy for depression among women with metastatic cancer: a single-case experimental study. J Behav Ther Exp Psychiatry. 2004;35:287–305.
35. Hrushesky WJ, Grutsch JF, Wood P, et al. Circadian clock manipulation for cancer prevention and control and the relief of cancer symptoms. Integr Cancer Ther. 2009;8:387–97.
36. Minton O, Richardson A, Sharpe M, Hotopf M, Stone PC. Psychostimulants for the management of cancer-related fatigue: a systematic review and meta-analysis. J Pain Symptom Manag. 2011;41(4):761–7.
37. Mantovani G, Macciò A, Madeddu C, Serpe R, Antoni G, Massa E, Dessì M, Panzone F. Phase II nonrandomized study of the efficacy and safety of COX-2 inhibitor celecoxib on patients with cancer cachexia. J Mol Med (Berl). 2010;88(1):85–92.
38. Monk JP, Phillips G, Waite R, Kuhn J, Schaaf LJ, Otterson GA, Guttridge D, Rhoades C, Shah M, Criswell T, Caligiuri MA, Villalona-Calero MA. Assessment of tumor necrosis factor alpha blockade as an intervention to improve tolerability of dose-intensive chemotherapy in cancer patients. J Clin Oncol. 2006;24(12):1852–9.
39. Minton O, Richardson A, Sharpe M, Hotopf M, Stone P. A systematic review and meta-analysis of the pharmacological treatment of cancer-related fatigue. J Natl Cancer Inst. 2008;100(16):1155–66.
40. Jones M, Schenkel B, Just J, Fallowfield L. Epoetin alfa improves quality of life in patients with cancer: results of meta-analysis. Cancer. 2004;101:1720–32.
41. Cella D, Dobrez D, Glaspy J. Control of cancer-related anemia with erythropoietic agents: a review of evidence for improved quality of life and clinical outcomes. Ann Oncol. 2003;14:511–9.
42. Littlewood TJ, Cella D, Nortier JW. Erythropoietin improves quality of life. Lancet Oncol. 2002;3:459–60.
43. Schmitz KH, Courneya KS, Matthews C, Demark-Wahnefried W, Galvão DA, Pinto BM, Irwin ML, Wolin KY, Segal RJ, Lucia A, Schneider CM, von Gruenigen VE, Schwartz AL, American College of Sports Medicine. American College of Sports Medicine roundtable on exercise guidelines for cancer survivors. Med Sci Sports Exerc. 2010;42(7):1409–26.
44. Speed-Andrews AE, Courneya KS. Effects of exercise on quality of life and prognosis in cancer survivors. Curr Sports Med Rep. 2009;8:176–81.
45. van Weert E, Hoekstra-Weebers J, Otter R, Postema K, Sanderman R, van der Schans C. Cancer-related fatigue: predictors and effects of rehabilitation. Oncologist. 2006;11:184–96.
46. Segal R, Evans W, Johnson D, et al. Structured exercise improves physical functioning in women with stages I and II breast cancer: results of a randomized controlled trial. J Clin Oncol. 2001;19(3):657–65.
47. Milne HM, Wallman KE, Gordon S, et al. Effects of a combined aerobic and resistance exercise program in breast cancer survivors: a randomized controlled trial. Breast Cancer Res Treat. 2008;108(2):279–88.
48. Courneya KS, Friedenreich CM, Sela RA, et al. The group psychotherapy and home-based physical exercise (group-hope) trial in cancer survivors: physical fitness and quality of life outcomes. Psychooncology. 2003;12(4):357–74.
49. Klika RJ, Callahan KE, Drum SN. Individualized 12-week exercise training programs enhance aerobic capacity of cancer survivors. Phys Sportsmed. 2009;39:68–77.
50. McAuley E, White SM, Rogers LQ, Motl RW, Courneya KS. Physical activity and fatigue in breast cancer and multiple sclerosis: psychosocial mechanisms. Psychosom Med. 2010;72: 88–96.
51. Basen-Engquist K, Scruggs S, Jhingran A, et al. Physical activity and obesity in endometrial cancer survivors: associations with pain, fatigue, and physical functioning. Am J Obstet Gynecol. 2009;200:288 e281–8.
52. Item F, Konrad D. Visceral fat and metabolic inflammation: the portal theory revisited. Obes Rev. 2012;13 Suppl 2:30–9.
53. Bruunsgaard H. Physical activity and modulation of systemic low-level inflammation. J Leukoc Biol. 2005;78:819–35.
54. Ross R, Després JP. Abdominal obesity, insulin resistance, and the metabolic syndrome: contribution of physical activity/exercise. Obesity (Silver Spring). 2009;17(Suppl 3):S1–2.
55. Pedersen BK, Fischer CP. Beneficial health effects of exercise—the role of IL-6 as a myokine. Trends Pharmacol Sci. 2007;28(4):152–6.
56. Fischer CP. Interleukin-6 in acute exercise and training: what is the biological relevance? Exerc Immunol Rev. 2006;12:6–33.
57. Hill EE, Zack E, Battaglini C, Viru M, Viru A, Hackney AC. Exercise and circulating cortisol levels: the intensity threshold effect. J Endocrinol Investig. 2008;31(7):587–91.
58. Warren JB, Dalton N, Turner C, Clark TJ, Toseland PA. Adrenaline secretion during exercise. Clin Sci (Lond). 1984;66(1):87–90.
59. Petersen AM, Pedersen BK. The anti-inflammatory effect of exercise. J Appl Physiol (1985). 2005;98(4):1154–62.
60. Surmi BK, Hasty AH. Macrophage infiltration into adipose tissue: initiation, propagation and remodeling. Future Lipidol. 2008;3(5):545–56.
61. Gleeson M, McFarlin B, Flynn M. Exercise and toll-like receptors. Exerc Immunol Rev. 2006;12:34–53.
62. Kruijsen-Jaarsma M, Révész D, Bierings MB, Buffart LM, Takken T. Effects of exercise on immune function in patients with cancer: a systematic review. Exerc Immunol Rev. 2013;19:120–43.
63. Jones SB, Thomas GA, Hesselsweet SD, Alvarez-Reeves M, Yu H, Irwin ML. Effect of exercise on markers of inflammation in breast cancer survivors: the Yale exercise and survivorship study. Cancer Prev Res (Phila). 2013;6(2):109–18.
64. Fu JB, Raj VS, Guo Y. A Guide to Inpatient Cancer Rehabilitation: Focusing on Patient Selection and Evidence-Based Outcomes. PM R. 2017;9(9S2):S324–S334.
65. Sabatino SA, Coates RJ, Uhler RJ, Pollack LA, Alley LG, Zauderer LJ. Provider counseling about health behaviors among cancer survivors in the United States. J Clin Oncol. 2007;25(15):2100–6.
66. Brown P, Clark MM, Atherton P, et al. Will improvements in quality of life (QOL) impact fatigue in patients receiving radiation therapy for advanced cancer? Am J Clin Oncol. 2006;29:52–8.
67. Nieman DC. Exercise, infection, and immunity. Int J Sports Med. 1994;15(Suppl 3):S131–41.
68. Courneya KS, Segal RJ, Mackey JR, et al. Effects of aerobic and resistance exercise in breast cancer patients receiving adjuvant chemotherapy: a multicenter randomized controlled trial. J Clin Oncol. 2007;25:4396–404.
69. Cristian A, Tran A, Patel K. Patient safety in cancer rehabilitation. Phys Med Rehabil Clin N Am. 2012;23(2):441–56. https://doi.org/10.1016/j.pmr.2012.02.015. Epub 2012 Apr 10.
70. van Weert E, Hoekstra-Weebers JE, May AM, Korstjens I, Ros WJ, van der Schans CP. The development of an evidence-based physical self-management rehabilitation programme for cancer survivors. Patient Educ Couns. 2008;71:169–90.
71. Jacobsen PB, Donovan KA, Vandaparmpil ST, Small BJ. Systematic review and meta-analysis of psychological and activity-based interventions for cancer-related fatigue. Health Psychol. 2007;26(6):660–7.
72. Barsevick AM, Whitmer K, Sweeney C, Nail LM. A pilot study examining energy conservation for cancer treatment-related fatigue. Cancer Nurs. 2002;25:333–41.
73. Barsevick AM, Dudley W, Beck S, Sweeney C, Whitmer K, Nail L. A randomized clinical trial of energy conservation for patients with cancer-related fatigue. Cancer. 2004;100:1302–10.

74. Danhauer SC, Tooze JA, Farmer DF, et al. Restorative yoga for women with ovarian or breast cancer: findings from a pilot study. J Soc Integr Oncol. 2008;6:47–58.
75. Bower JE, Greendale G, Crosswell AD, Garet D, Sternlieb B, Ganz PA, Irwin MR, Olmstead R, Arevalo J, Cole SW. Yoga reduces inflammatory signaling in fatigued breast cancer survivors: a randomized controlled trial. Psychoneuroendocrinology. 2014;43:20–9.
76. Zeng Y, Luo T, Finnegan-John J, Cheng AS. Meta-analysis of randomized controlled trials of acupuncture for cancer-related fatigue. Integr Cancer Ther. 2013;13:193–200.
77. Cohen M, Fried G. Comparing relaxation training and cognitive-behavioral group therapy for women with breast cancer. Res Soc Work Pract. 2007;17:313–23.
78. Danhauer SC, Tooze JA, Holder P, Miller C, Jesse MT. Healing touch as a supportive intervention for adult acute leukemia patients: a pilot investigation of effects on distress and symptoms. J Soc Integr Oncol. 2008;6:89–97.
79. Dietz JH. Rehabilitation of the cancer patient: its role in the scheme of comprehensive care. Clin Bull. 1974;4(3):104–7.

Physical Therapy

44

Monica Verduzco-Gutierrez, Roy Rivera Jr., and Prathap Jayaram

Introduction

Cancer survivorship has been increasing due to the successful treatments and aging population. Survivorship will continue to grow exponentially in relation to the number of new cancer cases and deaths. In the United States during 2010, there was an estimated 13.8 million cancer survivors compared to the estimated 1.5 million new cases and 569,000 cancer deaths [1]. It is estimated that the cancer survivorship will continue to grow to an estimated 18.1 million by 2020 [1]. Physicians should expect an increased number of cancer survivors in their practice regardless of specialization.

Preventing and addressing functional impairments of cancer and cancer-related treatments vary because of difficulty identifying patients who would benefit from physical therapy, planning inconsistent individualized physical therapy programs, and having a lack of healthcare resources. The American College of Sports Medicine has established guidelines demonstrating the efficacy of an exercise program after a cancer diagnosis which result in a reduction of fatigue, increased physical function, and overall improvements in quality of life. While it seems trivial that physical activity would be beneficial for cancer-related pain syndromes, it is challenging to have specific therapy programs based on certain therapeutic approaches to cancer. The healthcare provider should be knowledgeable about physical therapy precautions prior to establishing a formal therapy program. Such precautions include weight-bearing status due to increased risk of fractures from hormonal therapies, balance precautions due to chemotherapy-related neuropathy, and cardiac precautions due to treatment-related cardiotoxicity. This chapter will expand on the use of physical therapy for treatment of cancer-related pain syndromes.

M. Verduzco-Gutierrez (✉)
Department of Physical Medicine and Rehabilitation, University of Texas Health Science Center, Houston, TX, USA
e-mail: Monica.verduzco-gutierrez@uth.tmc.edu

R. Rivera Jr.
Crom Rehabilitation, LLC, Department of Outpatient Sports Medicine, Houston, TX, USA
e-mail: RRivera@cromrehab.com

P. Jayaram
Baylor College of Medicine, Department of Physical Medicine and Rehabilitation, Houston, TX, USA
e-mail: jayaram@bcm.edu

Physical Therapy

According to the American Physical Therapy Association (2015), physical therapists (PT) are state-licensed allied health professionals who help patients reduce pain and improve or restore functional mobility caused by disability from disease or trauma. They evaluate patients, assess their levels of disability via outcome measures, develop and implement appropriate plans of care based on short- and long-term goals, and evaluate the outcomes to determine effectiveness of their interventions. Physical therapists practice in a variety of settings, including hospitals, hospices, outpatient clinics, home health agencies, schools, sports and fitness facilities, work settings, industrial, workplace or other occupational environments, and nursing homes [2].

Therapy Throughout the Continuum of Cancer Care

It is widely accepted that patients living with cancer necessitate a multidisciplinary rehabilitation program. Cancer rehabilitation programs treat the physical complications of cancer and its treatment, both pain syndromes and the medical comorbidities that affect quality of a patient's life. Cancer survivors tend to have worse physical and emotional quality of life, 24.5% vs 10.2% compared to patients without a cancer history [3].

A. Gulati et al. (eds.), *Essentials of Interventional Cancer Pain Management*, https://doi.org/10.1007/978-3-319-99684-4_44

There has been long-standing literature discussing the necessity of therapy throughout the continuum of cancer care [4]. According to Dietz, all responsive patients should be considered for a rehabilitation program, no matter the prognosis. Goal setting and treatment planning for cancer patients can be divided into four stages: preventative, restorative, supportive, and palliative. Patients with active cancer pain tend to also have poorer function [5]. The patients with mild, well-controlled pain functioned similarly to individuals without pain; therefore, it is necessary to diagnose and intervene in cancer pain conditions.

Rehabilitation for cancer patients is most beneficial when it is started at the earliest possible time. It is important physicians diagnose potential or actual disability soon after the diagnosis of cancer and even offer preventive therapy prior to the initiation of cancer treatment (prehabilitation). Screening for physical impairments and pain can be done during initial diagnosis and at subsequent follow-up visits (see Table 44.1). Prehabilitation is intended to assess pretreatment impairments and prevent future impairments. An example would be a patient awaiting surgical resection and having a strengthening and conditioning program done by physical therapy in order to increase their function in anticipation of the upcoming stressor. This would buffer detrimental effects of postsurgical immobility. Furthermore, a physical therapist could improve a patient's balance and implement home safety strategies to prevent falls.

Rehabilitation during acute cancer care that incorporates a multidisciplinary approach leads to better outcomes. A retrospective study of esophagectomy patients [6] compared fast-track rehabilitation patients who had early mobilization, epidural analgesia control, fluid infusion volume control, and enteral nutrition to conventional care patients. The fast-track group had fewer complications, less postoperative pain, shorter length of stays, and earlier return to work.

According to Dietz' continuum of cancer care, restorative rehabilitation efforts are initiated when no long-term disability is expected. In contrast, supportive rehabilitation begins therapeutic efforts for patients with ongoing residual disability (examples include hemiparesis after glioblastoma resection or metastatic disease to the spinal cord causing paraparesis). For example, a patient with chemotherapy-induced peripheral neuropathy may have severe neuropathic pain that can be treated with oral analgesics or antiepileptic medications. Additionally, physical therapist may start sensory integration techniques, physical modalities, and work on gait and balance abnormalities. A similar approach may be beneficial in patients with head and neck cancer who suffer from trismus. A referral to both physical therapy and speech therapy for treatment with a dynamic jaw opening device while improving posture and cervical range of motion is often beneficial.

Table 44.1 Examples of functional assessment tools

Functional independence measure (FIM)
WeeFIM (pediatric measure)
Brief Pain Inventory
Visual analog scales
Numeric rating scale
McGill Pain Questionnaire
Canadian Occupational Performance Measure
Eastern Cooperative Oncology Group (ECOG)
National Institutes of Health Rehabilitation Medicine Department Performance Scale
6-min walk test
Timed Up and Go (TUG) test
Tinetti Balance Assessment Tool
Disability Assessment Scale for spasticity

Palliative rehabilitation focuses on reducing impairments and disabilities with the goal of improving the patient and caregiver's quality of life at the end stages of cancer. Physical therapy treatments would focus on controlling pain, maximizing strengths, training in the use of adaptive equipment, and maintaining safe locomotion.

Precautions When Treating Cancer Patients

It is now clear that exercise benefits cancer patients and plays a role in prevention and control. Evidence supports exercise may decrease the risk of developing cancer and may extend survival for breast and colon cancer [7]. Patients who undergo a physical therapy program will need to be evaluated for neuropathies and musculoskeletal morbidities secondary to treatment. For example, a patient who had been on hormonal treatment may have an elevated cancer risk, or a patient treated with cardiotoxic chemotherapy may have undetected cardiac disease. The American College of Sports Medicine in 2010 published a Roundtable Consensus Statement on Exercise Guidelines for Cancer Survivors [7] and delineates an exercise prescription for cancer survivors. These guidelines highlight precautions in the cancer patient population. There are general contraindications for starting an exercise program, including allowing adequate time to heal after surgery and not exercising patients with extreme fatigue, anemia, or ataxia.

It is important that rehabilitation facilities and associated professionals follow neutropenic precautions and use them to guide their treatment sessions. If a patient has a known low white cell count, they may require a mask or be placed in a private or semi-private area for their therapy (or should not attend a public gym until white blood cell count is at a safe level of $>0.5\times10^9$μl). Patients on certain chemotherapy regimens are at risk for spontaneous hemorrhaging from therapy-related thrombocytopenia. Some programs use the Winningham Contraindications for Aerobic Exercise Guidelines that were established in 1986 [8]. These guidelines indicate that exercise is contraindicated with an absolute neutrophil count less than 0.5×10^9μl and platelet count less than 50×10^9μl.

Physical Therapy Interventions

Physical therapists implement a variety of treatment techniques based on the patient diagnosis and expected goals. The most common treatment techniques include therapeutic exercise, manual therapy, modalities, and neuromuscular reeducation.

Therapeutic exercises are treatment techniques implemented by physical therapists and other rehabilitation professionals that increase muscle strength through resistance training, endurance, joint mobility, and/or flexibility by stretching both actively and passively. A meta-analysis by Strasser et al. demonstrated significantly positive effects of resistance training on upper and lower extremity muscle strength, lean body mass, and body fat percentage in individuals with cancer [9]. Likewise, a systematic review by Focht et al. reported that resistance exercise training was a promising intervention that resulted in clinically relevant physiologic and quality of life outcomes pre- and post-cancer treatment [10].

Manual therapy, also known as soft tissue mobilization, joint mobilization, and joint manipulation, is a hands-on approach that targets muscles, soft tissues, and joints to help modulate pain, increase range of motion, increase circulation, reduce or manage edema, and increase flexibility. Often, in combination with other forms of treatment approaches, manual therapy can prove to be a vital adjunct to physical therapy. Systematic reviews have suggested massage to reduce anxiety and relieve several cancer-related symptoms such as pain, nausea, depression, anger, stress, and fatigue [11, 12].

Neuromuscular reeducation (NMR) is a form of treatment that targets balance, coordination, proprioception, posture, and/or kinesthesia in an individual that has had an insult or trauma to the nervous system. Some of the most common conditions that warrant NMR are cerebrovascular accidents, ischemic events, or stroke. In the case of an individual with cancer, it would be beneficial to employ NMR techniques in those conditions that affect the central or peripheral nervous systems. There are a few clinical trials in the current literature that support the use of NMR techniques; however, the majority of them cannot rate NMR techniques superior to other physical therapy treatments available.

Specific Disease States

Upper Extremity

Shoulder Pain

Shoulder pain and more specifically rotator cuff pathology is a common disorder amongst cancer patients, especially breast cancer. Pre-existing cervical degenerative changes, metastases, and neurotoxic chemotherapy commonly damage the upper cervical brachial plexus (C5, C6) nerve roots resulting in rotator cuff weakness. The damage that results from radiation fields, specifically the mantle field (MF), allows for anterior translation of the humerus within the glenoid and subsequently causes rotator cuff impingement and adhesive capsulitis from the ongoing local inflammation within the shoulder capsule.

Rotator Cuff (Rct) Impingement

Range of motion (ROM), stretching, strengthening, and stabilizing exercises are important in successful rehabilitation of the rotator cuff as it will help correct muscle weakness, glenohumeral instability, and impaired scapulohumeral rhythm. ROM exercises should be performed daily with the goals of achieving painless full glenohumeral ROM through performing shoulder pendulum exercises, internal/external rotation stretches, adduction/abduction stretches, and biceps/triceps stretches [13].

Resistance exercises can be implemented once range of motion has improved and the patient's pain level allows for progression. Once better control and stabilization of scapular positioning is achieved, eccentric resistance exercises can be implemented. Concentric exercises should involve higher repetitions and less resistance. The kinematics of the program should involve closed chain exercises such as standing with hands on a wall, prone on elbows to four-point stance. To target the glenohumeral and scapulothoracic joints, exercises can include a plank position, or a physio ball may be positioned under the hands. Scapular stabilization exercises can be obtained from tossing a medicine ball from hand to hand with progression to around the back to trunk and trunk toss and catch. The therapy program can then be progressed to wall dribbles in various ranges of shoulder flexion and abduction.

Secondary prevention of rotator cuff dysfunction should be aimed at correction of muscular imbalances between internal and external rotators of the shoulder. External rotators are typically weaker and can be strengthened using resistance band therapy or isotonic side-lying external rotation (Fig. 44.1). To target the infraspinatus, external rotation exercises can be performed using low-load isometric contractions. Scapular instability and dyskinesis should be addressed through stretching of scapular muscles (pectoralis minor, levator scapula, rhomboids, and latissimus dorsi) through sleeper stretches (Fig. 44.2), crossarm stretch, and internal rotation stretches. Scapular stability can be achieved through scapular clock exercise.

Adhesive Capsulitis

Adhesive capsulitis results in functional impairments that include pain, loss of function, sleep disturbance, loss of motion due to pain, and secondary capsular tightness. The initial rehabilitation approach should involve decreasing the inflammatory response, pain, increasing range of motion,

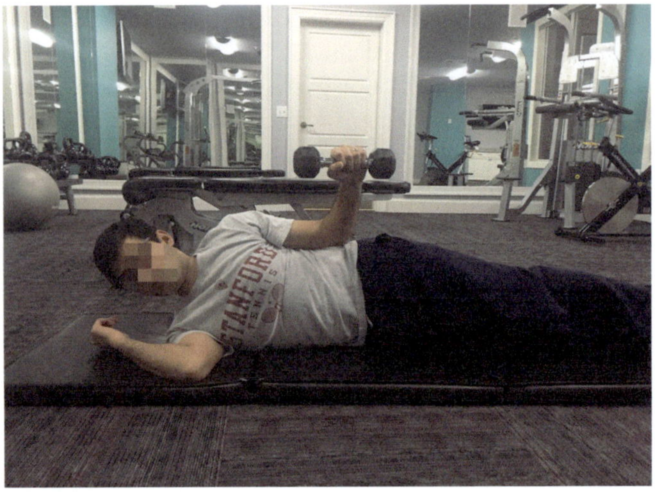

Fig. 44.1 Isotonic side-lying external rotation exercise for rotator cuff stabilization

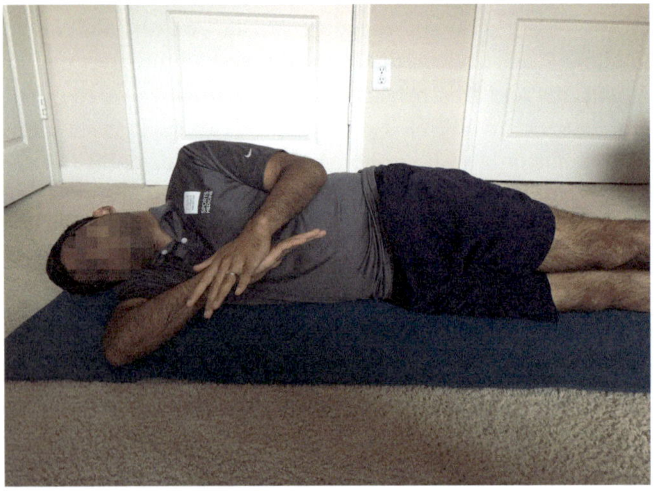

Fig. 44.2 Sleeper stretch

and reestablishing normal shoulder and scapular biomechanics. The focus of rehabilitation depends on the clinical stage of adhesive capsulitis. Therapeutic exercise will target biomechanical imbalances of soft tissues that are a result of disuse and capsular volume/contraction loss.

Pendulum exercises should be incorporated as they provide a pain-free active motion which stimulates deep heating of soft tissues and increases blood flow. Pulley exercises should be incorporated to further increase range of motion and to help with avoiding anterosuperior migration of the humeral head [14]. Strengthening will focus on periscapular musculature in the available range of motion with tolerable amounts of pain permitted. Closed chain exercises are beneficial in stimulating co-contracture of the stabilizing musculature [15].

Elbow/Forearm

Radiation therapy and chemotherapy effects on the extensor and flexor compartments of the forearm have not been exclusively studied; however, patients with breast cancer, melanoma, and lung cancer are more susceptible to upper extremity pain disorders [16]. Anatomically, the brachial plexus is most commonly affected by either direct tumor infiltration or through effects of radiation. Radiation can lead to progressive fibrosis, sclerosis, loss of elasticity, and shortening and contracture of the forearm compartment resulting in lateral and medial epicondylopathy and de Quervain's tenosynovitis.

Lateral Epicondylopathy

Therapeutic exercise should be aimed at decreasing pain and muscle atrophy. Initially it is imperative to restore symmetric flexibility of the involved site prior to strengthening exercises. Most literature to date supports eccentric strengthening in cases of lateral epicondylar tendinopathy [17]. Eccentric wrist extensor exercise (Fig. 44.3) can also be incorporated into a home exercise program. It is important to address muscle groups above and below the elbow. The well-accepted therapy program is initial forearm range of motion and gentle isometrics, followed by eccentric exercises.

Medial Epicondylopathy

Therapeutic exercises should target the flexor carpi radialis, pronator teres, and if present palmaris longus. After conservative precautions have been undertaken such as keeping forearm more prone during tasks, a stretching and range of motion program can be initiated. Stretching of the wrist flexors is performed with gentle movement into wrist extension. Each stretch should be held for 15–30 s. Once range of motion and flexibility have been obtained, a pain-free isometric exercise program can be initiated. It is recommended that the elbow should be flexed initially during these exercises than then be progressed to extension.

Wrist

The wrist is a commonly affected area in cancer and related therapies. The wrist is not usually affected because of direct radiation but at more proximal treatment regimens. The wrist compartment is equally susceptible to progressive fibrosis and sclerotic changes. Neuropathy-associated impairments are covered in nervous system section.

De Quervain's Tenosynovitis

Treatment is first addressed with immobilization to reduce pain and inflammation. Once immobilization has improved the inflammatory phase, a light active range of motion and isometric exercise program can be initiated without use of an immobilizer. Advancement to strengthening exercises can be initiated once the patient's pain level has improved.

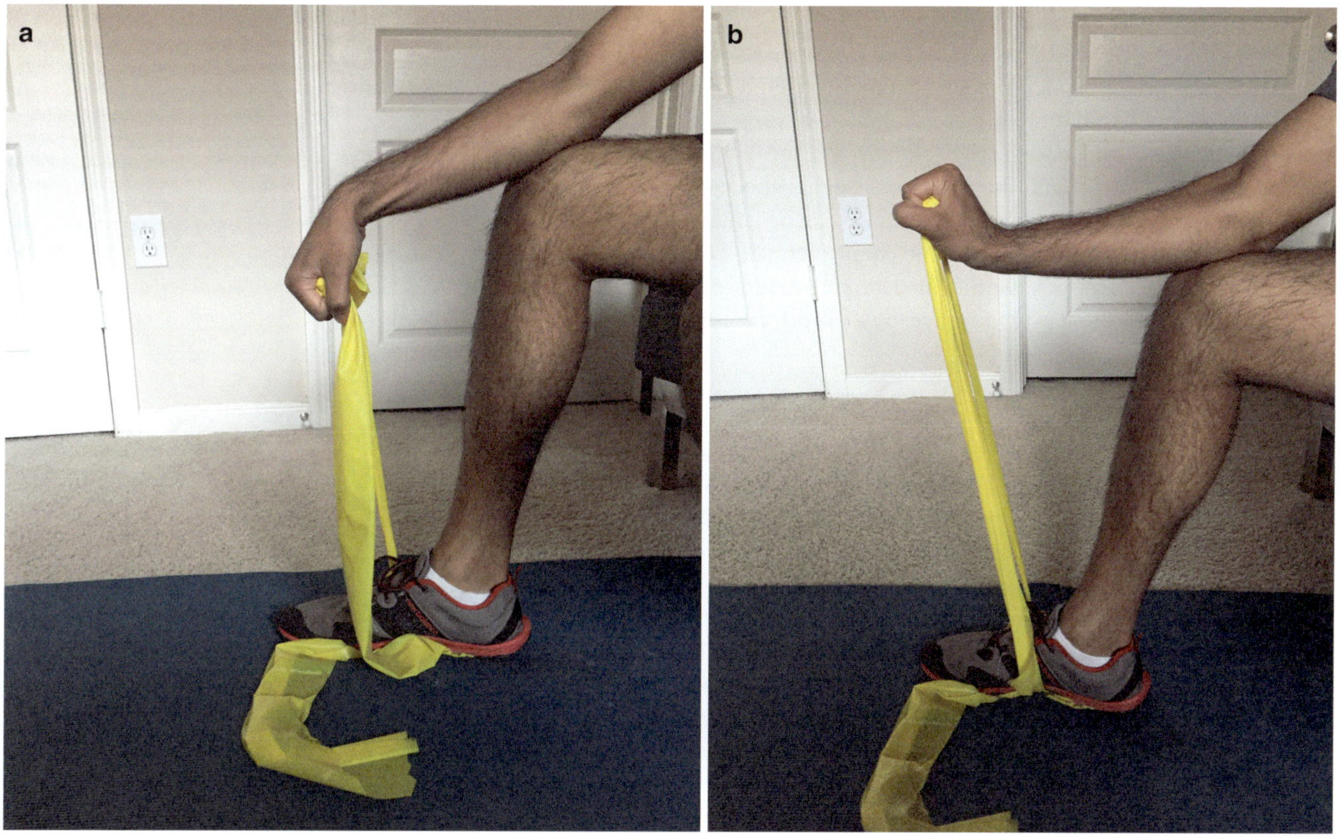

Fig. 44.3 Wrist extensor eccentric exercise with hand weight. (**a**) Wrist is in neutral position. (**b**) Then slowly lower wrist into flexion, and then use the uninvolved hand to bring the involved hand back to neutral and repeat

Strengthening of antagonistic muscles of the wrist can also improve overall wrist stability.

Lower Extremity

Lower extremity pathology in individuals with cancer is not uncommon, and the implications of this can be devastating. Losing the ability to ambulate, increasing the risk of falling, and decreasing overall functional mobility can all lead to decreased quality of life and psychological damage for individuals living with cancer. All joints in the lower extremities can be affected, and below are the most common conditions seen in individuals with cancer.

Hip

There is a wide differential when considering etiology of lower extremity pain in the cancer population. As with the upper extremity, pain is mediated through direct effects of tumor, or sequelae of surgery, chemotherapy or radiation.

The healthcare provider should also be aware that in addition to cancer-related pain of the lower extremity, underlying noncancer etiologies should be addressed. Mechanical changes and compensatory movement patterns because of surgical resection, radiation fibrosis, and/or chemotherapy-induced neuropathy may result in musculoskeletal pain indirectly related to cancer and its treatments. Many pain syndromes that are indirectly related to cancer and its treatments are due to repetitive strain injuries and degenerative changes.

Hip Osteoarthritis

Hip osteoarthritis is the most common form of arthritis seen in cancer population. The rehabilitation approach should focus on range of motion, flexibility, static and dynamic muscle strength, joint protection, and activity modification techniques. Therapies should follow the phases of rehabilitation continuum as with all therapies mentioned thus far; however due to the high recurrence of intra-articular hip flares, therapy activity should be downgraded appropriately. The initial approach should involve gentle range of motion, stretching, isometric strengthening with avoidance of high-impact aerobics, or isotonic lower limb exercises.

Stretching exercises can incorporate range of motion about the hip girdle in all planes by having a patient sit with legs abducted and progressive reach toward his or her toes, as this facilitates both hip adductors and extensors. Strengthening should focus on all hip girdle musculature but should specifically target the gluteus medius [18] preferably in with isotonic mechanics at first. It is important for the healthcare provider and therapy team to evaluate for muscle imbalances at the hip girdle, such as an overactive tensor fascia latae and underactive gluteus medius which lead to excessive loading on the hip joint itself [19]. Once the patient's strength has improved, resistance can be added, and further progression to closed kinetic chain exercises can be incorporated. Therapies should also target quadriceps strengthening and balance to improve any proprioceptive defects.

Greater Trochanteric Pain Syndrome

Greater trochanteric pain syndrome (GTPS) is defined as "tenderness to palpation over the greater trochanter with the patient in the side-lying position," and characteristically speaking, GTPS is typically not associated with signs of inflammation such as warmth, erythema, or swelling; likewise, the etiology is not fully known and may relate to myofascial pain rather than inflammation [20]. The goals of physical therapy treatment for GTPS involve increasing global hip strength and range of motion, decreasing local edema and inflammation, and modulating mechanical pain.

Individuals with GTPS have been found to have comorbid knee and low back pain secondary to compensatory strategies along the kinematic chain causing stresses in joints above and below the hip. Likewise, Segal et al. reported that individuals with GTPS have abnormal gait patterns with decreased velocities and difficulty rising from seated positions [20]. Because of these findings, physical therapy treatments directed at treating GTPS should include ensuring full pain-free range of motion in the hip joint with special attention to iliopsoas length. The Thomas test is one objective measure that can be used for determining iliopsoas pathology because of shortening.

Restoring hip range of motion can be achieved with stretching and manual therapy techniques. Therapies that focus on strengthening hip musculature will help restore lower limb coordination. Therapies should focus on stretching and strengthening opposing muscles to ideally obtain muscle balance. Flexibility achieved through stretching should focus on the iliotibial band (ITB) and tensor fascia latae (TFL); stretching can also correct underlying length deficits. Good examples of stretches that target ITB and TFL are standing stretches that put the hip in extension and adduction as seen in Fig. 44.4.

Strengthening of the hip abductors, gluteus medius, external rotators, and extensors will improve overall gait, hip biomechanics, and pelvic stability. Initial exercises can incorporate therapy bands or ankle weights and progress to side-lying hip abduction to target the gluteus medius and limb squats for the gluteus maximus.

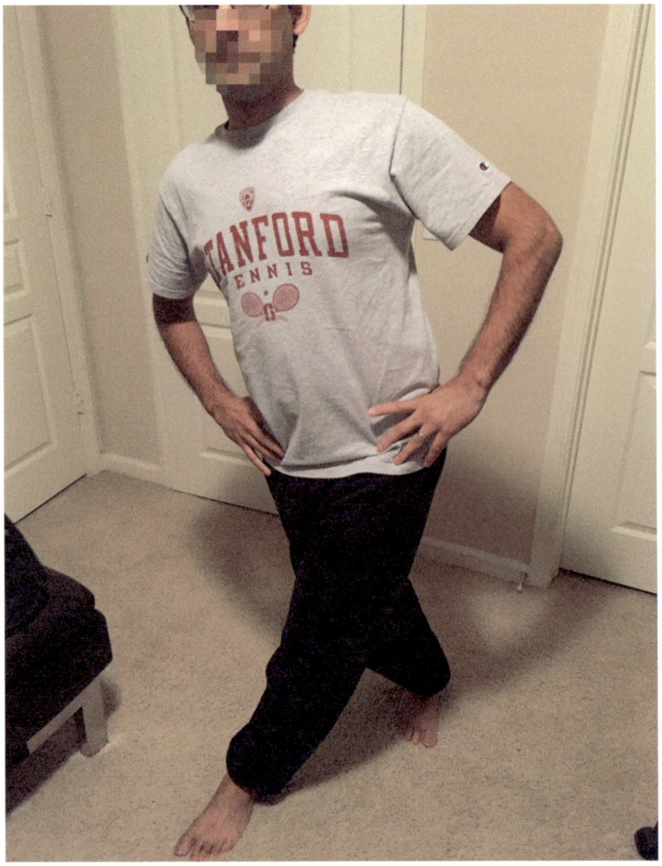

Fig. 44.4 Crossover standing stretch of ITB

Osteoporosis

Many studies have demonstrated that exercise in both pre- and postmenopausal women prevents bone loss; however, results of therapeutic exercise have fared more positive in premenopausal women, especially in the femoral neck of the hip joint [21, 22]. Individuals with cancer are often prescribed opioids for pain control; however, research shows that opioids have been reported to increase fracture risk in adults via falls secondary to dizziness and sedation and chronic opioid-induced hypogonadism [23]. The goals of physical therapy for individuals with cancer and osteoporosis are to increase global strength, especially around more proximal muscles and joints, e.g., shoulders, spine, and hips, and increase bone mineral density via appropriately supervised and indicated weight-bearing exercises.

A recent study by Pernambuco et al. demonstrated that an 8-month aquatic aerobic exercise program can increase levels of osteocalcin, a protein found in the extracellular matrix of bones involved in regulating mineralization [24]. This finding indicates that aquatic aerobic exercises could potentially help increase bone mineral density in individuals with osteoporosis.

Knee

Iliotibial Band Syndrome

Iliotibial band syndrome (ITBS) is a disorder of the lateral leg where the iliotibial band, a fibrous band of connective tissues, becomes irritated because of overdevelopment, shortening, or friction over bony prominences such as proximally over the greater trochanter or distally over the lateral tibial tubercle (Gerdy's tubercle). Goals of physical therapy for individuals with ITBS target hip and knee strengthening, stretching, edema management, and pain control.

Because the iliotibial band is a grossly superficial structure, the medical management of ITBS is largely conservative and employs the use of nonsteroidal anti-inflammatory drugs (NSAIDs), deep friction massage, immobilization, and corticosteroid injections. Therapeutic modalities are also other conservative approaches that physical therapists use for treating ITBS. These modalities include moist heat, ice massages, ultrasound, iontophoresis, and kinesiotaping.

Patellofemoral Pain Syndrome

Patellofemoral pain syndrome (PFPS) is a common ailment of the distal knee that affects people of all ages. Causes for PFPS are multifactorial but can include muscle weaknesses or imbalances, joint effusions or inflammation, overuse, or trauma. Goals of physical therapy are often global conditioning, postural strengthening, and pain management via modalities, such as therapeutic ultrasound, ice, heat, and topical analgesics.

The research has shown that conservative management of PFPS, such as exercise, manual therapy, taping, bracing, and pharmacology, has proven to be more beneficial than surgical options or approaches [25]. Focusing on the proximal muscles of the hip on the affected extremity and the quadriceps as well has proven to be effective in treating PFPS.

Ankle

Plantar Fasciitis

Plantar fasciitis is the inflammation of the plantar fascia or connective tissue made up mostly of collagenous substance found on the plantar aspect of the foot. Contributing factors to plantar fasciitis are often prolonged standing, improper footwear, and trauma. Physical therapy goals for treating plantar fasciitis are aimed at decreasing inflammation, addressing postural abnormalities via ergonomic assessments, and stretching out collagenous adhesions that are restricting range of motion of the foot. The research has shown that conservative measures such as orthotic insoles and plantar stretching exercises are more beneficial versus steroid injections or iontophoresis [26].

Achilles Tendinopathy

Achilles tendinopathy is a range of disorders that affect the Achilles tendon but mostly are inflammatory in nature. The mechanism of injury is usually secondary to chronic overuse in athletes, but it can also be traumatic in nature. Most rehabilitative evidence shows that eccentric loading exercises are superior to all other treatment modalities; however, a systematic review by Malliaras et al. recommends eccentric-concentric loading and questions the current literature [27]. Laser therapy and extracorporeal shock wave therapy are popular modalities in the treatment of Achilles tendinopathy, but the efficacy of each is questionable and definitively inconclusive.

Spine

Cervical Spine

Hodgkin's disease survivors are susceptible to cervical spine disorders due to neck atrophy and progressive weakness from mantle field (MF) radiation. The pathogenesis behind these affected areas can be better understood through radiation fibrosis syndrome [28]. Most of the atrophy seen in cervical musculature is not clearly understood but is related in part to the MF radiation that was previously delivered. While atrophy and surrounding muscle damage cannot be reversed, there is room for therapeutic interventions.

Cervical Extensor Weakness

The therapeutic approach to extensor weakness, like most cervical pathologies, should involve decreasing local inflammation and pain, opposing muscle tension, and improving range of motion in hypomobile planes. Therapeutic exercises should address muscular impairments with lower load initially to activate deeper cervical muscles [29]. Specific muscles that should be targeted include deep craniocervical flexors, deep lower cervical extensors, cervical extensors, cervical rotators, middle and lower trapezii, and latissimus dorsi. Strength training can begin with isometric exercises with an understanding that certain neck extensor musculature may not be active in certain planes due to atrophy and weakness. If the therapy team progresses the patient, then active with resistive strengthening should be incorporated. The role of cervical collars and adaptive equipment will be addressed in occupational therapy section.

Radiation-Induced Cervical Dystonia

Like cervical extensor weakness, cervical dystonia (CD) is also a common sequela of radiation fibrosis syndrome that can be a result from radiation that can involve many locations within the spine. Cervical dystonia is informally defined as a movement disorder that involves involuntary contractions of the head and shoulders which can involve aberrant positions such as torticollis [30]. Therapies should focus on improving ROM as much as possible in all neck planes; this can be limiting due to fixed contractures that have resulted in shortening of tendons and ligaments. Attempting to correct positional fault with scapular repositioning and muscle reeducation with corrective taping can improve muscle tension and pain. The benefits of facilitating cervical paraspinal unloading through interventional physiatry roles will be explained in other chapters.

Cervical Disc Pathology

Cervical disc pathology is responsible for over 20% of chronic neck pain [31]. Effects of radiation fibrosis syndrome along with cancers specific to the head and neck can disrupt the annulus fibrosus causing referred pain to the neck, shoulders, and arms. This type of discogenic pain could already preexist and can be further magnified with cancer-related pathology. Therapeutic exercise should involve stretching of the cervical paraspinals, scalenes, levator scapulae, and upper trapezii. Range of motion of the cervical spine with isometric strengthening exercises can be initiated in flexion, extension, lateral rotation, or lateral side bending. As mentioned in the cervical extensor weakness section, strengthening should aim to restore balance between the deep neck flexors and upper cervical extensors. This balance can be achieved with postural exercises which include chin tucks and scapular retractions.

Thoracic Spine

Back pain associated with cancer presents differently than nonmalignant back pain. One feature is that cancer-related back pain is not relieved with rest. The thoracic spine is a common location for metastases due to the surface area availability. Axillary dissections and breast reconstruction with implants after mastectomy can cause direct nerve injury at the time of surgery or progressive compression as scar tissue develops [16].

Postmastectomy Syndrome

Postmastectomy pain syndrome (PMPS) is defined as a chronic pain condition that follows surgery of the breast [32]. PMPS can include phantom breast pain, incisional pain, intercostobrachial neuralgia, and neuroma pain. Therapeutic management involves targeting active range of motion and passive range of motion of the pectoralis major, pectoralis minor, and latissimus dorsi. Stretching should be incorporated earlier on to minimize surgical scarring. A focused shoulder stretching program in all planes should be initiated with progression to strengthening.

Thoracic Spine Dysfunction

Various structures within the thoracic spine can be affected not just from primary tumor or metastasis but to effects from radiation fibrosis syndrome affecting the costovertebral articulations, facet joints, and intervertebral disc pathology. The thoracic spine due to its rigid architecture requires a more diverse therapeutic approach. The overall goal of a therapeutic program should be to improve mobility and function.

Once pain has been relatively controlled and measures have been taken to allow for bone healing, range of motion of the thoracic spine should be incorporated with stretching of the postural muscles. A strengthening program should incorporate dynamic stability through core strengthening and breathing [33]. Proximal crossed syndrome can occur when the tightness of the neck and scapula muscles causes protraction and shoulder elevation. Therapies should thus focus on scapular retraction exercises. Postural corrections should involve good pelvic and thoracic alignment. Other therapeutic exercises can include the sphinx exercise, which will allow for full extension and full flexion of the thoracolumbar spine. A patient who has a moderate degree of kyphoscoliosis can benefit from Swiss ball exercises, with a ball placed under them supporting the abdomen thoracic spinal muscles which can be activated.

Post-Thoracotomy Pain Syndrome

Post-thoracotomy pain syndrome (PTPS) is defined as pain that persists at incision site or in distribution of incised intercostal nerve for greater than 2 months after thoracotomy. Muscles involved with this pain-related syndrome are the serratus anterior and latissimus dorsi. This can alter scapulohumeral mechanics affecting scapular fixation, shoulder abduction, shoulder adduction, and elbow forward flexion. Initially therapies should aim at restoring range of motion; and once that has been achieved, strengthening around the shoulder can begin. To target the glenohumeral and scapulothoracic joints, exercises can include a plank position or a physio ball positioned under the hands. Scapular stabilization exercises can be obtained from simply tossing a medicine ball from hand to hand with progression to around the back to trunk and trunk toss and catch. The therapy program can then be progressed to wall dribbles in various ranges of shoulder flexion and abduction.

Lumbar Spine

Back pain is a common symptom for both cancer and noncancer patient population. Most people will experience an episode of back pain at some point in their lifetime, and it is estimated that 25% of the population will have low back pain in any given year [34]. The spine is the most common site for bony metastasis for breast, lung, prostate, colon, thyroid, and renal cancers. Amongst the most common primary malignancies include multiple myeloma, Ewing sarcoma, osteosarcoma, chondrosarcoma, and chondroma [30]. Cancer-related treatments that involve the lumbar spine include surgery, chemotherapy, and radiation therapy which all have deleterious functional impacts on patients with lumbar spine pain. Before a focused therapy can be implemented, patients who have an underlying cancer diagnosis with new symptoms of back pain should be presumed to have recurrence with spinal involvement pending oncologic evaluation.

Lumbar Radiculopathy

Radicular pain can result from direct compression of the nerve root from tumor, pre-existing degenerative changes, fibrosis related to prior surgery, radiation, paraneoplastic effects, and neurotoxic chemotherapy [30]. Therapeutic exercise should aim at early end-range lumbar extension range of motion as it has been suggested that this has a better prognosis when trying to avoid surgery [35]. The healthcare provider should also aim to understand the directional preference to begin the therapeutic program. Range of motion can be best restored through lower limb flexibility and spinal mobility. Examples of improving range of motion are standing forward trunk flexion and standing trunk extension. Core strengthening programs play a critical role in addressing lumbar radicular pain. Lower extremity strengthening including plantar flexor and evertor strengthening are also necessary. Balance and proprioceptive training can be beneficial in new radiculopathy assessments.

Lumbar Stenosis

Lumbar stenosis has an annual incidence of 5 cases per 100,000 [36]. It is by far the most common diagnosis leading to spinal surgery in patients above 65 years of age. Cancer-related surgeries, radiation, and chemotherapy can also alter architecture of the spinal canal, affecting multiple levels. The evidence for treatment of lumbar spinal stenosis with therapeutic exercises has been relatively poor; however, there have been small studies that have shown benefit from a therapeutic exercise program. The therapeutic program should aim at restoring range of motion. Flexion-based programs incorporate double knee to chest stretch, hip flexor stretches in supine, angry cat stretch, and pelvic tilts (Figs. 44.5, 44.6,

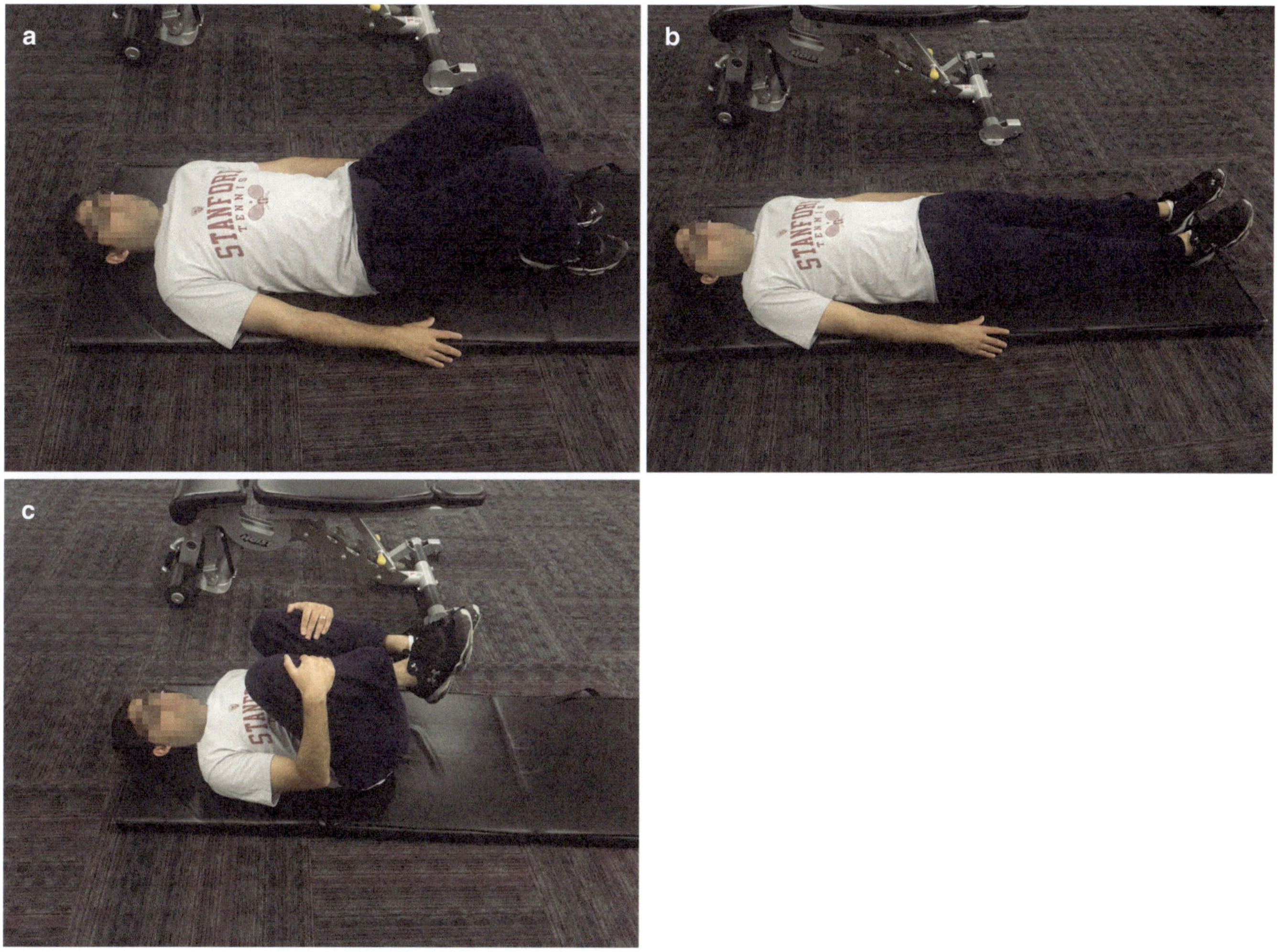

Fig. 44.5 (**a**) Starting position bilateral knee to chest for beginner with transverse abdominal brace (TvA). (**b**) Starting position bilateral knee to chest, advanced. (**c**) End pose for bilateral knee to chest

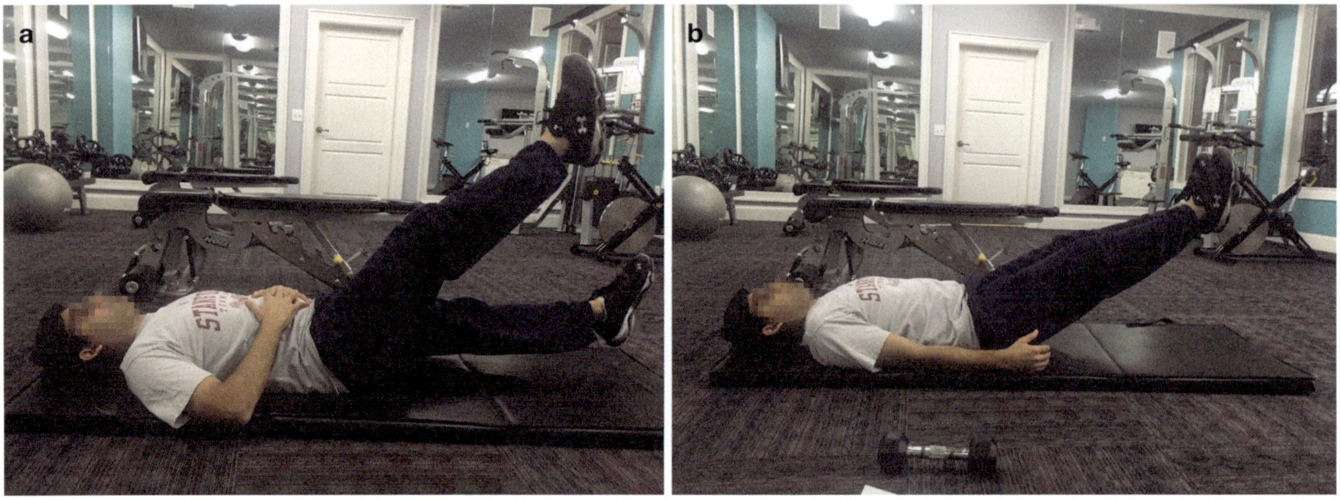

Fig. 44.6 (**a–b**) Straight leg raise with transverse abdominal brace with isometric hold

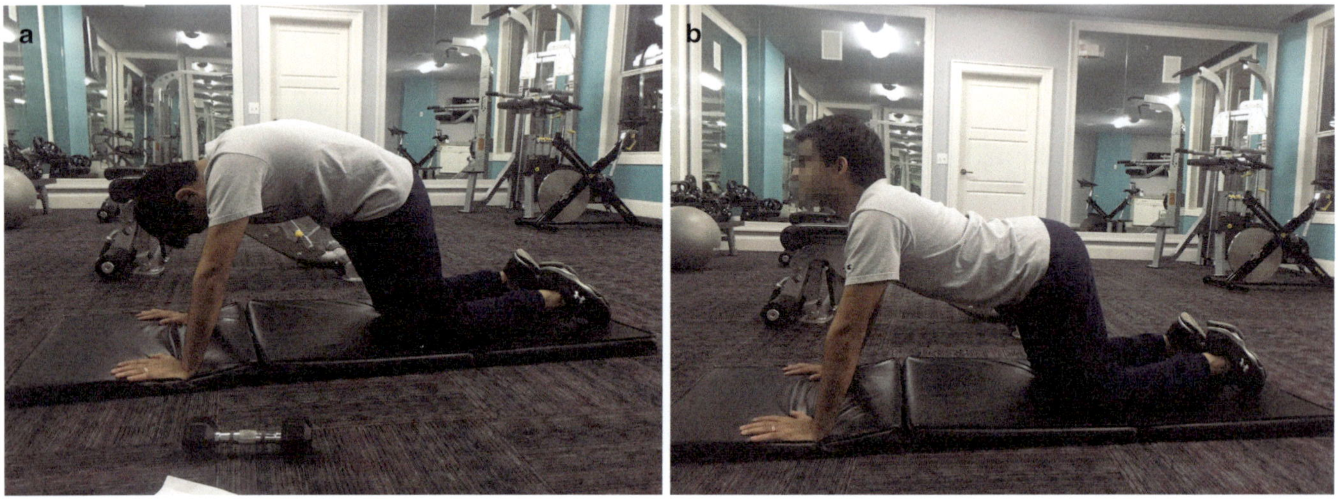

Fig. 44.7 (**a–b**) Cat camel stretch

44.7 and 44.8). Strengthening exercises should involve abdominal and gluteal muscles through pelvic tilt exercises, bridges in neutral spine, mini wall squats, and single leg standing. Conditioning exercises can incorporate an inclined treadmill or stationary bike to help improve cancer fatigue and related endurance.

Piriformis Syndrome

Mass lesions causing lumbar radicular pain can also affect the lumbosacral nerve root plexus and worsen nerve root compression in pre-existing lumbosacral dysfunction. Piriformis syndrome is a controversial diagnosis but is a contributing cause of sciatic pain. The therapy program should focus on piriformis stretching, either in the FAIR (flexion, adduction, and internal rotation) position or having the patient lying supine with the hip flexed greater than 90°, in abduction and external rotation [37]. Therapy strengthening should aim at core strengthening, lumbosacral stabilization, and hip strengthening exercises. Non-weight-bearing position exercises such as side-lying clamshell and supine bridge can be incorporated initially with gradual progression to weight-bearing exercises such as squatting or lunging. Exercises should also incorporate the transversus abdominis, multifidi, and internal and external obliques, as these help with lumbopelvic stabilization. Some examples include plank and side plank exercises. Therapeutic exercise should also incorporate pelvic tilt muscles such as hamstring stretching, iliotibial stretching, and hip extensor strengthening.

Gait and Balance Impairments

Individuals with gait and balance impairments also seek the assistance of physical therapists for rehabilitation to maxi-

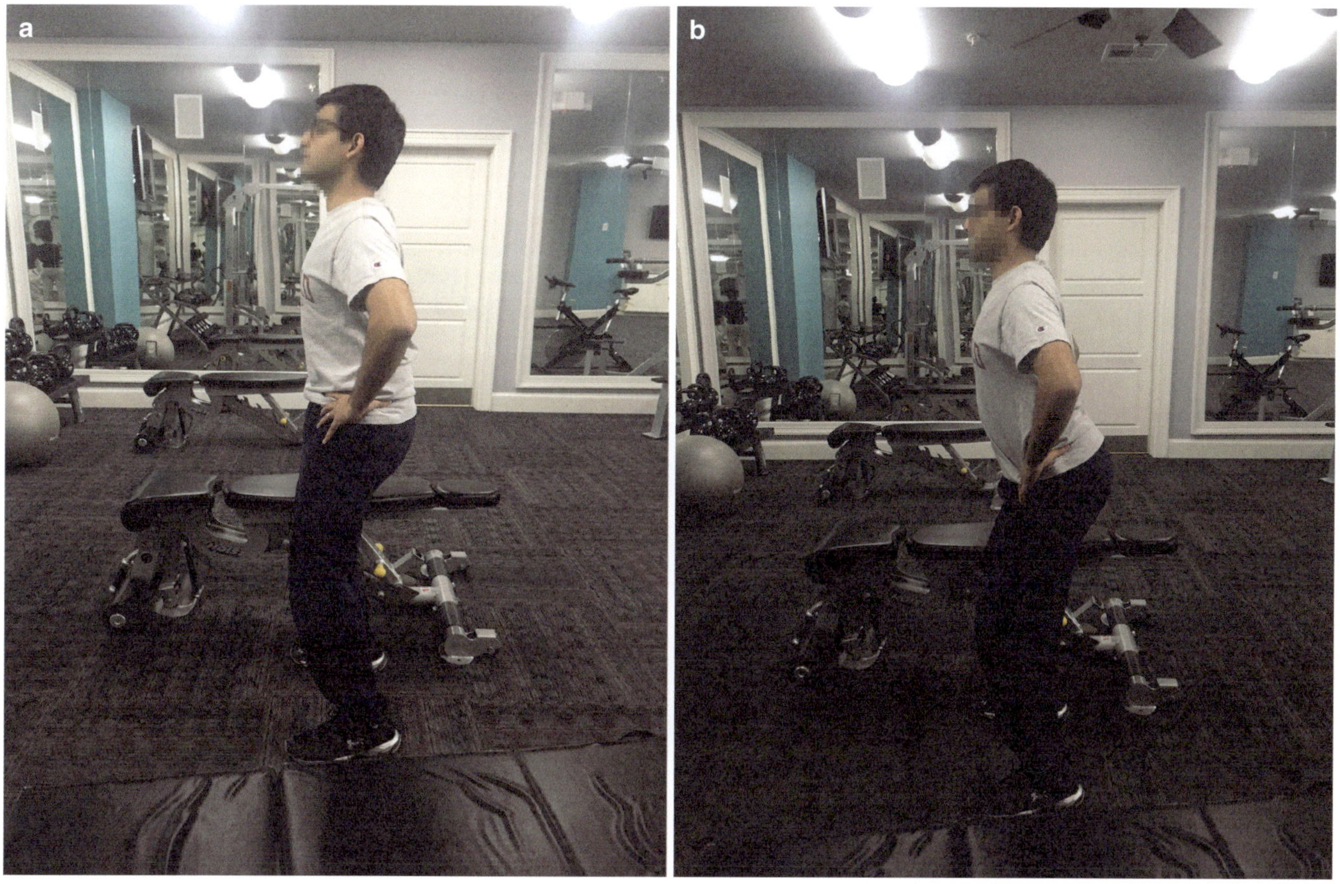

Fig. 44.8 Pelvic rotation (**a**) anterior pelvic tilt and (**b**) posterior pelvic tilt

mize functional mobility and increase balance and coordination. More specifically, there are physical therapists that specialize in vestibular rehabilitation, a type of rehabilitation technique aimed at individuals with balance disorders resulting from chronic inner ear infections, traumatic brain injuries, and vestibular neuritis to name a few.

Vestibular rehabilitation is indicated when an individual's equilibrium, proprioception, and balance are compromised as a result of the aforementioned conditions. Damage to the vestibular system may cause abnormal balance, dizziness, loss of coordination, and even vertigo. Vestibular physical therapists work with specific protocols targeted at the vestibular system which often incorporates eye movements, head and body positional changes, and acceleration and deceleration exercises. These exercises often provoke symptoms to desensitize the vestibular system and retrain or reset the brain to a baseline level. Assistive devices, such as durable medical equipment (DME), orthotics, and prosthetics, are also used by physical therapists to help individuals with gait and balance impairments. DME such as canes, crutches, walkers, and wheelchairs are often recommended and prescribed by physical therapists to assist with functional mobility.

Neurogenic Pain Disorders

Neoplastic lesions can result in poorly localized pain involving dysesthesias or allodynia. Direct infiltration of either a plexus or peripheral nerve can result in myotomal distribution weakness. Apart from neoplasia, effects from radiation and chemotherapy can be contributing causes. It has been shown that higher doses of cobalt radiation can lead up to 92% for brachial plexus injury [38]. Chemotherapy-induced neuropathy is commonly seen. In patients receiving taxanes, vinca alkaloids, or platinum-based compounds, 100% will develop symptoms of nerve dysfunction [39]. Common therapeutic approaches to neurogenic pain disorders are listed below.

Carpal Tunnel Syndrome

Carpal tunnel syndrome (CTS) is an assortment of clinical signs and symptoms that occur due to compression of the median nerve within the carpal tunnel. Treatment includes therapeutic exercise incorporating active range of motion in digits, increasing flexibility of the long finger flexors, and improving thenar muscle strengthening. Tendon and median nerve gliding can be of benefit in improving nerve mobility and tendon excursion. It should be noted that the strengthening programs, if causing reproducible symptoms, should be altered in intensity or range until the exercise no longer reproduces median nerve pain. Isometric strengthening of finger flexors and thenar muscles can be incorporated if median nerve pain is not reproducible. Hand ball and gripper type exercises should be avoided. Please refer to occupational therapy chapter for joint protection and ergonomic therapy interventions.

Ulnar Neuropathy

Ulnar neuropathy is also an entrapment neuropathy involving the ulnar nerve. Therapeutic exercise should incorporate neural glides and nerve mobilization after relative rest through immobilization, ideally in 45° elbow flexion. Active range of motion can be incorporated, and once pain-free range of motion has been achieved, tensioning exercises can be implemented. Intrinsic hand muscle strengthening can be included if it does not reproduce symptoms. Please refer to occupational therapy chapter for joint protection and ergonomic therapy interventions.

Peroneal Tendon Neuropathy

Therapeutic programs should aim at restoring lateral ankle pain stability due to the multiple avascular zones. Once pain-free range of motion has been restored, active passive range of motion can be incorporated to restore dorsiflexion with progressive resistance exercises. Therapeutic programs should incorporate proprioceptive training, neuromuscular reeducation and conditioning exercises. Please refer to occupational therapy chapter for joint protection, arch support, proper footwear, and ergonomic therapy interventions.

Summary

There has been an increase in number of cancer survivors, and the healthcare provider should at the very least know where and how to guide their functional recovery. This chapter aims to help meet those needs from a functional perspective that exist in the common cancer survivor population. As the field of cancer rehabilitation continues to grow and evidence-based protocols become more available, healthcare providers should feel comfortable in participating in basic functional therapy treatments. It is important to always evaluate therapy progression on a weekly or biweekly basis and have good communication with the therapy team to maximize functional outcome.

References

1. Stubblefield MD, Hubbard G, Cheville A, Koch U, Schmitz KH, Dalton SO. Current perspectives and emerging issues on cancer rehabilitation. Cancer. 2013;119(Suppl 11):2170–8.
2. American Physical Therapy Association. Who are physical therapists? 2015. Retrieved from: http://www.apta.org/AboutPTs/
3. Weaver KE, Forsythe LP, Reeve BB, et al. Mental and physical health-related quality of life among U.S. cancer survivors: population estimates from the 2010 National Health Interview Survey. Cancer Epidemiol Biomark Prev. 2012;21:2108–17.
4. Dietz JH. Adaptive rehabilitation of the cancer patient. Curr Probl Cancer. 1980;5(5):1–56.
5. Wang XS, Cleeland CS, Mendoza TR, et al. The effects of pain severity on health related quality of life: a study of Chinese cancer patients. Cancer. 1999;86:1848–55.
6. Cao S, Zhao G, Cui J, et al. Fast-track rehabilitation program and conventional care after esophagectomy: a retrospective controlled cohort study. Support Care Cancer. 2013;21:707–14.
7. Schmitz KH, Courneya KS, American College of Sports Medicine, et al. American college of sports medicine roundtable on exercise guidelines for cancer survivors. Med Sci Sports Exerc. 2010;7(42):1409–26.
8. Winningham ML, MacVicar MG, Burke MB. Exercise for cancer patients: guidelines and precautions. Phys Sportsmed. 1986;14:125–32.
9. Strasser B, Steindorf K, Wiskemann J, Ulrich CM. Impact of resistance training in cancer survivors: a meta-analysis. Med Sci Sports Exerc. 2013;45(11):2080–90. https://doi.org/10.1249/MSS.0b013e31829a3b63.
10. Focht BC, Clinton SK, Devor ST, Garver MJ, Lucas AR, Thomas-Ahner JM, Grainger E. Resistance exercise interventions during and following cancer treatment: a systematic review. J Support Oncol. 2013;11(2):45–60.
11. Wilkinson S, Barnes K, Storey L. Massage for symptom relief in patients with cancer: systematic review. J Adv Nurs. 2008;63(5):430–9. https://doi.org/10.1111/j.1365-2648.2008.04712.x.
12. Ernst E. Massage therapy for cancer palliation and supportive care: a systematic review of randomized clinical trials. Support Care Cancer. 2009;17(4):333–7. https://doi.org/10.1007/s00520-008-0569-z. Epub 2009 Jan 13.
13. Green S, Buchbinder R, Hetrick S. Physiotherapy interventions for shoulder pain. Cochrane Database Syst Rev. 2003;2:CD004258.
14. Neviaser AS, Hannafin JA. Adhesive capsulitis: a review of current treatment. Am J Sports Med. 2010;38(11):2346–56.
15. Kibler BW. Shoulder rehabilitation: principles and practice. Med Sci Sports Exerc. 1998;30(Suppl):S40–50.
16. Stubblefield MD, Custodio MD. Upper extremity pain disorders in breast cancer. Arch Phys Med Rehabil. 2006;87(3 Suppll):S96–9.
17. Crosier J-L, Foidart-Dessalle M, Tinant F, Crielaard J-M, Forthomme B. An isokinetic eccentric programme for the management of chronic lateral epicondylar tendinopathy. BMJ. 2007;41(4):269–75.
18. Stitik TP, Nadler SF, Foye PM, Smith R. Osteoarthritis of the knee and hip: practical non-drug steps to successful therapy. Consult Consultation Prim Care. 1999;39(6):1707–14.
19. Kummer B. Is the Pauwels' theory of hip biomechanics still valid: a critical analysis, based on modern methods. Ann Anat. 1993;175:203–10.
20. Segal NA, Felson DT, Torner JC, Zhu Y, Curtis JR, Niu J, Nevitt MC. Greater trochanteric pain syndrome: epidemiology and associated factors. Arch Phys Med Rehabil. 2007;88(8):988–92. https://doi.org/10.1016/j.apmr.2007.04.014.
21. Winters-Stone KM, Leo MC, Schwartz A. Exercise effects on hip bone mineral density in older, post-menopausal breast cancer survivors are age dependent. Arch Osteoporos. 2012;7(1–2):301–6. https://doi.org/10.1007/s11657-012-0071-6.
22. Saarto T, Sievanen H, Kellokumpu-Lehtinen P, Nikander R, Vehmanen L, Huovinen R, et al. Effect of supervised and home exercise training on bone mineral density among breast cancer patients: a 12-month randomized controlled trial. Osteoporos Int. 2012;23(5):1601–12. https://doi.org/10.1007/s00198-011-1761-4.

23. Li L, Setoguchi S, Cabral H, Jick S. Opioid use for noncancer pain and risk of fracture in adults: a nested case-control study using the general practice research database. Am J Epidemiol. 2013;178(4):559–69. https://doi.org/10.1093/aje/kwt013.
24. Pernambuco CS, Borba-Pinheiro CJ, Vale RG, et al. Functional autonomy, bone mineral density (BMD) and serum osteocalcin levels in older female participants of an aquatic exercise program (AAG). Arch Gerontol Geriatr. 2013;56(3):466–71.
25. Peters JS, Tyson NL. Proximal exercises are effective in treating patellofemoral pain syndrome: a systematic review. Int J Sports Phys Ther. 2013;8(5):689–700.
26. Lafuente GA, O'Mullony Munoz I, de la Fuente ME, Cura-Ituarte P. Plantar fasciitis: evidence-based review of treatment. Reumatol Clin. 2007;3(4):159–65. https://doi.org/10.1016/S1699-258X(07)73614-8.
27. Malliaras P, Barton CJ, Reeves ND, Langberg H. Achilles and patellar tendinopathy loading programmes: a systemic review comparing clinical outcomes and identifying potential mechanisms for effectiveness. Sports Med. 2013;43(4):267–86.
28. Stubblefield MD, O'Dell M. Cancer rehabilitation: principles and practice. 1st ed. New York: Demos Medical Publishing; 2009.
29. Hubbard TJ, Denegar CR. Does cryotherapy improve outcomes with soft tissue injury? J Athl Train. 2004;39(3):278–9.
30. Costa J, Espitito-Santo C, Borges A, et al. Botulinum toxin type A therapy for cervical dystonia. Cochrane Database Syst Rev. 2005;25:CD003633.
31. Braddom RL, editor. Physical medicine and rehabilitation. 4th ed. Philadelphia: Elsevier Saunders; 2011.
32. Macdonald et al. Long term follow up of breast cancer survivors with post-mastectomy pain syndrome. Br J Cancer. 2005;92(2):225–30.
33. Carriere B. Therapeutic exercises and self-correction programs. In: Flynn TW, editor. Thoracic spine and rib cage: musculoskeletal evaluation and treatment. Boston: Butterwork-Heinemann; 1996. p. 287–310.
34. Atlas SJ, Nardin RA. Evaluation and treatment of low back pain: an evidenced –based approach to clinical care. Muscle Nerve. 2003;27:265–84.
35. Wetzel FT, Donelson R. The role of repeated end-range/pain response assessment in the management of symptomatic lumbar discs. Spine J. 2003;3:146–54.
36. Siebert E, Pruss H, Klingebiel R, Failli V, Einhaupl KM, Schwab JM. Lumbar spinal stenosis: syndrome, diagnostics and treatment. Nat Rev Neurosci. 2009;5(7):392–403.
37. Robinson D. Piriformis muscle in relation to sciatic pain. Am J Surg. 1947;73:355–8.
38. Johansson S, Svensson H, Denekamp J. Timescale of evolution of late radiation injury after postoperative radiotherapy of breast cancer patients. Int J Radiat Oncol Biol Phys. 2000;48:745–50.
39. Hilkens PH, van den Bent MJ. Chemotherapy-induced peripheral neuropathy. J Peripher Nerv Syst. 1997;2:350–61.

Occupational Therapy

45

Meilani Mapa and Jason Chen

Philosophies, Principles, and Practice

"The practice of occupational therapy is based on the belief that occupation can be used to prevent and minimize dysfunction, and it can also bring forth beneficial adaptations in individuals" [1]. Occupation is commonly associated with a job or one's career. In the therapeutic sense, occupation refers to activities used by an occupational therapist with the intention to restore lost function caused by medical or psychological conditions. Occupational therapists evaluate a variety of factors that affect a patient's daily function: activities of daily living (ADLs), instrumental activities of daily living (iADLs), weakness, loss of range of motion (ROM), functional impairments because of disease, rest and sleep, education, work, play, leisure, and social participation. "An occupational therapist is someone who selects specific occupations to prevent the development of problems, improve performance and maintain a patient's existing abilities" [1].

According to the American Occupational Therapy Association, the practice of occupational therapy includes evaluating personal, medical, behavioral, and biopsychosocial factors that affect performance in areas of occupation (activities of daily living (ADLs), instrumental activities of daily living (iADLs), rest and sleep, education, work, play, leisure, and social participation) [2]. Evaluation starts with creating an occupational profile, which describes the patient's patterns of daily living, interests, values, and needs. This is followed by analysis of occupational performance in which a patient's problems or potential problems are identified and targeted outcomes are established as goals for therapy. Upon completing the assessment, occupational therapists utilize interventions that result in the "establishment, remediation, or restoration of a skill or ability that has not yet developed, is impaired, or is in decline." Interventions can include use of "occupations," exercises, activities, training in self-care, self-management, health management, home maintenance, community/work reintegration, and the use of physical modalities and modification of environments.

Broadly speaking, intervention strategies include remediation and compensation. Remediation is the "resolution of functional or structural deficits or the acquisition of new skills in an area of skilled movement, cognition or social function" [3]. Compensation is the performance of a task that can be adapted or performed by a caregiver within in the constraints of the patient's limitations. Models are domains that OTs examine and perform assessments of different areas, describing a patient's functionality. Some examples of models include biomechanical, cognitive, functional group, intentional relationship, human occupation, motor control, and sensory integration [4].

Purpose of Occupational Therapy

The role of occupational therapy in rehabilitation is to facilitate and enable an individual patient to achieve maximal functional performance, both physically and psychologically, in everyday living skills regardless of his or her life expectancy [5]. Occupational therapy aims to promote optimal functional independence and minimize the physical and psychological aspects of disability [6]. To formulate a treatment plan, the therapist must start with an evaluation of a patient.

Evaluation of a Patient

The evaluation of a patient for therapy services is based on the physiatric history and physical examination (H&P). The H&P includes the following components: chief complaint,

M. Mapa
Memorial Rehabilitation Institute, Memorial Healthcare Systems, Division of Physical Medicine and Rehabilitation, Hollywood, FL, USA

J. Chen (✉)
McGovern Medical School at UT Health, Department of Physical Medicine and Rehabilitation, The University of Texas Health Science Center at Houston, Houston, TX, USA
e-mail: Jason.Chen@uth.tmc.edu

A. Gulati et al. (eds.), *Essentials of Interventional Cancer Pain Management*, https://doi.org/10.1007/978-3-319-99684-4_45

history of present illness, past medical/social/family history, functional history, review of systems, physical exam, data review and assessment, and plan. Unique to the physiatric H&P is the focus on mechanism of injury, any prior history that may contribute to current deficits and identification of the individual's impairments, disability, and handicap. Furthermore, a functional history reveals baseline mobility, activities of daily living (ADLs), and instrumental activities of daily living (iADLs). According to Braddom et al. [7], the physiatric history and examination determines not only physical deficits but also the functional impact of these deficits. The identification of functional problems is the basis for developing a therapeutic plan. After reviewing the above, the occupational therapist will complete a variety of assessments with the patient to create a plan of care for the patient.

Disability/Impairment/Handicap

According to the World Health Organization (1980) in the International Classification of Impairments, Disabilities, and Handicaps, impairment is defined as any loss or abnormality of psychological, physiological, or anatomical structure or function. Disability is defined as any restriction or lack (resulting from an impairment) of ability to perform an activity in the manner or within the range considered normal for a human being. Handicap is defined as a disadvantage for a given individual that limits or prevents the fulfillment of a role that is normal. As traditionally used, impairment refers to a problem with a structure or organ of the body; disability is a functional limitation about a particular activity [8].

Functional History

A "functional history" refers to the level of independence at which the patient had with mobility and with ADLs, before their current diseased state. The functional history provides insight to determine what level of function a patient could potentially return to. This knowledge is essential in the formulation of therapeutic goals as a part of the patient's treatment plan. A commonly used objective functional measure is the Functional Independence Measure (FIM) instrument. The occupational therapist will use the FIM to assess their level of independence with ADLs.

Mobility

Mobility is characterized as the activities that allow person travel from one place to another. This includes ambulation, transfers (moving from one situation to another, i.e., transferring postings from a wheelchair to the bed), wheelchair mobility, and bed mobility. Mobility activities are rated with the FIM instrument, and a patient can range from dependent to independent. At times, patient may require assistive devices to maintain mobility. These include power wheelchairs, manual wheelchairs, scooters, walkers, crutches, canes, transfer board, bedside commode, tub bench, shower chair, and grab bars (for shower).

Activities of Daily Living

Activities of daily living are activities that are oriented toward taking care of one's own body; these activities are ordinary and familiar things that people do every day. In addition, they have purpose, value, and meaning to the performer and involve multiple tasks. According to Christiansen and Hammecker, these activities are fundamental to living in a social world; they enable basic survival and well-being. ADLs are also referred to as basic activities of daily living and personal activities of daily living. Examples include bathing, showering, bowel and bladder management, toileting, personal hygiene and grooming, dressing, and feeding oneself. An occupational therapist works in these areas during their therapeutic management plan to increase that person's independence [9].

FIM Instrument

FIM (Functional Independence Measure) is a tool used by therapists to indicate the patient's severity of disability. It is owned by Uniform Data System for Medical Rehabilitation (UDSMR), and practitioners who score FIMs must be certified prior to evaluating patients with the FIM. It is a 7-point ordinal scale that rates 18 items (13 motor tasks and 5 cognitive tasks) with functional scores ranging from dependence (0) to independence (7) [10]. This scale considers the level of assistance a patient requires to accomplish a task [5].

The following tasks are measured by the FIM:

- Eating
- Grooming
- Bathing
- Upper body dressing
- Lower body dressing
- Toileting
- Bladder management
- Bowel management
- Bed to chair transfer
- Shower transfer
- Locomotion (ambulation or wheelchair)
- Stairs
- Cognitive comprehension

- Expression
- Social interaction
- Problem solving
- Memory

The following describes the scoring of the FIM:

- 7: Complete independence – can safely perform all tasks 100% without assistive devices or modifications.
- 6: Modified independence – can safely perform 100% of the work with the use of aid or assistive device.
- 5. Supervision/setup – person performs 100% of the work, requires no physical contact, and can perform with a helper setting up the items or using cues or coaxing techniques.
- 4: Minimal assistance – person performs greater than 75% of the work.
- 3: Moderate assistance – person performs 50–74% of the work.
- 2: Maximal assistance – person performs 25–50% of the work.
- 1: Total assistance – person performs less than 25% of the work.
- 0: Activity does not occur.

The FIM has been validated by several research studies in the following populations: general rehabilitation, stroke, spinal cord injury (SCI), traumatic brain injury (TBI), orthopedic diagnoses, multiple sclerosis, and elderly adults.

Instrumental Activities of Daily Living (iADLs)

Instrumental ADLs describe the tasks required to function in the community independently. A common screening tool used to assess aids is the Lawton Instrumental Activities of Daily Living Scale. This is an ordinal scale that rates aids with total scores ranging from 0 (low function) to 8 (high function). The activities rated include using the telephone, shopping, preparing food, housekeeping, doing the laundry, using transportation, handling medications, and handling finances.

Evaluation of a Patient

After completing a thorough history of the patient including the functional history with mobility and ADLS, the therapist will complete a full physical examination focusing on the neurological and musculoskeletal exam.

The musculoskeletal exam consists of:

- Examining the muscle bulk, skin, and joints noting any deformities, edema, erythema, etc.
- Palpation of muscles and joints
- Manual muscle testing of the upper and lower extremity muscles
- Testing the range of motion of various joints and noting any spasticity or abnormal movements or abnormal end feels
- Measuring the angle of joints with a goniometer
- Evaluating the current level of ADLs including dressing, feeding, bathing, toileting, and transfers using the FIM instrument

The neurological exam consists of:

- Examining cranial nerves
- Testing sensation to light touch/pinprick in the dermatomes and peripheral nerve distribution
- Testing sensation; proprioception and kinesthesia
- Vision assessment
- Evaluating reflexes
- Cognitive evaluation using the Mini-Mental Status or MoCA exam
- Spasticity assessment using Modified Ashworth Scale and/or Tardieu Scale

*An occupational therapist's scope of practice includes upper extremities, ADLs, and cognition in comparison to a physical therapist that focuses on the lower extremities and mobility.

Treatment of a Patient

The therapist uses the information gathered in the history and physical examination to formulate the treatment plan and aids in setting the goals of what the therapist and patient wish to accomplish from the treatment. The therapist will formulate short-term goals and long-term goals and include personal goals of the patient and patient's family to create the plan of care. This process is client-centered and dynamic. Treatments consist of many domains ranging from hands-on therapy techniques to equipment considerations and family education.

Domains of Occupational Therapy (Table 45.1)

Neuromuscular Interventions

- This includes evaluation of joint range of motion, manual muscle strength testing, spasticity/tone, sensation, sensory deficits, and proprioception. The occupational therapist will evaluate the patient and then comment if any

Table 45.1 Domains of occupational therapy

Occupational therapy domains	Examples
Neuromuscular interventions	Balance training, manual muscle training, and postural awareness constraint-induced movement. Bobath/Brunnstrom techniques, serial casting, splint, positioning, neuromuscular reeducation concepts, NDT, PNF
Cardiopulmonary interventions	Breathing and endurance exercises to improve tidal volumes, aerobic and conditioning exercises, environmental changes
Musculoskeletal interventions	Strengthening, range of motion exercises, mobilization, manual therapy, edema control
Cognitive/ perceptual/ sensory interventions	Cognitive retraining; perceptual, visual, and sensory training; desensitization
Equipment	Durable medical equipment, splint fabrication, orthotics and prosthetics
Modalities	Hot/cold packs, whirlpool, contrast baths, electrical stimulation units (FES, NMES, TENS), fluidotherapy, paraffin baths, electrical stimulation (e-stim), ultrasound, iontophoresis
Education and training	Patient and family education

limitations exist. Once the limitations are identified, the OT will focus to improve those areas.

Cardiopulmonary Interventions

- This includes breathing and endurance exercises to improve tidal volumes and exercise tolerance. These interventions focus on aerobic and conditioning exercises and energy conservation techniques. The occupational therapist may teach the patient to grade their activity. Furthermore, these exercises can also better prepare the body prior to any surgical intervention. These exercises enhance and facilitate recovery. Occupational therapists will also assess the environmental demands or barriers, i.e., presence of stairs and airborne irritants.

Musculoskeletal Interventions

- These interventions include exercises or stretches to improve the strength and mobilization of affected muscles and the range of motion of tight or contracted joints. Therapist can also perform splinting, casting, manual therapy and edema control with massage therapy, retrograde massage, mobilizations, positioning, and kinesio taping.

Cognitive/Perceptual/Sensory Interventions

- In addition to the musculoskeletal interventions that OT can provide to patients, they are also trained in helping those with cognitive deficits. These interventions focus on exercises to improve cognitive retraining, perceptual, visual, and/or sensory training. The therapists can identify safety issues and help with return to work/school/driving.

Equipment

- The therapist will evaluate the current function of the patient and recommend any durable medical equipment such as a bedside commode, tub bench, wheelchair, sliding board, and assistive ambulatory devices such as walkers, canes, and crutches. Adaptive equipment can also be used to compensate weakness and increase independence with ADLs such as a sock aid, long-handled sponge, long-handled shoe horn, reacher, button hooks, etc. Therapist can also fabricate serial casts to help improve and maintain range of motion and splints to help maintain joint range of motion, maintain skin integrity, and prevent contractures. Finally, occupational therapists can trial and recommend orthotics and prosthetics for patients with bracing needs and amputations.

Modalities

- Therapist use a multitude of modalities in the treatment plan to help with desensitization of a painful limb, edema reduction, improvement of joint stiffness, spasticity and pain management, and delivery of medications. This includes hot/cold packs, whirlpool, contrast baths, electrical stimulation units (Functional Electrical Stimulation, Neuromuscular Electrical Stimulation, TENS), fluidotherapy, paraffin baths, ultrasound, and iontophoresis.

Education and Training

- Patient and family education is an integral part of the treatment plan. Occupational therapists provide strategies to compensate for their impairments. They also provide safety education in the home environment, i.e., home safety evaluation. With a home safety evaluation, the therapist can recommend equipment needed in the home – grab bars, ramp, and bathroom equipment.

Therapeutic Considerations in a Cancer Patient

To create a therapeutic treatment plan, it is important to understand the stage of the cancer or the disease status along the continuum of cancer care. This will help tailor treatment options, goals, duration, and treatment [9]. Goal setting and treatment planning for cancer patients can be separated in four categories: preventative, restorative, supportive, and palliative [9].

Patients with a diagnosis of cancer are at risk of developing permanent functional impairments involving multiple body systems. These adverse effects of cancer/cancer treatment include pain, fatigue, deconditioning, decreased physical strength, reduced range of motion, decreased cardiovascular capacity, lymphedema, mood disorder such as depression or anxiety, bone loss, and heart disease. Understanding these impairments and the role of occupational is imperative in formulating the treatment plan.

Continuum of Cancer Care

Before a therapist can formulate a therapeutic treatment plan, they must understand where the patient falls on the continuum of cancer care. Therapy prescriptions, the process, and progress of rehabilitation can vary depending upon what stage of the continuum of cancer care the patient is in. These stages include:

- Pretreatment: diagnosis of cancer has been established, but no treatment has begun.
- During treatment: Patient is receiving treatment for cancer. This can be the initial treatment course or treatment for a relapse. Patient can also be receiving long-term treatment antineoplastic treatment to keep disease in remission.
- Posttreatment/remission: patient has completed cancer treatments.
- Palliative: patient with incurable cancer is receiving treatment focused on relieving pain and preventing further suffering.

The focus of OT in the pretreatment stage is upon patient education and general strengthening and conditioning. The goal is to educate the patient about potential functional limitations that may arise as he or she progresses through the cancer continuum. General strengthening and conditioning prior to receiving antineoplastic treatment has been shown to "improve exercise capacity and preserve pulmonary function following surgery." In some cases, improving cardiopulmonary reserve through PT and/or OT is a major factor toward the decision for a patient to receive oncologic intervention [11].

OT during treatment stage focuses on general conditioning and addressing any specific treatment-related side effects and complications that may arise such as cancer fatigue, radiation fibrosis, chemotherapy-induced neuropathy, etc. Graded exercise is important at this stage since patient may be experiencing pronounced fatigue from the cancer and treatment.

OT during the posttreatment or remission stage focuses on improving the deficits and impairments that result from the disease process or from the oncologic treatment. OT will also focus on improving the overall strength and general conditioning of the patient.

OT during the palliative stage focuses on energy conservation, use of adaptive equipment as necessary for ADLs, family training, and maximizing the patient's strengths.

In general, OT interventions in the cancer continuum can be categorized as:

- Preventative interventions: attempt to decrease the effect of impairments caused by cancer and its treatment. This mainly occurs through patient education.
- Restorative interventions: attempt to return patient to previous level of function. For example, after lung resection, a patient participates in a graded exercise program to increased cardiopulmonary functioning.
- Supportive interventions: attempt to accommodate for impairments and disabilities. Occupational therapists play a central role with the use of assistive devices that can improve mobility and independence with ADL functions.
- Palliative interventions: attempt to provide both optimal function and comfort. Therapy goals here include pain control, prevention of contractures and pressure ulcers, prevention of reconditioning, and energy conservation.

Precautions/Considerations During Occupational Therapy

Orthopedic patients may have certain weight bearing restrictions through their limbs. This limits the amount of activity and type of activity in the therapeutic plan. Other patients may have postsurgical precautions, such as sternal precautions. When a therapist is evaluating a patient, they must establish the patient's baseline to detect changes and progression of disease over the treatment course. One should also monitor vital signs, fatigue levels, hydration status, and medication schedule. During treatments, a therapist should contact a physician immediately with any new onset or increase in symptoms of the following [12]:

- Fever
- Cardiac abnormalities
- Weakness or fatigue
- Leg pain or cramps
- Unusual joint pain
- Bruising and nausea
- Rapid weight loss
- Diarrhea or vomiting
- Changes in mental status
- Dizziness and blurred vision
- Fainting gray or pale appearance
- Night pain without a history of an injury

In regard to a cancer patient, symptoms a therapist should report [12]:

- Marked increase in lymphedema
- Sudden increase/change in pain symptoms
- New palpable mass/lymph node
- Change in continence
- Venous thromboembolic events

Conditions that are considered a contraindication to therapy or an emergency in cancer rehabilitation and that need acute medical management include [17]:

- Malignancy
  - Symptoms include pain paresthesia or paralysis. There might be swelling present and rapid onset of edema.
- Deep venous thrombosis
  - Symptoms include swelling of the leg, pain/tenderness of the leg, increased warmth or redness of the affected limb, and pain with ambulation.
- Pulmonary embolus
  - Symptoms include shortness of breath, pain with deep breathing, coughing of blood, and tachycardia.
- Malignant pericardial effusion
  - Symptoms include shortness of breath, cyanosis, anxiety, venous distention in neck, and orthopnea. This can lead to a life-threatening condition and cardiac tamponade.
- Superior vena cava syndrome
  - Symptoms include facial and neck swelling, ruddy complexion, and protruding eyes. This is a blockage of the superior vena cava from a tumor, swollen lymph node, or blood clot. It is associated with central venous catheters and cancers such as lymphoma and lung.
- Hypercalcemia
  - Symptoms include malaise, cognitive issues, nausea, frequent urination, and pain. It is associated with cancers such as lung, esophageal, head and neck, and cervical.
- Tumor lysis syndrome
  - Symptoms include polyuria, nausea, muscle weakness, joint pain, fatigue, lethargy, cardiac arrhythmias, and seizures. It is associated with fast-growing blood tumors, acute leukemia, and high-grade lymphoma. It is caused by a metabolic derangement with tumor breakdown following cytotoxic therapy.

Conditions that are considered a relative contraindication to therapy in a cancer patient are [13]:

Hematologic Consideration

- Anemia
  - Symptoms include fatigue, irritability, and light-headedness. Treatment should be modified on fatigue level.
- Thrombocytopenia
  - Symptoms include bruising, bleeding, and petechiae. Treatment should focus on functional mobility, and therapist should place the patient on fall precautions.
- Leukopenia/neutropenia
  - Symptoms include frequent infections, fevers, and throat/mouth sores. A patient with this is at risk for infection. The patient may need reverse or protective isolation or creative treatment interventions.

Musculoskeletal Consideration

- Bone metastases
  - During the treatment of patient in cancer rehabilitation, one must always consider if metastatic disease is present. Common primary tumors that metastasize to the bone include breast, prostate, lung, kidney, and thyroid [14]. This may change your course of rehabilitation and goals. For example, a weight bearing status may involve new ROM restrictions that necessitate assistive devices. Patients should avoid resistive exercises. Patients with spine metastases should avoid spinal loading.

Neurological Considerations

- Metastatic disease
  - SCI compression: Symptoms include bowel or bladder changes and pain at night [13]. In a patient that has a spinal cord injury due to a primary tumor or tumor progression, rehabilitation will focus on relief of symptoms, quality of life improvements, functional independence, and prevention of further complications
  - Brain tumor or metastases: In addition to the OT treatment aimed to help functional impairments, patients

with hemiparesis, spasticity, decreased range of motion, and pain may need cognitive retraining and safety awareness. A speech therapy consult may be warranted to evaluate cognition, communication, and swallowing difficulties.

Special considerations to oncologic cases are discussed below [13]:

- Chemotherapy
  - Chemotherapy can result in myelosuppression, specifically anemia and leukopenia. Leukopenic patients may require neutropenic precautions since they are susceptible to infections. Anemic patients with hemoglobin below 8 mg/dL may experience symptoms due to increased oxygen demand during therapeutic activities. Common presenting symptoms include fatigue, dizziness, light-headedness, and tachycardia. Anemic patients may require blood transfusions to tolerate therapies.
- Radiation therapy
  - During temporary brachytherapy, a patient may need to stay in isolation after implantation of radiation-emitting seeds. An occupational therapist should evaluate the patient beforehand to ensure they can perform ADLs at an independent level. If osseous structures are receiving radiation, weight bearing status can be changed to protect the bones since they can be prone to fractures. Radiation fibrosis can occur after completion of radiation therapy (6 months–5 years) and result in restricted range of motion. This restricted range of motion usually responds to soft tissue mobilization of the radiated area to maximize blood flow to the area. Mobilization of tissues prevents contractures which can result in permanent loss of range of motion.

Cancer-Related Pain

The occupational therapist is one member of an interdisciplinary team to treat a person's pain. According to the article written by McCormack, "the therapist promotes movement, alters mood, diverts the mind from pain, and provides a controlled amount of stress. These processes help the patient with chronic pain by stimulating natural physiological mechanisms in the endocrine, system, immune system, and nervous system." Occupational therapy can contribute to pain management by providing noninvasive techniques and purposeful activity that have been shown to potentiate physiological mechanisms associated with pain reduction.

Pain management techniques with occupational therapy include positioning strategies in the bed, wheelchair use to treat painful posture or movements, and casting or splinting of a painful limb to prevent contracture. Occupational therapists can also use modalities such as hot/cold compresses or ultrasound to help alleviate pain. Finally, massage, trigger point stimulation, and cognitive distraction techniques such as therapeutic relaxation and auditory distraction can be used [15].

Treatment Options

Massage

- Massage has been used as far back as 3000 BC when the Chinese used this technique to alleviate a sore muscle. Evidence suggests that deep pressure to specific sites on the skin can relieve chronic pain for long periods and even permanently [15].

Trigger Point Stimulation

- Trigger point stimulation is also known as acupressure, shiatsu, or myofascial release. The technique of trigger point stimulation is once the trigger point is located, the therapist applies pressure with his/her thumb or index finger over an area to locate a highly sensitive spot [15]. To discharge or release a trigger point, fingertip pressure is applied for 7 seconds with a pointed battery-operated vibrator (60 Hz) [15]. For large muscles of the extremities, Kraus recommends application of 15–20 lb. of pressure. Small facial muscles require 6 lbs. of pressure. After pressure has been applied for 7 s, the muscles should be stretched with active range of motion exercises. There are certain precautions one must consider before engaging in this technique. Releasing trigger points will cause some pain to the patient. Also, the therapist should have their fingernails trimmed to avoid injury. Skin surfaces that are infected or contused should be avoided. Contraindications include patients with a cardiac history, pregnant women, or patients with a full stomach because of autonomic or endocrine system imbalances. The treatment should be stopped if it aggravates the symptoms and brings no relief from pain [15].

Cognitive Distraction

- Cognitive distraction can activate the cortical modulation system as a way of "sensory shielding" and therefore distracting a patient away from his/her pain. Auditory distractions with the use of background music or music through headsets are an example of a cognitive distraction technique. Therapeutic relaxation is another type of cognitive distraction. Therapists can teach the patient certain breathing exercises such as deep breathing or rhythmic breathing to help alleviate the pain. Visualization techniques can also help one's pain. In this technique, a therapist uses visualization and metaphors to empower the patient to harness his or her natural ability to relieve pain [15].

Cancer Fatigue

Cancer fatigue is one of the most common symptoms that affect patients. Etiologies include side effects from cancer, oncologic treatment (radiation therapy, chemotherapy, and biologic therapies), or medical causes (deconditioning, anemia, hypothyroidism, etc.) [16]. Occupational therapists evaluate cancer fatigue with formal assessment tools and fatigue diaries. Treatment includes energy management strategies to conserve energy, relaxation and structured sleep, graded activity and exercise, structured psychological support, and assistance with lifestyle adaptation [17]. Graded activity and exercise is low to moderate intensity exercise that is progressive, initially starting at 15 min, 3 times per week, building up to a maximum of 30 min, 5 times per week. Energy conservation strategies include spreading out activities throughout the day, scheduling regular breaks between activities, and utilizing caregiver support or assistive devices. Furthermore, employing good sleep hygiene (maintaining a schedule of sleeping and waking hours, not using the bed for activities other than sleep, avoiding drinking caffeine prior to bedtime, etc.) can improve sleep quality which may decrease fatigue [17]. Occupational therapists can also address the performance of ADLs (activities of daily living).

Chemotherapy-Induced Peripheral Neuropathy

Chemotherapy-induced peripheral neuropathy is a significant, debilitating condition directly related to the administration of neurotoxic chemotherapy in the treatment of cancer. This neuropathy comprises quality of life and results in pain and discomfort. In addition to the pharmacologic interventions that have been studied to help prevent or improve CIPN, there are also non-pharmacologic interventions that may also prevent or improve CIPN. These non-pharmacologic treatments can be offered through occupational therapy; however, they have not been widely studied, and the effectiveness is unknown. Some of these non-pharmacologic interventions include physical activity and exercise, assistive devices, pulsed infrared light therapy, and transcutaneous nerve stimulation [18].

Treatment Options

Physical Activity and Exercise

- Physical activity and exercise interventions have not been exclusively studied in patients with chemotherapy-induced neuropathy. There are studies that show this is helpful in the diabetic neuropathy population.

Assistive Devices

- Occupational therapists can assist in identifying any equipment such as a bedside commode, tub bench/shower chair, wheelchair, shower chair, or splint fabrication. The occupational therapist may also provide the patient with adaptive equipment for energy conservation, i.e., long-handled sponge, long-handled shoe horn, sock aid, and/or a reacher.

Lymphedema

Lymphedema is a progressive disorder of the lymphatic system in which a buildup of lymph fluid can lead to adipose tissue hypertrophy and fibrosis. There are two types of lymphedema, primary and secondary. Primary lymphedema is caused by a genetic or inherited condition that causes issues with lymphatic flow [19]. Secondary lymphedema is due to an underlying disease or a complication to a prior treatment that interrupts lymphatic drainage [19]. Cancer and its related treatments such as surgery and radiation therapy are a common cause for secondary lymphedema in the United States. The incidence of lymphedema has been reported to be from 6% to 70% in breast cancer patients [20]. Cancer-associated lymphedema can occur in two ways: obstruction of lymphatic channels or node and infiltration of lymphatic vessels [19].

Symptoms of lymphedema include swelling, loss of range of motion, pain, and skin changes. There are three stages of lymphedema. Stage 1 presents with pitting. There is no increase of arm girth or heaviness. This stage is reversible. Stage 2 is characterized as brawny, fibrotic, and non-pitting. This stage is irreversible. Stage 3 is also known as advanced lymphedema. This stage is characterized by papillomatous outgrowths and hyperkeratosis of the skin [20].

Classification System

Taking preoperative and postoperative measurements of both arms can be useful in the assessment and diagnosis of lymphedema [20]. Measurements of the arm are taken in four locations: metacarpal phalangeal joint, wrist, 10 cm distal to the lateral epicondyle, and 15 cm proximal to lateral epicondyles [20]. According to the Harris et al. in the clinical practice guidelines of breast cancer: a difference of greater than 2.0 cm at any of the four measurements points may warrant treatment of the lymphedema, provided that the tumor involvement of the axilla or brachial plexus, infection and axillary vein thrombosis have been ruled out.

The classification of lymphedema is based on the American Physical Therapy Association [21]:

- Mild: girth difference < 3 cm
- Moderate: girth difference 3–5 cm difference
- Severe: girth difference > 5 cm

Treatment Options

Therapists may formulate a treatment plan for complete or complex decongestive therapy or CDT. In addition to splinting and positioning strategies, occupational therapists can also incorporate retrograde massage and manual drainage, prescribe compression garments, and help in improving quality of life. There are specialized courses that an occupational therapist can take to be certified in lymphedema management.

Complex decongestive therapy (CDT) is a technique that is designed to reduce the degree in lymphedema and to maintain the health of the skin and supporting structures. It is a two-phase program that can be used in children and adults. The first phase also known as the treatment phase includes skin care to avoid infection, manual lymph drainage compression garments, and serial measurements of the affected limb. This phase is usually 5 days per week for 2–4 weeks. The second phase also known as the maintenance phase focuses on the maintenance of benefits gained from the first phase. Again, compression garments, lymph drainage, and exercises are used in maintenance. Serial measurements of the affected limb are taken every 6 months. Contraindications to manual lymph drainage include active cellulitis, neoplasm, or other inflammations of the affected limb. Relative contraindications include uncontrolled hypertension, diabetes mellitus, asthma, or paralysis [22].

Manual lymph drainage is a massage technique that trained occupational therapists can perform. It is a massage technique that follows the anatomic lymphatic pathways along the surface of the skin [20]. Light pressure in used to mobilize fluid in a distal to proximal direction. This helps promote dilation and contractility of lymphatic conduits and create watershed pathways for limb flow. Contraindications to manual lymph drainage include active cellulitis, neoplasm, or other inflammations of the affected limb. Relative contraindications include uncontrolled hypertension, diabetes mellitus, asthma, or paralysis [22].

Compression garments with pressures from 20 mm Hg to 60 mm have been shown to be effective in the treatment of lymphedema. A randomized controlled study by Bertelli compared compression sleeve with electrical stimulated lymphatic drainage versus compression sleeve alone showed a 17% decrease in limb girth in both modalities. These garments can be custom-made or prefabricated, but all should be fitted by trained personal. Compression garments should be replaced every 4–6 months or when they lose their elasticity. Practitioners may want to encourage the long-term and consistent use of compression garments [20].

Brachial Plexopathy

The most common presenting symptom of a brachial plexopathy is pain in the shoulder or axilla [23]. Brachial plexopathies in a patient with cancer can be caused by the tumor itself or treatment for the tumor. Breast and lung cancers are the most frequent neoplasms leading to brachial plexopathy [23]. In comparison with radiation-induced plexopathies, neoplastic plexopathies more commonly produce pain as symptom onset, involve the lower plexus, and are frequently associated with a Horner's syndrome [23].

Radiation-induced brachial plexopathy (RIBP) results from radiation to the nerves and tissues adjacent to the clavicle and axilla, commonly treating lung and breast cancer [17]. Radiation-induced plexopathy frequently has less pain when compared to a neoplastic brachial plexopathy [23]. Pain also typically occurs later the course of cancer. The most common presenting symptom of RIBP is tingling and numbness of the forefinger and muscle wasting of the intrinsic hand muscles [17]. The pain associated with RIBP can be constant or intermittent. It can be characterized as burning, tingling/shooting, pins and needle-like, and/or cramp tightness [17].

A range of motion exercise program can be designed for the patient to be self-performed, or the therapist can train the family members to assist. This can help maintain joint mobility and prevent contracture. Occupational therapists can also fabricate splints or casts to help with positioning or maintain range or tape the shoulder to maintain proper anatomical alignment of the joints.

Radiation-Induced Fibrosis

Radiation-induced fibrosis is described as insidious pathologic fibrotic tissue sclerosis that occurs in response to radiation exposure [24]. Radiation can cause damage to the skin and subcutaneous tissue, lungs, gastrointestinal and genitourinary tracts, muscles, or other organs, depending upon the treatment site and dose. Radiation-induced fibrosis can cause both cosmetic and functional impairments and furthermore lead to death or a significant deterioration in the quality of life [25]. Radiation dose and volume, previous or concurrent treatments, genetic susceptibility, and comorbidities such as diabetes mellitus or an existing connective tissue disease or concurrent chemotherapy are risk factors for fibrosis [23]. Populations at risk of developing radiation-induced fibrosis include patients with Hodgkin's lymphoma, breast cancer, and head/neck cancers [24].

There are three stages of radiation fibrosis syndrome [24]:

- Acute: during or immediately after treatment.
- Early delayed: up to 3 months after completing treatment.
- Late/chronic: greater than 3 months to years posttreatment. This has a poorer prognosis.

The effects of radiation-induced fibrosis can be seen in multiple organ systems [24]:

- Cardiovascular
  Cardiomyopathy, conduction abnormalities, and pericardial disease
- Pulmonary
  Pulmonary fibrosis, pulmonary hypertension, and restrictive lung disease
- Gastrointestinal
  Dysphagia and esophageal motility
- Urinary
  Cystitis and proctitis
- Reproductive
  Vaginal stenosis
- Integumentary
  Dermatitis and skin atrophy
- Lymphatic endocrine
  Fatigue hypothyroidism xerostomia

Treatments may include manual therapy in the form of myofascial release and stretching to help with joint mobilization and improve range of motion. Occupational therapists can also develop an exercise program to help improve strength and can assist in developing splints to help maintain range of motion and positioning.

References

1. Punwar AJ. Occupational therapy: principles and practice. 3rd ed. Baltimore: Lippincott Williams & Wilkins; 2000. Print.
2. American Occupational Therapy Association. Occupational therapy practice framework: domain and process. Am J Occup Ther. 2002;56:609–39.
3. DeLisa JA, Gans BM. Physical medicine and rehabilitation: principles and practice. Philadelphia: Lippincott Williams & Wilkins; 2005. Print.
4. Kielhofner G. Conceptual foundations of occupational therapy practice. Philadelphia: F.A. Davis; 2009. Print.
5. Hugh CW, Godden D, Perkins CS. Splinting the radial forearm free flap donor site. Br J Oral Maxillofac Surg. 2003;41(3):193.
6. Cooper J. Occupational therapy intervention with radiation induced brachial plexopathy. Eur J Cancer Care. 1998;7(2):88–92.
7. Braddom R. Physical medicine and rehabilitation. 2nd ed. Philadelphia: WB Saunders; 2000.
8. International Classification of Impairments, Disabilities, and Handicaps. N.p.: n.p., 2003. Web. http://whqlibdoc.who.int/publications/1980/9241541261_eng.pdf
9. Cooper J. Occupational therapy in oncology and palliative care. Chichester: Wiley; 2006. Print
10. Rehab Measures – Functional Independence Measure. The rehabilitation measures database. N.p., n.d. Web. 21 July 2014.
11. Nagarajan K, Bennett A, Agostini P, Naidu B. Is preoperative physiotherapy/pulmonary rehabilitation beneficial in lung resection patients? Interact Cardiovasc Thorac Surg. 2011;13(3):300–2. Oxford Journals. Oxford Journals. Web.
12. Drouin J, Pfalzer C. Physical therapy precautions persons with cancer. Website of the National Center on Health, Physical Activity and Disability. 2009. http://www.ncpad.org.
13. Okeefe M. "Oncology basics: red flags and special considerations" Memorial Sloan Kettering Cancer symposium. Memorial Sloan-Kettering Cancer Center. May 2013. New York. Lecture.
14. Stubblefield MD, O'Dell MW. Cancer rehabilitation principles and practice. New York: Demos Medical; 2009. Print.
15. McCormack G. Pain management by occupational therapists. Am J Occup Ther. 1988;42(9):582–90.
16. National Cancer Institute. Fatigue (PDQ®) -. N.p., n.d. Web. 31 Oct. 2013. http://www.cancer.gov/cancertopics/pdq/supportivecare/fatigue/Patient/page1/AllPages
17. Cooper J. Occupational therapy in oncology and palliative care. Chichester: Wiley; 2006. Print
18. Visovsky C. Putting evidence into practice: evidence based interventions for chemotherapy induced peripheral neuropathy. Clin J Oncol Nurs. 2007;11(6):901–13.
19. Mohler III ER. Clinical manifestions and diagnosis of lymphedema. In: UpToDate, Post TW (Ed), UpToDate, Waltham. Accessed 21 Jan 2014.
20. Harris S. Clinical proactive guidelines for the care and treatment of breast cancer: 11 lymphedema. CMAJ. 2001;164(2):191–9.
21. American Physical Therapy Association. Guide to physical therapist practice. 2nd ed. Alexandria: APTA; 2001.
22. Mohler III ER. Prevention and treatment of lymphedema. In: UpToDate, Post TW (Ed), UpToDate, Waltham. Accessed 21 Jan 2014.
23. Bromberg MB. Brachial plexus syndromes. In: UpToDate, Post TW (Ed), UpToDate, Waltham. Accessed 23 Jan 2014.
24. Stubblefield M. "The radiation fibrosis syndrome" memorial Sloan Kettering Cancer symposium. Memorial Sloan- Kettering Cancer center. New York: Lecture; 2013.
25. Weiss E. Clinical manifestation and treatment of radiation-induced fibrosis. In: UpToDate, post TW (Ed), UpToDate, Waltham. Accessed 8 July 2014.

Cancer Pain and Physical Modalities

46

Joel Frontera and Amy Cao

Cancer pain can be quite debilitating, affecting not only quality of life and function, but mood and interpersonal social interactions as well. While medications play a large role in managing cancer pain, there are side effects to be considered such as constipation, sedation, and increased nausea. These side effects can exacerbate a patient's already depleted energy reserve. These side effects can exacerbate a patient's already depleted energy reserve. In addition to medications, physical and occupational therapy as well as physical modalities may be considered in combination to better control a patient's cancer-related pain. The literature and research into efficacy of many modalities are still young but promising. The use of electrophysical agents for therapeutic pain relief has been limited in cancer patients. It has primarily been used in palliative care [1]. Ahead, we discuss modalities and their role in cancer pain treatment.

Massage

According to the gate control theory, mechanisms in the dorsal horn of the spinal cord facilitate or inhibit the pain transmission from the periphery to the brain where it is then dynamically processed. Psychological factors can influence pain response and perception by acting on the gate control system. A painful stimulus will send a signal to the dorsal horn of the spinal cord which then travels to the central thalamic pain area of the brain. Non-painful stimuli can block or decrease the painful stimulus transmission to the dorsal horn. During massage, touch receptors are thought to decrease pain by decreasing the pain signal [2].

Therapeutic massage or therapeutic touch increases blood flow to local areas and stimulates nerve endings. There are several types of massage stemming from both Eastern and Western philosophies. Western philosophy includes effleurage, petrissage, tapotement, and Swedish massage. Effleurage is a stroking movement, petrissage is a kneading movement, and tapotement is a percussion type movement. Swedish massage is a combination of tapotement, petrissage, and deep tissue massage. Deep tissue massage helps by releasing chronic adhesion due to repetitive injury. Myofascial release is the use of controlled, prolonged, pressured massage to release tight fascia in the direction of the muscle fibers. Massage therapy has been shown to be effective in relieving pain. Other types of massage include Eastern methods such as shiatsu massage [3]. A number of texts report that massage is contraindicated in malignancy due to concern for seeding or spread local tumor. There are more studies emerging, however, that show massage may safely provide pain relief and benefits.

In one randomized controlled trial, 380 patients were randomized to either massage or simple touch. The study found that massage may have an immediate beneficial effect on both pain and mood in patients with advanced cancer [4]. Additional studies show that cancer pain can be reduced with therapeutic massage. Therapeutic touch as a form of massage can provide comfort and alleviate suffering; it also provides the patient with a sense of caring and empathy. Patients who have received massage have said that their stress levels improve, their muscles relax, and they feel calmer. Massage can improve quality of sleep, reduce pain, and decrease anxiety in cancer patients [5]. After a single 30- or 60-min massage treatment, both cancer patients and caregivers reported acute relief of self-reported symptoms [6]. However, the effect on tumor staging and progression was not followed in the above studies. Patients should consider massage therapy

J. Frontera (✉)
McGovern Medical School at The University of Texas Health Science Center at Houston (UTHealth), Houston, TX, USA
e-mail: joel.e.frontera@uth.tmc.edu

A. Cao
Baylor St. Luke's Medical Center, physical medicine and rehabilitation, Houston, TX, USA

A. Gulati et al. (eds.), *Essentials of Interventional Cancer Pain Management*, https://doi.org/10.1007/978-3-319-99684-4_46

as a therapeutic option to manage their pain. Massage therapy appears promising for reducing pain intensity, fatigue, and anxiety in cancer populations compared to the active comparators in a systematic review to assess function-related outcomes and health-related quality of life in cancer pain populations [7]. Overall, therapeutic massage appears to be a well-tolerated, noninvasive, cost-effective physical modality to manage cancer pain, though sustained effects have not been as well documented and the long-term safety in cancer patients has not been fully assessed.

Complex Decongestive Therapy

Lymphedema is a well-known side effect of mastectomy and lymph node dissection in women with breast cancer. This can cause emotional distress, pain, physical deformity, and impaired arm function and can increase risk of infection. Complex decongestive therapy is a combination of manual lymphatic drainage/massage, compression devices, wrapping, taping, exercise, and skin care.

Manual Lymphatic Drainage

Manual lymphatic drainage can be used as part of complex decongestive therapy. Theoretically, it can help drain local edema and relax the local musculature while bandaging prevents recurrence of the swelling.

There is unclear evidence for the use of manual lymphatic drainage for lymphedema in breast cancer patients. Dayes et al. [8] enrolled 103 women with breast cancer and lymphedema from six cancer centers and were unable to demonstrate significant improvement in lymphedema with complex decongestive therapy compared to a more conservative approach using only compression garments. The authors postulated that the lack of significant effect may have been due to small sample size [8]. An editorial review of this study emphasized that although it did not show a cost-benefit improvement of complex decongestive therapy compared to conservative therapy, there still may be a role for it in patients who have failed conservative therapy or who have advance, severe, long-standing lymphedema [9].

Taping

Kinesiology taping is the use of specialized tape that is porous and flexible to support an injured joint and the surrounding muscle. It is also used to theoretically decrease swelling, such as in cancer patients with lymphedema. Smykla et al. [10] looked at 65 women with breast cancer and lymphedema and found that kinesiology taping did not provide significant lymphedema relief compared to compressive bandaging. To date, there is not enough data to promote taping as first-line therapy in lymphedema cancer patients [10].

Cryotherapy

Cryotherapy, or therapeutic cold, is the use of topical cold to provide analgesia and pain relief. It also aids in reducing swelling. Cryotherapy is used for superficial depth penetration only. It works by triggering hemodynamic vasoconstriction, and results in slowing of nerve conduction, and reduces spasms and pain.

Kadakia et al. [11] assessed the effects of cryotherapy in prevention of oral mucositis in cancer patients. Oral mucositis can cause severe oropharyngeal pain, affecting swallow and thereby reducing oral intake. Oral intake is crucial to maintain in patients with cancer as they are at risk for cachexia and deconditioning. Oral mucositis has also been associated with increased hospitalization and increased need for total parenteral nutrition and sepsis. The use of cryotherapy with ice chips into the oral cavity during cytotoxic chemotherapy infusions induces vasoconstriction which may reduce the blood flow of the toxic agents to the oral mucosa, decreasing systemic side effects and providing local analgesia. In this study, the use of cryotherapy for 60 min compared to 120 min showed similar efficacy, and patients were more able to tolerate the shorter duration. Cryotherapy appeared to reduce the need for opioids and decreased the use of total parenteral nutrition [11]. Future studies are needed with focus on the effect of cryotherapy specifically on patient-reported pain and functional status.

Therapeutic Heat

Therapeutic heat is the application of heat to surface skin. The therapeutic range of heat in the general population is generally about 40–45 °C for a period of 5–30 min. Therapeutic heat depth is divided into superficial and deep. Heat that penetrates 1–2 cm is considered superficial, whereas heat that reaches a depth of 3.5–8 cm is considered deep penetration. There are various types of therapeutic heat: conduction, convection, and conversion. Conduction is the transfer of heat through direct contact such as in paraffin bath and hot packs. Convection is the flow of heat such as in fluid therapy, whirlpools, and moist air. Conversion is the use of nonthermal energy which is converted to heat [12]. This is discussed in more detail below. Therapeutic heat is being used more frequently in the treatment of cancer as it theoretically kills malignant cells above a certain temperature threshold; however, the use of heat for treatment of cancer pain is not as well studied. Overall, the role of therapeutic heat by conduction and convection in cancer patients has been controversial. The concern with this modality is that it may increase the risk of tumor growth and metastases, though this has been unproven by scientific research to date. Recommendations for therapeutic heat in this population cannot be given at this time.

Conversion Therapy

Conversion is the use of nonthermal heat which is then converted to heat to provide pain relief. The types of conversion are separated based on the frequency which is used. There is infrared, ultrasound, shortwave diathermy, and microwave diathermy. Diathermy is the use of high-frequency electromagnetic currents to provide deep heat. The goal of these modalities is to promote muscle relaxation and scar tissue release, increase range of motion, increase local metabolism, and provide pain control. They have been widely used in the general population. Below, we discuss the role of each in cancer patients.

Ultrasound

Ultrasound is the use of high-frequency acoustic vibration to deliver heat energy to targeted tissues. It delivers heat to a 3.5–8 cm depth penetration with the most heat being absorbed at the bone-tissue interface. Therapeutic low intensity ultrasound frequency is typically 0.8–1.1 MHz, intensity of 0.5–4 W/cm2, which is applied to a treatment area of around 100 cm2 for a period of 5–8 min. The energy is converted to heat in the body. Differential response of anatomic structures allows the user to focus on specific areas of interest. Ultrasound diathermy works particularly well on muscle tissue and less so on subcutaneous fat.

The literature on therapeutic ultrasound for cancer pain treatment is sparse. There is some evidence for MRI-guided high intensity focused ultrasound in treatment of painful bone metastases. In one prospective, single-armed study, researchers evaluated the effect of MRI-guided focused ultrasound for the primary treatment of painful bone metastases. They also assessed its potential for local control of bone metastasis in 18 patients. Researchers found significant pain palliation between baseline and at follow-up. They also found increased bone density with restoration of cortical borders in a third of the patients. There were no adverse events related to treatment. They concluded that MRI-guided focused ultrasound can be safely utilized and can provide effective pain control in patients with bone metastasis. It also has potential for local tumor control [13].

Shortwave Diathermy

Shortwave diathermy is the use of electromagnetic current derived from two condenser plates which are applied to the area being treated. The high-frequency waves are converted to heat deep in the body to a depth of about 4–5 cm, with a frequency of 27.12 MHz commonly being used. This is a particularly useful modality for areas with increased soft tissue coverage overlying area of interest for treatment. Shortwave diathermy works best on fat more than muscle. Johnson et al. [14] reported one case which studied the effects of shortwave diathermy combined with manual therapy techniques and joint/soft tissue mobilization for the treatment of pain after multiple surgeries for necrotizing fasciitis related to breast cancer chemotherapy treatment. The patient had significant hip and pelvic pain with severe scarring and limited hip and pelvis range of motion. After a 6-week course of shortwave diathermy, the patient's range of motion improved significantly, and she reported substantial pain relief and scar reduction [14]. This study highlights the possibility that shortwave diathermy may provide pain relief in cancer patients; however, larger studies with blinded placebo control are required before recommendations can be provided.

Microwave Diathermy

Microwave diathermy is the conversion of high-frequency waves to heat structures deep in the body. Common frequencies used include 915 MHz–2450 MHz. Microwave diathermy does not penetrate as deeply as shortwave diathermy. Of the diathermy types, microwave is the easiest to use, but it can cause local burns. It must be avoided on edematous tissue, wet dressing, or near metallic implants. It has been used in combination with radiation and chemotherapy for the treatment of superficial solid tumors. Storm et al. [15] examined the efficacy and safety of thermochemotherapy in patients who had failed chemotherapy alone. Thirty-four patients were selected having a variety of malignancies, including metastatic colon cancer, sarcoma, and hepatoma. They were treated with thermochemotherapy for 1 h daily for 5 days concurrently with their chemotherapy. Thermotherapy was administered using a magnetic-loop induction device (13.56 MHz, 400–1000 W) which provided a strong electromagnetic field into which the body area was exposed to. Tumor temperature was heated from 41 °C to 45 °C when possible. This was achieved in 89% of the tumors for which temperature could be measured safely. After 1–5 months, the authors found 15% tumor regression. After 1–9 months, they found 19% tumor stabilization with arrested development of previously progressive tumors. Eighteen percent of subjects reported improved activity and/or pain control, while 59% had no progression of symptoms during treatment. There was no significant increase in morbidity from thermochemotherapy and no evidence of increased chemotherapy toxicity [15]. This study reveals the potential for thermotherapy in combination with chemotherapy to provide improved pain control and symptom relief.

The known risks of diathermy include burns and hyperthermia. When applying diathermy, it is important to monitor the temperature of the area being treated. It is advisable to maintain tissue temperature less than 45 °C or 113 °F. Historically, having an implanted device has been an absolute contraindication for the use of diathermy due to concern that diathermy could traverse the lines and cause internal damage; however, the literature behind this is lacking. Seiger et al. [16] reported one case series study that looked at four patients with metal implants (e.g., internal fixators) and history of decreased ankle range of motion due to trauma. They employed cautious use of pulsed shortwave diathermy at 48 W in combination with joint mobilization therapy. Subjects previously received joint mobilization and therapeutic modalities such as moist heat and ice without improvement. After treatment with pulsed shortwave diathermy, there was a significant improvement in ankle range of motion, and the results were sustainable after a 4–6-week follow-up. Patients did not report discomfort, pain, or burning during or after treatment [16].

Currently, the presence of cardiac pacemakers and neurostimulators are absolute contraindications to diathermy use. Relative contraindications include patients with baseline neuropathy, impaired sensation, or with other implantable devices. More research is needed before more specific recommendations can be provided.

Traction

Traction is a relatively common manipulation technique used for pain from nonmalignant musculoskeletal and spinal origin. It is the use of controlled, manual force to increase intervertebral disc space with the intention of reducing pressure and pain. The use of traction is limited in cancer pain patients due to the increased number of patients who have bone metastases and malnutrition compared to the general population. Additionally, traction therapy is contraindicated in patients with spinal cord tumors or osteomyelitis.

Phonophoresis

Phonophoresis is the use of topical medications such as steroids or anesthetics coupled with an acoustic medium, which is then driven into the tissue by ultrasound. It is used regularly in practice for treatment of nonmalignant musculoskeletal pain. To date, there are no known studies assessing the use and safety of phonophoresis in cancer pain treatment.

Iontophoresis

Iontophoresis is the use of electrical current to drive medications, including opioids and chemotherapy, across biological membranes into targeted areas. This modality theoretically prevents systemic side effects of the medication being delivered. In cancer patients, it is not uncommon for patients to be unable to tolerate oral medications for a variety of reasons such as dysphagia, ileus, or altered mental status. Kumar et al. [17] looked at delivering hydromorphone by transdermal iontophoresis for the treatment of cancer pain. The study used full-thickness rat skin and found the dose of hydromorphone delivered to the tissue could reach therapeutic levels and the dose could be well controlled by adjusting the drug concentration and current strength [17]. The use of adjuvant iontophoresis for the delivery of topical opioids may be useful in cancer patients, but further research is needed.

Transcutaneous Electrical Neural Stimulation

Transcutaneous electrical neural stimulation also known as TENS has been used for the management of central pain in the general population for a variety of conditions. It is proposed to help alleviate hypersensitive skin via desensitization. Chronic regional pain syndrome has also been managed using TENS with some efficacy. The most common frequency used in TENS is between 50 and 100 Hz which is low amplitude with short duration. This frequency is well-tolerated and can be adjusted to various pulse widths and frequencies. A Cochrane Review of TENS for pain management in cancer patients assessed 3 randomized controlled trials with a total of 88 subjects. The reviewers found that the benefits of TENS continue are inconclusive due to lack of high quality research. TENS was noted to be well-tolerated in all the studies. Further research with well-designed, large, multicenter trials is needed to properly address the effects of TENS in patients with cancer pain [18].

Dance

Exercise as a treatment modality for cancer pain is discussed in more detail in other chapters, so it will be touched upon only briefly here. Sandel et al. [19] performed a randomized, controlled trial with 35 subjects to assess the effect of a dance and movement program on quality of life and shoulder function in women with history of breast cancer. They found that a 12-week dance movement program aimed at addressing the physical and emotional needs of women following breast cancer treatment may significantly improve quality of life and shoulder range of motion [19]. The major limitation of this study was its small sample size. A Cochrane Review done in 2011 looked at dance and movement therapy for improving psychological and physical outcomes in cancer patients. The review included two studies and found that dance and movement therapy may have a beneficial effect on quality of life and fatigue; however, the studies were limited by small sample size and risk bias, and recommendations for clinical practice could not be provided. They report that the current literature does not find clear evidence for the benefits of dance and movement therapy on mood, mental health, range of motion, or arm circumference. The review also mentions, given the nature of dance and movement studies, studies cannot be blinded. They recommend that future studies include an active control group to further differentiate the effects of different types of movement therapy [20].

Yoga

Yoga is a whole-body exercise which incorporates both spiritual and mind health with physical health. It is a combination of physical poses with controlled breathing and meditation. In non-cancer patients, it has been shown to improve cardiopulmonary function, motor skills, fitness, strength, flexibility, and pain. Yoga in cancer patients has been shown to improve sleep, quality of life, mood, and stress. A systematic review and meta-analysis of the effect of yoga in cancer patients in 13 publications found that yoga appeared to be a feasible intervention with beneficial effects on several physical and psychosocial symptoms. The effect on functional well-being was small, while the effect on psychosocial outcomes was moderate [21].

Weight Lifting

Weight lifting has been advised against particularly in breast cancer patients with lymphedema due to concern for exacerbating the lymphedema and causing increased pain and morbidity. However, Schmitz et al. [22] designed a randomized, controlled trial of 154 patients comparing a 1-year weight lifting intervention to no exercise. They found that weight lifting can be a safe modality for lymphedema breast cancer patients and that a program of slow, progressive weight lifting compared to no exercise did not increase incidence of lymphedema [22]. Further research into the effects of weight lifting on cancer pain is needed.

Conclusion

Overall, the modalities discussed above may be a safe and well-tolerated approach to assist in managing cancer-related pain. The hypothesized dangers of certain modalities have generally not been well researched, and there are numerous opportunities for further randomized, placebo-controlled studies. Currently, given the multifactorial nature of cancer pain, the widespread incidence of cancer pain affecting quality of life, and the lack of presently available literature on many modalities for cancer pain, we recommend use of modalities for cancer pain if there are no significant contraindications. The use of modalities is cost-effective and provides relief for some patients suffering from cancer-related paint. It is important to communicate the known and unknown risks and benefits of any modality with patients to allow them to make an informed decision before initiating any treatment.

References

1. Belanger A. Therapeutic electrophysical agents: evidence behind practice. Philadelphia: Lippincott Williams & Wilkins; 2010.
2. Choi H, Sugar R, Fish DE, Shatzer M, Krabak B. Physical medicine and rehabilitation Pocketpedia. Philadelphia: Lippincott Williams & Wilkins; 2003.
3. Kutner JS, Smith MC, Corbin L, Hemphill L, Benton K, Mellis BK, Beaty B, Felton S, Yamashita TE, Bryant LL, Fairclough DL. Massage therapy versus simple touch to improve pain and mood in patients with advanced cancer. Ann Intern Med. 2008;129:369–80.
4. Somani S, Merchant S, Lalani S. A literature review about effectiveness of massage therapy for cancer pain. J Pak Med Assoc. 2013;63:1418–21.
5. Pan YQ, Yang KH, Wang YL, Zhang LP, Liang HQ. Massage interventions and treatment-related side effects of breast cancer: a systematic review and meta-analysis. Int J Clin Oncol. 2014;19(5):829–41. https://doi.org/10.1007/s10147-013-0635-5. Epub 2013 Nov 26.
6. Lopez G, Liu W, Milbury K, Spelman A, Wei Q, Bruera E, Cohen L. The effects of oncology massage on symptom self-report for cancer patients and their caregivers. Support Care Cancer. 2017;25(12):3645–50.
7. Boyd C, Crawford C, Paat CF, Price A, Xenakis L, Zhang W. Evidence for massage therapy (EMT) working group. The impact of massage therapy on function in pain populations- a systematic review and meta-analysis of randomized controlled trials: part II, cancer pain populations. Pain Med. 2016;17(8):1553–68.

8. Dayes IS, Whelan TJ, Julian JA, Parpia S, Pritchard KI, D'Souza DP, Kligman L, Resise D, LeBlanc L, McNeely ML, Manchel L, Wiernikowski J, Levine MN. Randomized trial of decongestive lymphatic therapy for the treatment of lymphedema in women with breast cancer. J Clin Oncol. 2013;31:3758–63.
9. Javid SH, Anderson BO. Mounting evidence against complex decongestive therapy as a first-line treatment for early lymphedema. J Clin Oncol. 2013;21:3737–8.
10. Smykla A, Waleqicz K, Trybulski T, Halski T, Kucharzewski M, Kucio C, Mikusek W, Klakla K, Taradaj J. Effect of kinesiology taping on breast cancer-related lymphedema: a randomized single-blind controlled pilot study. Biomed Res Int. 2013;2013:1–7. [Epub ahead of print].
11. Kadakia KC, Rozell SA, Butala AA, Loprinzi CL. Supportive cryotherapy: a review from head to toe. J Pain Symptom Manag. 2014;47(6):1100–15. https://doi.org/10.1016/j.jpainsymman.2013.07.014. Epub 2013 Nov 7.
12. Choi H, Sugar R, Fish DE, Shatzer M, Krabak B. Physical medicine and rehabilitation Pocketpedia. Philadelphia: Lippincott Williams & Wilkins; 2003.
13. Napoli A, Anzidei M, Marincola BC, Brachetti G, Ciolina F, Cartocci G, Marsecano C, Zaccagna F, Marchetti L, Cortesi E, Catalano C. Primary pain palliation and local tumor control in bone metastases treated with magnetic resonance-guided focused ultrasound. Investig Radiol. 2013;48:351–8.
14. Johnson W, Draper DO. Case report: increased range of motion and function in an individual with breast cancer and necrotizing fasciitis – manual therapy and pulsed short-wave diathermy treatment. Case Rep Med. 2010;2010:1–4.
15. Storm FK, Silberman AW, Ramming KR, Kaiser LR, Harrison WH, Elliott RS, Haskell CM, Sarna G, Morton DL. Clinical chemotherapy: a controlled trial in advanced cancer patients. Cancer. 1984;53:863–8.
16. Seiger C, Draper DO. Use of pulsed shortwave diathermy and joint mobilization to increase ankle range of motion in the presence of surgical implanted metal: a case series. J Orthop Sports Phys Ther. 2006;36:669–77.
17. Kumar MG, Lin S. Transdermal iontophoresis of hydromorphone across hairless rat skin in vitro. Pharm Dev Technol. 2009;14(1):106–15. https://doi.org/10.1080/10837450802409479.
18. Hurlow A, Bennett MI, Robb KA, Johnson MI, Simpson KH, Oxberry SG. Transcutaneous electric nerve stimulation (TENS) for cancer pain in adults. Cochrane Database Syst Rev. 2012;(3):CD006276. https://doi.org/10.1002/14651858.CD006276. pub3.
19. Sandel SL, Judge JO, Landry N, Faria L, Ouellette R, Majczak M. Dance and movement program improves quality-of-life measures in breast cancer survivors. Cancer Nurs. 2005;28:301–9.
20. Bradt J, Goodill SW, Dileo C. Dance/movement therapy for improving psychological and physical outcomes in cancer patients. Cochrane Database Syst Rev. 2011;(10):CD007103. https://doi.org/10.1002/14651858.CD007103. pub2.
21. Buffart LM, Van Uffelen JGZ, Riphagen II, Brug J, Mechelen W, Brown WJ, Chinapaw MJM. Physical and psychosocial benefits of yoga in cancer patients and survivors, a systematic review and meta-analysis of randomized controlled trials. Biomed Cent Cancer. 2012;12:559.
22. Schmitz KH, Ahmed RL, Troxel AD, Cheville A, Lewis-Grant L, Smith R, Bryan CJ, Williams-Smith CT, Chittams J. Weight lifting for women at risk for breast cancer-related lymphedema: a randomized trial. J Am Med Assoc. 2010;304(24):2699–705.

Osteopathic Treatment for Cancer-Related Pain

47

Ryan K. Murphy and Jonas M. Sokolof

Part I: Osteopathic Manual Medicine (OMM)

Introduction

Osteopathic medicine traditionally approaches patient care holistically with the premise of reciprocal relationship between structure and function. The osteopathic foundation requires a comprehensive understanding of anatomy in conjunction with physiology and recognizing the subtle influences between organ systems when dysfunction is present. Osteopathic physicians use all conventional methods of diagnosis and treatment but are trained to place additional emphasis on restoring normal body mechanics for maintaining good health [1].

Osteopathic physicians place emphasis on a holistic view of the patient, with four key principles central to the care of all patients:

I. The person is a unit and all organ systems connected.
II. The body is capable of self-regulation, self-healing, and health maintenance.
III. Structure and function are reciprocally interrelated.
IV. Rational treatment is based on an understanding of these principles: body unity, self-regulation, and the interrelationship of structure and function [2].

R. K. Murphy (✉)
Valley Medical Group, Waldwick, NJ, USA
e-mail: murpry2@valleyhealth.com

J. M. Sokolof
Department of Rehabilitative Medicine, Weill College of Medicine Cornell University, New York, NY, USA

Department of Neurology – Rehabilitation Services, Memorial Sloan-Kettering Cancer Center, New York, NY, USA
e-mail: sokolofj@mskcc.org

An abbreviated review of osteopathic medical history, techniques, and how they may be used in the treatment of pain will follow.

History

Founding Father of Modern Osteopathy

Andrew Taylor Still, M.D., D.O. (1828–1917)

Andrew Still was born in Lee County, Virginia, in 1828, the son of a Methodist minister and physician. At an early age, Dr. Still decided to follow in his father's footsteps as a physician. After studying medicine and serving an apprenticeship under his father, he entered the Civil War as a hospital steward in the Army and was promoted to physician and surgeon [3].

After the war he practiced conventional medicine in the Midwest. Following the death of his wife, three of his children, and an adopted child from spinal meningitis in 1864, Still concluded that the orthodox medical practices of his day were frequently ineffective and sometimes harmful. He devoted the next 30 years of his life to studying the human body and finding alternative ways to treat disease [4].

Osteopathic manipulation treatment (OMT) is a core set of techniques, which rely on myofascial continuity – a tissue layer that connects all parts of the body. Physicians attempt to diagnose and treat somatic dysfunction by manipulating a person's bones and muscles and therefore address a variety of ailments. These OMT techniques are most commonly used to treat back pain and other musculoskeletal issues and are less commonly used to treat systemic conditions [5, 6].

Dr. Still founded the first school of osteopathy based on this new approach to medicine – the school was called the American School of Osteopathy (now A.T. Still University) in Kirksville, Missouri, in 1892 [7]. Dr. Still was also one of the first physicians to promote the idea of preventive medi-

A. Gulati et al. (eds.), *Essentials of Interventional Cancer Pain Management*, https://doi.org/10.1007/978-3-319-99684-4_47

cine and the philosophy that physicians should focus on treating the disease rather than just the symptoms [8].

He defined osteopathy as:

> *That science which consists of such exact, exhaustive, and verifiable knowledge of the structure and function of the human mechanism, anatomical, physiological and psychological, including the chemistry and physics of its known elements, as has made discoverable certain organic laws and remedial resources, within the body itself, by which nature under the scientific treatment peculiar to osteopathic practice, apart from all ordinary methods of extraneous, artificial, or medicinal stimulation, and in harmonious accord with its own mechanical principles, molecular activities, and metabolic processes, may recover from displacements, disorganizations, derangements, and consequent disease, and regained its normal equilibrium of form and function in health and strength.* [9]

Pathophysiology of Somatic Dysfunction

Tissue injury is followed by an inflammatory response with multiple chemical mediators from various cell types in the fascia. The purpose of these chemical mediators is to stimulate repair and cellular growth and subsequently stimulate nociceptive nerve endings. These nociceptive signals are transmitted through primary afferent fibers. Large caliber A fibers are well myelinated and therefore carry signals rapidly from the peripheral tissues to the spinal cord and finally to the somatosensory cortex. The small A and C fibers which are collectively the primary afferent nociceptors are minimally myelinated or not at all. Therefore, the transmission speeds of signals traveling on these nerve fibers are slow. However, these small fiber systems have the largest impact given the diffuse locations of these naked terminal nerve endings throughout the body such as the skin and fascia [10].

More relevant to osteopathic philosophy and treatment are the small fibers, which may make up to 50% of muscle nerve composition with these primary afferent nociceptors traveling throughout the connective tissue surrounding vasculature [11]. Many of these small fibers contain neuropeptides such as substance-P and calcitonin gene-related peptide which is consistent with their role as neurosecretory and sensory fibers [12].

Somatic dysfunction is defined as impaired or altered function of related components of the somatic system: skeletal and myofascial structures and their related vascular, lymphatic, and neural elements. Acute somatic dysfunction is an immediate- or short-term impairment or altered function of related components of the somatic framework. Somatic dysfunction during the early stages is characterized by vasodilation, edema, tenderness, pain, and tissue contraction. It is diagnosed by history and the palpatory assessment of tenderness, asymmetry of motion and relative position, and restriction of motion along with tissue texture change. Chronic somatic dysfunction is the impairment or altered function of related components of the somatic system. Tenderness, itching, fibrosis, paresthesia, and tissue contraction may characterize it [13]. Somatic dysfunctions could be caused by musculoskeletal restrictions involving only a single joint. However, more common restrictions involve more widespread changes in mobility and posture as compensatory alterations that develop in response to an initial restriction or injury [14].

Neuroanatomy of Pain

Small caliber primary afferent nerve fibers are unmyelinated or lightly myelinated and terminate with naked nerve endings in the peripheral tissue. A significant percentage of these small fibers carry information about potential or actual injury to the surrounding tissue to multiple areas of the brainstem, thalamus, and somatosensory cortex. Intensity of stimulation to small fiber afferents produces a variable response with low-intensity stimulation producing a sensation of light touch, whereas high levels of stimulation produce the sensation of pain possibly triggering immune and/or endocrine responses. In addition, this system has an inherent ability to become sensitized to repetitive stimuli and lower the threshold of activation [15].

Willard et al., Van Buskirk et al., Denslow and Korr, and several others have described several models of nociception and spinal facilitation with somatic dysfunction. Injury to tissue may modify pain-related sensory neurons resulting in changes of joint mobility and related visceral, autonomic, and immunologic systems. Under sustained afferent drive, pathologic changes can occur in the spinal cord, which may include inhibitory neuron cell death, windup, or sensitization of second-order neurons in the dorsal horn. If persistent for long enough periods of time, spinal facilitation may continue to occur despite cessation of the primary afferent nociceptive signal. Such facilitation from a chronically dysfunctional segment may progress further with altered global CNS activity including behavior, sleep, mood, and other manifestations seen in chronic pain syndromes.

Activation of nociceptors can produce guarding which results in abnormal positioning and range of motion of tissues. Autonomic reflexes and local inflammatory responses can further induce restriction. Maintaining joints, muscles, and other tissues in abnormal positions with guarding reinforces abnormal postural patterns. Sometimes, trying to stretch such modified tissues to normal positions or ranging a joint through its anatomic range can further stimulate the nociceptive response and reflexively reinforce an abnormal musculoskeletal response [15]. Osteopathic manual treatment (OMT) hopes to address some of these issues resultant from oncologic pain syndromes.

Part II: Osteopathic Manipulation Treatment (OMT) in Pain Medicine

Osteopathic Techniques

There are a wide variety of techniques used which all require hands-on approach. Most treatment sessions use a combination of several techniques based on individual findings and complaints from a structural exam. A sample of the common techniques employed in the cancer rehabilitation setting is listed below:

1. **Soft Tissue/Myofascial Release**

- Direct or indirect approaches treating the restrictive barrier.
- Both spine and joints are subject to rotational forces and restrictions.
- As gravity imposes a downward force on the spine, transitional zones are prone to rotation.
- At the transition zones, the spine is mechanically vulnerable due to conformational changes within the alignment of the facet joints.
- We have conformational changes in the facet joints because the axial support needs to transition from stable thoracic and sacral regions to the more mobile cervical and lumbar regions.
- Osteopathic treatment often begins with soft tissue techniques to decrease the overall tone which will enable the provider a more accurate diagnosis and customized treatment.
- Look for places where the rotation is inhibited.
- Paraspinal muscles are often treated.
- Technique involves traction, stretching, and pressure in longitudinal and lateral directions at varying depths, force, and angles.

Cervical Spine Soft Tissue/Myofascial Release

Position

The patient is prone. The practitioner sits to one side with the caudal arm underneath upper cervical spine. The practitioner's cephalad hand rests the forehead. See Fig. 47.1.

Action

The practitioner slowly moves the patient's head into positions of ease with varying traction, stretching, and pressure in longitudinal and lateral directions at varying depths, force, and angles. As muscle tension and tissue restriction decreases, the practitioner may slowly roll the head in an alternating rhythmic arching semicircle fashion along the caudal arm.

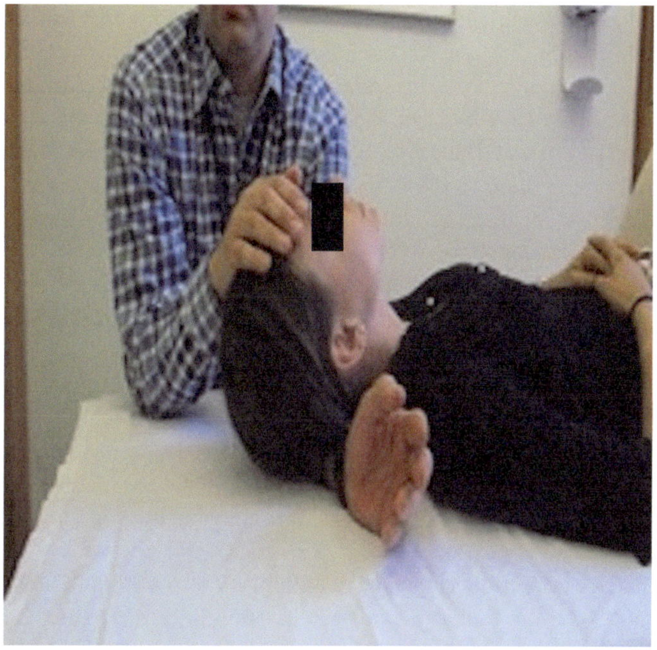

Fig. 47.1 Cervical spine soft tissue/myofascial release

Oncologic Setting

- Pain due to postsurgical or radiation changes in head and neck cancers or cervicothoracic anatomical changes due to disease or treatment such as postmastectomy syndrome
- Reduction in range of motion due to fibrosis, scar tissue, atrophy, and neuropathy related to cancer treatments or exacerbation of pre-existing musculoskeletal dysfunction

Thoracic Outlet Technique

Method 1

Position

The patient lies prone and the practitioner stands opposite the side to be treated. The practitioner's caudal hand grasps the anterior portion of the pelvis around the ASIS. The other hand is positioned posteriorly over the 11th and 12th ribs.

Action

The practitioner rolls the patient's pelvis posteriorly (toward practitioner) to maximum height without breaking restrictive barrier or discomfort. This is immediately followed by easing the pelvis back down toward the table, with the cephalad hand applying pressure over the 11th and 12th ribs, in an alternating rhythmic fashion. See Fig. 47.2.

This gentle kneading and stretching can be performed from the 11th rib down to L5 vertebral level. After the tension of the soft tissues has been released, a sudden brief force may be applied to the 11th and 12th ribs in an anterolateral direction. A slight articulatory sound may be audible during this maneuver.

A similar technique may be used along the full length of the thoracic spine. A pillow may be placed underneath the patient to protect the breasts.

Method 2

Position

The patient is supine with the knees flexed and the feet flat on the table. The practitioner stands opposite the side to be treated.

The practitioner grasps the patient's knees with one hand and, with the other, reaches across and under the patient to contact the hypertonic quadratus lumborum.

Action

The practitioner lifts these muscles taking up the slack while pushing the patient's knees away. The practitioner then relaxes the hand on the back muscles and brings the knees to their original position. This alternating rhythm is continued until a softening in tissue texture is appreciated. See Fig. 47.3.

To treat the 11th and 12 ribs, the practitioner places her hand on those ribs and takes up the slack. The patient is asked to cough. The intrinsic force of the cough along with the traction on the ribs may correct the motion restriction.

Oncologic Setting

- Pain due to postsurgical or radiation changes in thoracolumbar/abdominal regions and lower limb edema/lymphedema
- Reduction in range of motion due to fibrosis, scar tissue, atrophy, and neuropathy related to cancer treatments or exacerbation of pre-existing musculoskeletal dysfunction

2. **Muscle Energy**

- Is an active indirect technique which engages the restrictive barrier and was developed by Dr. Fred Mitchell.
- Requires active participation of the patient to contract a muscle in a specific direction and position against the counter force applied by the practitioner.
- The goal of this technique is to restore full range of motion while decreasing hypertonicity of muscles and improve overall symmetry of movement around a joint.
- Common applications:
  - Piriformis muscle which is often overactivated to compensate for weak gluteal muscles. Increased contraction may lead to irritation of the sciatic nerve leading to a "sciatica" pain pattern.

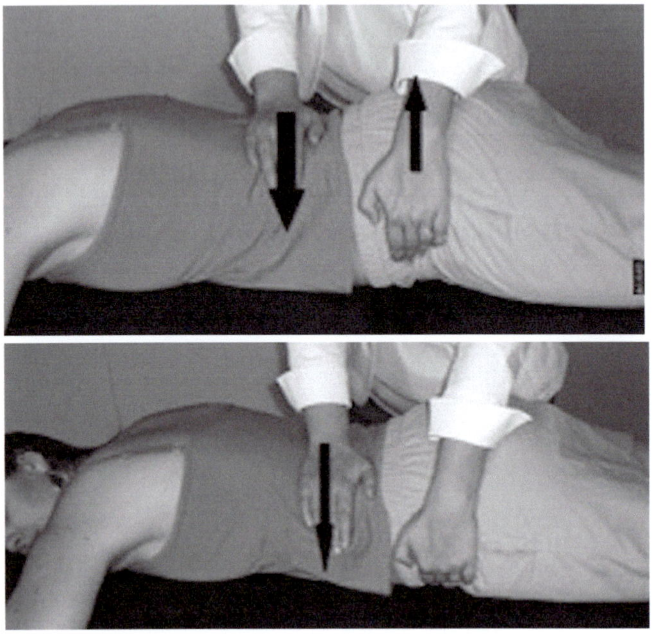

Fig. 47.2 Thoracic outlet/lumbar spine soft tissue/myofascial release, method 1

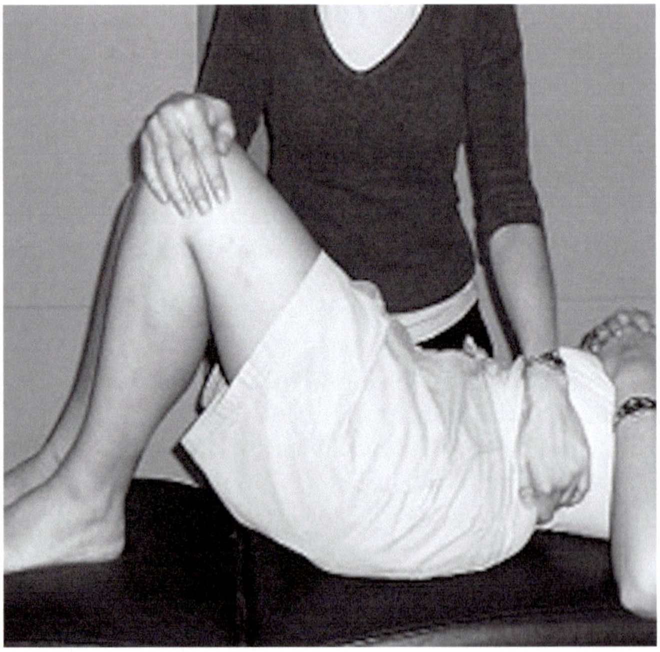

Fig. 47.3 Thoracic outlet/lumbar spine soft tissue/myofascial release, method 2

– Cervical paraspinals which are activated to compensate for rotation of each spinal segment and individualized motion resulting in counterforces and overuse of stabilizing muscles (see Fig. 47.4).

Psoas Imbalance

Position

The patient lies prone, and the practitioner stands on the contralateral side being treated for improved leverage but may be performed standing ipsilateral to side of treatment.

The practitioner flexes the patient's knee with one hand, while the other hand monitors the lumbosacral junction and ilium on the affected side. See Fig. 47.5.

Action

The practitioner lifts the patient's knee toward (hip extension) the ceiling until the motion barrier is reached. The patient is instructed to bring his knee down (hip flexion) to the table. The practitioner resists isometrically. Hold position for 3 s and then instruct the patient to relax.

Repeat/Recheck

Move the knee further toward the ceiling to engage the new motion barrier.

Repeat a total of three times or until the desired result is attained. Recheck psoas range of motion by extending at the hip.

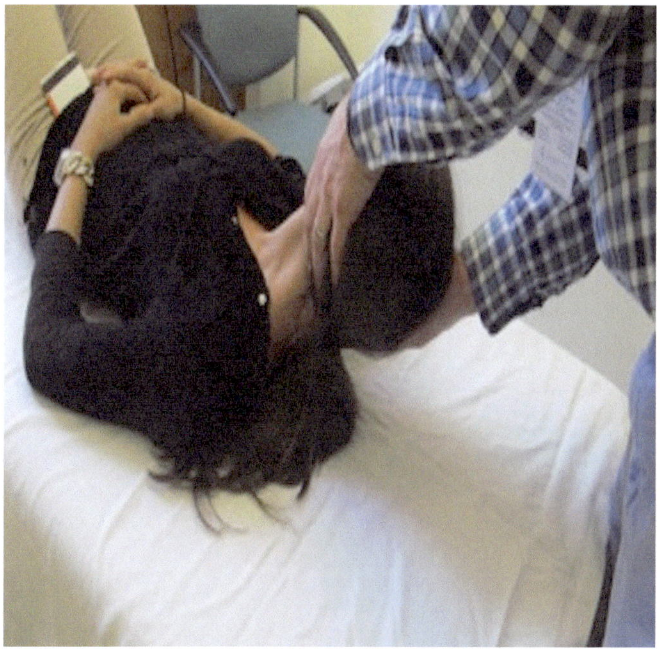

Fig. 47.4 Muscle energy to treat cervical paraspinals

Quadriceps Imbalance

Position

The patient is prone. The practitioner stands on restricted side. The involved knee is flexed and positioned against the operator's shoulder. See Fig. 47.6.

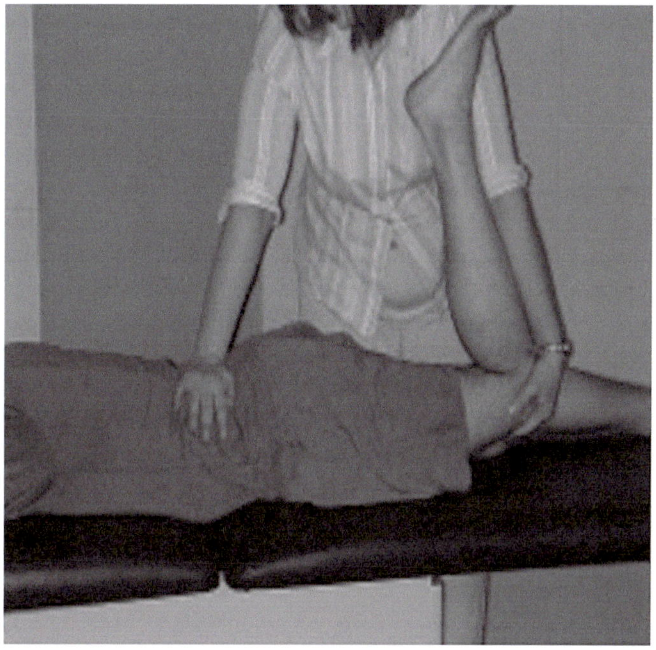

Fig. 47.5 Muscle energy to treat psoas muscle imbalance

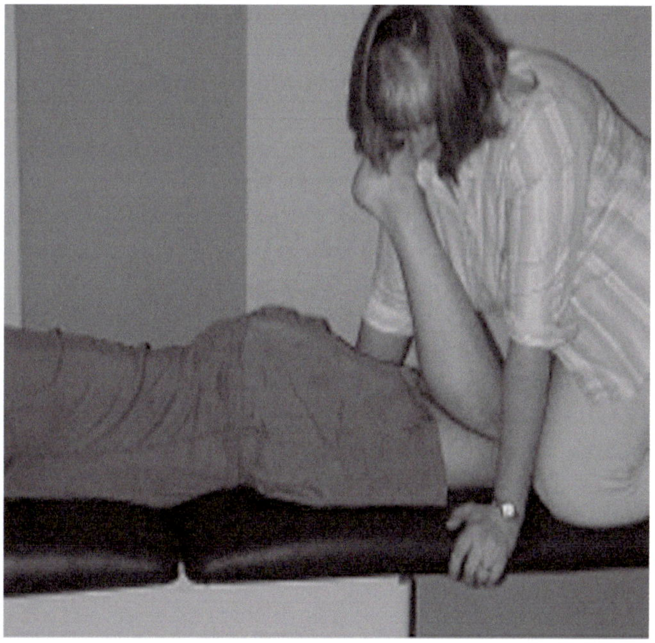

Fig. 47.6 Muscle energy for quadriceps muscle imbalance

Action

The practitioner moves the ankle toward the patient's gluteal region until the restrictive barrier is engaged. The patient is then instructed to straighten the leg (knee extension) as the practitioner resists isometrically.

Hold this position for 3 s and then instruct the patient to relax.

Repeat/Recheck

Move the ankle further cephalad to engage the quadriceps new motion barrier.

Repeat a total of three times or until the desired result is attained. Recheck by motion testing knee flexion.

Oncologic Setting

- Pain due to postsurgical or radiation changes in all cancers but most commonly used postmastectomy/breast cancer, post-radical dissection, and muscle imbalances related to tissue removal in limbs and joints
- Reduction in range of motion due to fibrosis, scar tissue, atrophy, and neuropathy related to cancer treatments or exacerbation of pre-existing musculoskeletal dysfunction

3. **Strain/Counterstrain**

- Is an indirect and passive technique discovered by Dr. Lawrence Jones to treat tender points at common locations.
- Passive technique is when the patient is relaxed and the practitioner is doing the manipulation.
- Indirect means the treatment technique involves moving away from the restrictive barrier.
- Placing the body into a position of maximum comfort can treat somatic dysfunction.
- Structure is related to function, and reciprocally function is related to structure.
- To maintain the network of physiological processes, feedback is obtained through neural and circulatory systems
- Afferent neural network: sensory nerve endings are embedded throughout the body to monitor various tissue conditions.
- When tissue is injured, the body adapts to reduce further irritation of the injured segments.
- While reducing aggravation at the injured site, there is further strain on other structures and alteration in muscular response.
- Longer-lasting functional imbalance can remain from this cascade of adaptations and positional compensation.
- A comprehensive osteopathic structural examination of tissues will reveal areas with restricted movement, altered orientation of paired anatomical structures, and variations in skin texture, temperature, and sensitivity to touch.
- The anterior and posterior aspects of the patient must be evaluated and treated to effectively treat somatic dysfunction.

Lumbosacral Strain

Position

Identify the tender point. Establish a pain scale from the patient with maximal tenderness at the location pretreatment which is to be considered a "10" out of 10. See Fig. 47.7. Position the patient so the muscle/area of tenderness being addressed is shortened. Continue positional adjustments until the patient-reported pain score improves by about 70% or a "3" out of 10.

Action

The practitioner holds the position for at least 90 s while monitoring the tender area of treatment with light contact, to appreciate for tissue change. The practitioner then slowly and passively returns the patient to a neutral position.

Repeat/Recheck

Palpate the tender point with the same pressure during the pretreatment examination. Inquire about the new patient-reported pain score. If less than 70% improvement, repeat treatment a total of three times or until maximal pain relief is achieved.

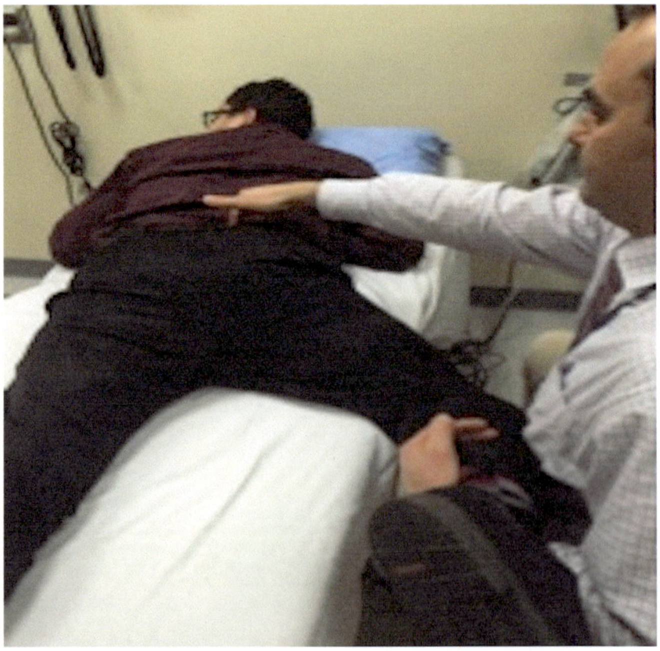

Fig. 47.7 Counterstrain technique to treat low back pain

Oncologic Setting

- Pain due to postsurgical or radiation changes in all cancers but most commonly used postmastectomy/breast cancer, post-radical dissection, and muscle imbalances related to tissue removal in limbs and joints
- Reduction in range of motion due to fibrosis, scar tissue, atrophy, and neuropathy related to cancer treatments or exacerbation of pre-existing musculoskeletal dysfunction

4. **Facilitated Positional Release** [16, 17]

- Technique which is indirect and active was developed by Dr. Stanley Schiowitz.
- A modification of indirect myofascial release technique.
- Identify the restricted region of the body.
- Keep the area of treatment in a neutral position to decrease tissue and joint tension in all planes to find the dynamic balance point of comfort.
- Modifying factors include placing treatment region into a neutral relaxed position which often involves shortening of the muscle then adding a facilitation force of compression and/or torsion.
- Traction force may be substituted for compression or torsion as indicated.
- Technique is usually to address hypertonic muscles both superficial and deep.
- Localization for areas of dysfunction often requires side-bending, rotation, flexion, and extension to find position for individual muscle belly shortening.
- Improvement in restriction often appreciated rapidly after treating for 3–4 s.
- Release from the treating position then reevaluate above, at, and below treatment areas.

Position

The patient is supine. The practitioner stands on restricted side. The involved upper extremity is flexed to 90° at the shoulder and then at the elbow along with internal rotation. The arm is then placed on the patient's chest at the level of the sternum. The practitioner's hands are positioned superiorly over the shoulder and palpating the first rib. The practitioner's other hand lies over the olecranon with fingers gripping the proximal forearm for leverage. See Fig. 47.8.

Action

The practitioner holds the area of treatment (right 1st rib) in the dynamically balanced position. The practitioner then adds an indirect guiding force adding compression and rotation to allow for spontaneous readjustment. The practitioner may need to hold treatment forces for 3–5 s or until the tissue relaxes or there is an articular release. Then slowly and passively return the patient to a neutral position.

Repeat/Recheck

Reexamine the range of motion and tissue texture of the area treated.

Oncologic Setting

- Pain due to postsurgical or radiation changes in all cancers but most commonly used functional scoliosis due to thoracic spine disease, postmastectomy/breast cancer, head and neck cancers, or muscle imbalances related to tissue removal in limbs and joints
- Reduction in range of motion due to fibrosis, scar tissue, atrophy, and neuropathy related to cancer treatments or exacerbation of pre-existing musculoskeletal dysfunction

Summary of Somatic Dysfunction Treatment in Cancer Rehabilitation

Osteopathic manipulation therapy (OMT) may be used in specialized disorders (neuropathy, radiation fibrosis, scar tissue mobilization, lymphedema, spinal alignment) within inpatient or outpatient settings, to provide effective and conservative therapy for complications or dysfunction due to medical and surgical treatment of the cancer patient.

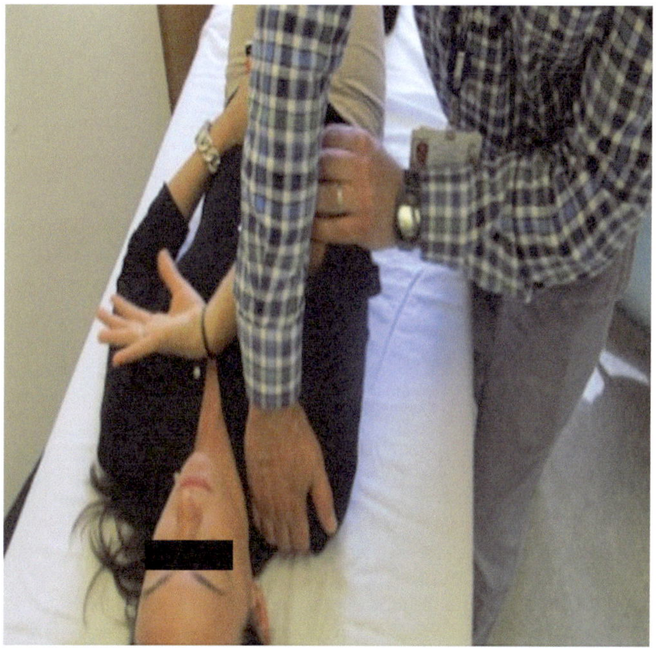

Fig. 47.8 Facilitated positional release of the first rib

Pain in the cancer patient is often multifactorial related to disease burden, chemotherapy, radiation, and other treatments. The most likely factors include:

- Increased mechanical stress from altered alignment and movement
- Degenerative muscle, bone, and synovial changes
- Muscle deconditioning and atrophy
- Scar tissue with fibrotic changes in the muscle, fascia, and soft tissue
- Surgical hardware placement
- Anatomical changes related to a tumor or surgery
- Fracture
- Delayed or poorly healing wound or surgical site
- Neuropathy
- Radiculopathy
- Plexopathy
- Myopathy
- Spasticity
- Avascular necrosis
- Lymphedema
- Premorbid conditions exacerbated by disease or treatment

Commonly Seen Pain Complaints Safely Treated with OMT

1. Headache
2. Trismus
3. Cervicalgia
4. Shoulder girdle/scapular pain
5. Pectoral/axillary pain (postmastectomy syndrome)
6. Thoracic spine/rib pain
7. Low back pain
8. Sacral/pelvic pain

General Contraindications to OMT

1. Osteoporosis
2. Impending pathologic insufficiency fracture
3. Exacerbation of symptoms
4. Local malignancy
5. Congenital malformations
6. Active infection

References

1. Lesho E. An overview of osteopathic medicine. Arch Fam Med. 1999;8:477–84. PMID 10575385.
2. Chila A. Osteopathic philosophy. In: Foundations of osteopathic medicine. 3rd ed. Philadephia: Lippincott Williams & Wilkens; 2011. p. 21.
3. http://cdm.sos.mo.gov/cdm4/document.php?CISOROOT=/atsu&CISOPTR=664&REC=2/
4. Still AT. The philosophy and mechanical principles of osteopathy. Kansas City: Hudson-Kimberly Pub Co; 1902. p. 9–20, 185, 210, 270.
5. HowellJD.Theparadoxofosteopathy.NEnglJMed.1999;341(19):1465–8. https://doi.org/10.1056/NEJM199911043411910. PMID 10547412.
6. Vincent C, Furnham A. Manipulative therapies: osteopathy and chiropractic. Complementary medicine: a research perspective. John Wiley & Sons; 1997. p. 15. isbn: 978-0-471-96645-6.
7. Trowbridge C. Andrew Taylor still, 1828–1917. Kirksville: Truman State University Press; 2007. isbn:1931112789.
8. Still AT. The true fountainhead of osteopathy. J Osteopathy. 1897;IV(1).
9. Still AT. In: Still AT, editor. Autobiography: publisher unknown; 1908. p. 402.
10. Julius D, Basbaum AI. Molecular mechanisms of nociception. Nature. 2001;413:203–10.
11. Mense S, Simons DG. Muscle pain: understanding its nature, diagnosis and treatment. Philadelphia: Lippincott, Williams and Wilkins; 2001.
12. Wall PD, Woolf CJ. Muscle but not cutaneous C-afferent input produces prolonged increases in the excitability of the flexion reflex in the rat. J Physiol (London). 1984;356:453–8.
13. http://www.aacom.org/resources/bookstore/Documents/GOT2011ed.pdf
14. Denslow JS. Soft tissues in areas of osteopathic lesion. 1947. J Am Osteopath Assoc. 2001;101(7):P406–9.
15. Willard F. Nociception, the neuroendocrine immune system, and osteopathic medicine. In: Ward RC, et al., editors. Foundation for osteopathic medicine. 2nd ed. Philadelphia: Lippincott Williams & Wilkens; 2003. p. 137–56.
16. Schiowitz S. Facilitated positional release. J Am Osteopath Assoc. 1990;90(2):145–6, 151–5.
17. Schiowitz S. Facilitated positional release. In: DiGiovanna E, et al., editors. An osteopathic approach to diagnosis and treatment. 3rd ed. Philadelphia: Lippincott Williams & Wilkins; 2004. p. 89–90.

Websites

http://www.powayusd.com/teachers/dsykes/MedicineFourHumoursMedievalWC.jpg

http://www.pcom.edu/Library/Internet_Guides/IG_osteopathic_resources/osteopathic_resource.html

Philadelphia College of Osteopathic Medicine (PCOM)

Journal

Korr I. Propriocepters and somatic dysfunction. J Am Osteopath Assoc. 1975;74(7):638–50.

Books

Digiovanna EL, Schiowitz S, editors. An osteopathic approach to diagnosis and treatment. 2nd ed. Philadelphia: Lippincott-Raven; 1997.

Greenman PE, editor. Principles of manual medicine. 3rd ed. Philadelphia: Lippincott Williams & Wilkins; 2003.

Groneymeyer J, Carayannopoulos A. Osteopathic medicine in chronic pain. In: Audette F, Bailey A, editors. Integrative pain medicine: the science and practice of complementary and alternative medicine in pain management. Totowa: Humana Press; 2008. p. 307–31.

Jones L, Kusunose R, Goering E. Jones Strain-Counterstrain. 1st ed. Boise: Jones Strain-Counterstrain, Inc.; 1995.

Schiowitz S. Facilitated positional release. In: DiGiovanna E, et al., editors. An osteopathic approach to diagnosis and treatment. 3rd ed. Philadelphia: Lippincott Williams & Wilkins; 2004. p. 89–90.

Ward RC, et al., editors. Foundations of osteopathic medicine. 2nd ed. Philadelphia: Lippincott Williams & Wilkens; 2003.

Willard F. Nociception, the neuroendocrine immune system, and osteopathic medicine. In: Ward RC, et al., editors. Foundation for osteopathic medicine. 2nd ed. Philadelphia: Lippincott Williams & Wilkins; 2003. p. 137–56.

Rehabilitation-Bracing as a Conservative Treatment Option

48

Lisa Marie Ruppert and Michelle Yakaboski

Introduction

Treatment of the cancer patient requires a multidisciplinary approach. Included in this approach are rehabilitation efforts which focus relieving symptoms, improving quality of life, enhancing functional independence, and preventing further complications. Rehabilitation goals may be achieved through medical and interventional management, physical and occupational therapies, and assessment for bracing and adaptive equipment.

Concept of Bracing

Bracing can represent a step in conservative care for selected patients. Existing literature offers conflicting advice on bracing in terms of mobilization and stabilization; however when considered as a compliment to rehabilitation efforts, its application has merit [1]. Orthotic intervention comes with the belief that there will be immobilization and may benefit patients. However, there are cases where orthoses can provide mild support and proprioceptive awareness and remind muscles to engage. Bracing has the potential to strengthen compromised muscles and stretch tight muscles [2].

Indications for Bracing

There are various indications for bracing in the oncologic population. These include supportive bracing for weakness, rigid bracing for stabilization of fractures, and flexible bracing postural correction. Bracing may also serve as an adjunct to medical and interventional pain management.

Vertebral Compression Fractures

Case 1 *Mr. George is a 76-year-old gentleman with history of metastatic prostate cancer treated with Lupron followed by external beam radiation therapy to the prostate and seminal vesicles. He subsequently developed castrate-resistant metastatic disease throughout the axial skeleton. Treatment for his metastatic disease included abiraterone, enzalutamide, and docetaxel. In addition, he completed radiation therapy to the lumbar spine. Mr. George also has a history of low back pain with lower extremity radicular symptoms related to disk disease treated with an epidural steroid injection 15 years ago.*

He notes localized thoracic back pain radiating to the chest wall in a band-like pattern. Cardiac causes for his symptoms are evaluated by his primary care physician. He completed an MRI of the total spine per his oncologist's recommendation which showed widespread metastatic disease and a new T7 compression fracture. He is referred to rehabilitation medicine for conservative management of his compression fracture. Bracing is considered as part of his treatment plan, and he is fitted with a thoracolumbosacral orthosis (TLSO).

Case 2 *Ms. Smith is a 59-year-old female with a history of multiple myeloma with lytic bone lesions involving the ribs, thoracolumbar spine, ischium, and bilateral iliac bones treated with carfilzomib, lenalidomide, and dexamethasone. She was diagnosed with compression fractures at L3 and L4 in the setting of an acute pain crisis. She is now status post two level kyphoplasty at the L3 and L4 levels. Kyphoplasty improved her pain significantly, but she continues to experience aching low back pain especially when fatigued. She is participating in physical therapy and spinal*

L. M. Ruppert (✉)
Memorial Sloan Kettering Cancer Center, New York, NY, USA
e-mail: rupperl1@mskcc.org

M. Yakaboski
Certified Prosthetist Orthotist at Boston Orthotics and Prosthetics, Stony Brook, NY, USA
e-mail: myakaboski@Hanger.com

A. Gulati et al. (eds.), *Essentials of Interventional Cancer Pain Management*, https://doi.org/10.1007/978-3-319-99684-4_48

precautions are in place. She inquires about a lumbar support to help with her pain. Based on her evaluation, a lumbosacral orthosis (LSO) is recommended.

Primary and metastatic spinal tumors alter normal bone architecture and can result in deformity or collapse of the affected vertebral body. This vertebral compression can lead to pain and potential spinal instability by increasing strain on the support and stability elements of the spine including muscles, tendons, ligaments, and joint capsules. This bony instability can also result in retropulsion of bone fragments into the epidural space, causing cord compression [3–5].

Oncologic treatment options, including chemotherapy, hormonal manipulation, and radiation therapy, result in tumor regression but may also result in peripheral neuropathies, myopathies, and osteoporosis, increasing the risk for fracture development. Corticosteroids, often used to palliate pain and reduce neurologic complications in individuals with spinal metastases, can accelerate bone loss and induce muscle weakness further increasing that risk.

Currently, many surgical approaches and instrumentation techniques for vertebral compression fractures are described as treatment options. Bracing had been a widely accepted mainstay for fractures in the traumatic and osteoporotic patient populations. It should also be considered in cancer patients with spinal involvement. When considering operative versus nonoperative treatment for a fracture, spinal stability, neurologic status, medical status, and oncologic status should be considered [6].

The primary goals of bracing in nonoperative management of thoracolumbar vertebral compression fractures are to prevent movement-related pain through stabilization of the spine, reduce spine fatigue, and provide an opportunity for early mobilization [7].

An ideal brace should provide adequate stabilization of the spine, reducing gross spinal motion as well as segmental motion at the injured level. It should promote neutral spine alignment to sagittal plane extension, if required. In addition, the ideal brace should be lightweight, easy to wear, prevent respiratory impairments, and ensure comfort to promote patient compliance. The type of brace may be chosen according to type and level of fracture or fractures, clinical status, and need for comfort and function [7].

Head cervical orthoses (HCO; Fig. 48.1) can be prescribed for cervical fractures. These orthoses are best at reducing flexion and extension but are limited in restricting rotation and lateral side bending. Dozens of different models are commercially available, including the Philadelphia, Miami J, and Aspen collars. Cervical thoracic orthoses (CTO) are the most effective at reducing cervical motion. They are useful in mid cervical injuries. Different styles include the Minerva, SOMI, Yale cervical orthosis, Aspen, and HCOs with thoracic extensions. Soft cervical collars provide tactile feedback, warmth, and comfort, but do not restrict movement in any plane. Soft collars may be used temporarily for psychological reassurance in patients who have completed their course in a more restrictive orthosis or in postoperative patients where there is no concern of mechanical instability [8, 9].

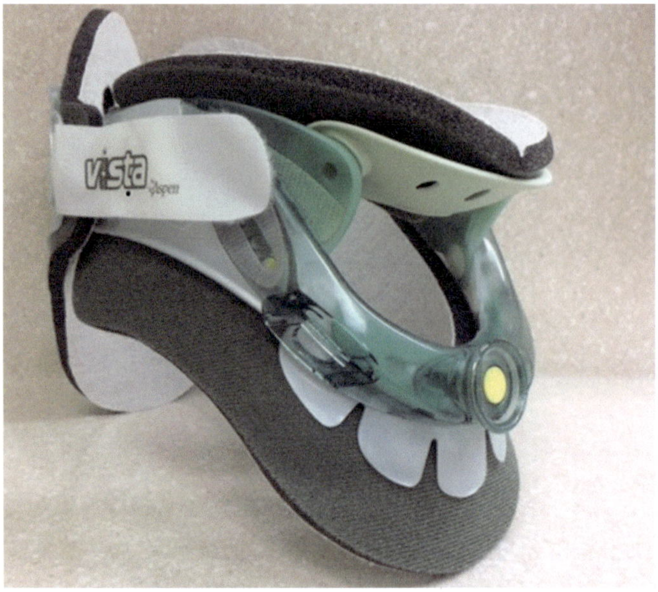

Fig. 48.1 Head cervical orthoses can be prescribed for cervical fractures

Thoracolumbar orthoses (TLOs) or thoracolumbosacral orthoses (TLSOs; Fig. 48.2) are usually prescribed for thoracic fractures. They are also considered for multilevel compression fractures involving the thoracic and lumbar spines. Several brace options are available including the Jewitt, cruciform anterior spinal hyperextension (CASH) orthosis, Taylor brace, Knight-Taylor brace, Spinomed brace, and custom-molded braces. For lower lumbar fractures, a lumbosacral orthosis (LSO; Fig. 48.3) is frequently adequate. Like the TLOs and TLSOs, there are multiple off-the-shelf and custom-molded options available [7].

Bracing may also be considered as an adjunct to surgical interventions to aid in pain management, muscle fatigue, and postural correction. Duration of bracing varies, but literature suggests continuation for 6–8 weeks after an acute vertebral compression fracture [7].

Spine Malalignment

Case 4 *Mr. Harris is a 71-year-old male with history of oropharyngeal squamous cell carcinoma. He is status post chemoradiation followed by a right modified neck dissection. He completed treatment 6 years ago. He presented complaining of poor posture that worsens as the day goes on and with increased activity. He notes that his posture results in*

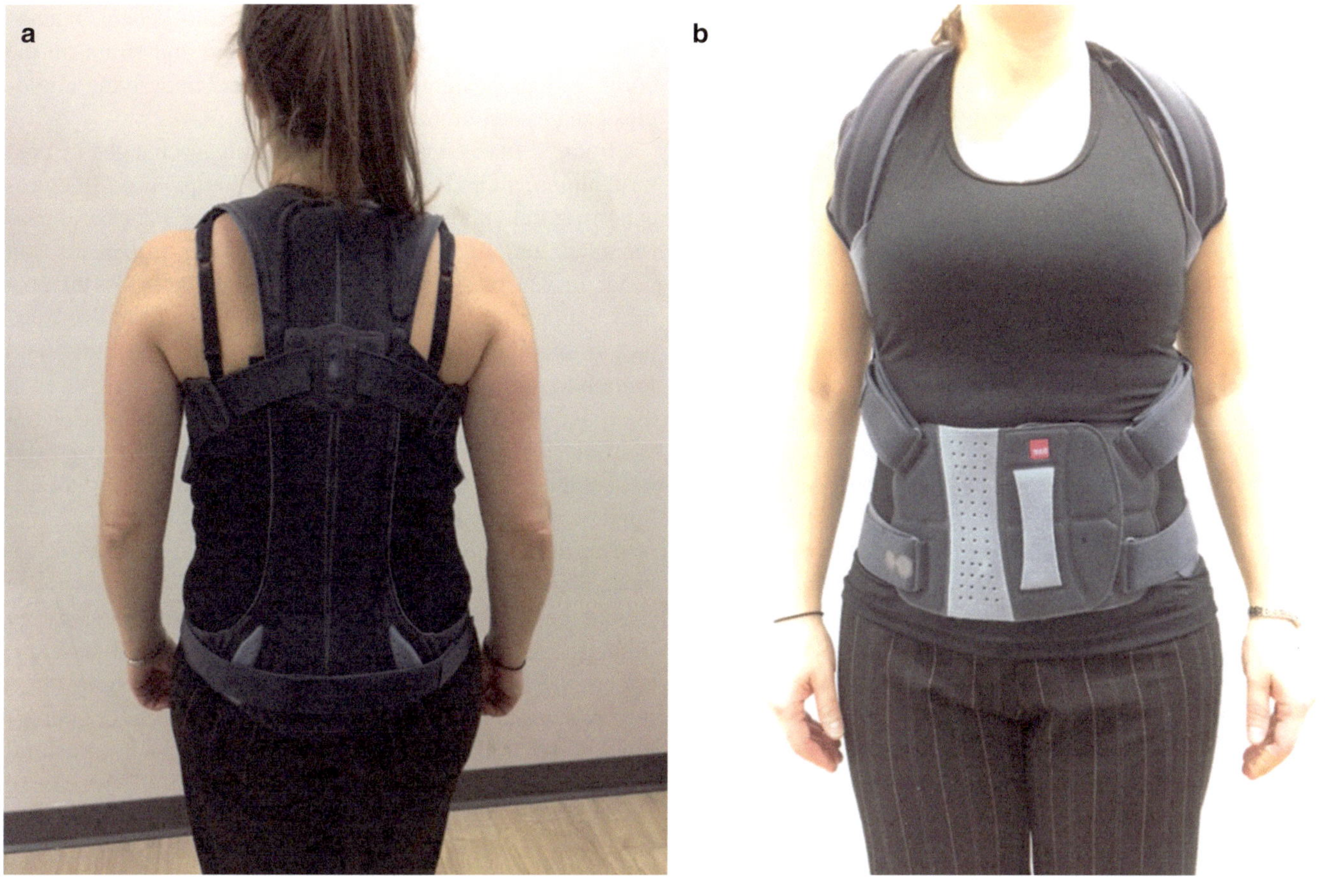

Fig. 48.2 Thoracolumbar orthoses or thoracolumbosacral orthoses are usually prescribed for thoracic fractures. Posterior view (**a**), Anterior view (**b**)

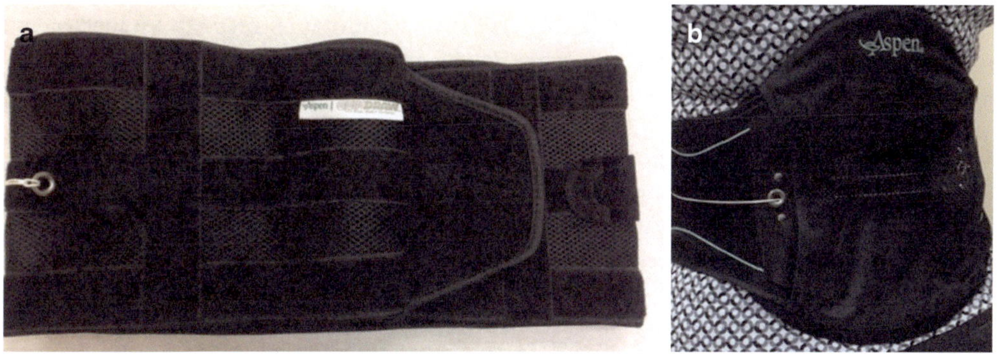

Fig. 48.3 For lower lumbar fractures, a lumbosacral orthosis is frequently adequate. Posterior view (**a**), Anterior view (**b**)

discomfort in the posterior aspect of his neck and shoulders. He reports no radiation of his pain and has no tingling, numbness, or weakness in the upper extremities. He feels his symptoms started shortly after completing his treatments, and symptoms have been worsening. He has been referred to physical therapy and presents for recommendations on postural correction. On examination he has trigger points throughout the bilateral trapezius muscles. He is noted to have forward head posture with ears anterior to the shoulder girdle. His posture corrects with tactile support about the shoulder girdle. Based on this recommendation, a clavicle collar is recommended.

Case 5 *Ms. Gold is a 70-year-old woman with a history of Hodgkin lymphoma diagnosed in 1971. She was treated with total nodal irradiation as well as MOPP chemotherapy. She finished treatment around 1973–1974. She is currently felt to be without evidence of disease. She reports neck pain, poor posture, and difficulty with standing balance and overhead activities. She has significant neck extensor weakness and* *scapular dysfunction resulting in dropped head posture. She underwent electrodiagnostic testing which demonstrated a left cervical polyradiculopathy, brachial plexopathy involving primarily the upper trunk, a mononeuropathy of the spinal accessory nerve, and myopathic changes in the cervical paraspinal muscles. A total spine MRI demonstrated old T2 and L1 vertebral compression fractures. She utilizes a soft cervical collar for pain relief and has participated in several courses of physical therapy.*

She was fitted with a TLSO at a prior visit. She presents for follow-up noting that since using the brace, she can achieve and transiently maintain an upright head posture without use of her hand as a support. She can water her plants and wash dishes without difficulty. She also notes her family has taken note of her improved posture.

Case 6 *Ms. Apple is a 70-year-old female with a history of breast cancer for which she is status post modified radical mastectomy and treatment with tamoxifen. She also has a history of scoliosis first noted in her 20s and osteoporosis. She has had no interventions for her scoliosis as it was felt to be mild. Due to her history of osteoporosis, she has participated in physical therapy for generalized strengthening and notes that she continues her exercises at home. She does not believe that her scoliosis has limited any of her daily functions, and she is quite active physically as an interior designer. She does however note that her posture has worsened over the past few years and she is more rounded. She notes intermittent aching back and neck pain. On examination she has protracted shoulders with thoracic kyphosis and a mild thoracolumbar scoliotic curve to the right.*

She dons a TLSO as recommended. Postural assessment when brace is donned reveals scapular retraction, head neutral posture, and a decrease in her thoracic curve.

Case 7 *Mr. Charles is a 60-year-old gentleman with a history of a traumatic spinal cord injury at the C4 level. He has tetraparesis and poor trunk control. Thirteen years ago, he was diagnosed with breast cancer. Earlier this year he developed nonspecific back pain and had a metastatic lesion at T9. He is undergoing active treatment with fulvestrant and trastuzumab. Despite treatment he notes ongoing back pain and worsening posture. He is leaning to the right and physical examination confirms a scoliotic posture. Imaging shows a Charcot deformity in the spine from T8–T10. His posture can be corrected by providing support to the trunk and spine. Weakness and sensory impairments from his spinal cord injury and his Charcot deformity are felt to contribute to his abnormal sitting posture. Based on this his physiatrist and orthotist recommend a custom-molded TLSO for him to use when sitting in his wheelchair.*

Proper posture is defined as a musculoskeletal balance which involves minimal amount of stress and strain on the body. Various postural abnormalities and underlying etiologies can be seen in the cancer setting.

Biologic pain from tumor can result in changes in postural alignment and body mechanics. Compression fractures can result in kyphotic and scoliotic postures. Peripheral neuropathies and myopathies from oncologic treatments can result in weakness, sensory impairments, and loss of proprioception impacting an individual's ability to utilize muscle to maintain a neutral spine posture. Inactivity and immobility during cancer treatments and comorbidities such as congenital abnormalities, diabetes mellitus, peripheral vascular disease, and neuromuscular disorders can also impact muscle strength and sensory function further increasing the risk for postural malalignment [10, 11].

The use of bracing for postural correction should promote neutral spine alignment. In addition, the ideal brace should be lightweight, easy to wear, prevent respiratory impairments, and ensure comfort to promote patient compliance. Bracing for this indication does not require 24 h use. Patients are educated on wearing their brace for approximately 4–6 h/day when upright and for activity. Postural bracing involves stretching muscles that are often tight or scarred down and strengthening muscles that are weak/have not been activated due to their abnormal mechanics. Furthermore, postural bracing may cause discomfort with initial use; therefore, patients are educated on donning their brace for 1 h on day of delivery and increasing time in brace in 1 h increments. Once postural correction is achieved and maintained when not in brace, patients are tapered out of their brace in 1 h increments with ultimate recommendation for as needed use [7].

Forward Head Posture

Forward head posture is the structural forward positioning of the head away from the centerline of the body, where the lower cervical vertebrae are bent and the upper vertebrae extended. In this posture, the weight of the head supported by the neck is increased [12]. Over time forward head posture may result in rounding of the shoulders and involuntary forward flexion of the thoracolumbar spine. These specific postural changes may lead to tension-type headaches, cervical headaches, neck pain, reduced cervical spine mobility, shoulder pain and decreased function, and back pain. They may also lead to functional and mobility impairments [12].

Braces such as the clavicle orthosis (Fig. 48.4) are designed to alter the posture of the shoulder and thoracic

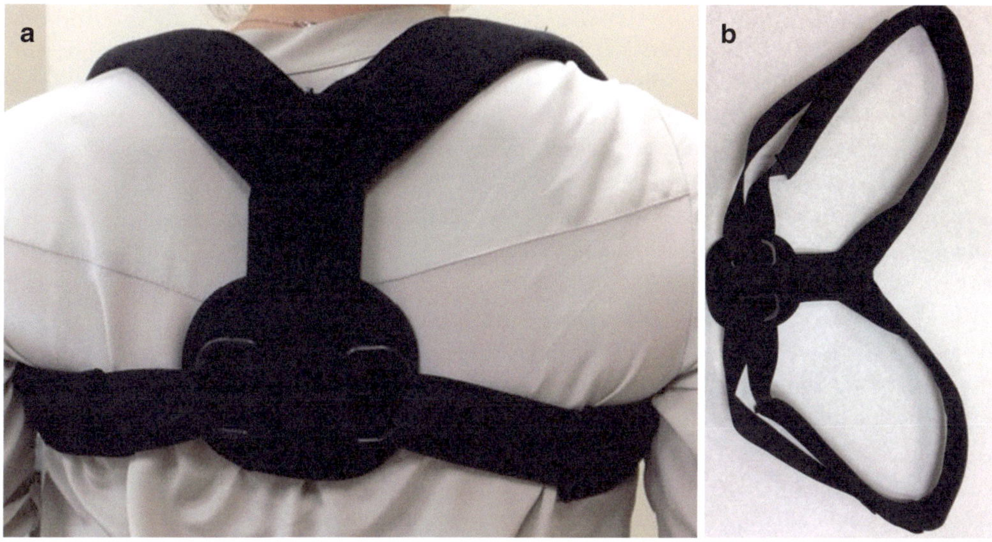

Fig. 48.4 Braces such as the clavicle orthosis are designed to alter the posture of the shoulder and thoracic spine, restoring a more normal posture and muscular activity around the scapula. Posterior view (**a**), Anterior view (**b**)

spine, restoring a more normal posture and muscular activity around the scapula. The restoration of a more optimal alignment involves the slow and gradual stretching of the anterior chest musculature and strengthening of the back musculature while providing a gentle reminder for the patient to retract their shoulders. Individuals with more significant core weakness and thoracic kyphosis in addition to forward head posture may benefit from use of clavicle collar in combination with an LSO or use of a TLSO for postural correction. When bracing individuals with unilateral shoulder protraction and postural malalignment, the Omotrain, Armadillo brace, and M-Brace Clavicle Support can be considered.

Dropped Head Syndrome

Dropped head syndrome is characterized by weakness of the neck extensors and an inability to extend the neck to achieve a head neutral posture. In severe cases, the head is fixed in a "chin on chest position." Patients with dropped head syndrome present with involuntary forward flexion of the thoracolumbar spine that typically increases with walking or standing [13]. Patients may report neck and back pain, balance impairments, and decreased functional status.

Given the extent of weakness and kyphosis in these individuals, a TLSO or clavicle collar with LSO can be considered. Using these orthoses will directly modify the thoracic kyphosis, with the goal of increasing neck extensor strength and ability to achieve head neutral posture. If patients require support to transiently hold their head up for activities and to provide comfort, consider use of a soft cervical collar or HCO. Once the patient achieves scapular retraction and decreases the extent of thoracolumbar kyphosis, a clavicle collar alone can be considered.

Kyphosis and Scoliosis

Patients with kyphosis but otherwise normal spinal alignment and good core strength may benefit from a clavicle collar. If there is core weakness, a provider may consider use of a TLSO to provide more support. If compensatory lordosis is present, a provider may consider the use of a clavicle collar and LSO to promote postural correction.

Patients who present with a scoliosis curvature and back pain pose a unique challenge. Evaluation of the patient's flexibility must be considered when recommending an appropriate orthosis. Patients with a mild flexible scoliosis can benefit from a TLSO such as a Spinomed with an additional back panel to provide some lateral stability. However, depending on the degree of curvature, a custom TLSO or LSO may be more appropriate. A custom design can strategically place areas of rigidity or padding to provide a corrective force to a flexible deformity. These designs have the potential to stretch musculature that has otherwise accommodated to the lateral flexion and rotation of the scoliotic spine. The goal of bracing the adult scoliosis patient is not to correct the curvature but rather to reduce pain associated with the malalignment and prevent further worsening of the curve.

Low Back Pain

Case 8 *Ms. Asche is a 70-year-old woman with a history of breast cancer for which she is status post lumpectomy followed by chemotherapy with doxorubicin, cyclophosphamide, and paclitaxel. She also completed radiation therapy to the breast, supraclavicular fossa, and axilla followed by 5 years of Arimidex. She had been doing well until last month when she developed low back pain. Workup of her symptoms including a total spine MRI revealed metastatic disease from T1–T3,*

T7–T8, and L1–L2. Imaging also revealed lumbar spinal stenosis worst at the L3–L4 levels. She is awaiting onset of a clinical trial for her metastatic disease. She is followed by the pain service for medical management of her pain and referred to rehabilitation for bracing recommendations. On evaluation she is noted to have loss of lumbar lordosis and pain with forward flexion as well as extension. Given her examination and imaging findings, an LSO is recommended.

Low back pain is common in the cancer setting. Pain may be localized, radicular, or mechanical in nature depending on the underlying etiology. Etiologies of pain include tumor, fractures, infection, and referred pain from pelvic organs. Age-related changes such as loss of intervertebral disk integrity, facet joint arthropathy, and weakness of the core musculature also play a role in the development of back pain in this population.

Depending on the etiology of pain, various oncologic and conservative treatments can be initiated. Lumbar support braces, such as a lumbosacral orthosis (LSO), can be considered as an adjunct to pain management and for injury prevention in both oncologic and non-oncologic etiologies. LSOs result in restriction of flexion-extension movements and lateral side bending, as well as reduction of intradiscal pressure on the lumbar vertebrae and decreased load on the trunk. LSOs also provide a physical and psychological reminder to utilize proper lifting techniques and voluntarily restricting motion and protecting the spine from assuming improper body mechanics [14].

Summary

The goals of rehabilitation efforts in the cancer setting include relieving symptoms, improving quality of life, enhancing functional independence, and preventing further complications. Incorporation of a bracing should also be included in these efforts. Many different off-the-shelf and custom bracing options are available. Selection of brace is based on a patient's needs, medical and oncologic status, surgical status, and stability, goals, and mobility.

References

1. Lee SH, Grant R, Kennedy C, Kilbride L. Positioning and spinal bracing for pain relief in metastatic spinal cord compression in adults. Cochrane Database Syst Rev. 2015;9:CD007609.
2. Lantz SA, Schultz AB. Lumbar spine orthosis wearing. II. Effect on trunk muscle myoelectric activity. Spine. 1986;11(8):838–42.
3. Kim DH, Chang UK, Kim SH, Bilsky MH, editors. Tumors of the spine. Philadelphia: Saunders Elsevier; 2008.
4. Sciubba DM, Gokaslan ZL. Diagnosis and management of metastatic spine disease. Surg Oncol. 2006;15(3):141–51.
5. Raj VS, Lofton L. Rehabilitation and treatment of spinal cord tumors. J Spinal Cord Med. 2013;36(1):4–11.
6. Chang V, Holly LT. Bracing for thoracolumbar fractures. Neurosurg Focus. 2014;37(1):E3.
7. Longo UG, Loppini M, Denaro L, Maffulli N, Denaro V. Osteoporotic vertebral fractures: current concepts of conservative care. Br Med Bull. 2012;102:171–89.
8. Spinal cord medicine. 2nd ed. Philadelphia: Wolters Kluwer/ Lippincott Williams and Wilkins; 2011.
9. Vaccaro A, editor. Fractures of the cervical, thoracic and lumbar spine. New York: Marcel Dekker Inc; 2002.
10. Wong CC, McGirt MJ. Vertebral compression fractures: a review of current management and multimodal therapy. J Multidiscip Healthc. 2013;6:205–14.
11. Sinaki M. Exercise for patients with osteoporosis: management of vertebral compression fractures and trunk strengthening for fall prevention. PMR. 2012;4(11):882–8.
12. Kim EK, Kim JS. Correlation between rounded shoulder posture, neck disability indices, and degree of forward head posture. J Phys Ther Sci. 2016;28(10):2929–32.
13. Seidel C, Kuhnt T, Kortmann RD, Hering K. Radiation-induced camptocormia and dropped head syndrome: review and case report of radiation-induced movement disorders. Strahlenther Onkol. 2015;191(10):765–70.
14. Walsh NE, Schwartz RK. The influence of prophylactic orthoses on abdominal strength and low back injury in the workplace. Am J Phys Med Rehabil. 1990;69(5):245–50.

Part IX

Complementary and Psycho-Behavioral Therapies

Psychosocial Assessment and Treatment for Patients with Cancer Pain

49

Laura M. van Veldhoven and Diane M. Novy

Introduction

With the shift from tumor-focused treatment to person-centered care in most large cancer centers, more attention has been focused on the individual's psychosocial reaction to his or her cancer experience and related treatments. Cancer patients with greater psychological distress are more likely to have poor adherence to treatment recommendations, less satisfaction with treatment received, and a poorer quality of life [1–4]. The role of the mental health clinician in an interdisciplinary pain team, which includes pain medicine physicians and nurses, is to help patients identify and manage psychological symptoms that can increase and maintain their pain experience. A mental health clinician on an interdisciplinary pain team may be a psychiatrist, psychologist, clinical social worker, or psychiatric nurse. The interdisciplinary pain team seeks to understand the relationships between pain and the cancer disease process, the types of mechanisms that might be sustaining the pain, and the extent to which the pain is accompanied by other symptoms or problems [5].

From relatively healthy outpatients to those at the end of life, the strong association between cancer pain and distress is evident across the disease spectrum [6–8]. The inherent uncertainty of cancer, and of the duration of pain, can intensify the pain experience and increase emotional distress. Psychological disorders are twice as prevalent among cancer patients with pain than those without [9]. Pain from cancer and its treatments can result in anxiety, depression, fear, anger, helplessness, and hopelessness, and those with both pain and depression have an amplification of disability and poor quality of life [7, 10, 11]. Cancer pain affects many facets of the individual's social support, as higher levels of pain are associated with decreased social activities, lower levels of social support, reduced social functioning, and lower resiliency of the social network, [7, 12]. Individuals with heightened cancer pain have a greater tendency to cope through catastrophizing [7, 13, 14]. Patients with unrelieved cancer pain are at high risk to consider and to commit suicide [15, 16]. The role of cancer pain in suicide appears to be intertwined with the reactionary psychological suffering to the pain [17].

Cancer pain is unlike "normal" pain, as a cancer diagnosis is linked with death, uncertainty, and loss of control [6, 18]. Further, cancer pain is also a predictor of survival: pain can signal tumor progression or be a pathogen that can further the progression of metastatic disease [19, 20]. The pain experience and level of suffering related to a cancer diagnosis, cancer pain, or treatment side effects can be heightened by high levels of depression and anxiety. For example, anxiety and tension can heighten sympathetic nervous system activity, which can lead to muscle spasm, vasoconstriction, and other physiological changes. These changes have the potential to decrease pain tolerance, to worsen the pain experience, and to increase total suffering [21].

Comprehensive Assessment of Psychosocial Factors Related to Cancer Pain

Numerous practice guidelines for the management of cancer pain include the thorough assessment of psychosocial factors [22–25]. The guidelines suggest that the assessors collect data along sensory/physical, affective, cognitive, and behavioral domains. As such, a psychosocial assessment should include the following:

L. M. van Veldhoven (✉)
Department of Physical Medicine and Rehabilitation, Baylor College of Medicine, Houston, TX, USA
e-mail: veldhove@bcm.edu

D. M. Novy
Department of Pain Medicine, The University of Texas MD Anderson Cancer Center, Houston, TX, USA
e-mail: dnovy@mdanderson.org

A. Gulati et al. (eds.), *Essentials of Interventional Cancer Pain Management*, https://doi.org/10.1007/978-3-319-99684-4_49

Sensory/Physical

- The patient's understanding of his or her cancer diagnosis
- The meaning of pain for both the patient and his or her family
- How pain influences relationships within the patient's family

Affective

- The relationship between the patient's mood and pain
- Current and preexisting affective functioning (i.e., anxiety, depression, anger, frustration, hopelessness, etc.)

Cognitive

- Cognition (i.e., expectations and preconceptions) related to pain management

Behavioral

- Preexisting and current coping strategies
- The impact of pain on the patient's sleep pattern
- The availability of social support

These psychosocial domains interact and are impacted by the underlying construct of suffering. Thus, when receiving information about one domain, the information will be influenced by the overall severity of suffering the patient is experiencing.

Psychosocial assessments are most often completed through a face-to-face interview with the patient and possible from one or more of the patient's family members and/or significant others. During these interviews, the mental health clinician gathers demographic and clinical information about the patient's background and current situation, as well as evaluating the psychosocial domains. From the oncologist's report, the mental health clinician can gain an understanding of the extent of the disease, medical treatment of disease and pain/symptom control, prognosis, and phase in the disease timeline. The pain medicine physician's report can provide the mental health clinician with an understanding of the initial assessment of the patient's pain syndrome and subsequent updated biomedical information.

Sensory/Physical Domain

Some cancer patients can be leery of interacting with the mental health clinician on the pain team. A patient may question if his or her pain is being taken seriously by the team, wonder if his or her pain physician believes that he or she is "crazy," or question how a mental health clinician could help him or her. We suggest that a mental health clinician begin his or her interaction with the patient by first focusing on the patient's understanding of his or her cancer diagnosis. Information gathered can help the mental health clinician to identify similarities and/or potentials gaps in the patient's understanding. In our clinical experience, this starting point helps the patient to tell his or her "story," and the mental health clinician can start to make initial impressions about the psychological impact of the cancer diagnosis and subsequent treatment course.

Following information gathered related to the patient's cancer diagnosis, we suggest focusing on the patient's pain experience. Numerous methods are available for gathering information on the patient's sensory/physical experience of pain. The mental health clinician can ask the patient to use a numeric rating scale (0, no pain, to 10 pain as bad as you can imagine) to rate his or her current, average, highest and lowest pain intensity during the past 24 h and to label various aspects of his or her pain experience with descriptors, such as stabbing, aching, or dullness. Specific questioning related to the impact of pain to the patient's daily life is encouraged. It is important to assess the range of behaviors a patient is physically capable of engaging in but restricts because of pain. Frequently when a patient is asked about how he or she paces activity level, it becomes apparent that there is the tendency to overdo activities during periods of diminished pain and then suffer consequences of increased pain afterward.

It is paramount that mental health clinician fully understands and appreciates the meaning of pain to the patient and his or her family. Some patients might believe that pain is part of the cancer experience and that pain is something he or she needs to endure. Others might fear that pain means a recurrence or spreading of cancer. Patients may avoid appearing a complainer or fear treatment of pain might complicate cancer treatment. There are also fears of addiction that can influence the meaning of pain. Understanding what pain means to the patient and to his or her family will help the clinician to identify and clarify inaccuracies and barriers to various treatment modalities.

Involvement of family member(s) and/or significant other(s) in the discussion of what pain means to the cancer patient allows the mental health clinician to understand how pain influences relationships within the family. Dynamics within a family can shift as the cancer patient's role becomes complicated by illness. For example, a family member who was not previously a caretaker may assume a caretaking role as a spouse becomes weakened with illness. Family members can have their own concerns about addiction and other misconceptions about cancer pain management. Although not usually the case among patients with cancer pain, pain behaviors can be inappropriately or excessively reinforced by family and/or significant others without their awareness of it. For example, a husband may encourage a wife to not engage in previously held household responsibilities at the first sign that she might be experiencing a mild degree of pain despite her functional capability to complete these tasks.

Affective Domain

While many patients with cancer adjust to the stress of the disease and its symptoms without a diagnosable psychological disorder, a significantly higher rate of depression and anxiety symptoms is found among cancer patients with higher levels of pain [26]. In general, depression and anxiety are among the most common psychological symptoms experienced by cancer patients [27–29]. The etiology of psychological symptoms in cancer patients, both with and without pain, is diverse and ranges from reactions to the diagnosis of cancer, concerns of disease recurrence or progression, diminished quality of life, interruptions with life plans, and preexisting psychological dysfunction [29]. Psychological distress can also arise in cancer patients in response to treatments, adverse disease symptoms, and/or treatment side effects. For example, cancer treatments often provide ample opportunity for anticipatory anxiety. Patients may worry about the next checkup, procedure, reaction to chemotherapy and/or radiation, call or office visit with test results, the cause of new or different pain, etc. While etiology of the psychological distress is important, the mental health clinician in a cancer pain center must also consider the influence of the comorbidity of pain and psychological distress, as the presence of depression is associated with the amplification of the experience of pain [30].

Standard affect assessment should include evaluation of suicidal ideation and intent. While relatively few patients with cancer pain commit suicide, the majority of those that do often experience severe, inadequately controlled, or poorly tolerated pain and depression [31]. In our clinical experience, it is not unusual that patients have some degree of passive thoughts of dying.

Cognitive Domain

In the context of cancer pain, the assessment of cognition includes gathering information about a patient's thoughts and beliefs about his or her disease/condition and his or her ability to manage the associated problems, including pain. A range of cognitive psychological factors has been identified as modulators of pain perceptions. Included among them are expectancy, perceived controllability, appraisal processes, perceived self-efficacy, and contingencies of reinforcement [32]. We focus on maladaptive patterns of thinking that are unrealistic or distorted. Such errors in thinking have the potential to impact the maintenance and exacerbation of pain and interfere with treatment (e.g., belief that there is nothing that they can do to reduce pain and belief that pain is inevitable and should be tolerated). It also is important to ask about a self-talk. This pertains to internal dialogues that reflect thoughts about the patient's condition or pain. Both the cognitive errors and self-talk can be assessed in the clinical interview and/or by asking the patient to monitor his or her pain and record any thoughts or feelings that accompany the pain [33].

Behavioral Domain

At the time of initial psychosocial assessment, a patient with cancer pain may or may not be using psychological coping strategies to help manage his or her pain. The mental health clinician will want to ascertain which, if any, behavioral strategies (e.g., distraction, relaxation, meditation, and prayer) and cognitive coping strategies (e.g., thought stopping, problem solving and positive self-statements) are currently being used and their effectiveness for cancer pain management. For a patient who already uses some techniques, subsequent treatment would build on the techniques that are effective.

Cancer pain is one of the primary factors that often precede sleep disruption in cancer patients [34]. A recent study found cancer patients actively receiving chemotherapy were three times more likely to meet criteria for insomnia than those in the general population [35], and approximately 30–50% of newly diagnosed cancer patients experience disrupted sleep [36]. Disrupted sleep can include difficulty falling asleep, maintaining sleep once asleep, and/or awaking up before desired. When a patient feels well rested, he or she can be better able to manage pain. Without a comfortable sleeping position, the cancer pain patient often experiences frequent nighttime waking. Further disruption to the patient's natural sleep cycle can be the lack of activity during the day because of pain. The mental health clinician is encouraged to first identify what aspect of the sleep cycle is disrupted and provide the patient with appropriate strategies that could promote good sleep habits.

Social support is important for anyone going through a cancer experience. Hence, we recommend asking about the extent and satisfaction of social support. Having stable and caring relationships for assistance with responsibilities and as outlets to "vent" are immensely helpful. In addition to family and friends, most people also benefit from connection to their faith and to other people who are going through similar medical experiences.

Other Areas to Be Included in the Assessment

"Chemobrain" and potential cognitive side effects associated with opioid medications are just two examples of possible sources of changes in cognition that a cancer patient may face. Cognitive deficits can be very troubling to a patient, and these deficits can have implications on the types of psychosocial interventions chosen (e.g., cognitive-behavioral techniques vs. mind-body techniques vs. supportive psychotherapy). The most commonly reported changes in cognition following and undergoing chemotherapy include reduction in attention span, short-term memory loss, and inefficient information processing speed. For some, declines in cognition might be transient and resolve once treatment has ended, but for others, declines in cognition can persist following the completion of treatments [37]. With respect to opioid medications, a cancer patient with pain might experience changes in cognition in the days immediately after starting an opioid medication or during the first few hours after taking a dose [38, 39]. Consultation with a neuropsychologist for assessment of cognitive strengths and weaknesses and for recommendations on strategies to address cognitive weaknesses might be of benefit. For example, if neuropsychological evaluation reveals deficits in short-term memory, it might be necessary to provide a written, step-by-step guide on how to use various pain management techniques.

An additional psychosocial factor of consideration is the economic impact of cancer and pain. Continuing to work can become too difficult for cancer patients in pain. Some cancer patients with pain must consider a leave of absence from his or her position or quitting his or her job. The reality of decision such as these can result in a major change in financial status of the family and impact a patient's ability to maintain insurance benefits. Should these present problems for a patient, it may be helpful to consult social services for guidance on disability or external government support.

Treatment Plan Formulation from the Psychosocial Interview

After gathering information from the psychosocial interview, we ask the patient what help is needed from the mental health provider. Some patients, particularly those who are psychologically minded, either from prior psychological treatment or personal introspection, may have a specific goal in mind (i.e., learning to be less reactive to pain, help for depression, end-of-life issues). Other patients may not have thought about specific goals and coping strategy needs. In the latter situation, we identify specific areas from the interview that the patient mentioned as being problematic and together with the patient assess whether those areas are ones they would like to address.

With a treatment goal established, we evaluate what strategy might best fit the patient's needs. In our clinical experience, selection of psychological coping strategies should be specific to the patient. Information from the psychosocial assessment informs the mental health clinician of the patient's preferences, available resources, and psychological coping strategies. If the patient has already utilized a strategy and is not happy with results, the clinician would critically evaluate and adapt a previously utilized strategy or suggest a new strategy. For some, treatment plans begin with learning a new psychological coping strategy in a step-by-step process with repetition for better retention. Due to the length of time that it can take for the successful implementation of a strategy, we provide significant reinforcement of the patient's efforts each visit and encourage caregivers and/or family members to support and aid the patient toward mastery.

Psychosocial Interventions for Cancer Pain

Clinical practice guidelines issued by the World Health Organization, American Pain Society, and National Comprehensive Cancer Network (NCCN) recommend both pharmacological and psychosocial interventions for effective management of pain in patients with cancer [25, 40, 41]. The origins of psychosocial interventions for patients with cancer pain come from well-researched interventions for patients with non-cancer pain syndromes [33]. Frequently, standardized psychosocial intervention protocols developed and utilized in research are customized to meet the specific needs, desires, and resources of the individual patient [42]. Psychosocial interventions for cancer pain fall into two major categories: (1) education and (2) skills training [43]. The focus of most education interventions is to provide the patient with skills to effectively communicate with clinicians regarding pain relief and instruction about analgesic medication use. The intent of skill training interventions, which includes cognitive-behavioral techniques, hypnosis and imagery, and mindfulness skills, is to provide an approach to manage and change the interpretation of pain [43].

A recent meta-analysis of psychosocial interventions to reduce pain in patients with cancer, which improved up previous meta-analyses through its comprehensive selection of randomized controlled trials and inclusion of both education and skill-based interventions, found medium-size effects on both pain severity and pain intensity [43]. While the findings were not statistically significant due to low power related to within-group heterogeneity, skill-based interventions relative to educational interventions demonstrated a slightly greater effectiveness in reducing pain severity. Additionally, the meta-analysis found that effectiveness of psychosocial interventions was the same across patient sociodemographic characteristics.

Cancer Pain Education

The Basics of Cancer Pain Education for Both Patients and Healthcare Providers

Cancer pain educational interventions generally teach patients about pain, the role of medications in the management of pain, and how to communicate with healthcare providers about their pain experience. By teaching patients about these topics, it is believed that cancer pain educational interventions can reduce barriers to effective pain management and address a patient's sense of helplessness, inadequacy, uncertainty, and unpredictability stemming from a lack of knowledge. Numerous reviews and randomized controlled trials have found that essential elements to effective cancer pain education include information that (1) clarifies myths/misconceptions about addiction and tolerance to pain medication, (2) teaches skills for communication with healthcare providers, (3) promotes pain-related coping skills, (4) fosters involvement of family members and caregivers in the educational sessions with the patient, and (5) uses preconstructed educational material that is suitable for individuals with low literacy and English as a second language [44–48]. Systematic review and meta-analysis by Cummings et al. [44] suggest that effective educational interventions are delivered in 30–60 min individualized, face-to-face coaching sessions, which include written material that is referenced during the session and taken home by the patient at its conclusion.

As Martin and colleagues [47] point out, it is necessary to customize cancer pain education programs to the phase of cancer survivorship. Individuals who are newly diagnosed with cancer may less likely discuss pain with their treatment providers due to concerns that it would detract from treatment and are potentially more focused on making treatment decisions rather than those related to pain management [49, 50]. Newly diagnosed individuals may be less likely to process and remember information as it is presented to them [51]. Given these characteristics, Martin and colleagues [47] suggest that cancer pain education for newly diagnosed include frequent opportunities for repetition and reinforce the idea that both treatment and optimal pain management can coexist. They also emphasize that providers need to remember that preferences for information and extent of involvement can change over the course of the cancer continuum and should be frequently assessed.

After the completion of cancer treatment, patients have fewer contacts with healthcare providers, and some are uncertain of when and how to seek further medical care [47]. During this phase, Martin and colleagues suggest that cancer pain education focuses on the patient's understanding of chronic pain symptoms and facilitates an understanding of when to access care for the management of chronic pain. Cancer pain education for patients with advance cancer should be designed to produce change quickly and be of relatively low burden to the patient [52]. Cancer pain education should explain adverse effects of analgesia and increase the patient's understanding of the service offered by palliative care and providers that address psychosocial issues related to end of life [47]. Effective cancer pain education interventions demonstrate consideration of content, format, timing, duration, follow-up, and the interaction of these factors [53].

Like cancer patients with pain, healthcare professionals also face barriers to effective pain management that educational interventions have been designed to address. The barriers that healthcare professionals face include inadequate knowledge, ineffective pain assessment, insufficient opioid prescription due to beliefs that opioids are addictive, prescribing "as needed" rather than on regular interval, lack of adjuvant analgesia or not titrating the dose, and ineffective management of opioid side effects [54]. Evidence suggests educating healthcare professionals results in improvement in their own knowledge and attitudes about cancer pain management but unfortunately does not translate into improvement on patients' experiences of pain [53]. Bennett and colleagues [53] point out that improved patient pain control and satisfaction can occur when focused educational interventions for healthcare professional, which take place within the clinical setting, are aimed at the following behaviors:

1. Stating pain control is of importance to the patient.
2. Regular assessment of pain and the use of these data to inform prescribing decisions.
3. The use and adherence to a prescribing protocol.
4. Identifying and clarifying patients' fears related to pain and analgesic use.
5. The provision of clear explanation of how and when to use their analgesic medications.
6. Appropriate monitoring of and response to adverse side effects.
7. Frequent reassessment of pain.

Examples of Cancer Pain Education Interventions

In many cultures, there is hesitancy among family members involved in a cancer patient's care to report pain and use analgesics [47, 54]. Some family members fear the report of pain will distract treatment from the cancer and use of opioid medication will result in addiction and experience fatalism with respect to pain relief [55]. Furthermore, many family members actively involved in the care of their loved one report receiving little instruction on how to manage pain [56]. Within this context, Lin and colleagues [57] sought to identify the long-term effectiveness of a patient and family cancer pain educational program that was aimed at reducing the barriers to both patient use and family-supported use of analgesics, as well as the effects of the education on adherence and use of prescribed analgesics, pain intensity, and pain interference for cancer patients. The pain education was based on previous research and consisted of a booklet that was culturally appropriate and used short descriptions and illustrations to address concerns related to fatalism, addiction, a desire to be good, fear of distracting physicians, disease progression, tolerance, side effects, religious fatalism, and use as need instructions (i.e., p.r.n. use).

Using a randomized controlled design, 31 patient-family pairs in the experimental group received a 30–40 min educational session during which the research assistant reviewed the information within the educational booklet and encouraged the patient-family pair to ask questions. The patient-family pair was provided with a copy of the booklet. Assessment data were collected prior to the educational session and at 2 and 4 weeks post-educational session. Those randomized to the control group received conventional care, and data were collected at the same time intervals. At both outcome assessments, those in the experimental group showed significantly lower barrier scores relative to those in the control group. Members of the experimental group also reported significantly better adherence to use of prescribed analgesics at both time points and at the 4-week follow-up only, they reported significantly lower levels of worst pain intensity and pain interference. These results support the effectiveness of cancer pain education programs for both patients and family members in improving pain management.

Kravitz and colleagues [46] compared the effectiveness of a tailored education and coaching (TEC) intervention for reducing pain misconceptions and enhancing self-efficacy for communicating with physicians about pain severity and impairment versus pain education without the coaching component. The results demonstrated significant benefits in communication self-efficacy of the TEC intervention over the control condition. The TEC intervention had small and temporary benefits on pain-related impairment and achieved its immediate aims of reducing pain-related misconceptions and increasing confidence in communicating about pain. However, misconceptions were reduced equally in the group that received pain management education only, and improvements in communication self-efficacy did not lead to consistent or sustained improvements in pain outcomes.

Meta-analyses of Cancer Pain Education Interventions

Most evidenced-based guidelines include the provision of cancer pain education [25, 45]. However, while systematic reviews of the effect of education on cancer pain have shown small to moderate effects on pain intensity and pain interference [44, 52, 58–61], recent data suggest that educational interventions do not work in the way naturally assumed by most healthcare professionals. Bennett and colleagues [52] found patient-based educational interventions improve knowledge and attitudes toward pain and the use of analgesics and reduce pain intensity, although the data did not support the relationship between improved knowledge and attitudes leading to improved medication adherence. It is likely that reduced pain intensity is the function of greater reporting of pain and adverse effects, improved sense of control, and reduced anxiety. Also, while their results demonstrated a positive effect on worst or maximum pain intensity, there was not an improvement on interference from pain in daily activities. The authors could not determine the optimal exposure type or the duration of the effect.

Using a theory-based approach to classifying and comparing educational interventions for cancer pain, a systematic review done by Marie et al. [61] found that inclusion of enabling functions in interventions was associated with a significant improvement in pain intensity. Enabling functions were defined as those that promote a sense of self-efficacy. Marie and colleagues [61] argue that results such as these suggest that cancer education interventions need to include strategies beyond knowledge transfer to be of benefit to the patient. Specifically, self-efficacy skills aimed at improving communication, promoting personalized pain management plans and the use of pillboxes, teaching cognitive-behavioral techniques for distraction and reframing, and improving confidence may help reduce barriers to effective pain management.

Consistent with other meta-analyses, Jho and colleagues [59] found small efficacy for pain education in cancer patients; however, unlike other meta-analyses, Jho and colleagues [59] only used randomized controlled trials and combined results with different measures of pain, which demonstrated no beneficial effect when an attention control group was used as a control. The authors argue the beneficial effect of education may be a placebo effect. Subgroup analysis demonstrated several key findings: (1) pain education was more effective for inpatients than outpatients; (2) pain education was effective within 2 weeks of first follow-up, but not at time intervals greater than this; (3) pain education was retained longer when multiple educational sessions were provided; and (4) pain education was significantly effective in studies reporting worst, average, and least pain intensity, but not effective in those reporting current and composite pain intensity.

Cognitive-Behavioral Techniques: Distraction, Cognitive Reframing, and Relaxation

Cognitive-behavioral approaches modify thoughts and behaviors contributing to the patient's experience of pain. These techniques can enhance the patient's sense of control and resourcefulness by providing the patient with coping skills that promote self-efficacy, minimize the tendency to negatively catastrophize, and enhance an overall sense of well-being. Research supports patients who have high self-efficacy and perceptions of control over pain often experience reduced pain, while in contrast, those patients who catastrophize frequently experience greater pain intensity [62].

Cognitive-behavioral interventions for cancer patients undergoing painful procedures and/or treatments may benefit those with chronic cancer pain [63]. Anderson and colleagues [63] suggest cognitive-behavioral techniques are ideally instructed to patients in either a one-to-one or small group setting; however, most oncology patients receive instruction through written or recorded media secondary to time constraints.

Distraction

The goal of distraction is to shift the patient's focus from pain to non-painful sensations such as positive thoughts, positive images, or other aspects of the environment [33]. Patients should have an appreciation of the role that attention plays in the amplification or reduction of pain. The mental health clinician can teach a patient to engage in distraction by encouraging the patient to experiment with his or her awareness of pain and other bodily sensations. This enables the patient to shift and control his or her attention focus away from pain sensations [33]. Frequently, distraction is taught via audio tracks of nature sounds or information on topics such as history, foreign language, geography, or vocabulary [63, 64].

Cognitive Reframing

Negative expectations, interpretations, and anticipatory fears such as unavoidable pain, loss of control, disfigurement, and subjective perceptions of rejection are common among patients with cancer. Cognitive reframing involves the reconceptualization of thoughts and feelings that have a negative effect on the patient's overall adjustment and experience of pain. Under conditions of stress and minimal coping resources, patients have the tendency to make global, extreme, one-sided, and absolutistic appraisals and judgments of a situation. In these situations, the behavioral response also tends to be extreme. For example, a person who is susceptible to fear reactions may interpret a bodily sensation deemed by a physician to be insignificant and unrelated to cancer in a catastrophic manner. A depression-prone person may interpret a concise and brief follow-up appointment with a healthcare provider as a rejection and may seek withdrawal from treatment.

Cognitive restructuring training seeks to bring awareness to the patient's evaluation process. The mental health clinician will query several things related to when pain was severe. These include what the situation was at the time of the pain; what thoughts the patient had before, during, and after the pain episode; what techniques were tried to decrease pain; and what resources are available to help deal with the pain. By examining the answers to these questions, the patient and clinician can identify negative thoughts and feelings that are not based on well-grounded evidence, and the patient can learn to develop alternative ways of responding [33].

Relaxation

Numerous relaxation exercises are available for utilization by patients with cancer pain. The most commonly used relaxation procedure is progressive muscle relaxation [65]. Progressive muscle relaxation is a group of techniques that vary in procedural detail, complexity, and length. Progressive muscle relaxation consists of systematically tensing and relaxing several of the 16 major muscle groups. Most relaxation techniques used by cancer patients with pain adhere to either an individual or group session format, with multiple sessions and supplemental learning via audiotape-guided home practice.

Examples of Cognitive-Behavioral Interventions

With an initial study sample of 131 patients, Dalton and colleagues [42] investigated the differential effects on cancer pain of a tailored cognitive-behavioral intervention vs. a traditional cognitive behavioral intervention vs. usual care. For those in the tailored cognitive-behavioral intervention, five 1-h treatment modules were selected and delivered based on participant responses to the Biobehavioral Pain Profile, which measures the biobehavioral factors related to the verbal report of pain, activity, medication, as well as the environmental and personal attributes that influence the experience of pain. Those in the standard cognitive-behavioral group were taught six to eight treatment strategies as part of a comprehensive program of cognitive and behavioral techniques that evaluated thoughts, feelings, and behaviors. Participants in the intervention groups were able to receive three out of the five treatment sessions over the phone, and the therapy materials were mailed to the participants in advance of the session. Participants randomized to usual care were treated using standard educational and supportive techniques. At the 1-month follow-up, those in the tailored cognitive-behavioral intervention experienced substantial improvement in worst pain, least pain, and less interference of pain. At the time of the 6-month follow-up, those in the standard cognitive-behavioral intervention had greater improvements in less average pain, and less pain now scores relative to those in the tailored cognitive-behavioral intervention. Participants in the tailored intervention demonstrated substantial improvements from baseline to 1-month post-intervention, but the degree of improvement decreased at 6 months. The authors concluded that the results supported the use of CBT to help patients with cancer pain and that the tailored intervention yielded better outcomes overall.

Kwekkeboom and colleagues [64] expanded upon a feasibility study and piloted a patient-controlled cognitive-behavioral intervention that included a variety of relaxation, distraction, and imagery recordings on a MP3 player that participants self-administered. Using a randomized controlled trial design, 86 patients receiving treatment for advanced lung, prostate, colorectal, or gynecologic cancer were randomized to either the intervention or waitlist control condition. Relaxation exercises consisted of progressive muscle relaxation, jaw relaxation, and focused breathing relaxation. Distraction was promoted through nature sound recordings of a rainstorm, sounds of surf and waves, and forest sounds. Symptom-focused imagery strategies consisted of (1) pain-focused imagery that instructed the participant to imagine a draining pain from the body and using a special glove to change any residual pain to a pleasant sensation, (2) fatigue-focused imagery that instructed participants to imagine a circulating ball of healing energy throughout their bodies, and (3) sleep-focused imagery that instructed participants to imagine floating through the sky into a peaceful sleep. At the end of a 2-week study period, participants in the intervention group showed statistically significant improvements in pain and fatigue scores compared to those in the waitlist control condition. The authors concluded that cognitive-behavioral strategies can be useful in the treatment of multiple related symptoms that are made worse by negative psychological reactions and that cognitive-behavioral strategies produce a sustained, beneficial effect when they are used frequently and routinely.

The efficacy of cognitive-behavioral strategies for pain control in cancer patients taking opioid medications for pain management was investigated by Anderson and colleagues [63] using a sample of 57 patients from a large cancer care center. Patients were randomized to one of four groups: a positive mood group, relaxation group, distraction group, or a waitlist control group. Those in the positive mood group received a 20-min audiotape that included positive mood statements and positive imagery suggestions. Patients in the relaxation group received a 20-min audiotape that provided instructions for standard progressive muscle relaxation. Patients in the distraction group selected an audiotape that provided information on history, geography, vocabulary, or foreign language instruction. Participants were instructed to practice the technique at least five times a week for 2 weeks for 20 min each time. Distraction and relaxation interventions yielded transient decreases in pain intensity; however, the dropout rate of participants enrolled in the study was high. The authors concluded the techniques provided in the intervention did not provide long-term pain relief and were not appealing to many cancer patients (over 50% patients approached for the study declined to participate).

Mind-Body Therapies: Hypnosis and Imagery

Hypnosis

Hypnosis is a formal induction of a state of sustained attention and concentration, reduced peripheral awareness, and openness to suggestion [66]. The five major hypnotic techniques that have been used for the treatment of cancer pain are anesthesia, direct diminution, sensory substitution, displacement, and dissociation [67, 68]. The technique of anesthesia refers to hypnotic suggestions that render a body area numb and insensitive to pain. Direct diminution and sensory substitution change the meaning of pain so that it is less important (e.g., turning down the volume; interpreting pain as coldness). Displacement suggestions change the location of the pain. Dissociation is used to separate pain from the patient's awareness. Posthypnotic suggestion and self-hypnosis are additional techniques that are used to extend pain relief [67, 68].

Imagery

Imagery involves having a patient develop a mental image associated with feelings of peacefulness and calmness. The patient is involved in the decision about the selection of the image. The inclusion and emphasis on various senses enhance the vividness of the image and facilitate the imagery process and relaxation [32]. When a patient is in a relaxed state, he or she can be instructed to focus on an image that symbolizes pain. The patient is taught to modify the image in a therapeutic manner. By so doing, he or she can experience a greater sense of control over pain [69]. The content of the image does not seem to be the important factor, rather the manner in which the imagery is presented, the involvement of the patient, and practice appear to be crucial.

Examples of Hypnosis and Imagery Interventions

Kwekkeboom and colleagues [70] conducted a review of mind-body interventions that have demonstrated efficacy in the treatment of two or more symptoms in the pain-fatigue-sleep disturbance cancer symptom cluster. Of the six studies where hypnosis/imagery was the primary treatment being tested, five demonstrated efficacies in the treatment of the cluster symptoms and in three of four studies in which hypnosis/imagery was an active comparison condition. Most of the studies reviewed used randomized or crossover designs with primarily hospitalized patients experiencing cancer-related pain. Interventions in these studies ranged from one 12-min session to 50-plus-min sessions plus daily practice over several weeks.

In a randomized controlled trial that compared the effects of hypnosis and empathic attention to standard care in 201 patients during percutaneous tumor treatments, patients treated with hypnosis experienced significantly less pain and anxiety than those in empathic attention and standard conditions at several time intervals [71]. Patients who received hypnosis also received fewer median drug units than patients in the other two conditions. The hypnosis script used in this trial suggested that patients roll their eyes upward, close their eyes, breathe deeply, focus on a sensation of floating, and experience a pleasant setting of choice. The authors argued that patients who received hypnosis were better able to utilize their own internal coping resources.

In a crossover design, individual difference variables on the effectiveness of progressive muscle relaxation and analgesic imagery were studied in 40 hospitalized patients with cancer-related pain [72]. The guided imagery, progressive muscle relaxation, and control condition interventions were done using recordings on a CD that was played for the participant. In the nearly 15-min imagery intervention, the participant was guided through a glove anesthesia technique that asked the listener to first scan his or her body for areas of pain and then imagine replacing the pain with comforting sensations. Afterward, the participant was asked to imagine soaking his or her hand in an anesthetic fluid that resulted in the hand feeling numb. The participant was then asked to transfer the numbness to other areas of pain in the body. In the progressive muscle relaxation condition, the participant was guided through the tensing and relaxing of 12 major muscle groups. The control condition consisted of information on the healthcare team, patients' rights and hospital services, as well as exercises and activities to maintain strength while in the hospital. While both the imagery and progressive muscle relaxation interventions were significantly more effective than the control condition, meaningful improvement in pain was limited to nearly half of the participants. Pain relief provided by the interventions was short term, and pain returned to pre-intervention levels before the next trial started and, in some cases, within an hour.

Mindfulness-Based Interventions

Mindfulness has its roots in Buddhist psychology, which posits that human suffering is often the result of a disproportionate focus on the past or planning for the future, and as a result, the present experience is lost [73]. Formal mindfulness meditation includes directing one's focus on breathing, body sensations, feelings, or thoughts and can also include the acknowledgment of whatever arises into consciousness at a given time [74]. Mindfulness encourages one to have feelings of universal acceptance, patience, openness, curiosity, kindness, and non-striving when focusing attention on the present experience [75].

The diagnosis of disease or illness can result in fear, terror, and challenges to beliefs about control and certainty. Mindfulness can teach an individual that the loss of control is inevitable in life and that by not engaging in an active process to address one's distress can be a liberating experience. While a situation can be extremely unpleasant, the situation can be tolerated and will pass with time [74]. Recently, mindfulness-based interventions have been used to address the psychological and physical effects of many diseases and conditions, including chronic pain. Chief among mindfulness-based interventions are Kabat-Zinn's mindfulness-based stress reduction (MSBR) and mindfulness-based cognitive therapy (MBCT) [76]. MSBR is often an 8-week program that trains participants in sitting meditation, body scan, walking meditation, loving kindness meditation, and gentle Hatha yoga. Interactive learning of mindfulness key elements of self-discovery and personal growth is also included in MSBR programs [74]. MBCT was first developed for the treatment of major depression and builds upon MSBR with the inclusion of identification of maladaptive thought patterns and other cognitive therapy techniques [77].

MSBR has been studied in cancer populations for its appropriateness to manage symptoms of stress, anxiety, depression, sleep disruption, and pain. Using a program modeled after Kabat-Zinn's Stress Reduction and Relaxation Clinic-Massachusetts Medical Center, Carlson and colleagues [78] investigated the effects of an 8-week MSBR intervention in 59 patients with breast and prostate cancer. Significant improvements in overall quality of life, symptoms of stress, and sleep quality were found post-intervention; however, no change was evident on a quality of life pain subscale. Pain was included as a quality of life indicator in an investigation of the effectiveness of MBSR for management of psychological distress and improvement in quality of life in breast cancer survivors [79]. Eighty-four breast cancer survivors were randomized to either a 6-week MBSR program or standard care. Improvements in physical functioning, pain, and emotional well-being were found in those who received the MBSR intervention. In a meta-analysis of MBSR and MBCT interventions for patients with breast cancer that included three randomized controlled trials with a total of 327 participants, Cramer and colleagues [80] found small effects of MBSR compared with standard of care in decreasing depression and anxiety.

Future Directions of Psychosocial Interventions for Cancer Pain

There is a developing field that involves use of the Internet to deliver behaviorally based interventions for pain [81]. This method of delivery allows patients to access the intervention at their pace with the convenience of not having to locate an appropriate mental health provider or to travel to obtain those services. Many pain physicians do not have comprehensive services that include mental health interventions, and using the Internet for this has appeal.

The available Internet-based behavioral pain management interventions can be classified into three types: (1) comprehensive programs guided by a professional therapist or other trained provider; (2) unguided or automated programs that do not include contact with a therapist; and (3) pain applications that provide targeted pain self-management tools specifically designed for mobile platforms [81]. These treatments vary in terms of user interfaces, treatment components, and degree to which they have been subjected to empirical testing. The next step in advancing these interventions is addressing barriers related to design, implementation, and assessing their effectiveness.

Summary

In this chapter, we presented literature that supports a person-centered approach to care for cancer patients with pain and psychological distress. This approach includes an interdisciplinary pain team to assess the relationships between pain and the cancer disease process, the types of mechanisms that might be sustaining the pain, and the extent to which the pain is accompanied by other symptoms or problems.

In a person-centered approach to care for cancer patients with pain, information from the psychosocial assessment is used to coordinate care with the medical members of the pain team to address the sensory-physical, affective, behavioral, and cognitive aspects of cancer pain. Depending on individual patient needs, goals, and resources, interventions should include components of well-researched psychological interventions. Interventions fit into two broad categories, education and skills training, and the technique to deliver this effectively has been a primary goal of pain practitioners.

References

1. Jacobsen PB, Ransom S. Implementation of NCCN distress management guidelines by member institutions. J Natl Compr Canc Netw. 2007;5:99–103.
2. Kennard BD, Smith SM, Olvera R, et al. Nonadherence in adolescent oncology patients: preliminary data on psychological risk factors and relationships to outcome. J Clin Psychol Med Settings. 2004;11:30–9.
3. Von Essen L, Larsson G, Oberg K, et al. 'Satisfaction with care': associations with health-related quality of life and psychosocial functioning among Swedish patients with endocrine gastrointestinal tumors. Eur J Cancer Care (Engl). 2002;11:91–9.
4. Skarstein J, Aass N, Fossa SD, et al. Anxiety and depression in cancer patients: relation between the Hospital Anxiety and Depression Scale and the European Organization for Research and Treatment of Cancer Core Quality of Life Questionnaire. J Psychosom Res. 2000;49:27–34.
5. Portenoy RK. Cancer pain management. Clin Adv Hematol Oncol. 2005;3(1):30–2.
6. Keefe FJ, Abernethy AP, et al. Psychological approaches to understanding and treating disease-related pain. Annu Rev Psychol. 2005;56:601–30.
7. Zaza C, Baine N. Cancer pain and psychosocial factors: a critical review of the literature. J Pain Symptom Manage. 2002;24(5):526–42.
8. Portenoy RK, Thaler HT, et al. Symptom prevalence, characteristics and distress in a cancer population. Qual Life Res. 1994;3(3):183–9.
9. Derogatis LR, Marrow GR, Fetting J, et al. The prevalence of psychiatric disorders among cancer patients. JAMA. 1983;249:751–7.
10. Glover J, Dibble SL, Dodd MJ, Miaskowski C. Mood states of oncology outpatients: does pain make a difference? J Pain Symptom Manag. 1995;10(2):120–8.
11. Kroenke K, Theobald D, Wu J, et al. The associations of depression and pain with health-related quality of life, disability, and health care use in cancer patients. J Pain Symptom Manag. 2010;40(3):327–41.
12. Green CR, Hart-Johnson T, Loeffler DR. Cancer-related chronic pain: examining quality of life in diverse cancer survivors. Cancer. 2011;117(9):1994–2003.
13. Jacobsen PB, Butler RW. Relation of cognitive coping and catastrophizing to acute pain and analgesic use following breast cancer surgery. J Behav Med. 1996;19:17–29.
14. Wilkie DJ, Keefe FJ. Coping strategies of patients with lung cancer-related pain. Clin J Pain. 1991;7:292–9.
15. Bolund C. Suicide and cancer: II. Medical and care factors in suicide by cancer patients in Sweden, 1973–1976. J Psychosoc Oncol. 1985;3:17–30.
16. Breitbart W. Suicide in cancer patients. Oncology. 1987;1:49–53.
17. Breitbart W. Cancer pain and suicide. In: Foley K, Bonica JJ, Ventafridda V, editors. Advances in pain research and therapy, vol. 16. New York: Raven Press; 1990. p. 399–412.
18. Turk DC. Remember the distinction between malignant and benign pain? Well, forget it. Clin J Pain. 2002;18(2):75–6.
19. Herndon JE, Fleishman S, Kornblith AB, et al. Is quality of life predictive of survival of patients with advanced nonsmall cell lung carcinoma? Cancer. 1999;85:333–40.
20. Page GG, Ben-Eliyahu S. The immune-suppressive nature of pain. Semin Oncol Nurs. 1997;13(1):10–5.
21. Otis-Green S, Sherman R, et al. An integrated psychosocial-spiritual model for cancer pain management. Cancer Pract. 2002;10(10Suppl 1):S58–65.
22. American Pain Society. Guideline for the management of cancer pain in adults and children. Glenview: Author; 2005.
23. American Society of Anesthesiologists Task Force on Pain Management, Cancer Pain Section. Practice guidelines for cancer pain management. Anesthesiology. 1996;84:1243–57.
24. British Pain Society. Cancer pain management: a perspective from the British Pain Society, supported by Association for Palliative Medicine and the Royal College of General Practitioners. 2010. Available at: http://www.britishpainsociety.org/book_cancer_pain.pdf. Accessed 13 Oct 2013.
25. National Comprehensive Cancer Network. NCCN clinical practice guidelines in oncology: adult cancer pain, version 2, 2011. Available at: http://www.nccn.org/professionals/physician_gls/PDF/pain.pdf. Accessed 13 Oct 2013.
26. Spiegel D, Sands S, Koopman C. Pain and depression in patients with cancer. Cancer. 1994;74(9):2570–8.
27. Newport DJ, Nemeroff CB. Assessment and treatment of depression in cancer patients. J Psychosom Res. 1998;45:215–37.
28. Stark DPH, House A. Anxiety in cancer patients. Br J Cancer. 2000;83:1261–7.
29. Jacobsen PB, Donovan KA, Swaine ZN, et al. Management of anxiety and depression in adult cancer patients: towards an evidenced-based approach. In: Chang AE, Ganz PA, Hayes DF, et al., editors. Oncology: evidence-based approach. New York: Springer; 2006. p. 1552–79.

30. Korff MV, Simon G. The relationship between pain and depression. Brit J Psychiatry. 1996;168(Suppl30):101–8.
31. Massie MJ, Gagnon P, et al. Depression and suicide in patients with cancer. J Pain Symptom Manag. 1994;9(5):325–40.
32. Turk D, Fernandez E. Pain and cancer: a cognitive-behavioral perspective. In: Watson M, Greer S, editors. Cancer patient care: psychosocial treatment methods. Cambridge: Cambridge University Press; 1991. p. 15–44.
33. Turk DC, Meichenbaum D, Genest M. Pain and behavior medicine: a cognitive behavioral perspective. New York: Guildford Press; 1987.
34. Theobald DE. Cancer pain, fatigue, distress, and insomnia in cancer patients. Clin Cornerstone. 2004;6(1SupplD):S15–21.
35. Palesh OG, Roscoe JA, Mustain KM, et al. Prevalence, demographics, and psychological associations of sleep disruption in patients with cancer: University of Rochester Cancer Center-Community Clinical Oncology Program. J Clin Oncol. 2010;28(2):292–8.
36. Savard J, Morin CM. Insomnia in the context of cancer: a review of a neglected problem. J Clin Oncol. 2001;19(3):895–908.
37. Meyers CA, Abbruzzese JL. Cognitive functioning in cancer patients: effect of previous treatment. Neurology. 1992;42(2):434–6.
38. Chapman SL, Byas-Smith MG, et al. Effects of intermediate- and long-term use of opioids on cognition in patients with chronic pain. Clin J Pain. 2002;18(4 Suppl):S83–90.
39. Strassels SA. Cognitive effects of opioids. Curr Pain Headache Rep. 2008;12(1):32–6.
40. Jadad AR, Browman GP. The WHO analgesic ladder for a cancer pain management: stepping up the quality of its evaluation. JAMA. 1995;274:1870–3.
41. Miaskowski C, Cleary J. Guidelines for the management of cancer pain in adults and children. Glenview: American Pain Society; 2005.
42. Dalton JA, Keefe FJ, Carlson J, Youngblood R. Tailoring cognitive-behavioral treatment for cancer pain. Pain Manag Nurs. 2004;5(1):3–18.
43. Sheinfeld Gorin S, Krebs P, Badr H, et al. Meta-analysis of psychosocial interventions to reduce pain in patients with cancer. J Clin Oncol. 2012;30:539–47.
44. Cummings CG, Olivo SA, Biondo PD, et al. Effectiveness of knowledge translation intervention to improve cancer pain management. J Pain Symptom Manag. 2011;41(5):915–39.
45. Green E, Zwaal C, Beals C, et al. Cancer-related pain management: a report of evidence-based recommendations to guide practice. Clin J Pain. 2010;26(6):449–62.
46. Kravitz RL, Tancredi DJ, Grennan T, et al. Cancer Health Empowerment for Living without Pain (Ca-HELP): effects of a tailored education and coaching intervention on pain and impairment. Pain. 2011;152(7):1572–82.
47. Martin MY, Pisu M, Kvale EA, Johns SA. Developing effective cancer pain education programs. Curr Pain Headache Rep. 2012;16:332–42.
48. Miaskowski C, Dodd M, West C, et al. Randomized clinical trial of the effectiveness of a self-care intervention to improve cancer pain management. J Clin Oncol. 2004;22(9):1713–20.
49. Gwede CK, Pow-Sang J, Seigne J, et al. Treatment decision-making strategies and influences in patients with localized prostate carcinoma. Cancer. 2005;104(7):1381–90.
50. Oldenmenger WH, Sillevis Smitt PA, van Dooren S, et al. A systematic review on barriers hindering adequate cancer pain management and interventions to reduce them: a critical appraisal. Eur J Cancer. 2009;45(8):1370–80.
51. Miller SM, Bowen DJ, Croyle RT, Rowland JH. Handbook of cancer control and behavioral science, a resource for researchers, practitioners, and policymakers. Washington, DC: American Psychological Association; 2009.
52. Bennett MI, Bagnall AM, Jose Closs S. How effective are patient-based educational interventions in the management of cancer pain? Systematic review and meta-analysis. Pain. 2009;143(3):192–9.
53. Bennett MI, Flemming K, Jose Closs S. Education in cancer pain management. Curr Opin Support Palliat Care. 2011;5:20–4.
54. Jacobsen R, Sjøgren P, Møldrup C, Christup L. Physician-related barriers to cancer pain management with opioid analgesics: a systematic review. J Opioid Manag. 2007;3:207–14.
55. Lin CC. Barriers to analgesic management of cancer pain: a comparison of attitudes of Taiwan patients and their family caregivers. Pain. 2000;88:1–7.
56. Lin CC, Lai YL, Lo EC. Life-extending therapies among patients with advanced cancer: patients' levels of pain and family caregivers' concerns about pain relief. Cancer Nurs. 2001;24(6):430–5.
57. Van Ryn M, Sanders S, Kahn K, et al. Objective burden, resources, and other sources of stressors among informal cancer caregivers: a hidden quality issue? Psycho-Oncology. 2011;20(1):44–52.
58. Lin CC, Chou PL, Wu SL, Chang YC, Lai YL. Long-term effectiveness of a patient and family pain education program on overcoming barriers to management of cancer pain. Pain. 2006;122:271–81.
59. Jho HJ, Myung SK, Chang YJ, et al. Efficacy of pain education in cancer patients. Support Cancer Care. 2013;21:1963–71.
60. Koller A, Miaskowski C, DeGeest S, et al. A systematic evaluation of content, structure, and efficacy of interventions to improve patients' self-management of cancer pain. J Pain Symptom Manag. 2012;44(2):264–84.
61. Marie N, Luckett T, Davidson PM, Lovell M, Lal S. Optimal patient education for cancer pain: a systematic review and theory-based meta-analysis. Support Care Cancer. 2013;21(12):3529–37.
62. Bishop SR, Warr D. Coping, catastrophizing and chronic pain in breast cancer. J Behav Med. 2003;18(12):1261–72.
63. Anderson KO, Cohen MZ, Mendoza TR, Guo H, et al. Brief cognitive-behavioral audiotape interventions for cancer-related pain. Cancer. 2006;107:207–14.
64. Kwekkeboom KL, Abbott-Anderson K, Cherwin C, Roiland R, et al. Pilot randomization controlled trial of a patient-controlled cognitive-behavioral intervention for pain, fatigue, and sleep disturbance symptom cluster in cancer. J Pain Symptom Manag. 2012;44:810–22.
65. Jacobsen P, Hann DM. Cognitive-behavioral interventions. In: Holland JC, editor. Psycho-oncology. New York: Oxford University Press; 1998. p. 717–29.
66. Weil A, Kabat-Zinn J. Meditation for optimum health: how to use mindfulness breathing to heal [Audio CD]. Louisville: Sound True Incorporated; 2003.
67. Barber J, Gitelson J. Cancer pain: psychological management using hypnosis. CA Cancer J Clin. 1980;30(3):130–6.
68. Barber J. Hypnotic analgesia. In: Holzman AD, Turk DC, editors. Pain management: a handbook of psychological treatment approaches. New York: Pergamon Press; 1986. p. 151–67.
69. Spiegel D, Bloom JR. Group therapy and hypnosis reduce metastatic breast cancer pain. Psychosom Med. 1983;45(4):333–9.
70. Kwekkeboom KL, Cherwin CH, Lee JW, Wanta B. Mind-body treatments for the pain-fatigue-sleep disturbance cluster in persons with cancer. J Pain Symptom Manag. 2010;39:126–38.
71. Lang EV, Berbaum KS, Pauker SG, Faintuch S, et al. Beneficial effects of hypnosis and adverse effects of empathic attention during percutaneous tumor treatment: when being nice does not suffice. J Vasc Interv Radiol. 2008;19:897–905.
72. Kwekkeboom KL, Wanta B, Bumpus M. Individual difference variables and the effects of progressive muscle relaxation and analgesic imagery interventions on cancer pain. J Pain Symptom Manag. 2008;36:604–15.
73. Germer CK. Mindfulness. In: Germer CK, Siegel RD, Fulton PR, editors. Mindfulness and psychotherapy. New York: The Guilford Press; 2005. p. 3–27.

74. Carlson LE. Mindfulness-based interventions for physical conditions: a narrative review evaluating levels of evidence. ISNR Psychiatry. 2012;2012:1–13.
75. Kabat-Zinn J. Full catastrophe living: using the wisdom of your body and mind to face stress, pain and illness. New York: Delacourt; 1990.
76. Baer RA. Mindfulness training as a clinical intervention: a conceptual and empirical review. Clin Psychol Sci Pract. 2003;10:125–43.
77. Segal ZV, Williams MG, Teasdale JD. Mindfulness-based cognitive therapy for depression: a new approach to preventing relapse. New York: The Guilford Press; 2002.
78. Carlson LE, Speca M, Patel KD, Goodey E. Mindfulness-based stress reduction in relation to quality of life, mood, symptoms of stress, and immune parameters in breast and prostate cancer outpatients. Psychosom Med. 2003;65:571–81.
79. Lengacher CA, John-Mallard V, Post-White J, et al. Randomized controlled trial of mindfulness-based stress reduction (MSBR) for survivors of breast cancer. Psycho-Oncology. 2009;18(12):1261–72.
80. Cramer H, Lauch R, Paul A, Dobos G. Mindfulness-based stress reduction for breast cancer- a systematic review and meta-analysis. Curr Oncol. 2012;19(5):343–52.
81. Rini C, Williams DA, Broderick JE, Keefe FJ. Meeting them where they are: using the internet to deliver behavioral medicine interventions for pain. Transl Behav Med. 2012;2:82–92.

50 Relaxation Techniques and Biofeedback for Cancer Pain Management

Asimina Lazaridou and Robert R. Edwards

Introduction

In this chapter we report on evidence for the effectiveness of relaxation and biofeedback therapy for managing cancer symptoms. A variety of views and techniques are presented as well as evidence to support the therapeutic underpinnings of relaxation-based therapies. In general, interventions such as these are grounded in the biopsychosocial model of cancer management which highlights the influence of many factors on the experience of cancer symptoms, ranging from genetics to physiological or pharmacological as well as psychological and social aspects. (Fig. 50.1). Psychosocial influences have been the focus of a number of recent studies assessing the influence of cognitive and affective processes on a range of clinical outcomes, from symptoms such as pain and fatigue to medical costs [1]. Mind-body therapies target reductions in depression and anxiety by facilitating acceptance as well as a diminution in the frequency or impact of negative thoughts that lead to a generally maladaptive cognitive and emotional mental state. These maladaptive processes usually include feelings of helplessness when in pain, rumination about illness, and magnification of cancer-related symptoms.

Mind-body therapies have been introduced into clinical settings and usually include meditation, relaxation, guided imagery, hypnosis, and biofeedback. In the present chapter, we focus exclusively on relaxation techniques which are part of CBT (cognitive-behavioral therapy) including guided imagery (GI), progressive muscle relaxation (PMR), biofeedback, and breathing techniques (e.g., abdominal, thoracic breathing). Even though similar practices are often used in other therapies (e.g., mindfulness-based cognitive therapy, dialectical behavioral therapy, acceptance and commitment therapy, etc.), the present chapter is restricted to CBT-based relaxation techniques for adults.

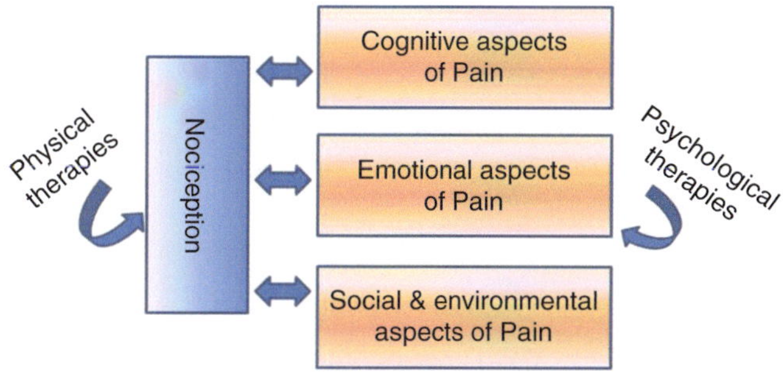

Fig. 50.1 Aspects of cancer pain

A good deal of evidence supports many biopsychosocial factors contributing to disease-related quality of life among cancer survivors [1]. For instance, depression, anxiety, and distress are tightly related to perceived patient difficulty in managing cancer symptoms. Recent studies have expanded on this research by examining how psychosocial factors relate to the development of chronic pain conditions as well as physical functionality for cancer survivors. The biopsychosocial model underscores the conceptualization and symptom management in cancer patients at all stages of the disease process.

Many cancer patients undergo chemotherapy and suffer unpleasant side effects. These may include weakened immune responses, peripheral neuropathy, changes in liver enzymes, hair loss, loss of appetite, fatigue, depression, anxiety, and sexual side effects. Psychological therapies such as relaxation, visual imagery, mindfulness, and hypnotherapy are among the most popular "alternative therapies" used in managing these symptoms, with more than 50% of Australian and up to a third of North American and European cancer

A. Lazaridou
Department of Anesthesiology, Brigham & Women's Hospital and Harvard Medical School, BWH Pain Management Center, Chestnut Hill, MA, USA
e-mail: alazaridou@mgh.harvard.edu

R. R. Edwards (✉)
Department of Anesthesiology, Perioperative, and Pain Medicine, Brigham & Women's Hospital and Harvard Medical School, BWH Pain Management Center, Chestnut Hill, MA, USA
e-mail: RREdwards@Partners.org

A. Gulati et al. (eds.), *Essentials of Interventional Cancer Pain Management*, https://doi.org/10.1007/978-3-319-99684-4_50

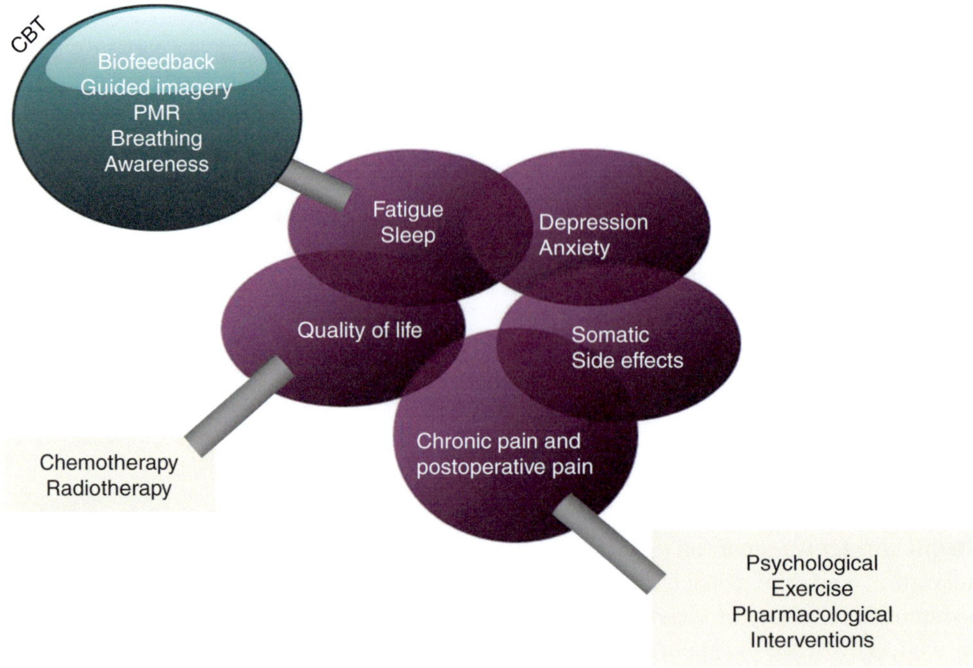

Fig. 50.2 Symptom management

patients reporting the use of at least one of these psychological therapies in the 1990s [2, 3]. More recent studies by Sparber and colleagues [4] have noted that relaxation techniques and spiritual practices are among the most commonly used approaches to cope with side effects of treatment. Public surveys have noted that many patients express a preference for, and seek out, noninvasive therapies which give the individual an active role in treatment (training), involving the body, mind, and spirit [5, 6]. Indeed, it may well be the case, as recent reviews have suggested [7], that since some physicians appear to disapprove the use of these therapies, many patients utilize them without reporting that use to their providers, resulting in underestimates of the total utilization of these treatment approaches (Fig. 50.2).

What Is Biofeedback?

Biofeedback is one of the most popular mind-body therapies focusing on a holistic understanding of disease and treatment. It uses physiological monitoring equipment, with real-time, continuous feedback (usually visual or auditory) to help individuals obtain awareness and control over a variety of aspects of their physiology (e.g., muscle tension, heart rate, etc.) [6, 8, 9]. Patients learn to gain voluntary control over physiological responses that are ordinarily involuntary and automatic. During biofeedback, patients typically connected to sensors (e.g., surface EMG electrodes, an external probe to monitor skin temperature); these sensors then "feedback" a continuous recording of such responses. This feedback allows patients to determine individualized approaches for altering those physiological states to achieve results such as reducing muscle tension, lowering heart rate, achieving physiological states of relaxation, etc. Biofeedback is widely used in psychiatric and psychological practice for the treatment for anxiety and stress-related disorders.

Although there are many different biofeedback procedures, they generally share a common goal: reduction in physiological stress responses. In addition to standard biofeedback techniques, neurofeedback is gaining popularity in the management of numerous medical and psychiatric conditions [10, 11]. Neurofeedback uses a feedback electroencephalogram (EEG) to show the patient current electrical patterns in their cortex. Many neurological and medical disorders are associated with abnormal patterns, or signatures, of cortical activity. Neurofeedback uses a baseline EEG assessment, and sometimes a multi-site quantitative EEG (QEEG), to identify these abnormal patterns [10]. Biofeedback and neurofeedback emphasize training individuals to self-regulate, gain awareness, increase control over their body and nervous system, as well as improve adaptability in physiological responding. To date, while there is fairly limited research on biofeedback for cancer management, one study examined the effect of electromyography (EMG) biofeedback-assisted relaxation on cancer-related pain in advanced cancer patients [12]. Findings suggested that six sessions of EMG biofeedback-assisted relaxation, compared to a usual care control group, were effective in reducing cancer-related pain in advanced cancer patients, possibly through a mechanism of attenuation of physiological arousal.

Another form of biofeedback targets voluntary changes in heart rate variability (HRV). The term RSA (respiratory sinus arrhythmia) predates the term HRV and refers to the increase and decrease of heart rate synchronized with each breath. The magnitude of this synchronized variability seems to reflect a healthy alternation between two types of autonomic impact on the heart rhythm: the sympathetic and parasympathetic. There has been substantial support for heart rate variability biofeedback (HRVB) for a variety of conditions, some of which are characterized by persistent pain [13]. Since conditions as widely varied as asthma and irritable bowel syndrome seem to respond to this form of cardiorespiratory feedback training, the issue of possible mechanisms becomes more salient. The most widely supported possible mechanism underlying the efficacy of HRVB is the facilitation of homeostatic balance in the baroreceptors, sensors located in the blood vessels [14–16].

Other popular forms of biofeedback training include skin conductance, skin temperature, and electromyography (EMG) training [17]. Skin conductance feedback provides information about sweat gland activity on the hands that is closely correlated with the sympathetic nervous system. This assessment process typically utilizes such terms as SCA (skin conductance activity), EDA (electrodermal activity), or GSR (galvanic skin response). Sensors are attached to two fingers or on the palm, and feedback is provided visually or through audio. Participants are instructed to relax themselves by physical or cognitive techniques that tend to lower skin conductance, while negative emotions such as anger and worry usually increase it. Individuals with mood or other affective disorders especially benefit from GSR biofeedback [18].

Temperature feedback training specifically has been applied with reported success in the clinic in several vascular-related disorders. Temperature training has been used in cardiovascular-related disorders because of its impact on the vasodilatation response (widening the blood vessels) increasing blood flow through the skin and consequently increasing skin temperature [19]. Conditions such as Raynaud's syndrome, which is characterized by inadequate peripheral blood flow in the extremities (particularly the hands), can be caused or exacerbated by cancer or cancer treatment, and in these cases skin temperature biofeedback may provide relief from symptoms such as pain by allowing patients to learn to increase peripheral blood flow.

Evidence on Biofeedback

We have witnessed a growing interest in using different biofeedback techniques for cancer management, providing encouraging results in a number of trials. In a recent study, the application of neurofeedback to breast cancer survivors resulted in improvements in psychosocial domains including cognitive abilities, fatigue, sleep quality, and measures of psychological distress [20]. In a similar study, guided imagery, with physiological monitoring and biofeedback, was implemented on patients undergoing radiation therapy for breast cancer [21]. Eligible patients were assessed before and after each session. Monitored measures included blood pressure, respiration rate, pulse rate, and skin temperature. Results showed decreases in respiration rate and pulse rate as well as systolic and diastolic blood pressure. Skin temperature increased, indicating more peripheral blood flow secondary to a decrease in the sympathetic response. Interestingly, biofeedback has also been applied in relation to motor abilities in cancer patients. In a recent study using visual feedback, head and neck cancer patients were trained to initiate swallows during the mid-expiratory phase of quiet breathing and to continue the expiration after swallowing. This study showed that improvements in respiratory-swallowing coordination can be trained using a systematic protocol and respiratory phase-lung volume-related biofeedback [22]. Overall, representative studies indicate improvements in care for patients with cancer and support the value of incorporating practices of biofeedback as well as guided imagery along with the standard treatment.

Breathing-Based Relaxation Techniques

Within the great diversity of relaxation practices, perhaps one of the most common elements is a focus on breathing awareness. These techniques generally aim to promote strong and flexible lung function, as well as the reduction of skeletal muscle tension and emotional distress [23, 24]. Many of these techniques confer physiological benefits such as increases in the efficiency of oxygen transfer and greater availability of oxygen in circulating blood [23]. In general, breathing is an automatic process to which individuals don't pay close attention. Breathing-based relaxation techniques aim at improving awareness over the breathing process, with eventual control of the rate and depth of breathing. Basic practices usually begin with awareness of breathing without controlling it. For instance, practitioners are asked to pay attention to the rhythm, depth, and sound of their breathing without any effort to control or change it. As practice develops, more advanced techniques are introduced, with practitioners learning to alter the duration of breaths, the inter-breath interval, etc. Many breathing techniques involve diaphragmatic breathing, characterized by deep and slow breaths through the nose [24].

Several studies have investigated the benefits of breathing training for patients with cancer. For instance, Rao and colleagues [25] assessed a relaxation program that included a breath work component among women with breast cancer receiving treatment. Results from this study suggested improvements in state anxiety within the breathing awareness group compared to a control group receiving supporting care. Danhauer and colleagues [26] conducted a randomized pilot study of a restorative yoga intervention, which included a strong breathing component. Forty-four women with breast cancer were randomized to 10-week program or a wait-list control. Statistically significant differences were shown favoring the experimental group on measures of quality of life, depressive symptoms, positive affect, and spirituality. In addition, several articles by Kim and colleagues reported on a breathing/exercise program for patients undergoing stem cell transplantation. These studies showed a benefit in fatigue, anxiety, and depressive symptoms among these patients [27, 28]. Collectively, these findings highlight the potential benefits (improvements in anxiety and quality of life measures) of breathing-based relaxation interventions, particularly for patients undergoing cancer-related treatments such as surgery, stem cell transplantation, etc.

Guided Imagery and Other Relaxation Techniques

Guided imagery (GI), or visualization, is often used as a cognitive-behavioral strategy to reduce pain, distress, and other unpleasant symptoms. Patients are guided by a therapist in imaging a relaxing scene or series of experiences. Patients are usually asked to select a personally relevant pleasant image that will generate positive feelings. In addition, patients may be asked to facilitate awareness of the senses (vision, hearing, touch, taste, and smell) during GI training to bring about relaxation. This practice can work as a distress tolerance skill, helping patients alleviate their stress and anxiety. As a related technique, depending on the relevant mental health condition (e.g., PTSD, GAD, anorexia) or medical condition (cancer or/and chronic pain), patients sometimes are asked to visualize aversive images that could work as exposure therapy. For example, in PTSD or phobias, bringing an unpleasant image into one's mind could potentially help individuals learn to tolerate those aversive feelings and reduce negative responses. However, some imagery techniques used in rational emotive therapy [29] can trigger high levels of anxiety in some clients. Thus, therapists are usually very careful before applying these techniques to assure patients' safety.

GI is often part of holistic nursing interventions, and it has been employed by healthcare professionals in the past two decades to promote improvements in many health-related outcomes. For instance, Yoo and collaborators [30] demonstrated that guided imagery significantly reduced pre- and post-chemotherapy nausea, vomiting, and negative affect among treated breast cancer patients. Results also showed some improvements in immune function, decreased anxiety, improved sleep, and a reduction in treatment-related side effects. Similarly, Eremin and colleagues [31] conducted a study with 80 women undergoing multimodality treatment for locally advanced breast cancer. These patients participated in a randomized control trial to evaluate the immune-modulatory effects of relaxation training and guided imagery. Participants in the intervention group were taught relaxation and guided imagery after diagnosis and before the first cycle of chemotherapy. Significant between-group differences were found in the number of CD25+ (activated T cells) and CD56+ (lymphocyte-activated killer cells) subsets and the number of CD3+ (mature) cells. These results expand upon earlier studies which also suggested relaxation and GI-based improvements in immune system functioning on parameters such as natural killer cell (NK) activity in stage 1 breast cancer patients [32]. Of note, there is evidence suggesting a relation between GI and physiological processes based on the ability of GI to stimulate the transmission of messages from the brain to the central nervous system [33]. According to Benson [34], GI can decrease autonomic nervous system responses with the consequence of relaxation in skeletal muscle tension often seen in cancer patients. Majority of GI studies were performed to study GI's impact on symptoms associated with cancer or cancer treatment [35, 36], as well as in the treatment of acute preoperative pain [37].

Progressive muscle relaxation (PMR) is a technique that is popular for managing pain and anxiety. PMR was originally introduced by Jacobson [38] and modified in 1973 by Bernstein and Borkovec [39]. Since then, many forms of PMR have been elaborated in textbooks, and this technique has been recommended as a management strategy, often for patients suffering from acute or chronic musculoskeletal pain conditions [40, 41]. PMR is a technique that involves sequentially tensing targeted muscles and then relaxing them to create a contrast and awareness between tension and relaxation. It is called "progressive" because it proceeds through all main muscles, relaxing them one at a time, and eventually leads to an overall muscle relaxation.

Managing Depression and Anxiety

Mental health represents an important concern in the treatment of cancer patients. Results from one recent study showed that nearly 2/3 of cancer patients may experience clinically significant feelings of anxiety and depression [42]. Anxiety and depression may impair the quality of the patient's lives as it may cause psychological and physical suffering, interfere with day-to-day functioning, delay return to work, and impair patients' abilities to engage productively in interpersonal relationships and decision-making [43]. Unfortunately, while efforts to promote cancer education are laudable, research shows that when patients know more about these tumors, they have more severe fear of these cancers [44]. The location of the cancer may also be an important consideration, as patients with gastric, cardiac, esophagus, and lung cancers have worse quality of life after surgery than those suffering from other tumors [45]. Relaxation exercises are often used as an intervention for reducing these mood symptoms [46].

Multiple lines of evidence support the contention that relaxation interventions such as abdominal breathing training can alleviate anxiety and adverse reactions in breast cancer patients who received adjuvant chemotherapy [47] and that PMR training can reduce oxygen consumption, heart rate, respiration rate, and muscle tension, as well as normalize the blood pressure and ease anxiety [48]. There are many studies that explored the effects of specific relaxation techniques on psychological distress, though fewer well-controlled studies have been conducted in populations of cancer patients [49–53]. Of note, a recent systematic review showed that RCT studies on relaxation and cancer patients had large effect sizes on perceived stress and state anxiety and medium effect sizes on symptoms of stress and mood disturbance [54]. Another promising randomized controlled trial comparing alprazolam (a benzodiazepine used for the treatment of anxiety disorders) to progressive muscle relaxation (PMR) demonstrated that both treatment arms led to similar reductions in observer- and patient-reported anxiety and depression levels [55], highlighting the potential benefits of such non-pharmacologic treatment approaches.

Pain Management and Psychosocial Aspects

Pain is one of the most common and bothersome symptoms of many cancers and may result from painful procedures, disease progression, or damage of nerves, tissues, or organs from tumors [56, 57]. High-quality evidence indicates that distraction, relaxation, and imagery can be effective in reducing pain when added to standard analgesic treatment. American Pain Society standards for pain management in cancer recommend a combination of pharmacologic and psychosocial approaches. This recommendation derives support from a recent review demonstrating that psychosocial interventions have medium-size effects on pain severity and interference in cancer patients and this review strongly supported use of quality-controlled psychosocial interventions in a multimodal approach to pain management [58]. The effect sizes and stability of effects for these methods are substantial enough to support their inclusion in standard care for cancer pain during treatment, and some recent laboratory-based research suggests that negative cognitive and emotional states promote amplifications of pain sensitivity in cancer survivors, suggesting that psychosocial interventions which reduce distress may have additional benefits in the reduction of pain sensitivity as well as daily clinical pain [59].

Multiple controlled trials support the efficacy of relaxation-based treatments in samples of patients suffering from cancer pain. For example, 40 hospitalized cancer patients received 2 trials of progressive muscle relaxation (PMR), 2 trials of analgesic imagery, and 2 trials of a control condition [60]. PMR and analgesic imagery produced greater short-term improvements in pain intensity, pain-related distress, and perceived control over pain compared to the control condition. In some other trials, such short-term benefits did not generalize to the long-term improvement in pain-related outcomes (e.g., [61]), but other GI-based work has reported lasting benefits of these techniques [62, 63]. For example, Syrjala and colleagues [64] conducted a trial with patients suffering from oral mucositis pain receiving bone marrow transplants (BMT). In this study, patients were randomly assigned to a treatment as usual control group, a therapist support intervention, relaxation and imagery training, and CBT including GI techniques. Results indicated that patients in both the relaxation/imagery group and the CBT groups had significantly less mucositis-related pain compared to the standard treatment group. Of note, Kwekkeboom and colleagues [65] explored patients' perceptions of these treatments and factors that contribute to their effectiveness through a qualitative study. Hospitalized patients with cancer pain who had completed trials of guided imagery and PMR were assessed through interviews. In most cases, participants' perceptions of treatment efficacy matched observed changes in pain scores. In addition, participants suggested that effectiveness of intervention is attributed to active involvement, providing a source of distraction, clear instruction, stimulating relaxation, and pain qualities [66, 67].

Overall, guided imagery has been broadly applied in cancer pain management, and GI techniques seem especially well-suited to help patients separate the sensory dimension of the pain experience from the affective and evaluative reaction to pain. However, as with most treatments, there are broad individual differences in the degree of benefit that patients report experiencing. To date, several studies have found that response to imagery interventions is highly associated with imaging ability [68, 69]. Therefore, assessing imaging ability at baseline is vital to predict the effectiveness of these treatments. While many reviews and meta-analyses [70–72] suggest that biofeedback and GI hold great promise for pain management, a sentiment with which we agree, it may be that future recommendations involve the tailoring of specific treatments to particular patient characteristics (e.g., patients with the most imagery ability receive GI training, etc).

Managing Chronic Pain Post-Surgery

In the last few years, several reviews have emerged, which have found moderate effect sizes for psychosocial interventions in cancer pain management after surgery [73]. Of note, a review presented evidence for the importance of various psychosocial factors in combination with surgical, medical, psychophysical, and demographic factors, which may also influence persistent pain after breast cancer surgery [74]. These findings are broadly consistent with a larger literature on postoperative pain, which suggests that GI and similar techniques can effectively decrease pain, stress, and anxiety after surgery [75, 76]. In a study with colorectal cancer patients after stoma surgery, the use of PMR significantly decreased state anxiety and improved generic quality of life in the experimental group especially in the domains of physical health, psychological health, social concerns, and environment [77]. A systematic review showed that relaxation and guided imagery when employed prior to surgery produced an averaged effect size of 0.85 for pain reduction and 0.61 for improved recovery time [78]. There is an interest in the use of guided imagery for chronic pain after cancer-related surgery, given the severe declines in quality of life suffered by many of these cancer patients [79]. One example of this work, Bartlett and collaborators explored the effects of biofeedback on quality of life in colorectal cancer patients who had recently undergone surgery, demonstrating improvements in lifestyle, coping, and feelings of embarrassment [80]. Interestingly, the quality of life of patients' family members is also strongly impacted by cancer and cancer-related surgery, and several studies have examined the effects of psychosocial treatments in the setting of a patient's immediate social environment (see below).

Relaxation Techniques for the Caregivers

Relaxation techniques could also be beneficial for caregivers in cancer clinics and units as well as families [81]. Keir and colleagues [82] conducted a study assessing distress in caregivers treating brain tumor patients and evaluating their interest in relaxation techniques. Most caregivers believed that stress reduction programs could indeed help them reduce their stress and sought learning more about these programs. When looking at gender, more male than female caregivers believed programs could help them reduce stress (95% vs 83%). More specifically, 30% of the participants expressed an interest in biofeedback and 35% in GI and a 48% in PMR. These results suggest the potential for the application of relaxation programs to both patients and healthcare providers. Oncology healthcare professionals usually demonstrate higher levels of burnout relative to colleagues working in other medical fields [83]. The process of recovery from work-related stress plays an important role in maintaining well-being, but it is poorly understood in cancer workers, though there are clear negative associates of burnout with psychological well-being and relaxation [84]. In line with these results, a 30-min relaxation training session was applied in hospital employees and cancer patients demonstrating improvements in perceived stress and adaptive effect on skin temperature [85]. Though these results are preliminary, it appears that relaxation training can be beneficial for employees in oncology settings, suggesting potential implications in quality of care as well. Therefore, there is a great need for the application of such relaxation programs in oncology settings that can be easily accessible and are cost-effective [86].

Relaxation Training for Cancer-Related Fatigue and Sleep

Fatigue is another common symptom of cancer and its treatment. A systematic review demonstrated prevalence rates for clinically significant fatigue ranging from 46% to 96% at the end of treatment (e.g., radiotherapy) in cancer patients [23]. While there is limited research in the impact of relaxation training on fatigue, several studies have demonstrated some interesting preliminary results. Findings suggest relaxation techniques as an adjunct therapy during radiotherapy reduce fatigue and increase sleep quality [59]. Interestingly, PMR training seems to potentially prevent chemotherapy-associated increases in fatigue following treatment [23, 87]. Of note, surgery studies have generally reported minimal relationships between surgical variables and fatigue-related outcomes [88–92], suggesting that psychosocial factors (which are modifiable by relaxation-based interventions) may be the predominant influences on the extent and impact of fatigue in cancer patients.

Studies have explored fatigue and sleep changes together in cancer management since a strong association has been previously demonstrated [93–95]. Sleep disturbances usually included difficulty falling asleep, poor sleep efficiency, and excessive daytime drowsiness. Such problems can become chronic in some patients, persisting for many months or years after completion of cancer therapy. In one clinical trial, Cohen and Fried found significant improvements in sleep parameters (e.g., a reduction in the reported difficulty falling asleep) in groups relaxation and imagery group compared to basic CBT and control groups [96]. Another study combining CBT and relaxation training demonstrated greater improvement in sleep immediately posttreatment and at 6 months compared to a control group [97], demonstrating that such interventions can have long-term benefits. Broeckel and colleagues [95] have suggested that patients with breast cancer in particular have a high risk of fatigue after chemotherapy is completed, and multiple studies have suggested that PMR treatments lead to reduced fatigue that is present before, throughout, and following chemotherapy in these patients [87, 95]. As a result, some recommendations have included the implementation of relaxation training just before the start of chemotherapy in order to decrease severity and occurrence of fatigue and sleep disruption [87].

Chemotherapy-Related Cognitive Impairment

Apart from sleep disturbance and fatigue, many cancer survivors completing chemotherapy have reported mild to moderate cognitive impairment which affects the ability to function at work and home [98, 99]. While some research has focused on pharmacologic management of these symptoms [100], non-pharmacological treatments may provide more effective alternatives with an emphasis on functional improvement. Cognitive-behavioral therapy treatment packages that include relaxation training and stress management have demonstrated promising outcomes (in the form of cognitive improvements in cancer patients undergoing chemotherapy), though effect sizes have been modest [101, 102]. Alvarez and colleagues [20] were the first to study neurofeedback for cognitive functioning in breast cancer survivors suggesting an approach for restoring full cognitive function during cancer treatment. EEG biofeedback training improved cognitive measures (e.g., cognitive impairment, cognitive abilities), quality of life, and fatigue as well as other psychological outcomes such as somatization and depression [20].

Conclusions

Overall, CBT-based relaxation therapies such as imagery, progressive muscle relaxation, breathing awareness, and biofeedback seem to positively affect various important clinical dimensions of patient functioning depression, anxiety, sleep, fatigue, cognitive function, and pain experience in cancer survivors. Unfortunately, some evidence suggests that oncologists use these therapies less than other specialties, even if cancer patients may have a higher rate of their use than that of the general public [103]. Patients may also devalue mind-body therapies and avoid discussing alternative treatments with their doctors for fear of offending them [104]. Such reluctance on the part of patients and providers is unfortunate, since in addition to the clear benefits on self-reported outcomes, it is notable that guided imagery and training in breathing techniques can enhance the immune response among breast cancer patients, providing a biological basis for future studies of the mechanisms by which psychosocial processes shape medical outcomes. Relaxation techniques also seem to be a promising approach for reducing side effects in chemotherapy including chemotherapy-related nausea and other somatic symptoms.

Future research directions in this area should focus on methodologically rigorous studies exploring the efficacy of relaxation techniques targeting at reducing these negative symptoms in cancer management and evaluating patient and provider characteristics that are associated with maximizing the benefits of these treatments. Overall, it is our contention that relaxation-based inventions should be applied to the same standards of quality and consideration as conventional interventions. Considering the growing interest in relaxation training for cancer symptom management, healthcare professionals should be informed and trained to communicate to their patients regarding the non-pharmacological options that are available. Taking into consideration the severe side effects that medications can cause in cancer survivors, the minimal risk of relaxation-based treatments and their potentially broad benefits, such as non-pharmacological treatments as adjuncts to mainstream cancer treatment, can be of great value.

References

1. Syrjala KL, Jensen MP, Mendoza ME, Yi JC, Fisher HM, Keefe FJ. Psychological and behavioral approaches to cancer pain management. J Clin Oncol. 2014;32(16):1703–11.
2. Montbriand MJ. Freedom of choice: an issue concerning alternate therapies chosen by patients with cancer. Oncol Nurs Forum. 1993;20(8):1195–201.
3. Warrick PD, Irish JC, Morningstar M, Gilbert R, Brown D, Gullane P. Use of alternative medicine among patients with head and neck cancer. Arch Otolaryngol Head Neck Surg. 1999;125(5):573–9.
4. Sparber A, Bauer L, Curt G, Eisenberg D, Levin T, Parks S, et al. Use of complementary medicine by adult patients participating in cancer clinical trials. Oncol Nurs Forum. 2000;27(4):623–30.
5. Jonas WB, Levin JS, Berman B. Essentials of complementary and alternative medicine. Philadelphia: Williams & Wilkins; 1999. xxi, 605 p.
6. Moss D. Handbook of mind-body medicine for primary care Thousand Oaks: Sage Publications; 2003. xix, 545 p.
7. Elkins G, Fisher W, Johnson A. Mind-body therapies in integrative oncology. Curr Treat Options in Oncol. 2010;11(3–4):128–40.
8. Schwartz GE. Biofeedback as therapy. Some theoretical and practical issues. Am Psychol. 1973;28(8):666–73.
9. Schwartz MS, Andrasik F. Biofeedback: a practitioner's guide 3rd ed. New York: Guilford Press; 2003. xiv, 930 p.
10. LaVaque TJ. Neurofeedback, neurotherapy, and QEEG. In: Moss D, McGrady A, Davies T, Wickramasekera I, editors. Handbook of mind body medicine for primary care. Thousand Oaks: Sage; 2003.
11. Evans JR, Abarbanel A. Introduction to quantitative EEG and neurofeedback San Diego: Academic Press; 1999. xxi, 406 p.
12. Tsai PS, Chen PL, Lai YL, Lee MB, Lin CC. Effects of electromyography biofeedback-assisted relaxation on pain in patients with advanced cancer in a palliative care unit. Cancer Nurs. 2007;30(5):347–53.

13. Reynard A, Gevirtz R, Berlow R, Brown M, Boutelle K. Heart rate variability as a marker of self-regulation. Appl Psychophysiol Biofeedback. 2011;36(3):209–15.
14. Lehrer P, Vaschillo E, Lu SE, Eckberg D, Vaschillo B, Scardella A, et al. Heart rate variability biofeedback: effects of age on heart rate variability, baroreflex gain, and asthma. Chest. 2006;129(2):278–84.
15. Vaschillo E, Lehrer P, Rishe N, Konstantinov M. Heart rate variability biofeedback as a method for assessing baroreflex function: a preliminary study of resonance in the cardiovascular system. Appl Psychophysiol Biofeedback. 2002;27(1):1–27.
16. Vaschillo EG, Vaschillo B, Lehrer PM. Characteristics of resonance in heart rate variability stimulated by biofeedback. Appl Psychophysiol Biofeedback. 2006;31(2):129–42.
17. Gaudette M, Prins A, Kahane J. Comparison of auditory and visual feedback for EMG training. Percept Mot Skills. 1983;56(2):383–6.
18. Nagai Y, Goldstein LH, Fenwick PB, Trimble MR. Clinical efficacy of galvanic skin response biofeedback training in reducing seizures in adult epilepsy: a preliminary randomized controlled study. Epilepsy Behav. 2004;5(2):216–23.
19. Bregman NJ, McAllister HA. Role of suggestions in digital skin temperature: implications for temperature biofeedback research. Int J Neurosci. 1985;27(1–2):115–20.
20. Alvarez J, Meyer FL, Granoff DL, Lundy A. The effect of EEG biofeedback on reducing postcancer cognitive impairment. Integr Cancer Ther. 2013;12(6):475–87.
21. Serra D, Parris CR, Carper E, Homel P, Fleishman SB, Harrison LB, et al. Outcomes of guided imagery in patients receiving radiation therapy for breast cancer. Clin J Oncol Nurs. 2012;16(6):617–23.
22. Martin-Harris B, McFarland D, Hill EG, Strange CB, Focht KL, Wan Z, et al. Respiratory-swallow training in patients with head and neck cancer. Arch Phys Med Rehabil 2015;96(5):885–93.
23. Prue G, Rankin J, Allen J, Gracey J, Cramp F. Cancer-related fatigue: a critical appraisal. Eur J Cancer. 2006;42(7):846–63.
24. Jerath R, Edry JW, Barnes VA, Jerath V. Physiology of long pranayamic breathing: neural respiratory elements may provide a mechanism that explains how slow deep breathing shifts the autonomic nervous system. Med Hypotheses. 2006;67(3):566–71.
25. Rao RM, Nagendra HR, Raghuram N, Vinay C, Chandrashekara S, Gopinath KS, et al. Influence of yoga on postoperative outcomes and wound healing in early operable breast cancer patients undergoing surgery. Int J Yoga. 2008;1(1):33–41.
26. Danhauer SC, Mihalko SL, Russell GB, Campbell CR, Felder L, Daley K, et al. Restorative yoga for women with breast cancer: findings from a randomized pilot study. Psychooncology. 2009;18(4):360–8.
27. Kim SD, Kim HS. Effects of a relaxation breathing exercise on fatigue in haemopoietic stem cell transplantation patients. J Clin Nurs. 2005;14(1):51–5.
28. Kim SD, Kim HS. Effects of a relaxation breathing exercise on anxiety, depression, and leukocyte in hemopoietic stem cell transplantation patients. Cancer Nurs. 2005;28(1):79–83.
29. Ellis A, Dryden W. The practice of rational emotive behavior therapy. 2nd ed. New York: Springer Pub. Co.; 1997. vii, 272 p.
30. Yoo HJ, Ahn SH, Kim SB, Kim WK, Han OS. Efficacy of progressive muscle relaxation training and guided imagery in reducing chemotherapy side effects in patients with breast cancer and in improving their quality of life. Support Care Cancer. 2005;13(10):826–33.
31. Eremin O, Walker MB, Simpson E, Heys SD, Ah-See AK, Hutcheon AW, et al. Immuno-modulatory effects of relaxation training and guided imagery in women with locally advanced breast cancer undergoing multimodality therapy: a randomised controlled trial. Breast. 2009;18(1):17–25.
32. Gruber BL, Hersh SP, Hall NR, Waletzky LR, Kunz JF, Carpenter JK, et al. Immunological responses of breast cancer patients to behavioral interventions. Biofeedback Self Regul. 1993;18(1):1–22.
33. Schaub BGaB, M. M. Imagery. In Dossey B, Keegan L, editors. Holistic nursing: a handbook for practice (6th ed.) Burlington: Jones & Bartlett Learning; 2013. 363–95 pp.
34. Benson H, Greenwood MM, Klemchuk H. The relaxation response: psychophysiologic aspects and clinical applications. Int J Psychiatry Med. 1975;6(1–2):87–98.
35. Kwekkeboom KL, Bumpus M, Wanta B, Serlin RC. Oncology nurses' use of nondrug pain interventions in practice. J Pain Symptom Manag. 2008;35(1):83–94.
36. Lee MH, Kim DH, Yu HS. The effect of guided imagery on stress and fatigue in patients with thyroid cancer undergoing radioactive iodine therapy. Evid Based Complement Alternat Med. 2013;2013:130324.
37. Sears SR, Bolton S, Bell KL. Evaluation of "Steps to Surgical Success" (STEPS): a holistic perioperative medicine program to manage pain and anxiety related to surgery. Holist Nurs Pract. 2013;27(6):349–57.
38. Jacobson E. Progressive relaxation; a physiological and clinical investigation of muscular states and their significance in psychology and medical practice, vol. xiii. Chicago: The University of Chicago Press; 1929. p. 428.
39. Bernstein DA, Borkovec TD. Progressive relaxation training: a manual for the helping professions Champaign: Research Press; 1973. viii, 66 p.
40. Snyder M, Lindquist R. Complementary & alternative therapies in nursing. 6th ed. New York: Springer; 2010. xxii, 511 p.
41. Potter PA, Perry AG. Basic nursing therapy and practice. St. Louis: Mosby-Year Book Inc.; 1995.
42. Lim L, Jin AZ, Ng TP. Anxiety and depression, chronic physical conditions, and quality of life in an urban population sample study. Soc Psychiatry Psychiatr Epidemiol. 2012;47(7):1047–53.
43. Maguire P. Improving the quality of life of cancer patients. In: Levy JA, Jasmin C, Bez G, editors. Cancer. AIDS, and quality of life. New York: Plenum Press; 1997.
44. Lin CC, Lai YL, Ward SE. Effect of cancer pain on performance status, mood states, and level of hope among Taiwanese cancer patients. J Pain Symptom Manag. 2003;25(1):29–37.
45. Hong JS, Tian J. Prevalence of anxiety and depression and their risk factors in Chinese cancer patients. Support Care Cancer. 2014;22(2):453–9.
46. D'Avanzato C, Martinez J, Attiullah N, Friedman M, Toba C, Boerescu DA, et al. Anxiety symptoms among remitted depressed outpatients: prevalence and association with quality of life and psychosocial functioning. J Affect Disord. 2013;151(1):401–4.
47. Kim KS, Lee SW, Choe MA, Yi MS, Choi S, Kwon SH. Effects of abdominal breathing training using biofeedback on stress, immune response and quality of life in patients with a mastectomy for breast cancer. Taehan Kanho Hakhoe Chi. 2005;35(7):1295–303.
48. Sheu S, Irvin BL, Lin HS, Mar CL. Effects of progressive muscle relaxation on blood pressure and psychosocial status for clients with essential hypertension in Taiwan. Holist Nurs Pract. 2003;17(1):41–7.
49. Fawzy FI, Cousins N, Fawzy NW, Kemeny ME, Elashoff R, Morton D. A structured psychiatric intervention for cancer patients. I. Changes over time in methods of coping and affective disturbance. Arch Gen Psychiatry. 1990;47(8):720–5.
50. Larsson G, Starrin B. Relaxation training as an integral part of caring activities for cancer patients: effects on wellbeing. Scand J Caring Sci. 1992;6(3):179–85.
51. Walker LG, Walker MB, Ogston K, Heys SD, Ah-See AK, Miller ID, et al. Psychological, clinical and pathological effects of relaxation training and guided imagery during primary chemotherapy. Br J Cancer. 1999;80(1–2):262–8.

52. Burish TG, Lyles JN. Effectiveness of relaxation training in reducing adverse reactions to cancer chemotherapy. J Behav Med. 1981;4(1):65–78.
53. Lyles JN, Burish TG, Krozely MG, Oldham RK. Efficacy of relaxation training and guided imagery in reducing the aversiveness of cancer chemotherapy. J Consult Clin Psychol. 1982;50(4):509–24.
54. Matchim Y, Armer JM, Stewart BR. Mindfulness-based stress reduction among breast cancer survivors: a literature review and discussion. Oncol Nurs Forum. 2011;38(2):E61–71.
55. Holland JC, Morrow GR, Schmale A, Derogatis L, Stefanek M, Berenson S, et al. A randomized clinical trial of alprazolam versus progressive muscle relaxation in cancer patients with anxiety and depressive symptoms. J Clin Oncol. 1991;9(6):1004–11.
56. Benitez Del Rosario MA, Perez Suarez MC, Fernandez Dias R, Cabrejas SA. Diagnosis and treatment of chronic cancer pain (I). Aten Primaria. 2002;29(6):374–7.
57. Mantyh PW. Cancer pain and its impact on diagnosis, survival and quality of life. Nat Rev Neurosci. 2006;7(10):797–809.
58. Sheinfeld Gorin S, Krebs P, Badr H, Janke EA, Jim HS, Spring B, et al. Meta-analysis of psychosocial interventions to reduce pain in patients with cancer. J Clin Oncol. 2012;30(5):539–47.
59. Decker TW, Cline-Elsen J, Gallagher M. Relaxation therapy as an adjunct in radiation oncology. J Clin Psychol. 1992;48(3):388–93.
60. Kwekkeboom KL, Wanta B, Bumpus M. Individual difference variables and the effects of progressive muscle relaxation and analgesic imagery interventions on cancer pain. J Pain Symptom Manage. 2008;36(6):604–15.
61. Haase O, Schwenk W, Hermann C, Muller JM. Guided imagery and relaxation in conventional colorectal resections: a randomized, controlled, partially blinded trial. Dis Colon Rectum. 2005;48(10):1955–63.
62. La Roche MJ, Batista C, D'Angelo E. A content analyses of guided imagery scripts: a strategy for the development of cultural adaptations. J Clin Psychol. 2011;67(1):45–57.
63. Roffe L, Schmidt K, Ernst E. A systematic review of guided imagery as an adjuvant cancer therapy. Psychooncology. 2005;14(8):607–17.
64. Syrjala KL, Donaldson GW, Davis MW, Kippes ME, Carr JE. Relaxation and imagery and cognitive-behavioral training reduce pain during cancer treatment: a controlled clinical trial. Pain. 1995;63(2):189–98.
65. Kwekkeboom KL, Hau H, Wanta B, Bumpus M. Patients' perceptions of the effectiveness of guided imagery and progressive muscle relaxation interventions used for cancer pain. Complement Ther Clin Pract. 2008;14(3):185–94.
66. Hadhazy VA, Ezzo J, Creamer P, Berman BM. Mind-body therapies for the treatment of fibromyalgia. A systematic review. J Rheumatol. 2000;27(12):2911–8.
67. Smarr KL, Parker JC, Wright GE, Stucky-Ropp RC, Buckelew SP, Hoffman RW, et al. The importance of enhancing self-efficacy in rheumatoid arthritis. Arthritis Care Res. 1997;10(1):18–26.
68. Johnsen EL, Lutgendorf SK. Contributions of imagery ability to stress and relaxation. Ann Behav Med. 2001;23(4):273–81.
69. Watanabe E, Fukuda S, Hara H, Maeda Y, Ohira H, Shirakawa T. Differences in relaxation by means of guided imagery in a healthy community sample. Altern Ther Health Med. 2006;12(2):60–6.
70. Redd WH, Montgomery GH, DuHamel KN. Behavioral intervention for cancer treatment side effects. J Natl Cancer Inst. 2001;93(11):810–23.
71. Meyer TJ, Mark MM. Effects of psychosocial interventions with adult cancer patients: a meta-analysis of randomized experiments. Health Psychol. 1995;14(2):101–8.
72. Devine EC, Westlake SK. The effects of psychoeducational care provided to adults with cancer: meta-analysis of 116 studies. Oncol Nurs Forum. 1995;22(9):1369–81.
73. Novy DM, Aigner CJ. The biopsychosocial model in cancer pain. Curr Opin Support Palliat Care. 2014;8(2):117–23.
74. Schreiber KL, Kehlet H, Belfer I, Edwards RR. Predicting, preventing and managing persistent pain after breast cancer surgery: the importance of psychosocial factors. Pain Manag. 2014;4(6):445–59.
75. Charette S, Fiola JL, Charest MC, Villeneuve E, Theroux J, Joncas J, et al. Guided imagery for adolescent post-spinal fusion pain management: a pilot study. Pain Manag Nurs. 2015;16(3):211–20.
76. Rejeh N, Heravi-Karimooi M, Vaismoradi M, Jasper M. Effect of systematic relaxation techniques on anxiety and pain in older patients undergoing abdominal surgery. Int J Nurs Pract. 2013;19(5):462–70.
77. Cheung YL, Molassiotis A, Chang AM. The effect of progressive muscle relaxation training on anxiety and quality of life after stoma surgery in colorectal cancer patients. Psychooncology. 2003;12(3):254–66.
78. Johnston MVC. Benefits of psychological preparation for surgery: a meta-analysis. Ann Behav Med. 1993;15:245–56.
79. Casso D, Buist DS, Taplin S. Quality of life of 5–10 year breast cancer survivors diagnosed between age 40 and 49. Health Qual Life Outcomes. 2004;2:25.
80. Bartlett L, Sloots K, Nowak M, Ho YH. Biofeedback therapy for symptoms of bowel dysfunction following surgery for colorectal cancer. Tech Coloproctol. 2011;15(3):319–26.
81. Hong MJ, Tae YS. Structural relationship of burnout and related variables among family caregivers of cancer patients. J Korean Acad Nurs. 2013;43(6):812–20.
82. Keir ST, Swartz JJ, Friedman HS. Stress and long-term survivors of brain cancer. Support Care Cancer. 2007;15(12):1423–8.
83. Mallett K, Price JH, Jurs SG, Slenker S. Relationships among burnout, death anxiety, and social support in hospice and critical care nurses. Psychol Rep. 1991;68(3 Pt 2):1347–59.
84. Poulsen MG, Poulsen AA, Khan A, Poulsen EE, Khan SR. Recovery experience and burnout in cancer workers in Queensland. Eur J Oncol Nurs. 2015;19(1):23–8.
85. Balk JL, Chung SC, Beigi R, Brooks M. Brief relaxation training program for hospital employees. Hosp Top. 2009;87(4):8–13.
86. Belletti M, Mallia L, Lucidi F, Reichmann S, Mastroianni C, De Marinis MG, et al. Complementary therapy and support services for formal and informal caregivers in Italian palliative care hospices: an exploratory and descriptive study. Support Care Cancer. 2011;19(12):1939–47.
87. Demiralp M, Oflaz F, Komurcu S. Effects of relaxation training on sleep quality and fatigue in patients with breast cancer undergoing adjuvant chemotherapy. J Clin Nurs. 2010;19(7–8):1073–83.
88. Can G, Durna Z, Aydiner A. Assessment of fatigue in and care needs of Turkish women with breast cancer. Cancer Nurs. 2004;27(2):153–61.
89. Jacobsen PB, Hann DM, Azzarello LM, Horton J, Balducci L, Lyman GH. Fatigue in women receiving adjuvant chemotherapy for breast cancer: characteristics, course, and correlates. J Pain Symptom Manage. 1999;18(4):233–42.
90. Donovan KA, Jacobsen PB, Andrykowski MA, Winters EM, Balducci L, Malik U, et al. Course of fatigue in women receiving chemotherapy and/or radiotherapy for early stage breast cancer. J Pain Symptom Manage. 2004;28(4):373–80.
91. Haghighat S, Akbari ME, Holakouei K, Rahimi A, Montazeri A. Factors predicting fatigue in breast cancer patients. Support Care Cancer. 2003;11(8):533–8.
92. Geinitz H, Zimmermann FB, Thamm R, Keller M, Busch R, Molls M. Fatigue in patients with adjuvant radiation therapy for breast cancer: long-term follow-up. J Cancer Res Clin Oncol. 2004;130(6):327–33.
93. Okuyama T, Akechi T, Kugaya A, Okamura H, Imoto S, Nakano T, et al. Factors correlated with fatigue in disease-free breast

cancer patients: application of the Cancer fatigue scale. Support Care Cancer. 2000;8(3):215–22.
94. Servaes P, Verhagen S, Bleijenberg G. Determinants of chronic fatigue in disease-free breast cancer patients: a cross-sectional study. Ann Oncol. 2002;13(4):589–98.
95. Broeckel JA, Jacobsen PB, Horton J, Balducci L, Lyman GH. Characteristics and correlates of fatigue after adjuvant chemotherapy for breast cancer. J Clin Oncol. 1998;16(5):1689–96.
96. Cohen MFG. Comparing relaxation training and cognitive-behavioral group therapy for women with breast cancer. Res Soc Work Pract. 2007;17:313–23.
97. Espie CA, Fleming L, Cassidy J, Samuel L, Taylor LM, White CA, et al. Randomized controlled clinical effectiveness trial of cognitive behavior therapy compared with treatment as usual for persistent insomnia in patients with cancer. J Clin Oncol. 2008;26(28):4651–8.
98. Vardy J, Dhillon H. The fog hasn't lifted on "chemobrain" yet: ongoing uncertainty regarding the effects of chemotherapy and breast cancer on cognition. Breast Cancer Res Treat. 2010;123(1):35–7.
99. Hede K. Chemobrain is real but may need new name. J Natl Cancer Inst. 2008;100(3):162–3, 9.
100. Kohli SFS, Tra Y, Wesnes K, Morrow GR. The cognitive effects of modafinil in breast cancer survivors: a randomized clinical trial. J Clin Oncol. 2007;25:9004.
101. Ferguson RJ, Ahles TA, Saykin AJ, McDonald BC, Furstenberg CT, Cole BF, et al. Cognitive-behavioral management of chemotherapy-related cognitive change. Psychooncology. 2007;16(8):772–7.
102. Ferguson RJ, McDonald BC, Rocque MA, Furstenberg CT, Horrigan S, Ahles TA, et al. Development of CBT for chemotherapy-related cognitive change: results of a waitlist control trial. Psychooncology. 2012;21(2):176–86.
103. Lee RT, Hlubocky FJ, Hu JJ, Stafford RS, Daugherty CK. An international pilot study of oncology physicians' opinions and practices on Complementary and Alternative Medicine (CAM). Integr Cancer Ther. 2008;7(2):70–5.
104. Eliott JA, Kealey CP, Olver IN. (Using) complementary and alternative medicine: the perceptions of palliative patients with cancer. J Palliat Med. 2008;11(1):58–67.

51 Mood and Anxiety in Cancer Pain

R. Garrett Key and William S. Breitbart

The Prevalence of Pain and Distressing Symptoms in Cancer Patients

Pain is a common problem for cancer patients, with approximately 70% of patients experiencing severe pain at some time in the course of their disease [4]. It has been suggested that nearly 75% of patients with advanced cancer have pain, 50% of terminally ill patients are in moderate to severe pain [5, 6], and 25% of cancer patients die in severe pain [7]. In addition to pain, cancer patients have been found to suffer from an average of three additional troubling physical symptoms [8]. With disease progression, the number of distressing physical symptoms increases. Patients with advanced disease report a median of 11 problematic symptoms [9]. A global evaluation of symptom burden allows for a more complete understanding of the patient's pain experience [10].

Optimal pain management for advanced-stage cancer is multimodal and includes pharmacological, psychotherapeutic, cognitive–behavioral (CBT), anesthetic, neurostimulatory, and rehabilitative approaches. This chapter will focus on the demographics and comorbidity of anxiety and depression in cancer-related pain followed by pharmacologic treatment of these symptoms. Biofeedback, CBT, deep relaxation, meditation, and complimentary therapies are an integral part of complete pain care and are covered in previous chapters of this text.

R. Garrett Key (✉)
University of Texas at Austin Dell Medical School, Austin, TX, USA
e-mail: garrett.key@austin.utexas.edu

W. S. Breitbart
Department of Psychiatry and Behavioral Sciences, Memorial Sloan Kettering Cancer Center, New York, NY, USA
e-mail: breitbaw@mskcc.org

An Integrated Experience: The Biopsychosocial Model of Pain

The perception of pain can be considered as a complex integration of somatosensory information, cognitive processes, affective and emotional state, and cultural or personal beliefs. Significant study has been devoted to the relationship between psychic state and pain, leading to the development and wide acceptance of a biopsychosocial model of pain [11, 12]. The biopsychosocial model is based on the concept of pain as a multifaceted experience generated in response to physiological and psychosocial factors [13]. Perhaps the most influential description of this integration is the gate control theory of pain, which offers an elegant neurological explanation of the processing of somatic input with influence from modifying factors such as experiences, memories, beliefs, and psychological state to produce perceived pain [14]. Effective management of pain in patients with advanced cancer requires a multidisciplinary approach, enlisting expertise from a wide variety of clinical specialties including neurology, neurosurgery, anesthesiology, psychiatry, and rehabilitation medicine [4, 15, 16]. Psychiatric interventions targeting psychological distress in the treatment of cancer pain have become an integral part of comprehensive pain management [17, 18]. A pain treatment plan must target physiologic sources of somatic pain and also include attention to the complete pain experience of the person as a whole, seen in the context of their life (Fig. 51.1).

Pain, and particularly pain related to advancing malignancy, is not only a somatic and nociceptive experience but also involves less concrete factors related to affect, personality, cognition, behavioral responses, and social relationships [19]. Cecily Saunders described the pain associated with terminal illness as "total pain" to reflect its consuming and enveloping nature [20]. Through the lens of "total pain," it can be seen how pharmacologic analgesia cannot completely extinguish cancer pain. Psychological factors have been found to play a modest but important role in pain intensity

A. Gulati et al. (eds.), *Essentials of Interventional Cancer Pain Management*, https://doi.org/10.1007/978-3-319-99684-4_51

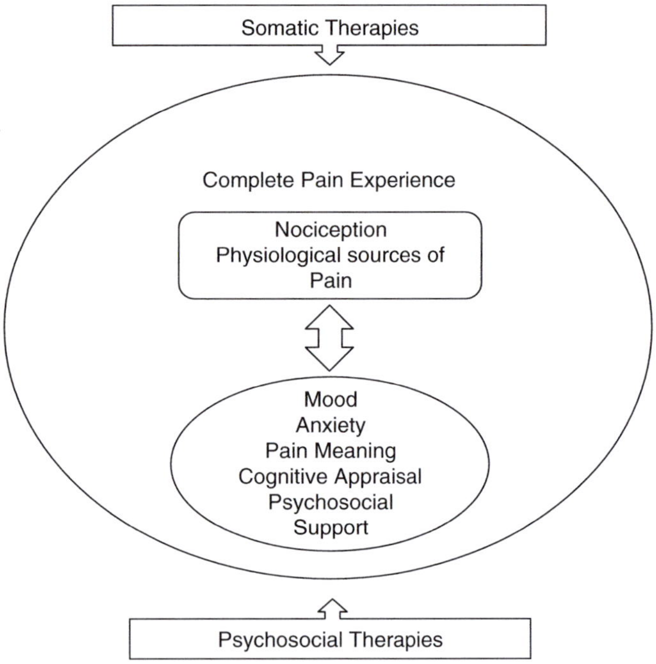

Fig. 51.1 A conceptual model of the interaction between physiological and psychosocial variables in pain. Somatic and psychosocial therapies have complimentary impact on the complete pain experience. The magnitude of the complete pain experience is determined by the interaction between somatic variables and psychosocial variables

[11, 21]. Therapies targeting psychic pain and the psychosocial impact of pain will decrease the overall pain experience of the patient. Reflexively, somatic treatments that reduce the nociceptive and physiological aspects of pain will positively influence the psychosocial well-being of patients. Ideally, psychosocial and somatic treatments are combined in a multidisciplinary pain management plan.

Depression and Anxiety as Exacerbating Factors in Pain Syndromes

Patients with pre-existing anxiety or mood disorders require ongoing attention and psychiatric support. It is important to screen for emergence of new disorders during illness for patients without any prior psychiatric history. The comorbidity between depression and chronic pain is the most studied relationship between pain and psychiatric disorders. Anxiety disorders, also occur with significant frequency in the context of pain and can affect a patient's ability to adapt to pain and manage it effectively [13, 22]. In a study done by McWilliams and colleagues, comorbid panic disorder in chronic pain was found at nearly twice the rate for depression (OR 4.27 vs 2.82) [22]. After adjusting for age, race, socioeconomic status, gender, and comorbid medical conditions, they found significantly increased risk of depression (OR 2.00) and anxiety disorders, including panic disorder (OR 2.66) and post-traumatic stress disorder (PTSD) (OR 2.45). Other studies have also found symptoms consistent with PTSD with relatively high frequency in cancer patients, estimated between 3% and 35% [23]. Different types of pain have variable associations with anxiety (i.e., low back pain is not closely associated, whereas facial pain syndromes are associated with PTSD) [22]. Screening for both anxiety and depression in pain populations is recommended.

Pain is a principal source of distress in cancer patients. Anxiety, depression, and the meaning of pain can intensify the cancer pain experience and overall level of distress [11, 12, 24]. Measures of emotional disturbance have been reported to be predictors of pain in late stages of cancer, and cancer patients with less anxiety and depression are less likely to report pain [25, 26]. The patient with cancer faces many stressors during the course of illness including dependency, disability, and fear of painful death. Virtually all people have these fears, but their level of psychological distress varies in response to medical factors, social supports, coping skills, and personality.

Surprisingly, beliefs about the meaning of pain and the presence of a mood disturbance are better predictors of level of pain than is the site of metastasis. As an example, women with metastatic breast cancer reported more intense pain if they believed the pain to be the result of disease progression and also if they were depressed [27]. Patients also find pain less functionally interfering and less severe when they believe it to be unrelated to their cancer [24, 28, 29]. Patients reporting poorly controlled pain or higher overall levels of pain also describe more existential concerns and fear about the future [30]. Patients with negative thoughts about personal or social competence also report increased pain intensity and emotional distress [25, 31]. Maladaptive coping strategies, lower sense of self-efficacy, and distress about treatment or progression of disease were predictors of pain intensity in one prospective study [11]. Unpredictable pain episodes are correlated with greater psychological distress [32].

Persistent cancer pain may be unjustifiably attributed to a psychological cause when it does not respond to treatment. Patients who report their pain as "severe" are sometimes dismissed as having a large psychological component to their pain. Grossman et al. [33] found that while there is a high degree of concordance between patient and caregiver ratings of patient pain intensity at the low and moderate levels, this concordance breaks down at high levels. In their study, clinician agreement with patient pain reports lost concordance when patients reported scores of 7 or higher on a visual analog rating scale of 0–10. This underscores the importance of accepting patient reports of pain and discussing differences in provider impression of the patient's pain in order to reach a mutual understanding.

The reflexive relationship between psychological variables and pain perception makes it necessary to exhaustively explore physiologic sources of pain before attributing poor pain control or limited treatment response to psychological causes. Psychological variables are too frequently proposed to explain continuing pain or lack of response to pain treatment when, on close examination, medical causes of pain have not been completely addressed. Pain can overwhelm a person's ability to adaptively cope, resulting in behavior suggestive of psychiatric disorders which disappear once the pain is relieved [34, 35]. Psychological distress in terminally ill patients with pain should initially be assumed to be the consequence of uncontrolled physiologic pain.

Psychiatric Disorders in Advanced-Stage Cancer

The relationship between psychiatric disorders, pain, and cancer is complex. A number of studies have explored the topic, but estimates of prevalence remain broad. There is consensus that both pain patients and cancer patients exhibit increased rates of depression and anxiety above what is found in the general population.

In the Psychosocial Collaborative Oncology Group Study [36] on the prevalence of psychiatric disorders in cancer patients, 39% of the patients who received a psychiatric diagnosis also reported significant pain while only 19% of patients without a psychiatric diagnosis reported significant pain. The psychiatric disorders seen in these cancer patients with pain included primarily Adjustment Disorder with Depressed or Anxious Mood (69%) and Major Depression (15%). An increased frequency of psychiatric disorders in cancer pain patients has also been reported by other investigators [37, 38]. A meta-analysis conducted by Mitchell and colleagues examining data from 94 studies found psychiatric disorders occurring in 30–40% of cancer patients in a hospital setting [39]. There was no effect seen for age or sex on the prevalence of disorders, and the data was insufficient to support conclusions about duration of illness or cancer type. A summary of their results is below (Table 51.1). Variable rates of depression have been seen related to cancer type in other analyses with particularly elevated prevalence in oropharyngeal (22–57%), pancreatic (33–50%), lung (11–44%), and breast (1.5–46%) cancers [40] (see Table 51.1).

Table 51.1 Depression and anxiety prevalence in palliative care and oncology/hematology settings (Adapted from Mitchell et al. [39] with automatic permission from Elsevier through STM signatory guidelines)

Psychiatric diagnosis	Prevalence in palliative care (95% CI)	Prevalence in hematology/oncology (95% CI)
Depression (DSM or ICD major depression)	16.5% (13.1–20.3)	16.3% (13.4–19.5)
Adjustment disorder	15.4% (10.1–21.6)	19.4% (14.5–24.8)
Anxiety disorders	9.8% (6.8–13.2)	10.3% (5.1–17.0)

Cancer, Pain, and Suicide

Suicide risk has been the subject of debate and much uncertainty around absolute risk exists. There is reasonable consensus that suicide risk is elevated in cancer patients in the first year after diagnosis and also in the terminal phase of illness [41]. Although relatively few cancer patients commit suicide, they are at increased risk [42, 43]. Suicide risk and suicidal ideation have been linked to uncontrolled pain in cancer patients [44, 45]. The majority of suicides seen in patients with cancer are in the context of severe pain, which may be inadequately controlled or tolerated poorly [46]. Patients with advanced illness are at highest risk and are the most likely to have the complications of pain, depression, delirium, and deficit symptoms. Filiberti and colleagues reviewed five suicides completed by patients in palliative home care programs in Italy and found common factors of uncontrolled physical symptoms including pain, previous psychiatric history and prior suicide attempts, isolation, and poor social support [41]. A review of the psychiatric consultations at Memorial Sloan Kettering Cancer Center (MSKCC) found that one-third of cancer patients evaluated for suicidality were diagnosed with major depression, approximately 20% were diagnosed with delirium, and over 50% met criteria for adjustment disorder [44]. Cancer is perceived to be a particularly painful disease which may promote consideration of suicide. In one study, 69% of respondents opined that cancer-related pain could cause a person to consider suicide [42].

Thoughts of suicide are not uncommon in patients with pain and cancer, particularly in advanced stages, and can represent a patient's way of maintaining a sense of control and defending against the fear of unavoidable, uncontrolled suffering. Data suggest that earnest suicidal ideation is relatively infrequent in cancer and is limited to those who are significantly depressed [10, 44, 47, 48]. A cancer patient's desire for hastened death is complex. Severity of clinical depression and hopelessness are associated with suicidal ideation and predictive of desire for hastened death. Social supports and physical function add significant but smaller contributions [49]. Interestingly, in a study population with cancer pain, suicidal ideation was not directly related to pain intensity but was strongly related to degree of depression and mood disturbance. Pain makes patients more vulnerable to suicide, but associated psychological distress, hopelessness, delirium, and depression are larger factors in the overall increase in suicide risk [46].

Screening for Anxiety and Depression

In routine clinical examination, assessment of tearfulness, social withdrawal, pessimism, lack of affective reactivity, loss of interest in activities, reported chronic low mood, or desire for hastened death are all suggestive of depression. Loss of appetite, fatigue, decreased concentration, and sleep disturbance are less reliable indicators of mood changes in medically ill patients, particularly in cancer patients where the disease and treatment can induce this symptom cluster [50].

A wide variety of screening instruments have been developed for assessing distress, anxiety, and depression in patients with pain and cancer. A practical approach is to use a brief self-report screen that can trigger a more involved and specific assessment or referral. Two commonly used self-report measures are the nine-item Patient Health Questionnaire (PHQ-9) and seven-item Generalized Anxiety Disorder Scale (GAD-7) which are both designed for ease of use, well validated, have well-defined clinical cutoffs, and are widely accepted [51, 52]. A positive screen should result in a more detailed assessment, attempt at initial treatment of symptoms, or referral to a mental health specialist.

Physiologic Causes of Psychiatric Symptoms

Medically compromised patients can exhibit psychiatric symptoms as a consequence of physiological abnormalities which must be investigated and corrected before symptoms can be safely attributed to primarily psychiatric causes.

Delirium is a common occurrence in the medically ill and patients or families may report psychological distress, fear, hopelessness, depression, rapid personality changes, or psychotic symptoms that can be misinterpreted as psychiatric illness. The hallmark of delirium is an altered state of arousal that is fluctuant over hours, frequently described as a waxing and waning level of alertness. The incidence of pain, depression, and delirium increases with greater debilitation and advanced stages of illness [53]. Delirium in cancer patients seen for psychiatric consultation in a hospital setting is estimated at 25–40% and up to 85% during the terminal stages of illness [54]. Suspicion of delirium should trigger immediate medical workup including a mental status exam, medication review, and evaluation for infection, metabolic abnormalities, new organ dysfunction, or evolving brain disease.

Other important medical causes of psychiatric symptoms include:

- Opioid-induced hypogonadism via suppression of GnRH can cause depression and anxiety which may be reversible with hormone replacement in men [55, 56].
- Cardiopulmonary problems including, pneumothorax, vocal cord dysfunction, pulmonary embolus, pneumonia, or hypercapnia/hypercarbia of any cause can induce anxiety [57].
- Thyroid dysfunction can produce anxious and depressive symptoms and should be evaluated by testing thyroid-stimulating hormone (TSH) initially and evaluation for abnormal results with repeat TSH and thyroxine (T_4) [58].
- Thiamine deficiency can occur in cancer patients, particularly in the context of cachexia/anorexia and can produce subtle cognitive problems, low mood, and a sense of decreased energy in addition to the more classically described and reversible Wernicke's encephalopathy. If thiamine deficiency is suspected, immediate supplementation with 200–500 mg intravenously three times daily is recommended [59, 60].
- Vitamin D deficiency is associated with depression, and there is evidence that supplementation improves depressive symptoms [61–63]. Testing for 25-OH Vitamin D is the appropriate screen.
- B12 deficiency is linked with depression and replacement is recommended [64].
- Inflammation and pro-inflammatory cytokines are causally linked to depression, although treatment strategies are less clear [65, 66]. A theoretical basis for NSAID treatment has been proposed, but clinical data is currently lacking [67].
- Epinephrine/norepinephrine-secreting pheochromocytomas in the multiple endocrine neoplasia syndrome, type IIA or IIB, can cause panic symptoms.

Pharmacologic Treatment of Anxiety and Depression in The Context of Cancer Pain

There are a number of psychotropic drugs with proven usefulness as adjuvant analgesics and they can provide an economy of function by addressing multiple problems with a single medication. They are valuable tools in the treatment of cancer pain through their utility in addressing mood, anxiety, pain, and other common symptoms like fatigue, nausea, low appetite, poor concentration, and poor sleep. These medications are not only effective in managing symptoms of anxiety, depression, insomnia, or delirium that commonly complicate the course of advanced disease in patients with cancer but also potentiate the analgesic effects of opioid drugs and have innate analgesic properties of their own [68].

The current literature supports the use of antidepressants as adjuvant analgesic agents in the management of a wide variety of chronic pain syndromes, including cancer pain [69–77]. The most commonly used adjuvant analgesics are antidepressants and anticonvulsants, but a number of other medications are useful and discussed below [78]. As to the time course of onset of analgesia or with antidepressants, there appears to be a biphasic process that occurs with immediate or early analgesic effects that occur within hours or days and later, longer analgesic effects that peak over a 4–6 week period [79–81].

Tricyclic Antidepressants (TCA)

Tricyclic antidepressants have the most well-established efficacy as adjuvant analgesics. Amitriptyline is the most studied and proven member of the class [79–83]. Imipramine [84–86], desipramine [87, 88], nortriptyline [89], clomipramine [90, 91], and doxepin [92] are other members of this category which have been found to have helpful analgesic properties. In general, the tricyclic antidepressants are most useful in cancer pain as adjuvant analgesics, potentiating the effects of opioid analgesics, and are rarely used as the primary analgesic [74, 93, 94]. Analgesic benefit independent of mood effect was found in a one study involving a group of chronic cancer pain patients [93]. Ventafridda et al. reviewed a multicenter clinical experience with trazodone and amitriptyline in patients with chronic neuropathic/deafferentation cancer pain and found that pain control was improved with antidepressants and follow-up study through a randomized, double-blind study found amitriptyline and trazodone to have similar analgesic benefit [74]. There is some evidence that there may be a subgroup of patients who respond differentially to tricyclics, and therefore if amitriptyline fails to alleviate pain, another tricyclic should be tried [94].

The tricyclic antidepressants are effective as adjuvants in cancer pain through a number of mechanisms that include direct analgesic effects [95], antidepressant activity [69], and potentiation of opioid analgesia [96–98]. In terms of appropriate dosage, there is evidence that the therapeutic analgesic effects of amitriptyline are correlated with serum levels just as the antidepressant effects are, and analgesic treatment failure is due to low serum levels [79, 80, 99]. A high-dose regimen of up to 150 mg of amitriptyline or higher is suggested if pain persists [82, 100].

Tricyclic antidepressants do have significant side effects which should be taken into account. Anticholinergic side effects like constipation, dry mouth, blurred vision, urinary retention, incoordination, worsened cognition, and tremor are not uncommon and typically are dose dependent. Anticholinergic delirium can be precipitated at higher doses. Elderly or medically compromised patients are more vulnerable to these side effects; thus slow and careful titration is advised.

Serotonin and Norepinephrine Reuptake Inhibitors (SNRI)

The newer antidepressants venlafaxine and duloxetine, members of the SNRI class, have been found to have good analgesic properties attributable to their similarity to TCAs in blocking reuptake of serotonin and norepinephrine. Their side-effect profile is significantly more tolerable than the TCAs, rendering them more widely useful in more medically compromised populations. Evidence indicates benefit from venlafaxine in chemotherapy-induced neuropathy, postmastectomy pain syndrome (PMPS), and also was found to decrease the development of PMPS when administered perioperatively [101–103]. Duloxetine is an effective treatment for depression and has also been found effective for chemotherapy-induced neuropathic pain [104, 105].

Selective Serotonin Reuptake Inhibitors (SSRI)

SSRIs may be useful as adjuvant analgesics for cancer patients with pain, but clinical trials of their efficacy as analgesics have been equivocal and do not clearly demonstrate the analgesic properties seen in TCAs and SNRIs [106–113]. There are several case reports that suggest that fluoxetine may be a useful adjuvant analgesic in the management of headache [114], fibrositis [115], and diabetic neuropathy [116]. One study of fluoxetine in women with fibromyalgia showed benefit to measures of illness impact and mood in women with fibromyalgia, but improvements in pain were small and statistically insignificant [117]. Paroxetine and citalopram demonstrated analgesic effect in neuropathic pain but have not been tested in cancer patients [118, 119]. Escitalopram, the separately marketed s-isomer of citalopram, is noteworthy in that it has the highest receptor selectivity in its class, no active metabolites, and does not significantly affect the CYP450 isoenzyme system [120].

Mirtazapine, Bupropion, and Trazodone

These three antidepressant medications are worthy of mention for their usefulness in cancer pain and general symptom management. All three are effective for treating depressive symptoms and have side-effect profiles that can be used advantageously.

Mirtazapine is less well studied but had some benefit for cancer patients in a small pilot study [121], increased the pain threshold in a small group of healthy subjects [122], and in mice demonstrated opioid receptor-mediated anti-nociception [123]. Mirtazapine significantly improved pain, sleep disturbance, irritability, and exhaustion in a study of 594 depressed chronic pain patients [124]. It has potent antiemetic effects related to $5HT_3$ antagonism, promotes appetite, and is also beneficial in treating insomnia. This has obvious implications in cancer patients for whom nausea, poor appetite, and poor sleep are a common symptom cluster.

Bupropion has been shown to have some benefit in neuropathic pain [125, 126]. There is some evidence that bupropion improves cancer-related fatigue [127, 128] and is effective in promoting smoking cessation for which it has an FDA indication. Bupropion, unlike most antidepressants, does not typically cause sexual dysfunction and was found to improve sexual function in a group of breast cancer patients being treated with adjuvant chemotherapy [129].

Trazodone is beneficial in the treatment of anxiety and depression, has been found to have some antinociceptive activity in mice, and theoretically should carry some of the benefits of SNRIs and TCAs because of similarity in receptor binding profile [130]. Clinical data in humans or focused study in cancer pain populations is lacking. It does have well-established benefit for sleep and can be used as an alternative to sedative-hypnotics and thereby reduce the risk of precipitating delirium, particularly in the context of concomitant opioid use (See Table 51.2).

Psychostimulants

Psychostimulants can be useful in treating depressed mood, potentiating analgesia, and also treating some of the side effects of opioid therapy. Broadly, there are amphetamines and non-amphetamine stimulants. The amphetamines dextroamphetamine and methylphenidate are useful as antidepressant agents for medically ill cancer patients with depression [131, 132]. Bruera et al. [133–135] demonstrated that methylphenidate taken twice daily significantly decreased sedation and potentiated narcotic analgesia in patients with cancer pain. Dextroamphetamine has been reported to have improved analgesia when used in conjunction with morphine in postoperative pain [136]. Psychostimulants given in a relatively low dose to cancer patients can stimulate appetite rather than decrease appetite as they do in healthy patients. They also can improve overall sense of well-being and decrease fatigue. Tolerance can develop, and adjustment of dose may be necessary. Side effects that can limit upward titration include a sense of overstimulation, anxiety, development of paranoia, and insomnia.

Non-amphetamine stimulants include modafinil and armodafinil, the separately marketed r-isomer of modafinil, and are described as wakefulness promoting agents, FDA approved for the treatment of excessive daytime sedation related to sleep disorders like narcolepsy and sleep apnea. They are used in a palliative setting for similar purposes [137]. DeBattista et al. [138] tested modafinil on subjects with major depression and incomplete response to antidepressants and found that addition of modafinil improved fatigue and depressive symptoms along with improved attention, concentration, and cognitive functioning. Modafinil has been shown to improve fatigue in cancer patients and also for people with multiple sclerosis [139, 140]. Modafinil is useful

Table 51.2 Antidepressants useful as adjuvant analgesics

–	Name	Dosing in mg	Route
Tricyclic antidepressants (TCA)	–	–	–
–	Amitriptyline	10–150 QHS	PO, IM, PR
–	Nortriptyline	10–50 QHS	PO
–	Imipramine	12.5–150 QHS	PO, IM
–	Desipramine	12.5–150 QHS	PO
–	Clomipramine	10–150 QHS	PO
–	Doxepin	12.5–150 QHS	PO, IM
Serotonin and norepinephrine reuptake inhibitors (SNRI)	–	–	–
–	Venlafaxine	37.5–225 daily or Q8-12H depending on form (extended vs immediated release)	PO
–	Duloxetine	20–60 daily or BID	PO
Selective serotonin reuptake inhibitors (SSRI)	–	–	–
–	Fluoxetine	20–60 daily	PO
–	Paroxetine	20–60 daily	PO
–	Citalopram	10–40 daily	PO
–	Escitalopram	10–20 daily	PO
–	Sertraline	50–100 daily	PO
H1,α2, and serotonin antagonist	–	–	–
–	Mirtazapine	7.5–60 QHS	PO
Serotonin antagonist and reuptake Inhibitor,H1, and α1 antagonist	–	–	–
–	Trazodone	25–100 QHS	PO
Norepinephrine and dopamine reuptake inhibitor (NDRI)	–	–	–
–	Bupropion	75–450 daily or BID depending on form (extended vs immediate release	PO
–	PO, oral; IM, intramuscular; PR, parenteral; QHS, every bedtime; Q8-12H, every 8 to 12H; BID, two times a day		

in palliative care to reduce fatigue and counteract opioid-related sedation. Modafinil is not a sympathomimetic agent, and its mechanism of action is distinct from amphetamines. There is some evidence that these newer psychostimulants have lower abuse potential in general; however caution is advised in patients with known substance misuse in the past [141, 142] (see Table 51.3).

Neuroleptics

Neuroleptic medications are prescribed for psychotic symptoms in the general population but have a very useful place in the treatment of pain and other symptoms in cancer patients, namely, nausea, vomiting, insomnia, and anxiety.

Phenothiazine neuroleptics are particularly helpful with nausea and vomiting and also can offer benefit for anxiety. Methotrimeprazine, which is not available in the United States, is a phenothiazine that is equianalgesic to morphine but without major effects on gut motility and thought to produce analgesia through alpha-adrenergic blockade [143]. It is also antiemetic and anxiolytic by virtue of dopamine blockade which makes it useful for advanced-stage cancer patients [144]. Sedation and hypotension can occur and slow intravenous infusion is recommended to minimize this effect. Chlorpromazine and prochlorperazine are useful as antiemetics in cancer patients but probably have limited use as analgesics [145]. Fluphenazine in combination with TCAs has been shown to be helpful in neuropathic pain [90].

Haloperidol, a butyrophenone, is the drug of choice in the management of delirium or psychosis in cancer patients, but evidence for effectiveness as analgesic or co-analgesic is inconsistent [145, 146]. Pimozide, also a member of the butyrophenone group, is effective as an analgesic in the management of trigeminal neuralgia but unproven specifically in cancer pain [147].

The newer atypical antipsychotics, including as olanzapine, risperidone, quetiapine, aripiprazole, and ziprasidone are primarily used to treat delirium in the palliative care setting. Boettger and Breitbart [148] suggest that olanzapine and risperidone are the atypical antipsychotics with the most demonstrated efficacy for managing the symptoms of delirium. Smaller studies and case series reports indicate potential benefit from quetiapine [149], ziprasidone [150], and aripiprazole [151, 152]. Olanzapine has been used to successfully treat refractory pain in the context of anxiety and mild cognitive impairment [153] (see Table 51.4).

Table 51.3 Psychostimulants useful in cancer pain

–	Name	Dosing in mg	Route
Amphetamines	–	–	–
–	Methylphenidate	2.5–20 BID (morning and early afternoon)	PO
–	Dextroamphetamine	2.5–20 BID (morning and early afternoon)	PO
Non-amphetamine psychostimulants	–	–	–
–	Modafinil	50–200 daily	PO
–	Armodafinil	150–250 daily	PO
–	PO, oral; BID, two times a day		

Benzodiazepines

Benzodiazepines can be helpful in the management of pain through unclear mechanisms, perhaps related to the reduction in overall pain experience that occurs when anxiety is reduced (see Table 51.5). Hydroxizine is a mild anxiolytic with sedating and analgesic properties that are useful in the anxious cancer patient with pain [154, 155]. Benzodiazepines have not been felt to have direct analgesic properties, although they are potent anxiolytics and can be helpful in reducing anxiety that is associated with painful procedures or other acutely painful events. Alprazolam offered some benefit in a series of cancer patients with phantom limb or deafferentation pain [156]. Clonazepam may be useful in the management of lancinating neuropathic pain and allodynia [157, 158]. The synergistic sedative effects of benzodiazepines when combined with opioids require caution and judicious use of both drugs, particularly in debilitated and elderly patients. Focus on pain as the primary symptom is vital as uncontrolled pain will continue to produce anxiety despite aggressive anxiolytic treatment. Efforts to reduce nociceptive pain input should be maximized before pursuing more aggressive anxiolytic treatment.

Table 51.4 Neuroleptics useful in cancer pain

–	Name	Dosing in mg	Route
Phenothiazines	–	–	–
–	Fluphenazine	1–3 Q6-8H	PO, IM
–	Methotrimeprazine	10–20 Q8-12H	PO, IM, IV, SC
Butyrophenones	–	–	–
–	Haloperidol	1–3 QHS to Q8H	PO, IM, IV, SC
–	Pimozide	2–6 BID	PO
Second generation antipsychotics (SGA)	–	–	–
–	Olanzapine	2.5–20 QHS	PO
–	Risperidone	5–6 QHS	PO
–	Quetiapine	25–300 QHS	PO
–	Aripiprazole	10–20 daily	PO
–	PO, oral; IM, intramuscular; IV, intravenous; SC, subcutaneous; QHS, every bedtime; Q8H, every 8 h; Q6-8H, every 6–8 h; Q8-12H, every 8 to 12H; BID, two times a day		

Table 51.5 Benzodiazepines useful in cancer pain

Name	Dosing in mg	Route
Lorazepam	0.25–1 daily to Q8H	PO, IV
Alprazolam	0.25–2 daily to Q8H	PO
Clonazepam	0.25–2 daily to Q12H	PO
Diazepam	2.5–10 daily to Q12H	PO, IV

PO, oral; IM, intramuscular; PR, parenteral; IV, intravenous; QHS, every bedtime; Q6H, every 6 h; Q4-6H, every 4–6 h; Q8-12H, every 8 to 12H; Q12H, every 12 h; BID, two times a day; TID, three times a day.

References

1. Gordon DB, Dahl JL, Miaskowski C, McCarberg B, Todd KH, Paice JA, et al. American pain society recommendations for improving the quality of acute and cancer pain management: American pain society quality of care task force. Arch Intern Med. 2005;165(14):1574–80.
2. Miaskowski C, Cleary J, Burney R, Coyne P, Finley R, Foster R, et al. Guideline for the management of cancer pain in adults and children. Glenview: American Pain Society; 2005.
3. Institute of Medicine. Committee on Advancing Pain Research C, Education. Relieving pain in America: a blueprint for transforming prevention, care, education, and research. Washington, DC: National Academies Press; 2011.
4. Foley KM. The treatment of cancer pain. N Engl J Med. 1985, 313:845.
5. Weiss SC, Emanuel LL, Fairclough DL, Emanuel EJ. Understanding the experience of pain in terminally ill patients. Lancet. 2001;357:1311–5.
6. Fitzgibbon DR. Cancer pain: management. In: Loeser JD, editor. Bonica's management of pain. 3rd ed. Philadelphia: Lippincott Williams & Wilkins; 2001. p. 659–703.
7. Twycross RG, Lack SA. Symptom control in far advanced cancer: pain relief. London: Pitman Brooks; 1983.
8. Grond S, Zech D, Diefenbach C, Bischoff A. Prevalence and pattern of symptoms in patients with cancer pain: a prospective evaluation of 1635 cancer patients referred to a pain clinic. J Pain Symptom Manag. 1994;9:372–82.
9. Walsh D, Donnelly S, Rybicki L. The symptoms of advanced cancer: relationship to age, gender, and performance status in 1000 patients. Support Care Cancer. 2000;8(3):175–9.
10. Achte KA, Vanhkouen ML. Cancer and the psych. Omega. 1971;2:46–56.
11. Syrjala KL, Chapko ME. Evidence for a biopsychosocial model of cancer treatment-related pain. Pain. 1995;61:69–79.
12. Gatchel RJ, Peng YB, Peters ML, Fuchs PN, Turk DC. The biopsychosocial approach to chronic pain: scientific advances and future directions. Psychol Bull. 2007;133(4):581.
13. Turk DC, Okifuji A. Psychological factors in chronic pain: evolution and revolution. J Consult Clin Psychol. 2002;70(3):678.
14. Melzack R, Wall PD. Pain mechanisms: a new theory. Science. 1965;150(3699):971–9.
15. Foley KM. Pain syndromes in patients with cancer. In: Bonica JJ, VV RBF, Jones LE, Loeser JD, editors. Advances in pain research and therapy, vol. 2. New York: Raven Press; 1975. p. 59–75.
16. Breitbart W, Holland J. Psychiatric aspects of cancer pain. In: Foley KM, editor. Advances in pain research and therapy, vol. 16. New York: Raven Press; 1990. p. 73–87.
17. Breitbart W. Psychiatric management of cancer pain. Cancer. 1989;63:2336–42.
18. Massie MJ, Holland JC. The cancer patient with pain: psychiatric complications and their mangement. Med Clin N Am. 1987;71:243–58.
19. Stiefel F. Psychosocial aspects of cancer pain. Support Care Cancer. 1993;1:130–4.
20. Saunders CM. The management of terminal illness. London: Hospital Medicine Publications; 1967.
21. Sheinfeld Gorin S, Krebs P, Badr H, Janke EA, Jim HS, Spring B, et al. Meta-analysis of psychosocial interventions to reduce pain in patients with cancer. J Clin Oncol. 2012;30(5):539–47.
22. McWilliams LA, Cox BJ, Enns MW. Mood and anxiety disorders associated with chronic pain: an examination in a nationally representative sample. Pain. 2003;106(1):127–33.
23. Akechi T, Okuyama T, Sugawara Y, Nakano T, Shima Y, Uchitomi Y. Major depression, adjustment disorders, and post-traumatic stress disorder in terminally ill cancer patients: associated and predictive factors. J Clin Oncol. 2004;22(10):1957–65.
24. Daut RL, Cleeland CS. The prevalence and severity of pain in cancer. Cancer. 1982;50:1913–8.
25. McKegney FP, Bailey CR, Yates JW. Prediction and management of pain in patients with advanced cancer. Gen Hosp Psychiatry. 1981;3:95–101.
26. Bond MR, Pearson IB. Psychological aspects of pain in women with advanced cancer of the cervix. J Psychosom Res. 1969;13:13–9.
27. Spiegel D, Bloom JR. Pain in metastatic breast cancer. Cancer. 1983;52:341–5.
28. Smith WB, Gracely RH, Safer MA. The meaning of pain: cancer patients' rating and recall of pain intensity and affect. Pain. 1998;78(2):123–9.
29. Padilla G, Ferrell B, Grant M, Rhiner M. Defining the content domain of quality of life for cancer patients with pain. Cancer Nurs. 1990;13:108–15.
30. Strang P. Existential consequences of unrelieved cancer pain. Palliat Med. 1997;11(4):299–305.
31. Payne D. Cognition in cancer pain. Unpublished dissertation 1995.
32. Portenoy RK, Payne D, Jacobsen P. Breakthrough pain: characteristics and impact in patients with cancer pain. Pain. 1999;81(1–2):129–34.
33. Grossman SA, Sheidler VR, Sweden K, Mucenski J, Piantadosi S. Correlations of patient and caregiver ratings of cancer pain. J Pain Symptom Manag. 1991;6(2):53–7.
34. Marks RM, Sachar EJ. Undertreatment of medical inpatients with narcotic analgesics. Ann Intern Med. 1973;78:173–81.
35. Cleeland CS, Tearnan BH. Behavioral control of cancer pain. In: Holzman AD, Turk DC, editors. Pain Mangement. New York: Pergamon Press; 1986. p. 93–212.
36. Derogatis LR, Morrow GR, Fetting J, Penman D, Piasetsky S, Schmale AM, Henrichs M, Carnicke CL Jr. The prevalence of psychiatric disorders among cancer patients. J Am Med Assoc. 1983;249:751–7.
37. Ahles TA, Blanchard EB, Ruckdeschel JC. The multi-dimensional nature of cancer related pain. Pain. 1983;17:277–88.
38. Woodforde JM, Fielding JR. Pain and cancer. J Psychosom Res. 1970;14:365–70.
39. Mitchell AJ, Chan M, Bhatti H, Halton M, Grassi L, Johansen C, et al. Prevalence of depression, anxiety, and adjustment disorder in oncological, haematological, and palliative-care settings: a meta-analysis of 94 interview-based studies. Lancet Oncol. 2011;12(2):160–74.
40. Massie MJ. Prevalence of depression in patients with cancer. J Natl Cancer Inst Monogr. 2004;2004(32):57–71.
41. Filiberti A, Ripamonti C, Totis A, Ventafridda V, De Conno F, Contiero P, et al. Characteristics of terminal cancer patients who

committed suicide during a home palliative care program. J Pain Symptom Manag. 2001;22(1):544–53.
42. Levin DN, Cleeland CS, Dan R. Public attitudes toward cancer pain. Cancer. 1985;56:2337–9.
43. Farberow NL, Schneidman ES, Leonard CV. Suicide among general medical and surgical hospital patients with malignant neoplasms. Washington, DC: US Veterans Administration; 1963. Contract No: Medical Bulletin 9.
44. Breitbart W. Suicide in cancer patients. Oncology. 1987;1:49–53.
45. Breitbart W. Cancer pain and suicide. In: Foley KM, editor. Advances in pain research and therapy, vol. 16. New York: Raven Press; 1990. p. 399–412.
46. Bolund C. Suicide and cancer: II. Medical and care factors in suicide by cancer patients in Sweden, 1973–1976. J Psychosoc Oncol. 1985;3:17–30.
47. Silberfarb PM, Manrer LH, Cronthamel CS. Psychological aspects of neoplastic disease, I: functional status of breast cancer patients during different treatment regimens. Am J Psychiatr. 1980;137:450–5.
48. Brown JH, Henteleff P, Barakat S, Rowe JR. Is it normal for terminally ill patients to desire death. Am J Psychiatr. 1986;143:208–11.
49. Breitbart W, Rosenfeld B, Pessin H, Kaim M, Funesti-Esch J, Galietta M, Nelson CJ, Brescia R. Depression, hopelessness, and desire for hastened death in terminally ill patients with cancer. J Am Med Assoc. 2000;284(22):2907–11.
50. Endicott J. Measurement of depression in patients with cancer. Cancer. 1984;53(10 Suppl):2243–9.
51. Spitzer RL, Kroenke K, Williams JB. Validation and utility of a self-report version of PRIME-MD: the PHQ primary care study. Primary care evaluation of mental disorders. Patient health questionnaire. JAMA. 1999;282(18):1737–44.
52. Spitzer RL, Kroenke K, Williams JB, Lowe B. A brief measure for assessing generalized anxiety disorder: the GAD-7. Arch Intern Med. 2006;166(10):1092–7.
53. Bukberg J, Penman D, Holland J. Depression in hospitalized cancer patients. Psychosom Med. 1984;43:199–212.
54. Massie JM, Holland JC, Glass E. Delirium in terminally ill cancer patients. Am J Psychiatr. 1983;140:1048–50.
55. Katz N, Mazer NA. The impact of opioids on the endocrine system. Clin J Pain. 2009;25(2):170–5.
56. Daniell HW, Lentz R, Mazer NA. Open-label pilot study of testosterone patch therapy in men with opioid-induced androgen deficiency. J Pain. 2006;7(3):200–10.
57. Smoller JW, Pollack MH, Otto MW, Rosenbaum JF, Kradin RL. Panic anxiety, dyspnea, and respiratory disease. Theoretical and clinical considerations. Am J Respir Crit Care Med. 1996;154(1):6–17.
58. Dickerman AL, Barnhill JW. Abnormal thyroid function tests in psychiatric patients: a red herring? Am J Psychiatry. 2012;169(2):127–33.
59. Isenberg-Grzeda E, Kutner HE, Nicolson SE. Wernicke-Korsakoff-syndrome: under-recognized and under-treated. Psychosomatics. 2012;53(6):507–16.
60. Benton D, Griffiths R, Haller J. Thiamine supplementation mood and cognitive functioning. Psychopharmacology. 1997;129(1):66–71.
61. Gloth FM 3rd, Alam W, Hollis B. Vitamin D vs broad spectrum phototherapy in the treatment of seasonal affective disorder. J Nutr Health Aging. 1999;3(1):5–7.
62. Holick MF. Vitamin D deficiency. N Engl J Med. 2007;357(3):266–81.
63. Jorde R, Sneve M, Figenschau Y, Svartberg J, Waterloo K. Effects of vitamin D supplementation on symptoms of depression in overweight and obese subjects: randomized double blind trial. J Intern Med. 2008;264(6):599–609.
64. Tiemeier H, van Tuijl HR, Hofman A, Meijer J, Kiliaan AJ, Breteler MM. Vitamin B12, folate, and homocysteine in depression: the Rotterdam study. Am J Psychiatry. 2002;159(12):2099–101.
65. Miller AH, Maletic V, Raison CL. Inflammation and its discontents: the role of cytokines in the pathophysiology of major depression. Biol Psychiatry. 2009;65(9):732–41.
66. Dantzer R, O'Connor JC, Freund GG, Johnson RW, Kelley KW. From inflammation to sickness and depression: when the immune system subjugates the brain. Nat Rev Neurosci. 2008;9(1):46–56.
67. Asnis GM, De La Garza R 2nd, Kohn S, Reinus J, Henderson M, Shah J. IFN-induced depression: a role for NSAIDs. Psychopharmacol Bull. 2002;37(3):29–50.
68. Breitbart W. Psychotropic adjuvant analgesics for cancer pain. Psycho-Oncology. 1992;1:133–45.
69. France RD. The future for antidepressants: treatment of pain. Psychopathology. 1987;20:99–113.
70. Getto CJ, Sorkness CA, Howell T. Antidepressants and chronic nonmalignant pain: a review. J Pain Symptom Control. 1987;2:9–18.
71. Walsh TD. Antidepressants and chronic pain. Clin Neuropharmacol. 1983;6:271–95.
72. Walsh TD, editor. Adjuvant analgesic therapy in cancer pain. Second international congress on cancer pain. New York: Raven Press; 1990.
73. Butler S. Present status of tricyclic antidepressants in chronic pain therapy. In: Benedetti C, Chapman CR, Moricca G, editors. Advances in pain research and therapy, vol. 7. New York: Raven Press; 1986. p. 173–96.
74. Ventafridda V, Bonezzi C, Caraceni A, DeConno F, Guarise G, Ramella G, Saita L, Silvani V, Tamburini M, Toscani F. Antidepressants for cancer pain and other painful syndromes with deafferentation component: comparison of amitriptyline and trazodone. Ital J Neurol Sci. 1987;8:579–87.
75. Magni G, Arsie D, DeLeo D. Antidepressants in the treatment of cancer pain. A survey in Italy. Pain. 1987;29:347–53.
76. Onghena P, Van Houdenhove B. Antidepressant-induced analgesia in chronic non-malignant pain: a meta-analysis of 39 placebo-controlled studies. Pain. 1992;49:205–19.
77. McQuay H, Tramer M, Nye B, Carroll D, Wiffen P, Moore R. A systematic review of antidepressants in neuropathic pain. Pain. 1996;68(2):217–27.
78. Farrar JT, Portenoy RK. Neuropathic cancer pain: the role of adjuvant analgesics. Oncology. 2001;15(11):1435–42, 45, 50–3.
79. Max MB, Culnane M, Schafer SC, Gracely RH, Walther DJ, Smoller B, Dubner R. Amitriptyline relieves diabetic-neuropathy pain in patients with normal and depressed mood. Neurology. 1987;37:589–96.
80. Max MB, Schafer SC, Culnane M, Smollen B, Dubner R, Gracel RH. Amitriptyline, but not lorazepam, relieves postherpetic neuralgia. Neurology. 1982;38:427–32.
81. Pilowsky I, Hallett EC, Bassett DL, Thomas PG, Penhall RK. A controlled study of amitriptyline in the treatment of chronic pain. Pain. 1982;14:169–79.
82. Sharav Y, Singer E, Schmidt E, Dione RA, Dubner R. The analgesic effect of amitriptyline on chronic facial pain. Pain. 1987;31:199–209.
83. Watson CP, Evans RJ, Reed K, Merskey H, Goldsmith L, Warsh J. Amitriptyline versus placebo in post herpetic neuralgia. Neurology. 1982;32:671–3.
84. Kvindesal B, Molin J, Froland A, Gram LF. Imipramine treatment of painful diabetic neuropathy. J Am Med Assoc. 1984;251:1727–30.

85. Young RJ, Clarke BF. Pain relief in diabetic neuropathy: the effectiveness of imipramine and related drugs. Diabet Med. 1985;2:363–6.
86. Sindrup SH, Ejlertsen B, Frøland A, Sindrup EH, Brøsen K, Gram LF. Imipramine treatment in diabetic neuropathy: relief of subjective symptoms without changes in peripheral and autonomic nerve function. Eur J Clin Pharmacol. 1989;37:151–3.
87. Max MB, Kishore-Kumar R, Schafer SC, Meister B, Gracely RH, Smoller B, Dubner R. Efficacy of desipramine in painful diabetic neuropathy: a placebo-controlled trial. Pain. 1991;45:3–10.
88. Gordon N, Heller P, Gear R, Levine J. Temporal factors in the enhancement of morphine analgesic by desipramine. Pain. 1993;53:273–6.
89. Gomez-Perez FJ, Rull JA, Dies H, Rodriquez-Rivera JG, Gonzalez-Barranco J, Lozano-Castañeda O. Nortriptyline and fluphenazine in the symptomatic treatment of diabetic neuropathy. A double-blind cross-over study. Pain. 1985;23:395–400.
90. Langohr HD, Stohr M, Petruch F. An open and double-blind crosover study on the efficacy of clomipramine (anafranil) in patients with painful mono- and polyneuropathies. Eur Neurol. 1982;21:309–15.
91. Tiegno M, Pagnoni B, Calmi A, Rigoli M, Braga PC, Panerai AE. Chlorimipramine compared to pentazocine as a unique treatment in post-operative pain. Int J Clin Pharmacol Res. 1987;7:141–3.
92. Hameroff SR, Cork RC, Scherer K, Crago BR, Neuman C, Womble JR, Davis TP. Doxepin effects on chronic pain, depression and plasma opioids. J Clin Psychiatry. 1982;2:22–6.
93. Walsh TD, editor. Controlled study of imipramine and morphine in chronic pain due to advanced cancer (Abstract). Los Angeles: ASCO; 1986.
94. Watson C, Chipan M, Reed K, Evans R, Birket N. Amitriptyline versus maprotiline in postherpetic neuralgia: a randomized double-blind crossover trial. Pain. 1992;48:29–36.
95. Spiegel K, Kalb R, Pasternak GW. Analgesic activity of tricyclic antidepressants. Ann Neurol. 1983;13:462–5.
96. Botney M, Fields HL. Amitriptyline potentiates morphine analgesia by direct action on the central nervous system. Ann Neurol. 1983;13:160–4.
97. Malseed RT, Goldstein FJ. Enhancement of morphine analgesics by tricyclic antidepressants. Neuropharmacology. 1979;18:827–9.
98. Ventafridda V, Bianchi M, Ripamonti C, Sacerdote P, De Conno F, Zecca E, Panerai AE. Studies on the effects of antidepressant drugs on the antinociceptive action of morphine and on plasma morphine in rat and man. Pain. 1990;43:155–62.
99. McQuay H, Carroll D, Glynn C. Dose-response for analgesic effect of amitriptyline in chronic pain. Anesthesia. 1993;48:281–5.
100. Watson CP, Evans RJ. A comparative trial of amitriptyline and zimelidine in post-herpetic neuralgia. Pain. 1985;23:387–94.
101. Tasmuth T, Hartel B, Kalso E. Venlafaxine in neuropathic pain following treatment of breast cancer. Eur J Pain. 2002;6:17–24.
102. Özdogan M, Samur M, Bozcuk HŠ, Aydin H, Çoban E, Savaš B. Venlafaxine for treatment of chemotherapy-induced neuropathic pain. Turk J Cancer. 2004;34(3):24–31.
103. Reuben SS, Makari-Judson G, Lurie SD. Evaluation of efficacy of the perioperative administration of venlafaxine XR in the prevention of postmastectomy pain syndrome. J Pain Symptom Manag. 2004;27(2):133–9.
104. Goldstein DJ, Lu Y, Detke MJ, Wiltse C, Mallinckrodt C, Demitrack MA. Duloxetine in the treatment of depression: a double-blind placebo-controlled comparison with paroxetine. J Clin Psychopharmacol. 2004;24(4):389–99.
105. Smith EML, Pang H, Cirrincione C, Fleishman S, Paskett ED, Ahles T, et al. Effect of duloxetine on pain, function, and quality of life among patients with chemotherapy-induced painful peripheral neuropathy: a randomized clinical trial. JAMA. 2013;309(13):1359–67.
106. Davidoff G, Guarracini M, Roth E, Sliwa J, Yarkony G. Trazodone hydrochloride in the treatment of dysesthetic pain in traumatic myelopathy: a randomized, double-blind, placebo-controlled study. Pain. 1987;29:151–61.
107. Costa D, Mogos I, Toma T. Efficacy and safety of mianserin in the treatment of depression of woman with cancer. Acta Psychiatr Scand. 1985;72:85–92.
108. Eberhard G, von Knorring L, Nilsson HL, Sundequist U, Björling G, Linder H, Svärd KO, Tysk L. A double-blind randomized study of clomipramine versus maprotiline in patients with idiopathic pain syndromes. Neuropsychobiology. 1988;19:25–32.
109. Feighner JP. A comparative trial of fluoxetine and amitriptyline in patients with major depressive disorder. J Clin Psychiatry. 1985;46:369–72.
110. Hynes MD, Lochner MA, Bemis KG, Hymson DL. Fluxoetine, a selective inhibitor of serotonin uptake, potentiates morphine analgesia without altering its descriminative stimulus properties or affinity for opioid receptors. Life Sci. 1985;36:2317–23.
111. Stockler MR, O'Connell R, Nowak AK, Goldstein D, Turner J, Wilcken NR, et al. Effect of sertraline on symptoms and survival in patients with advanced cancer, but without major depression: a placebo-controlled double-blind randomised trial. Lancet Oncol. 2007;8(7):603–12.
112. Fishbain D. Evidence-based data on pain relief with antidepressants. Ann Med. 2000;32(5):305–16.
113. Lussier D, Huskey AG, Portenoy RK. Adjuvant analgesics in cancer pain management. Oncologist. 2004;9(5):571–91.
114. Diamond S, Freitag FG. The use of fluoxetine in the treatment of headache. Clin J Pain. 1989;5:200–1.
115. Geller SA. Treatment of fibrositis with fluoxetine hydrochloride (Prozac). Am J Med. 1989;87:594–5.
116. Theesen KA, Marsh WR. Relief of diabetic neuropathy with fluoxetine. DICP, Ann Pharmacother. 1989;23:572–4.
117. Arnold LM, Hess EV, Hudson JI, Welge JA, Berno SE, Keck PE Jr. A randomized, placebo-controlled, double-blind, flexible-dose study of fluoxetine in the treatment of women with fibromyalgia. Am J Med. 2002;112(3):191–7.
118. Sindrup SH, Gram LF, Brosen K, Eshoj O, Mogenson EF. The selective serotonin reuptake inhibitor paroxetine is effective in the treatment of diabetic neuropathy symptoms. Pain. 1990;42:135–44.
119. Sindrup SH, Bjerre U, Dejgaard A, Brosen K, Aaes-Jorgensen T, Gram LF. The selective serotonin reuptake inhibitor citalopram relieves the symptoms of diabetic neuropathy. Clin Pharmacol Ther. 1992;52(5):547–52.
120. Sidney H, Kennedy HFA, Lam RW. Efficacy of escitalopram in the treatment of major depressive disorder compared with conventional selective serotonin reuptake inhibitors and venlafaxine XR: a meta-analysis. J Psychiatry Neurosci. 2006;31(2):122–31.
121. Theobald DE, Kirsh KL, Holtsclaw E, Donaghy K, Passik SD. An open-label, crossover trial of mirtazapine (15 and 30 mg) in cancer patients with pain and other distressing symptoms. J Pain Symptom Manag. 2002;23(5):442–7.
122. Arnold P, Vuadens P, Kuntzer T, Gobelet C, Deriaz O. Mirtazapine decreases the pain feeling in healthy participants. Clin J Pain. 2008;24(2):116–9.
123. Schreiber S, Rigai T, Katz Y, Pick CG. The antinociceptive effect of mirtazapine in mice is mediated through serotonergic, noradrenergic and opioid mechanisms. Brain Res Bull. 2002;58(6):601–5.
124. Freynhagen R, Muth-Selbach U, Lipfert P, Stevens MF, Zacharowski K, Tolle TR, et al. The effect of mirtazapine in patients with chronic pain and concomitant depression. Curr Med Res Opin. 2006;22(2):257–64.

125. Semenchuk MR, Sherman S, Davis B. Double-blind, randomized trial of bupropion SR for the treatment of neuropathic pain. Neurology. 2001;57(9):1583–8.
126. Semenchuk MR, Davis B. Efficacy of sustained-release bupropion in neuropathic pain: an open-label study. Clin J Pain. 2000;16(1):6–11.
127. Moss EL, Simpson JSA, Pelletier G, Forsyth P. An open-label study of the effects of bupropion SR on fatigue, depression and quality of life of mixed-site cancer patients and their partners. Psycho-Oncology. 2006;15(3):259–67.
128. McDowell I, Lindsay J, Sykes E, Verreault R, Laurin D, Hendrie HC, et al. Bupropion sustained release treatment reduces fatigue in cancer patients. Can J Psychiatr. 2004;49:139–44.
129. Mathias C, Mendes CC, de Sena EP, de Moraes ED, Bastos C, Braghiroli M, et al. An open-label, fixed-dose study of bupropion effect on sexual function scores in women treated for breast cancer. Ann Oncol. 2006;17(12):1792–6.
130. Davis MP. Does trazodone have a role in palliating symptoms? Support Care Cancer. 2007;15(2):221–4.
131. Fernandez F, Adams F, Holmes VF, Levy JK, Neidhart M. Methylphenidate for depressive disorders in cancer patients. Psychosomatics. 1987;28:455–61.
132. Kaufmann MW, Murray GB, Cassem NH. Use of psychostimulants in medically ill depressive patients. Psychosomatics. 1982;23:817–9.
133. Bruera E, Chadwick S, Brennels C, Hanson J, MacDonald RN. Methylphenidate associated with narcotics for the treatment of cancer pain. Cancer Treat Rep. 1987;71:67–70.
134. Bruera E, Brenneis C, Paterson AH, MacDonald RN. Use of methylphenidate as an adjuvant to narcotic analgesics in patients with advanced cancer. J Pain Symptom Manag. 1989;4:3–6.
135. Bruera E, Fainsinger R, MacEachern T, Hanson J. The use of methylphenidate in patients with incident cancer pain receiving regular opiates: a preliminary report. Pain. 1992;50:75–7.
136. Forrest WH Jr, Brown BW Jr, Brown CR, Defalque R, Gold M, Gordon HE, James KE, Katz J, Mahler DL, Schroff P, Teutsch G. Dextroamphetamine with morphine for the treatment of postoperative pain. N Engl J Med. 1977;296:712–5.
137. Morrow GR, Shelke AR, Roscoe JA, Hickok JT, Mustian K. Management of cancer-related fatigue. Cancer Investig. 2005;23(3):229–39.
138. DeBattista C, Lembke A, Solvason HB, Ghebremichael R, Poirier J. A prospective trial of modafinil as an adjunctive treatment of major depression. J Clin Psychopharmacol. 2004;24(1):87–90.
139. Kingshott RN, Vennelle M, Coleman EL, Engleman HM, Mackay TW, Douglas NJ. Randomized, double-blind, placebo-controlled crossover trial of modafinil in the treatment of residual excessive daytime sleepiness in the sleep apnea/hypopnea syndrome. Am J Respir Crit Care Med. 2001;163(4):918–23.
140. Rammohan KW, Rosenberg JH, Lynn DJ, Blumenfeld AM, Pollak CP, Nagaraja HN. Efficacy and safety of modafinil (Provigil) for the treatment of fatigue in multiple sclerosis: a two centre phase 2 study. J Neurol Neurosurg Psychiatry. 2002;72(2):179–83.
141. Myrick H, Malcolm R, Taylor B, LaRowe S. Modafinil: preclinical, clinical, and post-marketing surveillance-a review of abuse liability issues. Ann Clin Psychiatry. 2004;16(2):101–9.
142. Volkow ND, Fowler JS, Logan J, Alexoff D, Zhu W, Telang F, et al. Effects of modafinil on dopamine and dopamine transporters in the male human brain: clinical implications. JAMA. 2009;301(11):1148–54.
143. Beaver WT, Wallenstein SL, Houde RW, Rogers A. A comparison of the analgesic effect of methotrimeprazine and morphine in patients with cancer. Clin Pharmacol Ther. 1966;7:436–46.
144. Kennett A, Hardy J, Shah S, A'hern R. An open study of methotrimeprazine in the management of nausea and vomiting in patients with advanced cancer. Support Care Cancer. 2005;13(9):715–21.
145. Maltbie AA, Cavenar JO Jr, Sullivan JL, Hammett EB, Zung WW. Analgesia and haloperidol: a hypothesis. J Clin Psychiatry. 1979;40:323–6.
146. Patt RB, Proper G, Reddy S. The neuroleptics as adjuvant analgesics. J Pain Symptom Manag. 1994;9(7):446–53.
147. Lechin F, van der Dijs B, Lechin ME, Amat J, Lechin AE, Cabrera A, Gómez F, Acosta E, Arocha L, Villa S, et al. Pimozide therapy for trigeminal neuralgia. Arch Neurol. 1989;9:960–4.
148. Boettger S, Breitbart W. Atypical antipsychotics in the management of delirium: a review of the empirical literature. Palliat Support Care. 2005;3(3):227–37.
149. Sasaki Y, Matsuyama T, Inoue S, Sunami T, Inoue T, Denda K, et al. A prospective, open-label, flexible-dose study of quetiapine in the treatment of delirium. J Clin Psychiatry. 2003;64(11):1316–21.
150. Leso L, Schwartz TL. Ziprasidone treatment of delirium. Psychosomatics. 2002;43(1):61–2.
151. Boettger S, Breitbart W. An open trial of aripiprazole for the treatment of delirium in hospitalized cancer patients. Palliat Support Care. 2011;9(04):351–7.
152. Alao AO, Moskowitz L. Aripiprazole and delirium. Ann Clin Psychiatry. 2006;18(4):267–9.
153. Khojainova N, Santiago-Palma J, Kornick C, Breitbart W, Gonzales GR. Olanzapine in the management of cancer pain. J Pain Symptom Manag. 2002;23(4):346–50.
154. Rumore MM, Schlichting DA. Clinical efficacy of antihistamines as analgesics. Pain. 1986;25:7–22.
155. Hupert C, Yacoub M, Turgeon L. Effect of hydroxyzine on morphine analgesia for the treatment of postoperative pain. Anesth Analg. 1980;59(9):690–6.
156. Fernandez F, Adams F, Holmes VF. Analgesic effect of alprazolam in patients with chronic, organic pain of malignant origin. J Clin Psychopharmacol. 1987;3:167–9.
157. Caccia MR. Clonazepam in facial neuralgia and cluster headache: clinical and electrophysiological study. Eur Neurol. 1975;13:560–3.
158. Bartusch SL, Sanders JB, D'Alessio JG, Jernigan JR. Clonazepam for the treatment of lancinating phantom limb pain. Clin J Pain. 1996;12(1):59–62.

52 Acupuncture and Cancer Pain

Yan Cui Magram and Gary E. Deng

Introduction

Acupuncture is one of the oldest forms of medical treatment in the world. It originated in China more than 3000 years ago, with many of its philosophies rooted in the principles of Taoism. When performing acupuncture, the acupuncturist inserts filiform needles into certain points on the body, called acupoints. The acupuncturist then manipulates the needle by twisting, turning, advancing, or withdrawing the needles to stimulate the surrounding tissues. Heat may also be applied to the needles. Electroacupuncture is a relatively new variation on traditional acupuncture and involves needles placed in traditional acupuncture points connected to small devices that generate electrical pulses. The frequency and intensity of the electrical pulses may be adjusted based on each specific case. The choice of most acupoints is pre-defined by anatomical landmarks, while others are located according to symptoms, such as pain.

The practice of acupuncture is based on three principles. Firstly, "Qi," often described as the "vital energy" or "life force," travels through different meridians or pathways interconnecting points along the body and is connected to different organ systems [1]. The positions of acupoints are often based on the location of these meridians. Secondly, acupuncture is based on the principle that the body is in a dynamic balance between two opposing factors: "yin" – the cool, dense, material state of matter – and "yang," the warm, light, and immaterial state of matter [2]. Lastly, acupuncture meridians and their associated organs can be characterized by one of the five basic elements in Chinese medicine, wood, water, fire, earth, and metal, and are intricately related to the bodily balance [3].

Though the philosophy of acupuncture may not be rooted in human anatomy and physiology, recent neuroscience research suggests that acupuncture produces its clinical effects via modulation of the nervous system. Since its popularization in the United States in the 1970s, acupuncture has gained widespread use as a form of complementary medicine, with more than 2 million Americans cited as recent users according to a 2002 NHIS survey [4]. An increasing number of clinical trials have been conducted to evaluate acupuncture for its effectiveness in treating a myriad of clinical conditions. The strongest evidence came from studies for chronic pain, acute pain, and nausea and vomiting.

Evidence on Acupuncture and Noncancer Pain

Acute pain, such as that experienced in the postoperative period, and chronic pain such as long-standing back pain, joint pain, fibromyalgia, and headache disorders have all been indications for patients seeking acupuncture treatment. The efficacy of acupuncture for the treatment of pain focuses on multiple studies and meta-analyses. Studies on the efficacy of acupuncture often compare acupuncture to "sham" or placebo acupuncture or no acupuncture. Sham acupuncture may be performed by superficial needling without skin penetration, by inserting needles at non-acupuncture points, or by inserting needles at acupuncture points that are not indicated for the condition or type of pain being treated. In a recent meta-analysis of individual patient data obtained from high-quality trials, acupuncture was found to be associated with a reduction of chronic pain when compared to sham acupuncture or no acupuncture controls [5]. The studies included in this meta-analysis included studies on musculoskeletal pain, osteoarthritis, chronic headache, and shoulder pain. The meta-analysis data also suggest that there is a

Y. C. Magram (✉)
New York Presbyterian Hospital-Weill Cornell Medicine, Department of Anesthesiology, New York, NY, USA
e-mail: yac2005@nyp.org

G. E. Deng
Memorial Sloan Kettering Cancer Center, Department of Integrative Medicine Service, New York, NY, USA
e-mail: Dengg@mskcc.org

A. Gulati et al. (eds.), *Essentials of Interventional Cancer Pain Management*, https://doi.org/10.1007/978-3-319-99684-4_52

smaller difference in response rate between the acupuncture vs. sham acupuncture groups, when compared to the acupuncture vs. no acupuncture groups [5], suggesting a placebo or possible physiological effect of sham acupuncture.

Evidence on Acupuncture and Cancer Pain

Despite inconclusive evidence toward its effectiveness, acupuncture has been used frequently in the treatment of cancer pain. Whether acupuncture is efficacious in reducing pain associated with cancer has been the subject of several studies. However, comprehensive data from large-scale randomized controlled trials specifically looking at cancer pain and acupuncture are rare.

A recently updated Cochrane review article aimed to look at this subject in more detail [6]. The inclusion criteria were randomized controlled trials with either crossover or parallel groups that evaluated any type of invasive acupuncture for pain related to cancer (excluding pain related to treatments, such as neuropathic pain from chemotherapy or postoperative pain). Included were studies that assessed any type of invasive acupuncture such as a manual acupuncture, electroacupuncture, and auricular acupuncture. The comparison groups included conventional treatment, no treatment, sham non-penetrative acupuncture, and penetrative acupuncture at non-acupuncture points. The primary outcome measured was patient pain scores on scales such as the visual analogue scales (VAS), or numerical rating scales (NRS), or verbal reporting. Secondary outcomes included quality of life, patient satisfaction, decrease in analgesic consumption, hospital and hospice stay, and any adverse events. Five studies, including 285 participants, were ultimately included in their analysis.

The authors of the Cochrane review article pointed out that this review illustrates that there is a paucity of high-quality studies on acupuncture and cancer pain [5]. Three of the five studies were included in a previous version of the Cochrane review article by the same group published in 2011, and two were newer studies [7]. The Alimi 2003 study found a decrease in VAS at 1 and 2 months in the acupuncture group compared to the sham acupuncture group in patients who received auricular acupuncture for cancer-related neuropathic pain [8]. In Dang [9], the researcher compared gastric cancer patients in an acupuncture group to a Western medication group who received conventional medication based on the WHO analgesic ladder over a 2-month period and found that the conventional medication group experienced better pain control during the first 10 days of the study. However, by the final 10 days, results were similar between the two groups. Chen et al. [10] found that acupuncture was more effective than conventional medication based on the WHO analgesic scale in patients with late-stage, unspecified cancer pain [10]. Chen et al. [11] found a benefit of electroacupuncture over sham acupuncture after 3 days of treatment in patients with pancreatic cancer [11]. Finally, the Lu et al. [12] study compared women with ovarian or peritoneal cancer and uterine cancer who received electroacupuncture and sham electroacupuncture and found no significant difference in reported pain levels but an improvement in the quality of life measure of social functioning [12]. All of the included studies had small samples sizes, with the Alimi 2003 study having the largest number of participants at 90. Therefore, sample sizes were a source of high risk of bias [11]. Additionally, lack of adequate blinding was another source of high risk of bias among these studies. Since each study used a different cancer population and different methodologies, the authors could not pool the data to carry out a meta-analysis. The overall conclusion summarized by the Cochrane review is that there is not sufficient evidence to conclude whether acupuncture is effective in treating cancer pain in adult patients [5].

Mechanism of Action

Multiple hypotheses have been proposed and studied over the past several decades to understand the effects of acupuncture. Early hypotheses include the neurophysiological model of acupuncture, which suggests that stimulation of acupuncture points causes the release of centrally acting, endogenous opioids and neurotransmitters such as endorphins, enkephalins, and dynorphins, which play a role in its analgesic effect [13]. Newer studies implicate the involvement of other agents. One theory suggests that the release of adenosine triggered by the mechanical movements of the acupuncture needles and the activation of peripheral adenosine A1 receptors are involved in the analgesic effects of acupuncture [14].

Advances in neuroimaging techniques allow researchers to elucidate the effects of acupuncture on brain stimulation, with studies showing activation in the sensorimotor cortical network and deactivation in the limbic-paralimbic-neocortical network [15]. Additionally, recent functional imaging studies suggest that there is an interaction between the regions of the brain important to endogenous analgesia, affect, memory, and self-projective thinking (the default mode network) [16]. The default mode network (DMN) involves a network of connected brain regions including the prefrontal cortex, posterior cingulate cortex, precuneus, lateral parietal, and temporal cortex and is activated when a person focuses on its inner state, reasoning, introspective thinking, feeling, remembering, and prospecting [16]. These functional imaging studies suggest acupuncture is a “mind-body therapy” that helps the body find homeostasis [16]. All of these studies suggest that the mechanism of acupuncture is likely complex, involving the release of central and peripheral transmitters and activation and deactivation of specific brain regions.

Safety Profile

Complications from acupuncture are rare, and acupuncture is accepted as a highly safe practice when performed correctly. Possible complications include pneumothorax, pneumoperitoneum, infection, transmission of disease, nerve injury, bleeding, pain, and paresthesias.

Large prospective survey studies show that serious complications leading to permanent disability or death are almost nonexistent and that minor adverse events including bruising, local pain, mild bleeding, failure to remove needles, and nausea and vomiting occur at a rate of approximately 0.1% [17, 18]. A peer-reviewed article published in 2006 set out guidelines for the use of acupuncture for cancer patients [19].

Specific Application of Acupuncture to Cancer Pain

The acupuncture points and meridians used in the treatment of cancer pain are individualized to each patient based on the patient’s set of symptoms, location of pain, and limitations, instead of specific cancer diagnosis. Typical treatment routines involve treatment sessions once or twice a week for 6–8 weeks to determine if there is any benefit. Treatments are often altered and tweaked based on each patient’s specific needs.

Aromatase Inhibitor-Induced Musculoskeletal Pain

Aromatase inhibitors (AI) are commonly used adjuvant hormone treatment for women with hormone receptor-positive breast cancer. Musculoskeletal symptoms such as arthralgia and joint stiffness are serious side effects of AI and can be seen in 35–81% of AI users [20]. Of those who experience arthralgia and bone pain, 20% of patients discontinued AI because of this side effect [21]. In a systematic review of two RCTs on manual acupuncture and two RCTs on electroacupuncture, researchers found that acupuncture has potential benefits to improve arthralgia induced by AIs, although further studies are needed [20]. Standard acupuncture points (CV 4, CV 6, CV 12, and bilateral LI 4, MH 6, GB 34, ST 36, KI 3, BL 65 in the Bao et al. study) to improve pain and stiffness of arms, hands, legs, and feet are typically chosen [22, 23]. Needles are typically left in for 20–30 min, during which time, the acupuncturist may return to stimulate the needle and re-elicit *de qi* [23].

Chemotherapy-Induced Peripheral Neuropathy

Chemotherapy-induced peripheral neuropathy (CIPN) is a common side effect experienced by patients after treatment with alkaloids, platinum derivatives (cisplatin and oxaliplatin), taxanes, and bortezomib. Most CIPN is a sensory neuropathy, presenting as numbness or tingling sensations. When severe, it can reduce quality of life and result in discontinuation of treatment. Chemotherapeutic agents likely induce neuropathic pain by causing destruction of neural microtubules, axonal degeneration, and damage to the dorsal root ganglia (DRG) [24]. A systematic review of seven clinical studies on CIPN and acupuncture found that only one study (a randomized controlled trial) showed that acupuncture may be beneficial for CIPN [24]. However, the studies in this systematic review were heterogeneous, with methodological limitations, necessitating the need for further studies to investigate the effects of acupuncture and CIPN [24].

Cancer-Induced Bone Pain

Pain from bony metastases is a major symptom experienced by patients with advanced-stage cancer. Conventional treatments for cancer-induced bone pain (CIBP) may involve the use of bisphosphonates, radiation, and opioids. Acupuncture appears to provide a relatively safe alternative therapy for some of these patients. Most studies on acupuncture and CIBP to date have been on animal models, and several studies show promising results that electroacupuncture improves CIBP [25, 26]. Some proposed that special considerations should be taken for patients with CIBP who wish to undergo acupuncture. Since patients with bony metastasis already suffer from a high pain burden, and often exhibit hyperalgesia and allodynia, they may not tolerate additional stimulation from acupuncture needles [27]. Additionally, care must be taken as patients with advanced bone disease may also be undergoing chemotherapy and be severely immunosuppressed and thrombocytopenic and therefore be more susceptible to infection and bleeding.

Summary

Acupuncture is practiced worldwide, either alone or in conjunction with other forms of treatment. Research into the efficacy of acupuncture, and the underlying effects have extended several decades. While the exact mechanism of the analgesic effects of acupuncture is unclear, there is evidence that it may be effective in the treatment of certain noncancer and cancer pain and likely involves not only a neurophysiological component but also an interaction between brain regions responsible for endogenous analgesia, thinking, emotion, and homeostasis. Acupuncture is commonly used in several cancer-related pain syndromes including aromatase inhibitor-induced musculoskeletal pain, chemotherapy-induced peripheral neuropathy, and cancer-induced bone pain. Although much is still unknown about acupuncture, it is a relatively safe form of treatment that may present a significant form of pain treatment for patients with cancer-related pain.

References

1. Unschuld P. Medicine in China: a history of ideas. Berkeley: University of California Press; 1985.
2. Birtch S, Felt R. Understanding acupuncture. London: Churchill Livingstone; 1999.
3. Manioca G. The foundations of Chinese medicine. London: Churchill Livingstone; 1989.
4. Burke A, Upchurch DM, Chyu L. Acupuncture use in the United States: findings from the National Health Interview Survey. J Altern Complement Med. 2006;12(7):639–48.
5. Vickers AJ, Linde K. Acupuncture for chronic pain. JAMA. 2014;311(9):955–6.
6. Paley CA, Johnson MI, Tashani OA, Bagnall A. Acupuncture for cancer pain in adults. Cochrane Database Syst Rev. 2015;10:CD007753.
7. Paley CA, Tashani OA, Bagnall AM, Johnson MI. A Cochrane systematic review of acupuncture for cancer pain in adults. BMJ Support Palliat Care. 2011;1(1):51–5.
8. Alimi D, Rubino C, Pichard-Leandri E, Fermand-Brule S, Dubreuil-Lemaire M, Hill C. Analgesic effect of auricular acupuncture for cancer pain: a randomized, blinded, controlled trial. J Clin Oncol. 2003;21(22):4120–6.
9. Dang W, Yang J. Clinical study on acupuncture treatment of stomach carcinoma pain. J Tradit Chin Med. 1998;18(1):31–8.
10. Chen ZJ, Guo YP, Wu ZC. Observation on the therapeutic effect of acupuncture at pain points on cancer pain. Zhongguo Zhen Jiu [Chinese Acupuncture & Moxibusion]. 2008;28(4):251–3.
11. Chen H, Liu TQ, Zhu J, Wu CJ, Liu LM. Electroacupuncture treatment for pancreatic cancer pain: a randomized controlled trial. Pancreatology. 2013;13(6):594–7.
12. Lu W, Matulonis UA, Dunn JE, Lee H, Doherty-Gilman A, Dean-Clower E, et al. The feasibility and effects of acupuncture on quality of life scores during chemotherapy in ovarian cancer: results from a pilot-randomized sham-controlled trial. Med Acupunct. 2012;24(4):233–40.
13. Cabyoglu MT, Ergene N, Tan U. The mechanism of acupuncture and clinical applications. The mechanism of acupuncture and clinical applications. Int J Neurosci. 2006;116(2):115–25.
14. Goldman N, Chen M, Fujita T, Xu Q, Peng W, Liu W, Jensen TK, Pei Y, Wang F, Han X, Chen J, Schnermann J, Taano T, Bekar L, Tieu K, Nedergaard M. Adenosine A1 receptors mediate local anti-nociceptive effects of acupuncture. Nat Neurosci. 2010;13(7):883–8.
15. Chae Y, Chang DS, Lee SH, Jung WM, Lee IS, Jackson S, Kong J, Lee H, Park HJ, Lee H, Wallraven C. Inserting needle into the body: a meta-analysis of brain activity associated with acupuncture needle stimulation. J Pain. 2013;14(3):215–22.
16. Otti A, Noll-Hussong M. Acupuncture-induced pain relief and the human brain's default mode network—an extended view of central effects of acupuncture analgesia. Forsch Komplementmed 2012;19($):197–201.
17. Yamashita H, Tsukayama H, Tanno Y, Nishijo K. Adverse events in acupuncture and moxibustion treatment: a six-year survey at a national clinic in Japan. J Altern Complement Med. 1999;5(3):229.
18. MacPherson H, Thomas K, Walters S, Fitter M. The York acupuncture safety study: prospective survey of 34,000 treatments by traditional acupuncturists. BMJ. 2001;323(7311):486.
19. Filshie J, Hester J. Guidelines for providing acupuncture treatment for cancer patients- a peer-reviewed sample policy document. Acupunct Med. 2006;24(4):172–82.
20. Bae K, Yoo HS, Lamoury G, Boye F, Rosenthal DS, Oh B. Acupuncture for aromatase inhibitor-induced arthralgia: a systematic review. Integr Cancer Ther. 2015;14(6):496–502.
21. Presant CA, Bosserman L, Young T, Vakil M, Horns R, Upadhyaya G, Ebrahimi B, Yeon C, Howard F. Aromatase ingibitor-associated arthralgia and/or bone pain: frequency and characterization in non-clinical trial patients. Clin Breast Cancer. 2007;7(10):775.
22. Bao T, Cai L, Giles JT, Gould J, Tarpinian K, Betts K, Medeiros M, Jeter S, Tait N, Chumsri S, Armstrong DK, Tan M, Fokerd E, Dowsett M, Singh H, Tkaczuk K, Stearns V. A dual-center randomized controlled double blind trial assessing the effect of acupuncture in reducing musculoskeletal symptoms in breast cancer patients taking aromatase inhibitors. Breast Cancer Res Treat. 2013;138(1):167–74.
23. Crew KD, Capodice JL, Greenlee H, Brafman L, Fuentes D, Awad D, Tsai WY, Hershman DL. Randomized, blinded, sham-controlled trial of acupuncture for the management of aromatase-inhibitor-associated joint symptoms in women with early-stage breast cancer. J Clin Oncol. 2010;28(7):1154–60.
24. Franconi G, Manni L, Schroder S, Marchetti P, Robinson N. A systematic review of experimental and clinical acupuncture in chemotherapy-induced peripheral neuropathy. Evid Based Complement Alternat Med. 2013: Article ID 516917, 7 pages.
25. Zhang RX, Li A, Liu B, Wang L, Xin J, Ren K, Qiao JT, Berman BM, Lao L. Electroacupunctur attenuates bone-cancer-induced hyperalgesia and inhibits spinal preprodynorphin expression in a rat model. Eur J Pain. 2008;12(7):870–8.
26. Zhang RX, Li A, Liu B, Wang L, Ren K, Qiao JT, Berman BM, Lao L. Electroacupuncture attenuates bone cancer pain and inhibits spinal interleukin-1 beta expression in a rat model. Anesth Analg. 2007;105(5):1482–8.
27. Paley CA, Bennett MI, Johnson MI. Acupuncture for cancer-induced bone pain? Evid Based Complement Alternat Med. 2011: Article ID 671043, 8 pages.

53 Creative Therapies and Mind-Body Health Systems

Veena Sankar

Abbreviations

AATA	American Art Therapy Association
ACMT	Advanced certified
AMA	American Medical Association
AMTA	American Music Therapy Association
ATCB	Art Therapy Credentials Board
ATCS	Art Therapist Certified Supervisor
ATR	Art therapist registered
ATR-BC	ATR-Board Certified
CAM	Complementary and alternative medicine
CMT	Certified massage therapist
CMT	Certified music therapist
FDA	Food and Drug Administration
fMRI	Functional magnetic resonance imaging
IAYT	International Association of Yoga Therapists
JAMA	*Journal of the American Medical Association*
LMT/P	Licensed massage therapist/practitioner
MBAT	Mindfulness-based art therapy
MEG	Magnetoencephalography
MT-BC	Music Therapist Board Certified
NCBMTB	National Certification Board for Therapeutic Massage
NCCAM	National Center for Complementary and Alternative Medicine
NMTR	National Music Therapist Registry
PET	Positron emission tomography
RMT	Registered music therapist

V. Sankar (✉)
Austin Anesthesiology Group, Austin, TX, USA

Introduction

Between frequent doctor's visits and a bombardment of medical care and treatments, a diagnosis of cancer can swiftly besiege a patient's life and take over his/her identity. The physical and emotional impact of cancer on patients' quality of life is undeniable and ubiquitous. Further, with advances in oncology and greater efficacy of treatments, medical therapies have become increasingly technical, specific, and potentially more difficult for patients to fully understand. In this milieu of uncertainty, it is perhaps a sense of vulnerability and a desire for self-care that draws cancer patients to seek out complementary and alternative medicine (CAM), whose therapies tend to take a more holistic and intuitive approach to care [1]. These adjunctive therapies usually address the element of suffering involved in being diagnosed with cancer and, thus, have the potential to alleviate physical pain and the emotional pain and distress felt by the patient, their caregivers, and loved ones [2, 3].

What Is CAM?

CAM as defined by the National Center for Complementary and Alternative Medicine (NCCAM) is a group of diverse medical and healthcare systems, practices, and products that are not generally considered a part of conventional biomedicine [4]. Many complementary therapies, such as acupuncture and Ayurveda, are discussed in other chapters throughout this text. This chapter serves to cover the topic and to address the challenges, issues, and progress in this emerging field of study. A heterogeneous group of therapies will be explored for their potential value in the treatment of cancer pain syndromes. Many of the modalities discussed here are not covered in traditional allopathic mediums but may be adjuncts to integrative oncologic treatment and comprehensive pain management plans.

A. Gulati et al. (eds.), *Essentials of Interventional Cancer Pain Management*, https://doi.org/10.1007/978-3-319-99684-4_53

Why Should Physicians Consider CAM?

Whether due to a growing disillusionment with conventional biomedicine or a desire to exhaust all potential options of treatment, the use of complementary therapies should be considered by physicians. A recent meta-analysis and review estimates that approximately 40% of cancer patients are using some form of CAM [5]. In 2007, annual spending on complementary therapies amounted to 34 billion dollars, accounting for 11% of out-of-pocket expenditure on healthcare [6]. Pain was the most common reason for CAM treatment [6].

Due to the magnitude of CAM as a sociocultural movement and the potential therapeutic value of different modalities, the demand for thorough analysis has emerged along with a growing body of CAM research. In 1998, the National Institute of Health (NIH) created the National Center for Complementary and Alternative Medicine (NCCAM) to address this social phenomenon and "to define, through rigorous scientific investigation, the usefulness and safety of complementary and alternative medicine interventions and their role in improving health and health care" [4]. Table 53.1 defines the goals and objectives of NCCAM.

Surveys have shown that cancer patients often do not tell their physicians about the use of complementary therapies [7]. At worst, this is a health hazard. At best, it is a commentary on the current level of awareness, trust, and openness between patients and their healthcare providers. The primary reasons given were that patients did not know they should tell their providers and that their physician did not ask [7]. To address this communication gap, NCCAM launched the "Time to Talk" campaign to encourage patients and healthcare providers to discuss the usage of complementary medicine [7].

Table 53.1 Goals and objectives of NCCAM4

NCCAM: National Center for Complementary and Alternative Medicine
Goals
Advance the science and practice of symptom management
Develop effective, practical, personalized strategies for promoting health and well-being
Enable better evidence-based decision-making regarding complementary and alternative medicine use and its integration into healthcare and health promotion
Develop and disseminate objective, evidence-based information on complementary and alternative medicine interventions
Objectives
Advance research on mind and body interventions, practices, and disciplines
Advance research on complementary and alternative medicine natural products
Increase understanding of "real-world" patterns and outcomes of complementary and alternative medicine use and its integration into healthcare and health promotion
Improve the capacity of the field to carry out rigorous research

When discussing patients' CAM usage, it is important to be respectful while discussing patient's choices and beliefs. Similarly, when recommending CAM, it is important to note patient preferences and level of activity to make the most relevant suggestions [8]. For example, some CAM therapies are more passive (music listening, massage, acupuncture), while others are more active (yoga, t'ai chi, meditation, music entrainment). Knowing a patient's level of function, desired level of participation, and specific issues they hope to address should help guide the discussion. A list of credible sources for patient referral is given in Table 53.2.

In general, strong evidence for measurable benefits of CAM is still forthcoming [9]. Modalities that have been integrated into cancer treatment centers across the country are those that have an excellent safety profile, do not cause emotional or financial harm, and are done alongside (complementary and integrative medicine) not in lieu of conventional treatment (alternative medicine).

CAM and Cancer Pain

A 2006 systematic review of the efficacy of CAM therapies in relieving cancer pain concluded that, at best, the data was promising for the ability of some CAM therapies to positively impact cancer pain. Reviewers found very few rigorous trials, citing the following as potential reasons for the dearth of scientific evidence [9]:

- CAM is a new area of study, and many therapies are in the fledgling stages of development as academic disciplines.
- Practitioners have not developed a significant scientific framework for evaluating their discipline. This could be due to the above but also because many practitioners view their work in a more artistic framework and do not see a need for scientific validation.
- Funding for CAM research is poor – CAM therapies generally lack patent potential, and thus pharmaceutical companies have low incentive to invest in clinical trials.

Table 53.2 Patient resources for credible information regarding CAM

http://nccam.nih.gov/
http://www.mskcc.org/cancer-care/integrative-medicine
http://cam.cancer.gov/health_patients.html
NCCAM clearinghouse: Provides information on complementary health approaches, including publications and searches of federal databases of scientific and medical literature. Toll Free: 1-888-644-6226. Email: info@nccam.nih.gov
Music therapy: http://www.musictherapy.org/
Art therapy: http://www.arttherapy.org/
Massage therapy: http://www.ncbtmb.org/
Yoga: http://www.iayt.org/
T'ai Chi: http://www.americantaichi.org/

- While CAM therapies are increasingly being offered at cancer centers, CAM practitioners are typically not fully integrated within the oncology community making it difficult to accrue sizeable numbers of participants and/or conduct multi-institutional research.
- Because these therapies are not considered drugs, they are generally not subject to the strict regulation by the FDA. Therefore, there is no regulatory demand for strict and rigorous trials.

Creative (Expressive) Arts Therapies

Creative (expressive) arts therapy is the use of creative arts and process as a form of psychotherapy [10]. Creative arts therapists are professionals who utilize different modalities with the intent of improving patient/client outcomes and functionality [10]. Expressive arts therapists practice based on the belief that illness and its associated suffering can be explored and transformed through guided, creative self-expression, ultimately leading to deeper connections with one's self and others. The expressive arts include visual arts, movement, drama, music, writing, and other creative processes [10].

Distraction as Analgesia

High-attention endeavors are powerful distractions that have repeatedly demonstrated the ability to reduce pain perception [2, 11]. Patients often distract themselves from pain with everyday tasks and hobbies independent of any professional advice. Today, with advancements in neuroimaging and sophisticated study design protocols, neuroscientists are elucidating physiologic mechanisms by which cognitive processes, such as distraction, alter pain processes. Findings are suggestive that there may be a sound scientific explanation for the effectiveness of distraction as an analgesic [11–13].

Scientists have long been able to demonstrate that subjects report reduction in pain perception after painful stimulus while performing a high working memory load task [13], defined as complex tasks that require attention and, therefore, serve to distract [14]. Using high-resolution functional magnetic resonance imaging (fMRI), functional neuroimaging studies demonstrate modulation of pain by distraction. Current models of this pathway include regions of the cortical and subcortical brain (i.e., thalamus, insula, primary and secondary somatosensory cortices), as well as the dorsal horn of the spinal cord [11, 12]. In a 2012 study by Sprenger attempting to determine the mechanism of distraction modulation of pain, fMRI signal intensity decreased significantly at the level of the spinal cord corresponding to a painful stimulus in subjects performing a high working memory task. If the patient's arm in the C6 dermatome was subjected to painful stimuli while she was being distracted, the spinal cord at the corresponding level on fMRI showed decreased activity, which corresponded to a decrease in pain perception. Investigators were also able to reverse these effects with the administration of naloxone, suggesting an opioid mechanism involved in modulation [11].

Music Therapy

Music therapy is an established, evidence-based health discipline utilizing music interventions in a goal-directed fashion to improve clinical outcomes [15]. In an integrative oncology setting, music therapists are part of a multidisciplinary team. Through music and sound, music therapists are trained to assess and respond to physical, psychosocial, and spiritual needs via a therapeutic relationship rooted in compassion and direct communication with the patients, families, and caregivers [2, 15]. Music is selected either by the patient or by the therapist. Goals of treatment guide music selection and can be based on patient familiarity, tempo, pitch, frequency, volume, etc. [15–17]. Music therapists can also empower caregivers with methods to allay the patient's symptoms using soothing voices and hums. Table 53.3 highlights components of a typical musical therapy consultation to assess and address a patient's specific needs, set therapeutic goals, and develop a treatment plan [17, 18].

Music therapy techniques can broadly be divided into two categories: active (or entrainment) and passive (or receptive) [19]. Active applications include those treatments in which the patient and therapists play music together. Applications can be categorized by primarily vocal techniques (with or without accompanying instruments) and instrumental techniques (with or without vocals). Vocal techniques include sing-alongs to precomposed music, lyric improvisation and songwriting (also known as the entrainment method), chanting, and toning. Instrumental techniques include improvisation, drum and chime circles, and meditation and relaxation classes. Receptive (also known as passive) music therapy

Table 53.3 Music therapy consultation [17, 18]

Assessment and observations	Goals
Consultation with collaborating staff	Pain relief
Psycho-emotional status	Relaxation and stress management
Needs, values, preferences (cultural, social, spiritual)	Emotional support and expression
Patient decision-making capacity	Improved sense of control
Cognitive function	Distraction
Level of orientation	Improve communication
Prior and current coping strategies	Promote physical rehabilitation
Prior musical experience	
Social support	

involves patients listening to prerecorded or live music provided by the music therapist [17–19].

Scientific interest in music therapy has expanded over the last few decades. Historically, the majority of studies on music therapy focus on acute and postsurgical pain and involve patients passively listening to music [16, 20]. Music therapy has been demonstrated to reduce pain perception [16], reduce cortisol levels [21], reduce anxiety [16], improve fatigue [16], and show a variety of other positive outcomes [16]. Like with distraction and cognition studies, advances in neuroscience and neuroimaging, namely, magnetoencephalography (MEG) [19], positron-emission tomography(PET) [22], and functional magnetic resonance imaging (fMRI) [19], have greatly expanded the depth and breadth of research. Multiple basic science research studies have suggested that the specific link between music therapy, particularly the more active forms, and analgesia is more powerful and complex than previously understood [16, 19, 20, 23]. Current literature provides promising prospects regarding a theoretical and empirical scientific foundation for music therapy [23]. Music listening and producing have been shown to modulate activity in the same brain structures (the limbic and paralimbic structures, including the dorsomedial midbrain, amygdala, and hippocampus) via the same neuroanatomical pathways as those involved in pain, anxiety, and depression [20, 22]. These same structures are known to have a dense population of endogenous opioid receptors, suggestive also of an opioid mechanism of action for music-induced analgesia [20, 22]. These findings carry promise that active methods of music therapy, such as lyric writing and composing, have the potential for long-term analgesic effects and of reducing opioid requirements and use in pain patients [19, 22, 24].

Neurophysiologist Michael Hauck and his colleagues at the University of Hamburg used magnetoencephalography (MEG) to characterize the effects of music and music therapy on cortical activity. The 2012 study compared two different therapeutic concepts: receptive (passive) and entrainment (active). In the receptive form, patients were instructed to select music they associated with well-being to oppose the painful stimuli. In the entrainment form, the patient worked closely with a music therapist and actively participated in composing and performing the music. The control was a condition with no sound at all. Using EEG and MEG, the authors were able to delineate at least two different and separate mechanisms in which the two music therapies modulated pain perception and different stages in the brain's pain processing system. They connected music therapy with the effects of cognitive behavioral therapy in that treatment can empower the patient "to actively explore and learn individual pain coping capabilities" [19].

Thomas Hillecke, a professor of therapeutic sciences in Germany and a prominent figure in music therapy research, has developed a "heuristic working factor model for music therapy" that credits the therapeutic effects of music to five modulating factors: attention, emotion, cognition, behavior, and communication. Modulation, in psychotherapeutic terms, refers to purposeful regulation in therapy to reduce the intensity and/or duration of an undesired experience. In this model, the analgesic effects of music would be related to attention and behavior modulation. He promotes utilizing a variety of musical parameters (volume, rhythms, tempo, pitch) to attract and maintain a patient's attention and deflect the patient's symptoms to enhance alertness and arousal in an inactive or fatigued patient. Pleasant and unpleasant pieces of music are partly processed in different brain regions. He suggests using music (specifically rhythm and dance) to introduce new behavioral and action plans to alter patient's cognitive pain processes [23, 25].

Cancer pain patients stand to benefit both from long-term behavior modulation and short-term distraction/attention modulation-based music therapy. Many cancer centers and hospitals already utilize music therapy in an inpatient setting, which seems to fit into the attention modulation model. Further, for cancer patients and survivors, active music therapy that utilizes behavioral modulation has the potential to enhance coping mechanisms for long-term pain management. Advancements in the field highlight the high efficacy of using active music therapy as a form of creative psychotherapy utilizing a specific music therapy concept customized to meet the needs of individual patients [26–30].

If access to a music therapist is limited, combining the experiments of Hauck and working model of Hillecke and the following noninvasive, low-risk procedures can be recommended. In cases of patients receiving painful infusions, healthcare locales may equip themselves with low-cost means of providing relaxing and distracting music for patients to listen to with headphones. Further, if a patient has any musical background, simply encouraging them to reengage in musical activity can go a long way both in terms of helping to distract and allay pain and deepening the physician-patient relationship.

Art Therapy

Art therapy is a mental health profession with a well-established presence in integrative oncology. It has roots in both art and psychotherapy. Art therapists establish professional relationships with patients/clients using art media, the creative process, and resulting artwork to improve and enhance physical, mental, and emotional well-being and function.

Fundamental to art therapy is the belief that the self-expressive creative process enables people to reduce stress, develop coping strategies, resolve problems, improve cognition, and achieve insight [31]. Via free association and imagery, artistic expression provides a nonverbal platform for patients to process intense, unfamiliar emotions that may be difficult to articulate and understand. By creating distance between the patient and the experience, art therapy has the potential to convert feelings of isolation and distress into those of transformative integration and creative exploration [32]. At the very least, art therapy provides an opportunity for patients to relish in the pleasure of art making. While various art forms are used, drawing, painting, and sculpting are the mainstay of most research reports, particularly in oncology settings.

The Art Therapy Credentials Board (ATCB) is the credentialing body for the art therapy profession whose mission is "to protect the public by promoting the competent and ethical practice of art therapy through the credentialing of art therapy professionals" [33, 34]. The ATCB and AATA are separate organizations. Table 53.4 lists possible credentials/qualifications of art therapists. The AATA website also has an art therapist locator. Credentialing can be verified at the ATCB website (http://www.atcb.org).

Like music therapy, art therapy research has increased in recent years. Comparative studies have found that images created under the guidance of an art therapist expressed a wider range of emotions than those of art making alone [35]. Historically, most publications have been based on observational studies and/or patient case analysis that uses nonuniform narrative and experiential research methods. In terms of art therapy and cancer pain management, art has been used as a tool for patients to nonverbally and visually communicate their emotional and physical pain experience by filling out and coloring a body outline [32]. Practitioners are attempting to determine efficacy in alleviating pain or distress from pain, as well as other psychological and physical symptom management [35–38].

The art therapy community regards their work as highly individualized, and the process itself, which emphasizes free expression and release, seems diametrically opposed to the standardization and uniformity required in rigid, randomized controlled trials. To date, the most earnest attempts at fitting art therapy into the reductionist scientific method are self-admittedly "quasi-experimental" and difficult to randomize.

Table 53.4 Credentials of art therapists

Title (abbreviation)	Description
Art Therapist Registered (ATR)	Completion of graduate education and postgraduate supervised experience
Art Therapist Registered – Board Certified (ATR-BC)	Required passing a written examination Maintained through continuing education
Art Therapist Certified Supervisor (ATCS)	Board certified art therapists who have demonstrated substantial supervision qualifications

So, while art therapy research now is also shifting toward increased utilization of the scientific method, statistics, and controls in attempts to quantify and qualify the efficacy of art therapy, investigators are utilizing mixed methods to hopefully reach more applicable and accurate conclusions [35–39].

A 2004 randomized controlled trial by Monti et al. explored the efficacy of mindfulness-based art therapy (MBAT) in over 90 women with cancer in active treatment. MBAT consisted of an 8-week program that integrated mindfulness meditation methods and art therapy. The women reported improvements in bodily pain [39]. The primary finding of the study was improvement in distress levels [39]. A contemporaneous study by Nainis specifically examined the efficacy of a single session of art therapy in relieving physical symptoms in oncology inpatients and found a statistically significant reduction in eight of nine symptoms measured, including pain and pain-related fatigue, perhaps, in such an acute setting, by means of distraction [36].

Meeting the gold standards of research studies is notoriously difficult, and many of the problems with art therapy research may be explained by its relative nascence. Art therapy research is in a pioneer stage and is an undoubted valuable area to study given its viability as an economical and feasible adjunct in both the hospital and outpatient setting. A 2011 systematic review of research evidence by Wood et al. reached similar conclusions, also adding that most of published studies fail to report training of therapists, disease stage of participants, and absence of long-term follow-up. Among other specific suggestions, Wood recommended multicenter mixed methods randomized controlled trials with long-term follow-up with a focus on the replicability of current research [35].

Mind-Body Therapies

Mind-body therapies are those CAM interventions that are "based on a reciprocal relationship in every human being between the mind and the body" [40]. A universal definition for mind-body therapy is difficult, but these modalities emphasize the power and ability of the mind (or thoughts) to influence physical health and well-being. These therapies are gaining popularity in the integrative oncology community for their general safety and efficacy and potential to treat symptom clusters (pain, fatigue, sleep disturbances, mood disorders, etc.) that plague patients because of cancer and its treatment [41].

The belief that the mind and mental processes play a critical role in physical health and illness is one that has fascinated philosophers and scientists throughout history across societies and civilizations. Emphasis on this interconnectedness fell out of the popular conscience following scientific discoveries and technological breakthroughs of the Renaissance and Enlightenment, leading to the eventual predominance of allopathic medicine [42].

A Brief History of Allopathic and CAM Convergence

In the early twentieth century, due to general lack of standards, high rate of fraud, and dubious training of so-called healers and physicians, the government began regulating the practice of medicine and "any activity that potentially could be construed as diagnosis and treatment" [43]. Until 1983, the AMA Code of Ethics contained the following:

> A physician should practice a method of healing founded on scientific bases; and he should not voluntarily associate professionally with anyone who violates this principle. [44]

In 1963, the Committee on Quackery was established which, alongside the Coordinating Conference on Health Information, acted as a task force targeting vitamins, homeopathy, chiropractic, naturopathy, all alternative cancer treatments, and other practices which competed with the drug sales of pharmaceutical companies [45]. In 1976, this was challenged in court which ruled that the AMA had violated part of the Sherman Antitrust Act and had engaged in an unlawful conspiracy in restraint of trade "to contain and eliminate the chiropractic profession" [46]. The Committee has since been disbanded, and today, perhaps fueled by popular usage and a more open viewpoint on potential therapies, the *Journal of the American Medical Association* (JAMA) contains numerous scholarly articles on what would have once been considered quackery.

Massage Therapy

Massage is a well-known, popular modality utilized for a variety of potential health-related benefits. It refers to a group of systematic and scientific manipulations of body tissues typically performed with the hands to affect the nervous and muscular systems and general circulation [8]. It is offered in clinical settings to aid in relaxation, facilitate sleep, and relieve muscular aches and pains [40].

Historical references to massage appear in ancient texts and depictions from China, India, Japan, and Egypt, with the oldest references dating at least as far as 1600 BC. In the United States, two New York physicians introduced Swedish-type massage therapy to popular culture in the mid-nineteenth century. By the 1930s and 1940s, the influence of massage had declined with the rise and advancements of allopathic medicine. Massage regained popularity in the 1970s when it was frequently used among athletes. Today, massage therapy is a state-regulated profession generally requiring licensure and board certification. Massage therapists work in a variety of settings and are often a popular component of integrative cancer centers [47, 48].

There are many different styles of massage all of which use manual manipulation of soft tissue through contact, pressure, or movement with the intended purpose of enhancing well-being [49]. As a complementary treatment for cancer-related symptoms, the gentler Swedish massage, aromatherapy massage, manual lymphatic drainage, acupressure, and reflexology are the types most commonly implemented and the basis of most studies in cancer patients [47]. Swedish massage is simply called a "classic massage," as Swedish massage is a misnomer. Its development is historically credited to a Swedish physiologist Peter Henry Ling when in fact experts now credit the systemization of massage to a Dutch practitioner Johann Georg Mezger [48]. The style consists of five basic strokes: effleurage (sliding or gliding), petrissage (kneading), tapotement (rhythmic tapping), friction (cross fiber), and vibration. Oil or lotion is often used to reduce friction and facilitate stretching of muscles. Massage is often applied with the patient lying down (usually on a specialized massage table), but it can also be applied with the patient in a seated position. Massage can result in "blood vessel dilation, skin temperature rise, and a decrease in heart rate" [50]. Proposed, unproven mechanisms of action for massage include reduced lactic acid buildup in muscles, stimulation of healing of connective tissues, and increase in lymphatic and venous circulation [50, 51].

Perhaps due to its mainstream popularity, scientific research on massage therapy is considerably more voluminous than other areas of complementary medicine. The benefits of massage have been studied in pain, cancer, rehabilitation, cardiovascular, and mental health. Evidence suggests that massage may reduce anxiety, alleviate pain, improve sleep, and promote relaxation [50]. A large, retrospective observational study conducted on 1,290 inpatients and outpatients over a 3-year period found large, immediate statistical improvements in pain, fatigue, anxiety, nausea, and depression [52]. The Reducing End-of-life Symptoms with Touch (REST) study, a large multisite randomized trial funded by NCCAM to evaluate the efficacy of massage for decreasing pain and symptom distress and improving quality of life among patients with advanced cancer, concluded also that massage may have immediate beneficial effects on pain and mood [51]. Investigators also found improvements in control groups in which patients received simple touch and attention, acknowledging that this "control" group could also be perceived as an intervention with its own benefits. In general, it is believed the effects of massage are short term and maintenance therapy is necessary for benefits to persist [50, 51]. A 2008 literature review from the National Cancer Institute conducted by massage therapists assessing the value of massage therapy in cancer care concluded that "evidenced-based massage administered by properly trained individuals can provide a soothing and nurturing experience in the midst of stressful cancer treatment and should therefore be made available to patients to assist in the optimal prevention and control of cancer symptoms and treatment side effects" [53]. The National Comprehensive Cancer Network recommends the use of massage therapy in its treatment guidelines for refractory cancer pain [52].

Based on anecdotal evidence and outcome studies regarding feasibility [52], advocacy for massage therapy in medical settings by massage therapists, patients, and healthcare providers has led to greater access and increased utility. Oncology massage is an emerging subspecialty within the massage therapy profession. In 2007, the Society for Oncology Massage was formed; its mission is to link cancer patients and their families and caregivers with skilled oncology massage therapists. Today, massage educators have authored numerous texts and articles with guidelines and recommendations for therapists treating this unique patient population. When discussing massage with cancer patients, the following recommendations are in place [50–53]:

- Avoid open wounds, bruises, and areas with skin breakdown as these areas are at risk for infection. Catheters and ports should be avoided as well.
- Do not massage directly over the tumor site. Note: To date, there has been no evidence that massage causes tumor manipulation and spread of cancer.
- Do not massage areas with a known DVT or other blood clot.
- Avoid sensitive areas following radiation therapy as massage therapy could then exacerbate pain.

Certain cancer patients are at higher risk for massage-related adverse outcomes [50].

- In patients with a coagulation disorder (i.e., low platelet count, prolonged PT/PTT/INR) and/or on anticoagulation therapy, there is increased risk of bleeding (minor bruising, hemorrhage). Deep tissue massage should be avoided, and massage pressure should be lightened
- Patients with metastatic bone disease are at increased risk of fracture. Massage therapists should be aware of the location of bone metastases and lighten pressure over those areas.

It is important to note that even healthy patients may experience bruising, localized swelling over massaged muscles, temporary increase in pain, or an allergic reaction to lotion/oil used to aid in massage.

Given relative safety and efficacy in the hands of an appropriate massage therapist, massage therapy may be recommended for symptom management, particularly pain and anxiety. In general, cancer patients should be referred to a massage therapist experienced and trained in oncology massage. Therapists should have a minimum of 500 h of training and be from an accredited massage therapy school that meets the criteria set by the Commission on Massage Therapy Accreditation [50]. The National Certification Board for Therapeutic Massage and Bodywork (NCBTMB) is an independent, private, nonprofit organization that administers and oversees Board Certification and licensure for individual therapists; Table 53.5 lists common licenses or certifications for massage therapists in the United States [54–56].

Table 53.5 Common licenses or certifications for massage therapists [54, 55]

Title (abbreviation)	Description
Licensed massage therapist (LMT)	Licensure is a state designation. In 39 states and the District of Columbia, massage therapists are required to be licensed in order to practice. LMT are required to pass the NCBTMB exam and fulfillment of other criteria that vary by state. All administration and oversight of licensing are governed at the state level
Licensed massage practitioner (LMP)	Same as LMT
Certified massage therapist (CMT)	Certification is a professional designation. Precise requirements vary by organization, but in general certification requires completion of an approved massage training program, demonstration of competency in applying standard massage therapies, passage of a written exam testing theoretical knowledge, and an understanding of ethical requirements set forth by the organization
NCTMB/ NCTM	Denotes that a CMT has been specifically credentialed by the NCTMB, the largest professional organization of massage therapy certification

Yoga Therapy

Yoga therapy, as defined by the International Association of Yoga Therapists (IAYT), is the process of empowering individuals to progress toward improved health and well-being through the applied philosophy and practice of Yoga [57]. An over 5,000-year-old tradition, yoga is one of the oldest mind-body health systems with deep roots in classical Hindu philosophy and over a hundred different schools of practice.

The word yoga is derived from the Sanskrit word, *yuj*, or to yoke, referring to the unification of the individual self with the universal self. The *Yoga Sutras of Patanjali* is a 2000-year-old script that serves as the foundation for the modern-day practice of yoga. The Sutras are made up of 196 aphorisms delineating the path to reach *samadhi*, or pure awareness without distractions (enlightenment) via the cultivation of *prana* (vital energy or life force). The

Sutras define eight limbs, or disciplines of yoga: *yamas* (ethical disciplines), *niyamas* (individual observances), *asana* (postures), *pranayama* (breath control), *pratyahara* (withdrawal of senses), *dharana* (concentration), *dhyana* (meditation), and ultimately *Samadhi* (enlightenment) [58]. Broadly speaking, the present-day practice of yoga in the United States focuses on the third and fourth limbs. A *typical* Western yoga practice refers to sessions of non-aerobic exercise typically ranging from 15 to 90 min. Each session or class is composed of purposeful sequences of *asanas*, specific systematic traditional postures/poses (as outlined in the sutras and other yoga texts), *pranayama*, rhythmic awareness of breath, and guided meditation. Postures are generally classified as standing, sitting, twisting, balancing, inverting, and forward and back bending [59–61]. While equipment is not mandatory, yoga is typically performed on a stylized mat with or without the assistance of standard props, such as blocks, bolsters, blankets, straps, and eye masks (Fig. 53.1).

Because the breadth of yoga extends to both philosophy and the physical body, it is considered and being studied as both a psychosocial and exercise intervention. Current areas of investigation include the impact of yoga on both psychosocial factors (quality of life, mood, anxiety) and physical end points (increased strength and flexibility and reduction of pain scores) [59–64]. Yoga studies in noncancer populations have demonstrated a variety of positive effects such as improved perceptual and motor skills, cardiopulmonary function, and joint pain [65].

Yoga is recommended and studied specifically to help patients cope with the symptoms and side effects of cancer and its treatment [62]. Studies investigate varying stages of disease, including active and remission disease, varying extent of disease, and different cancer populations (lymphoma, breast, prostate) [61]. Outcomes vary depending on the type of cancer, stage of disease, and point in treatment trajectory [61]. Studies have shown promising preliminary findings in the following areas: reduced fatigue, self-reported physical health and quality of life, pain, mood, chemotherapy-induced nausea, and stress [63–67]. One study in India found reduced DNA damage in breast cancer patients receiving radiotherapy who completed an integrated yoga program as compared to control group, which was speculated to be a result of reduced psychological stress [67].

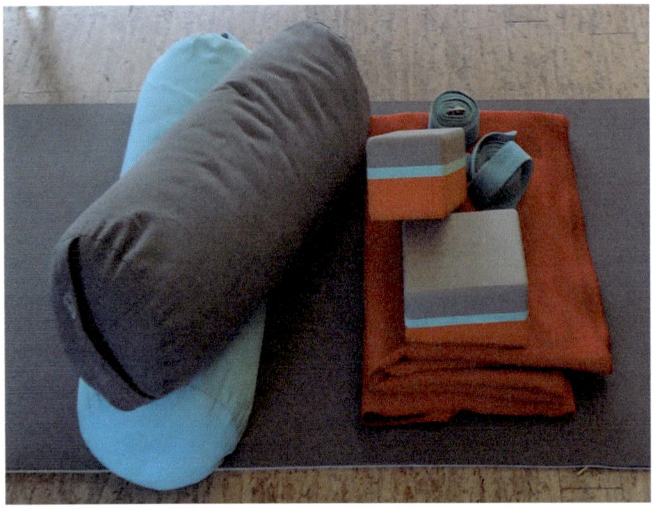

Fig. 53.1 Standard Yoga props utilized in a typical restorative yoga session. From left, bolsters, blankets, blocks, and straps. Props are supportive equipment that can increase safety, reduce strain, and optimize body alignment so that practitioners can maximize gain from specific poses

A 2012 meta-analysis of randomized controlled trials of yoga and cancer patients by Buffart concluded that there is strong evidence for beneficial effects of yoga on distress, anxiety, and depression, moderate effects for fatigue and general health-related quality of life and emotional and social function, and small effects on functional well-being [65]. Much of the current research has been limited by small sample size, lack of a control group, and inadequate statistical analyses [61]. In a 2005 review of yoga and cancer, Bower et al. suggest a more targeted approach for future study. For example, instead of examining general health and well-being, which is uniquely multifactorial in this population, a future study could examine the change in pain scores after a yoga program comprised of chest and shoulder asana sequences in patients who have had surgery on the breast, chest, and axilla [60, 61].

A 2008 study by Duncan et al. contextually demonstrates pluralism in complementary medicine research. The study investigated how an Iyengar yoga program affects the self-identified worst symptom in a group of patients during the course of and after a 6-week program. To measure outcome, the study utilized a medical outcome questionnaire that had been validated over several populations, as well as interviews with six participants (selected at random) using the instrumental case study method with the intent that these interviews would help elucidate and interpret quantitative findings. Qualitative results showed participants in the study had statistically significant improvements in their most bothersome symptom (including pain, fatigue, and anxiety). Qualitatively participants reported mental and physical invigoration, feelings of empowerment, and an increased ability to cope [62].

Many cancer centers now offer yoga classes and programs specifically designed for this patient population with different health and safety considerations than the public. Patients may feel more at ease with fellow cancer patients and specialized teachers as compared to a local gym or yoga studio. Teachers and instructors generally have experience with cancer and/or chronically ill patients to reduce chances of injury or adverse events. They typically utilize gentle poses and stretching that can safely be executed by persons with functional limitations. Chair yoga, in which participants perform yoga-based stretches and postures while seated, may be offered as well [60, 61].

If such specialized yoga instruction is not locally available, it is important to advise a patient on what to look for when starting a yoga practice.

- Most studios and gyms include in their contract that all persons with illnesses seek approval from their healthcare provider before initiating an exercise program. Therefore, a physician should have at least some awareness of yoga basics from which to base recommendations and concerns.
- Balancing poses may be challenging but helpful and recuperative for those with chemotherapy-induced neuropathy. Suggest standing near a wall for stability if attempting to balance.
- Patients with symptomatic anemia, postural hypotension, and/or lightheadedness should avoid long-standing poses and be instructed to move slowly when transitioning between postures.
- Patients with fever, systemic infection, or significant thrombocytopenia should avoid the more vigorous poses. Neutropenic patients should avoid crowded classes. Susceptible patients should be reminded of the importance of hygiene and maintaining sanitation and cleanliness of shared mats and props [60].

Instruct patients to inquire about a specific teacher's credentials and training history before taking a class as teacher training is widely variable and not standardized. The Yoga Alliance is a nonprofit national organization that registers and credentials individual yoga instructors and training programs. Registered Yoga Teacher (RYT) is the standard credential with the Yoga Alliance. Table 53.6 outlines Yoga Alliance credentials [68].

While yoga philosophy and fundamentals are universal, some types of yoga may not be safe or appropriate for oncology patients even under the supervision of a vetted instructor. It is safe to recommend a restorative yoga class at any stage of illness or recovery as they are designed to energize the weak, fatigued, or stressed practitioner. They involve gentle, multidirectional spinal movements and incorporate inversions (postures in which the head is below the heart which increases venous return and may improve heart function) [61]. Figure 53.2a–d shows examples of restorative asanas. Some facilities also offer chair yoga classes that are specifically designed for patients with limited exercise tolerance and/or mobility and likely safe for cancer patients.

T'ai Chi

T'ai chi ch'uan (commonly truncated to t'ai chi) is a Chinese mind-body exercise system which, like yoga, is deeply rooted in philosophy. Just as the physical practice of yoga emerged from Hindu philosophy, the principles of t'ai chi are derived from the Chinese philosophical schools of Buddhism, Taoism, and Confucianism collectively known as neo-Confucianism. Much of the origin of t'ai chi is based on legend; the first written reference of t'ai chi ch'uan is in a seventeenth-century text in which it was described as a new form of kung fu [69].

T'ai chi ch'uan is commonly translated to "supreme ultimate" or "supreme fist," a reference to the Taoist principle of

Table 53.6 Credentials with the Yoga Alliance

Credential	Training requirements	Teaching hours and time
RYT 200	Completed 200 h of training with Registered Yoga School (RYS 200) All training must be completed at the same school	None required
RYT 500	Completed a 500-h training program with an RYS 500 Completed a 200-h training program with a RYS 200 and an additional 300 h of training with either the same RYS or a different RYS registered as a RYS 300	Has >100 h of teaching experience since completing training with a RYS 200 or 500 RYT 500 is able to provide continuing education classes and workshops to other teachers
E-RYT 200, E-RYT 500®	Completed a 500-h training program with a RYS 500 Completed a 200-h training program with a RYS 200 and an additional 300-h training program with either the same RYS (if it is registered as a RYS 300) or a different RYS 300	>1,000 h of teaching experience since completing training with an RYS 200 or RYS 500 At least 2 years of teaching experience following training
E-RYT 500®	Completed a 500-h training program with a RYS 500 Completed a 200-h training program with a RYS 200 and an additional 300-h training program with either the same RYS (if it is registered as a RYS 300) or a different RYS 300	>2,000 h of teaching experience since completing training with a RYS 200 or 500 >500 of these hours must be taught after completing training with a RYS 300 or 500 At least 4 years of teaching experience following training

RYT Registered yoga teacher, *E* experienced [68]

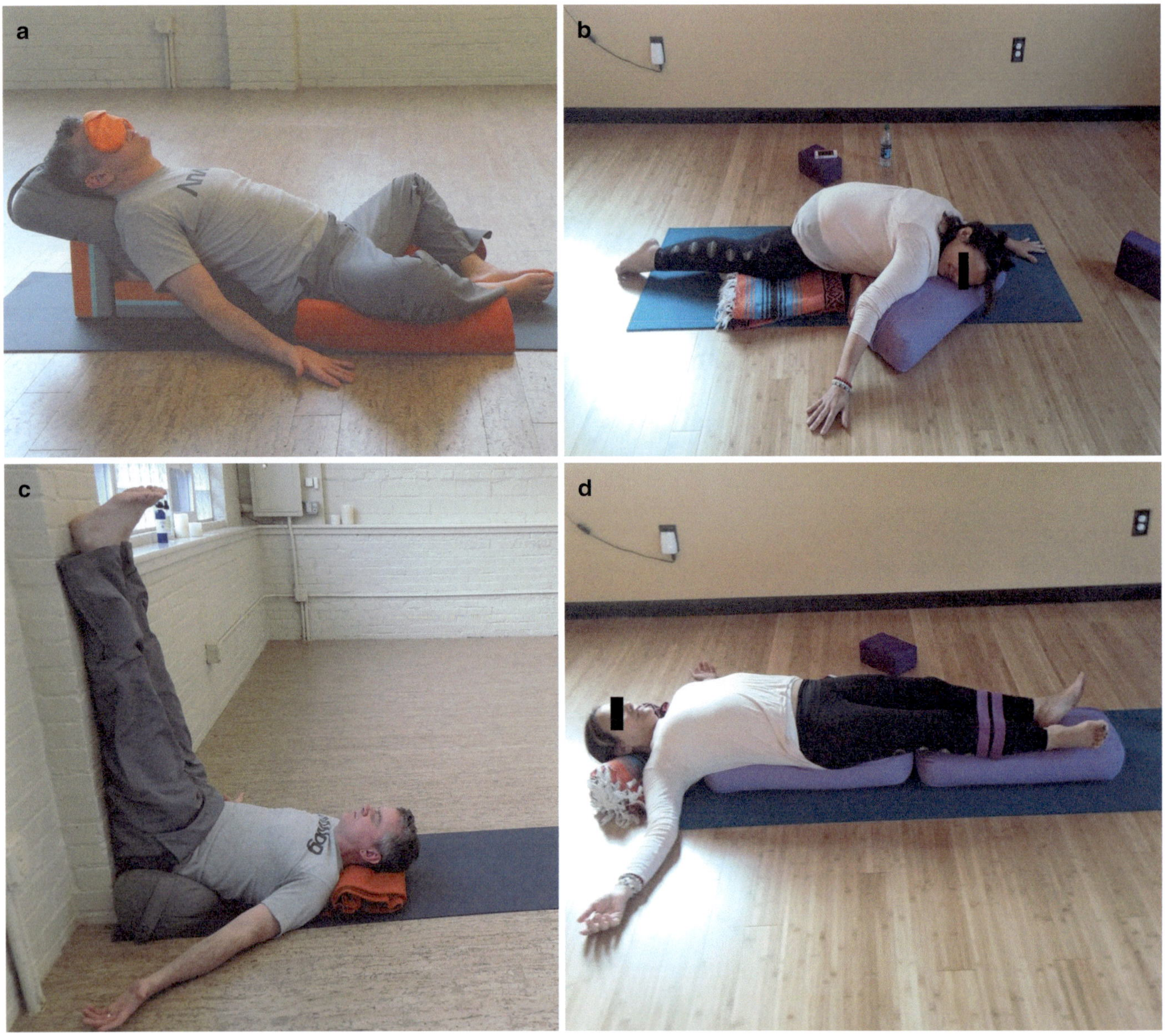

Fig. 53.2 Restorative Yoga is a passive form of yoga that utilizes props and bolsters to support and assist practitioners in a given pose. (**a**) Restorative supta baddha konasana (reclining bound angle pose), (**b**) supported half pigeon, (**c**) restorative viparita karani (legs-up-the-wall), (**d**) restorative savasana (corpse)

the union between Yin and Yang. T'ai chi is referred to as an internal martial art form, which refers to systems that use movement and stillness to cultivate awareness that is then used to guide the physical body to increase the natural flow of *qi*. *Qi* roughly translates to life energy and is philosophically comparable to the yogic term, prana. In practice, t'ai chi is comprised of slow purposeful movements that are coordinated with the breath and imagery. The sequences are intended to simultaneously strengthen and relax the physical body. After the body is controlled, the mind follows ultimately leading to heightened self-awareness and skill levels [69, 70].

There are five major schools, or styles, of t'ai chi which originate from different family lineages: Chen (the oldest school from which the other schools are derived), Yang (the most prevalent), Wu Hao, Wu Ch'uan-yu, and Sun. With time and geographical spread, new schools and branches have emerged from these original five schools that blend modern insights, progressions, and fusions with conventional wisdom. T'ai chi ch'uan was brought to the United States in 1939 by Choy Hok Peng of the Yang school. Over the years, several teachers immigrated to the United States and have popularized the practice of t'ai chi in the West with approximately 5 million Americans (as of 2008) having at least some exposure to the art form. Today, although its origins are within the martial arts, t'ai chi is currently integrated into traditional Chinese medicine principles and, like yoga, is taught as a philosophical exercise [69–71].

T'ai chi has been steadily increasing in popularity as a restorative and rehabilitative form of low-impact exercise both in the general population and in the integrative oncology community. With its intrinsic focus on balance and slow movements, it has been effectively used to reduce falls in the elderly [72]. Further, in cardiovascular studies, it has been shown to improve quality of life scores and exercise tolerance in chronic stable heart failure patients, decrease blood pressure, improve fasting lipid profiles, and improve physical functioning in rheumatoid arthritis and HIV patients [72].

The body of literature regarding t'ai chi and cancer patients is inconclusive. A 2012 systematic review by Lee evaluated the effectiveness of t'ai chi for supportive breast cancer care and concluded that the existing trial evidence is not convincing that t'ai chi is an effective modality [73]. Lee reports that his own review lacks statistical power due to a dearth of existing RCT and CCT and further that it is difficult to make any fast conclusions from the existing studies due to a lack of methodological rigor [73]. He recommends future trials to have larger sample sizes and clearly outline the t'ai chi protocol utilized and the use of standardized and validated statistical measures.

To date, no trials report negative or deleterious outcomes. Thus, perhaps due to its safety, positive outcome studies in other areas of study, and anecdotal reports of efficacy, t'ai chi ch'uan is commonly offered in integrative departments in major cancer centers throughout the United States. While specific recommendations for t'ai chi in cancer patients do not exist, the physical requirements are similar to that of restorative yoga. T'ai chi is primarily done standing, does not require bare feet or sharing of props, and, thus, perhaps poses less of a concern for infection than does the practice of yoga. Patient should have easy access to a chair in case of dizziness or fatigue.

CAM Research: Where Do We Go from Here? What Is Methodological Pluralism?

As discussed in his book and throughout this chapter, there is emerging popularity in utilizing mixed methods in the budding field of CAM research. Methodological pluralism is an approach to scientific study that promotes flexibility in the selection of social research methods. Complementary therapies have the healing intent of biomedicine and the intuitive, intangible elements of the social sciences which require different modalities for appropriate study. Flexibility and tolerance of nouveau research designs allow for the ethereal claims and nature of many complementary therapies to be appropriately studied [76, 77].

Studying Complexity: Whole-Systems Research, Cancer, and CAM

A diagnosis of cancer carries with it a whole host of lifestyle, physical, and emotional implications and burdens, making it difficult to study the effect of a single intervention with a singular outcome as is lauded in conventional scientific research [75]. This well-recognized phenomenon has led to the emergence of whole-systems research in oncology and, more recently, in CAM. Whole systems refers to multicomponent interventions, like those discussed in this chapter, which are arguably mismatched when being considered as akin to a medication that has a single mechanism of action [75]. In other words, many CAM therapies, like Ayurveda and t'ai chi, represent entire networks of approaches to care that are different from conventional biomedicine and, according to some CAM investigators, thus need to be studied in a different framework [69, 74, 75].

In 2008, Dr. Peter Wayne, research director of the Osher Center for Integrative Medicine, and Ted Kaptchuk, director of the Harvard-wide program in Placebo Studies and the Therapeutic Encounter, presented two companion paradigm papers outlining the difficulties and challenges of studying complex multicomponent interventions, like t'ai chi, using the conventional biomedicine model that is designed to study pharmaceuticals with a given effect [69, 74]. There is no "active ingredient" in t'ai chi or any of the complementary therapies discussed here in this chapter. It is impossible to blind patients and therapists and extremely difficult to construct a standard placebo, and randomization inherently may be at odds with desired outcome given the likelihood that the intention or belief is integral to the purported success of these therapies. Wayne et al. also note that the relationship between the t'ai chi instructor and practitioner is part of the t'ai chi system and thus cannot be removed as a variable – another factor at odds with current standards.

Complex systems, like yoga and t'ai chi, have cognitive, physical, and even ritualistic components that are fundamentally inseparable and potentially have synergistic effects. Wayne et al. suggest shifting research in t'ai chi toward a whole-systems research model, as used in disciplines such as epidemiology, sociology, and ecology that commonly deal with complex, multivariate phenomenon [69, 74–76].

Integrative Medicine Now

Combined with the discovery of the placebo effect and the effects of stress on health, many fields in allopathic medicine began exploring the significance of the interactions between the brain, the rest of the body, the mind, and behavior. Integrative medicine rotations and classes are now offered at major allopathic medical and nursing schools across the country and globe. Many medical schools, healthcare clinics, and research institutions are combining the best of high-tech

Table 53.7 Patient resources for critical information regarding CAM [77, 79]

http://www.sciencebasedmedicine.org	From website: SBM's authors are all medically trained and have spent years writing for the public about science and medicine, tirelessly advocating for high scientific standards in healthcare
http://www.quackwatch.com	Founded by Dr. Stephen Barnett in 1969 Activities (from website) Investigating questionable claims Answering inquiries about products and services Advising quackery victims Distributing reliable publications Debunking pseudoscientific claims Reporting illegal marketing Assisting or generating consumer-protection lawsuits Improving the quality of health information on the Internet Attacking misleading advertising on the Internet Consumer Health Digest, a free weekly e-mail newsletter The Health Fraud Discussion List, which has about 600 members

medicine with the wisdom of premodern medicine to transform the physician-patient relationship [78].

The Society for Evidence-Based Medicine (http://www.sciencebasedmedicine.org) is "dedicated to evaluating medical treatments and products of interest to the public in a scientific light, and promoting the highest standards and traditions of science and health care" [77]. Quackwatch (Quackwatch.com) is "an international network of people who are concerned about health-related frauds, myths, fads, fallacies, and misconduct" [79]. It was founded by Dr. Stephen Barnett in 1969 and has now expanded to 24 websites addressing specific areas of interest [79]. Table 53.7 provides more details regarding these watch sites which present dissenting viewpoints regarding the integration of complementary therapies into mainstream healthcare.

Conclusion

Keeping an open mind is an essential attribute of a sound and empathic physician, particularly in the fields of oncology and pain management. While the therapies discussed here may not be clinical requirements or part of the standard of care, these noninvasive interventions can be safe, low-cost, feasible adjuncts as part of a holistic oncologic treatment plan [40]. The majority of these therapies pose no appreciable harm to patients and potentially considerable gain. Mixed and new methods are being introduced by those seeking for holism in medicine. Awareness of these therapies will arm the physician with informed answers in the event of patient inquiry. A discussion or suggestion of any of these creative therapies, with selection based on the individual patient, could serve to deepen the doctor-patient relationship and overall satisfaction of the patient and the physician.

References

1. Barrett B, Marchand L, Scheder J, Plane M, Maberry R, Appelbaum D, et al. Themes of holism, empowerment, access, and legitimacy define complementary, alternative, and integrative medicine in relation to conventional biomedicine. J Altern Complement Med. 2003;9(6):937–47.
2. O'Callaghan CC. Pain, music creativity and music therapy in palliative care. Am J Hosp Palliat Med. 1996;13(2):43–9.
3. National Center for Complementary and Alternative Medicine (NCCAM). Get the facts: cancer and complementary health approaches [Internet]. Bethesda: NCCAM Pub No.: D453. c2005 September [updated 2013 May; cited 2014 July 19]. Available from: http://nccam.nih.gov/sites/nccam.nih.gov/files/CAM_Basics_Cancer_and_CHA_0.pdf
4. NCCAM. NCCAM facts-at-a-glance and mission [Internet]. Bethesda: NCCAM [last modified 2014 July 2; cited 2014 July 22]. Available from http://nccam.nih.gov/about/ataglance
5. Horneber M, Bueschel G, Dennert G, Less D, Ritter E, Zwahlen M. How many cancer patients use complementary and alternative medicine: a systematic review and metaanalysis. Integr Cancer Ther. 2012;11(3):187–203.
6. Nahin, RL, Barnes PM, Stussman BJ, Bloom B. Costs of complementary and alternative medicine (CAM) and frequency of visits to CAM practitioners: United States, 2007. National health statistics reports; no 18. Hyattsville: National Center for Health Statistics; 2009. Available from: http://www.nih.gov/news/health/jul2009/nccam-30.htm
7. NCCAM. Time to a talk [Internet]. Bethesda: [last updated 2012 March 14, cited 2014 July 22]. NCCAM Publication No.: D381-G. Available from http://nccam.nih.gov/timetotalk/backgrounder.htm
8. Deng G, Cassileth B. Integrative oncology: complementary therapies for pain anxiety, and mood disturbance. CA Cancer J Clin. 2005;55(2): 109–14. [Internet]. 2005 Mar/Apr [cited July 22, 2014]. https://doi.org/10.3322/canjclin.55.2.109 Available from: http://CAonline.AmCancerSoc.org
9. Bardia A, Barton DL, Prokop LJ, Bauer BA, Moynihan TJ. Efficacy of complementary and alternative medicine therapies in relieving cancer pain: a systematic review. J Clin Oncol. 2006;24:5457–64.
10. National Coalition of Creative Arts Therapists Associations (NCCATA) [Internet]. [place unknown] [cited July 22, 2014]. Available from: http://nccata.org
11. Sprenger C, Eippert F, Finsterbusch J, Bingel U, Rose M, Buchel C. Attention modulates spinal cord responses to pain. Curr Biol. 2012;22:1019–22.
12. Bantick SJ, Wise RG, Ploghaus A, Clare S, Smith SM, Tracey I. Imaging how attention modulates pain in humans using functional MRI. Brain. 2002;125:310–9.
13. Buhle J, Wager TD. Performance-dependent inhibition of pain by an executive working memory task. Pain. 2010;149:19–26.
14. Eccleseton C. Chronic pain and distraction: an experimental investigation into the role of sustained and shifting attention in the processing of chronic persistent pain. Behav Res Ther. 1995;33:391–405.
15. American Music Therapists Association (AMTA) [Internet]. Silver Spring: AMTA; 1998–2014 [cited July 22, 2014]. Available from: http://www.musictherapy.org/

16. AMTA [Internet]. Silver Spring: AMTA [cited July 23, 2014]. Available from: http://www.musictherapy.org/assets/1/7/MT_Pain_2010.pdf
17. Magill L. Role of music therapy in integrative oncology. J Soc Integr Oncol. 2006;4(2):79–81.
18. Mahon EM, Mahon SM. Music therapy: a valuable adjunct in the oncology setting. Clin J Oncol Nurs. 2011;15(4):353–6.
19. Hauck M, Metzner S, Rohlffs F, Lorenz J, Engel A. The influence of music and music therapy on pain-induced neuronal oscillations measured by magnetoencephalography. Pain. 2013;154(4):539–47.
20. Archie P, Bruera E, Cohen L. Music-based Interventions in palliative cancer care: a review of quantitative studies and neurobiological literature. Support Care Cancer [Internet]. 2013 May 30 [cited July 24, 2014];21:2609–2624. Available from: http://link.springer.com/article/10.1007/s00520-013-1841-4
21. McKinney CH, Antoni MH, Kumar M, Tims FC, McCabe PM. Effects of guided imagery and music therapy on mood and cortisol in healthy adults. Health Psychol. 1997;16(4):390–400.
22. Blood A, Zatorre R, Bermudez P, Evans A. Emotional responses to pleasant and unpleasant music correlate with activity in paralimbic brain regions. Nat Neurosci. 1999;2(4):382–7.
23. Hillecke TK, Nickel A, Bolay HV. Scientific perspectives on music therapy. Ann N Y Acad Sci. 2005;1060:1–12.
24. Wiech K, Ploner M, Tracey I. Neurocognitive aspects of pain perception. Trends Cogn Sci [Internet]. Available online 5 July 2008 [cited July 24, 2014];12(8): 306–13.
25. Koelsch S. A neuroscientific perspective on music therapy. Neurosciences and Music III-Disorders and Plasticity, Ann N Y Acad Sci. 2009;1169: 374–84.
26. Koenig, J, Warth M, Oelkers-Ax R, Wormit A, Bardenheuer HJ, Resch F. et al. I need to hear some sounds that recognize the pain in me: an integrative review of a decade of research in the development of active music therapy outpatient treatment in patients with recurrent or chronic pain. Music Med [Internet] 2013 [cited on November 10, 2013];5(3):150–61.
27. Kenny D, Faunce G. The impact of group singing on mood, coping, an perceived pain in chronic pain patients attending a multidisciplinary pain clinic. J Music Ther. 2004;XLI(3):241–58.
28. Burns D. Theoretic rationale for music selection in oncology intervention research: an integrative review. J Music Ther. 2012;49(1 Spring):7–22.
29. Wormit AF, Warth M, Koenig J, Hillecke T, Bardenheuer HJ. Evaluating a treatment manual for music therapy in adult cancer care. Music Med [Internet]. 2012;4(2):65–73.
30. Pothoulaki M, Macdonald R, Flowers P. An interpretive phenomenological analysis of an improvisational music therapy program for cancer patients. J Music Ther. 2012;49(1 Spring):45–67.
31. American Art Therapy Association [Internet]. Alexandria: AATA [cited July 24, 2014]. Available from: http://www.arttherapy.org/aata-aboutus.html
32. Luzzatto P, Sereno V, Capps R. A communication tool for cancer patients with pain: the art therapy technique with the body outline. Palliat Support Care. 2003;1:135–42.
33. AATA [Internet]. Alexandria: AATA [cited July 26, 2014]. Available from: http://www.americanarttherapyassociation.org/upload/LOCATOR2.15.11.pdf
34. Art Therapy Credential Board (ATCB) [Internet]. Greensboro: ATCB. [cited on July 26, 2014]. Available from http://atcb.org/home/find_a_credentialed_art_therapist/
35. Wood MJM, Molassiotis A, Payne S. What research evidence is there for the use of art therapy in the management of symptoms in adults with cancer? A systematic review. Psycho-Oncology. 2011;20:135–45. Epub 2010 Mar 24.
36. Singh B. The therapeutic effects of art making in patients with cancer. Arts Psychother. 2011;38:160–3.
37. Geue K, Goetze H, Buttstaedt M, Kleinert E, Richter D, Singer S. An overview of art therapy interventions for cancer patients and the results of research. Complement Ther Med. 2010;18:160–70. Epub 2015 May 15.
38. Nainis N, Paice J, Ratner J, Wirth J, Lai J, Shott S. Relieving symptoms in cancer: innovative use of art therapy. J Pain Symptom Manage. 2006;31(2):162–9.
39. Monti D, Peterson C, Kunkel EJS, Hauck W, Pequignot E, Rhodes L, Brainard GC. A randomized controlled trial of mindfulness-based art therapy (MBAT) for women with cancer. Psycho-Oncol. 2006;15:363–73. Epub 2005 Nov 15.
40. Cassileth BR, Keefe F. Integrative and behavioral approaches to the treatment of cancer-related neuropathic pain. Oncologist. 2010;15(suppl 2):19–23.
41. Kwekkeboom KL, Cherwin CH, Lee JW, Wanta B. Mind-body treatments for the pain-fatigue-sleep disturbance symptom cluster in persons with cancer. J Pain Symptom Manag. 2010;39(1): 126–38.
42. NCCAM. Mind-body medicine practices in complementary and alternative medicine [Internet]. Bethesda: NCCAM (page last updated March 29, 2013; cited on July 26, 2014). Available from: http://report.nih.gov/nihfactsheets/viewfactsheet.aspx?csid=102
43. Simpson CA. Complementary and alternative medicine. In: Fishman SM, Ballantyne JC, Rathmell JP, editors. Bonica's management of pain. 4th ed. Baltimore: Wolters Kluwer; 2010. p. P1365–74.
44. Hall H. The war on chiropractors. 2012 Oct 23 [cited 2014 Jul 26]. In: Science-based medicine blog [Internet]. Available from: http://www.sciencebasedmedicine.org/the-war-against-chiropractors
45. Kent M. False cry of quackery. Cited on July 27, 2014. Available from: http://campaignfortruth.com/Eclub/011101/FALSECRYOFQUACKERY.htm
46. Wilk v. American Medical Ass'n, 671 F. Supp. 1465, N.D. Ill. 1987. [Internet]. Available from: http://en.wikipedia.org/wiki/Wilk_v._American_Medical_Association
47. Government. Massage therapy [Internet]. New York: MedicineNet. 2014 Apr 2 [cited July 26, 2014]. Available from: http://www.medicinenet.com/massage_therapy/article.htm
48. Calvert RN. Pages from history: Swedish massage. Massage Magazine [Internet]. 2014 April 24 [cited July 26, 2014]. Available from: http://www.massagemag.com/magazine-2002-issue100-history100-24026/
49. NCCAM. Massage therapy: an introduction [Internet]. Silver Spring: NCCAM. [cited July 26, 2014]. Available from: http://nccam.nih.gov/sites/nccam.nih.gov/files/D327.pdf
50. Corbin L. Safety and efficacy of massage therapy for patients with cancer. Cancer Control. 2005;12(3):158–63.
51. NCCAM. Massage therapy for health purposes: what you need to know [Internet]. Silver Spring: NCCAM. [cited July 26, 2014]. Available from: http://nccam.nih.gov/sites/nccam.nih.gov/files/Get_The_Facts_Massage_Therapy_02-20-2014.pdf
52. Cassileth BR, Vickers AJ. Massage therapy for symptom control: outcome study at a major cancer center. J Pain Symptom Manag. 2004;28(3):244–8.
53. Myers CD, Walton T, Small BJ. The value of massage therapy in cancer care. Hematol Oncol Clin North Am. 2008;22:649–60.
54. NCBTMB [Internet]. Difference between licensure, national and board certification. Oakbrook Terrace: NCBTMB; [cited July 27, 2014]. Available from: http://www.ncbtmb.org/sites/default/files/files/Webinar_QA_Difference-between-Licensure-National-Board-Certification.pdf
55. AMTA [Internet]. Credentials for the massage therapy profession. Evanston: AMTA; c2014 [cited July 27, 2014]. Available from: http://www.amtamassage.org/findamassage/credential.html
56. California Massage Therapy Council [Internet]. Frequently asked questions. Sacramento; 2013 [cited July 27, 2014]. Available from: https://www.camtc.org/faq.aspx

57. Taylor MT. What is yoga therapy: an IAYT definition [Internet]. Little Rock: IAYT. 2007 [cited July 27, 2014]. Available from: http://c.ymcdn.com/sites/www.iayt.org/resource/resmgr/PDFs/IAYT_Yoga_therapy_definition.pdf
58. Satchidananda S. The yoga sutras of patanjali. 7th ed. Buckingham: Integral Yoga; 1999.
59. American Cancer Society [Internet]. Yoga. Atlanta: American Cancer Society; [updated 2008 Nov 1; cited July 27, 2014]. Available from: http://www.cancer.org/treatment/treatmentsandsideeffects/complementaryandalternativemedicine/mindbodyandspirit/yoga
60. DiStasio SA. Integrating yoga into cancer care. Clin J Oncol Nurs. 2008;12(1):125–30.
61. Bower JE, Woolery A, Sternlieb B, Garet D. Yoga for cancer patients and survivors. Cancer Control. 2005;12(3):165–71.
62. Duncan MD, Leis A, Taylor-Brown JW. Impact and outcomes of an Iyengar yoga program in a cancer centre. Curr Oncol. 2008;15(supp2):S72–7.
63. Danhauer SC, Mihalko SL, Russell GB, Campbell CR, Felder L, Daley K, Levine EA. Restorative yoga for women with breast cancer: findings from a randomized pilot study. Psycho-Oncology [Internet]. 2009 [cited July 28, 2014] [4p.]. doi:10.1002/pon.1503. Available from: http://www.ncbi.nlm.nih.gov/pmc/articles/PMC3930083/
64. Carson JW, Carson KM, Porter LS, Keefe FJ, Shaw H, Miller JM. Yoga for women with metastatic breast cancer: results from a pilot study. J Pain Symptom Manag. 2007;33(3):331–9.
65. Buffart LM, van Uffelen JGZ, Riphagen II, Brug J, van Mechelen W, Brown WJ, et al. Physical and psychosocial benefits of yoga in cancer patients and survivors, a systematic review and meta-analysis of randomized controlled trials. BMC Cancer [Internet]. 2012;12:559: [6p.]. Available from: http://www.biomedcentral.com/1471-2407/12/559
66. Lin KY, Hu YT, Chang KJ, Lin HF, Tsauo JY. Effects of yoga on psychological health, quality of life, and physical health of patients with cancer: a meta-analysis. Evid Based Complement Alternat Med [Internet]. 2011 Mar 9 [cited July 27, 2014];2011:659876 [12p.]. Available from: http://www.ncbi.nlm.nih.gov/pmc/articles/PMC3062158/
67. Banerjee B, Vadiraj HS, Ram A, Rao R, Jayapal M, Gopinath KS, et al. Effects of an integrated yoga program in modulating psychosocial stress and radiation-induced genotoxic stress in breast cancer patients undergoing radiotherapy. Integr Cancer Ther. 2007;6(3):n242–50.
68. Yoga Allliance [Internet]. Yoga teacher designations. Arlington: Yoga Alliance; c2015 [cited August 11, 2015].
69. Wayne PM, Kaptchuk TJ. Challenges inherent to t'ai chi research: part I. – t'ai chi as a complex multicomponent intervention. J Altern Complement Med. 2008;14(1):95–102.
70. Tai-chi.com [Internet]. Los Angeles: T'ai Chi: The International Magazine of T'ai Chi Ch'uan; c2009 [cited July 30, 2014]. Available from: http://www.tai-chi.com/taichi_info.php
71. Wikipedia contributors. T'ai chi ch'uan [Internet]. Wikipedia, the free encyclopedia; 2014 Jul 29, 21:07 UTC [cited 2014 Jul 30]. Available from: http://en.wikipedia.org/w/index.php?title=T%27ai_chi_ch%27uan&oldid=619029840
72. Mansky P, Sannes T, Wallerstedt D, Ge A, Ryan M, Johnson LL. Tai Chi Chuan: mind-body practice or exercise intervention? Studying the benefit for cancer survivors. Integr Cancer Ther. 2006;5(3):192–201.
73. Lee M, Choi TY. Tai chi for breast cancer patients: a systematic review. Breast Cancer Res Treat. 2010;120:309–16.
74. Wayne PM, Kaptchuk TJ. Challenges inherent to t'ai chi research: part II. – defining the intervention and optimal study design. J Altern Complement Med. 2008;14(2):191–7.
75. Bell IR, Kothan M. Models for the study of whole systems. Integr Cancer Ther. 2006;5(4):293–307.
76. Callahan D, editor. The role of complementary & alternative medicine: accommodating pluralism. Washington, DC: Georgetwon University Press; 2002.
77. Sciencebasedmedicine.org [Internet]. Science-based medicine; c2013 [cited July 29, 2014]. Available from: http://www.science-basedmedicine.org/about-science-based-medicine/
78. The New Medicine [Internet]. The New Medicine; c2005 [cited July 29, 2014]. Available from: http://www.thenewmedicine.org/about_the_show.html
79. Quackwatch.com [Internet]. Chapel Hill: Quackwatch; [updated August 1, 2014, cited August 1, 2014]. Available from: www.quackwatch.com

54 Botanical Treatments in Cancer Pain Management

Helen M. Blake

Introduction to Holistic, Alternative, and Complementary Medicine

Complementary and alternative medicine have become well-known terms for medical interventions and therapies that are distinct from conventional Western medicine. Complementary medicine refers to treatments that are used as an adjuvant to conventional treatment strategies. Alternative refers to those treatments that are used in place of conventional medicine. The focus of complementary and alternative medicine is on the whole person, rather than the disease. A patient's physical, mental, emotional, and spiritual health are addressed. Complementary medicine encompasses therapies such as meditation, acupuncture, reflexology, creative therapies, yoga, chiropractic care, massage therapy, herbal supplements, vitamins, and essential oils, among others (Table 54.1).

In 2007, the Center for Disease Control found in its National Health Statistics Survey that 38% of patients made use of complementary or alternative therapies [1]. Despite increasing interest and availability of these diverse interventions that facilitate healing and increase well-being, few patients in the United States are willing to completely substitute alternative medicine for their medical care. As such, the term integrative medicine has become preferred as it refers to a strategy which combines the best evidence-based practices in both conventional and complementary medical care.

In 1998, the National Institutes of Health (NIH) established the National Center for Complementary and Alternative Medicine (NCCAM). It has provided funding to numerous medical trials directed at evaluating the safety and efficacy of complementary and alternative medicine interventions. This research is conducted and monitored in the same rigorous manner as all other evidence-based medicine practiced in the United States.

H. M. Blake (✉)
Pain and Rehabilitation Specialists of Saint Louis, LLC, St. Louis, MO, USA
e-mail: hblake@prsstl.com

Ayurveda and Traditional Chinese Medicine

Ayurveda is the ancient medical principle native to the Indian subcontinent. Ayurveda is a blend of the Sanskrit word "Ayu" meaning life and "veda" meaning knowledge. Its literal translation is thus "the knowledge of life." Ayurveda is used both to treat illness and prevent it. The central philosophy of Ayurveda is to attain balance within the body and mind, which can be accomplished by restoring the balance of three basic factors. These represent three systems that make up the body: the nervous system (Vata or air), the venous system (Pitta or fire), and the arterial system (Kapha or water). Ayurvedic herbs and medicines are used to facilitate the restoration of balance along with massage, lifestyle change, detoxification, massage, meditation, and exercise.

By evaluating a person's physical and emotional ailments, a treatment strategy is developed. In addition to the prevention and resolution of disease, the effects include increased spiritual well-being, restored harmony with the world, and improved physical vitality. Some herbal medicines used in Ayurvedic practice have been purified into commercial drugs to treat cancer including vincristine, vinblastine, and taxol. In a controlled clinical trial of cancer patients suffering from opioid-induced constipation in India, researchers found that the Ayurvedic preparation Misrakasneham was as effective as senna at reducing opi-

Table 54.1 Complementary and alternative therapies

Acupuncture	Meditation
Ayurveda	Movement therapies
Biofeedback	Natural products
Chelation therapy	Naturopathy
Chiropractic or osteopathic manipulation	Progressive relaxation
Deep breathing exercises	Qi gong
Diet based therapies	Tai Chi
Energy healing therapy/Reiki	Traditional healers
Guided imagery	Yoga
Homeopathic treatment	Massage
Hypnosis	

A. Gulati et al. (eds.), *Essentials of Interventional Cancer Pain Management*, https://doi.org/10.1007/978-3-319-99684-4_54

oid-induced constipation [2]. The laxative effect of the herbal preparation was accompanied by a more tolerable taste, an acceptable side effect profile, and low cost.

Traditional Chinese medicine is also an ancient philosophy of medical care grounded in the value of restoring balance to the body. Good health can be attained and maintained by aligning energy, body, and spirit. In practice, the mind and the body are not viewed separately, but rather as one interconnected system. The vital force or energy responsible for controlling the human mind and body is known as the Qi. When Qi is out of balance, it causes disease and illness. When the flow is corrected, the body is restored to balance. To achieve balance in Qi two opposing forces, Yin and Yang, must achieve harmony. Herbal medicines are the cornerstone of traditional Chinese medicine and are used in conjunction with acupuncture, acupressure, exercise, massage, meditation, and lifestyle changes.

The potent effects of herbal preparations have been known for centuries, and the knowledge of various botanicals encompasses a body of knowledge far wider than the scope of this textbook. This introduction to the medicinal herbs used can augment the pain practitioner's armamentarium of possible adjuvant treatments.

Benefits of Botanicals

The significance of pain as it pertains to the patient fighting cancer is well documented throughout this work. Pain is often considered the most common complaint for which cancer patients seek treatment. Western medicine offers the patient a diverse selection of medications and interventional therapies to address a range of patient complaints. However, any physician devoted to the treatment of pain in the cancer patient has experienced inherent inadequacy of commonly accepted analgesic regimens.

Commonly used pain medications often cause untoward side effects like fatigue, sedation, constipation, and depression. To the patient and their family, these side effects can create anxiety and psychological distress in the context of ongoing cancer treatment. In fact, cancer patients often suffer from many symptoms prior to initiation of pain medication that are then exacerbated as a side effect of therapy (Table 54.2) [3]. Health-care providers often accept these worsening side effects in their patients and treat them symptomatically. The benefit of halting the ensuing and worsening experience of pain as cancer progresses often outweighs the risk of side effects related to the medication. We use adjuvant medications to supplement ongoing therapy or turn to interventional therapies to mitigate these side effects. Botanical treatments are effective when both used synergistically with traditionally accepted therapies and individually to facilitate pain control and manage symptoms related to cancer that traditional medication regimens tend to worsen.

Table 54.2 Symptom prevalence in cancer patients [3]

Lack of energy	73.7%
Worrying	70.7%
Feeling sad	65%
Feeling nervous	61.3%
Feeling drowsy	59.8%
Difficulty sleeping	52.3%
Lack of appetite	44.4%
Constipation	34.7%
Weight loss	27.1%
Dizziness	23.6%
Shortness of breath	23.5%
Nausea/vomiting	20.6%

More than 25% of drugs used during the last 20 years are directly derived from plants [4]. In many cases, they offer an opiate sparing effect that can reduce the requirement for morphine or other similar mu-opiate agonists. Many botanical therapies promote relaxation, which has a positive impact on the psychological distress experienced by cancer patients. The improvement of vital physiological processes of sleep, digestion, nutrient absorption, and elimination can lead to increased vitality and vigor.

Some botanical strategies also have an anti-inflammatory effect, inhibiting multiple pro-inflammatory cytokines including COX-2, IL-1, IL-6, and TNF-alpha. The coagulation cascade is also affected by some botanical therapies, which can limit patient risk in development of venous thromboembolism. Some herbal medicines have a direct effect on the prevention of tumor progression and metastasis. The use of these potent natural compounds can have a profound impact on the cancer patient suffering from pain. Botanical alternatives are not only well tolerated and effective, but their use can free the mind to better focus on the process of healing.

Application of Specific Botanical Therapies

Throughout history, perhaps one of the most widely known herbal medications is opium. Opium, isolated from the seeds of opium poppies, yields the recognizable and potent painkiller, morphine. By binding mu-receptors, the analgesics derived from morphine exert analgesia, but also affect respiration and gastrointestinal motility. These well-known effects of the medications are believed to decrease the "vital force." This suppression of the vital force can have deleterious effects of exacerbating tumor progression secondary to facilitation of angiogenesis [5].

Much of the following information was derived from information contained within the materia medica [6]. The materia medica is a body of collected knowledge translated and compiled from leading medical textbooks in China. It is an essential resource for the practice of traditional Chinese medicine and offers entries on more than 470 herbs and medicinal substances. Many of the herbal medicines that are particularly useful for cancer pain treatment are listed under Chapters 10 and 12: "Herbs That Invigorate the Blood" and "Herbs That Tonify the Blood." Angiogenesis and hemostasis are consistently associated with cancerous conditions and tumor progression. Invigoration of the blood can prevent undesired clotting and stasis within the tissues, and tonification of the blood strengthens the circulatory processes of the body and supplements substances and nutrients that may otherwise be insufficient. Several relevant herbs are discussed below, and their dosage and use are summarized in Table 54.3. Each of these herbs has also demonstrated antitumor activity that suggests potential synergism between the chemotherapeutic treatments of allopathic medicine and the herbal treatments of traditional Chinese medicine.

Table 54.3 Summary of important botanical therapies in cancer pain management

Botanical	Use	Dosage	Toxicity
Corydalis yanhusuo	Pain, especially that associated with blood stasis, and abdominal pain	Rhizome powder form: 4.5–12 g dl-THP pills: 300–600 mg for anti-arrhythmic 100–200 at bedtime for insomnia 75 mg daily for neuropathic pain	The LD_{50} for oral administration in mice ranges from 36–125.3 g/kg
Panax notoginseng	Acute pain and inflammation will stop minor bleeding	3–9 g (1–3 g direct as powder)	Very safe chemical minimal lethal intravenous dose in mice is 460 mg/kg
Radix Paeoniae Rubra	Pain, notably muscle pain from paclitaxel	4.5–9 g prepared from good quality root	Very safe LD_{50} for intravenous administration is 3530 mg/kg
Radix Angelicae Sinensis	Pain from inflammation and especially due to accesses and uterine sources	3 g daily in 3 divided doses Daily dosage range 3–15 g	No established LD50 well tolerated and safe Avoid in estrogen sensitive tumors
Boswellia carterii	Traumatic pain from blood stasis	3–9 g fried with vinegar	
Curcuma longa	Pain, especially neuropathic	3–9 g, combined with oil as an ointment, if desired	Contraindicated in blood deficiencies

Corydalis (*Corydalis yanhusuo*)

Corydalis is an herb native to China and used extensively in traditional Chinese medicine for pain control. It is particularly effective for pain related to blood stasis and gastrointestinal pain related to ulcers and obstruction. Corydalis appears to function through inhibition of the reticular activating system in the brain. In the body, it has an analgesic effect, approximately 1% the potency of pure opium. Extracts formulated with alcohol and acetic acid are approximately 40% as effective as morphine [6]. The herbal preparations are excreted by the kidneys.

Corydalis can treat insomnia and has potent anticonvulsant action. Through the reversal of stasis in the body, it increases cellular waste removal and improves nutrient uptake at a cellular level. *Corydalis yanhusuo* also has potent cytotoxic effects and has been shown to inhibit p-glycoprotein and multidrug resistance-associated protein 1 in cancer cell lines [7] and suppresses the oncogene N-ras mRNA [8]. These cytotoxic effects position corydalis as an effective adjuvant to many chemotherapeutic regimens in addition to the potential effects on pain control.

Panax notoginseng

Panax notoginseng is the drug of choice in traditional Chinese medicine to treat inflammatory pain due to traumatic injury such as falls, fractures, contusions, and sprains. It has potent effects on reversing blood stasis and can effectively treat joint pains due to blood stasis and chest pain such as angina. *Panax notoginseng* stops bleeding without causing blood stasis. It has potent effect on our circulatory system, dilating coronary arteries and restoring microcirculation to damaged cardiac muscle. Research studies have also shown antitumor effects [6].

Peony, Red and White (Radix Paeoniae Rubra, Radix Paeoniae Lactiflorae)

Peony is particularly effective at treating spasmodic conditions and muscular pain. Through its effects on reversing blood stasis, it can resolve liver pain and improve pain and swelling due to trauma. The spasmolytic effects appear to be mediated by interference with acetylcholine release into the neuromuscular junction [6]. Peony root extracts also have anticancer effects through antiproliferative and apoptotic effects [9].

Dong Quai (*Angelica sinensis*)

Dong quai is a potent tonifier of the blood and is commonly used for pain that is associated with blood stasis. Traditional uses are in menstrual disorders and dysmenorrhea [6]. The antitumor effects of dong quai may be due to its inhibitory effects on invasion and metastasis of carcinoma cells [10]. Injection of dong quai into acupuncture points can produce significant improvement of pain due to neuralgia, ischemic pain, occipital neuralgia, and arthritis. Dong quai can also function as an antispasmodic. It is also a source of vitamin B12 and can help facilitate improvement of anemias caused during chemotherapy.

Boswellia carterii (Frankincense)

Especially helpful for pain which arises from blood stasis, carbuncles, sores, swelling, and similar pain, Boswellia invigorates the blood and promotes movement of qi [6]. It can be applied topically as an ointment or powder to reduce swelling, promote healing, and relieve pain in these conditions. The familiar combination of "frankincense" and "myrrh" invigorates the blood and can alleviate chest pain associated with stasis in the cardiac system.

Boswellia inhibits COX-2 and 15-lipoxygenase. This function has potent antilipid effects that can serve to slow the progression of atherosclerosis as well as modulate the anti-inflammatory effects. Some studies have shown that the gumlike resins have potent antitumor and immune enhancing activity that prove particularly useful in the cancer patient.

Curcuma longa (Turmeric)

Turmeric is known for its culinary uses in curry powder. Prevalent in the Indian and Asian continents, turmeric has anticancer, antioxidant, anti-inflammatory, fibrinolytic, and liver-protective properties. The active compound is the yellowish-orange oil that gives the herb its deep color. Curcumin exerts its effects largely via the coagulation cascade. It activates plasmin, which breaks down fibrin. This is essential to the anticancer effects of curcumin.

Curcumin promotes the movement of qi and alleviates pain from stagnant qi, especially that in the epigastric and abdominal area [6]. In addition to anti-inflammatory and anticancer effects, curcumin can lower blood pressure and has antibiotic effects against *Staphylococcus aureus.*

Conclusion

There are diverse natural agents that can have a profound effect on patients with ongoing cancer pain. These adjuvants can complement a traditional medication regimen with minimal opioid medications and thus spare the cancer patient from myriad deleterious side effects. Hopefully, this chapter will inspire the reader to expand their knowledge further to implement botanical therapies in their practice of cancer pain. Certainly, the complementary therapies introduced have potential to improve patient's quality of life as they battle the fight of their life.

References

1. Barnes P, Bloom B, Nahin R. Complementary and alternative medicine use among adults and children. National health statistics reports; no 12. Hyattsville: National Center for Health Statistics; 2007.
2. Ramesh P, Kumar K, Rajagopal M, Balachandran P, Warrier P. Managing morphine-induced constipation: a controlled comparison of an ayurvedic formulation and senna. J Pain Symptom Manage. 1998;16(4):240–4.
3. Portenoy RK, Thaler HT, Kornblith AB, Lepore JM, Friedlander-Klar H, Coole N, Smart-Curley T, Kemeny N, Norton L, Hoskins W, Scher H. Symptom prevalence, characteristics and distress in a cancer population. Qual Life Res. 1994;3(3):183–9.
4. Cravotto G, Boffa L, Genzini L, Garella D. Phytotherapeutics: an evaluation of the potential of 1000 plants. J Clin Pharm Ther. 2010;35(1):11–48.
5. Gupta K, Kshirsagar S, Chang L, Schwartz R, Law P, Yee D, Hebbl R. Morphine stimulates angiogenesis by activating proangiogenic an survival promoting signaling and promotes breast tumor growth. Cancer Res. 2002;62(15):4491–8.
6. Bensky D, Gamble G, editors. Chinese herbal medicine: materia medica. Seattle: Eastland Press; 1993.
7. Lei Y, Tan J, Wink M, Ma Y, Li N, Su G. An isoquinoline alkaloid from the Chinese heal plant Corydalis yanhusuo W.T. Wang inhibits P-glycopotein and multi drug resistance-associate protein 1. Food Chem. 2013;15(136):1117–21.
8. Xu Z, Chen X, Zhang Q. Corydalis yanhusuo W.T. Wang extract inhibit MCF-7 cell proliferation by inducing cell cycle G2/M arrest. Am J Chin Med. 2011;39(3):579–86.
9. Li C, Yazawa K, Kondo S, Mukudai Y, Sato D, Kurihara Y, Kamatani T, Sinta I. The root park of Paeonia moutan is a potential anticancer agent in human oral squamous cell carcinoma cells. Anticancer Res. 2012;32(7):2625–30.
10. Shang P, Qian A, Yang T, Jia M, Mei Q, Cho C, Zhao W, Chen Z. Experimental study of anti-tumor effects of polysaccharides from Angelica sinensis. World J Gastroenterol. 2003;9(9):1963–7.

Integrative Therapies for Pain Modulation

55

Joan Pope and Aron Legler

Introduction

This chapter will focus on some non-pharmacological therapies that may support the first line of pain treatment, namely, morphine derivatives, especially opioids, anxiolytics, muscle relaxants, etc. Collectively, these therapies go under various group names: complementary, alternative, adjuvant, integrative, and others. Many of these techniques are now being sought by patients for both acute and chronic pain, such as meditation, mindfulness, reflexology, hypnotherapy, herbal medicine, acupuncture, music and art therapy, reiki therapy, and therapeutic touch.

In general, these techniques are ill-suited to hospital bedside applications. There are various reasons for this, for example, many of these methods are most efficacious in peaceful surroundings requiring at least 30 min without interruption: unfortunately, hospitals may have too many distractions. In fact, there are few, if any, medical schools or schools of nursing that teach these practices for relief of pain. And in most hospitals, there are few bedside caregivers who utilize these techniques. Because the delivery of these techniques is personal, the remainder of the chapter will highlight past experiences during treatment of patients suffering from severe cancer pain.

Choosing Patients for Adjuvant Pain Modulation

If the patient is not experiencing acute pain, a complete family, social, and medical history is obtained to develop a rapport with the patient. The length of stay will help decide how much time can be spent on these techniques and which would be most effective given time constraints. A patient's sense of anger and fear, for example, to chemotherapy, radiation, and surgery, may require more preparation and personal rapport prior to proceeding. Much of the relief of pain symptoms is dependent on personality qualities between the patient and practitioner. After developing trust and commitment with one another can practitioners proceed with image-guided techniques discussed below.

An assessment of a patient's mental status, such as memory loss, wakefulness, ability to concentrate, and level of fatigue, is invaluable for suitability. For example, can he/she participate in an experience of guided imagery or hypnosis? Patients with anemia, with fatigue after cancer treatment, and on multiple medications may suffer from fatigue preventing active participation. Physical symptoms such as nausea, emesis, or respiratory distress are obvious impediments to the planned treatment.

Perhaps overlooked is the practitioner's own mood and peacefulness. The art of image guidance requires a bond with the patient. Emotions that the practitioner feels will be interpreted by the patient. It is difficult to transmit images of relaxation if the practitioner is hurried and stressed. Both mental health of the practitioner to deliver a message and the patient's ability to absorb the treatment are important for success.

Case 1 *When I first met Ben, a 15-year-old boy who had been treated for leukemia at age 12, he had experienced a recurrence of disease and, during his hope for remission and a bone marrow transplant, had begun to exhibit signs of frustration. He and his mother were already practiced in meditation through prayer. I explained how we could use similar practices, techniques in relaxation and image-guided hypnosis, to assist him through chemotherapy and, eventually, posttransplant. After a few sessions developing a rapport, Ben shared his passions and dreams, and because he wanted to continue pursuing them, he accepted*

J. Pope (✉)
Memorial Sloan Kettering, New York, NY, USA
e-mail: popej@mscc.org

A. Legler
Memorial Sloan Kettering, Department of Anesthesiology, New York, NY, USA

A. Gulati et al. (eds.), *Essentials of Interventional Cancer Pain Management*, https://doi.org/10.1007/978-3-319-99684-4_55

the treatment. For several weeks we successfully used image-guided hypnosis to help with nausea and control his pain.

During the bone marrow transplant and posttreatment, we changed techniques, focusing on relaxation during each session. The initiation phase guided him into a light trance, closing his eyes, focusing on his breathing in and out, and slowly taking longer inhalations and exhalations. Using a part of his history, he remembered a happy time at his parents' garden. This is the focus of his hypnotic trance, having the patient focus on a more favorable environment to achieve a calmer state of mind. The following is an excerpt of the trance state.

As his body relaxed, I started with the suggestions to initiate the hypnotic state.

"We are going back to the garden you and your parents planted 4 years ago. It's spring now, the grass is light green, and buds are forming on the trees. Tell me what you see." (Here we are invoking patient participation so he can be actively engaged in becoming hypnotized). He described his surroundings.

"Those trees that were dry and leafless and seemed dead in February, March, and early April are forming buds, new growth. And the daffodils just pushing up out of the earth, the stems are growing tall out of the ground; your body, too, which had had leukemia cells die with the chemotherapy, is getting strong with the stem cells. New growth is taking place in your bone marrow. As the sap comes up from the roots of the trees into the branches, so the cells from your bone marrow transplant are maturing and coming into your blood vessels. The blood flowing through these vessels is bringing strength and health to your body. The strong red blood cells are carrying oxygen from your lungs to your heart and throughout your whole body. The healthy white blood cells are moving to clear the infection from your mouth and intestines. Your mouth sores are improving. Your taste buds are awakening; taking the apple juice on the table by you, you smell the aroma and as you sip it, you know its apple juice. This brings a smile to your face and heart. There is a slight memory of what it was like when you were a baby tasting apple juice for the first time. This joy you can take with you as you slowly come back from the garden to this room. You know that through the day you'll have other experiences of the healing taking place in you. I want you to take a slow deep breath and let it out. In the next minute, when you're ready, slowly open your eyes and come back to this room."

A year later I received a picture of Ben with his family in the garden. He is in his graduation cap and gown. His mother has a small bouquet of daffodils, grape hyacinths, and an iris in her hands. This is bond we hope to make with our patients, leading to a successful future.

Consciousness and Hypnosis

The first documented use of "mesmeric sleep" as a successful anesthetic during surgery was described by John Elliotson in the 1840s [1]. Since that time, a variety of methods and techniques have been employed with varying success. From the perspective of an image-guided therapist, pain follows an adage that it resides "in our head." While pain is defined as a perception in the brain of an unpleasant sensation created by a noxious stimulus or tissue damage from a point in the body, hypnosis and guided therapies aim to disrupt this perception and reduce patient suffering.

The effectiveness of hypnotic states has been shown in meta-analysis to be effective for pain management with a moderate to large effect size, though the hypnotic analgesic effects were found to differ based on participants level of susceptibility [2]. At this time, possibly due to difficulties associated with study design and conflicting results, there is no consensus as to whether complementary therapies should be included for pain control. However, even those who are unconvinced by current evidence concede it may improve patient well-being [3]. Further well-designed controlled research is needed to augment the wealth of anecdotal reports that exist.

New imaging modalities have been used to elucidate possible mechanisms for hypnotic modulation on pain perception. A study using positron emission tomography found "the hypnotic state, significantly enhanced the functional modulation between midcingulate cortex and a large neural network involved in sensory, affective, cognitive and behavioral aspects of nociception" [4]. fMRI studies have also been used in this regard and have shown that activations of the midbrain, cerebellum, thalamus, and midcingulate, primary and secondary sensory, inferior parietal, insula, and prefrontal cortices correlated with reported changes in pain with hypnotic and non-hypnotic suggestion; however these activations were of greater magnitude when suggestions followed a hypnotic induction [5].

The pain response to illness and treatment is variable in every individual, and it may change in the same individual from day to day. This accounts for the wide variability in pharmaceutical and/or psychological treatment response rates. It helps to describe why the psychological modulations for the relief of pain may be a daily experience for both the patient and the caregiver.

Since a large part of pain perception is emotional, when one's emotions change, for example, from a good mood to a bad mood, his or her pain will be more intense or less intense [6].

Case 2 *Of the six or so human emotions the one that has, the most negative effect on pain relief is fear. I come across this frequently in my practice as patients in cancer hospitals have* *a lot of fear, as epitomized by Carole, a 58-year-old woman status post 3 days from abdominal surgery for colon cancer. I called her name as I opened her bedroom curtain. At that time a surgical resident was beginning to remove her sutures and express fluid from the wound; she pulled the bed covers up to her eyes and trembled with anticipatory fear of pain. I went to her bedside, and as I took her hand, I said, "take my hand Carole, don't look at the doctor, and instead look at me. Slow down your breathing like this, smell the flowers now blow out the candles. Close your eyes and imagine the place where you most like to be. Where are you now Carole? In church, Sacred Heart Church. Sit down in the pew and describe what you see."*

She described the status, giving names to them, and then she talked about the stained-glass windows and the sunlight beaming through them. She said she wanted to pray, and we prayed together. When the surgeon announced that he was finished, she remarked with great surprise that the procedure had not taken long and that it had not hurt. I asked her to rate her pain. She said that out of 10 it was 2 and 1/2 and that she could not believe that it was so low.

On return visits by this patient, it was gratifying to learn that our 15-min encounter had been the beginning of a trusting relationship. Gradually, she got rid of her fear of further cancer. These quick interventions in the fast-moving situations of a cancer hospital may have long-term benefits with respect to modulating an individual's pain before it becomes chronic.

There is growing evidence that as pain becomes more chronic, it becomes more resistant to standard modulatory techniques. Evidence even exists for anatomical alterations in the signaling system for pain, in both emotional and cognitive parts, in patients with chronic pain. There appears to be a thickening of nerve fibers and opioid receptor damage or destruction in persons with chronic pain which intensifies the longer the pain endures. Such patients may require treatment with antidepressants and anxiolytics [6].

Relaxation

An individual's stress is almost as unique to that person as his or her fingerprints. Stress is the same biochemical experience for every human being; but when, how, or why it occurs in one person differs from another individual. Each person discovers by experience what relieves his or her own stress, for example, walking, exercise, reading, listening to music, and reciting a mantra; but for some individuals' repetitive stressful experiences, such as those encountered in a cancer hospital, stressors cause passivity and even depression. Understanding this relationship is an important skillset for providers wishing to provide adjuvant therapies for pain.

Guiding a patient who needs help to achieve a desirable level of relaxation may take as long as 60 min or as little as 5 min. Time is often a considerable restraint on applying this therapy for a patient. A typical session with a patient may follow this schema: Start by telling the person to sit or lie comfortably. Guide them to slowly inhale while counting 1–5; then exhale 6–12. Do this for 4 cycles. Next introduce visualizing the breath. Remind the patient that as he or she breathes and he or she can see the oxygen as a light blue color. Avoid leading the patient with a specific light blue such as baby blue; instead allow the person to pick his or her own blue. Instruct the patient to inhale through the top of his OR her head bringing the clear light blue oxygen to his or her scalp, brain, eyes, ears, nose, mouth, and throat. Remind the patient that as he or she exhales, the carbon dioxide takes away any impurities or illnesses in his or her brain, scalp, eyes, ears, nose, mouth, and throat. As the patient takes the next breath, the light blue oxygen comes through his or her shoulders, arms, fingers, and arteries. This is continued throughout the entire body.

This technique, which can be done by an individual alone for self-benefit, is modeled a course called "The Life You Save May Be Your Own" developed by D. Pachuta, MD. The following is an example of therapeutic relaxation.

Case 3 *Mary and I worked together for a 2-year period. She had been diagnosed with CNS lymphoma. She was 62 years old, widowed with four children and six grandchildren. Some of her presenting disabilities were memory loss, agitation, fear, swollen legs, and fatigue. During her 7 months of treatment, we got to know each other well. Assisting her in relaxation was challenged by her short-term memory loss. For the first few weeks, relaxation would start: "'Mary, I'm Joan; we met yesterday. We talked about your children, she smiles. Tell me, did you have a good night, how is your pain. 'BAD!' Where is the one place the pain is the worst. 'My low back.' Can we do the relaxation we did yesterday to help get rid of a little of the pain? 'I'd like that.'" She enjoyed having her hands held, so taking her right hand in mine we would continue. "I'd like you to close your eyes and we'll go back to the beach where we were yesterday." As she closes her eyes I continue; "you're walking down Ocean City Beach and you see a place on the beach that is a little bit away from the crowd. It is a warm sunny day. The water feels like bath water, you lay down on the beach and the first wave touches your toes and then your ankles, as the wave goes back out to sea it takes away any tightness and pain in your feet." Slowly I take her through her entire body to her chest, each wave bringing in warmth and relaxation, each receding wave removing stiffness, tightness, and pain.*

When her memory improved, I made a tape of the relaxation, and she began to practice at home. Mary was cured; however, a side effect of the chemotherapy caused her to have neuropathic pain in her legs from her knees to her toes. Periodically she would be hospitalized with increased pain. Over the years she has had a reduction in the pain. She was hospitalized for leg pain from her knees to her mid calves. Similar to many people with chronic pain, she tends to dwell on the pain and forgets the things she can when she has less pain. Today she was out of the bed in the chair, and as soon as we saw each other, we smiled; I hugged her, saying, "Wow your feet no longer hurt. You have happy feet." This surprised her, and she said "YES that is right." I do feel a bit better. We talked about adjusting her medications and hoped for further improvement.

In this last encounter, I used distraction as part of the therapy. When I returned the next day, we were able to evaluate if she was any better with the medication adjustments. I reminded her that she still had happy feet and gave her the task of getting the video of "Happy Feet" to watch with her young grandchildren. This might help her to remember that she is feeling better.

Reflexology

This non-pharmacological therapy consists of massaging a patient's hand or feet, based on the theory that the human body contains ten zones of biologic activity for which there exists a corresponding pressure point on each person's hands or feet. After locating the zone in which pain is felt, the therapist massages the corresponding pressure point on the patient's hands or feet. It can be done quickly, and if any change or improvement results in the pain, it may be repeated. Systematic reviews for a variety of medical conditions failed to demonstrate convincingly that reflexology is effective; this may be due to poor-quality studies with low sample sizes [7, 8]. Despite this, reflexology is considered a very low-risk and inexpensive adjunct that many patients will pursue. One benefit for patients with metastatic cancer, whose partners were taught reflexology and used the technique on the patient, is having immediate decrease in pain intensity and anxiety [9].

Case 4 *Gerald was a patient of mine, while I worked at Hospice of Connecticut. He was 56 years old, suffering from severe bone pain in his low spine due to metastatic prostate cancer. I had given him his morphine sulfate pills and began to talk with him about hand reflexology. At that time, I had been practicing reflexology with people who had colds, toothaches, headaches, sinusitis and stomachaches, and general tiredness. I prefer hand reflexology to foot reflexology because our hands are readily accessible. I showed Gerald on my hand where the spine was located, in particular the sacrum and coccyx which was were his pain was most severe, noting that these are located on both hands since they are central in the body. Placing his left hand in mine, he told me to give it a try. Originally, I put pressure on the point with too much force. Yelling "OUCH my back," he pulled his hand away. Mortified, I apologized and got another order for a STAT rescue of IV morphine sulfate. After the medicine took effect, I explained that I had put too much pressure on the point. I did not start gently and go slow. Unfortunately, at Gerald's expense I learned a lesson I've never forgotten, I can't take away all of a patient's pain and "Slow is beautiful."*

The next day to my surprise, Gerald asked me to teach him the entire body reflex points on the hands. More surprisingly, he requested I work with him using less pressure. Gerald was discharged from in-patient hospice to home hospice care. He had me teach his wife reflexology, so they could treat each other. I continue to practice reflexology, often massaging the nervous system of a patient after I shake their hands during morning rounds.

Conclusion

In a 2008 survey of the literature on integrative therapies for pain management, the investigators found that nurses do not utilize nondrug pain control methods as a routine [10]. Some factors in this omission may be a lack of time; nonacceptance by patients, physicians, or administrators; and so forth.

On the other hand, the 2007 National Health Interview Survey found that 38% of all Americans used integrative therapies and 32% of these used them for various kinds of pain [11]. A Harvard survey in 2013 of the literature on chronic pelvic pain management reported a study of 22 women enrolled in a mindful meditation program for 8 weeks with daily assessments of pain and symptoms of depression. Barely half of the women finished the program, and the investigators found that these 12 showed significant reductions in pain scores. The same survey concluded that women in general, more than men, tend to seek out mind-body complementary therapies, while men sought out and preferred herbal medicine and acupuncture [11].

In the Harvard analysis of the literature of nondrug therapies for chronic pelvic pain, it was reported that many of the studies were not blinded or randomized and that the data they presented is difficult to replicate. Another critique of the same studies was their small sample size. Scientifically, they concluded, future studies should "improve external validity," that is, be blinded and randomized with larger cohorts of subjects [11].

It is irrefutable that the physiological evidence of brain function points to an important, but not well defined, contribution of an individual's emotions, as well as his or her idiosyncratic psychology, in the experience of pain perception and sensitivity. Yet, there are few accepted objective measurements for these subjective phenomena. One measure that attempts objectivity is the quantitative sensory testing (QST) [12]. QST assess patients' sensitivity to different pain stimuli, for example, heat and cold, and it is routinely used to calculate sensory loss or gain in patients suffering from neuropathic pain. A high pain sensitivity may accurately predict a negative outcome for an individual's pain management program.

Physiologically, human brains and nervous systems are very similar from one individual to another, but the mind and subjective experience of an individual is very different. This may emphasize the challenge to future investigators who seek to quantify and objectify the emotional and psychological factors in pain perception and the effect of pain modulatory techniques on the experience of pain, both pharmacologic and non-pharmacologic.

References

1. Elliotson J. Numerous cases of surgical operations without pain in the mesmeric state: with remarks upon the opposition of many members of the Royal Medical and Chirurgical Society and others to the reception of the inestimable blessings of mesmerism. Philadelphia: Lea & Blanchard; 1843.
2. Montgomery GH, DuHamel KN, Redd WH. A meta-analysis of hypnotically induced analgesia: how effective is hypnosis? Int J Clin Exp Hypn. 2000;48(2):138–53.
3. Raphael J, Ahmedzai S, Hester J, et al. Cancer pain: part 1: pathophysiology; oncological, pharmacological, and psychological treatments: a perspective from the British pain society endorsed by the UK Association of Palliative Medicine and the Royal College of General Practitioners. Pain Med. 2010;11(5):742–64.
4. Faymonville M-E, Boly M, Laureys S. Functional neuroanatomy of the hypnotic state. J Physiol Paris. 2006;99(4–6):463–9.
5. Derbyshire SWG, Whalley MG, Oakley DA. Fibromyalgia pain and its modulation by hypnotic and non-hypnotic suggestion: an fMRI analysis. Eur J Pain. 2009;13(5):542–50.
6. Bushnell MC, Ceko M, Low LA. Cognitive and emotional control of pain and its disruption in chronic pain. Nat Rev Neurosci. 2013;14(7):502–11.
7. Ernst E. Is reflexology an effective intervention? A systematic review of randomised controlled trials. Med J Aust. 2009;191(5):263–6.
8. Quattrin R, Zanini A, Buchini S, et al. Use of reflexology foot massage to reduce anxiety in hospitalized cancer patients in chemotherapy treatment: methodology and outcomes. J Nurs Manag. 2006;14(2):96–105.
9. Stephenson NLN, Swanson M, Dalton J, Keefe FJ, Engelke M. Partner-delivered reflexology: effects on cancer pain and anxiety. Oncol Nurs Forum. 2007;34(1):127–32.
10. Kwekkeboom KL, Bumpus M, Wanta B, Serlin RC. Oncology nurses' use of nondrug pain interventions in practice. J Pain Symptom Manag. 2008;35(1):83–94.
11. Carinci AJ, Pathak R, Young M, Christo PJ. Complementary and alternative treatments for chronic pelvic pain. Curr Pain Headache Rep. 2013;17(2):316.
12. Baad-Hansen L, Abrahamsen R, Zachariae R, List T, Svensson P. Somatosensory sensitivity in patients with persistent idiopathic orofacial pain is associated with pain relief from hypnosis and relaxation. Clin J Pain. 2013;29(6):518–26.

Suggested Readings

Bonadonna R. Meditation's impact on chronic illness. Holist Nurs Pract. 2003;17(6):309–19.

Dossey BM, Keegan L. Holistic nursing: a handbook for practice. Burlington: Jones and Bartlett Publishers IIC; 2008.

Felman J, editor. Hands-on healing: massage remedies for hundreds of health problems. Prevention magazine health books. Emmaus: Rodale Press; 1989.

Krieger D. The therapeutic touch: how to use your hands to help or to heal. New York/Upper Saddle River: Simon and Schuster/Prentice Hall Press; 1979.

Kwekkeboom KL. Music versus distraction for procedural pain and anxiety in patients with Cancer. Oncol Nurs Forum. 2003;30(3):433–40.

Levy MH, et al. Management of chronic pain in cancer survivors. Cancer J. 2008;14(6):401–9.

Orme-Johnson DW, et al. Neuroimaging of meditation's effect on brain reactivity to pain. Cogn Neurosci Neuropsychol. 2006;17(12):13591363.

Pachuta D. The life you save may be your own: a comprehensive course in the mastery of stress, health and well-being in yourself and others. Baltimore: Self Published; 1987.

Roffe L, Schmidt K, Ernst E. A systematic review of guided imagery as an adjuvant cancer therapy. Psycho-Oncology. 2005;14:607–17.

Running A, Thurnbeaugh E. Oncology pain and complementary therapy: a review of the literature. Clin J Oncol Nurs. 2011;15(4):374–9.

Villemure C, Bushnell MG. Cognitive modulation of pain: how do attention and emotion influence pain processing? Int Assoc Study Pain. 2002;95:195–9. Elsevier Science B.V.

Index

A

Abdominal nerve plexus, 301
Ablative techniques
  chemical ablation, 314
    advantages, 314
    application, 314
    limitations, 314
    procedure, 314
  chemical neurolysis
    cryoneurolysis, 143
    ethyl alcohol, 142
    glycerol, 143
    phenol, 142, 143
  cryoablation
    advantage, 312
    application, 313, 314
    chemical ablation, 314
    description, 312, 313
    limitations, 312
  diagnostic *vs.* therapeutic block, 141
  hepatocellular carcinoma and painful metastasis, 311
  HIFU, 143
    advantages, 315
    application, 315
    limitations, 315
    procedure, 315
  hyperintense lesion, 309
  literature of, 310
  lytic lesion with cortical destruction, 313
  MWA
    advantages, 310, 311
    application, 311, 312
    description, 311
    limitations, 311
  percutaneous image-guided ablation, considerations, 307
  radiofrequency ablation
    continuous thermal radiofrequency ablation, 141
    cooled, 141, 142
    pulsed radiofrequency treatment, 142
  RFA
    advantages, 308
    application, 308, 309
    description of, 308
    limitations, 308
Acceptance and commitment therapy (ACT), 52
Achilles tendinopathy, 409
Activities of daily living (ADL), 418
Acupoints, 485
Acupuncture
  application of
    aromatase inhibitors, 487
    CIBP, 487
    CIPN, 487
  and cancer pain, 486
  mechanism of action, 486, 487
  and noncancer pain, 485, 486
  philosophy of, 485
  practice of, 485
  safety profile, 487
Acute somatic dysfunction, 434
Acute toxicities, 347
Adhesive capsulitis, 68, 69, 405, 406
Adjuvant analgesics, 478
Aerobic exercises, 398
Affective domain, 453
Alcohol, 278
Alkyl bioreductives, 19
Alkyl sulfonate, 19, 20
Alkylating agents, 19, 21, 22, 365
Allopathic convergence, 494
American College of Radiology (ACR), 348
American Society for Radiation Oncology (ASTRO), 348
Amitriptyline, 477
Amputation, 364
Analgesic therapy, 129
Anatomic cancer-related pain, pathophysiology for, 14
Anchoring device, 281
Anemia, 422
Angiogenesis, 505
Anterior abdominal wall pain, 99
Anterior cingulate cortex (ACC), 225
Anterior paratracheal fluoroscopic technique, 149, 150
Anthracyclines, 21, 24, 135, 365
Antibiotics, 21
Anticholinergic delirium, 477
Anticoagulation
  cancer pain syndromes, 213
  pump implantation technique, 277
Antidepressants, 478
Antigen-presenting cells (APCs), 133
Antimitotic drugs, 24, 25
Anxiety, 466, 467, 474
  palliative care and oncology/hematology settings, prevalence in, 475
  pharmacologic treatment of, 476, 477
    benzodiazepines, 479
    mirtazapine, bupropion and trazodone, 477, 478
    neuroleptics, 479
    psychostimulants, 478, 479
    SNRI, 477
    SSRIs, 477
    TCA, 477
  psychiatric disorders, 476

A. Gulati et al. (eds.), *Essentials of Interventional Cancer Pain Management*, https://doi.org/10.1007/978-3-319-99684-4

Arachnoiditis, 248, 253
Armodafinil, 478
Aromatase inhibitor-induced musculoskeletal pain, 487
Aromatase inhibitors (AI), 48
Art therapists, 493
Art therapy, 492, 493
Art Therapy Credentials Board (ATCB), 493
Arthralgias, 48
ATRA-induced headaches, 125
Atrophy, 390
Authorized agent controlled analgesia (AACA), 114
Autonomic nerve block
  celiac plexus block, 176–178
  ganglion of impar block, 177, 178, 180
  stellate ganglion block, 175–177
  superior hypogastric plexus block, 177, 179
Autonomic nervous system, 145
Autonomic neuropathy, 26
Axillary web syndrome (AWS), 74
Ayurveda, 503
Aβ fibers, 32

B
B12 deficiency, 476
Baclofen, 289, 294
Bean bag, 278
Behavioral domain, 453
Benzodiazepines, 479, 480
Bertelli compared compression, 425
Bevacizumab, 25
Bilateral percutaneous occipital nerve stimulators, 257
Bilateral transpedicle access, 206
Biobehavioral Pain Profile, 457
Biofeedback, 464
  evidence on, 465
  temperature feedback training, 465
  training, 465
Biologically equivalent dose (BED), 320
Biopsychosocial model, 463, 473, 474
Bioreductive, 20
Bisphosphates, 15
Bisphosphonates, 86, 109, 124, 340, 355, 356
Bladder cancer, 108
Bleomycin, 24, 365
Blood-related cancers (BRC)
  bone lesions, 124, 125
  bone pain, 124
Bone lesions, hematologic malignancies, BRC, 124
Bone marrow transplant, 129, 130
Bone metastases
  EBRT, 339, 340
    dose fractionation, 341, 342
    highly conformal therapy, 345
    planning and delivery, 342–344
    re-treatment with, 343, 345
    side effects of, 342, 343
    surgical evaluation, impending or pathologic fracture, spinal instability, and need for, 340
  randomized clinical trials, treatment of, 330
Bone pain, 15
  gastrointestinal cancer pain, 99
  genitourinary somatic pain syndromes, 108, 109
  hematologic malignancies, BRC, 124
Bone remodeling, 15
Bone tumor pain, pathophysiology of, 13
Bortezomib, 48, 127
Boswellia carterii, 506
Botanicals
  benefits of, 504
  therapies, application of, 504
    Boswellia carterii, 506
    corydalis, 505
    Dong quai, 505, 506
    Panax notoginseng, 505
    peony, red and white, 505
    turmeric, 506
Botulinum toxin, 215, 221
Bowel obstruction, 98
Brachial plexopathy, 14
  malignancy-associated neuropathic pain syndromes, 88
  NCS and EMG findings of, 379
  nervous system, 70
  radiation-induced, 71
  RIBP, 425
Brachial plexus block
  anatomy, 173
  benefits, 174, 175
  complications, 175
  incidence, 172, 173
  interscalene approach, 174
  supraclavicular approach, 174
  technique, 173, 174
Brachytherapy, 324, 327
Bracing, 443
  dropped head syndrome, 447
  forward head posture, 446, 447
  indications, 443
    spine malalignment, 444–446
    vertebral compression fractures, 443, 444
  kyphosis and scoliosis, 447
  low back pain, 447, 448
Brain metastases
  graded prognostic assessment, patients with, 331
  palliation for, 330, 331
  recursive partitioning analysis, patients with, 331
Brain radiation therapy, 330
Brain tumor, 56, 321, 325, 331, 422, 468
Breast cancer, 63, 446
  acute, subacute, and chronic pain disorders, 65
  anatomical treatment paradigm, 78
  breast, innervation of, 64
  conservative treatment
    medication management, 74
    physical therapy, 74
    preventative strategies, 75
    trigger point injection, 75
  epidemiology, 64
  integumentary system, 74
  interventional treatment options, 75, 78
    chemodenervation, 76, 77
    dorsal root ganglia, pulsed radiofrequency of, 76
    intercostal nerve block, 76
    intrathecal pump placement, 77
    neuroma injection, 77
    paravertebral block, 75, 76
    Pecs block, 76
    serratus plane block, 75
    spinal cord stimulation, 77
    SSNB, 75

stellate ganglion blockade, 76
intraoperative brachytherapy for, 328
lymphatic system
AWS, 74
lymphedema, 72, 73
musculoskeletal, 64
adhesive capsulitis, 68, 69
contractures, 69, 70
costochondritis, 66
hormonal therapy-induced arthralgias, 66
MTPs, 66
radiation-induced fibrosis, 69
rotator cuff tendonitis, 67, 68
scapulothoracic bursitis, 69
surgical pain, 67
tumor-related pain, 66
nervous system, 70
brachial plexopathies, 70
cervical radiculopathy, 70
CRPS, 72
intercostobrachial neuralgia, 71
leptomeningeal metastases, 72
mononeuropathies, 71
neuroma pain, 72
phantom breast pain, 71
polyneuropathies, 70
radiation-induced brachial plexopathy, 71
organ system, 65
pain syndromes, 73
pathophysiology, 15
side effects, myriad of, 63
treatments, 63
Breathing-based relaxation techniques, 465, 466
Bupivacaine, 288–290
Bupropion, 478
Busulfan, 19
Butyrophenone, 479

C

C7-T1 syndrome, 87
Cancer bone pain, pathophysiology of, 201–203
Cancer fatigue, 396, 399, 412, 424
Cancer-induced bone pain (CIBP), 487
Cancer management
biofeedback, 464, 465
biopsychosocial model of, 463
breathing-based relaxation techniques, 465, 466
chemotherapy and suffer unpleasant side effects, 463, 464
chemotherapy-related cognitive impairment, 469
chronic pain post-surgery, managing, 468
depression and anxiety, managing, 466, 467
guided imagery, 466
mind-body therapies, 463
pain management and psychosocial aspects, 467
relaxation
for caregivers, 468
training, cancer-related fatigue and sleep, 468, 469
symptom management, 464
Cancer pain, 13
acupuncture and, 486
advanced-stage cancer, optimal pain management for, 473
advanced-stage cancer, psychiatric disorders in, 475
anxiety and depression, screening for, 476
pharmacologic treatment, anxiety and depression, 476–479
and suicide, 475
symptoms, physiologic causes of, 476
anatomic cancer-related pain, pathophysiology for, 14
anxiety and tension, 451
aspects of, 463
biopsychosocial model of, 473, 474
bone tumor pain, pathophysiology of, 13
CAM and, 490, 491
celiac plexus and splanchnic nerve block
anatomy, 154
computed tomography, 156, 157
evidence, 154, 155
fluoroscopic celiac plexus/splanchnic nerve block, 155, 156
indications, 154
side effects and complications, 157, 158
chemical mediators, 14
breast cancer, pathophysiology, 15
multiple myeloma, pathophysiology, 15
cognitive-behavioral techniques, 456, 457
cognitive reframing, 457
distraction, 457
effects of, 457, 458
efficacy of, 458
relaxation, 457
depression and anxiety, 474, 475
diagnosis, community setting, 5, 6
epidemiology of, 5
ganglion impar block
anatomy, 162
evidence, 162
fluoroscopic technique, 162
indications, 162
side effects and complications, 162
lumbar sympathetic block
anatomy, 158
evidence, 158
fluoroscopic lumbar sympathetic block, 158, 159
indications, 158
side effects and complications, 159, 160
mind-body therapies
hypnosis, 458
imagery, 458
interventions, 458, 459
mindfulness-based interventions, 459
neuropathic pain, etiologies of, 14
novel therapies, 15, 16
oncologic patients
changing pain states in, 7
intrathecal drug delivery in, 7–9
peripheral nerve stimulation for, 255, 256
specific devices, 258, 259
techniques, 256, 257
person-centered care, 451
and physical modalities (*see* Physical modalities)
psychosocial factors, comprehensive assessment of, 451, 452
affective domain, 453
behavioral domain, 453
cancer pain education, 455, 456
chemobrain, 454
cognitive domain, 453
cognitive strengths and weaknesses, assessment of, 454
psychosocial factor, 454
psychosocial interview, treatment plan formulation from, 454
sensory/physical domain, 452, 453
sphenopalatine ganglion block

Cancer pain (*cont.*)
- anatomy, 147
- evidence, 147
- indications, 147
- infrazygomatic fluoroscopic technique, 147, 148
- intranasal technique, 147
- side effects and complications, 148

spinal neuroablation for (*see* Spinal cord ablation)
stellate ganglion block
- anatomy, 148, 149
- anterior paratracheal fluoroscopic technique, 149, 150
- evidence, 149
- indications, 149
- oblique fluoroscopic technique, 150
- side effects and complications, 150
- ultrasound-guided technique, 150

superior hypogastric plexus block
- anatomy, 160
- evidence, 160
- fluoroscopic technique, 160, 162
- indications, 160
- side effects and complications, 162

symptom management in, 6, 7
tCDS and rTMS, 263
- benefit, 264
- mechanism of action, 263, 264
- risks/limitations, 264

TENS for
- application and use, 262
- benefit, 262, 263
- mechanism of action, 261
- risks/limitations, 263

thoracic sympathetic ganglion blocks
- anatomy, 151, 152
- evidence, 152
- fluoroscopic T2–T3 technique, 152, 153
- indications, 152
- side effects and complications, 154

Cancer pain management
- ayurveda and traditional Chinese medicine, 503, 504
- botanicals, therapies, application of, 504, 505
  - benefits of, 504
  - *Boswellia carterii*, 506
  - corydalis, 505
  - Dong quai, 505, 506
  - *Panax notoginseng*, 505
  - peony, red and white, 505
  - turmeric, 506
- symptom prevalence in, 504

Cancer pain syndromes, 271
- chemotherapy-induced peripheral neuropathy, 213, 214
- coagulopathy and anticoagulation, 213
- concurrent chemotherapy, 213
- insufficiency fractures, 217
  - kyphoplasty and vertebroplasty, 217
  - sacroplasty, 217
- post radical neck dissection pain, 217–220
- radiation therapy-induced pain
  - cervical dystonia, 215
  - oral mucositis, 214
  - osteonecrosis of the jaw, 214–217

Cancer rehabilitation
- chemotherapy, complications of, 364
  - cardiomyopathy, 365
  - cognitive disorders, 365
  - neuropathy, 364, 365
  - pulmonary toxicity, 365, 366
- palliative rehabilitation, 371
- preventative therapy, 370
- radiation, complications of, 366
  - cerebral atrophy, 366
  - encephalopathy, 366
  - RFS, 366–368
- somatic dysfunction treatment in, 439, 440
- supportive therapy, 371
- surgery, complications of, 363
  - amputation, 364
  - donor graft surgeries, 363
  - dysphonia, 364
  - spinal accessory nerve palsy, 363
- treatments, impairments caused by, 363
- vocational rehabilitation and disability, 368, 369
  - comprehensive inpatient rehabilitation, 370
  - general strategies, 369
  - lymphedema, 369
  - pathological fractures, 369, 370

Cancer-related fatigue (CRF), 395
- causes and pathophysiology of, 396
- exercise, on deconditioning, 397
- identification and evaluation of, 395, 396
- patient evaluation, history and physical during, 398
- treatment of, 396
  - exercise mechanism, 396, 397
  - treating with exercise, 397, 398

Cancer-related pain
- occupational therapy, 423
- OMT
  - cancer rehabilitation, somatic dysfunction treatment in, 439, 440
  - osteopathic techniques, 435
  - thoracic outlet technique, 435–439
- osteopathic medicine, 433
  - founding father of modern osteopathy, 433, 434
  - pain, neuroanatomy of, 434
  - somatic dysfunction, pathophysiology of, 434
- pain syndromes, 48, 49

Cancer-related pelvic pain, 385
- anatomy, pelvis, 385, 386
- cancer treatment, sequelae of, 389
- cervical cancer, 388, 389
- endometrial cancer, 388
- history and physical exam, 386, 388
- interventional management
  - nerve blocks, 391
  - neuromodulation, 392
  - pelvic floor botulinum toxin injections, 391
  - pelvic floor trigger point injections, 391
- ovarian cancer, 389
- prostate cancer, 389
- treatment, 389
  - pharmacology, 391
  - physical therapy, 390
  - psychotherapy, 390
  - vaginal dryness, stenosis, and atrophy, 390
- vulvar cancer, 389

Cancer survivorship, 403
Capecitabine, 23
Capillary leak syndrome (CLS), 23
Carboplatin, 24
Cardiac tumors, 85, 86
Cardiomyopathy, 365

Carmustine, 21
Carnett's sign, 100
Carpal tunnel syndrome (CTS), 413, 414
Cat camel stretch, 412
Caudal epidural injections, 216
Caudal injection, 216
CCL2 cells, 15, 34, 35
Celiac plexus and splanchnic nerve block, 101, 157, 176–178, 302
  anatomy, 154
  computed tomography, 156, 157
  evidence, 154, 155
  indications, 154
Central inflammatory responses in spinal cord, 35
Central sensitization, 34
Cerebral atrophy, 366
Cervical cancer
  cancer-related pelvic pain, 388, 389
  genitourinary visceral pain syndromes, 108
Cervical disc pathology, 410
Cervical dystonia, 215, 368
Cervical extensor weakness, 409
Cervical paraspinals, 437
Cervical plexopathy, 14
Cervical plexus block
  anatomy, 197, 198
  clinical indications, 198
  procedure
    deep cervical plexus, 198, 199
    superficial cervical plexus, 198
  risk/complications, 199
Cervical radiculopathy, 70
Cervical spine, 89, 185, 195, 231, 232, 409, 410
  soft tissue, 435
Cervical thoracic orthoses (CTO), 444
Cetuximab, 25
C fibers, 128
Charcot deformity, 446
Chassaignac's tubercle, 215
Chemical ablation, 314
  advantages, 314
  application, 314
  limitations, 314
  procedure, 314
Chemical neurolysis, 153
  cryoneurolysis, 143
  ethyl alcohol, 142
  glycerol, 143
  phenol, 142, 143
Chemobrain, 454
Chemodenervation, 70, 76, 77, 381
Chemoradiation, 388
Chemotherapeutic agents, thoracic cancer pain, 89
Chemotherapeutic pain, 25
Chemotherapy, 19
  alkylating agents, 19, 21, 22
  anthracyclines, 24
  antimitotic drugs, 24, 25
  cancer rehabilitation, 364
    cardiomyopathy, 365
    cognitive disorders, 365
    neuropathy, 364, 365
    pulmonary toxicity, 365, 366
  folates, 22
  monoclonal antibodies, 25
  nucleotide and platinum analogs, 22–24
Chemotherapy-associated neuropathies, 100
Chemotherapy-induced peripheral neuropathy (CIPN), 48, 49, 126, 127, 213, 214, 380, 381, 424, 487
Chemotherapy-related cognitive impairment, 469
Chest wall pain, 7, 40, 43, 59, 77, 86, 90
Chlorhexidine, 278
Chlorpromazine, 479
Chronic cancer pain syndromes, 52
Chronic graft *vs.* host disease (GVHD), 49
Chronic pain post-surgery, managing, 468
Chronic pain rehabilitation programs (CPRPs), 47
Chronic pelvic pain, 385, 387
Chronic postamputation pain, 30, 31
Chronic postmastectomy pain, 29, 30
Chronic postsurgical pain (CPSP)
  incidence of, 29
  and neuroinflammation, 32
    DRG, 35
    emerging preventive therapeutics, 35
    neuroinflammatory modulation, 35
    neurotransmission modulation, 35
    pro-resolution lipid mediators, 35, 36
    spinal cord, central inflammatory responses in, 35
  and neuronal plasticity
    central sensitization, 32
    peripheral sensitization, 32
  risk factors for, 30
Chronic somatic dysfunction, 434
Cingulotomy, 227
  operative technique, 225, 226
  outcomes, 226
  rationale and patient selection, 225
Cisplatin, 23, 127
Clavicle orthosis, 446, 447
Clonazepam, 479
Clonidine, 289
Coagulopathy, 213
Coasting, 48, 100
Coaxial technique, 304
Cognitive-behavioral techniques, 52, 456
  cognitive reframing, 457
  distraction, 457
  effects of, 457, 458
  efficacy of, 458
  relaxation, 457
Cognitive-behavioral therapy (CBT), 47
Cognitive disorders
  cerebral atrophy, 366
  chemotherapy, 365
  encephalopathy, 366
  RFS, 366–368
Cognitive distraction, 423
Cognitive domain, 453
Colorectal cancer, 98
Combination therapy, 293, 294
Complementary and alternative medicine (CAM), 119, 489, 499, 503
  and cancer pain, 490, 491
  convergence, 494
  measurable benefits, 490
  patient resources, 490, 500
  physicians, 490
  whole-systems research, cancer, and, 499, 500
Complex decongestive therapy, 425
  manual lymphatic drainage, 428
  taping, 428

Complex regional pain syndrome (CRPS), 72, 100, 247
Compounded sterile preparation (CSP), 294
Comprehensive inpatient rehabilitation, 370
Computed tomography (CT), 156, 157, 307
Cone beam computerized tomography (CBCT), 236
Consciousness, 508, 509
Continuous thermal radiofrequency ablation, 141
Continuum of cancer care, occupational therapy, 421
Contractures, 69, 70
Conversion therapy, 429
  microwave diathermy, 429, 430
  shortwave diathermy, 429
  ultrasound, 429
Cooled radiofrequency ablation, 142
Cordotomy, 231, 232
Corticosteroids, 137
Corydalis, 505
Corydalis yanhusuo, 505
Costochondritis, 66
Counterstrain technique, 438
Cranial electrotherapy stimulation (CES), 263, 264
Cranial nerve targets
  gasserian ganglion block, 176
    location, 175
    nerve root block, 175
    neurolytic glossopharyngeal nerve block, 175
  glossopharyngeal nerve (*see* Glossopharyngeal nerve block)
  trigeminal nerve (*see* Trigeminal nerve)
  vagus nerve (*see* Vagus nerve)
Creative (expressive) arts therapy
  distraction, 491
  music therapy, 491, 492
Cryoablation, 91, 192
  advantage, 312
  application, 313, 314
  description, 312, 313
  limitations, 312
Cryoneurolysis, 143
Cryotherapy, 428
Curcuma longa, 506
Curcumin, 506
CXCL1 chemokine, 34
Cyclophosphamide, 21, 366
Cytarabine, 23

D
Dacarbazine, 22
Dance, physical modalities, 431
De Quervain's tenosynovitis, 406
Decongestive lymphatic therapy (DLT), 73
Deep brain stimulation (DBS), 241, 242, 255
Deep venous thrombosis, 422
Default mode network (DMN), 486
Delirium, 476
Denosumab, 86, 358
Depression
  palliative care and oncology/hematology settings, prevalence in, 475
  pharmacologic treatment of, 476, 477
    benzodiazepines, 479
    mirtazapine, bupropion and trazodone, 477, 478
    neuroleptics, 479
    psychostimulants, 478, 479
    SNRI, 477
    SSRIs, 477
    TCA, 477
  psychiatric disorders, 476
Depth-dose curves, 320
Dermatologic cancer pain syndromes
  pain syndromes and management
    injection site reactions, 134, 135
    PHN, 135, 136
    PPE, 136, 137
    trichodynia, 137
  skin, anatomy and physiology of, 133, 134
Dermis, 133
Dexmedetomidine, 289
Dexrazoxane, 135
Dextroamphetamine, 478
Diarrhea, 157
Diffuse spinal vertebral metastasis, 202
Dihydropyrimidine dehydrogenase (DPYD), 136
Disability/impairment/handicap, 418
Distraction, creative (expressive) arts therapy, 491
Docetaxel, 365
Docosahexaenoic acid (DHA), 35
Dong quai, 505, 506
Donor graft surgeries, 363
Dorsal Root Entry Zone (DREZ) surgery, 233
Dorsal root ganglia (DRG), 34, 35, 76, 127, 145
Dose fractionation, 320, 341, 342
Dose-limiting organs, 322
Douleur Neuropathique (DN4), 4
Doxorubicin, 24
Dropped head syndrome, 367, 447
Ductal carcinoma in situ (DCIS), 251
Dysesthesia, 186–189, 195, 197
Dyspareunia, 388–390, 392
Dysphonia, 364

E
Eccentric wrist extensor exercise, 406
Effective dose-fractionation, 329
Eicosapentaenoic acid (EPA), 35
Elbow/forearm, physical therapy, 406
Electroacupuncture, 485
Electrodes, 247, 250
Electrodiagnostic tools, 375
Encephalopathy, 366
Endometrial cancer, 388
Energy conservation and activity management (ECAM), 398
Epidural drug delivery systems, 102, 111
Epidural motor cortex stimulation (MCS), 243, 244
Estrogen therapy, 390
Ethyl alcohol neurolysis, 142
Excitatory synaptic transmission, 33
Exercise, 396–398
External beam radiation therapy (EBRT), 339
  dose fractionation, 341, 342
  fractionation schemes and response rates, 342, 346
  highly conformal therapy, 345
  planning and delivery, 342–344
  re-treatment with, 343, 345
  side effects of, 342, 343
  surgical evaluation, impending or pathologic fracture, spinal instability, and need for, 340
Extralemniscal myelotomy (ELM), 233
Extravasation, 135

F
Facial pain, 88
Failed back surgery syndrome, 253
Fatigue, 395, 468
Fentanyl, 288
Fibrosis, radiation-induced, 69
Filtration, 295
Fluoroscopic celiac plexus/splanchnic nerve block, 155, 156
Fluoroscopic lumbar sympathetic block, 158, 159
Fluoroscopic technique, 149, 150, 160, 162
Fluoroscopy, 302
5-Fluorouracil (5-FU), 23
Fluphenazine, 479
Folates, 20, 22
Frequency, 262
Functional history, 418
Functional independence measure (FIM), 404, 418, 419
Functional status assessment, 50
Funicular pain, 367

G
GABAergic, 33
Gait and balance impairments, 412, 413
Gamma Knife technique, 229
Ganglion impar block, 101, 177, 178, 180, 216
  anatomy, 162
  evidence, 162
  fluoroscopic technique, 162
  indications, 162
  side effects and complications, 162
Ganglionopathy, 378
Gasserian ganglion block, 176
  location, 175
  nerve root block, 175
  neurolytic glossopharyngeal nerve block, 175
Gastric cancer, 98
Gastrointestinal cancer pain
  gastrointestinal nociceptive pain syndromes
    anterior abdominal wall pain, 99
    bone pain, 99
    malignant perineal pain, 99
  gastrointestinal visceral pain syndromes
    bowel obstruction, 98
    colorectal cancer, 98
    gastric cancer, 98
    liver cancer, 97, 98
    pancreatic cancer, 97
    peritoneal carcinomatosis, 98
    retroperitoneal pain syndrome, 98
    ureteric obstruction, 98
  infusion therapies
    ketamine, 102, 103
    lidocaine, 103
  interventional pain control options
    celiac plexus block, 101
    ganglion impar block, 101
    splanchnic nerve block, 101
    superior hypogastric plexus block, 101
    visceral pain, sympathetic blocks for, 100
  malignancy-associated neuropathic pain syndromes
    malignant mononeuropathy, 100
    malignant plexopathy, 99, 100
    malignant radiculopathy, 99
  neuraxial pain control systems
    intrathecal, epidural drug delivery systems, 102
    SCS, 102
  neuropathic pain, 103
  somatic nerve blocks
    TAP block, 102
    thoracic intercostal/paravertebral block, 101, 102
  treatment-associated pain syndromes
    chemotherapy-associated neuropathies, 100
    postsurgical pain, 100
    radiation-associated pain, 100
Gastrointestinal malignancy pain syndromes, 97
Gastrointestinal nociceptive pain syndromes
  anterior abdominal wall pain, 99
  bone pain, 99
  malignant perineal pain, 99
Gastrointestinal visceral pain syndromes
  bowel obstruction, 98
  colorectal cancer, 98
  gastric cancer, 98
  liver cancer, 97, 98
  pancreatic cancer, 97
  peritoneal carcinomatosis, 98
  retroperitoneal pain syndrome, 98
  ureteric obstruction, 98
Gate control theory (GCT), 247, 261, 427
Gemcitabine, 23
Genitofemoral neuralgia, 160
Genitourinary cancer pain syndromes
  interventional pain treatments, 109, 110
  neuraxial pain techniques, 110, 111
  neuroablative procedures
  neuropathic pain syndromes, 109
  punctate midline myelotomy, 110
  somatic pain syndromes, 108, 109
  visceral pain syndromes
    bladder cancer, 108
    cervical cancer, 108
    ovarian cancer, 108
    prostate cancer, 107
    renal cell carcinoma, 107, 108
    testicular cancer, 108
    uterine cancer, 108
Glossopharyngeal nerve block
  anatomic considerations, 193
  clinical indications, 192, 193
  procedure
    intraoral approach, 193
    percutaneous approach, 193
  side effects/complications, 193
Glycerol, 143
Glycinergic interneurons, 33
Granulomas, 297
Greater and lesser occipital nerves
  anatomy, 195
  nerve stimulation
    anatomic considerations, 197
    clinical indications, 197
    procedure, 197
    risk/complications, 197
  radiofrequency ablation, and cryoablation
    anatomic considerations, 196
    clinical indications, 195, 196
    procedure, 196
    risk/complications, 197
Greater trochanteric pain syndrome (GTPS), 408
Guided imagery (GI), 466, 507
Gynecologic cancers, 385

H

Haloperidol, 479
Hand-foot skin reaction (HFSR), 136
Hand-foot syndrome (HFS), 136
Head and neck nerve cancer
  cervical plexus (*see* Cervical plexus block)
  greater and lesser occipital nerves (*see* Greater and lesser occipital nerves)
  isodose plan for, 323
  palliation for, 331
  sphenopalatine ganglion (*see* Sphenopalatine ganglion block)
  TMJ (*see* Temporomandibular joint (TMJ))
Head cervical orthoses (HCO), 444
Heart rate variability (HRV), 464
Heart rate variability biofeedback (HRVB), 465
Hematologic malignancies
  ATRA-induced headaches, 125
  BRC
    bone lesions, 124, 125
    bone pain, 124
    pain in, 123, 124
  CiPN, 127
  herpes zoster and postherpetic neuralgia
    bone marrow transplant, 129, 130
    cord compression, back pain from, 129
    oral mucositis, 128, 129
    procedure-related pain, 129
  pegfilgrastim, bone pain, 125
  PPN, 126
  procedure-related headaches, 125, 126
Hematopoietic stem cell transplant (HSCT), 129
Hemolytic uremic syndrome (HUS), 23
Hemorrhage, 160
Hemostasis, 277, 505
Hepatic cancers, 331, 332
Hepatic plexus, 98
Hepatic sinusoidal obstruction syndr, 21
Hepatosplenic T-cell lymphomas (HSTCL), 23
Herpes zoster (HZ)/shingles
  bone marrow transplant, 129, 130
  cord compression, back pain from, 129
  oral mucositis, 128, 129
  procedure-related pain, 129
High-intensity focused ultrasound (HIFU), 143, 314
  advantages, 315
  application, 315
  limitations, 315
  procedure, 315
Hip osteoarthritis, 407, 408
Hodgkin lymphoma, 445
Hormonal therapy-induced arthralgias, 66
HRQol, 48
Hydromorphone, 288
Hydroxizine, 479
Hydroxyurea, 23
Hypercalcemia, 422
Hypersensitivity, 381
Hyperuricemia, 23
Hypnosis, 458, 508, 509
Hypnotherapy, 507
Hypofractionation, 320, 330, 332
Hypophysectomy
  operative technique, 229, 230
  outcomes, 230
  rationale and patient selection, 229
Hypotension, 157, 289, 479
Hypoxanthine-guanine phosphoribosyl transferase (HGPRT), 22

I

Ilioinguinal neuralgia, 253
Iliotibial band syndrome (ITBS), 408, 409
Image guidance
  anatomy, 301
  lumbar sympathetic block, 303–306
  mapping strategies, 302
  radiologic modalities, 302
  vascular, 301
Imatinib, 25
Immobilization devices, 322
Immunomodulatory agents, 127
Impar ganglion block, 110, 163
Implantable intrathecal pump systems, 102
Infections, 396
Inflammatory cytokines, 15
Infraorbital nerve block
  anatomic considerations, 191
  clinical indications, 191
  procedure, 191, 192
Infrazygomatic fluoroscopic technique, 147, 148
Infrazygomatic sphenopalatine block, 148
InfusAid pump, 270
Infusion related chemotherapeutic pain, 25
Infusion therapies
  ketamine, 102, 103
  lidocaine, 103
Injection site reactions, 134, 135
Instrumental ADLs, 419
Insufficiency fractures, 217
Integumentary system, 74
Intensity-modulated radiation therapy (IMRT), 323
Intercostal nerve, block, 76, 218, 219
  anatomy, 170, 171
  benefits, 171
  complications, 171
  indications, 170
  technique, 170–172
Intercostal neuropathy, 88
Intercostobrachial nerve block, 218
Intercostobrachial neuralgia (ICN), *see* Postmastectomy pain syndrome
Interdisciplinary chronic pain management, 48
International Association of Yoga Therapists (IAYT), 495
International Organization for Standardization, 295
Interventional Cancer pain management, 3, 4
Interventional pain services, 117
Intracranial neuroablation
  cingulotomy
    operative technique, 225, 226
    outcomes, 226
    rationale and patient selection, 225
  hypophysectomy
    operative technique, 229, 230
    outcomes, 230
    rationale and patient selection, 229
  thalamotomy
    operative technique, 228, 229
    outcomes, 229
    rationale and patient selection, 228
  trigeminal nucleotractotomy

operative technique, 227, 228
outcomes, 228
rationale and patient selection, 227
Intractable inguinal pain, 258
Intrathecal (IT) pumps
baclofen, 289
clonidine, 289
dosing, 290
intrathecal medications, titration and bolus of
bupivacaine, 290
opioid, 290
ziconotide, 290
ketamine, 290
local anesthetics
bupivacaine, 288, 289
dexmedetomidine, 289
ropivacaine, 289
maximum concentration, 290
opioids, 287
fentanyl, 288
hydromorphone, 288
morphine, 287, 288
sufentanil, 288
ziconotide, 288
Intrathecal access, 279, 280
Intrathecal catheter tip, 281
Intrathecal drug delivery systems (IDDS), 7–9, 102
history of, 269, 270
implantation without trial, 274, 275
indications
comorbid conditions, 271
inadequate analgesia, 270, 271
intolerable side effects, 271
life expectancy, 271
localized pain, 271
pain, type of, 271
neuraxial pain techniques, 111
trials, drugs used in, 273–275
types of, 269
Intrathecal neurolysis, 110
Intrathecal pump (ITP), 9
indications, 270
relative and absolute contraindications for, 270
Intrathecal pump placement, 77
Intrathecal use
agents and sterile technique, preparation of, 294
compounding labs, responsibility of, 295
compounding therapy, 293, 294
device, insertion of, 296
filtration, 295
high-risk level requirements, 294
inflammatory mass formation, 297
International Organization for Standardization, 295
medication problems, 296
microbial contamination risk level, 294
pain transmission and FDA approval, receptors for, 293
pump stability and failure, 296
solubility and pKa coefficients, 296
stability and solubility, 295, 296
therapy, risks of, 296
Intravenous alcohol, 355
Intravenous infusions, 219
Inverse planning, 323
Ioban®, 278
Iontophoresis, 430

K
Ketamine, 102, 103, 219, 290, 353, 354
Knee, 409
Kyphoplasty, 201, 207, 208
complications, 209, 210
insufficiency fractures, 217
procedure, 209
Kyphosis, 447

L
Langerhans cells, 133
Lateral branch blocks, 109
Lateral epicondylopathy, 406
Leeds assessment of neuropathic symptoms and signs (LANSS), 4
Leptomeningeal disease, 72, 330, 331
Leukemia, 319
Leukopenia, 422
Lidocaine, 75, 103, 116, 219, 354, 355, 390
Ligaments, 367
Limb amputation, phantom pain after, 115
Linear accelerator, 320
Liver cancer, 97, 98
Liver radiation therapy, 332
Long thoracic nerve (LTN), 64
Low back pain, 447
Lower extremity
ankle, 409
GTPS, 408
hip osteoarthritis, 407, 408
knee, 409
osteoporosis, 408
Lower lumbar fractures, 445
Low-level laser therapy (LLLT), 73
Lumbar pedicle access, 205
Lumbar plexus, 14
Lumbar radiculopathy, 411
Lumbar spine, 410, 411
Lumbar splanchnic nerve blockade, 109
Lumbar stenosis, 411, 412
Lumbar sympathetic block, 159, 303
anatomy, 158
evidence, 158
fluoroscopic lumbar sympathetic block, 158, 159
image guidance, 303
agents, confirmation and injection of, 306
anatomy under fluoroscopy evaluation, 304
engaging target site, 305
needle insertion, 305
review radiological studies, 304
indications, 158
side effects and complications, 159, 160
Lumbar sympathetic blocks, 103
Lumbar sympathetic chain neurolysis, 158
Lumbosacral orthosis (LSO), 445, 448
Lumbosacral plexopathy, 379
Lumbosacral strain, 438, 439
Lumpectomy, 447
Lung cancer, 85
Lymphatic system
AWS, 74
lymphedema, 72, 73
Lymphedema, 68, 72, 73
brachial plexopathy, 425
cancer rehabilitation, 369

Lymphedema (*cont.*)
- occupational therapy, 424
- treatment options, 425

Lymphoma, 319

M

Macrophages, 134
Magnetoencephalography (MEG), 492
Major histocompatibility complexes (MHCs), 134
Malignancy-associated neuropathic pain syndromes
- mononeuropathy, 100
- plexopathy, 99, 100
- radiculopathy, 99
- sequence of interventions for, 104

Malignancy-associated visceral pain syndromes, 104
Malignant mononeuropathy, 100
Malignant pain
- deep brain stimulation, 241, 242
- epidural MCS, 243, 244

Malignant pericardial effusion, 422
Malignant perineal pain, 99
Malignant plexopathy, 99, 100
Malignant radiculopathy, 99
Malignant radiculopathy/plexopathy, 109
Mandibular nerve block and radiofrequency ablation
- anatomic considerations, 189
- clinical indications, 189
- procedure, 189
- side effects/complications, 189

Manual lymphatic drainage (MLD), 73, 425, 428
Manual therapy, 405
Massage therapy, 427, 428, 494, 495
Materia medica, 504
Maxillary nerve block and radiofrequency ablation
- anatomic considerations, 188
- clinical indications, 188
- procedure, 188
- side effects/complications, 188

McGill Pain Questionnaire, 4
Mechanical allodynia, 33
Meckel's cave, 175, 183, 187
Medial branch blocks, 109
Medial canthus skin cancer, 335
Medial epicondylopathy, 406
Meditation, 510
Medtronic 3387 DBS electrode, 256
Medtronic 3987A On-Point Peripheral Nerve Stimulator, 258
Megavoltage photon x-ray beams, 319
Meissner's corpuscles, 134
Melanomas, 335
Memorial Pain Assessment Card (MPAC), 307
Memorial Sloan Kettering Cancer Center (MSKCC), 339
Mental nerve block
- anatomic considerations, 192
- clinical indications, 192
- procedure, 192
- side effects/complications, 192

Mercaptopurine, 22
Merkel cells, 134
Metastatic epidural spinal cord compression (MSCC), 340, 341
Methotrexate, 22
Methotrimeprazine, 479
Microglia, 34
Microwave ablation (MWA)
- advantages, 310, 311
- application, 311, 312
- description, 311
- limitations, 311

Midazolam, 294
Mimic, 22
Mind-body therapies, 463, 487, 493
- allopathic and CAM convergence, 494
- hypnosis, 458
- imagery, 458
- interventions, 458, 459

Mindfulness-based art therapy (MBAT), 493
Mindfulness-based interventions, 459
Mirtazapine, 477
Mitomycin C, 19–21
Modafinil, 478
Modified Pecs block, 76
Monoclonal antibodies, 25
Mononeuropathy, 71, 380
Morphine, 270, 287, 288, 297
Motivational interviewing (MI), 52
Motor cortex stimulation (MCS), 241, 255
Motor neuropathies, 26
M phase, 19, 24
Multimodal analgesia, 75
Multiple hypotheses, 486
Multiple myeloma (MM), 15, 124
Multiple system types, 269
Muscle energy, 437
Music therapy, 491, 492
Myalgias, 48
Myelogram, 281, 282
Myeloma bone disease, 16
Myofascial trigger points (MTPs), 66
Myokymia, 380
Myopathy, 381

N

National Center for Complementary and Alternative Medicine (NCCAM), 489, 490, 503
National Certification Board for Therapeutic Massage and Bodywork (NCBTMB), 495
National Comprehensive Cancer Network, 395
National Quality Forum (NQF), 348
Neck extensor weakness, 367, 368
Needle electromyography, 375–377
Neoplastic plexopathy, 14
Nerve blocks, 7, 391
Nerve conduction studies (NCS), 375–377
Nerve growth factor (NGF), 146
Nerve root block, 175
Nerve tissue destruction, 142
Nervous system, 70
- brachial plexopathies, 70
- cervical radiculopathy, 70
- CRPS, 72
- intercostobrachial neuralgia, 71
- leptomeningeal metastases, 72
- mononeuropathies, 71
- neuroma pain, 72
- phantom breast pain, 71
- polyneuropathies, 70
- radiation-induced brachial plexopathy, 71

Neuralgias, 49
Neuraxial nerve blocks, 117
Neuraxial pain techniques, 92, 93

intrathecal and epidural drug delivery systems, 111
spinal cord stimulation, 110, 111
Neurectomy, 70
Neuroablative procedures, 141
Neurofeedback, 464
Neurogenic pain disorders
CTS, 413, 414
peroneal tendon neuropathy, 414
ulnar neuropathy, 414
Neuroinflammation, CPSP and, 32
DRG, 35
emerging preventive therapeutics, 35
neuroinflammatory modulation, 35
neurotransmission modulation, 35
pro-resolution lipid mediators, 35, 36
spinal cord, central inflammatory responses in, 35
Neuroinflammatory modulation, 35
Neuroleptics, 479
Neurolysis, 218
Neurolytic blocks, 51
Neurolytic celiac plexus block (NCPB), 154
Neurolytic glossopharyngeal nerve block, 175
Neuroma, 33
Neuroma injections, 77, 218
Neuroma pain, 72
Neuromodulatory techniques, 91, 92, 255, 381, 392
Neuromuscular dysfunction, 375
Neuromuscular junction, 381
Neuromuscular medicine
abnormal MUAP, morphology and firing pattern of, 378
abnormal spontaneous activity, 377
brachial plexopathy, NCS and EMG findings of, 379
CIPN, 380, 381
clinical and pathophysiology neuromuscular pain, 375
ganglionopathy, 378
lumbosacral plexopathy, NCS and EMG findings of, 379
mononeuropathy, 380
nerve conduction studies and needle electromyography, 375–377
neuromuscular junction and myopathy, 381
peripheral neuropathy, 380
plexopathy, 378–380
radiculopathy, 377, 378
treatment, 381, 382
Neuromuscular pain, 375
Neuromuscular reeducation (NMR), 405
Neuromuscular RFS, 366
Neuronal plasticity, 32
Neuropathic cancer pain, 115
Neuropathic pain, 103, 241
etiologies of, 14
malignant radiculopathy/plexopathy, 109
RFS, 367
Neuropathy, 23, 25, 364, 365, 367
Neurosurgical techniques, 93
Neurotransmission, pharmacological modulation of, 31, 32
Neutropenia, 422
Nitrogen mustards, 19, 20
Nitrosoureas, 19, 20
N-methyl-D-aspartate (NMDA) receptors, 15, 102, 290
Nociceptive fibers, 101
Noncancer pain, acupuncture and, 485, 486
Noncompetitive N-methyl-D-aspartate (NMDA) receptor antagonist, 353
Non-opioid intravenous infusions
bisphosphonates, 355, 356
denosumab, 358
ketamine, 353, 354
lidocaine, 354, 355
radium-223, 357, 358
strontium-89, 356, 357
Non-spinal bone metastasis, 236
Non-steroidal anti-inflammatory drugs (NSAIDs), 13, 123
Nucleotide analogs, 22–24

O

Oblique fluoroscopic technique, 150
Oblique stellate ganglion block, 151
Obstructive uropathy, 98
Occipital nerve stimulation (ONS), 255
Occipital neuralgia, 195, 196
Occupational therapy, 370
activities of daily living, 418
cancer fatigue, 424
cancer patient, therapeutic considerations in, 421
cancer-related pain, 423
cardiopulmonary interventions, 420
chemotherapy-induced peripheral neuropathy, 424
cognitive/perceptual/sensory interventions, 420
continuum of cancer care, 421
disability/impairment/handicap, 418
domains of, 420
education and training, 420
equipment, 420
evaluation of patient, 417, 418
FIM, 418, 419
functional history, 418
hematologic consideration, 422
instrumental ADLs, 419
lymphedema, 424
brachial plexopathy, 425
classification system, 424, 425
treatment options, 425
mobility, 418
modalities, 420
musculoskeletal interventions, 420
neurological considerations, 422, 423
neuromuscular interventions, 419
patient, evaluation and treatment of, 419
philosophies, principles, and practice, 417
precautions/considerations during, 421, 422
purpose of, 417
radiation-induced fibrosis, 425, 426
treatment options, 423, 424
Olanzapine, 479
Oncologic pain, 250
implantable pulse generators, effects of radiation, 251
MRI compatibility, 251
Open caudalis DREZ ablation, 233
Operant-behavioral therapy (OBT), 47
Opioids, 99, 136, 271, 287, 353
fentanyl, 288
hydromorphone, 288
intrathecal pumps, 290
morphine, 287, 288
sufentanil, 288
ziconotide, 288
Oral mucositis, 128, 129, 214
Oropharyngeal squamous cell carcinoma, 444
Orthostatic hypotension, 157
Orthovoltage therapy unit, 320
Osphena, 390

Osteoclast-activating factors (OAF), 124
Osteoclastogenesis, 15
Osteonecrosis, , 15, 124, 214, 215
Osteopathic manipulation treatment (OMT), 433–435
  cancer rehabilitation, somatic dysfunction treatment in, 440
  osteopathic techniques, 435
  thoracic outlet technique, 435–439
Osteoporosis, 408
Osteoradionecrosis, 89
Ovarian cancer
  cancer-related pelvic pain, 389
  genitourinary visceral pain syndromes, 108
Oxaliplatin, 24, 25

P

Pacinian corpuscles, 134
Paclitaxel, 25, 365
Pain control, 236
Pain management
  assessment process, 48
  clinical practice of, 5
  physical therapy management, 50, 52, 53
  physician assessment, 49, 50
  program structure, 47
  psychological assessment, 50–52
  survivors, cancer-related pain syndromes in, 48, 49
  treatment, 51
Pain modulation
  choosing patients for, 507, 508
  consciousness and hypnosis, 508, 509
  reflexology, 510
  relaxation, 509, 510
Pain services, integration of, 119, 120
Pain syndromes
  chronic cancer-related, 49
  sequence of interventions, 104
Palifermin, 129
Palliative care, 119, 120
Palliative radiation therapy (PRT), 119, 329
  brain metastases and leptomeningeal disease, palliation for, 330, 331
  head and neck cancers, palliation for, 331
  pelvic tumors, palliation for, 332
  primary/metastatic hepatic cancers, 331, 332
  re-irradiation, 335, 336
  skin cancers, palliation, 333, 335
  SVC syndrome, palliation, 333
  vertebral and bone metastases, palliation for, 329, 330
Palliative rehabilitation, 404
Palliative sedation therapy (PST), 119
Palmar-plantar erythrodysesthesia (PPE), 23, 136, 137
Pancoast syndrome, 86
Pancreatic cancer, 97
Paraneoplastic syndromes, 87
Paraproteinemic PN (PPN), 126
Paravertebral block, 75, 76, 91, 219
Paravertebral space, 101
Patellofemoral pain syndrome (PFPS), 409
Pathological fractures, 369, 370
Pecs block, 76
Pediatrics, 113
  AACA, 114
  anesthetic agents, 116
  assessment of pain, 114
  complementary therapies, 119
  pain services, integration of, 119, 120
  procedural cancer pain management, 114
  PRT, 119
  PST, 119
  regional anesthesia interventional procedures, 116, 118
  treatment-related pain, 115
    limb amputation, phantom pain after, 115
    neuropathic cancer pain, 115
    pain after limb-salvage procedures, management of, 115
Pegfilgrastim, 125
Pelvic floor botulinum toxin injections, 391
Pelvic floor dysfunction (PFD), 385
Pelvic floor muscles (PFM), 385, 386, 388
Pelvic floor physical therapy, 390
Pelvic floor trigger point injections, 391
Pelvic rotation, 413
Pelvic tumors, 332
Pemetrexed, 22
Percutaneous electrodes, 256
Periaqueductal (PAG) gray, 241
Peripheral nerve block, 117
  autonomic nerve block (*see* Autonomic nerve block)
  brachial plexus block
    anatomy, 173
    benefits, 174, 175
    complications, 175
    incidence, 172
    interscalene approach, 174
    supraclavicular approach, 174
    technique, 173
  neurolytic block agents, 168
  non-neurolytic block agents, 167, 168
  phantom limb pain and stump pain, 220, 221
  pudendal nerve, 175
  somatic blocks (*see* Somatic nerve block)
Peripheral nerve injury, 34
Peripheral nerve stimulation (PNS), 255
Peripheral neuropathy (PN), 126, 213, 380
Peripheral sensitization, 32, 34
Peripheral sympathetic nervous system, 146
Perirectal pain, 8
Peritoneal carcinomatosis, 98
Periventricular (PVG) gray, 241
Peroneal tendon neuropathy, 414
Phantom breast pain, 71
Phantom limb pain (PLP), 247, 364
  botulinum toxin injections, 221
  peripheral nerve blocks, 220, 221
  scar injection, 221
  SCS, 221
  sympathetic nerve blocks, 220
Pharmacological multimodal therapy, 4
Pharmacological pain therapy, 4
Pharmacology, 391
Phenol neurolysis, 142
Phenothiazine neuroleptics, 479
Phlebitis, 135
Phonophoresis, 430
Photon *vs* proton beam targeting, 321
Physical modalities
  complex decongestive therapy, 428
    manual lymphatic drainage, 428
    taping, 428
  conversion therapy, 429
    microwave diathermy, 429, 430
    shortwave diathermy, 429
    ultrasound, 429

cryotherapy, 428
dance, 431
iontophoresis, 430
massage, 427, 428
phonophoresis, 430
TENS, 430
therapeutic heat, 428, 429
traction, 430
weight lifting, 431
yoga, 431
Physical therapy, 74, 370, 403
assessment, 50
cancer care, continuum of, 403, 404
interventions, 405
lower extremity, 407
ankle, 409
GTPS, 408
hip osteoarthritis, 407, 408
knee, 409
osteoporosis, 408
management, 52, 53
neurogenic pain disorders, 413
CTS, 413, 414
peroneal tendon neuropathy, 414
ulnar neuropathy, 414
precautions, 404
spine
cervical disc pathology, 410
cervical extensor weakness, 409
lumbar spine, 410–412
PMPS, 410
PTPS, 410
radiation-induced cervical dystonia, 409
thoracic spine dysfunction, 410
upper extremity
adhesive capsulitis, 405, 406
De Quervain's tenosynovitis, 406
elbow/forearm, 406
lateral epicondylopathy, 406
medial epicondylopathy, 406
rotator cuff impingement, 405
shoulder pain, 405
wrist, 406
Piriformis syndrome, 412
Plantar fasciitis, 409
Platin compounds, 364
Platinum agents, 25
Platinum analogs, 20, 22–24
Platinum compounds, 127
Plexopathies, 49, 378–380
Pluralism, 496
Pneumatic compression devices (PCDs), 73
Pneumonitis, 21
Pneumothorax, 170, 171, 175, 177
Polyanalgesic Consensus Conference (PACC), 273
Polyanalgesic therapy, 295
Polymethylmethacrylate (PMMA), 204
Post-augmentation breast pain, 69
Posterior cingulate cortex (PCC), 225
Postherpetic neuralgia (PHN), 135, 136, 253
bone marrow transplant, 129, 130
cord compression, back pain from, 129
oral mucositis, 128, 129
procedure-related pain, 129
Postmastectomy pain syndrome (PMPS), 71, 218, 410, 477
Postsurgical pain syndromes, 89, 100, 217
clinical studies, prevention in
nerve blockade with regional and neuraxial anesthetic techniques, 30, 31
neurotransmission, pharmacological modulation of, 31, 32
preventive strategies, limitations of, 32
incidence
chronic postamputation pain, 30
chronic postmastectomy pain, 29, 30
PTPS, 30
phantom limb pain and stump pain
botulinum toxin injections, 221
peripheral nerve blocks, 220, 221
scar injection, 221
SCS, 221
sympathetic nerve blocks, 220
post radical neck dissection pain
intercostal nerve block, 218, 219
intercostobrachial nerve block, 218
intravenous infusions, 219
neuroma injections, 218
paravertebral block, 219
postmastectomy pain, 218
post-thoracotomy pain syndrome, 218
scar injections, 218
SCS, 219, 220
TENS, 219
Post-thoracotomy pain syndrome (PTPS), 30, 31, 218, 253, 410
Potential sympathetic blocks, 163
Premature ovarian failure, 389
Primary chest wall pain, 86
Procedural cancer pain management, 114
Procedure-related headaches, 125, 126
Procedure-related pain, 129
Prochlorperazine, 479
Prognostic index for spine metastasis (PRISM) model, 346
Progressive muscle relaxation (PMR), 466, 467
Prometra, 270
Propofol, 116
Pro-resolution lipid mediators (PRLMs), 35, 36
Prostaglandin E_2 (PGE2), 13
Prostate cancer
cancer-related pelvic pain, 389
genitourinary visceral pain syndromes, 107
Proteasome inhibitors, 127
Protectin D1/neuroprotectin D1 (PD1/NPD1), 35
Psoas imbalance, 437
Psychiatric disorders
anxiety and depression, screening for, 476
cancer, pain and suicide, 475
pharmacologic treatment, anxiety and depression, 476, 477
benzodiazepines, 479
mirtazapine, bupropion and trazodone, 477, 478
neuroleptics, 479
psychostimulants, 478, 479
SNRI, 477
SSRIs, 477
TCA, 477
symptoms, physiologic causes of, 476
Psychological assessment, 50, 51
Psychological distress, 453
Psychosocial therapies, 474
Psychostimulants, 478, 479
Psychotherapy, 390
Pterygopalatine ganglion, 147
Pudendal nerve block, 110, 168, 175
Pulmonary embolus, 422

Pulmonary fibrosis, 366
Pulmonary toxicity, 365, 366
Pulse width, 262
Pulsed radiofrequency, 91
  dorsal root ganglia, 76
  treatment, 142
Pump implantation technique
  anticoagulation and hemostasis, 277
  drug, 278
  imaging, 277
  marking, 278
  operating room, 278
  presurgical considerations, 277
  procedure
    anchor placement, 279, 282, 283
    catheter anchoring, 281
    catheter placement, 280
    draping, 278, 279
    follow-up, 285
    intrathecal access, 279, 280
    lumbar incision and dissection, 278, 279
    myelogram, 281, 282
    positioning, 278
    postoperative period, 285
    pump insertion, 283, 284
    pump pocket creation, 281, 282
    skin closure, 284, 285
    skin preparation, 278
    tunneling, 282, 283
Punctate midline myelotomy, 110
Purine analog, 20, 22, 23
Pyrimidine analog, 20, 21, 23

Q
Quadriceps imbalance, 437, 438
Quality of life, 428, 431

R
Radiation dose, 319
Radiation fibrosis syndrome (RFS)
  clinical dysfunctions
    cervical dystonia, 368
    neck extensor weakness, 367, 368
    shoulder pain, 368
    trismus, 368
  neuromuscular
    funicular pain, 367
    neuropathic pain, 367
    neuropathies, 367
    spasms, 367
    tendons, ligaments and bones, 367
  pathogenesis, 366
Radiation myelopathy (RM), 347
Radiation proctitis, 215, 216
Radiation therapy, 319
  brachial plexopathy, 71
  brachytherapy, 324, 327
  conformality in, 322, 323
  radiation biology, 319, 320
  radiation physics, 319
  treatment planning and dosimetry, 322
  treatment process, 320, 321
Radiation therapy-induced pain
  cervical dystonia, 215
  oral mucositis, 214
  osteonecrosis of the jaw, 214–217
Radiation-associated pain, 100
Radiation-induced brachial plexopathy (RIBP), 425
Radiation-induced cervical dystonia, 409
Radiation-induced dermatitis (RID), 74
Radiation-induced fibrosis, 69, 425, 426
Radiation-induced liver disease (RILD), 332
Radiation-induced neuritis, 15
Radiation-induced neuropathy, 217
Radiculopathy, 204, 377, 378
Radiofrequency ablation (RFA)
  advantages, 308
  application, 308, 309
  continuous thermal radiofrequency ablation, 141
  cooled radiofrequency ablation, 141, 142
  description of, 308
  limitations, 308
  pulsed radiofrequency treatment, 142
Radiosensitivity, 319
Radiotherapy, 89, 109
Radium-223, 357, 358
Raynaud's syndrome, 87, 465
Rectal tumor, 324
Reducing End-of-life Symptoms with Touch (REST), 494
Reflexology, 510
Regional and neuraxial anesthetic techniques, 30, 31
Regional anesthesia interventional procedures, 116, 118
Registered Yoga Teacher (RYT), 497
Rehabilitation, 404
Re-irradiation, 335, 336
Relaxation
  for caregivers, 468
  pain modulation, 509, 510
  training, cancer-related fatigue and sleep, 468, 469
Renal cell carcinoma, 107, 108, 235–237, 320
Repetitive transcranial magnetic stimulation (rTMS), 263
  benefit, 264
  mechanism of action, 263, 264
  risks/limitations, 264
Resiniferatoxin (RTX), 35
Resistive exercises, 398
Respiratory motion control methods, 235
Restorative yoga, 498
Retroperitoneal pain syndrome, 98
Risperidone, 479
Rituximab, 25
Robust inflammatory response, 34
Ropivacaine, 289
Rotator cuff impingement, 405, 406
Rotator cuff tendonitis, 67, 68
Ruffini cells, 134

S
Sacral kyphoplasty, 217
Sacral plexus, 14
Sacroplasty, 201
  complications, 209, 210
  insufficiency fractures, 217
  procedure, 208, 209
  sacral lesions, 208

Scapulothoracic bursitis, 69
Scar injection, 218, 221
Scoliosis, 446, 447
Sedation, 479
Selective norepinephrine reuptake inhibitors (SNRI), 381, 477, 478
Sensory nerve action potential (SNAP), 376, 379, 381
Sensory/physical domain, 452, 453
Serratus plane block, 75, 91
Sexual dysfunction, 388
Sham acupuncture, 485
Shingles vaccine, 128
Shortwave diathermy, 429
Shoulder pain, 368, 405
Skeletal metastatic disease, 86, 87
Skin cancers, 133, 134, 333, 335
Skull metastatic disease, 87
Social support, 453
Sodium channels, 32
Somatic dysfunction, 434
Somatic nerve block
  cranial nerve block (*see* Cranial nerve block)
  infection risk, 168
  peripheral nerve block (*see* Peripheral nerve block)
  principles, 168
  procedure-related challenges, 168
  TAP block, 102
  thoracic intercostal/paravertebral block, 101, 102
  truncal block (*see* Truncal block)
  ultrasound-guided technique, 169
Somatic therapies, 474
Spasm, 367
Speech language pathology, 370
Sphenopalatine ganglion block
  anatomic considerations, 194
  anatomy, 147, 194
  clinical indications, 194
  evidence, 147
  indications, 147
  infrazygomatic fluoroscopic technique, 147, 148
  intranasal technique, 147
  procedure
    lateral approach, 194, 195
    transnasal approach, 194
  side effects and complications, 148, 195
Spinal accessory nerve palsy, 363
Spinal cord ablation
  cordotomy, 231, 232
  DREZ surgery, 233
  extralemniscal myelotomy, 233
  trigeminal tractotomy-nucleotomy, 232, 233
Spinal cord stimulation (SCS), 92, 102, 214, 247
  application, placement, patient selection and contraindications, 247, 248
  burning and shooting pain, 252
  case report data, 252
  comprehensive review, 252
  cost-effectiveness of, 253
  dermatomal distribution, 248
  efficacy, 251
  implant, indications, 248
  implantation, 252, 253
  interventional treatment, 77
  osteonecrosis of the jaw, 217
  phantom limb pain and stump pain, 221
  placement, 248, 249
  post radical neck dissection pain, 219, 220
  step-by-step placement, 250
Spinal metastasis
  AP/PA plan, treatment of, 325
  SBRT, 236, 238, 239, 345
    acute toxicity, 347
    clinical applications, 346, 347
    guidelines and quality measures, 348
    late toxicity, 347, 348
    prognostic prediction, 346
    spine stereotactic body radiation therapy techniques, 347
Spinal paralysis, 157
Spinal tumor, 322
Spindle neuromas, 72
Spine
  cervical spine, 409
  cervical disc pathology, 410
  cervical extensor weakness, 409
  lumbar spine, 410–412
  PMPS, 410
  PTPS, 410
  radiation-induced cervical dystonia, 409
  thoracic spine, 410
  thoracic spine dysfunction, 410
Spine malalignment, 444–446
Spine stereotactic body radiation therapy techniques, 347
Splanchnic nerve block, 101, 156
Src molecule, 15
Standard affect assessment, 453
Stellate ganglion block, 76, 175–177, 220
  anatomy, 148, 149
  anterior paratracheal fluoroscopic technique, 149, 150
  evidence, 149
  indications, 149
  oblique fluoroscopic technique, 150
  side effects and complications, 150
  ultrasound-guided technique, 150
Stenosis, 390
Stereotactic body radiation therapy (SBRT), 235, 324
  for bone, spinal, and adrenal metastases with pain control, 237
  isodose plan, 336
  non-spinal bone metastasis, 236
  spinal metastases, 236, 238, 239, 345, 346
    acute toxicity, 347, 348
    clinical applications, 346, 347
    guidelines and quality measures, 348
    prognostic prediction, 346
    spine stereotactic body radiation therapy techniques, 347
  technical aspects of, 235, 236
  toxicities associated with, 239
Stereotactic radiosurgery (SRS), 235, 324, 330
Stimulation is spinal cord stimulation (SCS), 255
Stocking-glove pattern, 100
Streptozocin, 21
Strontium-89, 356, 357
Stump pain
  botulinum toxin injections, 221
  peripheral nerve blocks, 220, 221
  scar injection, 221
  SCS, 221
  sympathetic nerve blocks, 220
Subcostal plane block, 102
Subcutaneous peripheral nerve stimulation (SPNS), 255, 257, 258

Sufentanil, 288
Suicide, 475
Superficial cervical plexus block, 215
Superior hypogastric plexus block (SHPB), 101, 109, 110, 161, 177, 179, 301, 302, 391
  anatomy, 160
  evidence, 160
  fluoroscopic technique, 160, 162
  indications, 160
  side effects and complications, 162
Superior mesenteric artery (SMA), 101
Superior vena cava (SVC) syndrome, 333, 422
Supraorbital and supratrochlear nerves
  local anesthetic block and pulsed radiofrequency ablation
    anatomic considerations, 189
    clinical indications, 189
    procedure, 189, 190
    side effects/complications, 190
  stimulation
    anatomic considerations, 190
    clinical indications, 190
    procedure, 190, 191
    side effects/complications, 191
Suprascapular entrapment, 88
Suprascapular nerve blocks (SSNB), 75
Surgical pain, 67
Sympathetic coupling, 33
Sympathetic nerve blocks, 109, 220
Sympathetic nervous system (SNS), 145
SynchroMed infusion system, 270

T
T'ai Chi, 497–499
Tachyphylaxis, 118
Taoism, 485
Taping, 428
Taxanes, 21, 24, 25, 48
Temozolomide, 22
Temperature feedback training, 465
Temporomandibular joint (TMJ)
  anatomic considerations, 195
  clinical indications, 195
  procedure, 195
  risk/complications, 195
Tendons, 367
Testicular cancer, 108
TGF-β, 15
Thalamotomy
  operative technique, 228, 229
  outcomes, 229
  rationale and patient selection, 228
Therapeutic heat, 428, 429
Thermal radiofrequency ablation, 91, 141, 187
Thiamine deficiency, 476
Thioguanine, 23
Thiopurine methyltransferase (TPMT), 23
Thoracic cancer pain, 85
  interventional pain control options
    neuraxial techniques, 92, 93
    neuromodulatory techniques, 91, 92
    neurosurgical techniques, 93
    targeted and diagnostic nerve blockade, 90, 91
    treatment algorithm and relevant anatomy, 90
  thoracic nociceptive pain syndromes
    brachial plexopathy, 88
    C7-T1 syndrome, 87
    facial pain, 88
    intercostal neuropathy, 88
    pancoast syndrome, 86
    paraneoplastic syndromes, 87
    primary chest wall pain, 86
    skeletal metastatic disease, 86, 87
    skull metastatic disease, base of, 87
    spinal cord compression, 88, 89
    superior vena cava obstruction, 86
    suprascapular entrapment, 88
  thoracic visceral pain syndromes
    cardiac tumors, 85, 86
    lung cancer, 85
  treatment-associated pain syndromes
    chemotherapeutic agents, 89
    postsurgical pain, 89
    radiotherapy, 89
Thoracic cavity, 85
Thoracic intercostal/paravertebral block, 101, 102
Thoracic nociceptive pain syndromes
  C7-T1 syndrome, 87
  pancoast syndrome, 86
  paraneoplastic syndromes, 87
  primary chest wall pain, 86
  skeletal metastatic disease, 86, 87
  skull metastatic disease, base of, 87
  superior vena cava obstruction, 86
Thoracic outlet technique, 435–439
Thoracic outlet/lumbar spine soft tissue/myofascial release, 436
Thoracic paravertebral block (TPVB)
  anatomy, 169
  benefits, 170
  complications and side effects, 170
  incidence, 169
  technique, 169–171
Thoracic spine dysfunction, 410
Thoracic sympathetic ganglion blocks
  anatomy, 151, 152
  evidence, 152
  fluoroscopic T2–T3 technique, 152, 153
  indications, 152
  side effects and complications, 154
Thoracic visceral pain syndromes
  cardiac tumors, 85, 86
  lung cancer, 85
Thoracolumbar orthoses (TLOs), 444, 445
Thoracolumbosacral orthoses (TLSOs), 444, 445
Thrombocytopenia, 422
Thrombophlebitis, 134
Thymidylate synthase (TYMS), 136
Thyroid dysfunction, 476
Tietze's syndrome, 66
Tissue injury, 434
Toxicity related chemotherapeutic pain, 25
Traction, physical modalities, 430
Traditional Chinese medicine, 504
Transcranial direct current stimulation (tCDS), 263
  benefit, 264
  mechanism of action, 263, 264
  risks/limitations, 264
Transcutaneous electrical nerve stimulation (TENS), 261
  application and use, 262

benefit, 262, 263
mechanism of action, 261
physical modalities, 430
post radical neck dissection pain, 219
risks/limitations, 263
Transcutaneous splanchnic nerve block, 301
Transverse abdominal brace (TvA), 411
Transversus abdominis plane block (TAP block), 102
anatomy, 172, 173
technique, 172
Trastuzumab, 25, 365
Traumatic spinal cord injury, 446
Trazodone, 477, 478
Triazene, 20, 22
Trichodynia, 137
Tricyclic antidepressants (TCA), 271, 355, 477
Trigeminal ganglion balloon compression
anatomic considerations, 187
clinical indications, 187
complications/side effects, 187
procedure, 187
Trigeminal ganglion neurolysis
anatomic considerations, 185
clinical indications, 185
procedure, 185, 186
side effects/complications, 186
Trigeminal ganglion radiofrequency
anatomic considerations, 187
clinical indications, 187
procedure, 187
side effects/complications, 187
Trigeminal nerve
anatomy, 183, 185
cryoablation, 192
infraorbital nerve (*see* Infraorbital nerve)
mandibular nerve block (*see* Mandibular nerve block and radiofrequency ablation)
maxillary nerve block (*see* Maxillary nerve block and radiofrequency ablation)
mental nerve (*see* Mental nerve block)
procedural interventions, 185
supraorbital and supratrochlear nerves (*see* Supraorbital and supratrochlear nerves)
trigeminal ganglion balloon (*see* Trigeminal ganglion balloon compression)
trigeminal ganglion neurolysis (*see* Trigeminal ganglion neurolysis)
trigeminal ganglion radiofrequency (*see* Trigeminal ganglion radiofrequency)
Trigeminal nucleotractotomy
operative technique, 227, 228
outcomes, 228
rationale and patient selection, 227
Trigeminal spinal nucleus, 231
Trigeminal tractotomy, 228
Trigeminal tractotomy-nucleotomy, 232, 233
Trigger point injections, 75, 215
Trigger point stimulation, 423
Trismus, 368
Truncal block
intercostal block
anatomy, 170
benefits, 171
complications, 171
indications, 170
technique, 170, 171
TAP block, 171
anatomy, 172, 173
technique, 172
TPVB
benefits, 170
complications and side effects, 170
incidence, 169
anatomy, 169
technique, 169, 170
Tumor lysis syndrome, 422
Tumor microenvironment (TME), 14
Tumor-related pain, 66, 201
Tunneled epidural catheter placement, 102
Tunneling, 282, 283
Tuohy needle, 256
Turmeric, 506

U

Ulnar neuropathy, 414
Ultrasound-guided stellate ganglion block, 152
Ultrasound-guided technique, 150
United States Pharmacopeia (USP), 294
Upper body swelling, 333
Upper extremity
adhesive capsulitis, 405, 406
CT scan of, 6
elbow/forearm, 406
lateral epicondylopathy, 406
medial epicondylopathy, 406
rotator cuff impingement, 405
shoulder pain, 405
wrist, 406
Ureteric obstruction, 98
USP-National Formulary (USP-NF), 294
Uterine cancer, 108

V

Vagal neuralgia, 194
Vaginal dryness, 390
Vagus nerve
anatomic considerations, 194
anatomy, 193
clinical indications, 193, 194
procedure, 194
side effects/complications, 194
Valsalva maneuver, 100
Varicella-zoster virus (VZV), 128, 135
Vertebral and bone metastases, palliation for, 329, 330
Vertebral augmentation, 124, 208
Vertebral compression fracture (VCF), 201, 239, 347, 443, 444
Vertebroplasty, 201, 203–207, 210
complications, 209, 210
insufficiency fractures, 217
pathological fracture during, 206
procedure, 209
Vestibular rehabilitation, 413
Vinblastine, 25
Vinca alkaloids, 21, 24, 26, 48, 127, 364
Vincristine, 24
Visceral pain, sympathetic blocks for, 100
Visual analog scale (VAS), 252, 253
Vitamin D deficiency, 476

Vocational rehabilitation, 368
  comprehensive inpatient rehabilitation, 370
  general strategies, 369
  lymphedema, 369
  pathological fractures, 369, 370
Vulvar cancer, 389

W

Wallerian degeneration, 34
Walther's ganglion, 110
Weight lifting, 431
Western yoga, 496
Wong-Baker FACES® Pain Rating Scale (WBFPRS), 114
Wrist, 406

X

Xanthine oxidase (XO), 22

Y

Yoga Alliance, 497
Yoga therapy, 431, 495–497

Z

Ziconotide, 287, 288, 290, 296
Zoledronic acid, 124, 356

MIX
Papier aus verantwortungsvollen Quellen
Paper from responsible sources
FSC® C105338

If you have any concerns about our products,
you can contact us on
ProductSafety@springernature.com

In case Publisher is established outside the EU,
the EU authorized representative is:
Springer Nature Customer Service Center GmbH
Europaplatz 3, 69115 Heidelberg, Germany

Printed by Libri Plureos GmbH
in Hamburg, Germany